W. HARRY ARCHER, B.S., M.A., D.D.S.

University Professor, School of Dental Medicine, University of Pittsburgh

Formerly Professor of Oral Surgery and Anesthesia, Chairman, Department of Oral Surgery, School of Dental Medicine, Professor, Graduate Faculty (Dentistry), Formerly Lecturer, School of Nursing and School of Public Health, University of Pittsburgh

Active Staff, Department of Dentistry (Oral Surgery Division), Presbyterian-University Hospital, Pittsburgh

Medical Staff, Emeritus, Department of Oral Surgery, Magee-Women's Hospital, Pittsburgh

Senior Staff, Emeritus, Odontology (Oral Surgery), Children's Hospital of Pittsburgh

Medical Staff, Emeritus, (Oral Surgery), Eye and Ear Hospital of Pittsburgh

Emeritus Staff, Department of Surgery, Section of Oral Surgery, St. Clair Memorial Hospital

Senior Attending, Emeritus, Division of Oral Surgery, The South Side Hospital

Diplomate of the American Board of Oral Surgery

Fellow of the American College of Dentists

Fellow of the International College of Dentists

Honorary Member of the Horace Wells Club of Connecticut

Senior Consultant in Oral Surgery, Veterans Administration Hospital,

Chief of the Dental Department, Falk Clinic, University of Pittsburgh

Chief Oral Surgeon, Western State Psychiatric Institute and Clinic, Pittsburgh

Fulbright Professor, Facultad de Odontologia, Universidad Central del Ecuador, Quito, Ecuador, S.A.

Fulbright Professor, Facultad de Odontologia de Guayaquil, Santiago de Guayaquil, Ecuador, S.A.

Visiting Professor

Facultad de Odontologia, Universidad de Buenos Aires, Republica de Argentina, S.A.

Tokyo Medical and Dental University, Tokyo, Japan

La Facultade de Odontologia, Universidade Federale de Minas Gerais, Belo Horizonte, Brasil, S.A.

Faculty of Dentistry, University of Istanbul, Turkey

Faculty of Dentistry, The University of Sydney, Australia

College of Dentistry, University of the Philippines, Manila

School of Dentistry, Mahidol University, Bangkok, Thailand

Facultades de las Odontologia de las Universidades Javeriana, Bogota, Colombia, S.A.

Facultad de Odontologia, San Marcos Universidad, Lima, Peru, S.A.

Faculty of Dentistry, University of Singapore, Singapore

Dental School, University of Athens, Athens, Greece

Facultad de Odontologia, Universidad de San Carlos de Guatemala, Guatemala, C.A.

Facultad de Odontologia, Universidad de Antioquia Medina, Colombia, S.A.

Facultad de Odontologia, Universidad Central de Venezuela, Caracas, Venezuela, S.A.

Escuela de Odontologia, Universidad Technologica de Mexico, Mexico City, Mexico

Faculdade de Odontologia, Universidade de Sao Paulo, Sao Paulo, Brasil, S.A.

Faculty of Dentistry, National Defense Medical Center, Taipei, Taiwan.

Oral and Maxillofacial Surgery

Volume One

by W. HARRY ARCHER, B.S., M.A., D.D.S.

FIFTH EDITION

1975

W. B. SAUNDERS COMPANY

Philadelphia   London   Toronto

W. B. Saunders Company: West Washington Square
Philadelphia, Pa. 19105

12 Dyott Street
London, WC1A 1DB

833 Oxford Street
Toronto, Ontario M8Z 5T9, Canada

Listed here is the latest translated edition of this
book together with the language of the translation
and the publisher.

Spanish (*4th Edition*), (2 Vols.) — Editorial Mundi S.R.L.,
Buenos Aires, Argentina.

German (*3rd Edition*) — Medica Verlag,
Stuttgart, West Germany.

Japanese (*4th Edition*), (Vol. I, II, & III.) — Kenshin Imada,
Tokyo, Japan.

Italian (*4th Edition*), (Vol. I & II.) — Piccin Editore,
Padova, Italy.

Chinese — Shanghai, China.

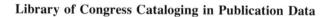

Library of Congress Cataloging in Publication Data

Archer, William Harry.

Oral and maxillofacial surgery.

First and 2d editions published in 1952 and 1956 under title:
A manual of oral surgery. Third and 4th editions published in
1961 and 1966 under title: Oral surgery.

1. Mouth — Surgery.   I. Title. [DNLM: 1. Face — Surgery.
2. Maxilla — Surgery.   3. Surgery, Oral. WU600 A672m]

RK529.A7 1975   617'.522   73–89931

ISBN 0–7216–1362–4 (v. I)

ISBN 0–7216–1363–2 (v. II)

Oral and Maxillofacial Surgery

Volume I: ISBN 0-7216-1362-4
Volume II: ISBN 0-7216-1363-2

Last digit is the print number: 9   8   7   6   5   4   3   2   1

To My Wife

LOUISE E. ARCHER

CHAPTER AUTHORS

RAMIRO ALFARO A., D.D.S., Professor of Oral Surgery, University of San Carlos, Facultad de Odontologia, Guatemala.

Rotation-Advancement Principle for Use in Wide Unilateral Cleft Lips

OSCAR ASENSIO DEL VALLE, D.D.S., Oral Surgeon and Director of Centro Infantil of Estomatologia, Antigua, Guatemala.

Rotation-Advancement Principle for Use in Wide Unilateral Cleft Lips

WILLIAM H. BELL, D.D.S., Associate Professor of Oral Surgery, Department of Surgery, University of Texas Health Science Center—Dallas. Staff, Parkland Memorial Hospital, Children's Medical Center, and Presbyterian Hospital, Dallas. Diplomate, American Board of Oral Surgery.

Orthognathic Surgery

HERBERT J. BLOOM, D.D.S., M.S., PhD., F.A.C.D., Adjunct Professor, Department of Speech and Hearing, and Adjunct Associate Professor, School of Medicine, Wayne State University, Detroit. Formerly Chief and now Consultant, Department of Oral and Maxillofacial Surgery, Sinai Hospital of Detroit. Chairman Emeritus, Department of Oral Surgery, Mount Carmel Mercy Hospital. Staff, United Hospitals of Detroit, Providence Hospital, and St. Joseph Mercy Hospital. Diplomate, American Board of Oral Surgery.

Surgical Repair of Cleft Lip and Palate

PHILIP J. BOYNE, D.M.D., M.S., F.A.C.D., Dean, Dental School, University of Texas Health Science Center—San Antonio. Staff, Department of Surgery, Bexar County Hospital, Santa Rosa Hospital, and Audie Murphy Veterans Administration Hospital. Diplomate, American Board of Oral Surgery.

Transplantation and Grafting Procedures

DONALD DAVIDSON, B.S., D.D.S., M.S., Consultant and Visiting Lecturer, West Virginia University Dental School and Medical Center, Morgantown. Chief of Oral Surgery, Uniontown Hospital, Uniontown, Pa. and Brownsville General Hospital, Brownsville, Pa. Staff, Connellsville State Hospital, Connellsville, Pa. and Mon Valley Hospitals, Charleroi and Monongahela Divisions, Charleroi and Monongahela, Pa. Diplomate, American Board of Oral Surgery.

Diagnosis and Treatment of Pain

CHARLOTTE P. DONLAN, M.D., F.A.C.R., Assistant Clinical Professor of Radiology, George Washington University Medical School, and Radiation Therapist and Consultant, St. Elizabeth's Hospital, Washington, D.C. Consultant in Radiation Therapy for Fairfax Hospital, Northern Virginia Doctors Hospital, and Arlington Hospital, Arlington, Va.

Radiation Therapy

J. CLIFTON ESELMAN, D.D.S., F.A.C.D., Formerly Associate Dean and Professor of Oral Roentgenology, University of Pittsburgh School of Medicine. Consultant in Oral Roentgenology, Veterans Administration Hospital, Pittsburgh, Pa.

Radiographs and Localization

LEWIS E. ETTER, M.D., F.A.C.R., Professor of Radiology, University of Pittsburgh School of Medicine, Falk Clinic, Presbyterian-University Hospital, University of Pittsburgh Medical Center. Consultant in Radiology, Western Psychiatric Institute and Clinic and C. Howard Marcy State Hospital, Pittsburgh, Pa.

Anatomy of Facial Bones and Jaws

JOHN COLLYER GAISFORD, M.D., F.A.C.S., Chief, Division of Surgery and Director, Burn Center, The Western Pennsylvania Hospital, Pittsburgh, Pa.

Oral Malignant Disease

T. CRADOCK HENRY, F.D.S., L.R.C.P., M.R.C.S., Consultant Oral Surgeon, The Hospital for Sick Children, Great Ormond Street, London, and Consultant Oral and Maxillo Facial Surgeon, Royal Surrey County Hospital, Guildford, Surrey, England.

Segmental Surgery

WILLIAM B. IRBY, D.D.S., M.S., F.A.C.D., Professor and Chairman, Department of Oral Surgery, and Assistant Dean for Postdoctoral Affairs, Medical University of South Carolina, College of Dental Medicine, Charleston. Consultant, U.S. Navy Hospital, Charleston, Fort Jackson, Fort Bragg, and Veterans Administration Hospital, Columbia. Staff, Medical University of South Carolina, Charleston County Hospital, and Veterans Administration Hospital, Charleston. Diplomate, American Board of Oral Surgery.

History of Oral Surgery and *Cast or Acrylic Splints*

A. D. MACALISTER, E.D., D.D.S.(N.Z.), F.D.S.R.C.S.(Eng.), F.R.A.C.D.S., Professor and Chairman, Department of Oral Medicine and Oral Surgery, University of Otago Dental School, Dunedin, New Zealand.

The Child Patient

ANDREW E. MICHANOWICZ, B.S., D.D.S., F.I.C.D., Associate Professor and Chairman of Graduate Endodontics, University of Pittsburgh School of Dental Medicine. Consultant in Endodontics, Children's Hospital, Pittsburgh. Staff, Montefiore Hospital, Pittsburgh, Pa.

Surgical Endodontics

MARVIN E. PIZER, D.D.S., M.S., F.I.C.D., Chief of Oral Surgery, Alexandria Hospital, Alexandria, Va. Consultant, National Orthopedic and

Rehabilitation Hospital, Arlington, Va. Courtesy Staff, Circle Terrace Hospital and Northern Virginia Doctors Hospital, Arlington, Va. Diplomate, American Board of Oral Surgery.

Diagnosis and Management of Oral Malignant Disease

H. B. G. ROBINSON, D.D.S., M.S., D.Sc.(Hon.), Dean Emeritus and Professor Emeritus of Oral Pathology and Diagnosis, School of Dentistry, University of Missouri—Kansas City.

Cysts of the Oral Cavity

MARSH ROBINSON, D.D.S., M.D., F.A.C.D., F.A.C.S., Professor and Chairman of Oral Surgery, School of Dentistry, University of Southern California, Santa Monica. Diplomate, American Board of Oral Surgery.

Orthognathic Surgery

VIKEN SASSOUNI, D.D.S., D.Sc., Professor of Orthodontics, University of Pittsburgh School of Dentistry. Chief Orthodontist, Children's Hospital and Western Pennsylvania Hospital, Pittsburgh, Pa.

Dentofacial Orthopedics

SIDNEY S. SPATZ, D.D.S., F.A.C.D., F.I.C.D., Professor and Chairman, Department of Oral Surgery, University of Pittsburgh School of Dental Medicine. Chief of Dentistry and Oral Surgery, Montefiore Hospital, Pittsburgh. Chief of Oral Surgery, Eye and Ear Hospital, Magee-Women's Hospital, Children's Hospital, and Central Medical Pavilion, Pittsburgh. Consultant, Veterans Administration Hospitals of Pittsburgh, Pa. Diplomate, American Board of Oral Surgery.

Antibiotic Therapy

CONRAD J. SPILKA, D.D.S., F.I.A.O.S., F.A.C.D., F.I.C.D., Clinical Professor of Oral Surgery and Anesthesia, Case Western Reserve University, Cleveland, Ohio. Chief, Department of Oral Surgery, Fairview General Hospital and Lutheran Medical Center, Cleveland, Ohio. Diplomate, American Board of Oral Surgery.

Orthognathic Surgery

IRVIN V. UHLER, D.D.S., F.A.C.D., F.I.C.D., Chief of Oral Surgery, Lancaster General Hospital, and Oral Surgeon, Lancaster Cleft Palate Clinic, Lancaster, Pa. Diplomate, American Board of Oral Surgery.

The Geriatric Patient

W. J. UPDEGRAVE, D.D.S., Professor Emeritus and Former Chairman, Department of Dental Radiology, Temple University School of Dentistry, Philadelphia, Pa.

Radiographs and Localization

YOSHIO WATANABE, D.D.S., M.D., D.Med.Sc., F.A.C.D., M.I.A.C., Director of Clinics and Professor and Chairman, Department of Oral Surgery, Tsurumi University School of Dentistry, Yokohama City, Japan.

Surgical Correction of Ankylosis of the Temporomandibular Joint

G. WREAKES, B.Ch.D., F.D.S., DIP.Orth., Consultant Orthodontist to the

Westminster Group of Hospitals and South West Thames Health Authority, Guildford, Surrey, England.

Segmental Surgery

HAROLD J. ZUBROW, A.B., D.D.S., F.A.C.D., Associate Professor of Oral Surgery, University of Pittsburgh School of Dental Medicine. Staff, Department of Oral Surgery, Montefiore Hospital, Eye and Ear Hospital, Magee-Women's Hospital, and Central Medical Pavilion, Pittsburgh, Pa.

Antibiotic Therapy

CONTRIBUTORS

JOSEPH ANDREWS, D.D.S., Departments of Oral Diagnosis and Oral Surgery, University of Pittsburgh School of Dental Medicine.

ABDEL K. EL-ATTAR, D.M.D., Assistant Professor, Department of Oral Surgery, University of Pittsburgh School of Dental Medicine.

STANLEY J. BEHRMAN, D.M.D., Clinical Assistant Professor of Surgery, Cornell University Medical College. Attending Oral Surgeon, The New York Hospital.

CARL J. BENDER, D.D.S., Formerly Senior Staff Dentist, Veterans Administration Hospital, Pittsburgh, Pa.

C. RICHARD BENNETT, D.D.S., Ph.D., Associate Professor and Chairman, Department of Anesthesia, University of Pittsburgh School of Dental Medicine.

JOSEPH L. BERNIER, D.D.S., M.S., Professor and Chairman, Department of Oral Pathology, Georgetown University School of Dentistry, Washington, D.C.

THOMAS C. BITHELL, M.D., Associate Professor of Internal Medicine, University of Virginia School of Medicine, Charlottesville.

HARRY BLECHMAN, D.D.S., Dean, College of Dentistry, New York University, New York, N.Y.

GERALD H. BONNETTE, D.D.S., School of Dentistry, University of Michigan, Ann Arbor.

JAMES L. BRADLEY, D.D.S., M.S.D., M.Sc., Oral Surgeon, St. John's Hospital, Memorial Hospital, and Passavant Hospital, Springfield, Ill.

PAUL M. BURBANK, D.M.D., M.S., Attending Oral Surgeon, Genesee Hospital and Highland Hospital, Rochester, N.Y.

D. LAMAR BYRD, D.D.S., M.S.D., Professor and Chairman, Department of Oral Surgery, Baylor College of Dentistry, Baylor University Medical Center, Dallas, Texas.

LESTER R. CAHN, D.D.S., President, New York Institute of Clinical Oral Pathology, New York, N.Y.

NOAH R. CALHOUN, D.D.S., M.S.D., Professor, Oral Surgery, Howard University. Professorial Lecturer, Georgetown University. Director of Oral Surgery Training, Veterans Administration Hospital, Washington, D.C.

RALPH J. CAPAROSA, M.D., Formerly Clinical Assistant Professor of Otolaryngology, University of Pittsburgh School of Medicine.

RICARDO CUESTAS CARNERO, M.D., Assistant Professor, Department of Oral Surgery, Part 2, Cordoba National University, Cordoba, Argentina.

A. P. CHAUDHRY, B.D.S., Ph.D., Professor of Oral Pathology, State University of New York at Buffalo School of Medicine.

LLOYD E. CHURCH, D.D.S., M.S., Ph.D., Assistant Professor of Anatomy, George Washington University School of Medicine, Washington, D.C.

LEON J. COLLINS, JR., M.D., Associate in Medicine, School of Medicine; Assistant Professor of Medicine, School of Dental Medicine, University of Pennsylvania, Philadelphia.

MARTIN P. CRANE, M.D., Quondam Chief Physician, The Misericordia Hospital and The Nazareth Hospital, Philadelphia, Pa.

THEODORE H. DEDOLPH, D.D.S., M.S.D., F.A.C.D., Staff, St. Cloud Hospital, and Veterans Administration Hospital, Minnesota.

EDWARD J. DEGNAN, D.D.S., Staff Oral Surgeon, Veterans Administration Hospital, Bay Pines, Fla.

B. F. DEWEL, D.D.S., Orthodontist, Evanston, Ill. Editor, American Journal of Orthodontics.

REED O. DINGMAN, D.D.S., M.D., Professor and Head, Section of Plastic Surgery, University of Michigan Medical School, Ann Arbor.

E. LLOYD DUBRUL, D.D.S., M.S., Ph.D., Professor and Head, Department of Oral Anatomy, University of Illinois College of Dentistry, Chicago.

EUGENE R. ELSTROM, R.T., Chief X-Ray Technician, Illinois Eye and Ear Infirmary, Chicago.

SALVATORE J. ESPOSITO, A.B., D.D.S., Chief of Dental Service, Veterans Administration Hospital, Boston, Mass.

WILLIAM EVANS, D.D.S., M.S., Instructor, Ohio State University College of Dentistry (Oral Surgery). Chairman, Oral Surgery Department, St. Anthony Hospital. Chairman, Maxillofacial Department, Grant Hospital of Columbus. Oral Surgeon, University Hospital, Children's Hospital, St. Anthony Hospital, and Grant Hospital of Columbus.

VICTOR H. FRANK, D.D.S., Emeritus Attending Chief of Oral Surgery Department, Albert Einstein Medical Center. Emeritus Staff, Graduate Hospital, University of Pennsylvania, Philadelphia.

EDUARD G. FRIEDRICH, D.D.S., Formerly Professor of Oral Surgery, Northwestern University Dental School, Chicago, Ill.

GEORGE E. FULLER, JR., D.D.S., Professor and Chairman, Department of Oral Surgery, Emory University School of Dentistry, Atlanta, Ga.

ITALO H. A. GANDELMAN, D.D.S., Associate Professor of Oral Surgery, Faculdade de Odontologia da U. F. R. J., Rio de Janeiro, G. B. Brazil.

ROBERT J. GORLIN, D.D.S., M.S., Professor and Chairman, Department of Oral Pathology, University of Minnesota, Minneapolis.

JAMES GUGGENHEIMER, D.D.S., Departments of Oral Diagnosis and Oral Surgery, University of Pittsburgh School of Dental Medicine.

ROGER A. HARVEY, M.D., Head, Department of Radiology, University of Illinois College of Medicine, Chicago.

FREDERICK A. HENNY, D.D.S., Formerly Chief, Division of Dentistry and Oral Surgery, Henry Ford Hospital, Detroit, Mich.

MATTHEW J. HERTZ, D.D.S., Assistant Attendant in Prosthetics, Bronx-Lebanon Hospital, New York, N.Y.

DANIEL J. HOLLAND, D.M.D., Formerly Professor of Oral Surgery, Tufts University School of Dental Medicine, Boston, Mass.

PETER J. JANNETTA, M.D., Professor and Chairman, Department of Neurosurgery, University of Pittsburgh School of Medicine.

JOSEPH H. JOHNSON, D.D.S., Late Emeritus Professor of Oral Surgery, Faculty of Dentistry, University of Toronto.

SHREE C. JOSHI, M.S., D.O.M.S., Scientific Officer, Medical Division, Bhabha Atomic Research Center, Trombay, Bombay-85.

SAMUEL I. KAPLAN, D.D.S., Chief Oral Surgeon, Mount Sinai Hospital, Hartford, Conn.

V. H. KAZANJIAN, C.M.J., D.M.D., M.D., Formerly Professor of Plastic Surgery, Harvard University, Boston, Mass.

P. L. KHURANA, L.R.C.P.(Edin.), L.R.C.S.(Edin.), L.D.S., R.C.S.(Edin.), F.I.C.D.(U.S.A.), F.I.O.A.S., Hon. Professor, Maulana Azad Medical College. Hon. Dental Surgeon, Irwin Hospital, N. Rly. Central Hospital, Shroff's Charity Eye Hospital, Jawahar Lal Nehru Institute of Physical Medicine and Rehabilitation. Hon. Dental Surgeon to the President of India.

STUART N. KLINE, D.D.S., Associate Professor, Department of Surgery, Division of Oral Surgery, University of Miami School of Medicine. Chief, Oral Surgery Section, Miami Veterans Administration Hospital and Jackson Memorial Hospital, Miami, Fla.

W. B. KOUWENHOVEN, M.E., M.D.(Hon.), Johns Hopkins University School of Medicine; D.Sc.(Hon.), Syracuse University; Doktor Ingenieur, Karls Ruhe Technische Hochschule, Baden, Germany.

BRUNO W. KWAPIS, D.D.S., M.S., Professor and Chairman of Oral Surgery, Southern Illinois University School of Dental Medicine, Edwardsville.

DANIEL M. LASKIN, D.D.S., M.S., Professor and Head, Department of Oral and Maxillofacial Surgery, University of Illinois College of Dentistry, Chicago.

FRANCIS M. S. LEE, D.D.S., Professor and Head, Department of Oral Surgery and Oral Medicine, Faculty of Dentistry, University of Singapore.

T. A. LESNEY, D.C., U.S.N., Formerly Consultant-Instructor to Dental Training Programs, U.S. Naval Hospital, Portsmouth, Va.

JACK E. McCALLUM, M.D., Department of Neurological Surgery, University of Pittsburgh School of Medicine.

CHARLES F. McCANN, A.B., D.M.D., Chief of Oral Surgery Section, Veterans Administration Hospital, Boston, Mass.

FRANK M. McCARTHY, D.D.S., M.D., Professor and Chairman, Department of Anesthesiology, University of Southern California Dental School, Los Angeles.

A. E. McDONALD, D.D.S., Associate Professor, Department of Oral Surgery, University of Pittsburgh School of Dental Medicine.

STEPHEN B. MALLETT, D.M.D., Consultant in Oral Surgery, Veterans Administration Hospital, Boston, Mass.

MARIA JULIANA MALMSTROM, Dr. Odont., Instructor, Department of Oral Surgery, Institute of Dentistry, University of Helsinki, Finland.

LEO D. C. MARCH, L.D.S., R.C.S.(Eng.), F.I.O.A.S., F.A.C.D., Consultant and Associate Lecturer in Oral Surgery, University of the West Indies, Kingston, Jamaica. Chief of Oral Surgery Division, Kingston General Hospital, Jamaica.

IRVING MEYER, D.M.D., M.Sc., D.Sc., Research Professor of Oral Pathology, Tufts University School of Dental Medicine; Lecturer on Oral Pathology, Harvard University School of Dental Medicine, Boston, Mass.

SANFORD M. MOOSE, D.D.S., Clinical Professor of Oral Surgery, School of Dentistry, College of Physicians and Surgeons, University of the Pacific, Stockton, Calif.

JOE HALL MORRIS, D.D.S., Professor and Chairman, Department of Oral Surgery, University of Tennessee College of Dentistry, Memphis.

ROBERT L. MOSS, D.D.S., Chief, Oral Surgery Section, Veterans Administration Hospital, Phoenix, Ariz.

NORMAN R. NATHANSON, D.D.S., Chief of Oral Surgery, Framingham Union Hospital, Framingham, Mass.

PAUL NATVIG, D.D.S., M.D., Assistant Clinical Professor of Plastic and Reconstructive Surgery, Marquette University School of Medicine, Milwaukee, Wisc.

K. ODENHEIMER, D.D.S., Ph.D., Professor of Pathology (Oral), Louisiana State University School of Dentistry, New Orleans.

VALLE J. OIKARINEN, M.D., D.D.S., Department of Oral Surgery, Institute of Dentistry, University of Helsinki, Finland.

THEODORE R. PALADINO, D.D.S., Assistant Professor, Department of Oral Surgery, University of Pittsburgh School of Dental Medicine.

HAROLD J. PANUSKA, D.D.S., M.S.D., Staff, Department of Oral Surgery, Fairview Hospital, Methodist Hospital, and Memorial Hospital, Minneapolis, Minn.

JACK L. PECHERSKY, D.M.D., Assistant Professor of Pedodontics, University of Pittsburgh School of Dental Medicine.

OTTO C. PHILLIPS, M.D., Clinical Professor of Anesthesiology, University of Pittsburgh School of Medicine. Chief, Division of Anesthesiology, Western Pennsylvania Hospital, Pittsburgh.

ROBIN M. RANKOW, D.D.S., M.D., Assistant Clinical Professor of Anatomy, College of Physicians and Surgeons, Columbia University, New York, N.Y.

GUILLERMO RASPALL, D.D.S., M.D., Chairman, Department of Oral and Maxillofacial Surgery, Hospital de la Cruz Roja, Barcelona, Spain.

H. SERRANO ROA, D.D.S., Chief of Estomatology, Roosevelt Hospital, Guatemala.

SHELDON ROVIN, D.D.S., M.S., Dean, School of Dentistry, University of Washington, Seattle.

NORMAN L. ROWE, F.D.S.R.C.S., L.R.C.P., M.R.C.S., L.M.S.S.A., H.D.D.R.C.S., Consultant, Oral Surgery Department, The Westminster Hospital and The Institute of Dental Surgery, London.

H. CLAYTON SATO, D.D.S., M.D., Assistant Professor and Head of Dentistry and Oral Surgery, The Tokyo Jikeikai University School of Medicine.

WILLIAM G. SHAFER, B.S., D.D.S., M.S., Distinguished Professor and Chairman, Department of Oral Pathology, Indiana University-Purdue University School of Dentistry, Indianapolis.

ROBERT B. SHIRA, D.D.S., Dean, Tufts University School of Dental Medicine, Boston, Mass.

HARRY SICHER, M.D., D.Sc., Late Emeritus Professor of Anatomy and Histology, Loyola University School of Dentistry, Chicago, Ill.

N. P. J. B. SIEVERINK, D.D.S., Professor of Oral Surgery, Catholic University Dental School. Staff, Department of Oral Surgery, St. Radboud Hospital, Catholic University, Nijmegen, Holland.

N. H. SMITH, M.D.S., Senior Lecturer, Department of Oral Medicine and Oral Surgery, Faculty of Dentistry, The University of Sydney, Australia.

LAKANA SRIVIROJANA, D.D.S., Assistant Professor, Department of Oral Surgery, School of Dentistry (Pratum Wan), Mahidol University, Bangkok, Thailand.

EDWARD C. STAFNE, D.D.S., Emeritus Chief of Dental Radiography, Mayo Clinic, Rochester, Minn.

CHARLES W. SUMMERS, D.D.S., Oral Surgeon, U.S. Army. Formerly Chief of Oral Surgery and Professional Training, U.S. Army Hospital, Ft. Carson, Colo.

CHEVKET O. TAGAY, Late Professor and Director, Maxillo-Dental Surgery Clinic, Dental Faculty of the University of Istanbul, Turkey.

RICHARD W. TIECKE, B.S., D.D.S., M.S., Professor, Department of Oral Pathology, University of Illinois, Chicago.

RICHARD G. TOPAZIAN, D.D.S., Professor and Head, Department of Oral and Maxillofacial Surgery, School of Dental Medicine, University of Connecticut Health Center, Farmington.

PORUS S. TURNER, M.D.S., Scientific Officer, Dental Services, Bhabha Atomic Research Centre, Trombay, Bombay-85.

CHARLES A. WALDRON, D.D.S., M.S.D., Professor of Oral Pathology, School of Dentistry, Emory University, Atlanta, Ga.

ROBERT V. WALKER, D.D.S., Professor and Chairman, Division of Oral Surgery, The University of Texas Southwestern Medical School at Dallas.

KJELL WALLENIUS, M.D., L.D.S., Professor and Head, Department of Oral Surgery, University of Lund School of Dentistry, Malmo, Sweden.

JERROLD I. WASSERMAN, D.D.S., Assistant Adjunct in Periodontics, Bronx-Lebanon Hospital, New York, N.Y.

SAM WEINSTEIN, D.D.S., Formerly Chairman, Department of Orthodontics, University of Nebraska. Now Professor, Orthodontics Department, University of Connecticut Health Center, Hartford.

MAXWELL M. WINTROBE, B.A., M.D., B.Sc.(Med.), PhD., Professor of Internal Medicine, University of Utah College of Medicine, Salt Lake City.

PREFACE TO THE FIFTH EDITION

THIS BOOK is intended for the oral surgeon, for the general dental practitioner and for the dental student. Its aim has been, where possible, to present a step-by-step technique of the various oral surgical procedures. The illustrations have been chosen to illuminate and graphically expand the text.

Oral surgery is but one division of the whole field of dentistry, yet in itself it deals with such a diversity of conditions and employs such a variety of operations for the cure or alleviation of those conditions that it is of necessity a highly specialized sphere of practice. It demands of its practitioners diagnostic acumen based on a thorough knowledge of pathology, physiology, bacteriology, normal and abnormal roentgenographic appearance of the facial bones, and anatomy. It requires highly trained technical skill and patient, thoughtful perseverance in the management of difficult traumatic, abnormal or pathologic conditions found in the oral cavity.

Ferrer has said it very well indeed:

Surgery is not an exact science, but it is closer to being exact than any other branch of medicine [or dental medicine]. The surgical discipline can be divided into two broad areas—the art and the science. Surgical judgment is based on the accumulated body of clinical knowledge about diseases and their treatment. It involves diagnosis, the understanding of disease processes, the timing and choice of the operative procedure, the preoperative evaluation and preparation of the patient, and postoperative care. Experience plays a major role in all these aspects of surgical judgment. This judgment is not an exact science and is sometimes called the "Art of Surgery."

The "Science of Surgery" requires a precise knowledge of anatomy and of pathology, as well as physiology and biochemistry. This knowledge is essential for the scientific management of the surgical patient and for the most exact facet of surgery—surgical technic. This requires further that the young surgeon train himself in the exacting technical details of performing surgical operations. There are no shortcuts to the achievement of technical proficiency. Manual dexterity alone is not enough. There must be careful attention to learning all the minute details of technic plus constant practice in performing each surgical maneuver and in the handling of each surgical instrument.

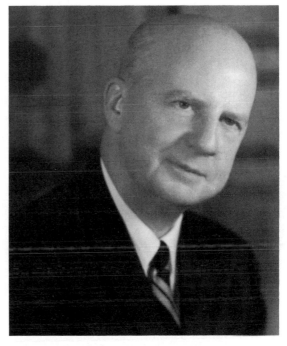

The perfection of his technic enables the surgeon to achieve his therapeutic end most efficiently, with the greatest dispatch consistent with safety, and with the greatest gentleness in the handling of living tissues. It must be recognized that at every operation the surgeon inevitably injures the patient; this injury can and must be minimized by the use of careful, gentle, and accurate surgical technic.*

The oral surgeon also makes his contribution as a member of the health team in the care of many of those conditions which require the combined skills of one or more of the following specialties: internal medicine, hematology, general surgery, neurosurgery, plastic surgery, otolaryngology, prosthodontics and roentgenology. For this reason there is material included that has been written by well-qualified specialists in these fields. Such knowledge

---

*From Ferrer, J. M.: Preface. *In* Zikria, B. A.: Manual of Surgical Knots. Somerville, N.J., Ethicon, Inc., 1970.

xvii

Preface to the Fifth Edition

makes the oral surgeon aware of the allied problems associated with complicated cases and thus better able to cooperate in the total management.

The scope of this subject, therefore, is very large, but an attempt has been made to keep this book within a reasonable size. Though it is not possible to avoid completely the theoretical aspects, for the most part all contributors have tried to give specific and concrete details, whether of etiology, diagnosis or treatment. Case histories, a number of them prepared by some of the many graduate students and residents who have trained in oral surgery at our University of Pittsburgh Health Center, have been included to illustrate the sometimes perplexing problems of diagnosis and treatment.

The reader of this book will find that in order to avoid duplication of material, much specific information not found in the text is contained in the legends of the illustrations. Therefore, he should study not only the text but the legends as well. Special effort has been made to place illustrations with their legends near the corresponding discussion in the text.

Seven new chapters have been added in this edition: "Segmental Surgery in the Treatment of Dental and Facial Disharmony," "Transplantation and Grafting Procedures in Oral Surgery," "Oral Surgery and the Geriatric Patient," "Surgical Correction of Ankylosis of the Temporomandibular Joint," "Oral Surgery for the Child Patient," "History of the Development of Oral Surgery in the United States," and "A Variation of the Rotation-Advancement Principles for Use in Wide Unilateral Cleft Lips." Authors of some of these new chapters are from Japan, Guatemala, New Zealand, and England.

Entirely rewritten are the chapters entitled "Surgical Repair of the Cleft Lip," "Surgical Repair of the Cleft Palate," "Radiation Therapy of Lesions of the Oral Cavity," "The Diagnosis and Management of Oral Malignant Disease," and "Surgical Endodontics."

Other chapters have been extensively revised with both new text and new illustrations. Special attention has been given to the chapters on the extraction of teeth, impactions, oral surgery for dental prosthesis, cysts, tumors, complications, fractures, and oral surgery in the hospital.

W. HARRY ARCHER

ACKNOWLEDGMENTS

Oral and maxillofacial surgery is a vast subject, and I acknowledge with gratitude the help I have had from my colleagues and co-workers in this field. Particularly do I wish to thank those who generously wrote chapters or made other major contributions to this book. These are all listed on earlier pages. In addition, many other individuals have helped in one way or another in the preparation of this edition.

All authors owe a debt of gratitude to librarians for their patient, painstaking help. To Carroll F. Reynolds, Ph.D., Director; Ms. Laurabelle Eakin, Assistant Director; Mrs. Madlynne Harris and Ms. June Bandemer, Reference Librarians; and Mrs. Janet Sondecker, Curator of Historical Collections, Falk Library of the Health Professions, University of Pittsburgh, go my heartfelt thanks.

My profound thanks go to Mrs. Marvin Sniderman for her knowledgeable skill in helping with the proofreading.

The illustrative material is a most important part of this book. Miss Margaret Croup, medical artist, played a major role in the creation of the oral surgery drawings used in illustrating the first four editions, and now again her superb line drawings enhance this, the fifth edition.

Also with sincere thanks, I acknowledge the help given in the preparation of the photographic prints for this fifth edition by Howard E. Sweitzer and Melvin H. Coles and for new drawings by Christine Trcynski of the Department of Illustrations, School of Dental Medicine, University of Pittsburgh.

I particularly express grateful appreciation to my secretary of many years, Mrs. Elizabeth D. Albrecht, for her ever available and invaluable help.

I also wish to acknowledge the many helpful suggestions that were made by many friends and teachers of oral surgery who use this book as their classroom text.

Special thanks are due the staff of the W. B. Saunders Co., whose help and guidance have been of inestimable value in the production of this and previous editions.

A partial list of former graduate students and residents who have prepared case reports or helped in other ways follows:

Archer, Fred
Baurle, James E.
Bruno, Carman C.
Cafaro, Ross P.
Campbell, George W.
Cerroni, A. P.
Cirlone, A. E.
Cohen, Bernard M.
Clark, Charles A.
Davidson, Donald
Deckman, Dalton H.
Donaldson, William B.
Eilderton, T. A.
El-Attar, Moneim A.
Federbusch, Melvin D.
Fischer, George
Fox, Lewis S.
Fuller, George E.
Ganley, Charles J.
Gould, A. J.
Hall, Robert M.
Hoffmaster, F. E.
Irby, W. B.
Iverson, Paul H.
James, William
Kaplan, Samuel I.
Kiem, Richard P.
King, Richard J.
Mangie, A. S.
Mashberg, Arthur
Mellaci, Louis F.
Mercier, Herbert A.
McDonald, Alonzo E.
Mintz, Sheldon M.
Mohnac, A. M.
Moore, C. H.
Nardozzo, Thomas M.
Novak, Charles J.
Pasqual, H. N.
Petitto, William J.
Pizer, Marvin E.
Reynolds, Amzie G.
Simms, William
Smith, John W.
Spatz, Sidney S.
Stern, Arnold
Sotereanos, George C.
Stoner, Charles E.
Thompson, Henry L.
Tucker, Charles J.
Wagner, Donald E.
Waltrip, Maurice
Whittaker, John E.
Zahm, Richard
Zubrow, Harold J.
Zwicker, Hollis W.

The author is indebted to Robert E. Silva, Editor of Dental Radiography, for his ready willingness to supply information and artwork.

And last but by no means least, I wish to thank the various hospital staffs and the members of the Oral Surgery Department at the University of Pittsburgh, in particular, Sidney S. Spatz, D.D.S., Sidie R. Bononi, D.D.S., Anthony W. Parella, D.D.S., A. E. McDonald, D.D.S., and Moneim A. El-Attar, D.D.S., for their support and encouragement.

The expert, authoritative oral histopathological diagnoses and consultative advice of our Professor of Oral Pathology, Robert S. Verbin, D.D.S., Ph.D., was always freely and quickly available and is gratefully acknowledged.

Of great help to an author associated with a university dental school is the ease with which he can consult with authorities in all phases of dentistry, and so it is with grateful appreciation that I acknowledge the advice and information given so freely by my colleagues at the University of Pittsburgh:

EDWARD J. FORREST, D.D.S., Ph.D., F.A.C.D. Dean of the School of Dentistry, Professor and Head of the Department of Orthodontics, Member of the Graduate Faculty.

SIDNEY S. SPATZ, D.D.S. Professor and Head of the Department of Oral Surgery, Member of the Graduate Faculty.

MOLLIE DAVIDSON FOSTER, D.D.S., F.A.C.D. Professor of Pedodontics, Member of the Graduate Faculty.

C. RICHARD BENNETT, D.D.S. Professor and Head of the Department of Anesthesia, Member of the Graduate Faculty.

VIKEN SASSOUNI, D.D.S., D.Sc. Professor and Co-Chairman of the Department of Orthodontics.

SIDIE BONONI, D.D.S. Professor of Oral Surgery and Anatomy.

ROBERT S. RAPP, D.D.S., M.S. Professor and Head of the Department of Pedodontics.

ROBERT MUNDEL, Ph.D. Professor and Head of the Department of Anatomy.

YAHIA ISMAIL, D.D.S., M.S. Professor and Head of the Department of Prosthodontics.

RUTH S. FRIEDMAN, D.D.S. Professor and Director of the Department of Oral Hygiene.

ANDREJS BAUMHAMMERS, D.D.S., M.S. Professor and Head of the Department of Periodontics.

JAMES W. SMUDSKI, D.D.S., Ph.D., Professor and Head of the Department of Pharmacology.

ANTHONY F. PARELLA, D.D.S. Associate Professor of Oral Surgery.

HAROLD J. ZUBROW, D.D.S., F.A.C.D. Associate Professor of Oral Surgery.

CARL J. BENDER, D.D.S. Assistant Professor of Prosthodontics.

ANDREW E. MICHANOWICZ, D.D.S. Assistant Professor of Oral Medicine.

DANIEL M. MAZZOCCO, D.M.D. Assistant Professor, Department of Radiography.

W. HARRY ARCHER

CONTENTS

Volume I

Volume II

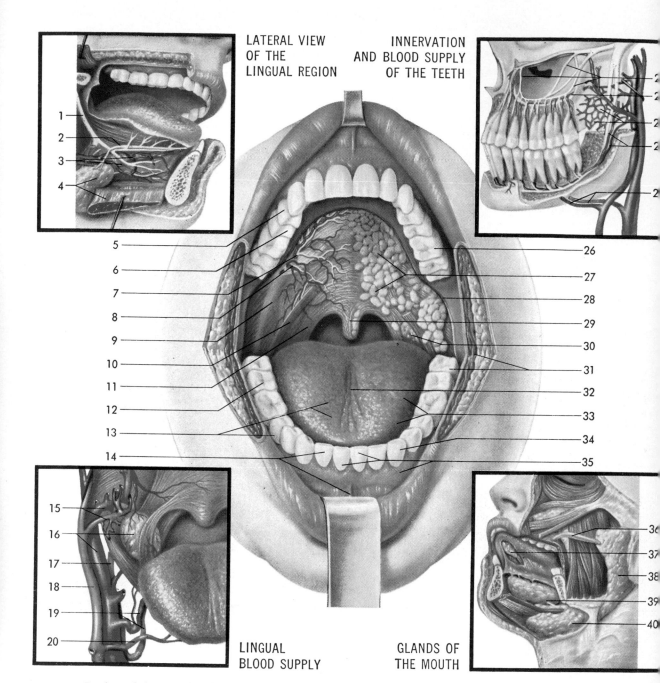

LATERAL VIEW OF THE LINGUAL REGION

INNERVATION AND BLOOD SUPPLY OF THE TEETH

LINGUAL BLOOD SUPPLY

GLANDS OF THE MOUTH

Region of the mouth. (Courtesy of Lederle Laboratories Division, American Cyanamid Company.)

1. Lingual nerve
2. Submandibular duct
3. Sublingual branches of lingual artery and vein
4. Submandibular gland; mylohyoid muscle
5. First bicuspid
6. Second bicuspid
7. Greater palatine artery and nerve
8. Lesser palatine artery and nerve
9. Pterygomandibular raphe
10. Glossopalatine muscle
11. Pharyngopalatine muscle
12. Second molar
13. Filiform papillae; second bicuspid

14. Lateral incisor; frenulum of lower lip
15. Internal maxillary artery and vein
16. External carotid artery; palatine tonsil
17. Internal jugular vein
18. Posterior facial vein
19. Lingual artery and vein
20. Ranine vein
21. Anterior, middle and posterior superior alveolar nerves
22. Posterior superior alveolar artery
23. Pterygoid venous plexus
24. Inferior alveolar nerve and artery
25. External maxillary artery; anterior facial vein

26. First molar
27. Palatine glands
28. Cut edge of mucous membrane
29. Uvula
30. Palatine tonsils
31. Third molar; buccinator muscle
32. Median sulcus of tongue
33. Fungiform papillae
34. Cuspid
35. Central incisors; gingiva
36. Parotid duct
37. Anterior lingual gland
38. Parotid gland
39. Sublingual gland
40. Submandibular gland

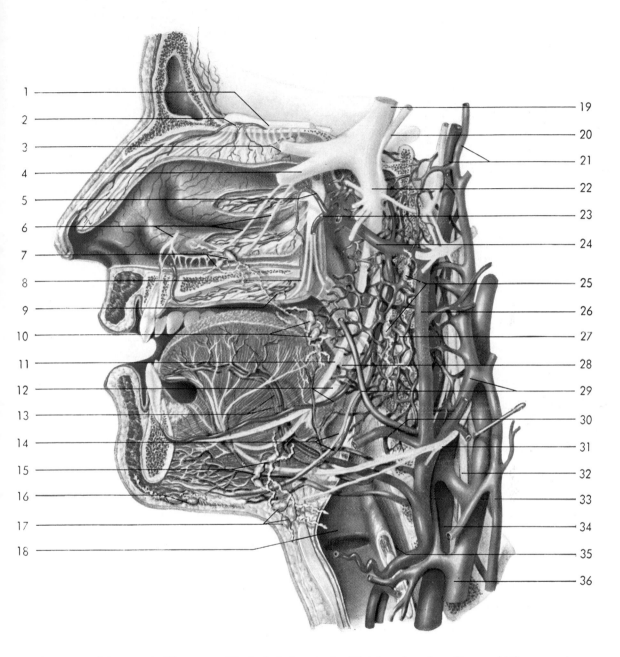

Anatomy of the mouth. (Courtesy of Lederle Laboratories Division, American Cyanamid Company.)

1. Olfactory nerve
2. Anterior ethmoidal artery
3. Ophthalmic nerve
4. Maxillary nerve
5. Sphenopalatine ganglion
6. Anterior, middle and posterior superior alveolar nerves
7. Maxillary lymph nodes
8. Anterior palatine nerve
9. Great palatine artery
10. Buccinator lymph nodes
11. Lingual nerve
12. Inferior alveolar nerve and artery
13. Lingual artery and vein
14. Mylohyoid nerve and artery
15. Supramandibular lymph nodes
16. Submental lymph nodes
17. Submaxillary lymph nodes
18. Trachea
19. Sensory root of trigeminal nerve
20. Motor root of trigeminal nerve
21. Superficial temporal artery and vein
22. Mandibular nerve
23. Sphenopalatine artery
24. Internal maxillary artery
25. Parotid lymph nodes
26. External carotid artery
27. Pterygoid venous plexus
28. Oropharynx
29. Anterior and posterior facial veins
30. External maxillary artery
31. Hypoglossal nerve
32. Vagus nerve
33. External jugular vein
34. Internal carotid artery
35. Esophagus
36. Internal jugular vein

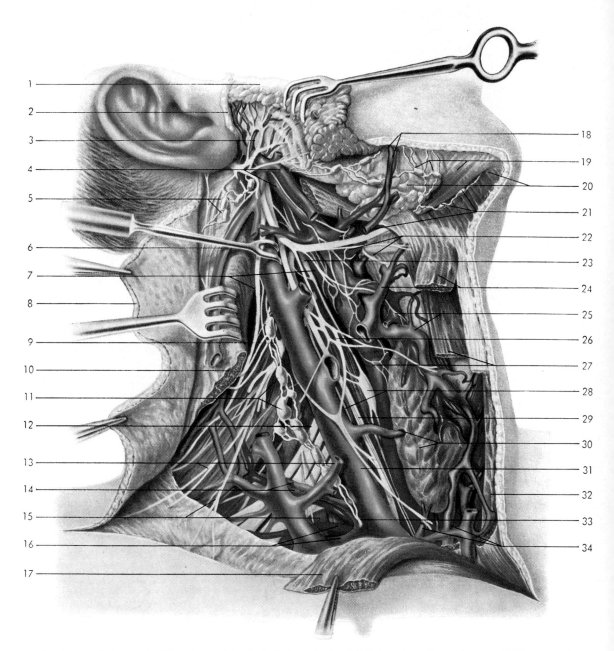

Anatomy of the neck. (Courtesy of Lederle Laboratories Division, American Cyanamid Company.)

1. Parotid gland
2. Superficial temporal artery and vein
3. Temporal branch of facial nerve
4. External carotid artery and posterior facial vein
5. Superficial cervical lymph nodes
6. External jugular vein
7. Accessory nerve and internal carotid artery
8. Platysma muscle
9. Fourth cervical nerve
10. Superior portion of sternocleidomastoid muscle
11. Deep cervical lymph nodes
12. Fifth cervical nerve
13. Posterior supraclavicular nerve and anterior jugular vein
14. Superficial cervical artery and vein
15. Middle supraclavicular nerve and subclavian artery
16. Transverse scapular artery and vein
17. Inferior portion of sternocleidomastoid muscle
18. External maxillary artery and anterior facial vein
19. Submandibular lymph nodes and digastric muscle
20. Submandibular gland and mylohyoid muscle
21. Submental lymph nodes and hypoglossal nerve
22. Superior laryngeal artery and nerve
23. Superior cervical ganglion
24. Superior laryngeal vein and omohyoid muscle
25. Superior thyroid artery and vein
26. Ansa hypoglossi
27. Common carotid artery and sternothyroid muscle
28. Middle cervical ganglion and phrenic nerve
29. Vagus nerve
30. Thyroid gland and middle thyroid vein
31. Internal jugular vein
32. Sternohyoid muscle
33. Jugular lymphatic trunk
34. Inferior thyroid veins

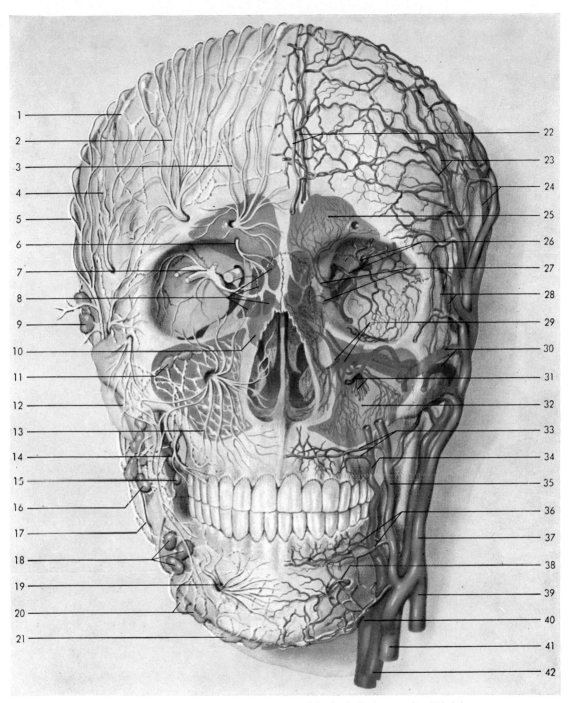

Anatomy of the facial sinuses. (Courtesy of Lederle Laboratories Division, American Cyanamid Company.)

1. Lymphatic vessels of scalp
2. Rami of supraorbital nerve
3. Rami of supratrochlear nerve
4. Rami of zygomaticotemporal nerve
5. Rami of auriculotemporal nerve
6. Infratrochlear nerve
7. Ophthalmic nerve
8. Ethmoidal cells
9. Posterior auricular lymph node
10. Sphenoidal sinus
11. Maxillary lymph node
12. Rami of zygomaticofacial nerve
13. Rami of infraorbital nerve
14. Buccal nerve
15. Buccinator lymph node

16. Parotid lymph node
17. Great auricular nerve
18. Supramandibular lymph nodes
19. Rami of mental nerve
20. Submandibular lymph nodes
21. Submental lymph node
22. Frontal artery and vein
23. Frontal branch of superficial temporal artery and vein
24. Parietal branch of superficial temporal artery and vein
25. Frontal sinus
26. Ophthalmic artery and vein
27. Anterior and posterior ethmoidal arteries

28. Deep temporal arteries
29. Sphenopalatine artery and vein
30. Internal maxillary artery and vein
31. Infraorbital artery and vein
32. Maxillary sinus
33. Superior labial artery and vein
34. External maxillary artery
35. Anterior facial vein
36. Inferior labial artery and vein
37. Posterior facial vein
38. Mental artery
39. External jugular vein
40. Internal carotid artery
41. Internal jugular vein
42. External carotid artery

CHAPTER 1

HISTORY OF THE DEVELOPMENT OF ORAL SURGERY IN THE UNITED STATES*

WILLIAM B. IRBY, D.D.S., M.S.

Oral surgery, as it is known and practiced today, did not exist slightly over 100 years ago.[12] Dentistry was a young profession not too highly considered by the medical profession, and surgical procedures of the jaws and associated structures were traditionally performed by the physician. However, a new era in dentistry, and more specifically oral surgery, was initiated with the opening of the Baltimore College of Dental Surgery in 1840. This historic event in dentistry was associated with an increased demand for oral care, and it stimulated dentists, whose previous interest had been directed primarily toward mechanical skills, to expand their interest gradually to diseases, injuries and malformations of the jaws and associated structures. Thus began the modern practice of oral surgery, which has developed over a period of time into its present status with well-trained dentists whose interest is directed not only to the specific oral surgical problem but also to the general health and supportive care of the patient.

ANCIENT HISTORY

Scientific progress through the ages has not been marked by an orderly progression; instead, it has been characterized by spurts of brilliance and depths of recession. This is true of all medical science and certainly applies to the development of oral surgery, which was practiced with rising knowledge and skill in a period extending to 1700 B.C. The accomplishments of the ancient surgeons must be recorded in any treatise dealing with the history of oral surgery, for their achievements became the cornerstone upon which oral surgery sporadically developed over the centuries.

The history of oral surgery begins with the Egyptians, dating from 1600 or 1700 B.C., and follows with the Greeks, who introduced scientific medicine around 500 B.C. It is of interest that the first account of oral surgical procedures was the treatment of facial injuries and is found in the Edwin Smith Papyrus, now in the New York Academy of Medicine Library. This manuscript, which dates from the Egypt of 1600-1700 B.C., described 27 head injuries, "including descriptions of fractures and dislocations of the jaw and injuries to the lip and chin, generally with diagnosis, treatment, and prognosis."[33]

Hippocrates, who was born around 460 B.C., also described the treatment of jaw fractures and advised the removal of decayed teeth. It is known that the Greeks used a type of dental forceps.[33]

---

*Revised and updated from Irby, W. B.: Chapter 12: History of the development of oral surgery in the United States. *In* Archer, W. H. (Ed.): Oral Surgery Directory of The World. 4th ed. Pittsburgh, 1971.

The highly developed civilization of the Roman empire was next to make its contribution to the treatment of pathologic processes of the oral regions, as well as jaw fractures. The fall of this empire plunged the Christian world into a scientific void, from which it only began to recover in the 10th and 11th centuries A.D. Beginning in Italy, this renaissance spread throughout Europe and reached its scientific and cultural maturity in the 14th, 15th and 16th centuries. While scientific advancement is generally conceded to have been outstripped by the great cultural or artistic achievements, anatomical and surgical advancements were noteworthy. It should be of especial interest to the oral surgeon that the celebrated French surgeon Ambroise Paré (1510–1590) described methods of transplanting and reimplanting teeth, described obturators for cleft or perforated palates, extracted teeth, drained dental abscesses and set jaw fractures.[33]

EARLY AMERICAN HISTORY

After the Renaissance little advancement occurred which could be credited to the field of oral surgery until the 19th century, when the scene dramatically switched to America and focused upon several great pioneers in the specialty of oral surgery, including Simon P. Hullihen and James E. Garretson. Following these great men in oral surgery came distinguished pioneers in surgery of the oral regions, such as Truman W. Brophy, Thomas L. Gilmer, George V. I. Brown, John Sayre Marshall and Matthew H. Cryer. These outstanding men, to whom oral surgery owes so much, seemed to have had many rather consistent characteristics; they all held M.D. and D.D.S. degrees, were authors, were affiliated with dental schools, and had the imagination and incentive to develop new techniques and instruments with which to perform surgical procedures. So great were the contributions of these pioneers that a listing of their major achievements was recorded in the May, 1966, *Journal of Oral Surgery* by a truly great oral surgeon, Robert H. Ivy.

Simon P. Hullihen (1810–1857). Born in Florida and self-trained, Dr. Hullihen practiced surgery and dentistry in Ohio and West Virginia. He is believed to be the first man designated an oral surgeon. His contributions to the literature were many; he described treatment of cleft lip and palate, treatment of maxillary sinus infections, resection of a part of the mandible and construction of a metal cap splint for treatment of a fracture of the mandible. A developer of numerous dental instruments, he also bequeathed a fair bibliography, including papers on prognathism and cleft palates, and a formidable list of operations performed.

James E. Garretson (1820–1895). Dr. Garretson is known as the "Father of Oral Surgery." He was professor of oral surgery in the Philadelphia Dental College, now School of Dentistry, Temple University, and established a surgery clinic in connection with the school. In 1869 Dr. Garretson published a monumental work, *A Treatise on Disease and Surgery of the Mouth, Jaws and Associated Parts.*[21] In the second edition, the title was changed to *System of Oral Surgery,* with original title as a subtitle. The sixth and last edition was published in 1898.

Truman W. Brophy (1848–1928). Dr. Brophy is best known for the so-called "Brophy operation" for cleft palate. He attained world fame as an oral surgeon, was a constant contributor to dental and medical literature and was a leader in the development of dental education. He was one of the organizers of the Chicago College of Dental Surgery, serving for 40 years as professor of oral surgery and as dean.[60] His book, *Oral Surgery, A Treatise on the Diseases, Injuries and Malformations of the Mouth and Associated Parts,*[8] published in 1915, was a 1100-page outstanding text.

Thomas L. Gilmer (1848–1931). Dr. Gilmer also ranks among the celebrated oral surgeons of America. He is especially well known for his development of new methods and procedures in oral surgery that were practiced by surgeons throughout the world.[36] He was first associated with the Chicago College of Dental Surgery and later served as professor of oral surgery at Northwestern University Dental School.

George V. I. Brown (1863–1948). Dr. Brown was a contemporary of Dr. Brophy but differed radically with Brophy as to techniques in treatment. He published a textbook, *The Surgery of Oral and Facial Diseases and Malformations,*[9] which appeared in four editions, the last of which was published in 1938.

John Sayre Marshall (1846–1922). Dr. Marshall is perhaps best known as the founder of the U.S. Army Dental Corps in 1901,[28] although he might be equally well known as a pioneer in dental pathology. He was professor of dental pathology and oral surgery at Northwestern University and, in 1897, published an excellent book entitled *Manual of Injuries and Surgical Diseases of the Face, Mouth and Jaws*.[39] This book was published in three editions, the last dated 1909.

Matthew H. Cryer (1840–1921). In a careful analysis of the skills and contributions of the early American pioneers in oral surgery Dr. Cryer must certainly rank as one of the greatest. Not only was he an outstanding oral surgeon, but his research in the anatomy of the facial bones, his remarkable ability in photography and his development of a surgical engine, operated by electricity, and of other surgical instruments served to enhance greatly the stature of oral surgery. Dr. Cryer was a profound student of anatomy of the head and face, and, while professor of oral surgery at the University of Pennsylvania, he sectioned hundreds of human heads. From these sections he made beautiful photographs and lantern slides. These were finally published in a widely acclaimed book, *Studies of Internal Anatomy of the Face*,[16] in 1901. It is also worthy of recording that Dr. Cryer founded the first complete hospital dental service in America, in 1901, at the Philadelphia General Hospital.

MEDICINE AND ORAL SURGERY

It is of special interest to note that, early in the last quarter of the 19th century, great controversy arose in the medical world concerning oral surgery. First, there was the question of whether oral surgery should be recognized as a separate specialty, many physicians believing that it was a part of general surgery. As an example, an editorial in *Dental Cosmos*, 1873, entitled "What is Oral Surgery?" replied as follows to an inquiry made by a medical journal: "An oral surgeon is one who, having received a general medical and surgical education, is drawn by interest or inclination to the special duty and treatment of all abnormal conditions of the mouth." In 1881, in a meeting of the American Medical Association, a motion was made and adopted that a section in oral surgery be added to other sections of that body. This was recognition of the claims of oral surgeons to a position of specialists of medicine but not that of the profession of dentistry.[32]

Thus, it became clear that medicine of that era held the position that an M.D. degree was mandatory for the practice of oral surgery. It is both interesting and ironical that Dr. Garretson, who is generally recognized as the "Father of Oral Surgery" and who was professor of oral surgery in the Philadelphia Dental College, was quoted by the *Medical Times*, 1875, as saying that he was "most decidedly in favor of the abolishment of the degree D.D.S. One degree in medicine is enough; the greater covers the lesser and includes it."[32]

DENTISTRY AND THE ERA OF CHANGING CONCEPT IN ORAL SURGERY

With the passing of this era in the history of oral surgery a change gradually took place which was to influence the specialty of oral surgery profoundly, that being the acceptance of the position that a dentist must not necessarily hold an M.D. degree in order to practice oral surgery. As previously stated, this change was gradual, and many of the fine oral surgeons, such as Louis Schultz, Herbert A. Potts, Carl W. Waldron and V. H. Kazanjian, held both degrees.[28] Concurrently, there emerged a group of great oral surgeons who, without the benefit of an M.D. degree, became recognized nationally and were accepted by their medical colleagues as having special talents in treating facial fractures and pathologic conditions affecting the mouth and jaws. Particular reference must be made to Chalmers J. Lyons, Thomas P. Hinman, Samuel L. Silverman, Kurt H. Thoma, James R. Cameron and W. Harry Archer.

Chalmers J. Lyons (1874–1935). Dr. Lyons was instructor in oral surgery from 1907 to 1915 in both the medical and dental schools of the University of Michigan and in 1915 assumed the rank of professor of oral surgery in the two schools. He made notable contributions to the literature, among which was a chapter entitled "Cleft Palate and Harelip," which was published in Mead's *Oral Surgery*.[43]

Thomas P. Hinman (1870–1934). Dr. Hinman was a dedicated dental educator, having served on the faculty of not only the Atlanta Dental College but also the Southern Dental College. As a professor, he taught oral surgery, operative dentistry, orthodontics, and dental ceramics at various times in his career. Following the consolidation of these two schools in 1917, Dr. Hinman became Dean of the Atlanta-Southern Dental College, a position he held the 14 years before his death. He was the author of many articles concerning dentistry, including oral surgery, a field in which he was greatly interested and quite proficient.

Samuel L. Silverman (1889–1934). Dr. Silverman was Clinical Professor of Oral Surgery, Atlanta-Southern Dental College; Associate Professor of Surgery (Oral), Emory University School of Medicine; and formerly Special Lecturer on Oral Surgery at Columbia University, New York. He was also Oral Surgeon to the City (Grady) Hospital, Scottish Rite, Piedmont and St. Joseph Hospitals, and Consulting Oral Surgeon to U.S. Veterans Hospital, Atlanta, Georgia. In 1926 he published a textbook, *Principles and Practice of Oral Surgery*.[58]

Kurt H. Thoma (1883–1972). No history of oral surgery is complete without recognition of the contributions of one of the truly great men of oral surgery who, while holding only a D.D.S. degree, made a lasting imprint on the practice of oral surgery as it is known today. Dr. Thoma truly paved the way and set a goal for every practitioner of oral surgery, and his surgical skill and literary ability are known throughout the world. His textbook, *Oral Surgery*,[61] published in 1969 (fifth edition), was a monumental treatise of this era. Of equal importance is the fact that his work and publications in pathology of the oral regions became the corner-stone upon which the modern specialty of oral pathology was built. For over 50 years he was in the active practice of oral surgery. (See the Appendix to this chapter for more details.)

James R. Cameron (1892–1969). Dr. Cameron was widely acclaimed for his surgical skill and teaching ability. He held the rank of Professor of Oral Surgery at Temple University from 1933 to 1964 and was professor and chairman of the course in oral surgery at the Graduate School of Medicine, University of Pennsylvania, from 1945 to 1959. He was one of the founding members of the American Board of Oral Surgery. His residents trained at the Episcopal and Pennsylvania hospitals in Philadelphia, and many are in practice throughout this country and several foreign nations.

W. Harry Archer (1905–　　). Dr. Archer, formerly Professor of Oral Surgery and Anesthesia, and Chairman of the Department of Oral Surgery at the University of Pittsburgh, now a Distinguished University Professor and in his 48th year as an educator, author, practitioner and worldwide lecturer in oral surgery, has made many valuable contributions in all phases of oral surgery. His numerous publications deal not only with oral surgery but also with dental anesthesia, hospital-dental school teaching relationships,

hospital dental service, the history of anesthesia, and the life of Horace Wells, the discoverer of anesthesia. Dr. Archer's textbook, *Oral and Maxillofacial Surgery* (now in its fifth edition) has been printed in seven languages (and is presently being translated into two more), a record in this field, and is used throughout the world. His textbook on dental anesthesia[2] has gone through two editions and is printed in two languages.

Hundreds of his former students have specialized in oral surgery. Nine of them are now professors and chairmen of departments of oral surgery* in dental and medical schools in the United States, and many others are members of oral surgery faculties, or are chiefs of oral surgery in hospitals or the armed forces.

TEXTBOOK AUTHORS IN EXODONTIA AND ORAL SURGERY

In a review of the development of oral surgery there is an all-too-common tendency to consider the so-called major aspects of the specialty and forget that the removal of teeth comprises a high percentage of procedures accomplished by the oral surgeon. Credit is largely due to two men, Wilton W. Cogswell of Colorado Springs, Colorado, and George B. Winter of St. Louis, for their untiring efforts in development of scientific principles in the removal of teeth, both erupted and impacted, and in surgery of the alveolar process. Through their scientific publications, surgical clinics for the general practitioner, and training of interns and residents, they have profoundly influenced the techniques presently employed in this country. Dr. Winter's book, *Principles of Exodontia As Applied to the Impacted Mandibular Third Molar*,[67] was a widely used and respected text for years.

Dr. Cogswell is probably the foremost developer of step-by-step techniques for the removal of teeth. Over half a century of time he carved, from a combination of soap and wax, classic models illustrating the position of teeth in the alveolus and the technique for

---

*Stanley J. Behrman, Cornell University Medical College; George E. Fuller Jr., Emory University; J. Frank Hall, University of Indiana (retired); William B. Irby, Medical University of South Carolina; Francis M. S. Lee, University of Singapore; Alex M. Mohnac, Temple University; Sidney S. Spatz, University of Pittsburgh; Donald B. Osbon, University of Iowa; and Stuart N. Klein, University of Miami.

their removal. His work was first published in a textbook entitled *Dental Oral Surgery*[14] in 1932. Since that time, Dr. Cogswell has continued with his work and conducted innumerable clinics concerned especially with the sectioning technique in the removal of impacted third molars.

Other prominent clinicians and authors of well-known textbooks on the extraction of teeth, or exodontia, as this surgical procedure became known in the early 1900's, were: William J. Lederer,[34] Leo Winter,[68] M. Hillel Feldman[20] and Frank W. Rounds.[56] Beginning in 1923 books on oral surgery by dentists began to appear: 1923, Adolph Berger; 1926, Samuel L. Silverman; 1936, Sterling Mead; 1943, Leo Winter; 1948, Kurt H. Thoma; 1948, W. Harry Archer; 1949, J. R. Bourgoyne; 1955, Henry C. Clark; 1968, Gustav O. Kruger; 1968, Walter C. Guralnick; and 1972, Daniel F. Waite.

In 1938 the *American Journal of Orthodontia and Oral Surgery* began publication, with Kurt H. Thoma as editor of the oral surgery section. In 1943 the *Journal of Oral Surgery,* with Carl W. Waldron as editor, began publication. In 1948 the *Journal of Oral Surgery, Oral Medicine and Oral Pathology,* with Kurt H. Thoma as editor of the oral surgery section, was launched.

IMPACT OF COMBAT SURGERY UPON THE DEVELOPMENT OF ORAL SURGERY

In an excellent article entitled "The History of Oral Surgery and Its Influence on the Profession of Dentistry,"[36] written by Chalmers J. Lyons and published in *Dental Cosmos* in 1934, Dr. Lyons made the following observations:

"As I reflect back over my own experience of over a quarter of a century in oral surgery, there are four distinct factors that have stood out in the development of this specialty during that period.

First.   The great advancements that have been made in both general and local anesthesia.

Second. The progress that has been made in the use of the x-ray.

Third.   The development of knowledge concerning the relation of the mouth to systemic involvements.

Fourth. The experiences and observations gained in major and minor surgery of the mouth as a result of the World War."

Dr. Lyons' profound observations most certainly summarize the factors responsible for the development of oral surgery. One additional factor should be added: the dedication and skill of the great men of oral surgery. Without them, the remarkable progress of the specialty would most certainly not have occurred.

Since the time of Dr. Lyons' observations, the United States has been engaged in three wars, with World War II fought on a global basis. Thus, in a period encompassing slightly more than a century, and beginning with the War between the States, surgeons have derived an untold amount of experience in the treatment of battle casualties. Without doubt, World War II served as the single greatest stimulus to the training of oral surgeons, and the lessons learned in these wars have produced a group of oral surgeons who know no peer in the skillful and definitive treatment of facial injuries. Because of this, it seems appropriate to begin with the War between the States and trace the development of the oral surgeon as related to combat.

WAR BETWEEN THE STATES

With the advent of the War between the States a few skilled, ingenious and dedicated dentists began to take an active and vital part in treatment of facial wounds. Their contribution was, for the most part, the reduction and fixation of jaw fractures. These pioneers, who possessed a knowledge of occlusion and of jaw function and who were skilled in the utilization of available materials, lent refinement and accuracy to the reduction of jaw fractures. Through persistence, and by continuously demonstrating their skills, these men became accepted as valuable additions to the surgical team. Thus they established the basis upon which the oral surgeon has gradually refined and improved his techniques in the management of facial injuries over the ensuing years.

Mass casualties unparalleled in any prior military encounter were seen in this war. These were due primarily to the introduction of rifled arms, fixed ammunition and conical bullets. The ferocity of the military engagements is indicated by the approximately 10,000 facial wounds treated by the Union Medical Service alone.

Attention to the effectiveness of proper splints in the treatment of jaw injuries and the ability of dentists to provide such treatment was dramatically demonstrated by Thomas B.

Gunning when, in April, 1865, William H. Seward, then Secretary of State under President Abraham Lincoln, fell from his carriage and suffered bilateral fractures of the body of the mandible in the premolar areas. The initial treatment of this injury was rendered by a physician who attempted to reduce and support these fractures by the application of ligatures on the mandibular teeth as well as a supporting bandage. This method proved unsuccessful and resulted in a compounding of the fracture into the mouth on the right side. On the ninth day after injury, April 14, 1865, the day of Lincoln's assassination, Seward was attacked while asleep, and a severe cut was inflicted on his face, extending from under the right zygoma to the left of the trachea. This wound resulted in exposing externally the fracture of the right body of the mandible, which was previously compounded intraorally. Aware of the success attained by Dr. Gunning with the use of vulcanite splints, Benjamin F. Bache, a surgeon and Chief of the Naval Laboratory in New York City, requested that he come to Washington to treat the patient. Upon his arrival in Washington on April 16, 1865, Dr. Gunning's examination of the patient disclosed that only the ten anterior mandibular teeth, the right third molar, and root of the left third molar remained. An open bite existed, with wide separation at the fracture sites. The right posterior fragment was markedly elevated. Pus discharged profusely from both fracture sites; the gums were pale and flaccid; and the general condition of the patient was poor. Opposition to the construction and application of the splint at this time was voiced by both the patient and his attending surgeon. Dr. Gunning refused to treat the patient on this basis, but upon request from Surgeon General Barnes, he returned to Washington on April 28, 1865, to complete the treatment. On May 2, the first of a series of three vulcanite splints was inserted. These splints were held in position by passing screws into the natural teeth. Upon removal of the splints, after a total of four months of splinting, it was determined that a firm union existed bilaterally and that function of the jaw was satisfactory.

The success of this treatment did much to enhance the reputation of both Dr. Gunning and the dental profession. Of great significance was the establishment of the fact that custom-built, rigid, interdental splints provided a most effective method of reducing and stabilizing displaced mandibular jaw fractures.

In the Southern states James Bean, another dentist, achieved prominence from his skill in splint construction and the application of these splints in the treatment of jaw fractures. He was interested in dental materials, and when he observed the inadequate methods by which facial injuries were being treated, he soon directed his attention to utilization of dental materials in order to improve treatment of these injuries. As Brooks[6] expressed it in referring to surgical advances in the War between the States, "Most importantly, face surgery brought the talents of the dentist to the fore, particularly in the Confederate medical service.... An important accomplishment in this area was the invention of the interdental splint by James Bean of Atlanta to correct fractures of the maxilla and mandible. Bean's success attracted so much attention that Surgeon General Moore directed all hospitals to set aside a ward to employ the device, and finally a hospital was set up in Atlanta, the first of its kind, to perform maxillo-facial surgery. Thus, Drs. Bean and Moore did a tremendous job in elevating the fledgling profession."

The contributions of Drs. Gunning and Bean not only resulted in better patient care but also succeeded in achieving recognition of the ability of the dentist to manage complicated maxillofacial surgery. This is well illustrated by the inclusion of the Bean and Gunning interdental splints by J. B. Stern[59] among his examples of discoveries and inventions in the history of medicine.

WORLD WAR I

World War I resulted in over 5000 dentists' being called to active duty. Although no precedent existed as to the requirements of organized dental support in combat, dentists as a group rose to the challenge and rendered a magnificently effective performance in many spheres of activity other than routine dental treatment. This included the care of facial injuries, assistance of the physicians in debridement and closure of wounds, administration of anesthetics and sorting of casualties. Statistics of facial injuries were less than adequate. It is recorded that 2000 fractures of the facial bones were treated, and of the 1123 gunshot fractures of the mandible, 125 required bone grafting.

During World War I, Douglas B. Parker, D.D.S., M.D., served in a base hospital in France, where he treated great numbers of traumatic injuries of the face and jaws. His superb work in this field was noted and commended.

Because of his World War I experience and 30 years of hospital and teaching experience in the field of maxillofacial surgery, he was urged by Brigadier General Fairbanks of the Army Dental Corps to write a "small concise volume adequately dealing with the many phases of traumatic injuries—of sufficient value to a young dentist or physician entering the military service without specialized training." And so, in 1942 with World War II in progress, Dr. Parker published his "concise" book, *Synopsis of Traumatic Injuries of the Face and Jaws.*[46]

WORLD WAR II

World War II caused a great need for qualified oral surgeons and the medical departments of the respective armed services were faced with the problem of caring for a heavy influx of casualties on an international basis.

Maxillofacial surgical teams were formed which could be placed at different field hospital locations as required. These teams, consisting of a plastic surgeon, an oral surgeon, a surgical nurse, an anesthetist and supporting personnel proved to be a sound and wise approach to the problem of caring for facial injuries. In many locations plastic surgeons were not available, and oral surgeons, adhering to fundamental surgical principles and common sense, provided exemplary early care. Much credit must be given to John B. Erich, D.D.S., M.D., for the training of both medical and dental officers in the treatment of facial injuries. Collaborating with Louis T. Austin, D.D.S., he published in 1944 the excellent book entitled *Traumatic Injuries of the Facial Bones.*[19]

KOREAN CONFLICT

Great progress was made in oral surgery during the Korean Conflict, 1950–1953, and oral surgeons proved capable of rendering complete and effective treatment for the nearly 3000 maxillofacial injuries incurred. The achievements and devotion to duty of these oral surgeons in their support is exemplified by the writings of those stationed in Korea and in the chain of evacuation in Japan. [13, 27, 31, 35]

VIETNAM CONFLICT

The Vietnam Conflict brought an important change in the method of evacuation of the wounded. Helicopters were effective in lifting the wounded from the field of battle and transporting them to well-staffed hospitals, sometimes within minutes after injury. When further evacuation was required, the injured man could be transported directly to a major installation in the continental United States by jet aircraft.

A classic article by James E. Chipps, "Intermediate Care of Maxillofacial Injuries,"[13] reporting some of his surgical experiences and observations during the Korean Conflict, makes an interesting comparison with the 1965–1967 reports from the conflict in Vietnam. In Vietnam, fully qualified oral surgeons were assigned to hospitals supporting the combat troops, and, because of the spectacularly rapid helicopter evacuation, casualties were seen within one or two hours, often within just a few minutes, of the time of their injuries. This made it possible to stabilize maxillofacial fractures very early in the treatment phase and markedly decreased the need for tracheostomies.

Thus, it has been clearly illustrated that the oral surgeons, in the support of combat operations, have performed in such a manner as to bring great credit to their specialty. Statistics regarding the treatment of facial injuries resulting from combat operations also reveal conclusive proof that the oral surgeon has assumed the major role in the treatment of these cases.

ORGANIZATIONAL DEVELOPMENT OF ORAL SURGERY

Histories of the development of oral surgery have tended to emphasize the scientific development of the profession and ignore, in large part, the activities of dedicated men who have striven valiantly to upgrade the status of oral surgery through better organization, expanded dental school–hospital teaching relationships and improved residency training programs. This is unfortunate, for it is because of these activities that oral surgery has been able to grow professionally and attain recognition by the medical profession as playing an important role in patient care.

Prior to the end of World War I, there was no organization devoted to the specialty of oral surgery, excepting the section on Oral Surgery, Anesthesia and Radiology in the American Dental Assocation. In 1918 the American Society of Exodontia was formed and also the American Association of Oral and Plastic Surgeons.[36] The latter organization was composed largely of men holding both medical and dental degrees. Growth of the

American Society of Oral Surgery and Exodontia, so named in 1921, was gradual, and, for many years, there were no specific training requirements, the chief criterion for membership being that of a limited practice of oral surgery. In 1938 this group appointed a committee to study the need for the creation of a certifying board to establish the qualifications for the practice of oral surgery. In 1943 the name of this organization was changed to the American Society of Oral Surgeons, and at their 1945 meeting, they enlarged the committee to seven members and authorized this committee to proceed with the formation of the American Board of Oral Surgery and to conduct examinations for the certification of specialists in oral surgery. In 1946 the American Board of Oral Surgery was incorporated under the laws of the State of Illinois, and requirements for qualification for examination were established. This certifying board was founded with the stipulation that the members be elected by the House of Delegates of the American Society of Oral Surgeons.*

In April, 1947, the American Board of Oral Surgery was approved by the Council on Dental Education of the American Dental Association and authorized to proceed in the certification of specialists in Oral Surgery. The original members of the Board were James R. Cameron of Philadelphia; Leslie M. FitzGerald of Dubuque; Athol L. Frew of Dallas; Frank B. Hower of Louisville; Aubrey L. Martin of Seattle; Howard C. Miller of Chicago, and Carl W. Waldron of Minneapolis. At the organization meeting of the Board of Directors it was decided that an Advisory Committee composed of representatives of various organizations in the specialty of Oral Surgery, be appointed to counsel and assist the Board of Directors. The original members of the Advisory Committee were Donald H. Bellinger of Detroit; Orlan K. Bullard of San Diego; Malcolm W. Carr of New York City; Thomas Conner of Atlanta; J. Orton Goodsell of Saginaw; Stephen P. Mallett of Boston; and Douglas B. Parker of New York City.

---

*In 1968 the American Dental Association adopted revisions to the Requirements for the National Certifying Board for Special Areas of Dental Practice (A.D.A. Transactions, *45, 46,* 1968). In the section "Organization of Boards," it states in part, "Although the Council does not prescribe the specific method for the selection of the Directors of the Board (A.B.O.S.), membership on the Board should not be self-perpetuating."

In 1955 the educational requirements were three years of advanced study and training in oral surgery. This requirement was confirmed in 1968 by the Council on Dental Education of the A.D.A., who stipulated that the programs must have their approval. By 1975 there were over 1600 board certified oral surgeons practicing in the United States.

HOSPITAL DENTAL SERVICE, INTERNSHIPS AND RESIDENCY TRAINING PROGRAMS

According to Asbell[3] and Archer,[1] "The establishment of dental services and dental departments came very slowly during the early decades of this century. Hospital administrators were not quick to affirm the importance of this type of service. Some hospital dental services were started on a personal appeal of the dentist vis-à-vis the medical director or even the oral surgeon of the hospital.

"John V. Shoemaker, Surgeon-General of the State of Pennsylvania at the turn of the century, was also the President of the Board of Charities and Corrections of the City of Philadelphia. His broad experience in these positions brought him to the realization that dental services were not being adequately rendered and that a fully organized service should be established in the Philadelphia (General) Hospital.

"It was upon his recommendation that a dental staff including a dental interne was organized" in December, 1900. The chief of oral surgery was Matthew H. Cryer, Professor of Oral Surgery of the Department of Dentistry at the University of Pennsylvania.

"The first oral surgical interne was W. David Easton, who served until June, 1902, at which time Robert H. Ivy was appointed. Actually, Dr. Ivy served from June, 1901, to June, 1903, having completed his course in dentistry in June, 1901, but did not receive his D.D.S. degree until 1902, when he became 21 years of age.

"The duties of the staff and interne were 'to take care of the teeth and maxillary bones' of the patients in the hospital, and to give public clinics for students attending the various colleges of Philadelphia. Thus a pattern for hospital dentistry and hospital orientation for dental students was established."

However, "hospital dental service, dental internships and residencies, teaching relationships between dental schools and hospitals, like 'Topsy,' 'just growed.' No one was quite certain what the dental staff, the dental department, the dental intern or resident, if any, were supposed to do. As late as 1941 it was frankly recognized that 'all too often the function of the dental department in a hospital [was] limited to that of becoming an adjunct to its emergency service in order to relieve dental pain in ambulatory patients.'[38] Many physicians believed that the only time a dentist should be allowed in a hospital was to visit a sick relative or friend, and then only during visiting hours,"[1] Unfortunately, many dentists and dental school deans had the same attitude.

Credit is given to W. Harry Archer for identifying and establishing officially the status of dentists, dental departments and internship and residency programs in oral surgery in the hospitals of the United States by his work as chairman of several historic committees: Committee on Hospital Dental Service of the American College of Dentists,* Special Committee on Hospital Dental Service of the American Dental Association† and the Committee on Hospital Dental Care and Internships in Hospitals of the American Association of Dental Schools‡ in the 1940's and 1950's.

Dr. Archer's motion—presented to the House of Delegates of the American Dental Association in 1944[62] and calling for the appointment of a Special Committee on Hospital Dental Service both to establish the Basic Requirements for Hospital Dental Service and to examine and approve hospitals meeting those requirements—was unanimously approved and the Special Committee† was appointed. The adoption of this resolution was of paramount importance to oral surgery, for it established a mechanism whereby the quality of hospital dental departments and hospital dental internships and residency programs might be evaluated and improved. This Spe-

cial Committee was made a standing council on Hospital Dental Service in 1948,[66] with Dr. Archer continuing as chairman. The first hospital dental departments were approved in 1947.

As a member of a special three-man Committee on Hospital Dental Internships and Residencies* appointed by the Council on Dental Education in 1945,[64] he helped formulate the Requirements for Hospital Dental Internships and Residencies.

Early in 1946 these requirements were approved by the Council on Dental Education, and at its request, the Council on Hospital Dental Service assumed the additional responsibility of examining dental internship and residency programs, as well as hospital dental departments. The first internship and residency programs in oral surgery were approved by the Council on Dental Education in 1948 on the recommendation of the Council on Hospital Dental Service.

Another major "breakthrough" in 1947 was the action of the Committee on Hospital Dental Care and Internships in Hospitals† of the American Association of Dental Schools in opening negotiations with the Veterans Administration that led to the establishment of dental residency programs in V.A. hospitals.[48]

In 1947 the first pilot oral surgery residency program was started at the V.A. Hospital in Pittsburgh in cooperation with the School of Dentistry, University of Pittsburgh, under Dr. Archer's supervision. Today the V.A. has the largest oral surgery residency training program in the United States.

Thus, for the first time, the American Dental Association assumed its responsibility for dental care and the graduate education of dentists in hospitals. Unsuccessful attempts had been made prior to 1944 to stimulate the A.D.A. to fulfill its responsibility in this area of health care for the patient. McCluggage in his *A History of The American Dental Association* states: "As early as 1922, a Special Committee [of the A.D.A.] recommended action to encourage establishment of hospital dental services. The duty was assigned to the Standing Committee on Education, where it

---

*Members of the Committee on Hospital Dental Service of the American College of Dentists, 1945: W. Harry Archer, Chairman, J. W. Kemper, S. P. Mallett, L. H. Meisburger, Howard C. Miller.

†Members of the Special Committee on Hospital Dental Service of the American Dental Association: W. Harry Archer, Chairman, J. Frank Hall, Secretary, Sam H. Brock, B. Lucien Brun, James O. Cameron, Malcolm W. Carr, Milburn M. Fowler, Charles W. Freeman, Paul Hamilton, Frank J. Houghton, Daniel F. Lynch, Stephen P. Mallett, Stanford Moose, Douglas Parker, Hamilton B. G. Robinson, Reed O. Dingman, Roy Stout, Sidney L. Tiblier, Carl W. Waldron, W. T. Wright.

‡Members of the Committee on Hospital Dental Care and Internships in Hospitals of the American Association of Dental Schools: W. Harry Archer, Chairman, Charles W. Freeman, J. Ben Robinson, Gerald L. Timmons.

---

*Council on Dental Education—Committee on Hospital Dental Internships and Residencies: Frank J. Houghton, Chairman, W. Harry Archer, W. N. Hodgkin.

†Members of the Committee on Hospital Dental Care and Internships in Hospitals of the American Association of Dental Schools: W. Harry Archer, Chairman, Charles W. Freeman, J. Ben Robinson, Gerald L. Timmons.

apparently languished."[40] In addition, the A.D.A. itself had been lethargic, because the groundwork for this major step forward was laid in the 1930's by Howard C. Miller and Malcolm W. Carr, the first chairmen of the American College of Dentists Committee on Hospital Dental Service and Committee on Oral Surgery, respectively. Dr. Carr was also chairman of a New York Committee on Dental Standards and Services in Hospitals and Institutions, whose proposals were published in J.A.D.A. in 1939.[52]

At present there is an active review of all oral surgery training programs by the Council on Dental Education of the American Dental Association. Currently (1975), 125 oral surgery programs are listed as having been granted either preliminary approval or full accreditation.

SUMMARY AND CONCLUSIONS

As one reviews the history of oral surgery in the United States, he must be impressed with several facts, the first of which is that the specialty has sailed a stormy course, especially in its relationship with the medical profession on the national level. It has previously been emphasized that the great men in oral surgery practicing in the latter part of the 19th century were holders of M.D. degrees. Additionally, it was the conviction of these surgeons and, in fact, the medical profession that an M.D. degree was mandatory for the practice of oral surgery. This feeling was even carried over into the 20th century; as late as 1948, for example, Malcolm T. MacEachern, Associate Director of the American College of Surgeons, wrote to the chairman of the A.D.A. Council on Hospital Dental Service, "The only criticism of the Basic Standards for Hospital Dental Service Required of Approved Hospitals by our group is the doing of oral surgery by dentists without an M.D. degree." To this Dr. Archer replied, "Since oral surgery has been established as the first specialty in dentistry and has been practiced by men with only the dental degree, the Committee will not consider any changes that affect the rights of qualified dentists to practice oral surgery in hospitals."[49]

This philosophy, on the part of medicine, changed very little from the 19th century until the oral surgeons, with their outstanding contributions during World War I, demonstrated to the medical profession that they possessed great skill in the treatment of facial injuries.

New training programs in oral surgery were organized and came of age following World War II. The impetus for more oral surgery training programs came from dentists who wanted to meet the requirements of the American Board of Oral Surgery (organized in 1946), which only could be met in hospital residency programs. For example, in 1950 Major General Thomas L. Smith, Chief of the Dental Division, stated, "The Department of Army is entering the field of oral surgery residency training slowly and cautiously... time is necessary to prepare qualified staffs... residency programs will be expanded as soon as the staffs are prepared." Recognizing the need to increase their staffs of qualified oral surgeons who could in turn head training programs in oral surgery in their service hospitals, the Army and Air Force sent many of their young oral surgeons to the University of Pittsburgh School of Dentistry and affiliated hospitals for graduate training to fill this need.

As already noted, programs were established in many Veterans Administration hospitals in cooperation with dental schools, and medical schools, with their accompanying hospitals, appointed dentists to their faculties as professors of oral surgery in the department of surgery. Oral surgery training programs have gradually improved to their present stage of excellence. Yet, in spite of continual demonstrations of professional qualifications, the Joint Commission on Accreditation of Hospitals agreed upon and published in June, 1963, a ruling that a physical examination must be done by a physician on the staff of the hospital before dental treatment of oral surgery was performed. Bulletin No. 36 (J.C.A.H. August, 1964) further stipulated that every dental inpatient must have a staff physician who is available and will be responsible for the medical aspects of the patient's care throughout the hospital stay. This ruling continues in effect in spite of continual improvements in oral surgery residency programs, both in quality and length of training. Conversely, the American Medical Association has approved, and there have been implemented, programs to train "physician's assistants." Graduates of these programs are allowed to perform both histories and physical examinations and to sign them. Ironically, the minimal educational requirement for admittance to such programs (some of which are only two years in length) is a high school diploma, and the only justification offered for allowing a physician's assistant to assume these responsibilities is that he is working under the overall supervision of a physician.

In 1969 the Board of Regents, American College of Surgeons, issued a statement without previous consultation with either the American Society of Oral Surgeons or the American Dental Association to the effect that "Those who perform major surgical procedures should be doctors of medicine with adequate graduate education in surgery." Naturally, this raises the question as to what constitutes "major surgery." Additionally, it poses the question of whether many doctors of medicine who perform major surgical procedures are adequately trained. Through long and persistent negotiations between representatives of the American College of Surgeons, the American Society of Oral Surgeons and the American Dental Association this statement was modified as follows:

"All specialties in the head, neck and oral area should work progressively toward the team approach in the total care of patients with injuries in multiple regions or extensive and complicated medical-surgical problems. The oral surgeon may be an essential member of the team and may act independently in his own area of special competence. In instances requiring a team approach for the management of injuries in multiple regions or extensive and complicated medical-surgical problems, the surgeon who is 'captain of the team' and has final responsibility for the care of the patient must be a Doctor of Medicine."

In 1968 the Washington State Supreme Court ruled in a case involving an oral surgeon that "as a matter of law, a hospital must have a medical doctor present and supervising any surgical procedure performed on a patient under general anesthesia and if the hospital fails in this regard, the hospital will be liable for any injury which might result from this failure." In an editorial, "An Undeserved Slur upon Dentistry from the Joint Commission on Accreditation of Hospitals" (J.A.D.A., July, 1968), it was stated, "For the editor of the J.C.A.H. bulletin to comment on the Washington Supreme Court case as though the only issue was one involving a dentist is disturbing. The physician's conduct, as well as that of a nurse anesthetist, also called forth some strong criticism by the court.

The liability of hospitals for negligence occurring during surgery performed by physicians is a far greater problem than that caused by dentists. One need only read the reported court cases for one month to determine from what source the hospitals' major legal problems stem." Although this decision applied only to the State of Washington, it received extensive publicity and caused many oral surgeons throughout the country to suffer restrictions in operating room privileges. Again, after considerable negotiations between representatives of the Joint Commission and the American Dental Association, the following statement of policy was issued:

"Requirements for the presence of a physician in the operating room during procedures involving oral surgery performed by dentists, not required by the Joint Commission, should be determined locally by those professionally involved in such procedures under the responsibility of the chief of surgery or chief of staff, as in other surgical specialties. Such a determination is to be made after careful evaluation of the condition of the patient, the complexity of the procedure proposed and the competence of the surgical practitioner."

Still another rebuff of the A.D.A. by the Joint Commission on Accreditation of Hospitals occurred in December, 1972. Although the J.C.A.H. at its April, 1972, meeting had "approved in principle the concept of joint accreditation," which was initially conceived in a cooperative manner over several months by representatives of the A.D.A. and J.C.A.H., the Board of Commissioners of the Joint Commission in Accreditation of Hospitals on December 9, 1972, voted to "postpone until some future time the request from the American Dental Association" for representation on the Commission.

The increase in numbers and organizational strength of plastic surgeons and otorhinolaryngologists has also posed a threat to the activities of the oral surgeon, for there is much interest among these groups in many procedures traditionally performed by the oral surgeon. A second change has gradually taken place in the practice of oral surgery, this being an increased emphasis on certain procedures in oral surgery, among which are orthodontic surgery, preprosthetic surgery, the correction of congenital and acquired abnormalities of the jaws and the refinement of outpatient anesthesia.

It is apparent that this area of specialization is one of great need, one in which the oral surgeon is most competent and skillful, and one which he should therefore pursue with vigor.

In summary, it may be stated that the development of oral surgery in the United States has been sporadic and turbulent, but, in spite of this, great progress has been made. An excellent quality of oral surgery is being practiced throughout the United States and Canada, and the specialty continues to grow, although the future is clouded by definite gray areas. The future can be bright, but it will necessitate not only the continued demonstration of competence by the oral surgeon but also leadership, wisdom and persistence.

These qualities will all be necessary to bring about changes, so that oral surgeons may practice their specialty free of some of the restrictions under which they are presently required to operate.

APPENDIX

KURT HERMANN THOMA, D.M.D., ORAL SURGEON*

Kurt H. Thoma died in Newton, Massachusetts, on June 5, 1972, after a long illness. Born in Basel, Switzerland, on December 2, 1883, he attended private schools and studied architecture at the Institute of Technology in Burgdorf, Switzerland. Dr. Thoma came to the United States in 1908 and graduated from Harvard Dental School in 1911. Thus began a long and most distinguished career in the specialties of oral surgery, oral medicine and oral pathology.

He climaxed his academic career by serving as Charles A. Brackett Professor of Oral Pathology and Professor of Oral Surgery at Harvard University. Though Professor Emeritus at Harvard, he was intensely concerned with graduate oral surgery programs and became Professor of Oral Surgery at the Graduate School of Dentistry, Boston University, and profoundly influenced scores of oral surgery trainees. In addition, he was long affiliated with the graduate oral surgery program at the Graduate School of Medicine, University of Pennsylvania, and was Honorary Professor of Odontology at San Carlos University in Guatemala. Dr. Thoma was a Fellow in Dental Surgery, Royal College of Surgeons, England, and was awarded honorary degrees of Doctor of Medical Dentistry, University of Zurich, and Fellow in Dental Surgery, Royal College of Surgeons, Edinburgh. He represented Harvard University at the quincentenary celebration of Basel University in 1950.

Kurt Thoma's contributions to the medical and dental literature in this country and abroad were voluminous, and perhaps no other author is as frequently referred to in previous and contemporary stomatologic scientific papers, journals and texts as Thoma. The textbook publications that he authored

alone represent a prodigious feat in the lifetime of a diligent teacher, sedulous surgeon and generous lecturer: *Oral Anesthesia,* 1914 (M. C. Cherry); *Oral Abscesses,* 1916; *Oral Roentgenology,* 1917 (Ritter & Co.); *Teeth, Diet and Health,* 1923; *Clinical Pathology of the Jaws,* 1925; *Oral Diagnosis,* 1936; *Oral Pathology,* 1941 (The C. V. Mosby Co.); and *Oral Surgery,* 1948 (The C. V. Mosby Co.).

Contemplate periodic revisions of the above texts (the two-volume *Oral Surgery* had a fifth edition in 1969) and add approximately 300 scientific articles over a 50-year period, and the extent and significance of the Thoma legacy may be partially appreciated.

Professor Thoma originated the oral surgery section in the *American Journal of Orthodontics and Oral Surgery*—the precursor to *Oral Surgery, Oral Medicine and Oral Pathology.* The "Triple O" first appeared in 1948, and Dr. Thoma remained its editor-in-chief until 1970.

Kurt Thoma formerly was oral surgeon and chief of the Dental Service at Massachusetts General Hospital. The case reports from the M.G.H. clinic and the Department of Oral Surgery at the Harvard School of Dental Medicine (1943 to 1948) were instrumental in establishing the definition of oral surgical diseases and oral surgical boundaries under the aegis of dentistry—ultimately accepted by most large hospitals and oral surgery training centers in the United States. His articles on the history of oral surgery and advances in the specialty, published in the *New England Journal of Medicine,* helped arbitrate many a controversy and gave significant support to struggling hospital dental services.

Dr. Thoma was actively involved in the International Association of Oral Surgeons, the American Society of Oral Surgeons, the American Academy of Dental Science (past-president), the American Board of Oral Surgery, the American Board of Oral Pathology, the Harvard Odontological Society (past-president), the Harvard Dental Alumni Association (past-president), the American Academy of Oral Pathology (past-president), Omicron Kappa Upsilon (past-president) and Sigma Xi.

A partial list of awards and honors includes the Fauchard Medal, the Callahan Medal, the Jarvie Fellowship Medal, the American Society of Oral Surgeons Award, the Fones Medal, the Gies Award, the Maislen Memorial Award, Charles Tomes Lecturer, Royal College of Surgeons, England, and honorary membership in Psi Omega, the Dental Society of New South Wales, Australia, the Dental Society of Guatemala and the Odontologic Society of Cuba.

Dr. Thoma was a consultant to the United States Public Health Service, the Veterans Administration, Walter Reed Army Medical Center and the Armed Forces Institute of Pathology in Washington, D.C. He was oral surgeon to the Brooks Hospital in Brookline, Massachusetts, for 50 years and was on the staff of many Greater Boston hospitals.

In 1912, Dr. Thoma married Louise Bird, who died a few years ago. He is survived by a son, Kurt Richard Thoma, and a daughter, Mrs. Richard S. Alles, six grandchildren and two great-grandchildren. Memorial services were held on June 8 at the First Parish Unitarian Church in Weston, Massachusetts.

Dr. Thoma was an expert horticulturist, and his West Newton garden was a source of much pleasure and beauty. He was an authority on bees and in times past found relaxation in showing and riding horses, hunting, fishing and frequent trips to Europe.

In the fields of oral surgery, oral medicine and oral pathology, Dr. Thoma has perpetuated himself admirably. Historically, in every specialty there have been a handful of strong, determined, resourceful men who set the pace, defined the goals, defended the boundaries and, undaunted by obstacles, thus made it infinitely easier for succeeding generations to follow. Kurt H. Thoma has long been recognized as the father of oral pathology, the defender of oral surgery, and the great teacher of oral medicine. He raised the standards, originated surgical techniques and encouraged several generations of oral surgeons to high levels of professional stature.

Such a legacy is difficult to match, such accomplishments difficult to comprehend, but certainly Kurt H. Thoma's influence will long endure.

REFERENCES

1. Archer, W. H.: The American Dental Association and hospital dental service—A critical historical review 1920–1950. J. Hosp. Dent. Pract., 5(2):53–66 (Apr.), 1971.
2. Archer, W. H.: A Manual of Dental Anesthesia. 2nd ed. Philadelphia, W. B. Saunders Co., 1958.
3. Asbell, M. B.: Hospital dental service in the United States—A historical review. J. Hosp. Dent. Pract., 3(1):9–11 (Jan.), 1969.
4. Berger, A.: Principles and Technique of the Removal of Teeth. Brooklyn, Dental Items of Interest Publishing Co., Inc., 1929.
5. Bourgoyne, J. R.: Surgery of the Mouth and Jaws. Brooklyn, Dental Items of Interest Publishing Co., Inc., 1949.
6. Brooks, S.: Civil War Medicine, p. 103. Springfield, Ill., Charles C Thomas, 1966.
7. Brophy, T. W.: Evolution of oral surgery in the past seventy-five years. Dent. Cosmos, 62:42–55, 1920.
8. Brophy, T. W.: Oral Surgery, A Treatise on the Diseases, Injuries and Malformations of the Mouth and Associated Parts. Philadelphia, P. Blakiston's Sons & Co., 1915.
9. Brown, G. V. I.: The Surgery of Oral and Facial Diseases and Malformations. Philadelphia, Lea & Febiger, 1912.
10. Buxton, J. L.: Dudley, Dental Surgery. New York, Wm. Wood, 1927.
11. Cahn, L. R.: The Modern Practice of Tooth Extraction. New York, The Macmillan Co., 1924.
12. Cameron, J. R.: Development of the specialty of oral surgery. J. Oral Surg., 17:14–19 (Sept.), 1944.
13. Chipps, J. E., Canham, R. G., and Makel, H. P.: Intermediate treatment of maxillofacial injuries. U.S. Armed Forces Med. J., 4:951–976, 1953.
14. Cogswell, W. W.: Dental Oral Surgery. Colorado Springs, Press of Out West Printing and Stationery Co., 1932.
15. Cooksey, D. E.: History of oral surgery in the United States Navy. J. Oral Surg., 20:365, 1962.
16. Cryer, M. H.: Studies on Internal Anatomy of the Face. Philadelphia, S. S. White Dental Manufacturing Co., 1901.
17. Cryer, M. H.: Contributions of dentistry to surgery. Dent. Cosmos, 39:102, 1897.
18. Durbeck, W. E.: The Impacted Lower Third Molar. Brooklyn, Dental Items of Interest Publishing Co., Inc., 1943.
19. Erich, J. B., and Austin, L. T.: Traumatic Injuries of Facial Bones: An Atlas of Treatment. Philadelphia, W. B. Saunders Co., 1944.
20. Feldman, M. H.: Exodontia. 3rd ed. Philadelphia, Lea & Febiger, 1941.
21. Garretson, J. E.: A Treatise on Disease and Surgery of the Mouth, Jaws and Associated Parts. Philadelphia, J. B. Lippincott Co., 1869.
22. Garrison, F. H.: Notes on the history of military medicine. Mil. Surg., 50:7.2, 1922.
23. Gwinn, C. D.: A Text-book of Exodontia. Philadelphia, Lea & Febiger, 1927.
24. Holland, D. J.: In memoriam: Kurt Hermann Thoma, D.M.D., Editor Emeritus. Oral Surg., 34(3):374–376 (Sept.), 1972.

25. Hornor, S. S.: The Medical Student's Guide in Extracting Teeth. Philadelphia, Lindsay & Blakiston, 1851.

26. Howe, G. L.: The Extraction of Teeth. Baltimore, The Williams & Wilkins Co., 1961.

27. Irby, W. B., and Gavin, G. P.: A new head appliance for maxillofacial injuries. J. Oral Surg., 13:297–299, 1955. Abstracted, J.A.D.A., (Sept.), 1955.

28. Ivy, R. H.: Some early history in the development of oral surgery as a specialty. J. Oral Surg., 24:201–208 (May), 1966.

29. Ivy, R. H., and Curtis, L.: Fractures of the Jaws. 3rd ed. Philadelphia, Lea & Febiger, 1945.

30. Jeffcott, G. F.: United States Army Dental Service in World War II. Washington, D.C., U.S. Government Printing Office, 1955.

31. Kapis, B. W.: Early management of maxillofacial war injuries. J. Oral Surg., 12:292–303, 1954.

32. Koch, R. E. (assisted by Brophy, T. W.): History of Dental Surgery. Chicago, National Articles Publishing Co., 1909.

33. Leake, D.: Chapter 1: History of oral surgery. In Guralnick, W. C.: Textbook of Oral Surgery. Boston, Little, Brown & Co., 1968.

34. Lederer, W. J.: The Principles and Practice of Tooth Extraction and Local Anesthesia of the Maxillae. New York, The Rebman Co., 1915.

35. Lighterman, I. I.: The division oral surgeon in Korea. Oral Surg., 9:239–252, 1956.

36. Lyons, C. J.: The History of Oral Surgery and Its Influence on the Profession of Dentistry. Dent. Cosmos, 76:27–40, 1934.

37. Malgaigne, J. F.: Treatise on Fractures. (Translated from French by J. H. Packard.) Philadelphia, J. B. Lippincott Co., 1895.

38. Manual on Dental Care and Dental Internships in Hospitals. Chicago, American Hospital Association, 1941.

39. Marshall, J. S.: Manual of Injuries and Surgical Diseases of the Face, Mouth and Jaws. Philadelphia, S. S. White Dental Manufacturing Co., 1897.

40. McCluggage, R. W.: A History of The American Dental Association. Chicago, The American Dental Association, 1959.

41. McCurdy, S. L.: Oral Surgery, A Textbook on General Surgery and Medicine As Applied to Dentistry. 2nd ed. Pittsburgh, Pittsburgh Dental Publishing Co., 1923.

42. McDaniel, D. J.: A New Technique and Instrumentation for the Removal of Impacted Teeth. Chicago, 1934.

43. Mead, S. V.: Oral Surgery. St. Louis, The C. V. Mosby Co., 1940.

44. The Medical and Surgical History of the War of the Rebellion (1861–1865), Part First, Surgical Volume. Second Issue, p. 321. Washington, D.C., U.S. Government Printing Office, 1875.

45. Officers and Standing Committees. J. Am. Coll. Dent., 13(1), 1945–46.

46. Parker, D. B.: Synopsis of Traumatic Injuries of the Face and Jaws. St. Louis, The C. V. Mosby Co., 1942.

47. Personal Communication from Shailer Peterson, Secretary, Council on Dental Education, American Dental Association, October 28, 1948.

48. Proceedings of the American Association of Dental Schools. 24th Annual Meeting, pp. 56–64, 81–82. June 23–25, 1947.

49. Proceedings of the American Association of Dental Schools, 24th Annual Meeting. Report of the Committee on Hospital Dental Care and Internships in Hospitals, pp. 105–107, 1948.

50. Proceedings of the American Association of Dental Schools. 26th Annual Meeting. Report of the Committee on Hospital Dental Care and Internships in Hospitals, pp. 60–62. June 27–29, 1949.

51. Proceedings of the American Association of Dental Schools, 27th Annual Meeting. Report of the Committee on Hospital Dental Care and Internships in Hospitals, p. 54. March 27–29, 1950.

52. Proposed basic standards of hospital dental service as a fundamental requirement of approved class "A" hospitals. Malcolm W. Carr, Chairman. J.A.D.A., 26:1016 (June), 1939.

53. Report of the Committee on Hospital Dental Service. W. Harry Archer, Chairman. J.A.D.A., 16(1):35–38 (Mar.), 1949.

54. Report of the Committee on Hospital Dental Service. W. Harry Archer, Chairman. J.A.D.A., 18:108–114, 1950–1951.

55. Robertson, A.: A Manual on Extracting Teeth. Philadelphia, Lindsay & Blakiston, 1868.

56. Rounds, F. W., and Rounds, C. E.: Principles and Techniques of Exodontia. St. Louis, The C. V. Mosby Co., 1953.

57. Schwartz, L.: The development of the treatment of jaw fractures. J. Oral Surg., 2:193–221 (July), 1944.

58. Silverman, S. L.: Principles and Practice of Oral Surgery. Philadelphia, P. Blakiston's Sons & Co., 1926.

59. Stern, B. J.: Social factors in medical progress. New York, Columbia University Press, 1927.

60. Thoma, K. H.: The history of oral surgery. Oral Surg., 10:1–10, 1957.

61. Thoma, K. H.: Oral Surgery, 5th ed. St. Louis, The C. V. Mosby Co., 1969.

62. Transactions of The American Dental Association. 84th Annual Meeting. House of Delegates Minutes, p. 354. October 16–18; 1944.

63. Transactions of The American Dental Association. 87th Annual Meeting. Report of the Committee on Hospital Dental Service, pp. 247–255. October 14–16, 1946.

64. Transactions of The American Dental Association. 87th Annual Meeting. Report of the Council on Dental Education, pp. 259–260. October 14–16, 1946.

65. Transactions of The American Dental Association. 88th Annual Meeting. Committee on Hospital Dental Service, p. 105. August 4–8, 1947.

66. Transactions of The American Dental Association. 89th Annual Meeting. Committee on Hospital Dental Service, p. 234. September 13–17, 1948.

67. Winter, G. B.: Principles of Exodontia as Applied to the Impacted Mandibular Third Molar. St. Louis, American Medical Book Co., 1926.

68. Winter, L.: Exodontia, Oral Surgery and Anesthesia. 5th ed. St. Louis, The C. V. Mosby Co., 1943.

CHAPTER 2

DENTOALVEOLAR SURGERY: THE EXTRACTION OF TEETH

The extraction of teeth, however accomplished, is a surgical operation involving bony and soft tissues of the oral cavity, access to which is restricted by the lips and checks, and further complicated by the movement of the tongue and mandible. An additional hazard is that this cavity communicates with the pharynx, which in turn opens into the larynx and esophagus. Furthermore, this field of operation is flooded by saliva and is inhabited by the largest number and greatest variety of microorganisms found in the human body. Finally, it lies close to the vital centers.

The number of teeth that can be "safely" extracted at one time depends upon the physical status of the patient and upon the extent and type of infection present. It is true that serious postextraction systemic complications such as, for example, subacute bacterial endocarditis, acute nephritis or a thyroid crisis can be and have been precipitated by a single extraction. Of course there is a greater possibility of producing acute exacerbations of various systemic disturbances by multiple extractions, which mean more trauma and the possibility of an increased bacteremia. The latter is particularly true where the indication for extraction is advanced suppurative periodontal disease.

It is essential, therefore, that this phase of oral surgery be given the same careful study and application of sound surgical principles as is given to surgery in any other part of the human body. No operation performed by the dentist is fraught with such great danger to the patient as those of oral surgery, a large part of which is the extraction of teeth.

While the great majority of extractions can be safely done in the dental office, some patients require hospitalization for this surgery, either because of systemic conditions which make them poor surgical risks, or because of the extent of the surgery and anticipated difficulties. A maxillary and mandibular odontectomy and alveolectomy (or alveoplasty) (see Plate I, page 55) involves both soft tissue and bone. It requires not only as much time and skill as many of the "major surgery" procedures performed daily in hospitals but also the same special services provided, including the anesthesiologist. The reader is also referred to Chapter 9, "Oral Surgery in the Hospital," beginning on page 419, for further discussion.

INDICATIONS FOR THE EXTRACTION OF TEETH

Dentists are frequently besieged by patients requesting, "Take out all my teeth," because these persons: (a) are seeking impossible cures for a myriad of diseases, (b) want a "set of beautiful white teeth," or (c) are tired of "always going to the dentist," plus many other equally foolish "reasons." No ethical dentist would extract teeth for such reasons any more than a surgeon would arbitrarily amputate a limb. If, following a complete oral examination employing all possible diagnostic aids, such as radiographs, vitality tests, and so forth, a dentist finds that a patient should not have "all his teeth out," then it is the dentist's responsibility to try to convince the patient that his teeth should not be extracted. In many cases this is not an easy task, but a dentist's refusal to carry out these wishes should make a strong impression on the patient. If the reason was, "My doctor (anyone of the health professions) said I needed my teeth out," the patient is informed that the "doctor" will be advised of the results of the oral examination before any surgery is performed. The "doctor" is called and diplomatically advised of the results of the oral examination, and hopefully the conflicts of opinion are resolved in the patient's best interests.

The following are indications for the extraction of teeth: (a) teeth that are hopelessly carious; (b) teeth with nonvital pulps, or acute or chronic pulpitis when root canal surgery is not indicated; (c) in cases of severe periodontoclasia in which excessive bony support of the teeth is destroyed; (d) teeth not treatable by apicoectomy; (e) teeth mechanically interfering with the placement of restorative appliances; (f) teeth not restorable by operative dentistry; (g) impacted teeth and unerupted teeth (there are exceptions — not all impacted or unerupted teeth should be removed — and these are discussed in Chapter 5); (h) supernumerary teeth; (i) retained primary teeth when a permanent tooth is present, and in normal position to erupt; (j) teeth with fractured roots (exceptions to this rule are discussed later in this chapter); (k) malposed teeth not amenable to orthodontic treatment; (l) roots and fragments (exceptions are discussed in Chapter 25); (m) teeth that are traumatizing soft tissues, if other treatment will not prevent this trauma; (n) all teeth before radiation therapy for oral malignancy (teeth should be extracted and a very extensive alveolectomy performed — study pages 106 to 110 for a detailed discussion of this subject before operating on these patients). There are "exceptions" to all "rules." Some specific references to this fact were noted above.

ORTHODONTIC TREATMENT AND THE EXTRACTION OF TEETH

The extraction of permanent teeth for the purpose of orthodontic treatment should not be carried out without expert advice by an orthodontist who is well experienced and qualified in this form of treatment. It would appear that all too frequently this is not so. According to De Angella (1973), "Indications for extraction and the [choice of] teeth to be extracted depend on specific aspects of the malocclusion. The decision to correct a malocclusion by the extraction of teeth should be based on the ratio of arch size to tooth size, facial appearance and other factors derived from the diagnosis. Selection of the teeth is determined by the location of the dentoalveolar dysplasias."[12]

CONTRAINDICATIONS TO THE EXTRACTION OF TEETH OR OTHER ORAL SURGICAL OPERATIONS

Before any oral surgical procedure, including the removal of teeth, is undertaken, a thorough oral examination and physical survey of the patient is mandatory. The specific details in making this survey are in Chapter 9, pages 422 to 425, and should be studied at this time. The results of this preliminary survey will be the determining factor as to whether a more exhaustive and detailed physical examination should be made by the patient's physician, or an internist, or a specialist in the area of particular concern, before the dentist proceeds with the surgery. This survey will give the dentist sufficient information to enable him, in discussing the case with the patient's physician, to present intelligently his findings and concerns, if any, about the patient's physical ability to undergo the proposed surgery safely, and if so, whether or not the proposed surgery (which includes the extraction of teeth) should be performed in the office or in the hospital, and the type of anesthesia. This latter question, however, actually should be decided in consultation with the anesthesiologist.

SYSTEMIC CONTRAINDICATIONS BEFORE CONSULTATION WITH THE PATIENT'S PHYSICIAN

Cardiac Disease. A brief history will indicate which patients should have further investigation. (a) Breathlessness is one of the first and most reliable signs of cardiac disease. (b) Chronic fatigue is a frequent indication of heart failure. Other contraindications are (c) palpitation of recent origin, induced now by activities which heretofore were tolerated without fatigue; (d) sleep which is disturbed unless the head is elevated; (e) headache from cerebral congestion; (f) vertigo from relative cerebral anemia.

In addition to this short history, the patient should be carefully scrutinized to ascertain whether there is (g) cyanosis of the lips, tongue or fingernails; (h) dyspnea on exertion; (i) engorged cervical veins; (j) edema of the ankles; (k) exophthalmos, with goiter, nervousness or sweating; (l) tachycardia, pulse markedly accelerated; (m) petechiae in the mouth or elsewhere; (n) blood pressure within normal limits.

Case Report No. 1

SUBACUTE BACTERIAL ENDOCARDITIS FOLLOWING THE EXTRACTION OF TWO TEETH

Past History. Miss F. G., age 18, was admitted to the hospital June 21. She had had her first attack of rheumatic fever at the age of 9. She had been in bed 3 months, with no cardiac involvement. At the age of 13, she had been hospitalized for two months for rheumatic fever and confined to bed for one year. Patient had been in good health since that time.

Present Illness. On May 1, she had had two teeth extracted in a dental office in a neighboring town. No history was taken or antibiotics given prior to extractions. On June 1, she had had a recurrence of rheumatic fever with aching joints and thought she had "grippe." Weakness, easy fatigability, anorexia, fever and malaise have been progressive. At present there are petechiae on the skin and oral mucosa.

Blood Counts and Cultures. On June 22, the white blood count was 20,000. Blood culture showed streptococci on June 23. Urine culture was negative.

The white blood count was 11,000 on June 24; 12,800 on July 1; 9400 on July 7.

Temperature Readings. On June 21, her temperature was 102° F.; on June 22, 102° F.; on June 23, 101° F.: on June 24, 98° F.; temperature was normal during the rest of her stay in the hospital.

Chest X-ray Conclusions.
1. Enlargement of the heart shadow, with left auricular and left ventricular preponderance.
2. Slight hilar vascular concentration.
3. Lung fields are clear.

Electrocardiograph Summary.
1. Sinus tachycardia with normal conduction time.
2. Magnitude of QRS complexes suggests left ventricular hypertrophy and minimal nonspecific ST-T changes are indicative of early left ventricular strain.

Treatment. Penicillin, 1,000,000 units every 8 hours, to a total 49,000,000 units, was given; also Meticorten, 5 mg. every 6 hours, to a total of 275 mg.

RHEUMATIC HEART DISEASE. Patients with a history of rheumatic heart disease should have, in consultation with their physicians, prophylactic administration of penicillin prior to and after the extraction of teeth or other oral surgical procedures. Heart valves which have been previously damaged from bouts with the disease are susceptible to invasion by *Streptococcus viridans,* which is frequently present in the blood stream after the extraction of teeth, thus inciting subacute bacterial endocarditis.

About one third of patients who have had rheumatic fever suffer chronic deforming valvular disease of the heart. These patients are in danger of contracting endocarditis every time a bacteremia occurs, because the roughened endocardium provides a place for the bacterial organisms to lodge, vegetate and eventually interfere with normal valvular function.

ANTIBIOTIC PROPHYLAXIS OF SUBACUTE BACTERIAL ENDOCARDITIS BEFORE ORAL SURGERY. Bacterial endocarditis is a disease due to bacterial infection of the valvular and mural endocardium. This infection can originate with the transient bacteremia which

occurs in approximately 50 to 80 per cent of the oral surgical procedures performed in septic mouths, and in about 43 per cent of oral surgical procedures performed in normal mouths.

The following program is suggested as an aid in the prevention of subacute bacterial endocarditis as a sequel to oral surgical procedures:
1. All patients should be questioned as to a history of rheumatic fever, congenital heart disease or persistent heart murmurs.
2. All patients having a positive history should receive antibiotic therapy as described in Chapter 8.

The following facts are pertinent: (*a*) In about 85 per cent of subacute bacterial endocarditis cases, the causative organism is *Streptococcus viridans.* (*b*) Antibiotic therapy reduces the incidence of bacteremia but does *not* prevent it entirely.

ANTIBIOTIC PROPHYLAXIS OF THE PATIENT WHO HAS HAD PROSTHETIC VALVULAR SURGERY OF THE HEART. Heart patients who have had prosthetic valvular surgery need extremely large doses of antibiotics before and after oral surgery. Each cardiologist has his own preference and should be consulted prior to surgery.

PATIENTS ON ANTICOAGULANT THERAPY. Patients on prolonged anticoagulant therapy who require oral surgical procedures are faced with two problems: (a) prolonged postoperative hemorrhage, or (b) if the anticoagulant therapy is discontinued until the prothrombin level returns to near normal, they risk a possible serious or fatal thromboembolic accident. However, it has been demonstrated that with close cooperation between the cardiologist, the internist and the oral surgeon, minor oral surgical procedures such as extractions, multiple extractions with the insertion of immediate dentures, alveolectomies, excision of hyperplasias, and incision and drainage of abscesses can be performed without much postoperative hemorrhage even though the anticoagulant therapy is continued. It is obvious that minimal trauma should accompany the surgery and hemorrhage-controlling techniques should be carried out as described in Chapter 25, pages 1560 to 1579. Major oral surgery requires thorough preoperative and postoperative care of the patient by personnel on the three services just mentioned.

Blood Dyscrasias. These include anemia, leukemia, hemorrhagic purpura and hemophilia. Collins and Crane[10] list the following diagnostic points.

ANEMIA. *Symptoms.* The principal symptoms, whether in reduction of hemoglobin or erythrocytes, or both, are as follows: (a) pallor (especially in the lips, fingernails, conjunctivae, tongue, and mucosa of the mouth); (b) dyspnea on exertion (breathlessness); (c) drowsiness or vertigo; (d) edema of the extremities (if severe anemia is present). In addition, certain less important symptoms may be present which include (e) circulatory symptoms—palpitation, tachycardia, fainting attacks, precordial distress, and a heart murmur; (f) nervous symptoms—irritability, restlessness, mental depression, insomnia, headaches, spots before the eyes, and nervousness; (g) gastrointestinal symptoms—poor appetite, abdominal discomfort, constipation or diarrhea; (h) decreased or absent menstruation and loss of sexual desire; (i) low-grade fever.

Dental Aspects. These patients frequently consult their dentists because of sore tongues. The presence of a glossitis, with a raw, smooth or bald tongue (with atrophy of the papillae), should raise the suspicion of Addisonian (pernicious) anemia.

The mucous membranes of the mouth may appear pale; small petechial hemorrhages may often be seen.

If there is a doubt concerning atrophy of the papillae of the tongue, a quick stroke with the edge of a tongue blade along the side of the tongue will cause the papillae to stand out, unless they have become atrophied (as is the general rule in pernicious anemia).

Extreme care must be used in handling patients with pernicious anemia, since they are easily disturbed by an unusual circumstance, such as fright, worry or surgical procedure, and may as a result show a sudden and often marked drop in the blood count. ✓

MYELOGENOUS LEUKEMIA. The symptoms of myelogenous leukemia are (a) a gradually progressive weakness and loss of weight; (b) the symptoms of anemia (described previously); (c) a sense of fullness or discomfort in the abdomen (due to an enlargement of the spleen), or a sensation of an intra-abdominal mass; (d) periods of irregular fever; (e) gastrointestinal symptoms—loss of appetite, flatulence, recurrent attacks of diarrhea and occasional vomiting; (f) itching of the skin; (g) hemorrhages from various parts of the body; (h) disturbances of vision or of hearing because of leukemic infiltrations; (i) occasional pains over the long bones; (j) excessive bleeding following minor trauma, including tooth extraction.

The physical findings of these patients will include (a) evidence of loss of weight; (b) pallor; (c) spongy, easily bleeding gums; (d) enlargement of the spleen (often marked); (e) enlargement of the liver (less marked than that of the spleen); (f) hemorrhagic phenomena (petechiae, bleeding gums and the like); (g) tenderness over the sternum and long bones (occasionally).

LYMPHATIC LEUKEMIA. The symptoms are (a) gradually increasing weakness and fatigue; (b) the symptoms of anemia (which usually develop earlier than in chronic myeloid leukemia); (c) enlargement of lymph nodes throughout the body; (d) hemorrhagic phenomena (bleeding from the gums, petechiae, hemorrhage following tooth extraction or tonsillectomy, and the like); (e) cough (due to enlargement of bronchial lymph nodes); (f) pruritus (itching).

Physical examination reveals (a) a discrete enlargement of lymph nodes throughout the body (neck, axillae, groin, mediastinum, retroperitoneum, and elsewhere); (b) moderate enlargement of the liver and spleen (less marked than in chronic myeloid leukemia); (c) the signs of anemia (pallor, cardiac murmurs, decreased exercise tolerance, lowered blood pressure and so forth).

Examination of the blood discloses (a) a secondary type of anemia, the severity of which depends on the stage of disease; (b) a marked increase in the total leukocyte count, averaging approximately 100,000 cells, although much higher counts may be found. (c) More than 90 or 95 per cent of the white cells are immature lymphocytes; during acute stages, lymphoblasts appear in the blood stream. (d) The neutrophils form only 5 or 10 per cent, or less, of the total white blood cells; eosinophils, basophils, and monocytes are usually not seen. (e) The platelets are usually somewhat reduced.

HEMORRHAGIC PURPURA AND HEMOPHILIA. Hemorrhage into or from the gum is also a common finding in advanced scurvy. Likewise petechial hemorrhage and ecchymosis following extravasation of blood into the tissues are the result of increased capillary fragility due to an ascorbic acid deficiency.

Always inquire as to the amount of postoperative bleeding the patient has had following previous extractions. If this is the first extraction, question him concerning the length of bleeding when he accidentally cuts himself. If the history is suspicious, a bleeding and coagulation time test as well as a prothrombin concentration test is ordered and evaluated before operating.

A dentist may be the first professional person consulted by a patient with a serious hemorrhagic disease resulting in purpuric bleeding into the gums (scurvy, idiopathic thrombopenia, leukemia), or because of prolonged bleeding following a simple extraction (idiopathic bleeding, hemophilia). Other causes of bleeding are lack of fibrinogen due to cirrhosis of the liver or due to a congenital deficiency, and increased antithrombin or fibrinolysin. The afibrinogenemia which occurs as a dramatic complication of pregnancy at the time of delivery is not a dental problem. For further information on bleeding see Chapter 25, pages 1560 to 1579.

POLYCYTHEMIA. There are two types of polycythemia: (a) *relative,* due to loss of fluid, which causes a hemoconcentration, and (b) *polycythemia vera,* a condition due to excessive production of red blood cells (RBC's) by bone marrow. The latter may cause excessive bleeding during oral surgery. Prior consultation with the patient's physician is recommended.

Diabetes. *Symptoms.* The symptoms of diabetes are (a) passage of large amounts of urine; (b) increased thirst and excessive appetite; (c) loss of weight and strength; (d) skin disturbances, furuncles, carbuncles, localized or generalized pruritus, and slowly healing ulcers; (e) disturbance of vision; (f) numbness and tingling; (g) pain (neuritis, especially in the lower limbs); (h) sugar in the urine; (i) a blood glucose well above its normal value.

Effects. Uncontrolled diabetes is a contraindication to oral surgery, because this disease predisposes to the development of infection in the wound with extension into the surrounding tissues in the following ways: (a) Peripheral circulation is reduced somewhat as a result of the deposition of cholesterol into the peripheral vessels (premature arteriosclerosis). (b) The high percentage of sugar in the body fluids helps bacterial growth by supplying the organisms with a rich source of food. Hence before either the extraction of teeth or other forms of oral surgery the diabetic patient should have his blood sugar controlled by diet or insulin. Again, consultation with the patient's physician is necessary.

Nephritis. *Symptoms.* The symptoms of nephritis include (a) decreased urinary output or dysuria; (b) hematuria; (c) fever; (d) albuminuria; (e) chills; (f) xerostomia (dryness) and burning in the mouth; (g) a generalized stomatitis in uremia; (h) a urinous odor to the patient's breath in renal failure.

Effects. The extraction of a large number of chronically infected teeth may precipitate an acute nephritis. If there is any indication of nephritis in a patient requiring extraction of teeth, refer the patient to his physician for diagnosis and treatment before instituting oral surgery.

Toxic Goiter. *Symptoms.* The symptoms are (a) nervousness, tremors and emotional instability; (b) tachycardia and palpitation; (c) excessive perspiration; (d) a diffuse enlargement of the thyroid gland (occasionally absent); (e) exophthalmos (increased prominence of the eyeballs) in 60 to 70 per cent of patients; (f) loss of weight; (g) elevation of the basal metabolic rate; (h) increase in the pulse pressure; (i) menstrual disturbances; (j) excessive appetite; (k) early fatigue and muscular weakness; (l) gastrointestinal symptoms—diarrhea in about 30 per cent of patients and at times nausea and vomiting; (m) pressure symptoms in some instances (such as dyspnea, dysphagia, hoarseness, and the like).

Effects. A thyroid crisis may be precipitated by oral surgery. The patient with a thyroid crisis is semiconscious, very restless, uncontrollable even with heavy sedation, cyanotic, and at times delirious, with an extremely rapid, thready pluse and a high temperature. No oral surgery procedure, including the extraction of teeth, should be performed on a patient with a toxic goiter, since such trauma may precipitate a crisis of thyroid activity with cardiac embarrassment and heart failure. Refer the patient for treatment before undertaking surgery.

Syphilis. The syphilitic patient's resistance is lowered, so that he is more liable to the development of postoperative infection because of delayed healing. These patients should be on antisyphilitic treatment before oral surgery is performed.

Jaundice. *Symptoms.* The symptoms include yellowish or bronzed skin and conjunctiva, yellow mucous membranes, and yellowish body fluids (the yellowish tint is caused by bile pigments).

Types. Jaundice comprises several types. One classification is as follows:

1. Obstructive jaundice.
2. Hemolytic or nonobstructive jaundice.
3. Jaundice due to infectious hepatitis.

In addition to the possibility of aggravating the etiologic factor responsible for the jaundice by the extraction of teeth, there is the danger of prolonged hemorrhage. If extraction is imperative, the patient should receive prophylactic doses of vitamin K before the operation. Patients with jaundice should be referred to their physicians for treatment before undergoing oral surgery.

Corticosteroid Therapy. Patients who have been on steroid therapy may have a suppression of output of adrenocorticotrophic hormone from the anterior pituitary gland, with resultant adrenal cortical atrophy. Several deaths have been reported in these patients after the stress of surgery.

At the Lahey Clinic, Fernandez-Herlily reports that unless a patient coming to surgery under general or spinal anesthesia gives a certain negative answer regarding prior cortisone therapy, he is given a "cortisone prep." "The patient undergoing a short, simple operation, such as tooth extraction, under general anesthesia is given 50 to 100 mg. of cortisone orally 2 hours preoperatively. During the operation, 100 mg. of hydrocortisone sodium succinate in 500 cc. of 5 per cent dextrose in water is available as an intravenous drip. Twelve hours postoperatively the patient receives 50 mg. of cortisone orally, or 100 mg. intramuscularly.

"Experience has shown that the most critical period for patients with adrenal unresponsiveness is that within 20 or so hours after operation. The clinical picture is that of sudden collapse, hypotension, tachycardia and very often a high fever."[16]

Oral Surgery during Pregnancy. CONTROVERSIAL CONSIDERATIONS. The question of whether the pregnant woman who presents herself for treatment should be subjected to oral surgery is a vexing one for many practitioners. While prevalent lay opinion now generally recognizes the need for dental care of the expectant mother, many persons feel that such care should extend only to prophylaxis and restorations and defer any necessary surgery until after the birth of the child. This is based primarily upon a fear of causing an abortion or premature labor, and secondarily upon a fear of causing actual physical damage to the child. Nothing could be further from the truth.

In an analysis by Davidson[11] of 1000 pregnancies during which oral operations had been performed, it was revealed that there was not a single case in which the operation was proved to cause or aggravate any complication of pregnancy. The incidence of pregnancy complications in all patients had no relationship to the question of whether an oral operation had been performed. What was revealed, however, was the reason for lay opinion's being what it is.

In many cases, extractions had been performed, and abortions followed some time afterward. The time period was variable, being anywhere from several hours to several days. These abortions, according to the obstetricians and pathologists, would have occurred regardless of whether the oral operation had been performed. The fetuses in many cases showed pathologic changes far antedating the time of the operation. The juxtaposition of the time of oral surgery and abortion was a mere coincidence. Herein lies the fire behind the smoke screen of opinion against operation during pregnancy.

People find it necessary to assign some cause to abortion, and conveniently seize upon this excuse if extractions or other oral operations have been done prior to the misfortune. The practitioner should not allow lay misconceptions to deter him in his role of eliminating oral sepsis and safe-guarding the health of the mother and the fetus. There are other considerations, however.

How much and what type of operation should be performed? What about impactions? These questions can be best answered by dividing all oral surgery into three classifications:

1. Emergency treatment—pain present.
2. Nonemergency but necessary treatment, *e.g.*, chronic periapical abscess.
3. Elective treatment.

There should be no compunction about performing the first two types of surgery during pregnancy. As to the last, one must decide whether or not the patient's general health is adequate, and measure the benefits against the operative discomforts and possible complications. In other words: Treat the pregnant woman with the same consideration that a cardiac or a diabetic patient would get because of altered physiology.

When should the work be done? In emergency cases there is no question: immediately. In the other cases the optimum time is probably the middle trimester of pregnancy. Later than this the patient has begun to be uncomfortable and cannot sit for any protracted period. Prior to this trimester, nausea and vomiting may still be present, making the dentist's work difficult.

ANESTHETIC CONSIDERATIONS.* With the exception of the muscle relaxants, all anesthetic drugs given to the pregnant patient cross the placenta and enter the blood stream of the fetus; these drugs have the same effect on the fetus as they do on the mother. A well-managed anesthesia for an oral surgical procedure, however, should offer no serious concern, since the operation will most certainly have been accomplished long enough before delivery for any anesthetic drugs to have been completely detoxified or eliminated.

Specific consideration must be given, however, to the time during pregnancy that the operation is done. As has already been pointed out, if the procedure is urgent because of pain, infection or other acute problems, it must be accomplished at the time the problem occurs. If the problem is not urgent, we have more latitude in the selection of time—that is, we choose the period least likely to be associated with any complications of anesthesia. In this aspect, the obstetric patient presents different considerations during each trimester.

First Trimester. Spontaneous or induced abortion is the most frequent complication oc-

curring during the first trimester. Recent data have suggested that the incidence of abortion is significantly higher among operating room personnel than in those working in other areas of a hospital; this incidence seems to be related to exposure to volatile anesthetic agents, such as Fluothane. In addition, differentiation and development of man's major organ systems occur during the first trimester. Drugs and infection during this period can interfere with this process and lead to grave congenital anomalies. Fluothane and other volatile agents have been shown to cause anatomic anomalies in lower species of animals. Although a similar effect has not been documented in the human, these studies cannot be ignored.

If an oral surgical procedure is necessary during the first trimester of pregnancy, a local anesthetic would be the method of choice, if possible. If a general anesthesia is necessary, the combination of an intravenous short-acting barbiturate (Pentothal or Surital), muscle relaxant (succinylcholine) and nitrous oxide is the method of choice, airway and ventilation being insured with an endotracheal tube. In some patients, these agents may not offer adequate analgesia and anesthesia, and they can be supplemented with small increments of intravenous narcotic, such as morphine or Demerol. At this point in our knowledge, it would probably be safest to avoid all halogenated hydrocarbons, such as Fluothane, Penthrane and so forth.

Second (Middle) Trimester. This is the time during pregnancy associated with the lowest incidence of obstetrical complications, and it is the period of choice for elective operations that yet need to be done. A properly conducted local or general anesthetic is as little likely to present problems to the parturient as to the same patient in the nonpregnant state.

Third Trimester. The blood volume of the parturient is at its peak at about the thirtieth week, remaining at an elevated level until the time of delivery. It is thus during this period that the pregnant patient is most likely to get into difficulty. If an operation is indicated, we should select the anesthetic management least likely to depress the heart. Again, local anesthesia should be considered if at all possible. If general anesthesia is needed because of infection or because of the magnitude of the operation, the same management proposed during the first trimester would be that of choice.

Toxemia (eclampsia or pre-eclampsia) is

---

*Otto C. Phillips, M.D.

one of the frequent complications of the third trimester, and it is often associated with depressed liver function. Since postoperative liver failure after a Fluothane anesthesia is usually associated with pre-existing liver disease, shock, or systemic infection, this drug is best avoided in the toxemic patient. The lowest incidence of postanesthetic hepatitis has followed the intravenous barbiturate, muscle relaxant, nitrous oxide sequence already described, and this would certainly be the first choice for general anesthesia in this group of patients.

Oral surgical problems needing treatment certainly do occur in the pregnant patient, and many of these can be managed only with the help of an anesthetic. The decision regarding the time of the operation and the anesthetic management should follow a conference between the oral surgeon, the anesthesiologist and the obstetrician; a safe approach for both the mother and the fetus is practically always available.

LOCAL CONTRAINDICATIONS TO THE EXTRACTION OF TEETH

Among the local contraindications to the extraction of teeth may be mentioned *(a) acute gingival infections* (Fig. 2–1), such as fusospirochetal or streptococcal infections; *(b) acute pericoronal infection,* such as is frequently found around partially erupted third molars. These infections must be treated and the tissues brought to normal before extraction. *(c)* Extraction of maxillary bicuspids and molars is contraindicated during *acute maxillary sinusitis.*

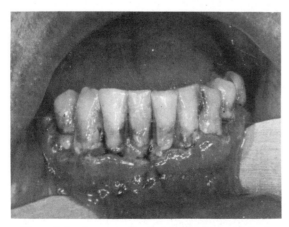

Figure 2–1   An example of an acute gingival infection of long duration, which contraindicates extraction until infection is treated.

SELECTION OF THE ANESTHETIC AGENT OR TECHNIQUE

Contraindications to the proposed oral surgery having been ruled out, the next problem is the selection of the anesthetic agent or technique. The choice is determined by the patient's preference; the patient's physical condition; the age of the patient; the type or extent of the operation; the condition of the operative site (is there local infection which would prevent injections of local anesthetic solution?); the place of operation, *e.g.,* the office, or hospital operating room; the patient's temperament. All these factors have to be studied carefully, and the final decision must be the one which offers the greatest safety to the patient and still permits careful, thorough surgery without psychic shock to or interference by the patient.

Frequently the final decision is reached by a three-way consultation between the operating surgeon, the anesthesiologist and the patient's physician. If I, or any of my family, were to undergo surgery, I would exercise as much care in selecting the anesthesiologist as I would the surgeon, and this would certainly be true of oral surgery.

PREMEDICATION

C. RICHARD BENNETT, D.D.S., PH.D.

Premedication is a valuable, well-established procedure prior to almost every general anesthetic and to many local analgesic administrations. As a matter of fact, premedication could be considered an integral part of the anesthetic. The drugs of choice should be prescribed or administered by the dentist with definite objectives in mind. The proper selection of premedicating agents plays a vital role in the overall success of the anesthetic, be it general or local.

Before the premedicating drugs are selected and administered, the anesthesiologist should be thoroughly familiar with the patient's history, his physical status, any previous information about the patient and the planned surgery. After reviewing all available information and formulating an anesthetic procedure, the anesthesiologist should order the premedication to implement the preplanned procedure.

Premedication should not be a fixed routine, but should be ordered as to specific drugs and dosages to fit the needs of the individual patient. The medication selected should be ordered on a pharmacologic basis with consideration for drug interaction as well as drug action.

Local Analgesia. The vast majority of dental procedures can be managed quite nicely with local analgesia alone. However, fear of pain and patient apprehension over the impending surgery make this procedure difficult in a significant number of cases. With the judicious use of premedication in combination with local analgesia, an ideal operating condition is provided for both patient and surgeon.

The premedicating drugs may be administered by a variety of routes. The intravenous route is preferred since it provides the most predictability in time of onset, duration, effect and drug dose. Other routes of administration may be chosen, based on the requirements of surgeon and patient.

In all cases where local analgesia is to be used, it should be stressed that the cooperation of the patient will be required, and the medication should not depress the patient's cerebral cortex to the degree that the patient becomes unresponsive or loses consciousness. If this is allowed to occur, operative or surgical procedures become most difficult, if not impossible. In addition, rendering the patient unconscious produces a state of general anesthesia which requires the attention of an anesthetist to safeguard the life and welfare of the patient.

For allaying fear and apprehension the barbiturates administered orally would be the first choice of the average general practitioner. For the more experienced individual the intravenous route should be considered for premedication, as the dosage can be controlled more accurately, thus increasing the drug's overall effectiveness. The operator should bear in mind that these drugs in other than anesthetic doses lower, rather than raise, the pain threshold. Therefore, when barbiturates are used, steps must be taken to be sure the local analgesia is complete.

The role of the barbiturates in preventing toxic reactions to local analgesic agents is controversial. They may mask the early central nervous system stimulation, which may be considered a disadvantage. It is my opinion that these drugs should not be used primarily as premedication to prevent any possible toxicity to local analgesic agents.

The ataractic drugs may be used alone or in combination with barbiturates or narcotics. By themselves, they produce a calming effect with only minimal sensory or motor function changes. Their chief advantage lies in their ability to potentiate other central nervous system depressants, thereby allowing smaller doses to be used.

As premedicating drugs for local analgesia the narcotics have a great deal to offer. They not only induce a state of euphoria and wellbeing, which is advantageous, but they also raise the pain threshold, a desirable factor in local analgesia. An uncooperative and restless patient is most unusual when the narcotics are used.

It is my opinion that the narcotics as premedication for local analgesia should be used more often. The intimated disadvantages—addiction, nausea and respiratory and circulatory depression—are not valid, as they do not occur when the drugs are used properly; that is, in weak concentrations and small doses. Here again, the intravenous route is desirable, but narcotics can be given by the intramuscular or oral route.

Some suggested dosages of the previously discussed drugs are shown in Table 2–1.

General Anesthesia. As previously stated, preanesthetic medication is a vital factor in the preparation of a patient for general anesthesia. It should be stressed that the medication should not be routine but should vary from patient to patient as dictated by the requirements of the individual patient.

The main reasons for premedication for general anesthesia are:

1. To afford a restful night before anesthesia and surgery.
2. To allay apprehension and to produce a degree of amnesia immediately prior to the anesthetic.
3. To depress reflex irritability.
4. To lessen metabolic activity.
5. To check excess salivation.
6. To raise the pain threshold when indicated.

The drugs most commonly used by us for premedication are shown in Table 2–2.

In the administration of these drugs, each has its indicated purpose. The barbiturates allay apprehension and fear; the narcotics elevate the pain threshold and provide the patient with a feeling of euphoria; the psychosedative drugs have a calming effect and potentiate the barbiturates and narcotics; and the belladonna derivatives depress parasympathetic nervous system activity. The aforementioned drugs may be used together with excellent results.

It should be understood that the hospital-

Table 2–1   *Suggested Premedication for Local Analgesia*

	BARBITURATES	
✓Pentobarbital (Nembutal)	50–100	mg. (Oral, IM or IV) (short-acting)
Secobarbital (Seconal)	50–100	mg. (Oral, IM or IV) (short-acting)
✓Methohexital sodium (Brevital)	10–40	mg. (IV) in divided doses, 10 mg./ml. (ultra-short-acting)
	NARCOTICS	
✓Morphine sulfate	8–16	mg. (IM or IV) in divided doses
✓Meperidine (Demerol)	40–75	mg. (IM or IV) in divided doses, 10 mg./ml.
Alphaprodine (Nisentil)	10–40	mg. (IM or IV) in divided doses, 6 mg./ml.
Anileridine (Leritine)	25–50	mg. (IM or IV) in divided doses, 5–10 mg./ml.
	ATARACTICS (PSYCHOSEDATIVES)	
✓Promethazine hydrochloride (Phenergan)	25–50	mg. (Oral, IM or IV) in divided doses
Hydroxyzine (Vistaril)	25–100	mg. (Oral or IM) in divided doses
✓Diazepam (Valium)	5–15	mg. (Oral, IM or IV) in divided doses

ized patient can be more heavily premedicated than the outpatient. Also, when premedication or general anesthesia is used for the outpatient, definite precautions must be observed. They are: *(a)* The patient must be accompanied by a responsible adult. *(b)* The patient should not be permitted to drive an automobile for 24 hours. *(c)* Alcohol intake must be restricted for 24 hours. *(d)* At home, the patient should be with a responsible person long enough to allow a wide margin of safety for elimination of any drugs.

DETAILED EXAMINATION OF THE TEETH AND CONTIGUOUS TISSUES BEFORE EXTRACTION

Having established that the necessity for the proposed extraction is valid, the dentist who is to perform the surgery must plan the operation itself.

Purpose.   The purpose of this detailed ex-

amination is to determine what technique to use in removing the tooth or teeth: whether forceps and elevators will be used; whether elevators alone will be used; if so, what elevators and what forceps are indicated; whether odontectomy (surgical removal) of the tooth or teeth is indicated; whether odontectomy plus sectioning is required; to determine whether there is a possibility of fracturing the tooth or teeth, of fracturing a large segment of alveolar process or tuberosity, of fracturing the mandible, or of tearing the floor out of the maxillary sinus.

If there is any possibility of a fracture of the tooth, always warn the patient. Explain to him why this might happen and your planned steps in attempting to prevent this complication. To attempt to explain to a patient why the tooth fractured, after it has occurred, puts the dentist in an awkward, defensive position. The average patient feels that the dentist is alibiing for what the patient considers faulty technique on the part of the dentist. This is

Table 2–2   *Suggested Premedication for General Anesthesia*

	BARBITURATES	
Secobarbital (Seconal)	50–150	mg. (IM or IV)
Pentobarbital (Nembutal)	50–150	mg. (IM or IV)
	NARCOTICS	
Morphine	8–15	mg. (IM or IV)
Meperidine (Demerol)	50–100	mg. (IM or IV)
	ATARACTICS (PSYCHOSEDATIVES)	
Hydroxyzine (Vistaril)	50–100	mg. (IM)
Promethazine hydrochloride (Phenergan)	25–50	mg. (IM or IV)
Diazepam (Valium)	5–15	mg. (IM or IV)
	BELLADONNA DERIVATIVES	
Atropine	0.2–0.5	mg. (IM or IV)
Scopolamine	0.2–0.5	mg. (IM or IV)

particularly true when the patient has previously had teeth extracted (without their breaking) by another dentist. More will be said about this later.

Components. THE TOOTH OR TEETH TO BE EXTRACTED. Note the following points: Is the tooth carious? Is it abraded? Does it contain a large filling? Does the tooth have an artificial crown? Is the tooth vital or nonvital? What is the size of the tooth? What are the formation, size and number of the roots? Is hypercementosis present on the root or roots? Is there an area of condensing or infective osteitis about the root or roots? Are the roots widely divergent? Are the roots in normal position buccolingually and mesiodistally? What is the relationship of the roots to the adjacent teeth? What is the relationship of the tooth to the tuberosity? What is the relationship of the roots to the maxillary sinus or to the mandibular canal? Is there a root canal filling in the tooth?

DENTAL RADIOGRAPHS AND THE EXTRACTION OF TEETH. Many of the foregoing questions can be answered only by careful study of good radiographs of the tooth or teeth to be extracted and their investing bony tissue. Radiographs are an invaluable aid to the oral surgeon in preventing untoward accidents, such as fracturing the mandible, tearing out the floor of the maxillary sinus, and so forth. They also permit the intelligent planning of the proposed operation before its start. This results in much less trauma to the tissues, reduction of operating time, and less chance of postoperative infection, with improved healing and with little postoperative pain.

In addition to the small dental intraoral films, it is sometimes necessary to take extraoral views to visualize impacted third molars completely. Occlusal films are also necessary to aid in the localization of unerupted teeth in either the maxilla or the mandible.

While the panoramic films are very helpful, the periapical films are mandatory for accurate

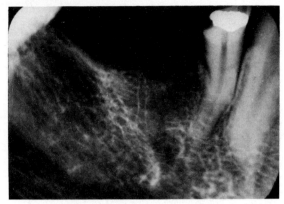

Figure 2–2 Normal cancellous bone.

evaluation of osseous changes, of tooth structure and (in conjunction with the occlusal films), of the relationships of impacted or unerupted teeth to adjacent teeth, as well as their labial, buccal or lingual relationship in either the maxilla or the mandible.

Radiographs should also be made of edentulous areas in both the maxilla and the mandible, no matter how long the teeth have been absent from those areas. Many retained roots, unerupted teeth, foreign bodies and residual cysts, or areas of infection, are discovered by radiographing these areas.

EXAMINATION OF THE SUPPORTING HARD TISSUES. Note the thickness of the labial, lingual and buccal cortical plate of bone by examining these areas visually and digitally.

Are there nodular areas of exostosis overlying the roots of the teeth?

Estimate the density of the bone. The age of the patient is a clue to density of bone: the older the patient, the denser the bone. Also note the general skeleton. Is the patient a "big-boned" individual? In general a massive skeleton means difficult extractions.

OSTEOSCLEROSIS, OSTEOPETROSIS (MARBLE BONE). Study the cancellous bone as revealed in the dental radiographs. Are the reticulations or cross-lines which form the

Figure 2–3 Mandibular bone in which there is very little osseous tissue, as is indicated by the large radiolucent areas seen between the fine, wide-apart radiopaque lines outlining the trabeculations.

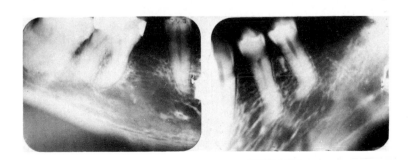

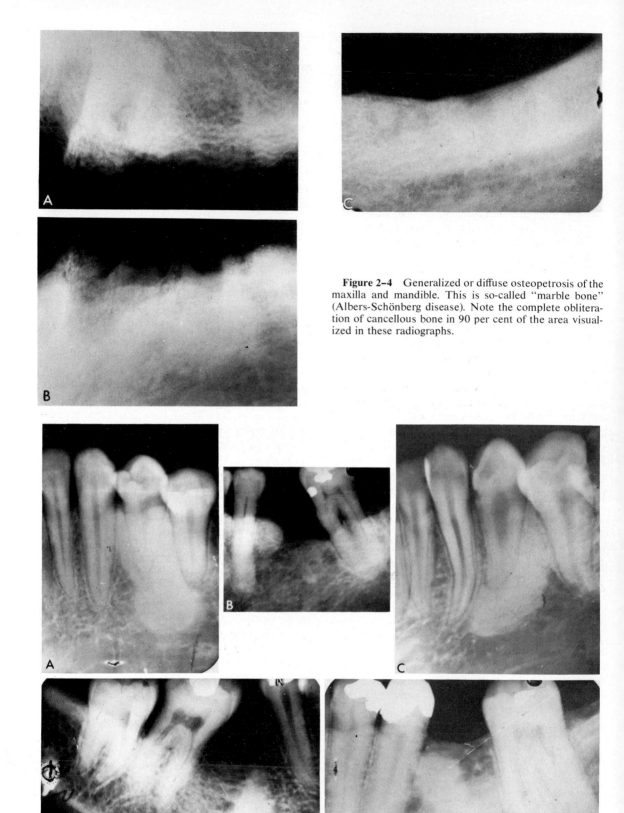

Figure 2-4 Generalized or diffuse osteopetrosis of the maxilla and mandible. This is so-called "marble bone" (Albers-Schönberg disease). Note the complete obliteration of cancellous bone in 90 per cent of the area visualized in these radiographs.

Figure 2-5 Examples of osteosclerosis about the roots of the teeth or body of the mandible.

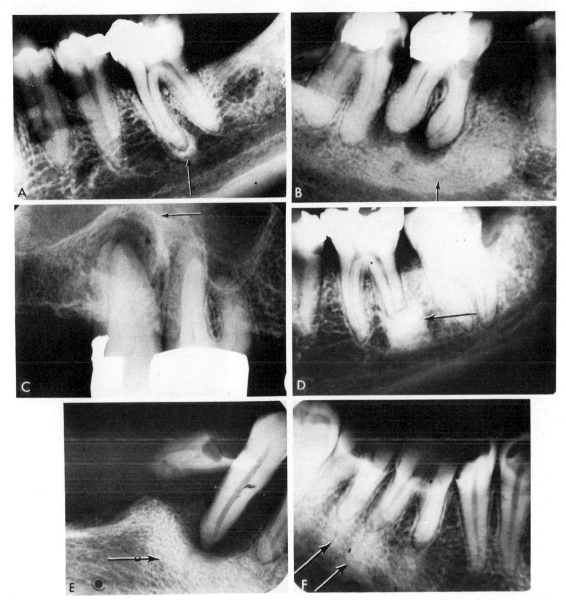

Figure 2–6 Examples of condensing osteitis. In these cases periapical pathosis has stimulated the sclerotic bone formation.

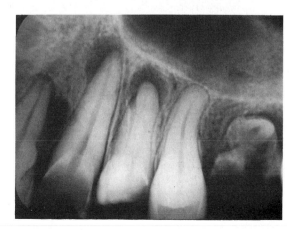

Figure 2–7 Periapical radiolucent areas produced by noxious stimuli that have passed from these root canals into the periapical tissues. All periapical radiolucent areas are not indicative of infection, a so-called "abscess" or a cyst, and they should not be so diagnosed by the radiograph alone. Grossman[20] has demonstrated that 85.3 per cent of these areas are sterile!

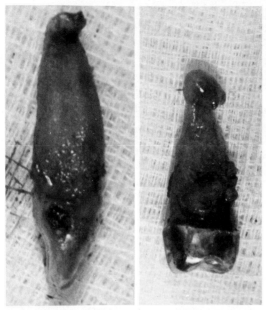

Figure 2–8 Nonvital teeth with apical inflammatory tissue, the "dental granuloma," attached.

spongy tissue of the bone spaced far apart or are they close even to the point of nonexistence? The latter condition indicates osteosclerosis. (See Chapter 13, pages 863 to 867 and Figures 13–166 to 13–171.)

In patients with this abnormal hardening and thickening of the maxilla or mandible, not only is the difficulty of the extraction of teeth markedly increased, but resistance to infection is reduced and there is a good possibility of at least a localized osteomyelitis postoperatively. The patient is advised of these facts, and if complications develop he understands why.

AGE OF THE PATIENT. In older patients osseous tissue and tooth structure are brittle and dense. In these cases it is impossible to expand the cortical plate. In younger patients the osseous tissue is less dense, the cortical plates of bone are more readily expanded and the cancellous bone compresses comparatively more easily. The teeth are usually nonbrittle.

PREVIOUS EXTRACTIONS. Ask the patient about previous extraction experiences. Explain to him the present operation, so that he will know what to expect.

POINTS TO REMEMBER IN EXTRACTION OF TEETH

Never refer to the extraction of a tooth or teeth as "a simple extraction (or extractions)."

You may find yourself in the embarrassing position of trying to explain to the patient why this simple extraction (or extractions) is taking so much time and effort to complete.

Anticipate breakage by knowing all the reasons that roots break and crowns fracture.

Forewarn the patient of the possibility of breakage or fracture, but in such a manner as to reassure rather than alarm him.

Never try to cover up breakage of roots; tell the patient.

After the root has broken off, remove the remaining root fragments from the socket. There are a few exceptions to this rule (see Chapter 4). When a root should not be removed, the patient should be explicitly told why and his consent obtained. This must appear in the patient's record.

Many fractures of roots, crowns, large segments of bone, tuberosities, and even the mandible itself can be prevented by odontectomy.

Radiographs of the jaws and teeth to be extracted are essential for intelligent performance of odontectomies.

REASONS FOR ROOT BREAKAGE

There are many reasons that roots break. Among them may be noted the following:
A. Improper application of beaks of forceps.
   1. Beaks placed on enamel instead of on cementum.
   2. Beaks not parallel to long axis of tooth.
B. Wrong type of forceps.
C. Extensive caries.
D. Brittleness due to age or nonvitality of the tooth: root canal fillings indicate the possibility of root fracture.
E. Peculiar root formation.
   1. Curved roots.
   2. Hypercementosis.
   3. Supernumerary roots.
F. Excessive density of surrounding bone due to:
   1. Condensing osteitis.
   2. Osteopetrosis (marble bone, Albers-Schönberg disease).
   3. Defensive osteitis.
   4. Isolated tooth, because of extraction of adjacent teeth some years previously.
   5. Bridge abutments, fixed or removable, subjected to great stress.
   6. A coarse diet stimulating osteoblastic activity.

7. Chewing of tobacco.
8. Low-grade chronic gingivitis, giving rise to periostitis, with resultant exostosis of labial or buccal cortical plate (see Figure 2–2).
G. Incorrect application of force in extraction of teeth.
1. Wrong direction.
2. Jerking a tooth (sudden, violent application of force in one direction).
3. Use of twisting motion when not indicated.
4. Pulling on a tooth.

LOOSE TEETH

Loose teeth may be due to advanced chronic suppurative periodontoclasia, a cyst, central hemangioma, neoplasm, hyperparathyroidism, eosinophilic osteomyelitic granuloma, osteomyelitis or fracture. The roentgenogram is an aid in ascertaining the cause of loose teeth and should be taken in all cases before extraction is undertaken. A biopsy is also taken when indicated. The patient is informed about the radiographic and histologic findings before any oral surgical procedure is performed.

In advanced destruction of the supporting alveolar process, nature compensates by increasing the density of bone about that portion of the root which is still held in bone. This is why we frequently are surprised when we fracture the apices of these teeth. They should be luxated with care to avoid this accident.

Dentists have inadvertently been involved in lawsuits, accused of fracturing the mandible or maxilla, because they extracted "a loose tooth." Subsequently it has been demonstrated that the mandible or maxilla was already fractured before the extraction, and the tooth was loose because it was in the line of the fracture. A history prior to extraction would have revealed that the patient had either fallen and struck his jaw, or had been struck with a blow. Of course teeth can be and have been loosened by trauma without an accompanying fracture. It is imperative in these cases that the jaw be carefully examined for movement and crepitus, and that a thorough radiographic examination be made to rule out the possibility of a fracture before proceeding with the extraction. Furthermore, as will be seen in Chapter 18, in many cases it is not desirable to extract the tooth in the line of fracture.

The injudicious extraction of teeth in an acute osteomyelitis may help spread the infection. Here again both the history and a roentgenographic examination are necessary. However, it must be remembered that in early osteomyelitis there will not be any osseous changes on the radiographs.

ODONTECTOMY AND TOOTH DIVISION

Odontectomy is the surgical removal of a tooth or teeth by the reflection of an adequate mucoperiosteal flap and the removal of overlying bone, and also bone from between the buccal roots of molars, by means of chisels, burs and/or rongeurs. After the removal of bone, in many cases of multirooted teeth, tooth division is indicated. In tooth division one or more roots are separated from the crown by crosscut fissure burs (see Figure 2–140), or the crown is entirely separated from the roots, and the roots are then cut apart (see Figure 2–145). Tooth division is also used in the removal of impacted teeth and will be discussed further in Chapter 5. This is followed by the application of forceps and/or elevators for the extraction of the tooth and then the roots.

The advantages of odontectomy are: the reduction in the number of fractured crowns or roots of teeth during extraction, less danger of creating an antro-oral fistula or injuring the neurovascular bundle in the mandible, smaller possibility of a fracture of the mandible or maxilla, and less chance of tearing out large areas of cortical and cancellous bone with the tooth during extraction.

INDICATIONS FOR ODONTECTOMY AND TOOTH DIVISION

The indications for odontectomy and tooth division may be briefly summarized as follows:
A. Hypercementosis of the roots.
B. Widely divergent roots of mandibular or maxillary molars.
C. "Locked roots"—lower or upper molars whose roots bow out from the gingiva to a point midway to the apices, where they then curve toward each other and touch, or nearly so; thus a portion of bone is "locked" between the roots.
D. Teeth with apices at right angles to the long axis of the teeth.
E. Teeth with post crowns.
F. Extensively decayed teeth, particularly those with deep gingival cavities.
G. Teeth with root canal fillings.
H. When a thick, dense buccal or labial cortical plate or multinodular exostosis is

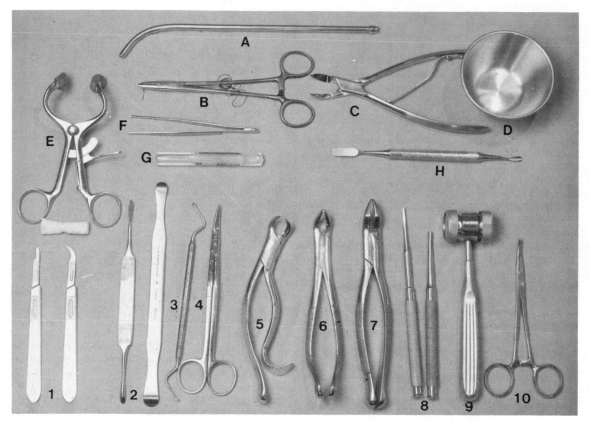

Figure 2–9   Basic tray set-up for maxillary and mandibular odontectomy and alveolectomy. Additional forceps, if needed, are added.

A, A universal suction tip; small apical suction tips are added if roots are fractured. (See Figure 2–24.) *B*, Needle holder with a threaded needle. *C*, Bone shear. *D*, Basin for extracted teeth. *E*, Mouth prop. *F*, Tissue forceps. *G*, Suture material. *H*, Double-end bone file.

1, Knives: one with a No. 15 blade and one with a No. 12 blade.

2, Small double-end periosteal elevator and a large double-end flap retractor also used as a periosteal elevator.

3, Medium double-end periapical curette; larger or smaller curettes are added if needed.

4, No. 9 Dean's Scissors.

5, No. 16, the so-called "cowhorn," forceps for the extraction of mandibular molars whose roots are not fused.

6, The No. 151 Universal mandibular forceps, which is extremely efficient for the extraction of all mandibular teeth, including mandibular molars with fused roots.

7, The No. 286 maxillary forceps for the extraction of the maxillary six anterior teeth and bicuspids. While some dentists use it for maxillary molars, I prefer either a No. 24 (see Figure 2–75) or a No. 10H (see Figure 2–79), which is also a "bayonet-type" forceps. Both have much broader beaks to distribute the pressure and thus are not so likely to fracture the crowns.

8, Chisels. *9*, Mallet. *10*, Mosquito forceps.

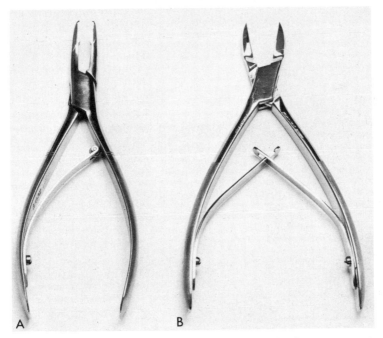

Figure 2-10 *A*, Universal bone rongeurs for postextraction trimming of alveolar process. *B*, Bone shears No. 5C designed for cutting in any part of the upper or lower jaw. Its blades are crescent-shaped and so arranged as to enable the operator to see clearly what and how much bone he is cutting. Excellent for alveolectomies.

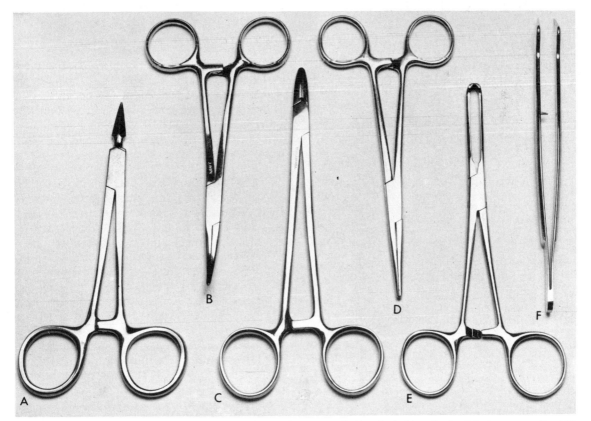

Figure 2-11 *A*, Apical fragment forceps. *B*, Curved hemostat. *C*, Needle holder. *D*, Straight hemostat. *E*, Allis forceps. *F*, Treatment pliers.

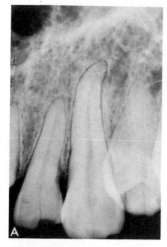

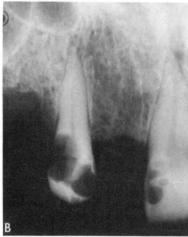

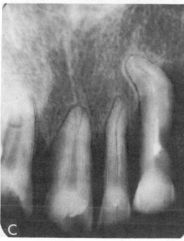

Figure 2–12 Abnormal root formations which indicate the need for surgical removal of these teeth.

present on the maxilla or mandible (Figs. 2–14 to 2–16).

I. When a low antral floor dips between the buccal and lingual roots of the maxillary molars.

J. When the maxillary alveolar tuberosity is hollow because the antral cavity extends into this area.

K. Thin mandibles in which excessive force is required to luxate the teeth. This excessive force may result in the fracture of the mandible.

L. Malposed teeth, impactions, unerupted teeth and supernumerary teeth.

M. When the forceps pressure on a mandibular tooth, in the attempt to luxate it for removal, results in dislocation of the condyles of the mandible from the glenoid fossae despite manual efforts to retain the condyles in their fossae.

N. Ankylosed roots (found only in elderly persons, and then rarely).

O. When the customary force fails to produce any luxation.

USE OF THE BONE BUR AND CHISEL

Johnson* succinctly and correctly states:

"There has been much dogmatizing as to how bone should be removed and teeth sectioned, with the protagonists of both the bur and the chisel technics forming traditional battle lines. Apparently, much can be said in favor of each technic as there are applications where one technic is better than the other.

"If a bur is used, it is essential that the handpiece be sterile, the bur sharp and flushed constantly during use with sterile normal saline solution to prevent overheating, to keep the cutting edges from becoming clogged with bone or tooth substance, and to keep the operative site clean and visible. Constant use of the suction and good retraction by a trained assistant is imperative. In addition to the above, visibility is dependent on the source of light and while a good overhead light is necessary for general illumination of the oral cavity, for specific and brilliant spot lighting of the actual operative site, nothing equals a good headlight. Given these factors, the postoperative results cannot be improved upon by any other method. Dentists are accustomed to using a handpiece and are skilled in its manipulation, which cannot always be said for the manner in which they use a mallet and chisel.

"The average operator can resect bone more easily and with less discomfort to the patient if he uses a bur and handpiece. The prolonged pounding to which patients are

---

*Johnson, J. H.: The fundamentals of oral surgery. J. Ont. Dent. Assoc., *34*:18–23 (June), 1957.

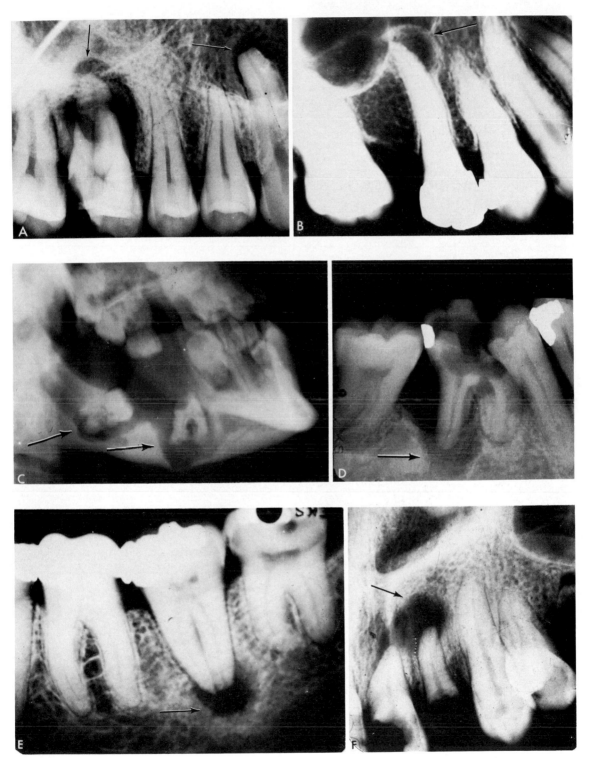

Figure 2–13 Examples of pathosis in periapical regions and beyond.

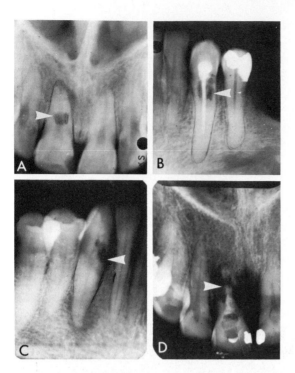

Figure 2–14 Examples of internal resorption in teeth. Frank and Weine[18] have described in detail a "nonsurgical therapy for the perforative defect of internal resorption" by which extraction can be avoided in many of these cases. However, when extraction is indicated, it must be remembered that internal resorption of the dentin, pointed to by the white arrows, weakens these teeth so that they will readily fracture when they are luxated by the forceps. An additional factor increasing the possibility of fracture is the nonvitality of these teeth. Note the evidence of periapical radiolucency.

Before applying forceps to these teeth, a flap should be reflected and buccal or labial cortical bone should be removed with a chisel. Preparation should be made for the removal of the roots because of the near certainty of the fracture of the crowns, as seen in radiographs *A, B* and *D*. In *C* the crown should be cut through the bifurcation from buccal to lingual, as shown in Figure 2–14O, and the tooth removed in sections.

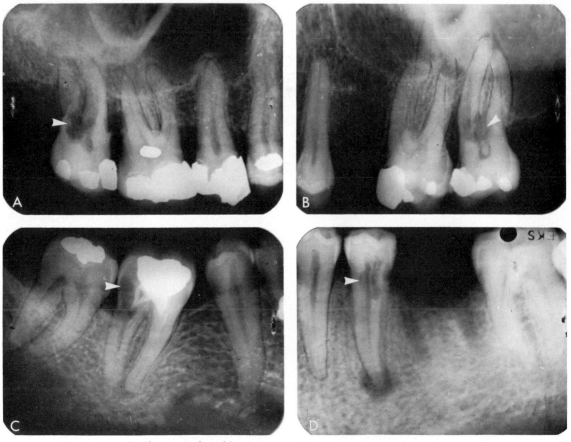

Figure 2–15 Further examples of internal resorption in teeth. See Figure 2–14 and legend.

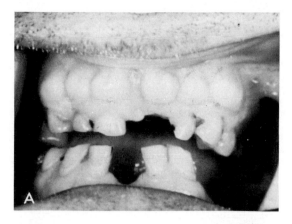

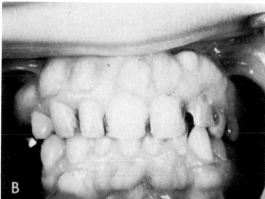

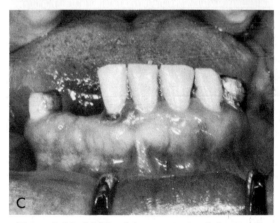

Figure 2–16 Multinodular exostosis of the maxillary and mandibular cortical bone. The etiologic factor in the patient shown in *A* was probably trauma. Note the extensive abrasion of the teeth. In *B* perhaps periodontal disease was a factor. In both these cases the mucoperiosteal membrane must be reflected and the exostosis planed off with a chisel before luxation and extraction of the teeth. *C,* The teeth in this figure were not extracted. They were used to illustrate the necessity of removing exostosis before tooth extractions in cases in which extraction is indicated.

Conservation of bone is always practiced, but more bone can be preserved by the judicious excision of some bone, which ultimately prevents the fracturing of large segments of bone, as will be shown in subsequent illustrations.

sometimes subjected during the removal of sclerotic bone is both unnecessary and unwise, since the same objective may be accomplished by use of bone drills with no distress to the patient.

"The suggestion that it is good practice to section maxillary teeth in the region of the antrum with a chisel and mallet is a clinical fallacy.* Such teeth are better and more easily sectioned with a bur.

"However, chisels have their indications and are extremely useful instruments for sec-

---

*AUTHOR'S NOTE: This technique has driven more than one impacted maxillary third molar into the maxillary sinus.

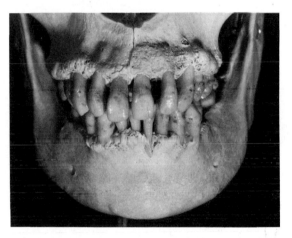

Figure 2–17 In this case there is a general exostosis of the alveolar process throughout the maxilla, which produces a marked bulging. Again it can be seen that this patient had periodontoclasia, with the loss of the gingival third of the alveolar process. Two factors again were at work in producing this exostosis: first, chronic infection, and second, nature's compensating effort to give additional support to the teeth, thus offsetting the loss of support around the necks of the teeth because of periodontoclasia.

This exostosis should be removed at the time of extraction for the following reasons: (*a*) It will interfere with the extraction of teeth. If brute force is used, a large segment of the bone will be fractured off with the tooth, or the roots of the tooth will be fractured. (*b*) If the teeth are extracted without either occurring, then it will be difficult, if not impossible, to construct a denture over this ridge, owing to the marked undercuts. Note the molar regions in particular. (*c*) If a denture could be made in such a case, there would be rapid resorption of this alveolar process, and the bone would be replaced by hypertrophied soft tissue. Note the many nutrient canals passing through this bony outgrowth. After the teeth are removed, and the infection has cleared, this ridge "melts away" because of rapid osteoclastic activity. Note the absence of exostosis on the mandible.

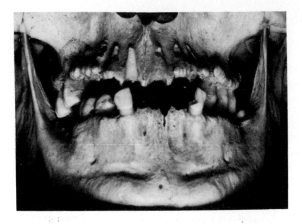

Figure 2–18 Multiple exostosis of the alveolar process of the maxilla. Note that these are localized nodular outgrowths of bone. In the left molar region there is a continuous series of these nodules. In this case a low-grade infection stimulated osteoblastic activity. This was probably nature's attempt to compensate for the loss of bone that is evident around the necks of the molar teeth. Note that there is not any exostosis on the mandible. It is rare to see exostoses on the buccal or labial surface of the mandible; why, I do not know. Exostosis on the lingual cortical bone is called mandibular tori.

tioning many impacted mandibular teeth prior to their removal. Many of these teeth may be sectioned with a light tap on a sharp chisel and without disturbing the patient, provided the mallet is correctly used. Unfortunately, such is often not the case.*

"To be effective, the mallet should be used with a loose, free-swinging wrist motion that gives maximum speed to the head of the mallet without introducing the weight of the arm or body into the blow.

"The formula for kinetic energy is $KE = \frac{1}{2}MV^2$, where KE is the energy possessed by a moving body, M the mass of the moving body and V its velocity. It will be noted that since the velocity is squared, it is a highly important factor. It would be futile to attempt to drive a golf ball with a sledge hammer. The same principle applies to the sectioning of teeth.

"When an assistant 'freezes' on the mallet, thus adding the weight of the hand and arm, and sometimes even of the shoulder, the mass

---

*AUTHOR'S NOTE: It is imperative that the chisels be "razor sharp" and kept that way. Multinodular exostosis of the maxillary or mandibular cortical bone and tori mandibularis can be planed off with a minimum of trauma. In conjunction with the bur, large tori palatini are efficiently removed.

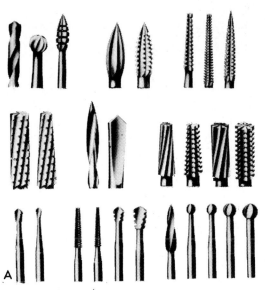

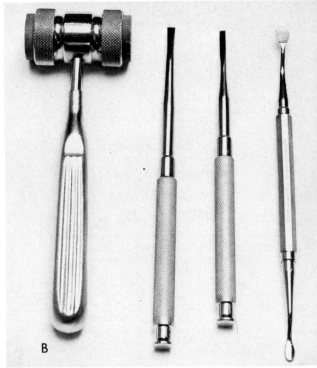

Figure 2–19 *A*, Burs for bone removal and tooth sectioning. *B*, Surgical mallet, chisels and bone file. See text for description of technique.

is increased, but there is a great reduction in the velocity. The net result is that the patient is severely jarred, but the blow may be totally ineffective from a clinical standpoint."

To *plane* bone with a chisel, have the bevel turned toward the bone. To *penetrate* bone, turn the bevel away from the bone.

REASONS FOR REMOVAL OF ROOTS

Fractured roots should be removed at the time of extraction. Large roots left in the alveolus will be a localized source of inflammation and soreness as the alveolar process resorbs and the denture strikes this prominence in the ridge.

Roots are removed to *eliminate a possible residual infection.* Even if the original tooth is noninfected, some roots may become infected at the time of extraction because of the decomposition of contents of the root canal plus the invasion of oral bacteria.

Remaining roots or fragments of root structure may act as *mechanical irritants.* These may set up an inflammatory reaction, which can give rise to neuralgic pains of obscure origin that are difficult to diagnose.

An exception to the general rule of removing all roots is the very small root tip located near anatomical structures into which the fragment may inadvertently be forced when removal is attempted. The technique for removing roots at the time of extraction, and the *indications* and *contraindications* of removal of roots in healed alveolar ridges, is discussed in Chapter 4.

MUCOPERIOSTEAL FLAPS

For the performance of odontectomy, or the removal of roots, it is necessary to expose adequately the labial or buccal cortical plate of bone overlying the operative site. To do so, the covering soft tissue must be incised and reflected. Some authors advocate simply incising the soft tissue about the neck of the tooth to be extracted, and about the necks of the immediate anterior and posterior teeth, and then elevating the tissue away from the gingival margin (the so-called "envelope flap"). It has been my experience that such a technique does not give adequate exposure, and that the mucoperiosteum is torn before the operation is completed. For that reason all my flaps are made with one or two semivertical incisions.

Two exceptions to the rule will be illustrated later in the text.

Steps in Preparing Mucoperiosteal Flaps

1. Mentally review the nerve and blood supply of the soft tissue to be included in the flap, and plan the lines of incision so that the flap will have a maximum blood supply and yet sever a minimum number of nerve filaments.

2. With a No. 12 Bard-Parker (BP) blade, cut through the junction of the periodontal membrane and the mucoperiosteum around the neck of the tooth or teeth to be extracted. It is at this point that the periosteum is most tightly adherent to the alveolar bone. If this attachment is not carefully severed, when an attempt is made to reflect the flap the mucoperiosteal tissue will be split, with the periosteum still attached to bone, and only the mucosa stripped free. Extreme care must be taken to prevent this. The periosteum is a very thin membrane at

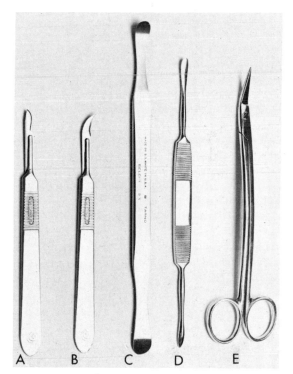

Figure 2–20 *A,* No. 15 blade on a No. 3 handle, for cutting flaps and making incisions on edentulous ridges. *B,* No. 12 blade is ideal for severing the attachment of the mucoperiosteal membrane around the necks of teeth so that this tissue can be reflected. *C,* Broad mucoperiosteal flap retractor. *D,* Excellent mucoperiosteal membrane elevator. See text for a description of this technique. *E,* No. 9 Dean's serrated cutting edge surgical scissors for general use in oral surgery.

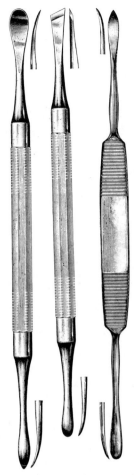

Figure 2–21 Examples of mucoperiosteal tissue elevators used to separate the attachment of this membrane and reflect it.

the gingival line. It can be compared to the thin membrane beneath the shell of a hard-boiled egg. Failure to reflect the periosteum will result in postoperative slough of the flap, pain and delayed healing. Epithelialization of exposed bone is a slow process.

3. Next, with a No. 15 BP blade, starting at the crest of the mesial interdental papillae, make an incision through the mucoperiosteum toward the mucobuccal fold (fornix of the vestibule) mesially at a 45-degree angle to the long axis of the tooth for a distance of 1.5 cm., or longer if the flap is to be elevated more than usual. If adequate exposure is not obtained when the mucoperiosteum is reflected, then make a second incision, starting at the crest of the distal interdental papillae, and extend this incision distally toward the mucobuccal fold at a 45-degree angle to the long axis of the tooth to be re-

moved. Starting the incision at the crest of the interdental papillae aids materially in the normal reattachment of the gingival tissues around the necks of the adjacent teeth. If the incision is started at the gingival line, there frequently follows a V-shaped exposure of the cementum at the necks of these teeth when the tissues have healed.

4. When planning flaps, always make certain that the base is wider than its free margin. A large number of blood vessels enter a wide base, thus insuring a good blood supply to the flap.

5. Always have the flap wider than the bone cavity which will be present at the conclusion of the operation, to insure that the sutured edges of the flap rest on a solid bony base, which means quick and painless healing. Otherwise the flap will drop into the cavity, exposing bone and resulting in pain, and healing will be retarded.

6. Make certain in planning and preparing your flap that the operative site is adequately exposed. Not only is the oral surgeon handicapped by being confined to a small space, but the flap is usually severely traumatized by efforts to retract it, or the edges are traumatized by instrumentation. Such flaps do not heal by first intention, and they are a source of pain.

7. Always use a sharp blade. Cut through the soft tissue at the starting point until bone is contacted; then with the knife edge held firmly in contact with bone, make your planned incisions with one cut. Repeated cuts in an incision needlessly traumatize the periosteum and jeopardize primary healing.

Reflecting Buccal, Labial and Lingual Mucoperiosteum for Multiple Extractions. Buccal or Labial Mucoperiosteum. After the soft tissues have been incised around the necks of the teeth and through the interproximal space, the fibers of the periodontal membrane being severed where they enter the periosteum, the spear point of the periosteal elevator is inserted into the interproximal space with the concavity of the instrument facing bone. The point of the instrument should touch the interproximal bone at a point midway between the labial or buccal and lingual surfaces. Then, using the mesial, labial or buccal surface of the tooth as a fulcrum, elevate the mucoperiosteal tissue from bone and

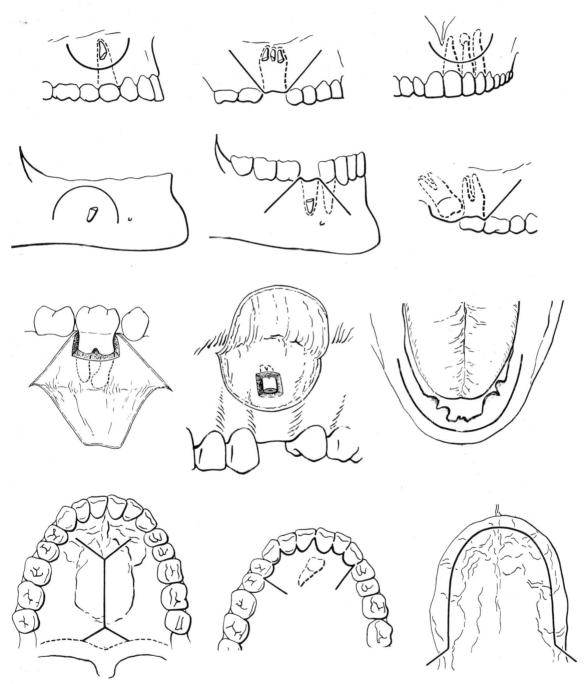

Figure 2–22 Examples of lines of incisions for flaps for various surgical procedures and the reflection of two types of flaps. The specific details of these flaps will be described in the text at the appropriate places.

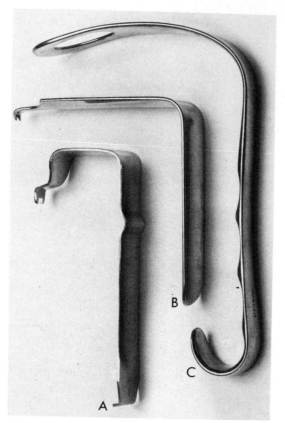

Figure 2–23 *A* and *B,* Third molar flap retractors. *C,* Cheek or tongue retractor.

traction of teeth. We merely loosen it with a periosteal elevator to make a pathway for the beaks of the forceps.

A pathway for the beaks of the forceps on the lingual surface of each tooth to be extracted is made by forcing the pointed end of the periosteal elevator between the necks of the maxillary teeth and the palatal mucoperiosteum, or between the necks of the mandibular teeth and the lingual mucoperiosteum until the lingual cortical bone is contacted, at which time a mesial-distal loosening of the mucoperiosteum is carried out.

REMOVAL OF BLOOD AND SALIVA FROM THE ORAL CAVITY

During operations in the oral cavity it is imperative that the operating field be well illuminated and freed from blood so as to be clearly visible at all times.

slide the edge of the elevator beneath the periosteum continuing around the neck of the tooth to the distal interproximal space.

Teeth should not be used as fulcrums unless they are to be extracted.

If more than one tooth is to be removed, continue this reflection of mucoperiosteum to include all teeth to be extracted.

After the gingival mucoperiosteal membrane is loosened, as described above, the surgeon reflects it further by contacting bone with the concave curved edge of the periosteal elevator turned toward the cortical plate, then pushing the elevator under the full thickness of the mucoperiosteal membrane, until the flap is reflected from the operative site for a distance of at least 1½ cm. The attachment of periosteum to bone is looser, the greater the distance from the gingival line.

LINGUAL MUCOPERIOSTEUM. Incise around the neck of the tooth on the palatal or lingual surface with a No. 12 BP blade. Do not cut through the interproximal tissue on the palatal or lingual surface. We do not reflect tissue on the lingual after incising for routine ex-

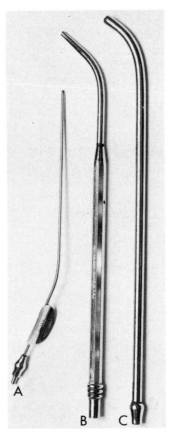

Figure 2–24 Suction tips. *A,* Very fine suction tip ideal for the apical third region of the alveolus. *B,* Cogswell suction used for tooth sockets. *C,* Yankauer suction tip for general use in the oral cavity.

To illuminate the operating field, a well-adjusted headlight which can be regulated to throw a 3-inch diameter beam of intense light is preferable. This is in addition to the usual overhead operating light.

For removal of blood from the oral cavity one of two methods is usually used:

Sponging. In operations in the oral cavity, conventional sponging, mopping and expectorating have many disadvantages. They are time-consuming. They interrupt the operating procedure. They seldom provide adequate elimination of blood to give a clear view of the operation. They tend to push foreign material into the wound. They tend to traumatize the tissues.

Suction Apparatus. There are two types of suction apparatus. In one a suction is created by a running stream of water; in the other a suction is created by a vacuum pump run by an electric motor. The first has the advantage of automatically discharging blood and saliva into the waste drain, thus eliminating a collection bottle which must be emptied periodically to prevent fouling the pump. It has the disadvantage, however, of being noisy and requires special plumbing if it is installed permanently.

The electrically operated suction pump is quieter and is readily moved about. However, it requires more care and attention than the water suction apparatus and is subject to mechanical breakdowns.

A suction apparatus is a *must,* and doubly so when operating under general anesthesia, because of the increased bleeding and the possibility of the patient's aspirating blood. It is wise to have an extra suction pump in good working order always available because these devices have a constant tendency to become clogged during surgery.

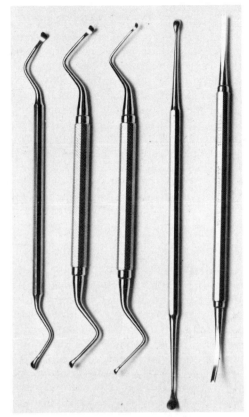

Figure 2–25 Curettes of various sizes and, on the extreme right, a gauze "packer" to aid in the insertion of drains and dressings. See the text for indications for, and techniques in the use of curettes.

USE OF THE CURETTE

The term "curette" comes from the French word *curer,* meaning "to cleanse." Through usage, unfortunately, it has come to mean vigorous scraping in order to remove dental granulomas or cystic walls, and even worse, to stimulate bleeding in the so-called "dry sockets." Some dental surgeons use a high concentration of a vasoconstricting agent in their local anesthetic solutions for infiltration anesthesia in order to have a "dry field" in which to operate, and then vigorously curette the operative site at the completion of the oral surgery in an attempt to induce bleeding so as

to assure the formation of a firm clot. This practice is injurious. It creates unnecessary trauma, predisposes to postoperative pain, and induces localized osteitis and in some cases osteomyelitis.

Indications for Use of the Curette. The curette may be used as an exploratory instrument, and to remove tooth particles or debris from sockets at the time of extraction, to enucleate cysts, dental granulomas, intraosseous tumors, or cystic neoplasms, and to remove small sequestra, which may develop, from sockets during healing.

Contraindications to Use of the Curette. Do not use the curette in acute infections (periapical or residual), in the presence of pus, to stimulate bleeding or to remove periapical granulomas following the extraction of primary (deciduous) teeth.

Technique for Use of the Curette. The curette is used primarily as an exploratory instrument. After a tooth or teeth have been removed, and the process has been trimmed and smoothed, and before the mucoperiosteal tissue is ironed back into place, a small-bowled double-end curette is carefully passed into each socket, and the periapical space is gently explored for small particles of bone, tooth structure or particles of amalgam fillings. If any are found, they are removed. Dental radiographs reveal periapical radiolucency.

The presence of periapical inflammatory tissue is revealed by a soft, rubbery feeling transmitted through the curette to the fingers of the surgeon. The curette must be held lightly in a pen grasp during this gentle exploratory process; otherwise the sense of touch is blunted. Whenever possible, direct visualization of the periapical space is obtained by the use of small suction tips and a strong source of light.

If a small apical granuloma or radicular cyst is located, it can be peeled from its bony crypt through the root socket by means of the curette. (See technique in Chapter 12.) If it is a large area of destruction, radiographs of the area should be made before the dental surgeon attempts to remove the cyst or granuloma.

The operator must always keep in mind, when exploring the sockets of maxillary molars, maxillary bicuspids and occasionally cuspids, that there is the possibility of the maxillary sinus' dipping down until there is nothing separating the apices of these teeth from the maxillary sinus proper, except the lining membrane of the maxillary sinus. Hence the surgeon is unable to tell, without a radiograph, whether the soft, rubbery feeling he encounters when exploring these sockets is a granuloma, a cystic wall, or the lining membrane of the maxillary sinus. He has another clue to guide him, and that is to determine preoperatively whether these teeth are vital. If nonvital, he can suspect that he has a periapical granuloma or radicular cyst if he encounters a soft, rubbery feeling when exploring this area. This can be misleading, however, in too many cases. From this discussion it becomes apparent again that having good dental radiographs carefully studied before the operation is the best way to determine with reasonable accuracy whether a dental granuloma or radicular cyst is present. There are entirely too many maxillary sinuses infected through carelessness at the time of extraction or by the injudicious use of the curette after extraction.

When the curette is used to remove dental granulomas or small cyst membranes, those tissues are not scraped from the bone. The thin edge of the curette, with its concavity turned toward the bone, is gently inserted between the soft tissue and the hard, bony crypt, and with a pushing, sliding motion all about the circumference of the granuloma or cystic sac, the soft tissue is peeled in toward the center of the cavity in the bone. Then, with the concavity of the curette turned toward the center of the bone cavity, it is placed in the space just created and the granuloma or small cyst is enucleated. (See Figures 12–6 and 12–22.)

After the removal of impacted, unerupted teeth by the sectional method, the curette is invaluable in removing small spicules of bone and segments of tooth structure. It is used to cut away sections of the tooth follicle which obscure the crown as the overlying bone is removed.

The curette is a great help in outlining the exposed coronal portions, and in determining just where there is bony tissue covering the crown. To do this, place the thin edge of the curette on that enamel surface which has been exposed, and slide it toward the bone. The edge will pass beneath the bone; if it is thin, the bone will be deflected away from the crown. Do this completely around the exposed area of enamel, and, now that you are oriented, and have a mental picture of the amount of bone still overlying the coronal portion, take the bone chisels or burs and proceed to remove this bone. As more of the bone is exposed, it will be necessary to use the curette again, or a hemostat, to remove small portions of bone and sections of tooth follicle, and to outline the exposed portion of the crown.

When a crown is sectioned by a chisel or bur, the curved bowl of the curette can be slipped around and between the section of the crown and its bony crypt, and by manipulation can remove the crown. Do not attempt to use the curette as an elevator or lever, since it is not made for this purpose and will break.

POSITION OF THE PATIENT

After the patient is seated, there are three adjustments to be performed, as outlined in the following three sections:

Head, Neck and Trunk. The back and the headrest of the chair are adjusted so that the head, neck and trunk are in one line. This will obviate any strain on the patient's neck caused by stretching it backward or pushing it forward.

Chair Angulation. The back of the chair is

angulated to adjust the operative field, when the mouth is opened, to the most visible and accessible position. When the dentist is injecting medications or operating on the mandibular teeth and standing in front of the patient, the occlusal plane of the mandibular teeth should be parallel, or at a 10-degree angle to the floor. When he is standing behind the patient, the angle of the occlusal plane of the mandibular teeth should be increased until the tooth or teeth can be grasped without placing the dentist, or his arm and hand, in an awkward position.

When making injections or operating on the maxilla, position the patient so that the occlusal plane of the teeth is between a 45- and a 60-degree angle to the floor.

Chair Height. For mandibular procedures, the occlusal plane of the mandibular teeth should be at, or slightly below, the level of the dentist's elbow. For maxillary procedures, the chair is elevated so that the occlusal plane of the maxillary teeth is above the level of the dentist's elbow, toward his shoulder. These positions will prevent undue muscular fatigue to the dentist's shoulder by allowing the upper arm to hang loosely from the shoulder girdle.

POSITION OF THE DENTIST

Posture. The dentist, by occupation, is subject to a certain amount of physical strain, more in some ways than persons in other professions. The reason for this is the necessity of prolonged standing in the same position, sometimes in an awkward position. This results in an abnormal strain at the weight-bearing articulations, which gives him trouble with his feet, his knees, at the lumbosacral angle, and at the sacroiliac joints.

The dentist should stand as nearly erect as possible, with his weight equally distributed to each foot. Any other position will eventually result in curvature of the spine, and sacroiliac strain, with attending discomfort and incapacitating effects. See Figures 2–165 to 2–167.

Relation to Patient. For all maxillary procedures, the dentist stands on the right side and in front of the patient.* (See Figures 2–37, 2–55 and 2–71.) When operating on mandibular teeth, he also stands on the right side, but whether in front of or behind the patient will depend on the tooth or teeth to be extracted and the type of forceps used. (See Figures 2–112, 2–117 and 2–133.) A position behind the patient is preferred for extraction of mandibular anterior teeth by means of American-type forceps and is a must for extractions of mandibular right posterior teeth with English-type forceps.

Dentist's Left Hand.* When extracting maxillary anterior teeth and teeth on the left side of the maxilla, the dentist places the thumb palatally and the index finger buccally or labially around the region of the tooth to be extracted. When extracting the teeth on the right side of the maxilla, he places the thumb buccally and the index finger palatally. The operator may use the three free fingers to stabilize the patient's head during the extraction movements. The operator should be aware not to injure the patient's eyes by the three free fingers. When extracting the mandibular anterior teeth, the operator should stand behind the patient and place the thumb of the left hand lingually and the index finger labially. The mandible is supported by the three free fingers. In case the operator prefers to stand in front of the patient, the middle finger is placed lingually and the index finger labially, and the thumb is used to support the mandible.

When extracting the teeth on the right side or the left side of the mandible, the operator should place the left hand in the most convenient position, depending on whether he prefers to stand in front of or behind the patient. The left hand performs most or all of the following functions:

A. During forceps application.
   1. Retraction of lip, cheek and tongue.
   2. Guiding the beaks of the forceps onto the tooth to be extracted.
   3. Stabilizing the patient's head during operations on the maxillary teeth and stabilizing the mandible during operations on the lower teeth.

B. During tooth luxation.
   1. Supporting the buccal and lingual cortical plates.
   2. Estimating the amount of pressure applied and the amount of alveolar bone dilatation.
   3. Counteracting the pressure applied. Unless the mandible is supported,

---

*These positions are designed for right-handed dentists. Left-handed dentists should reverse these positions.

the forces exerted through the forceps to the tooth and hence to the mandible will result in subluxation of the temporomandibular joint, tearing of the intercapsular fibers and in many cases result in chronic unilateral spontaneous dislocation and eventually chronic painful dysarthrosis of the temporomandibular joint.

4. Prevention and protection against slipping of forceps and elevators.
5. Removal of broken fillings, tooth fragments or a whole tooth before it reaches the oropharynx.

C. After tooth extraction.
1. Compressing the buccal and lingual cortical plates back into position.
2. Examination of the surgical field and detection of sharp, bony edges, bony undercuts or loose bone fragments.

Oral Visibility. The patient should be so positioned that the dentist can clearly see what he is doing without stooping, crouching, bending or twisting. This presupposes that he has a good source of light. For proper illumination of the oral cavity, a good headlight properly adjusted is essential. Overhead lights are at best inefficient. The slightest movement on the part of the patient, and the light must be readjusted. It is a good plan to have the room darkened with only sufficient light to enable the assistants to see the instrument tray. The only reflected light then is that from the field of operation.

Surgeon's Preparation. After the patient and chair or operating table are properly adjusted, the dentist dons his cap and mask, places and adjusts his headlight, and if he does not wear glasses, puts on a pair of plain shatter-resistant glasses as "goggles" to protect his eyes from flying debris. This is extremely important, as the author personally knows of two dentists, each of whom lost the sight of an eye as the result of injury in one case and infection in the other. The injury was the result of a carious lower bicuspid which shot out of the mouth, when forceps pressure was exerted on the neck of the tooth, and struck the dentist in the eye. The infection resulted from flying oral debris. The need for protective eyeglasses with use of the air turbines is clearly demonstrated by the splash sprayed on the glasses. This is not so with the conventional handpiece. Likewise, it has been shown that the spread of organisms by the air rotor makes mandatory the use of glasses to reduce the number of microorganisms blown directly into the eyes.*

The dentist removes rings and his watch and scrubs his hands and arms and puts on a sterile gown and gloves. The reader is referred to Chapter 9, page 426 for the details of this procedure as well as instruction on hospital operating room technique.

Draping the Patient. The patient's head, shoulders and chest should be covered with a green drape 30 inches wide by 48 inches long with an oblong opening 6 inches by 4 inches in the center, and 20 inches from the top.

FORCEPS TECHNIQUE

The extraction of teeth requires force to separate the tooth from its soft tissue and bony environment. In the great majority of extractions the ideal instrument to transmit the force exerted by the operator to the tooth is the forceps designed for that particular tooth. One might say that actually the tooth is the continuation of the instrument to effect its own removal, provided one does not use the barbaric technique of actually "pulling" the tooth out of its socket by brute force. To understand how the "tooth extracts itself," note that the force exerted by the muscles of the operator's arm and hand through the handles of the forceps to the beaks, and then to the firmly grasped tooth, moves that tooth—for example, a lower first molar—against the buccal plate, springing and compressing it. As the flow of force is reversed towards the lingual, the lingual plate is compressed; these forces are repeated again and again in a slow steady pressure, not a jerking action, and the alveolus in which the tooth is held is gradually enlarged until the tooth can be freely lifted, not pulled, from the socket.

Teeth in general are either single-rooted or multirooted. Roots are either conical or flattened; *i.e.,* the labiolingual diameter is larger than the mesiodistal diameter. Labiolingual or buccolingual movements are indicated for the extraction of both single-rooted and multirooted teeth, while mesiodistal movements are only limited to single-rooted teeth. Mesiodistal rotation is indicated for single conical roots, while mesiodistal pressure is indicated for single flattened roots. To exert mesiodistal

---

*Bissell, S. L.: Study of air turbine versus conventional handpiece on odontectomies. J.A.D.A., *72*:645–647 (Mar.), 1966.

pressure (with strictly limited rotary pressure), the forces are alternately applied mesially and then distally, with the major pressures applied buccolingually.

Before studying the following text, the reader should examine the sectional roentgenograms of the maxilla and mandible in Figure 16–4 and Figure 16–6 of Chapter 16, and note the relative thickness of the labial, buccal, and lingual cortical bone opposite the roots of the maxillary and mandibular teeth. The reason for the main direction of force in the luxation and removal of the various teeth will then become evident.

Sequence of Extractions. When extractions of the remaining teeth or multiple maxillary and mandibular extractions are indicated and are to be accomplished at the same appointment, the maxillary extractions are completed first. This will prevent broken or dislodged calculus, fillings, tooth fragments, bone chips and debris from falling into the mandibular alveoli, which might happen if the lower teeth were removed first. Extractions should be completed a quadrant at a time, starting from the most posterior tooth and moving anteriorly toward the midline.

EXTRACTION OF MAXILLARY AND MANDIBULAR TEETH

Pre-extraction Tissue Treatment. This is as follows:

1. Spray the mouth thoroughly with an antiseptic solution, taking care to flush out, in particular, the interproximal spaces.
2. Remove large deposits of salivary calculus which will be dislodged by the forceps and may drop into the open sockets.
3. Scrub the gingival tissues and the buccal and lingual tissues with germicidal solution.
4. Incise the gingival tissue with a No. 12 BP scalpel, using the gingival line as the incising guide and carrying the incision interproximally to the crest of the interdental papillae. Make certain that alveolar bone is contacted by the tip of the scalpel.
5. Reflect the mucoperiosteum with a periosteal elevator to the extent necessary to prevent damage to soft tissues by forceps, when the beaks are forced beneath this tissue, and so that the tissue will not be split by the buccal-lingual movement of the root of the tooth.

Application of Forceps. Certain rules must be observed in the application of forceps:

1. The correct forceps must be selected.
2. Do not grasp the forceps near the beaks. Instead, hold them so that the ends of the handles are almost covered by the palm of the hand.
3. The long axis of the forceps beaks must be parallel to the long axis of the tooth.
4. Forceps beaks must be placed on sound root structure and not on the enamel of the crown.
5. The root structure must be grasped firmly so that, when pressure is applied, the beaks do not move on the cementum; otherwise, breakage may occur.
6. Make certain that the beaks of the forceps will not impinge on adjacent teeth during the application of force.

Basic Forces Exerted in the Extraction of Maxillary Teeth in Normal Position in the Arch. The first pressure applied for the extraction of all maxillary teeth is apical force, until the beaks of the forceps engage the neck of the tooth, resting on cementum. Then apply pressure as follows:

CENTRAL INCISORS. Labial pressure, then lingual pressure, then labial pressure, with mesial rotation.

LATERAL INCISORS. Labial pressure, with mesial rotation.

CUSPIDS. Labial pressure, then lingual pressure, then labial pressure, with mesial rotation.

FIRST BICUSPIDS. Buccal pressure, lingual pressure, and removal in the buccal direction.

SECOND BICUSPIDS. Buccal pressure, lingual pressure, and removal in the lingual or buccal direction.

FIRST MOLARS. Buccal pressure, lingual pressure, and removal in the buccal direction.

SECOND MOLARS. Buccal pressure, lingual pressure, and removal in the buccal direction.

THIRD MOLARS. Buccal pressure and distal rotation.

Basic Forces Exerted in the Extraction of Mandibular Teeth in Normal Position in the Arch. The first pressure applied for the extraction of all mandibular teeth is apical force, until the beaks of the forceps engage the neck of the tooth, resting on cementum. Then apply pressure as follows:

CENTRAL INCISORS. Labial pressure, lingual pressure; also slight mesial to distal force, and removal in the labial direction.

LATERAL INCISORS. Labial pressure, lingual pressure; also slight mesial and distal force, and removal in the labial direction.

CUSPIDS. Labial pressure, with mesial rotation.

FIRST BICUSPIDS. Buccal pressure, with slight mesiodistal rotation.

SECOND BICUSPIDS. Buccal pressure, with slight mesiodistal rotation.

FIRST MOLARS. Buccal pressure, lingual pressure, and removal in the buccal direction.

SECOND MOLARS. Buccal pressure, lingual pressure, and removal in the buccal direction.

THIRD MOLARS. Buccal pressure, and removal in the buccal or lingual direction.

Specific Technique. EXTRACTION OF MAXILLARY TEETH. See Figures 2–26 to 2–99.

Maxillary Incisors and Cuspids. See Figures 2–26 to 2–46.

Maxillary Bicuspids. See Figures 2–47 to 2–60.

Maxillary Molars. See Figures 2–61 to 2–99.

EXTRACTION OF MANDIBULAR TEETH. See Figures 2–100 to 2–155.

Mandibular Incisors and Cuspids. See Figures 2–100 to 2–116.

Mandibular Bicuspids. See Figures 2–117 to 2–120.

Mandibular Molars. See Figures 2–121 to 2–155.

Variations in Pressure to Extract Teeth. Though the tooth to be extracted is in a normal position in a normal arch and there may not be any overlapping by adjacent teeth, the adjacent teeth may have restorations of metal, porcelain or synthetic porcelain whose proximal contours may be traumatized by the buccal, lingual or rotary movements of the tooth to be extracted, to the extent that the filling or restoration may be fractured or displaced.

Always carefully examine teeth to determine whether the adjacent teeth will be injured by the basic movements for the extraction of this tooth, and whether there are any restorations in the adjacent teeth that may be fractured or dislodged by the movements for the extraction of this tooth. If such a situation obtains, then study the tooth to be extracted, and its neighbors, to determine whether the basic luxating movements for that tooth may be changed, even reversed, so as to avoid encroaching on its neighbors.

If this is possible, then these new pressures are applied to the tooth, either by forceps or elevators, to dislodge it from the alveolus.

If this is impossible, then the proximal surfaces of the tooth to be extracted should be cut away with a carborundum disk. Whenever there is any doubt as to the possibility of avoiding injury to adjacent teeth, or restorations in adjacent teeth, always cut away the proximal surfaces of the tooth to be extracted before applying the forceps.

(Text continued on page 100)

EXTRACTION OF MAXILLARY TEETH

Extraction of Maxillary Incisors and Cuspids

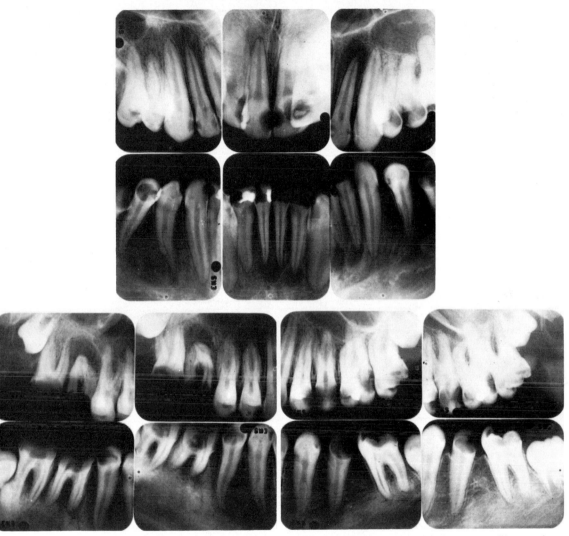

Figure 2–26   An example of extensive caries in the teeth of both the maxilla and mandible, which will necessitate care in extracting to avoid fracture of the crowns. Note also the many teeth with apical pathosis that will require thorough curettement.

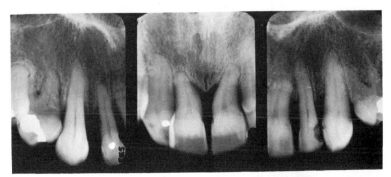

Figure 2–27   These maxillary incisors have lost two thirds of their bony support as a result of periodontal disease. However, they must be luxated and rotated slowly because the apices (still held tightly in bone) will easily fracture.

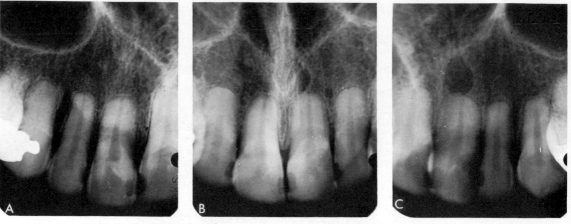

Figure 2–28 Resorption of roots as a result of orthodontic treatment. (See text.)

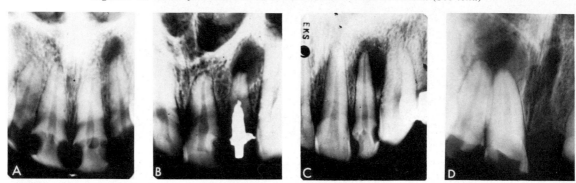

Figure 2–29 The extent and location of caries in the teeth to be extracted should be studied so that the technique for removal will reduce as much as possible the probability of fracture of the crowns. The presence of posts or fillings in the root canals almost mandates the removal of investing bone and the use of elevators to remove the roots. The apical radiolucent areas indicate periapical pathosis whose removal is a necessity to prevent the possibility of residual cyst development.

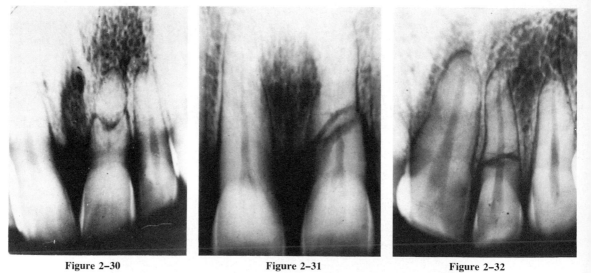

Figure 2–30   **Figure 2–31**   **Figure 2–32**

Figures 2–30, 2–31 and 2–32 In most cases of root fractures the vitality of the pulp is maintained. While fractures of the roots of the anterior teeth can occur in any area, the most common is in the middle third.

The most favorable fractures for healing are those of the apical and middle thirds; coronal fractures have the poorest prognosis because they are the most mobile and have the poorest, if any, bony support. Generally the middle and apical fragments are in reasonable approximation; if not, an attempt should be made to bring them closer together by finger pressure while they are splinted.

A periodontal pack is applied as a splint. This will support the tooth for the usual 3 or 4 weeks that it should be immobilized. It can be splinted again if necessary. (Quick-curing acrylic can be molded around the traumatized and adjacent teeth as a splint. It should be cooled with water while curing.)

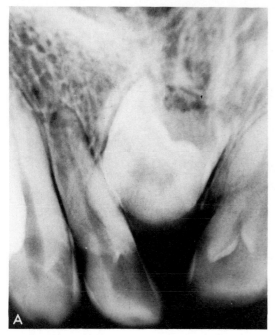

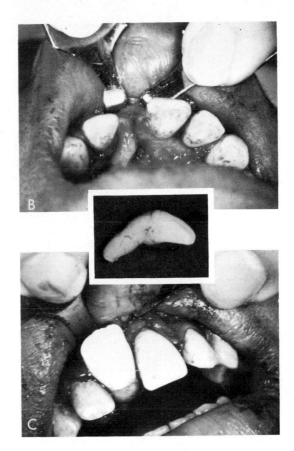

Figure 2–33 *A*, Dilaceration of the right maxillary central incisor. *B*, Labial and palatal flaps were reflected, and overlying bone was removed with chisels and burs with care not to injure the roots of the adjacent teeth. *C*, Tooth removed (*inset*) and partially replaced to illustrate its former position.

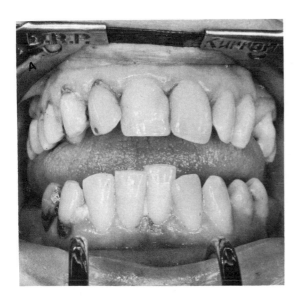

Figure 2–34 Irregularity and crowding in the maxillary and mandibular anterior teeth are frequent complications in their extraction. To prevent injury to adjacent teeth when luxating the tooth to be removed, it may be necessary to cut away a slice of the mesial and distal surfaces of the tooth to be removed before applying the forceps or the elevator. The elevators must be used with considerable caution for the removal of lower anterior teeth or roots because of the small amount of interseptal bone which can be used as a fulcrum. This means that the fulcrum will be compressed and injurious pressure will then be exerted on the adjacent tooth or teeth. See Figures 2–105 and 2–106 and legends for more discussion about overlapping of the mandibular six anterior teeth.

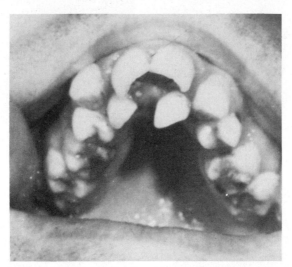

Figure 2–35   The gross malposition of these teeth makes it impossible to apply forceps in the normal position. These teeth could best be removed by the use of the No. 301 (81) Apexo elevator used as a wedge along the longitudinal axis of these teeth.

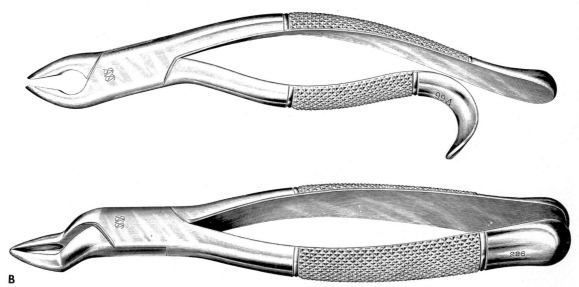

B

Figure 2–36   *A*, Forceps No. 99A. For the extraction of the six upper anterior teeth the straight forceps No. 99A is used. Forceps No. 286 is also a good instrument for the removal of maxillary central and lateral incisors. The soft tissue having been freed around the necks of the teeth to be extracted, the beaks are applied to the cementum well under the gum tissue and parallel to the long axis of the tooth. Central incisors are removed by strong labial-lingual pressure and mesial rotation; the same pressure is applied to the laterals. The cuspids are moved labially, then lingually, then labially with mesial rotation.

B, Forceps No. 286. For the extraction of upper bicuspids the "bayonet-type" forceps No. 286 is most suitable. The beaks are forced beneath the loosened soft tissue and are closed firmly on the cementum covering the neck of the bicuspid. This shape permits the parallel application of the beaks to the root of the tooth, and the handles avoid pinching the lip during the application of pressures (buccal-lingual-buccal and out of the buccal side) in the extraction of these teeth. This is an excellent forceps for the removal of primary and permanent anterior maxillary teeth.

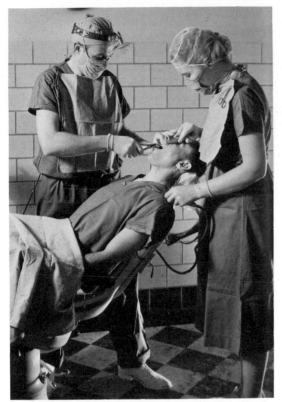

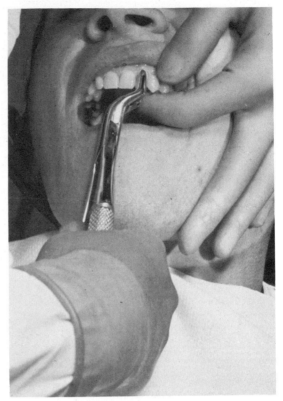

Figure 2-37 Positions of the dentist and the patient for the extraction of the maxillary six anterior teeth. The drape has been lowered so that the correct position of the patient in the chair is visible. Note that the head, neck and chest are all in a straight line. The chair is then tilted to an angle of 45 degrees to the floor; this gives good visibility and access to the maxilla. The dentist, who stands erect with his legs spread apart, distributing his weight equally on both feet, can see the operating field without bending of twisting his back.

Figure 2-38 Application of the No. 286 forceps to a maxillary lateral incisor. Note the position of the thumb and fingers of the left hand to reflect the lip and support the maxilla. The ends of the handles of this forceps are in the palm of the hand. Never grasp a forceps high up on the handles near the joints. The beaks are parallel to the long axis of the tooth and are engaging cementum. To extract this tooth, labial pressure with mesial rotation is applied.

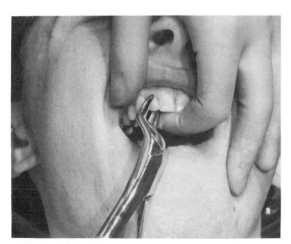

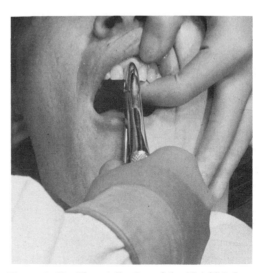

Figure 2-39 This shows the incorrect application of the beaks of the forceps; they are not parallel to the long axis of the tooth. If this tooth were rotated, the beaks would injure the adjacent teeth.

Figure 2-40 The application of the No. 99A forceps to a central incisor. To extract this tooth, labial pressure with mesial rotation is applied.

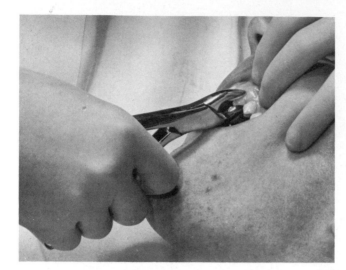

Figure 2–41 Side view of the application of the No. 99A forceps for extraction of a left maxillary cuspid. Pressures to extract this tooth are labial-lingual with mesial rotation.

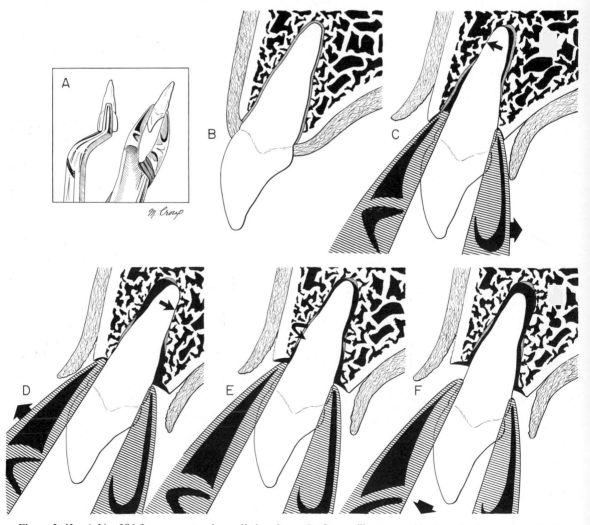

Figure 2–42 *A*, No. 286 forceps correctly applied to the neck of a maxillary central incisor. Study text for technique. *B*, Tooth in position in the alveolus. *C* and *D*, Pressures are alternated lingually and labially, thus enlarging the alveolus. *E*, The tooth is rotated mesially. *F*, Tooth is lifted from the alveolus.

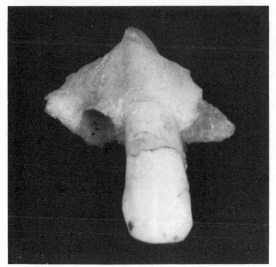

Figure 2–43

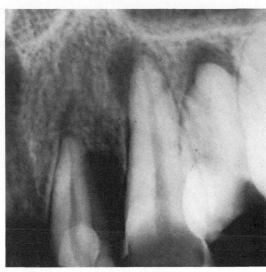

Figure 2–44

Figure 2–43   A standard technique in the extraction of maxillary or mandibular teeth in the past was to extract the teeth on either side of the cuspids so that presumably there would be less difficulty in enlarging the cuspid alveolus, thereby reducing the possibility of fracturing the cuspid during its extraction. The danger, however, is illustrated here; a large portion of the alveolar bone containing not only the cuspid but the first bicuspid alveolus and a portion of the lateral incisor's alveolus was segmentally fractured from the maxilla.

Figure 2–44   Illustrated here is a cuspid that has a carious crown and apical pathosis, a deep periodontal pocket mesially and carious first bicuspid with apical pathosis distally. In order to facilitate the removal of these teeth without fracturing them, as well as the removal of the periapical pathosis by means of the curette, a buccal flap should be reflected and buccal bone excised from the gingival third area of both teeth.

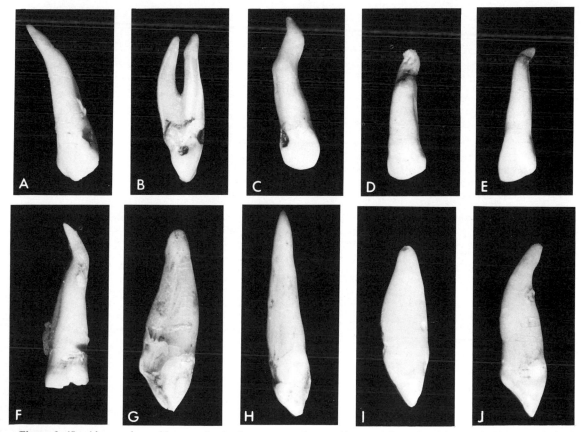

Figure 2–45   Abnormal cuspid roots. In the bottom row, the cuspid second from the right margin is a normal-sized and -shaped maxillary cuspid.

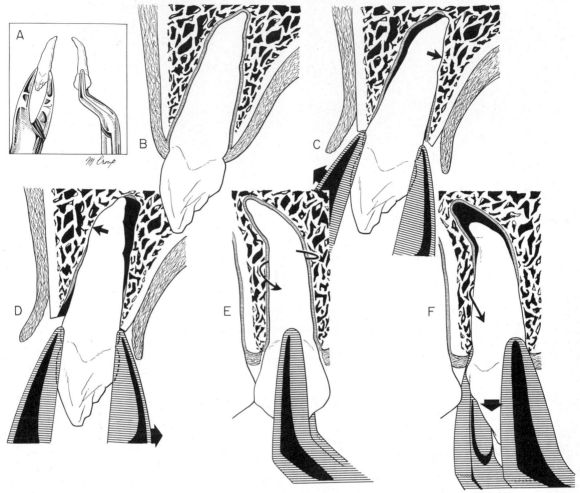

Figure 2–46 A No. 286 forceps correctly applied to the neck of a maxillary cuspid and the direction of forceps applied to luxate and remove this tooth. Study the text.

Plate I Technique for complete maxillary anterior extractions and alveoplasty. (For more on alveoplasty, see Chapter 3, page 181.)

A, Unibevel chisel used to remove the labial cortical bone, thus permitting easier luxation of the cuspid and preventing tearing out a large segment of bone with the tooth.

B, Extent of the removal of bone.

C, Extraction of the maxillary first bicuspid. Dr. Byrd, who contributed these illustrations, prefers the No. 151 forceps. My preference is the No. 286 forceps.

D, The mucoperiosteum is retracted, and the maxillary six anterior teeth are extracted by means of the No. 99A forceps. (The No. 286 forceps is also a very fine instrument for extraction of maxillary anterior teeth.)

E, With the No. 10 rongeur or the No. 5C bone shear the alveolar ridge is contoured.

F and *G*, Small, sharp projections of bone are removed with either a bone bur or a hand file.

H, A curette small enough to reach the apex of the alveolus is used to remove any small particles of bone or foreign material, such as filling materials or enamel, and, if the radiographs revealed a periapical radiolucent area, to explore this area and remove any so-called "granuloma" (which is actually a mass of chronic inflammatory tissue) that might be present.

I, Excess mucoperiosteal tissue is removed with the Dean's scissors. Care must be taken not to remove *too much,* or the buccal and labial vestibule will be decreased when the flap is sutured into place.

J, A half-circle cutting-edge needle with 000 black silk is passed through the loose labial mucoperiosteum, 3 to 4 mm. from the edge.

K, The needle is drawn through the labial flap and the tip then inserted through the palatal tissue.

L, The soft tissues are held in place with a running lock stitch, as illustrated in Figure 2–157.

(Photographs courtesy of D. Lamar Byrd, D.D.S., Professor and Chairman, Department of Oral Surgery, College of Dentistry, Baylor University, Dallas. From Byrd, D. L.: Exodontia: Modern concepts. Dent. Clin. North Am., *15*[2]:273–298, 1971.)

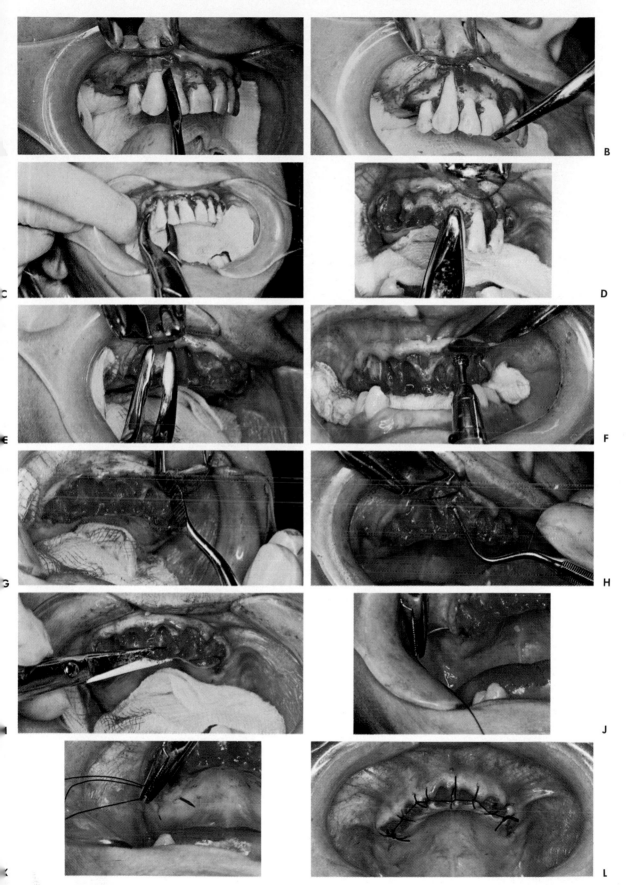

Plate I *See opposite page for legend.*

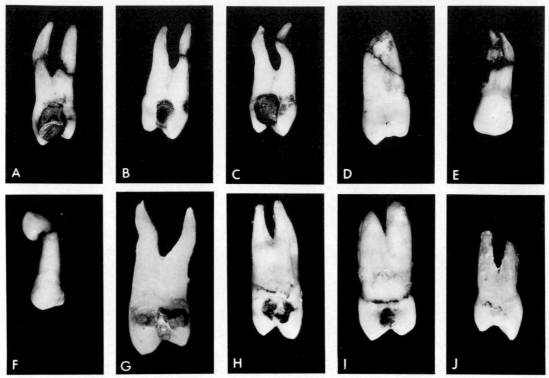

Figure 2–47   Unusual bicuspid and cuspid roots. The fractured roots have been reattached with black wax. Study Chapter 4, "The Use of Elevators in Oral Surgery," for the techniques used in the removal of these root fragments.

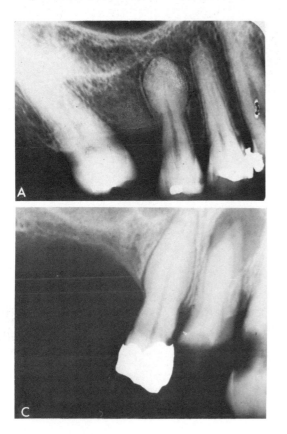

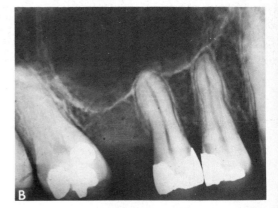

Figure 2–48   *A*, Large excementosis of the apical third of the maxillary second bicuspid root. Complete surgical exposure of this entire root would be necessary if extraction were ever indicated. Fortunately, there is adequate bone between the apex of this tooth and the maxillary sinus.

B, Note the very close relationship of the apices of the bicuspids and molars to the floor of the maxillary sinus. Note also the excementosis of the second bicuspid root.

C, The excementosis of the second bicuspid root is confined to the midportion of the root. There is a well circumscribed area of radiolucency about the apices of the first bicuspid.

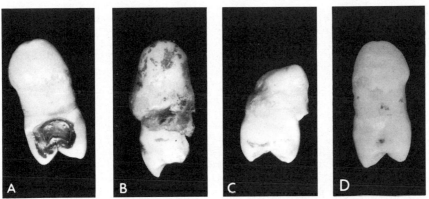

Figure 2–49 Excementosed maxillary bicuspids. Buccal, mesial and distal bone should be removed before the extraction of these teeth. Extreme care must be used not to injure the roots of adjacent teeth.

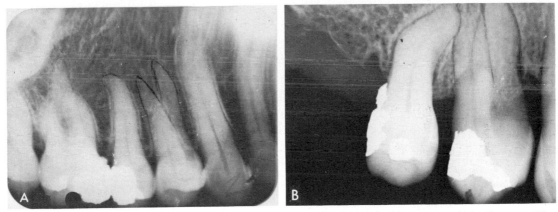

Figure 2–50 *A,* Maxillary bicuspids with thin, pointed apices. The first bicuspid roots are widely divergent. These apices frequently fracture during extraction. Removal of buccal bone and slow and deliberate buccal-then-lingual pressures are indicated to enlarge the alveolus. The second bicuspid in radiograph *A* has a single root with distal curvature of the apex. Buccal-lingual pressures with the No. 286 forceps are indicated with alternate moderate *mesial rotation.*

B, Maxillary bicuspids with round, thick roots and apices. The first bicuspid's buccal and lingual roots are not widely divergent, and these roots generally withstand the pressures exerted on them at the time of extraction without fracturing. The maxillary second bicuspid has a 45-degree mesial curvature of the apex, which is in close proximity to the first bicuspid roots. Buccal bone should be removed to prevent fracture during removal of such a tooth. In addition to buccal-lingual luxation with the No. 286 forceps, slight *distal rotation* should be alternately applied. Distal rotation takes advantage of the inclined plane of the root curvature to lift the tooth in the alveolus. Mesial rotation would drive the apex into the wall of the alveolus and if continued would result in the fracture of the apical third and probably injury to the first bicuspid roots; it is *definitely contraindicated.* If the roots are curved distally, then, and then only, is slight mesial rotation indicated.

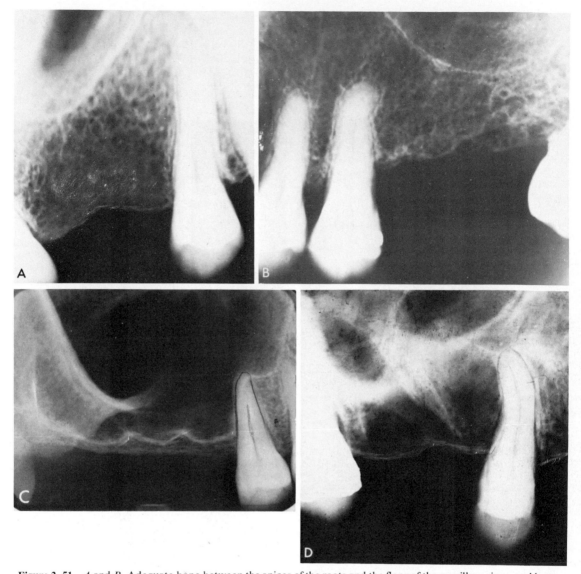

Figure 2–51 *A* and *B*, Adequate bone between the apices of the roots and the floor of the maxillary sinus, and between the crest of the ridge and the sinus.

C and *D*, Only a thin layer of cortical bone separates the roots of these bicuspids or the crest of the ridge. Extreme care must be exercised to prevent opening into the maxillary sinus. A buccal flap should be reflected and buccal and mesial bone excised before applying the forceps. Pressures indicated were previously described to remove these teeth. Obviously the problem here is to remove such teeth, when removal is indicated, as is not the case here, so that the maxillary sinus is not opened into. A buccal flap is reflected, buccal and some mesial bone is removed from over the root and then the teeth are carefully luxated with the No. 286 forceps and removed.

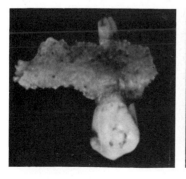
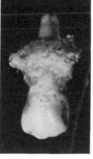

Figure 2–52 When thick cortical buccal or labial bone overlies the roots of teeth that are to be extracted, the possibility of fracturing the crown at the neck of the tooth or fracturing a segment of the bone is always present. The latter accident is illustrated in both these cases. This bone will not be replaced when the ridge heals. The excision of a comparatively small portion of this bone with a chisel before application of the forceps would have prevented this large loss of bone in both examples. This is known as an odontectomy, the surgical excision of a tooth.

If these teeth had had the relationship to the maxillary sinus that is shown in Figure 2–51C and D, the maxillary sinus would have been entered, creating an antro-oral fistula.

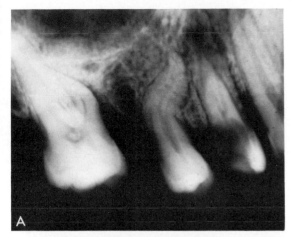

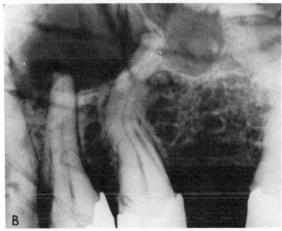

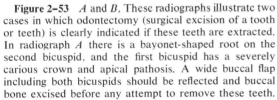

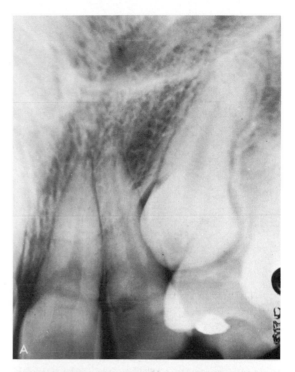

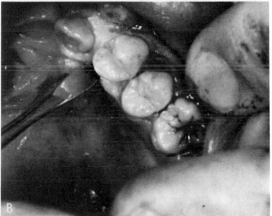

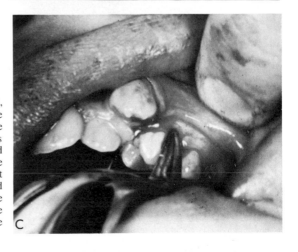

Figure 2-53 *A* and *B*, These radiographs illustrate two cases in which odontectomy (surgical excision of a tooth or teeth) is clearly indicated if these teeth are extracted. In radiograph *A* there is a bayonet-shaped root on the second bicuspid, and the first bicuspid has a severely carious crown and apical pathosis. A wide buccal flap including both bicuspids should be reflected and buccal bone excised before any attempt to remove these teeth.

B, The same surgical procedure is indicated here for the additional reason of the intimate relationship of the maxillary sinus to the apices of the bicuspids. The radiolucent area about the apex of the first bicuspid strongly suggests pathosis, and the absence of a sclerotic line of bone around the radiolucent area may indicate that there is antral involvement.

Figure 2-54 *A*, Malposition of the maxillary cuspid, which the orthodontist decided could be moved into a space created by the extraction of the first bicuspid. *B*, Soft tissue about the neck of the first bicuspid was incised to sever its connection with the periodontal ligament and then loosened buccally and lingually with a periosteal elevator. *C*, The beaks of a No. 286 forceps, placed beneath the loosened soft tissue, engage the cementum of the neck of the bicuspid and with *lingual pressure only* expand the alveolus and remove the tooth palatally. Buccal pressures would probably have resulted in the dislodgement of the cuspid, and so they were not used.

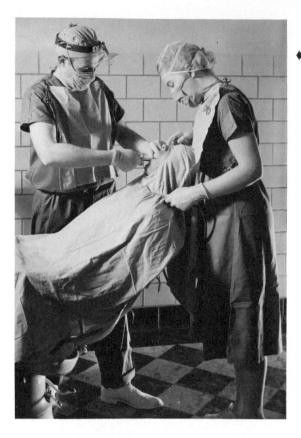

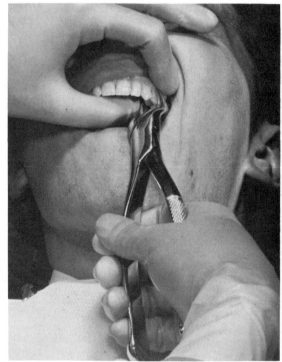

◆ **Figure 2–55** Positions of the dentist and the patient for extraction of the maxillary bicuspids and molars. Note that the patient and the chair are tilted back at a 45-degree angle to the floor. This permits good visibility and accessibility without the necessity of the dentist's bending and twisting his back in order to see.

Figure 2–56 Front view of the application of the No. 286 forceps for extraction of an upper first bicuspid. Note the simultaneous reflection of the lip and finger bracing of the forceps and maxilla by the fingers of the left hand. The proper position of the handles of the forceps in relationship to the hand is also illustrated here. ◆

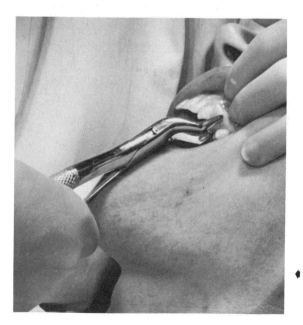

Figure 2–57 Correct application of the No. 286 forceps for extraction of upper bicuspids. Note that the beaks are parallel to the long axis of the first bicuspid. When the forceps move the tooth lingually, do not inadvertently compress the lower lip between the forceps and the lower teeth. If the lower lip is anesthetized, severe trauma to lip could result. ◆

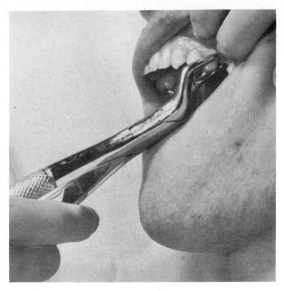

Figure 2–58 Incorrect application of the No. 286 forceps. Note that the forceps is reversed so that the joint is compressing the lip against the buccal surface of the mandibular teeth; note also that the beaks of the forceps are not parallel to the long axis of the second bicuspid. Actually the beaks would traumatize the first bicuspid so severely when the second bicuspid was luxated that this tooth also would most likely have to be extracted.

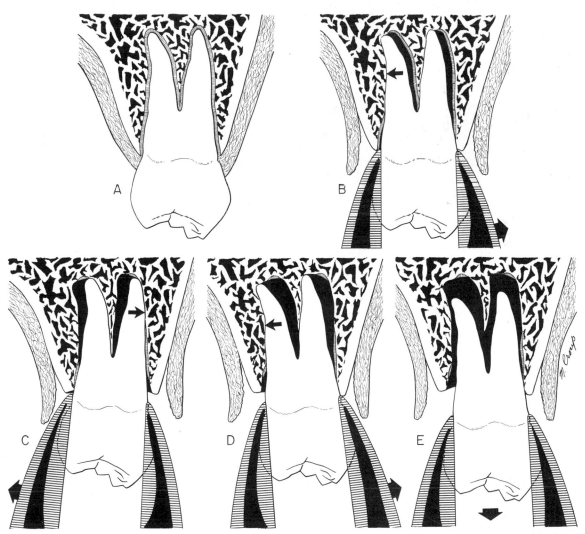

Figure 2–59 Application of the No. 286 forceps to the neck of the maxillary first bicuspid. Forces exerted in alternate directions, buccally and lingually, in order to luxate the tooth, free it from its periodontal attachment and expand the alveolus so that the tooth can be lifted out. The presence of two roots contraindicates rotary pressures. Study the text.

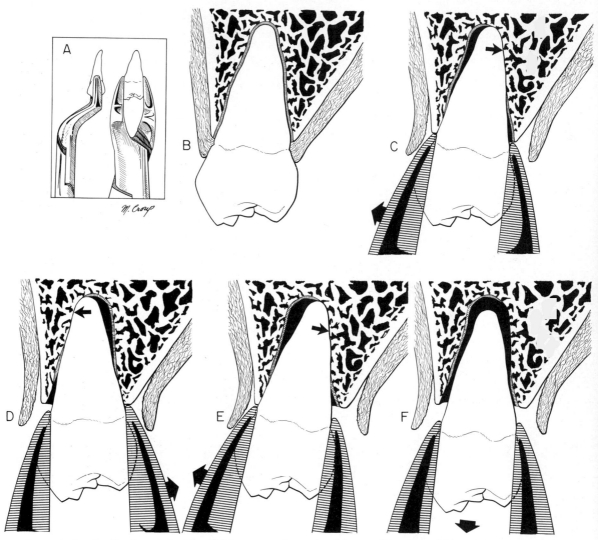

Figure 2–60 Application of the No. 286 forceps to the neck of the maxillary second bicuspid. *C,* Buccal pressure compresses lingual bone and expands gingival buccal bone. *D,* Lingual pressure compresses buccal bone and expands gingival lingual bone. *E,* Both buccal and lingual pressures are repeated. *F,* Tooth is lifted from the alveolus.

Second maxillary bicuspids are usually single-rooted; if the radiograph indicates this fact, then, although these roots are flat buccolingually, *very minimal* mesial and then distal rotary pressure can be exerted with the forceps, but only *if* the bicuspid is isolated or the adjacent teeth have been or are to be extracted. This pressure will help expand the alveolus.

Extraction of Maxillary Molars

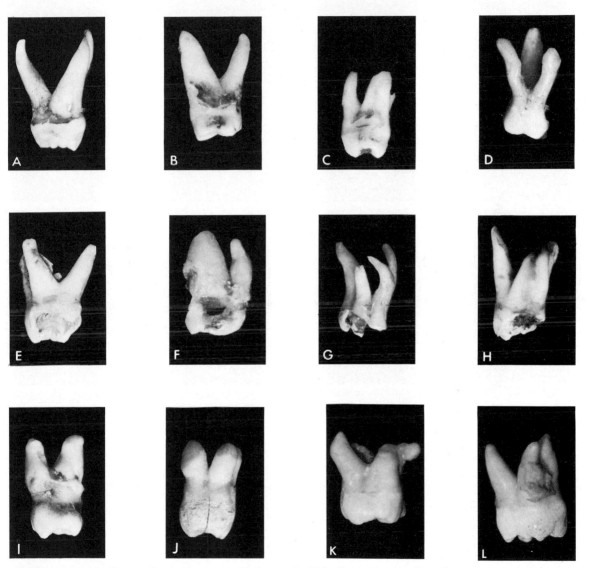

Figure 2–61 Maxillary molars with abnormally long and widely divergent roots. Some have one or more excementosed roots, or long and finely tapered roots. While these were removed by odontectomy (*i.e.,* surgical removal of bone), in retrospect bone could have been saved if a moderate portion of gingival bone had been excised, the buccal roots cut free from the crowns and the tooth removed as shown in Figure 2–86. *Note:* Tooth *C* is a normal-sized maxillary molar.

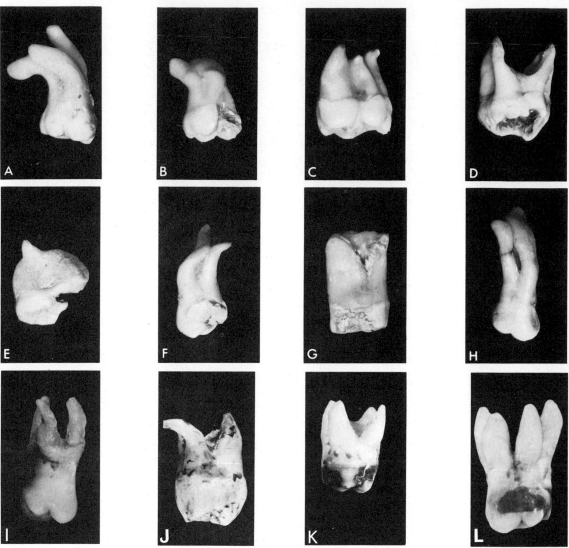

Figure 2–62 Maxillary molars with grossly abnormal roots either by number or formation. These teeth did not lend themselves to the root sectioning technique and so were surgically exposed (by odontectomy) and removed with forceps or elevators or both.

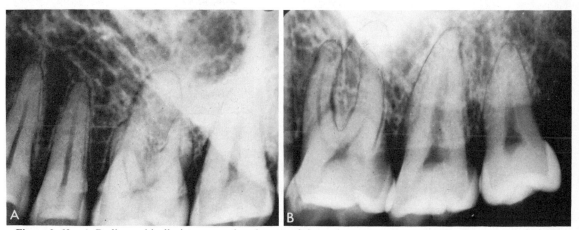

Figure 2–63 *A*, Radiographically it appears that these teeth have three normal roots. *B*, The second and third molar roots appear to be fused in a tapered solid unit. See specimen *A* in Figure 2–64. When such teeth have to be extracted, in addition to the standard buccal-then-lingual forceps pressures to enlarge the alveolus, mesial-then-distal rotary pressures can also be used.

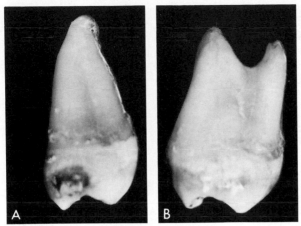

Figure 2–64 *A,* An example of a maxillary molar in which all three roots are fused. These teeth are easily extracted. *B,* Maxillary molar with buccal roots fused with the lingual root for 95 per cent of its length. Because of the superimposition of the buccal roots over the lingual on the radiographs, this slight separation of the lingual root tip is not seen. It usually is bulky enough that it does not fracture during extraction.

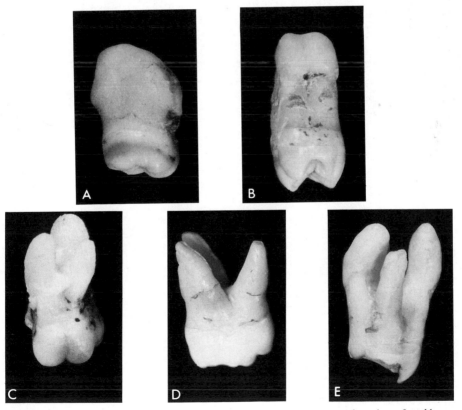

Figure 2–65 *A* and *B,* Examples of maxillary molars with fused roots that appear to have been fused by excementosis. *C* and *D,* Maxillary molars with three excementosed roots. *E,* An unusual maxillary molar with apical excementosis on two of its three roots. An odontectomy was performed to remove these teeth.

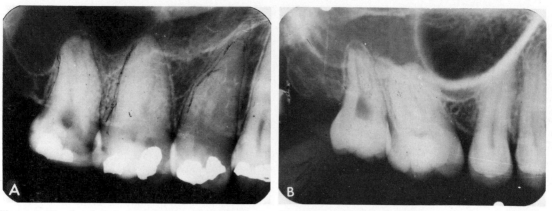

Figure 2–66 *A* and *B,* In both these radiographs the maxillary molar roots project into the sinus, but the sinus does not dip down to the crest of the ridge between the molar and second bicuspid.

If there is not any radiographic evidence of a periapical radiolucent area, then periapical curettage is contraindicated, and particularly in those cases in which there is root-antral relationship, such as is illustrated in these radiographs.

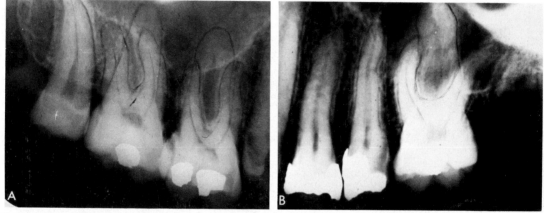

Figure 2–67 *A,* Maxillary molars in which the floor of the maxillary sinus dips slightly between the lingual and buccal roots. In the second molar the buccal bone is partially locked by the buccal roots. This indicates the need to use the sectional technique (see Figure 2–86), should this or a similar tooth require extraction.

B, The floor of the maxillary sinus dips deeply between the lingual and buccal roots in this case. In addition there is marked curvature of the apex of the distobuccal root. An odontectomy is indicated, with buccal bone being removed from both buccal roots before the application of forceps.

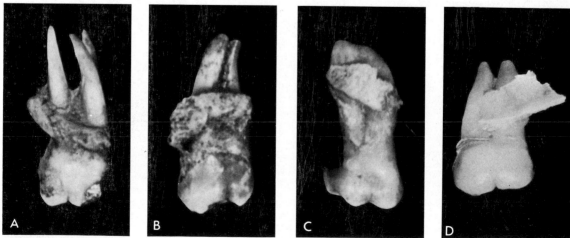

Figure 2–68 Maxillary molar specimens again illustrating bone torn out at the time of extraction. This bone could have been saved and the extraction simplified if an odontectomy had been performed.

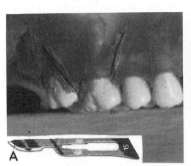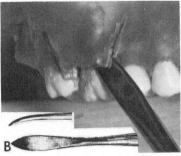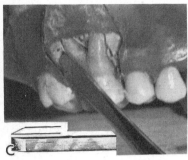

Figure 2–69 *A*, Incisions made through the mucoperiosteal membrane at a 45-degree angle to the gingival line by means of a No. 15 blade. *B*, The full thickness of the mucoperiosteal membrane is reflected by the subperiosteal elevator. *C*, Buccal cortical and cancellous bone is excised with a unibevel chisel prior to luxation of the tooth.

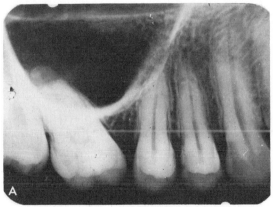

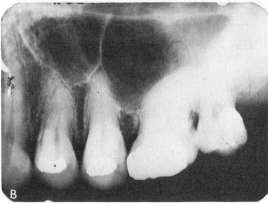

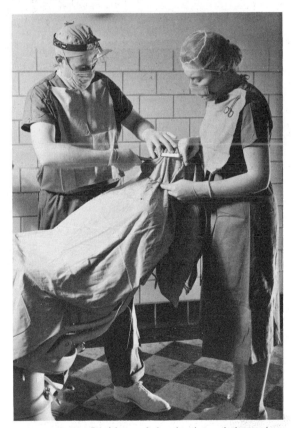

Figure 2–70 *A*, Maxillary sinus dips down between the buccal and lingual roots of the molars.

B, Maxillary sinus not only occupies the space between the molar roots but approximates the apices of the bicuspids as well.

Figure 2–71 Positions of the dentist and the patient for extraction of the maxillary bicuspids and molars. Note that the patient and the chair are tilted back at a 45-degree angle to the floor. This permits good visibility and accessibility without the necessity of the dentist's bending and twisting his back in order to see.

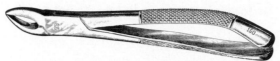

Figure 2–72 Forceps No. 150. For extensively decayed upper molars, the crowns of which are liable to fracture, forceps No. 150 is indicated. The narrow beaks permit the buccal beak to penetrate well up between the bifurcation of the buccal roots, so that if the tooth fractures, the roots will also be separated through the pulp chamber; then each root may be removed individually with the No. 286 forceps. The No. 150 forceps is an ideal instrument for extraction of maxillary deciduous molars.

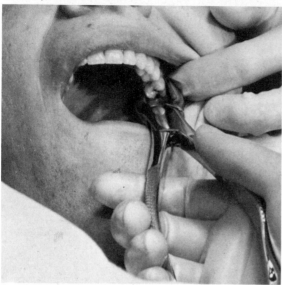
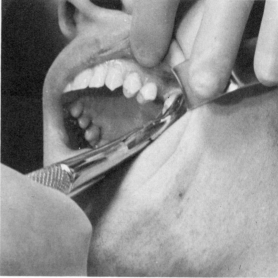

Figure 2–73   **Figure 2–74**

Figure 2–73 Front view of the application of the No. 150 forceps for extraction of the maxillary left second molar. Note that the handles of this forceps are above the mandible, thus permitting lingual movement of the forceps and tooth.

Figure 2–74 Lateral view of the No. 150 Universal upper forceps applied for extraction of the left maxillary first molar. Note that the beaks parallel the long axis of the crown.

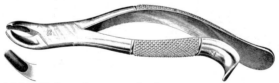

Figure 2–75 Forceps No. 24 is a Universal upper molar forceps with broad beaks to be used in the extraction of right and left maxillary molars with good crowns. As in all extractions, after the soft tissue around the neck has been freed, the lingual and buccal beaks are forced up on the cementum covering the roots—the beaks being parallel to the long axis of the tooth—buccal-lingual-buccal pressure is applied, and the molar is removed in the buccal direction.

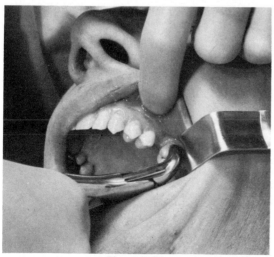
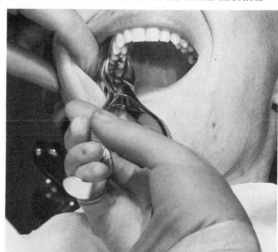

Figure 2–76   **Figure 2–77**

                     See opposite page for legend.

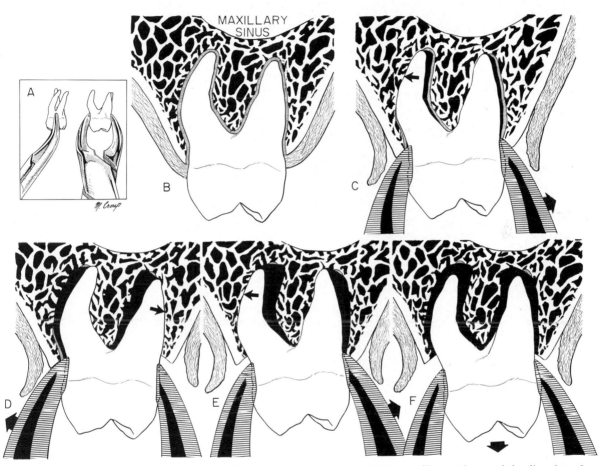

Figure 2–78   Universal maxillary forceps No. 150 applied to the neck of the maxillary molars, and the direction of force applied to extract maxillary molars. The same technique is followed when using forceps No. 24 to extract maxillary molars. Study the text.

Figure 2–76   Lateral view of the application of the No. 24 Universal upper molar forceps for extraction of a maxillary second molar. This forceps, as well as the Universal forceps No. 150, permits the operator to apply greater lingual pressure when luxating maxillary molars than is possible with the No. 10H forceps. The handles of the No. 10H strike the lower jaw when the tooth is moved lingually.

Figure 2–77   Front view of the application of forceps No. 24 for extraction of a right maxillary first molar. Note that the handles are above the mandible, permitting lingual movement of the tooth and the forceps. This forceps can be used for the extraction of all maxillary molars.

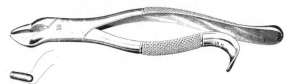

Figure 2–79 Forceps No. 10H. For upper third molars the "bayonet molar" forceps No. 10H can be used. This forceps can be also be used for the extraction of any maxillary molar with good crowns, but lingual force is limited because the handles will strike the lower jaw when the tooth is luxated lingually. Hence, when this forceps is used, only slight lingual force can be exerted, the main force being in the buccal direction.

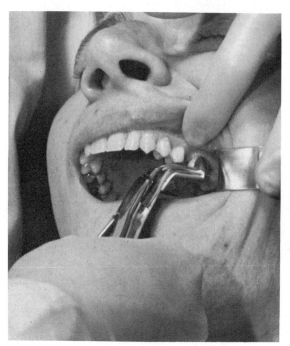

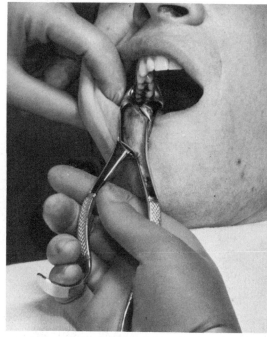

Figure 2–80   **Figure 2–81**

Figure 2–80 Lateral view of the No. 10H forceps for extraction of the left maxillary second molar. This "bayonet-type" forceps is used for the extraction of all maxillary molars. Lingual movement, however, is restricted.

Figure 2–81 Front view of the application of the No. 10H forceps for extraction of the upper right first molar. Note that the lingual movement is restricted because the handles strike the mandible.

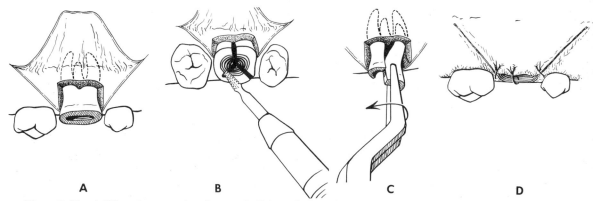

A   **B**   **C**   **D**

Figure 2–82 *A*, When the crown has fractured off through the pulp chamber, the same flap as in *A* is used and the buccal bone is removed. *B*, The roots are separated by a crosscut fissure bur. *C*, Each root is removed with forceps. *D*, The flap is sutured back into place.

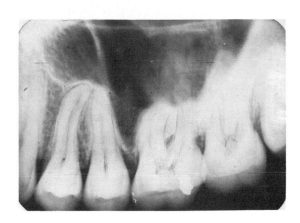

Figure 2–83 The maxillary sinus bears a close relationship to the roots of the molars and to the bicuspids as well. Note how it dips down to the crest of the ridge between the second bicuspid and first molar. If the first molar is to be extracted, an odontectomy should be performed.

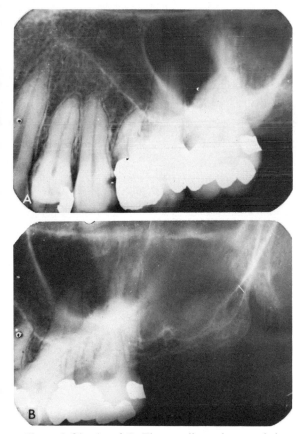

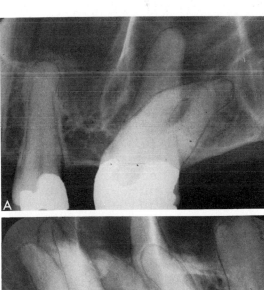

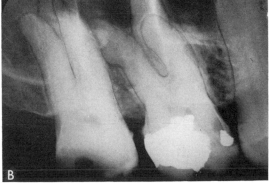

Figure 2–84 *A* and *B*, These radiographs reveal the floor of the maxillary sinus dipping deeply between the buccal and lingual roots and into the tuberosity, with only a millimeter or two of overlying bone. These are the cases in which the floor of the antrum and/or the tuberosity is torn out. (See Figures 2–91, 2–92 and 2–93.) Surgical odontectomy is indicated.

Figure 2–85 *A* and *B*, Because of the shape of these roots and their relationship to the maxillary sinus, a sectioning odontectomy is indicated when these teeth are removed (see Figure 2–86).

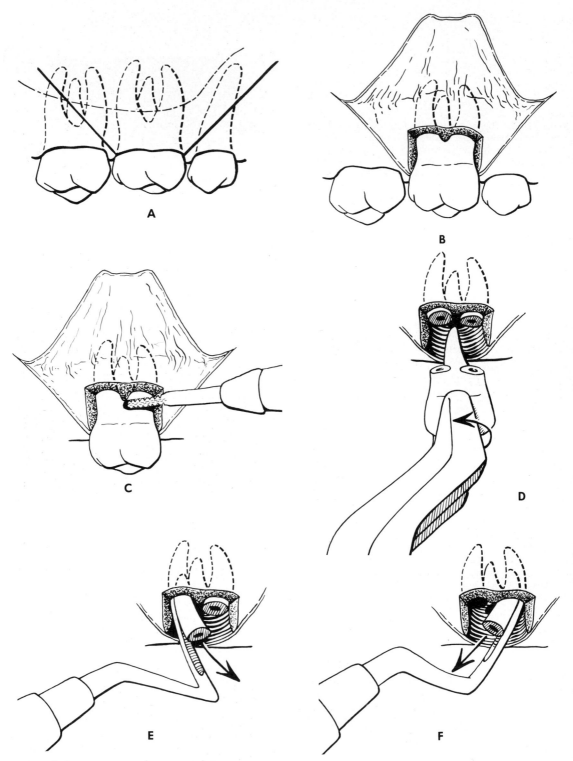

Figure 2–86 When radiographs of the maxillary molars show the floor of the maxillary sinus dipping down between the buccal and labial roots, as shown in *A*, the roots should be sectioned and the tooth and roots removed as shown in *B* through *F*. This prevents tearing out the floor of the sinus and creating an antro-oral fistula.

A, The relation of the floor of the maxillary sinus to the roots and the flap used. *B*, The buccal flap is turned back and the alveolar process is removed to the bifurcation of the roots. *C*, The two buccal roots are cut from the crown with a crosscut fissure bur. *D*, The remaining crown and lingual root is removed with forceps. *E*, The proximal root is elevated from the socket. *F*, The distal root is elevated from the socket.

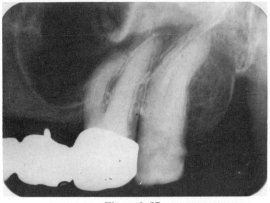

Figure 2–87

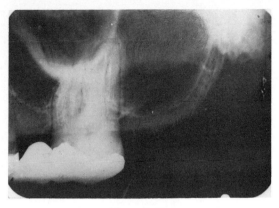

Figure 2–88

Figure 2–87 Floor of the maxillary sinus dipping down mesially to the crest of the ridge. Note that the tuberosity is normal.

Figure 2–88 The floor of the maxillary sinus dipping down to the crest of the ridge anteriorly and posteriorly to the second molar. There is a great possibility of tearing out the tuberosity and floor of the maxillary sinus when extracting this tooth. An odontectomy is indicated.

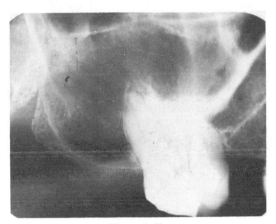

Figure 2–89

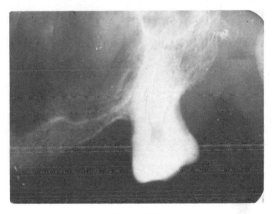

Figure 2–90

Figure 2–89 This molar's roots are completely surrounded by the maxillary sinus. Careful surgical removal would be required to prevent an antro-oral fistula or the tearing out of the osseous floor and tuberosity of the maxillary sinus. See Figure 25–42 on page 1584 for examples of this complication.

Figure 2–90 Although there is less danger of creating an antro-oral fistula by the extraction of this third molar, there is a good possibility that the tuberosity and a portion of the distal wall of the maxillary sinus will be torn out unless an odontectomy (surgical removal) is performed. See Figures 2–86 and 3–42 for a description of this technique.

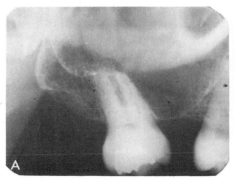
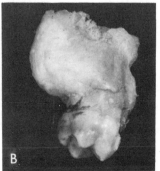

Figure 2–91 *A,* This radiograph reveals approximation of the maxillary sinus with the surface of the mesial root and the apices of all three roots. The floor of the sinus also invades the tuberosity. If this tooth were to be extracted without preliminary surgery to remove buccal and distal bone, the accident illustrated in *B* would in all probability occur.

B, Second molar with enveloping bone, tuberosity and floor of the maxillary sinus fractured from the maxilla when the second molar was extracted. This could have been avoided as previously described.

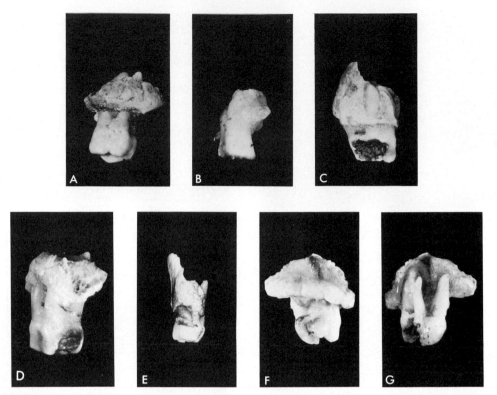

Figure 2–92 *A, B, C* and *D*, Large segments of alveolar bone torn out with maxillary molars at the time of extraction. See radiographs in Figures 2–87 to 2–90, which reveal situations in which the dentist can anticipate these bad results unless he uses the sectioning surgical technique to remove these teeth.

E, F and *G*, Buccal wall and floor of maxillary sinus torn out when these second molars were extracted. Had these teeth been surgically removed by sectioning the crowns and removing the roots individually, these iatrogenic osseous mutilations would not have occurred.

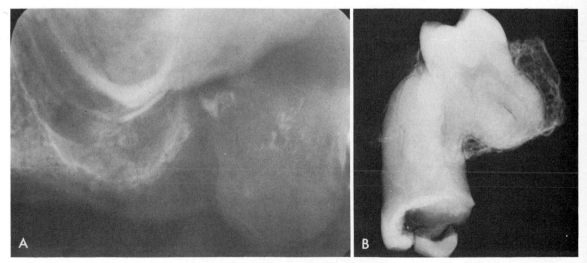

Figure 2–93 Failure to take a pre-extraction roentgenogram resulted in the dentist's tearing out the floor of the maxillary sinus together with a fused maxillary third molar. *A*, Postextraction radiograph reveals the large antro-oral fistula. *B*, Radiograph of second molar with its fused third molar and the maxillary tuberosity.

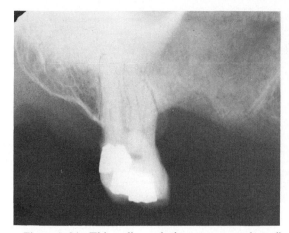

Figure 2–94 This radiograph shows an unusual maxillary molar and area surrounding the tuberosity, that is solid osseous tissue, devoid of any portion of the maxillary sinus. There would be very little, if any, danger of tearing out this tuberosity if extraction were ever necessary.

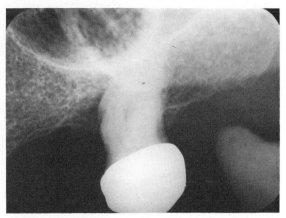

Figure 2–95 Isolated maxillary third molar with loss of the gingival third of the alveolar bone. There is moderate sinus approximation, but the tuberosity is not invaginated by the maxillary sinus. This tooth could be removed with very little danger of tearing out the tuberosity and the floor of the maxillary sinus. The buccal roots approximate each other and should offer little resistance to luxation.

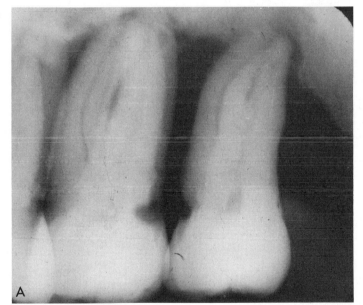

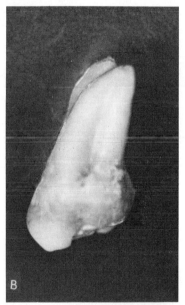

Figure 2–96 Extensive loss of osseous support (*A*) as a result of periodontal disease, where the roots are fused as in *B*, makes the extraction of teeth easy. However, in situations such as that shown in *C*, with widely separated roots whose apices are held firmly in bone, extraction frequently results in the fracturing of the apices, unless these teeth are slowly luxated.

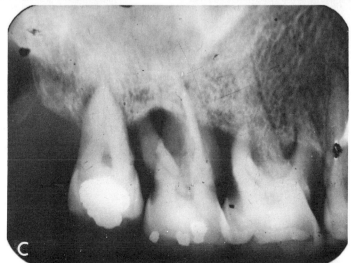

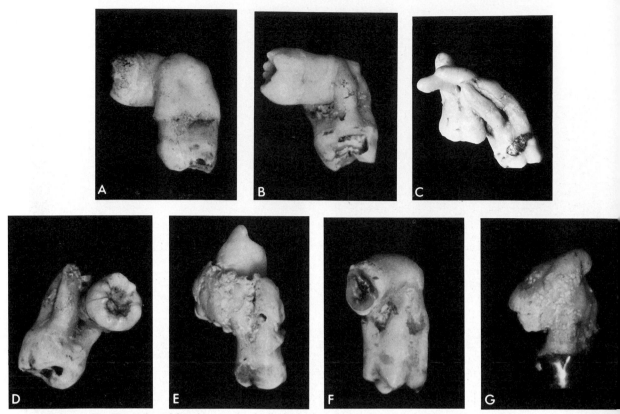

Figure 2–97 Examples of fused or mechanically locked second and third maxillary molars.

A, B and *C,* These third molars are mechanically locked to the second molars by the growth of the third molar roots between those of the second molar, as shown in *A,* or by the enveloping bone, as shown in *B* and *C.* In *D, E, F* and *G,* there is actual fusion between the roots of the second and third molars.

Just because unerupted maxillary third molars are fused or locked to the maxillary second molar, *their removal is not necessarily indicated.* If because of infection removal is necessary, surgical sectioning of the teeth is required to prevent tearing out the floor of the maxillary sinus and tuberosity, as shown in Figure 2–93.

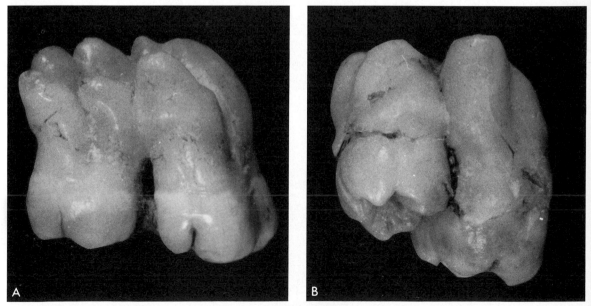

Figure 2–98 Two examples of concrescence: the roots of these maxillary second and third molars became fused during development (compare with Figure 2–99). This is another indication of the need for pre-extraction radiographs.

76

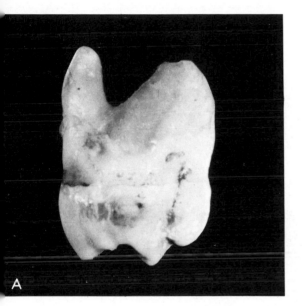 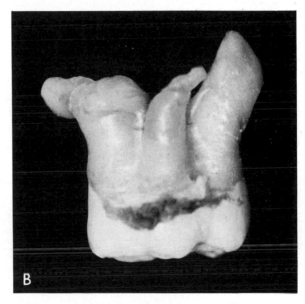

Figure 2–99 *A* and *B*, Geminous maxillary second and third molars, with fusion of their crowns. In *A* the buccal and lingual roots have fused in a symmetrical large mass, simulating an abnormally large root. In *B* the roots are bizarre and grotesque. These teeth developed in the same sac, the follicle containing twin germs. Each germ could have developed a single complete tooth. (See Chapter 13 for differentiation between concrescence and geminous teeth.)

These teeth should *only be removed* if there is a *specific reason for doing so*. When it is necessary, the radiographs should be carefully studied to determine how to remove these teeth with the least loss of osseous tissue and to prevent fracture of the mandible or maxilla, or the invasion of the maxillary sinus or mandibular canal. It may be necessary to section the geminous teeth with burs and remove them in several parts.

EXTRACTION OF MANDIBULAR TEETH

Extraction of Mandibular Incisors and Cuspids

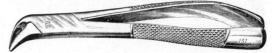

Figure 2–100 Forceps No. 151. The Cryer Universal lower No. 151 forceps can be used for the extraction of all lower teeth. It is of particular value for the extraction of lower anteriors, bicuspids and second and third molars. After loosening the mucoperiosteal tissue labially or buccally and lingually, the beaks are placed on the cementum so that they parallel the long axis of the tooth to be extracted. The lower incisors are moved labially and lingually with slight mesial and distal rotation and out to the labial side. The cuspids are moved by buccal pressure with mesial and distal rotation. The same pressures are applied to the bicuspids. To extract the molars the pressure is buccal, then lingual, and out to the buccal side, except the lower third molar, which needs the main force directed lingually, buccally, and out to the lingual side. Lower bicuspids and occasionally cuspids are sometimes shot upward with considerable force during extraction. Cases are known in which the dentist was struck in the eye by carious bicuspids, causing such extensive injury that loss of the eyeball occurred. Protective shatter-resistant eyeglasses should be worn at all times when operating in the oral cavity. This forceps is also well designed for the extraction of mandibular deciduous molars.

Fused mandibular molar roots, which are somewhat conical in shape (as illustrated in Figures 2–123 and 2–124), in addition to these buccal-lingual pressures should also have mesial-then-distal rotational pressures applied, as is used in the extraction of cuspids.

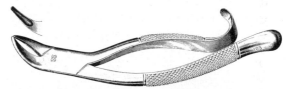

Figure 2–101 Forceps No. 103. For crowded lower anterior teeth the narrow-beaked forceps No. 103 can be used advantageously to extract mandibular incisors without danger of loosening adjacent teeth. It is also used to remove roots of lower incisors, cuspids, and bicuspids broken at the gingival line. This is a good forceps for the extraction of mandibular deciduous anterior teeth.

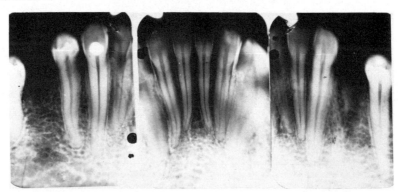

Figure 2–102 Long, thin mandibular incisor roots with extremely fine apices.

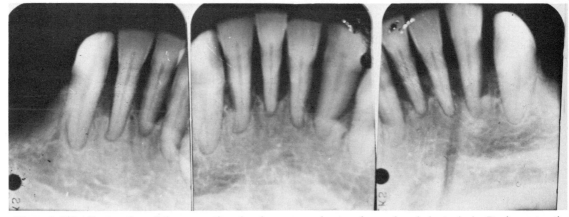

Figure 2–103 Destruction of the supporting alveolar process due to advanced periodontoclasia. During extraction frequently the apices of these teeth fracture because of the increased density of bone about the apices, which is nature's attempt to compensate for the loss of interseptal bone.

Figure 2–104 Geminous mandibular central incisors. If the necessity for the extraction of these teeth ever arose, the crowns should be cut apart with separating disks until the point of bifurcation of the roots. Then each tooth would be extracted individually.

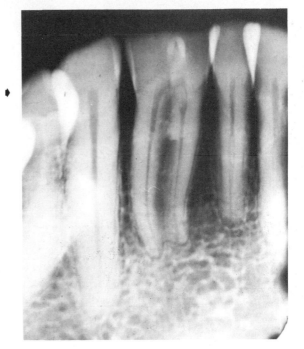

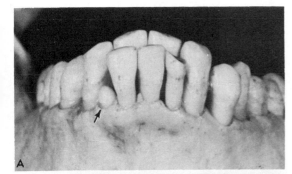

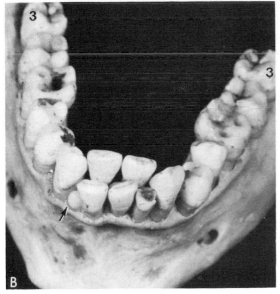

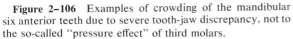

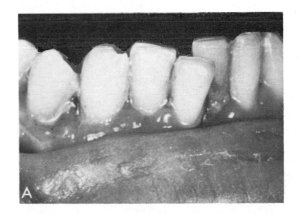

Figure 2–105 Crowding of the lower anterior teeth (*A*) in this jaw cannot be blamed on the mandibular third molars (*3* in *B*), which were not impacted and erupted normally.

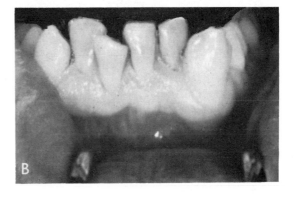

Figure 2–106 Examples of crowding of the mandibular six anterior teeth due to severe tooth-jaw discrepancy, not to the so-called "pressure effect" of third molars.

In both this figure and Figure 2–105, a study of the positions of the teeth will reveal the necessity of varying the basic forces in order to prevent injury to adjacent teeth when extracting any one of these. To prevent injury to adjacent teeth when luxating the tooth to be removed, it may be necessary to cut away a slice each of the mesial and distal surfaces of the crown of the tooth to be removed before applying the forceps.

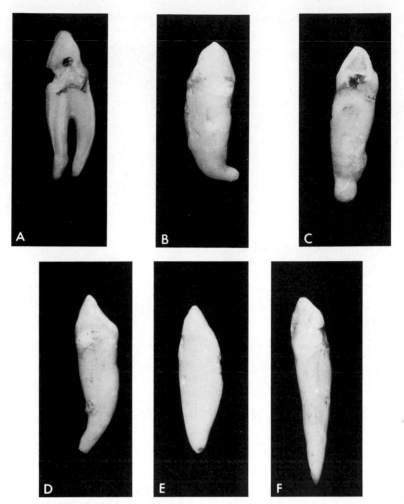

Figure 2–107 Examples of mandibular cuspids with irregular root structures. Careful study of good periapical radiographs taken from different angles will reveal variations from the normal shapes which indicate the necessary alterations in extraction techniques. Tooth *E* is the normal size and shape for a mandibular cuspid.

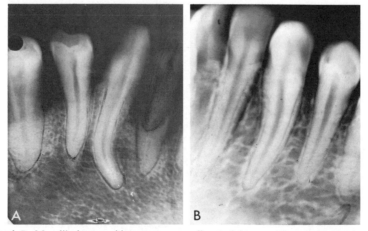

Figure 2–108 *A* and *B*, Mandibular cuspid roots are usually straight or with a slight distal curvature. The marked mesial curvature of these long cuspid roots is most unusual. The technique for the luxation and removal of these teeth would have to be modified by using a mesial rotation rather than distal as well as labial pressure. It would also be advisable to reflect a labial flap and remove the gingival third of the cortical bone before applying the No. 151 forceps. The technique for extraction of the apical third root tip is described in Chapter 4.

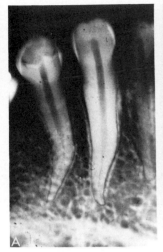
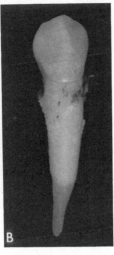
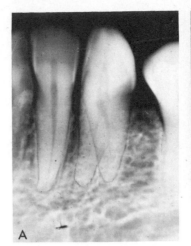
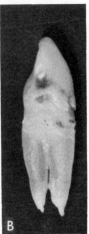

Figure 2–109 *A,* Radiograph reveals a long mandibular cuspid with an apical third that curves slightly distally, as is normal, but that has a small, sharp tip of 3 to 4 mm. curving mesially. Surgical removal (odontectomy) with a buccal flap, as illustrated in Figure 2–111, is indicated for the cuspid if extraction is ever required. The first bicuspid apical third has a sharper and greater than average distal inclination. If extraction is ever indicated, an odontectomy would be required.

B, This is not the cuspid shown in *A.* It is shown as a contrast in apical thirds, this one being long but straight and with a rounded apex. Normal pressure technique, as described in the text, will suffice for the extraction of these teeth.

Figure 2–110 *A,* This radiograph shows an unusual bifurcated mandibular cuspid root whose apices are straight, heavy and rounded. When extraction is indicated, it should be done by odontectomy.

B, This cuspid is not the one shown in *A.* Its removal, because of the very fine tips on each root, required more removal of labial bone and more slow and careful luxation.

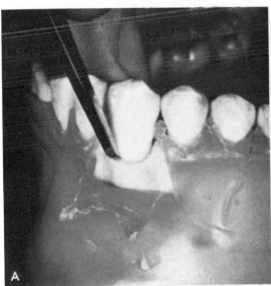
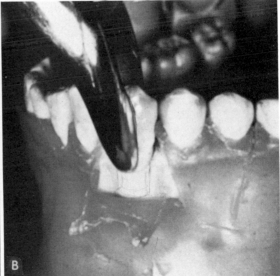

Figure 2–111 Removal of cortical bone from the gingival third of a mandibular cuspid to facilitate its extraction without fracture of the crown or root or the "tearing out" of a large section of bone, which might result in the loss of bone around the necks of the adjacent lateral incisor and first bicuspid roots. If lost, this bone would not be regenerated.

A, Mesial and distal incisions made beginning at the crest of the interseptal soft tissues and angled 45 degrees to the long axis of the tooth are extended as far as the area of bone to be excised. The flap is reflected and bone is removed with a *sharp* chisel and mallet.

B, The bone has been removed, and the beaks of the forceps, parallel to the long axis of the tooth, grasp the cementum at the neck and then the tooth is luxated and removed.

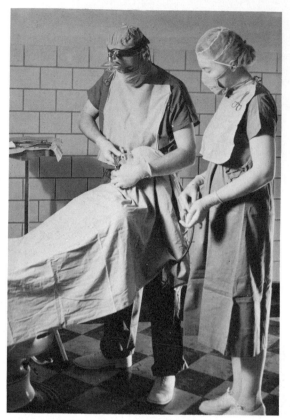

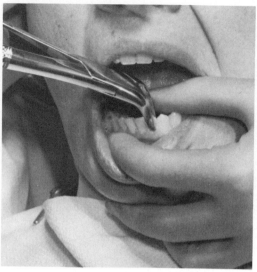

Figure 2–113 Forceps No. 151 applied to the mandibular left lateral incisor. Note how the lip is retracted, and at the same time the mandible is braced and supported by the thumb and fingers of the left hand.

Figure 2–112 The most frequently used position for extraction of the mandibular anterior teeth. Note again the erect position of the dentist, distribution of his weight equally on both feet, the support of the patient's mandible by the left hand, the fingers of which also reflect the lips.

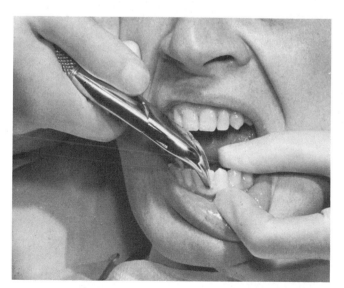

Figure 2–114 Forceps No. 103 applied to the lower left lateral incisor. This forceps is particularly advantageous for the removal of crowded or lower anteriors that are lapped lingually or labially by approximating teeth, such as those shown here, and in Figure 2–106*B*, after the overlapping portions have been cut away with discs.

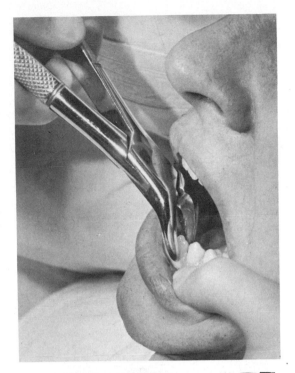

Figure 2–115 Forceps No. 151 applied to the lower left anteriors. Note that the beaks of the forceps are parallel to the long axis of the tooth and the handle must be kept at a 20 degree angle to the occlusal plane, in order to keep the beaks parallel to the long axis of the tooth. A frequent mistake is that the dentist forgets this fact and lowers the handles until they are almost parallel with the occlusal plane, thus changing the angle of the beaks on the tooth and thereby reducing the effectiveness of the instrument and increasing the possibility of fracturing the tooth and/or injuring proximal teeth.

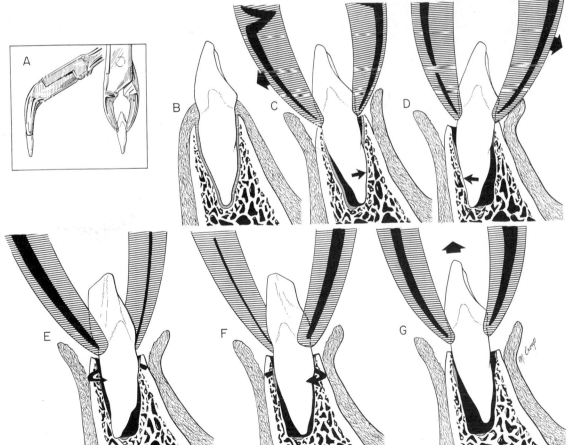

Figure 2–116 Application of the Universal mandibular forceps No. 151 to a lower central incisor and the direction of forces necessary to extract this tooth. Study the text.

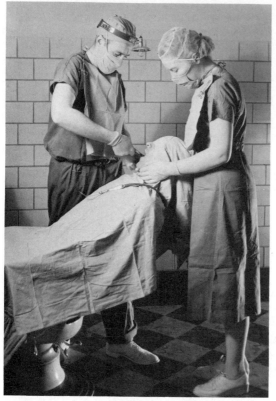

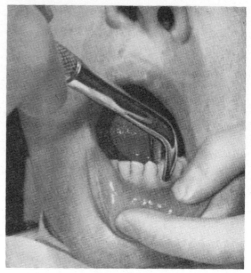

Figure 2–118   Lateral view of the application of the beaks of the No. 151 forceps to the mandibular left first bicuspid.

Figure 2–117   Position of patient and dentist for extraction of the mandibular right and left bicuspids and molars. Note that the dentist stands erect and squarely on both feet with his weight equally distributed. The patient's mandible is supported by the denist's left hand. The patient is adjusted in the chair so that when his mouth is open, the occlusal plane of the mandibular teeth is parallel to the floor.

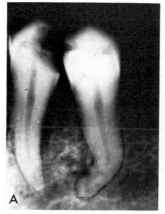
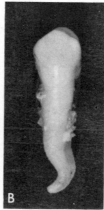
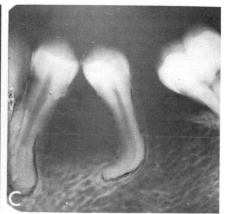

Figure 2–119   Right-angled curvature of the apical thirds of mandibular bicuspid roots. Odontectomy for surgical removal of the buccal cortical bone and cancellous bone above the right angle of the apical third is indicated before forceps are applied to luxate and extract these teeth.

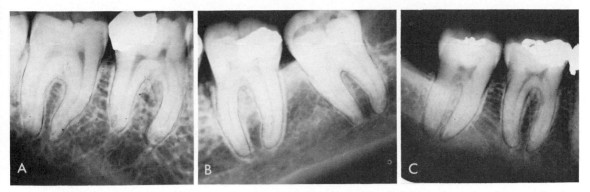

Figure 2–129 *A, B* and *C,* Radiographs of mandibular first molars with apical thirds that approximate each other, locking around the intraradicular bone. When such teeth have to be extracted, to prevent fracture of the crowns, tearing out of this bone, or destroying its vitality by compression from the roots, the crown should be sectioned and each root removed separately, as shown in Figure 2–140 (or if excementosed, Figure 2–145). The second molars in *A, B* and *C* would not require sectioning of the crowns for their extraction, if removal were indicated.

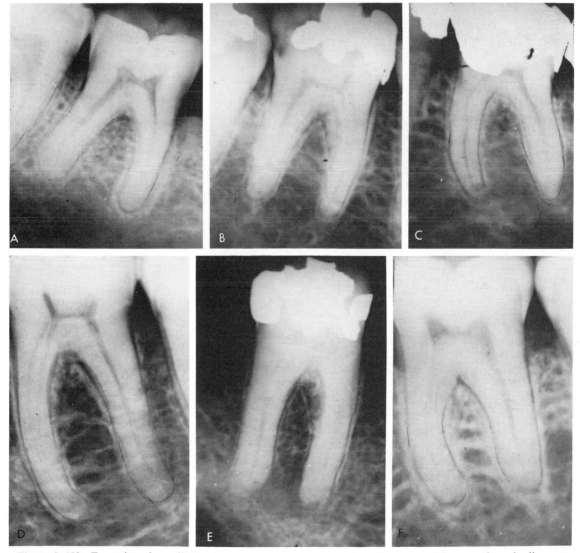

Figure 2–130 Examples of mandibular first molars whose two well-formed roots, straight or moderately divergent, indicate the use of the No. 16 "cowhorn" mandibular forceps when extraction of such teeth is required.

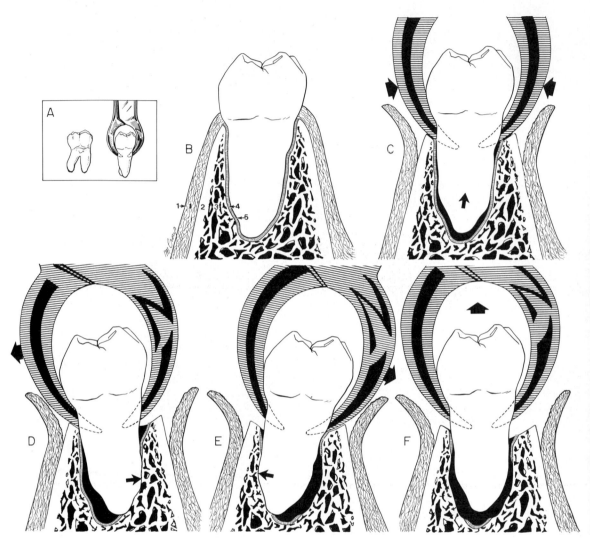

Figure 2–131   *A*, Mandibular first molar with the beaks of the No. 16 "cowhorn" forceps properly positioned. *B, 1,* The buccal mucoperiosteal tissue; *2,* the buccal cortical bone; *3,* cancellous bone; *4,* periodontal ligament; *5,* cementum.

    C, Buccal and lingual mucoperiosteal tissue loosened and reflected, exposing the edge of the cortical bone and the bifurcation of the roots. The beaks of the forceps are inserted lingually and bucally into the bifurcation of the roots and rest on the cortical plates of bone. The forceps handles are closed, driving the "cowhorn" beaks into the bifurcation, where the double wedging action of the inclined planes of the beaks lifts the tooth in its alveolus.

    D, The molar is moved lingually, compressing and expanding the lingual osseous tissue. *E*, Now the molar is moved buccally, expanding and compressing the osseous tissue. *F*, The molar is now lifted from its expanded alveolus.

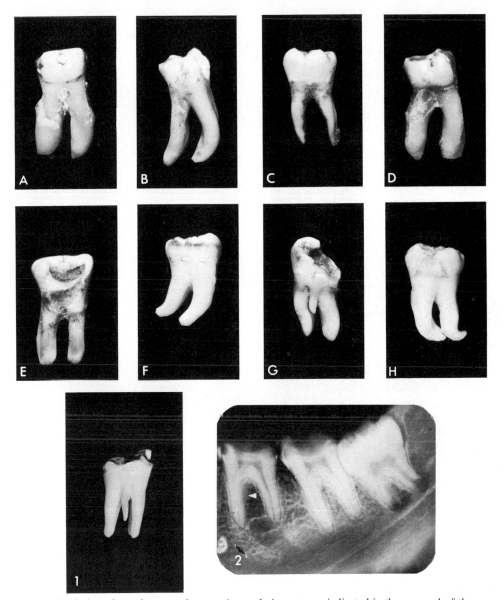

Figure 2–132 Variations from the normal extraction techniques were indicated in the removal of these mandibular molars. Odontectomy, forceps and elevators were used, according to the conditions indicated in each case.

A to *H*, Unusual root shapes, *A*, Mandibular first molar with 50 per cent of the roots heavily excementosed. *B*, Long, heavy, widely separated roots with distal curvature of the apical thirds. *C*, Normal size and shape of roots for a mandibular first molar. *D*, Mandibular molar with completely excementosed roots. *E*, Moderate excementosis. *F*, Distal and apically curved roots. *G*, Mandibular first molar with a short rudimentary root arising at the bifurcation and heavily excementosed distal root. *H*, First molar with "locked roots" and 45-degree angle of the apical thirds. Extraction technique is illustrated in Figure 2–140.

1 and *2*, Supernumerary rudimentary root. *1*, Photograph clearly showing supernumerary rudimentary root in bifurcation of the mandibular first molar. Where is the image of this small root in the radiograph (*2*) of this first molar? The answer is that there was just enough transverse angulation of the central x-rays to superimpose part of the mesial root over part of the mesial surface of the rudimentary root. In *2*, see white arrowhead for the distal lamina dura of this root. While rudimentary roots are not rare, they are frequently overlooked or are not readily visible on the radiograph. To avoid the embarrassment of having such roots fracture and be discovered in subsequent radiographic examinations, all teeth that are extracted should be carefully examined to make certain that an extra root, rudimentary or larger, was not fractured and left behind in the alveolus.

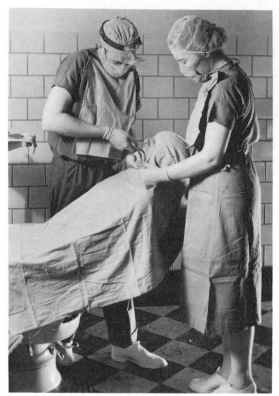

Figure 2–133 Positions of the dentist and patient for extraction of the mandibular left bicuspids and molars.

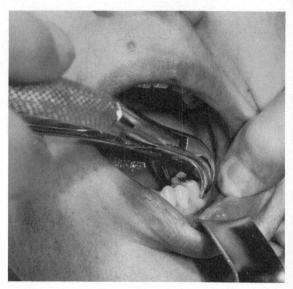

Figure 2–134 Front view of the application of the beaks of the No. 16 forceps to the mandibular first molar.

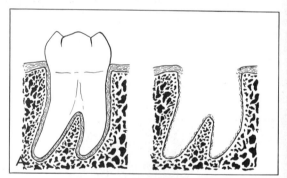

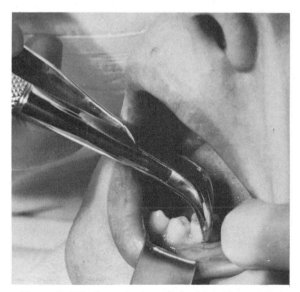

Figure 2–135 Lateral view of the No. 16, so-called "cowhorn," forceps applied to the mandibular first molar.

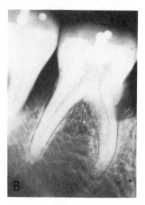

Figure 2–136 When extracting molars with widely divergent roots, do not remove the intraradicular bone. This intraradicular bone has a broad base and a good blood supply and will help clot organization.

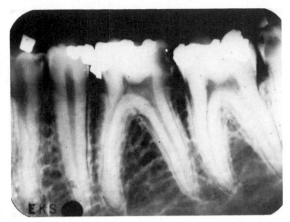

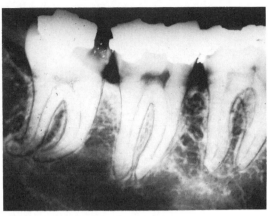

Figure 2–137 The mandibular first molar in this radiograph reveals the mesial and distal roots to be so widely divergent from the neck of the tooth, at the crest of the alveolus, that they could not possibly be withdrawn from the alveolus without either (1) compressing mesial and distal cancellous bone and possibly dislodging the second bicuspid and/or the second molar, or (2) fracturing the molar crown from the roots. In cases like this when extraction is indicated, the crown is sectioned with a bur from the buccal to the lingual edge, down to and through the bifurcation of the roots. Each segment of the crown with its attached root is grasped at the neck with a No. 151 Universal mandibular molar forceps and, with buccal-then-lingual pressure, is loosened and then lifted from the alveolus. (See Figure 2–140.)

Figure 2–138 If extraction of the three mandibular molars in this radiograph were indicated, they would all require the sectioning of the crown, as described in Figure 2–137 and illustrated in Figure 2–140 because the roots of all three lock the intraradicular bone between their roots, and in addition the third molar roots have sharp, almost 90-degree distal curvature of the apices. Certainly many teeth like these have been torn out of the alveolus by brute force, along with the trapped intraradicular bone, or the crowns have been fractured from the roots and the roots dug out with elevators, but this is not oral surgery. It is crude, barbaric, mutilating and traumatic "butchering." See Figures 2–139 and 2–141.

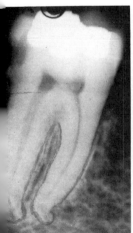

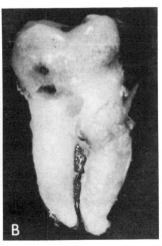

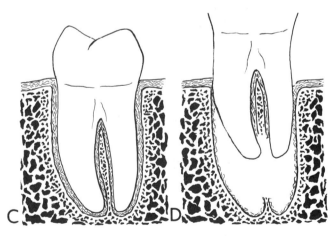

Figure 2–139 *A,* The intraradicular bone was locked in by this root formation. *B,* It was torn out when the tooth was extracted, as illustrated in *C* and *D.* Frequently this bone, locked through the roots from the buccal to the lingual cortical plate, prevents extraction, and the crown is fractured from the roots. When this condition is seen in the radiograph, the crown should be sectioned, as illustrated in Figure 2–140.

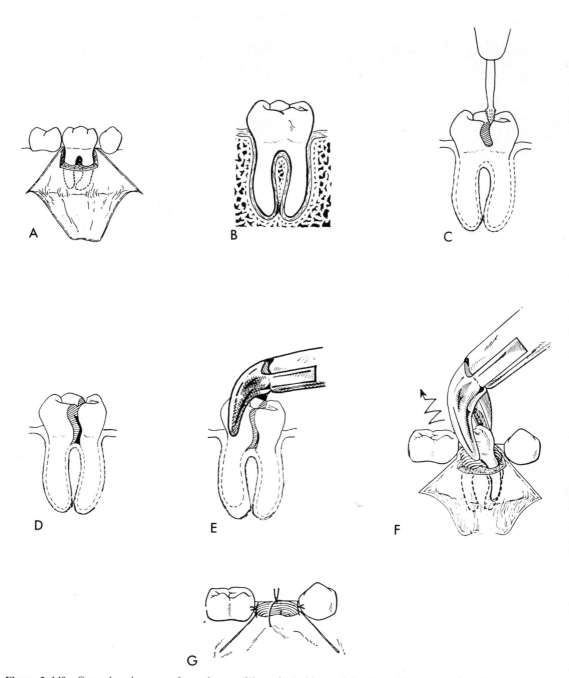

Figure 2–140 Curved molar roots formed around bone lock this tooth in place. To prevent the following possible complications: (*a*) fracturing of the crown or roots, (*b*) tearing out of the intraradicular bone and possibly also a portion of the cortical bone, and (*c*) fracturing of the mandible during the attempted extraction of this tooth, it is advisable to section the crown as shown in these illustrations.

A, Flap extends around the neck of tooth, then onto the buccal mucosa both mesially and distally at a 45-degree angle. Mucoperiosteal flap reflected. Removal of gingival third of cortical bone with mallet and chisel. *B*, Tooth with bone locked between the roots. *C*, Cutting through crown buccolingually with crosscut fissure bur. *D*, Crown cut through the bifurcation. *E*, Removal of the distal half of the molar with No. 300 or No. 151 forceps, bringing the fragment mesially. *F*, Removal of mesial half with No. 300 or No. 151 forceps, bringing the fragment distally. *G*, Approximation and suturing of the flap.

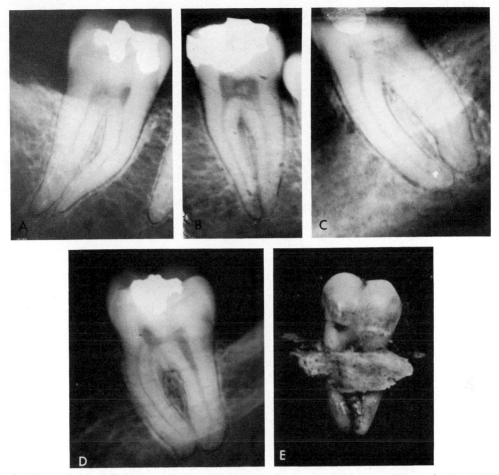

Figure 2–141   *A, B, C* and *D,* These are teeth with intraradicular bone locked between their roots. The complications that can result from the extraction of these teeth when such might become necessary have already been pointed out. These will occur unless the correct technique, which has been described in Figure 2–137 and illustrated in Figure 2–140, is followed.

E, Unfortunately, as illustrated by this specimen, many times a large section of buccal and mesial and distal bone is also torn out. This bone will not regenerate around the necks of the adjacent teeth, and so a surgically produced periodontal pocket results, reducing the life expectancy of these teeth.

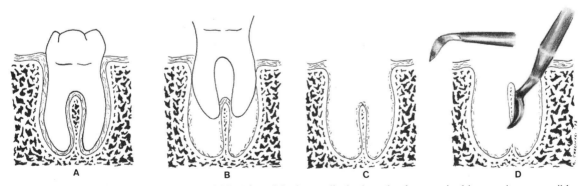

Figure 2–142   *A,* While there was a partial locking of the intraradicular bone by the roots in this case, it was possible, by excessive luxation of the tooth buccally and lingually, for the apices of the roots eventually to compress this intraradicular bone, permitting the extraction of this molar.

B and *C,* Obviously, the blood supply to this compressed bone has been severely curtailed. The possibility is very great that this bone would become nonvital, thus interfering with normal healing and becoming in fact a "localized area of osteomyelitis."

D, A very good way to remove this bone is shown here — by the use of a No. 14R or No. 14L elevator, depending on whether it is a right or left mandibular molar.

95

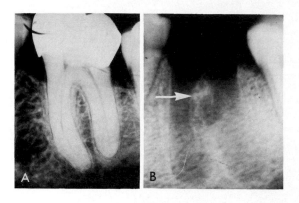

Figure 2–143 These radiographs illustrate the "localized osteomyelitis" which developed for the reason stated in the previous legend, namely compressed and devitalized intraradicular bone that was not removed.

A, This radiograph reveals the partially locked intraradicular bone that was severely compressed and traumatized by the roots when this molar was luxated and removed.

B, The arrow points to the "sequestrum," a nonvital portion of the intraradicular bone. Free pus exudes from the surrounding inflammatory tissue. When the sequestrum was freely movable by a curette, it was removed and normal healing followed.

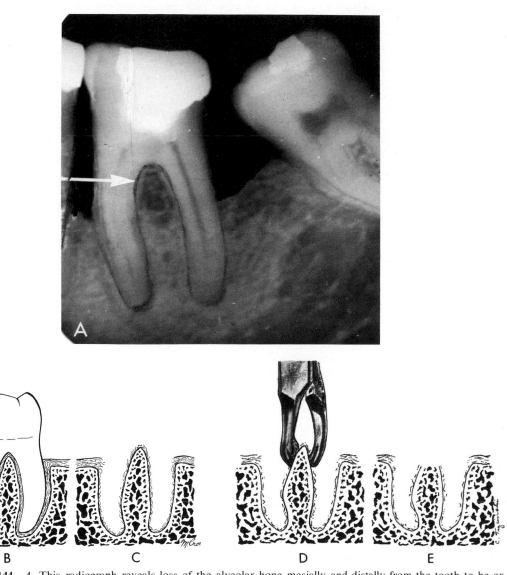

Figure 2–144 *A,* This radiograph reveals loss of the alveolar bone mesially and distally from the tooth to be extracted. *B* and *C,* This leaves the intraradicular bone projecting above the surrounding bone. *D* and *E,* This bone is reduced to the level of the surrounding bone by a hand-cutting rongeur, so that the alveolus heals smoothly. The same situation is seen occasionally following the extraction of upper molars. This projection of bone is best removed with rongeurs or bone shears.

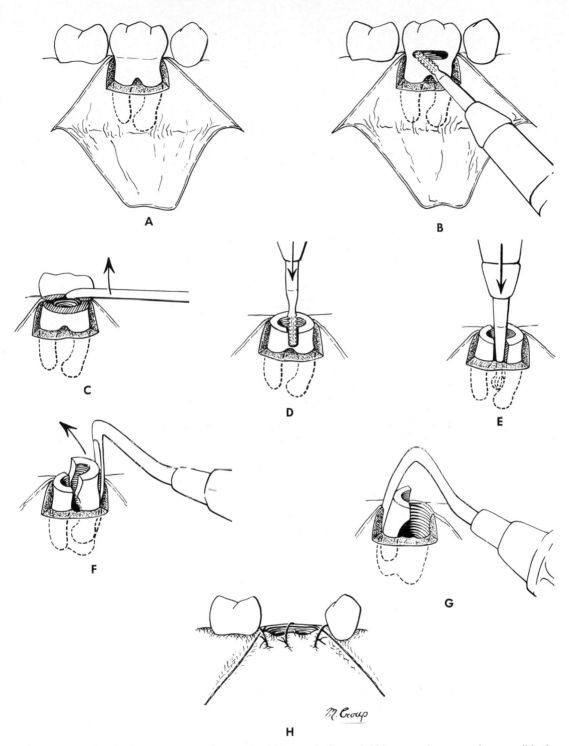

Figure 2–145 Teeth with excementosed roots should be surgically excised by removing as much as possible the enveloping bone from around the excementosis of the root. These drawings illustrate the odontectomy of a mandibular molar not only having excementosis of the apical third of the mesial root, but whose roots also lock around the intraradicular bone.

A, The buccal flap is turned back, and the alveolar process is removed to the bifurcation of the roots. *B*, A groove is cut at the neck of the tooth with a crosscut fissure bur. *C*, The crown is separated from the roots with a chisel. *D*, A crosscut fissure bur cuts down to the bifurcation of the roots on the buccal and lingual sides. *E*, The intraradicular bone is removed with a round bur. *F*, The distal root is elevated from the socket. *G*, The proximal root is elevated from the socket. *H*, The buccal flap is sutured back in place.

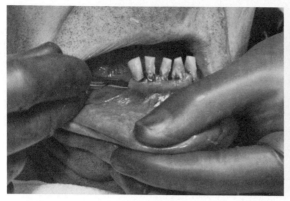

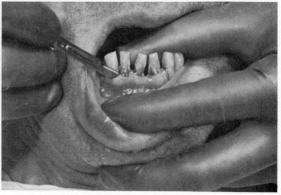

Figure 2–146

Figure 2–147

Figure 2–146 The mucoperiosteum is incised, starting 10 mm. distally and buccally from the cuspid, and contacting the midpoint of the distal surface of the cuspid.

Figure 2–147 The attachment of the periodontal membrane to the mucoperiosteum is severed around the necks of the teeth and through the interproximal spaces. This must be done carefully and thoroughly, or it will be impossible to reflect the full thickness of the mucoperiosteal flap.

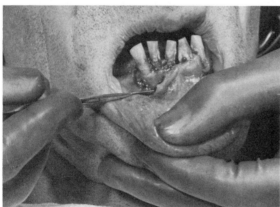

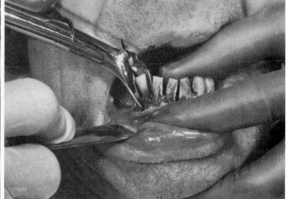

Figure 2–148

Figure 2–149

Figure 2–148 The mucoperiosteal flap is reflected, exposing the labial cortical plate of bone.

Figure 2–149 The teeth are luxated and removed with a No. 151 forceps.

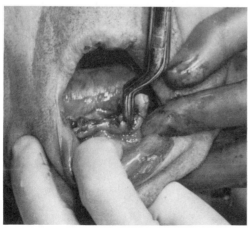

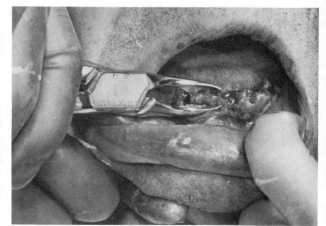

Figure 2–150

Figure 2–151

Figure 2–150 With the patient in a horizontal position, such as on an operating table, the No. 286 forceps can be used effectively for the removal of not only the lower six anterior teeth but the bicuspids as well.

Figure 2–151 The undercuts are removed by the bone shears. Note that one blade is placed on the crest of the ridge and one is below the undercut. This removes not only the undercut but this diseased portion of bone as well.

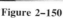

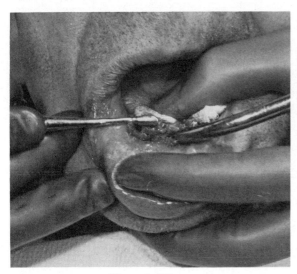

Figure 2–152

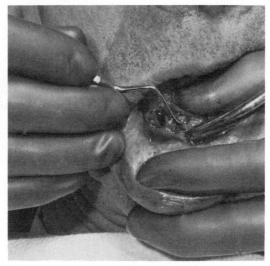

Figure 2–153

Figure 2–152 The alveolar process is filed to remove small, sharp spicules of bone. Suction should be used continuously.

Figure 2–153 Each socket is explored by a small-bowled curette. Periapical granulomas, if any, are removed. Also, any small particles of bone, tooth structure or calculus are removed.

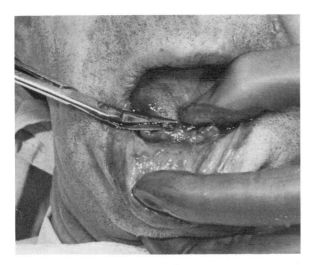

Figure 2–154

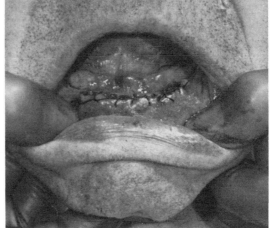

Figure 2–155

Figure 2–154 That portion of the mucoperiosteal tissue which overlaps is trimmed so that there is edge-to-edge contact.

Figure 2–155 The soft tissues are sutured back into place with a 000 continuous black silk suture.

Case Report No. 2

ODONTECTOMY WITH ALVEOLECTOMY

Patient.　E.B., a woman aged 65 years.

Preoperative Diagnosis.　Extensive caries of remaining maxillary and mandibular teeth; chronic suppurative pericementitis; periapical infection.

Operation.　　$\dfrac{3\ 2\ 1\ /\ 1\ 2\ 3}{3\ 2\ 1\ /\ 1\ 2\ 3\ 4}$

Maxillary and mandibular odontectomy and alveolectomy, with the insertion of immediate full upper and lower dentures.

Anesthetic.　Intravenous thiopental sodium with nasoendotracheal nitrous oxide and oxygen.

Technique.　The face and mucous membrane were prepared with tincture of Merthiolate, and the lips coated with petrolatum. A Molt mouth prop was inserted in the mouth, and the jaws were separated. An oropharyngeal gauze partition was then placed. Block and infiltration injections were made with a local anesthetic solution with a vasoconstrictor.

An incision was made with a No. 15 Bard-Parker blade, starting on the distal gingival tissue of the upper right cuspid and carried through the mucoperiosteal tissue toward the mucobuccal fold (fornix of the vestibule) at a 45-degree angle to the long axis of the cuspid for a distance of 10 mm. The same incision is made from the distal gingival tissue of the upper left cuspid. Then with a No. 12 BP blade the junction of the periosteum with the periodontal fibers around the neck of each tooth was severed, as was each interdental papilla. This mucoperiosteal tissue was then reflected labially with the periosteal elevator, the spear point of the instrument being used first to free the interseptal tissue, then its rounded edge, to strip the tissue away from the alveolar bone.

This mucoperiosteal tissue in the upper arch was stripped up for a distance of 10 mm. The labial bone was removed with the single-bevel chisel. The upper anterior teeth were extracted with a No. 99A forceps, the teeth being rotated mesially and removed in a labial direction.

The mandibular mucoperiosteal tissue was reflected by means of the technique just described. The lower anterior teeth were extracted with a No. 151 forceps, lingual labial pressure being applied and the teeth being removed in a labial direction. Sharp, bony projections were removed with the bone rongeurs by placing one edge of the cutting instrument on the crest of the ridge, and then placing the other edge on the labial plate, and cutting the bone in this fashion. Small projections were then trimmed down with the bone file, in a draw-cut manner.

The alveoli were explored thoroughly with a small-bowl curette. The mucoperiosteal flaps were then replaced and overlapping portions excised. Clear acrylic splints (baseplates) were inserted. Where the tissue blanched (showing pressure on the soft tissue from a bone protuberance), the flap was reflected and the bone in this area removed. By means of the continuous lock stitch with 000 silk, the soft tissues were sutured into place.

The full upper and lower dentures were immediately inserted. The oropharyngeal partition was removed, and the jaw closed in centric. The patient was removed from the operating room in good condition.

IMMEDIATE POSTEXTRACTION SURGICAL PROCEDURES

1. Trim osseous structures with bone shears or rongeurs. Smooth with a bone file. This is necessary (a) to remove the diseased bone and excessive bone, (b) to promote normal healing, and (c) to promote healing and a good base for subsequent prosthetic restorations.

   If multiple extractions are done, see page 181 in Chapter 3 for a description and detailed illustration of the technique for alveoplasty (partial alveolectomy). Plate I, page 55, also illustrates alveoplasty, and Case Report No. 2 describes odontectomy with alveolectomy.

2. The excision of excessive alveolar mucoperiosteum, the removal of interdental papillae to promote "line healing of the ridge," the removal of abnormal frenums, and the excision of abnormal muscle attachments are necessary to aid the dentist in securing a good result when the dentures are constructed.

3. If the periapical radiograph showed a radiolucent area about the apex, after extraction explore this area with a small curette and remove any soft tissue which might be present. If all areas cannot be reached with the curette through the alveolus, reflect a mucoperiosteal flap and open into this area through the cortical bone. The retention of this tissue may retard healing, or cause the formation of a residual cyst or of residual infection. Use the proper size of curette; if soft tissue is not felt with the curette, do not scrape bone with the curette.

4. Remove loose alveolar spicules, tooth fragments and debris, if present, gently from the alveoli with a curette.

5. In tooth sockets which are bleeding excessively, cut a piece of Gelfoam slightly smaller than the socket. Saturate the Gelfoam with 100 units of thrombin per cubic centimeter of normal saline solution, insert it in the socket, and suture across the socket to approximate as closely as possible the soft tissues, and to secure the Gelfoam. If bleeding continues, remove the Gelfoam and tightly pack ¼-inch iodoform gauze in the alveolus and firmly hold it in place 5 minutes before releasing the pressure. Then suture the soft tissue over the gauze; do not remove for 48 hours.

6. When a chronically infected tooth has been removed, or when a socket has been subjected to considerable trauma incidental to the removal of difficult molars or an impacted third molar, or

any other tooth, it was, and still is by some oral surgeons, considered to be good practice to insert various medicaments immediately into the alveolus. Time and experience have demonstrated that drugs, antiseptics, germicides and any other type of dressing do not aid healing or reduce the incidence of postoperative complications. The most frequent, alveolalgia (the so-called "dry socket") will require analgesic dressings in those with acute pain. The "best dressing" in the postextraction alveolus is a normal blood clot. However, do not try to stimulate bleeding by scraping the walls of the alveolus with a curette. This adds insult to injury. The same practice is followed in bony crypts from which cysts have been enucleated.

7. Replace soft tissues over the osseous tissue, and insure bone coverage by the use of sutures; use 000 black silk or 000 catgut.

(Text continued on page 105)

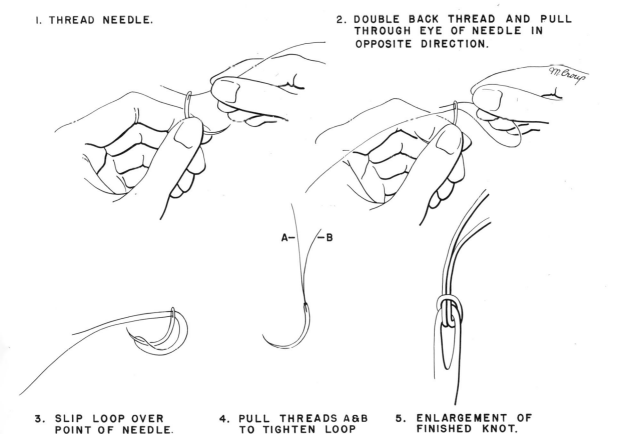

1. THREAD NEEDLE.

2. DOUBLE BACK THREAD AND PULL THROUGH EYE OF NEEDLE IN OPPOSITE DIRECTION.

A— —B

3. SLIP LOOP OVER POINT OF NEEDLE.

4. PULL THREADS A&B TO TIGHTEN LOOP ABOVE EYE.

5. ENLARGEMENT OF FINISHED KNOT.

Figure 2–156 A method of "locking" the suture material to the needle.

TECHNIQUE FOR CONTINUOUS SUTURE WITH LOCK STITCHES

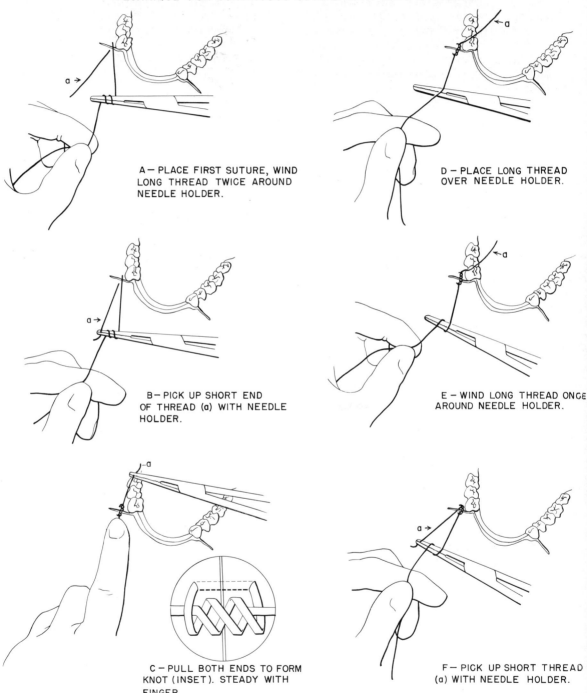

A — PLACE FIRST SUTURE, WIND LONG THREAD TWICE AROUND NEEDLE HOLDER.

B — PICK UP SHORT END OF THREAD (a) WITH NEEDLE HOLDER.

C — PULL BOTH ENDS TO FORM KNOT (INSET). STEADY WITH FINGER.

D — PLACE LONG THREAD OVER NEEDLE HOLDER.

E — WIND LONG THREAD ONCE AROUND NEEDLE HOLDER.

F — PICK UP SHORT THREAD (a) WITH NEEDLE HOLDER.

Figure 2–157   Technique for continuous suture with lock stitches.

(Figure 2–157 continued on opposite page)

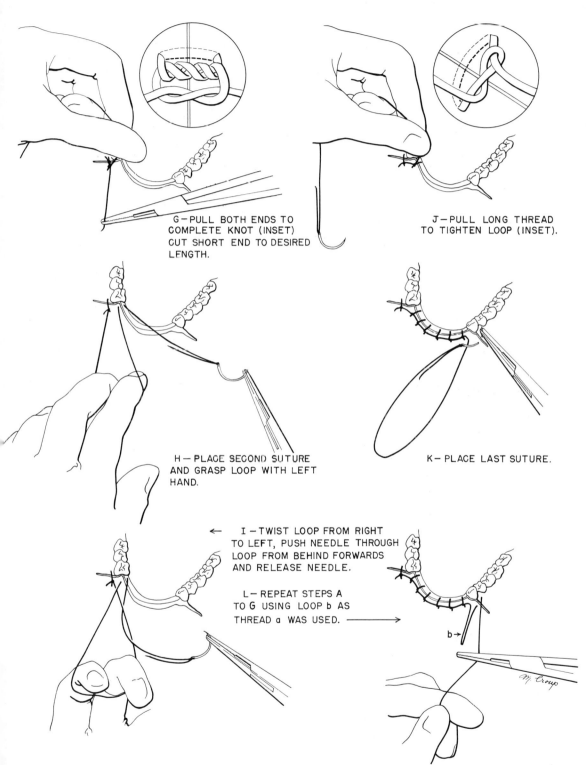

G—PULL BOTH ENDS TO
COMPLETE KNOT (INSET)
CUT SHORT END TO DESIRED
LENGTH.

J—PULL LONG THREAD
TO TIGHTEN LOOP (INSET).

H—PLACE SECOND SUTURE
AND GRASP LOOP WITH LEFT
HAND.

K—PLACE LAST SUTURE.

I—TWIST LOOP FROM RIGHT
TO LEFT, PUSH NEEDLE THROUGH
LOOP FROM BEHIND FORWARDS
AND RELEASE NEEDLE.

L—REPEAT STEPS A
TO G USING LOOP b AS
THREAD a WAS USED. ⟶

b→

Figure 2–157 *(Continued.)*

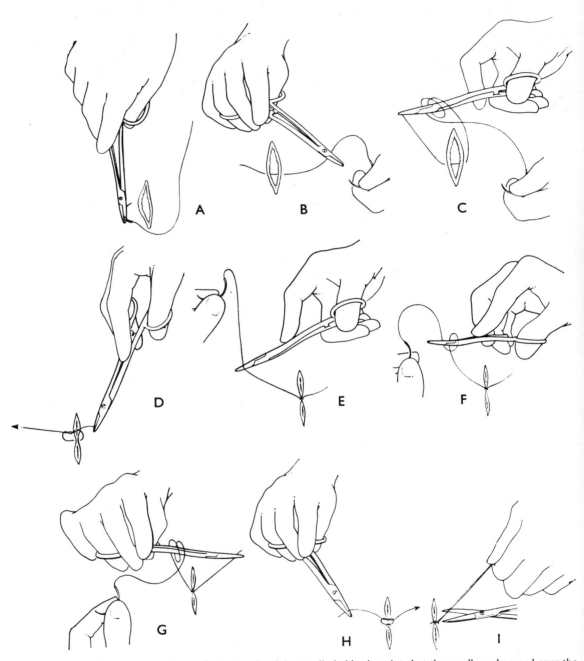

Figure 2–158 "Instrument tie." *A* and *B*, The tip of the needle-holder is pointed at the needle and passed over the silk twice. *C* and *D*, The tip of the short end of the silk is grasped and drawn through the loops. *E* and *F*, The needle-holders are pointed toward the needle once again and passed *under* the silk once or twice. *G*, The tip of the short end is then grasped and pulled through the loops, thus completing the knot. *H*, The loose ends are used to draw the knot to one side of the incision and, *I*, then cut with scissors. (From Howe, G. L.: Minor Oral Surgery. Bristol, England, John Wright & Sons, Ltd., 1971.)

8. Place gauze mouth packs and sponges over the operative field to prevent the entrance of saliva into the sockets, to act as a pressure pack after operation, and to check bleeding and aid in clot formation.

SUTURING

Mucoperiosteal flaps, small or large, are ironed back into position with the index finger, upon completion of the operation, and they are held in position by the insertion of sutures. Even when the soft tissue only has been incised and loosened around the necks of the teeth before extraction, it is ironed back into position, the buccal and lingual osseous cortical plates are compressed by squeezing between the thumb and index finger, and sutures are passed through the soft tissues on both sides of the dental ridge, and tied over the interdental bone. This is done for single extractions as well as in cases of multiple extraction.

Reasons for Suturing. Suturing of mucoperiosteal flaps is done because:

1. It holds the soft tissues in apposition with bone and the fixed soft tissues, thus aiding healing.
2. It prevents postoperative bleeding, particularly that most frequent type, capillary bleeding.
3. Holding the soft tissue over the sockets (alveoli) after extraction aids in the formation and maintenance of a good clot.
4. Good clot formation means less postoperative pain, especially that which originates from exposed bone.
5. The entrance of food debris into the wound is prevented.

Rules for Suturing. The following rules should be observed in suturing:

Do not use suture material larger than 000. The author uses catgut or surgical silk which is serum- and moisture-proof.

Use small half-circle needles, either round or with a cutting edge. The author uses the 5/8-inch half-circle atraumatic cutting needle to which is swaged 18 inches of 000 black braided silk, or the 5/8-inch half-circle Hu-Friedy No. 4 cutting-edge needle.

For suturing along the buccal edge of the tuberosities or the maxillary molars, where space is limited, or in the palate, use the 1/2-inch half-circle needle with a cutting edge, such as the J. & J. No. 18 or the Hu-Friedy No. 2.

When using cutting-edge needles, be careful not to apply any lateral pressure when passing the needle through the soft tissue, as the needle will slice through the edge of the incision. This is one of the two disadvantages of the cutting-edge needle; the second is that it makes a larger hole in the tissues than the tapered-point round half-circle needle.

When the oral tissues are thick and dense, a cutting-edge needle requires less force to penetrate the tissues; for example, in the closure of cartilaginous tuberosities which have been surgically reduced in size. Less pressure means less danger of needle breakage.

For suturing through the interseptal spaces — for example, when closing the palatal flap after the surgical removal of a palatally impacted cuspid — use a half-circle 5/8-inch round needle with a tapered point, such as the intestinal needle. Use this same needle for routine closure of the ridges after multiple extractions and alveolectomy.

When using a needle holder, never grasp the needle over its eye. This is the weakest part of the needle, and frequently it breaks at this point when being inserted through the mucoperiosteal tissue. (In some areas this tissue is very tough.) Always grasp the needle a short distance in front of its eye.

Hold the needle holder mounted with the needle and suture in a pen grasp.

Insert the needle into the loose reflected mucoperiosteal tissue 2.5 mm. from the free edge, and rotate the hand, forcing the needle through the tissue.

When the needle appears through the tissue, release the needle holder and grasp the needle on the other side. Rotate the needle through the tissue.

If the edges of the soft tissue are close, it is possible to pass the needle through both sides of the incision, *i.e.,* through the loose reflected mucoperiosteum and the firm, unreflected tissue, at the same time. If there is considerable distance, it is better to pass the needle completely through the reflected soft tissue on one side of the ridge and then through the unreflected soft tissue on the opposite side of the ridge as a two-step procedure. If an attempt is made to stretch the reflected tissue to reach the opposite side of the ridge, the needle frequently tears through the tissue.

Do not place the sutures closer than 5 mm. apart. If they are placed too closely, they strangulate the tissue and interfere with the escape of serum or inflammatory exudate.

Do not tie too tightly. The sutures will

produce ischemia of the edges of the incision, thus preventing normal healing because of the reduced blood supply. Eventually the sutures will cut through the tissues. Tied sutures should do no more than allow the tissues to fall into place. The purpose of the sutures is to prevent displacement of the tissues.

EXTRACTION OF TEETH FOR PATIENTS WITH ORAL MALIGNANT DISEASE

PRERADIATION EXTRACTION

Jaws in the "line of fire" of radiation therapy for malignant conditions have a reduced cellular activity in the bone and so lessened resistance to infection. Extraction of teeth in these areas is frequently followed by osteoradionecrosis of the jaw. Even in irradiated edentulous jaws the mucoperiosteum occasionally sloughs off, exposing bone which sometimes sequestrates locally. In other cases the osteoradionecrosis is so extensive that lateral jaw resection is necessary.

If the treatment selected for an oral neoplasm is radiation therapy, then at least all those teeth in the direct line of radiation should be extracted prior to treatment. Many authorities believe that all teeth in patients with oral malignant disease should be extracted before heavy radiation which will pass through the jaws.

Technique. The objective is to extract the teeth and perform a complete alveolectomy in this area, practically obliterating the alveolus.

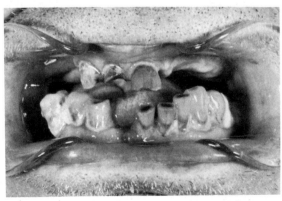

Figure 2–159 Patient with a "frozen tongue" due to invasive epidermoid carcinoma scheduled for radiation therapy. The remaining teeth were extracted and a radical alveolectomy was performed, as shown in Figure 2–160, prior to radiation. The same extensive surgery was carried out on the maxilla.

To do so, wide mucoperiosteal flaps are reflected, in the area to undergo surgery, to the mucobuccal or labial fold. The chisel and mallet are used to remove all labial or buccal bone from the roots and interseptal areas, and the teeth are luxated and extracted. Then, with bone rongeurs, chisels, large bone burs and rotary files, all the remaining alveolar process and lingual cortical plate are removed to at least the apical third of the alveolus. The flaps are then replaced, the overlapping portions are excised with scissors until the edges meet freely without tension and the soft tissues are sutured together with 000 silk. Healing in these cases is rapid, and radiation treatment can be started within a week. See Figures 2–159 and 2–160.

EFFECTS OF RADIATION ON ERUPTED TEETH

Robert L. Moss, D.D.S.

Radiation caries may develop in adult teeth as a sequela of radiation therapy administered in or near the oral cavity. The process is characterized by a progressive disintegration of enamel from the tooth crown. The enamel becomes chalky in appearance and porous in consistency. Frequently, dissolution begins in the cervical areas and then spreads to the occlusal surfaces, leaving discolored dentin stumps (see Figure 2–162). The patient may suffer severe discomfort from thermal and chemical stimulation. Oral hygiene fails.

The etiology of radiation caries is unknown. It has been suggested that radiation produces changes in the oral flora and in salivary pH, consistency and flow that favor caries activity. However, experimental data have been reported from our laboratory which indicate that gamma radiation of teeth will cause calcium and phosphorus demineralization of enamel.

Observations of the dentition of a limited number of patients who have received megavoltage therapy suggest that the latent radiation effects are much less catastrophic than those seen in low-voltage therapy.

Prevention. Prevention of "radiation caries" would be the ideal course of action. Thus, preradiation odontectomy and subsequent delay for initial healing of soft tissues would be eliminated. The patient could undergo immediate radiation treatment.

Recently, the practice of applying fluoride-containing compounds to the dentition before, during and after radiation has seemed to reduce the incidence of enamel disintegration.

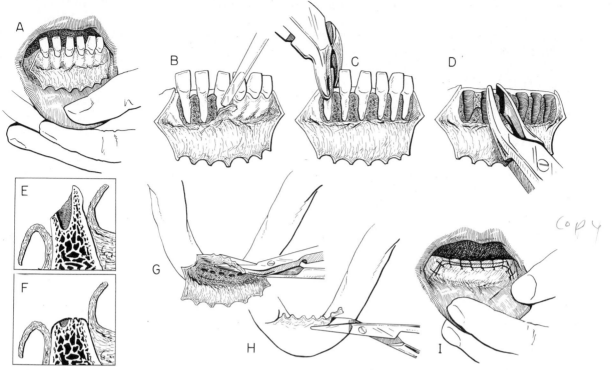

Figure 2–160 Extraction of remaining maxillary and mandibular teeth and an extensive radical alveolectomy performed before radiation for cancer in the oral cavity, where the teeth will be "in the line of fire."

A, Wide and deep reflection of the mucoperiosteal membrane.

B, Labial and buccal cortical bone removed with a chisel.

C, Teeth luxated and removed.

D, Interseptal bone removed with a bone shear.

E, Lingual mucoperiosteal membrane reflected.

F, Lingual cortical plate removed with bone shears and endcutting roengeurs. Bone carefully smoothed with hand and rotary files so that there are not any sharp ledges or points of bone left.

G and *H*, Excess lingual and labial soft tissue is cut off so that the edges of the flaps meet without tension.

I, Wound is closed with a continuous suture and lock stitches.

Figure 2–161 *A*, Panoramic radiograph of a patient's dentition before radiation for cancer of the hypopharynx. Teeth were not extracted because "the primary radiation did not involve the teeth." *B*, Twenty months after radiation therapy was completed. Note the extensive loss of tooth structure due to "radiation caries." (See Figure 2–162.)

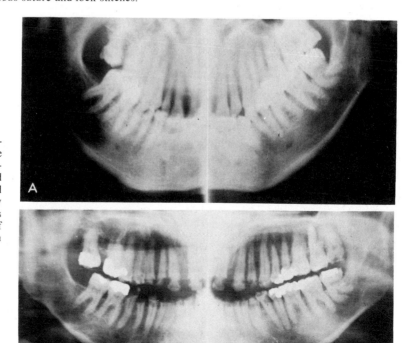

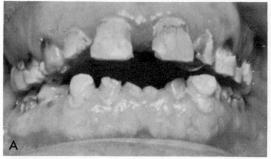

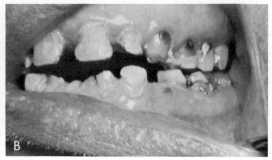

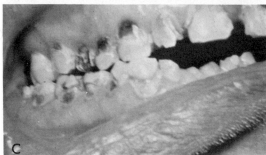

Figure 2–162 "Radiation caries" shown in Figure 2–161. *A,* Note the extensive loss of tooth substance in the mandibular anterior teeth and the "chalky enamel" in the maxillary anterior teeth.

B and *C,* Gingival and other areas of disintegration of the enamel of the bicuspid and molar teeth in both the maxilla and mandible are readily apparent.

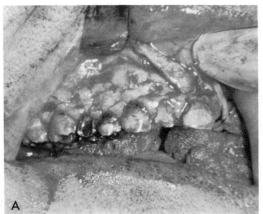

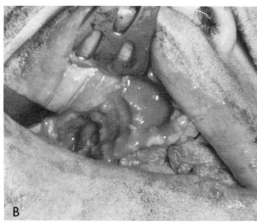

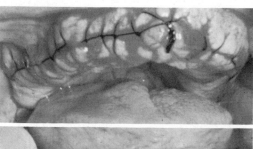

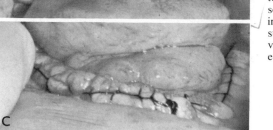

Figure 2–163 *A,* The mucoperiosteal membrane was raised and widely reflected in preparation for odontectomy and radical alveolectomy. *B,* Appearance of this segment after gross reduction of the alveolar bone. Bleeding from the bone was brisk. *C,* In spite of the extensive surgery, there is considerable bone remaining. The gingival tissues were carefully reapproximated for edge-to-edge contact and secured by continuous black silk suture.

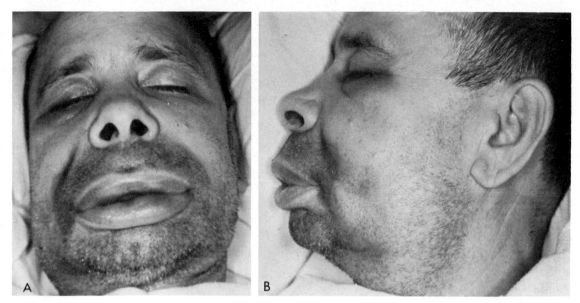

Figure 2–164 Appearance 24 hours postoperatively. There is edema and ecchymosis that is not excessive following the radical oral surgery.

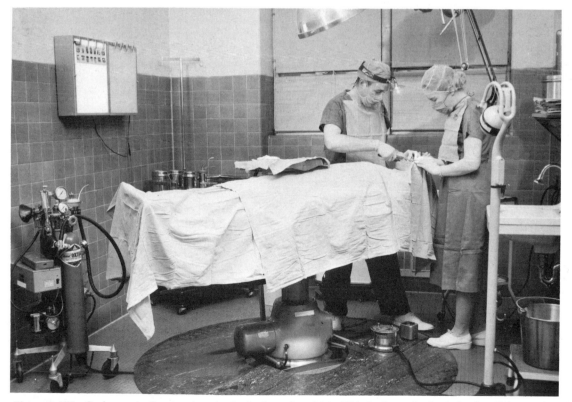

Figure 2–165 Oral surgery for a patient in the horizontal position. This is the author's choice for all forms of oral surgery. Access and visibility are excellent, postional strain on the surgeon is eliminated and the patient is comfortable. Maxillary teeth are being extracted.

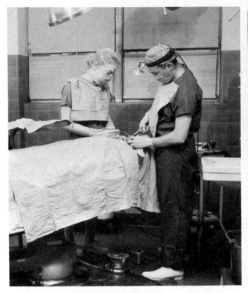

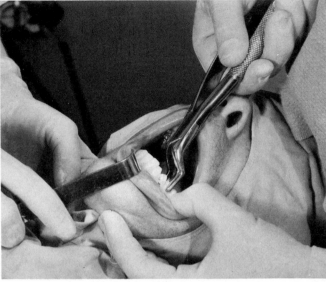

Figure 2–166   Figure 2–167

Figure 2–166   The position of the surgeon and assistant for the extraction of the mandibular ten (anterior and bicuspid) teeth.

Figure 2–167   A close-up view of the use of the No. 286 forceps for the extraction of mandibular bicuspids as well as the mandibular cuspids and central and lateral incisors.

Meticulous oral hygiene must be maintained by the patient

Treatment. When clinical signs of "radiation caries" develop, a conservative treatment method is the preparation of all residual crowns for full metal or resin crown prostheses. Root canal therapy may be necessary in selected teeth.

Odontectomy following radiation therapy is advocated by some, shunned by others. The patient must be advised of the possible sequelae and must sign an informed consent for surgery. Extractions and alveolectomy may be performed under local or general anesthesia, depending upon the physical condition of the patient. If the patient can tolerate oral lavage, frequent flushing of the mouth is ordered for the 24 hours preceding surgery. Antibiotic therapy is planned for establishing a high blood level immediately before surgery and then given in sufficient doses to maintain blood levels until there is evidence of complete mucous membrane seal. Following extraction of teeth, a radical alveolectomy is made in order to approximate the buccal and lingual flaps for tight closure (See Figures 2–161 to 2–164). Continuous loop sutures are preferred. Bleeding from the alveolar bone may be brisk but usually is controlled by tissue closure. The surgeon may order intraoral gauze pressure tampons and cold packs to the face to reduce postoperative bleeding and tissue edema.

EXTRACTION OF PRIMARY (DECIDUOUS) TEETH

Indications for the Extraction of Primary Teeth.

1. When there is extensive decay which has resulted in death of the dental pulp. This is controversial. Some dentists believe in attempting to treat the tooth, depending on a favorable general history; others extract at once. Certainly teeth have been saved through treatment without apparent detrimental effects to the child. However, primary teeth with infected pulps or periapical infection, in patients with rheumatic fever and its sequelae, such as rheumatic heart disease, or with kidney disorders, should *not be extracted until consultation with their physician.* The use of antibiotics in these cases is described in Chapter 8, "Antibiotic Therapy." In addition, primary extractions are contraindicated in patients with blood dyscrasias, such as hemophilia, until consultation with the hematologist and preoperative treatment is instituted.

(Text continued on page 125)

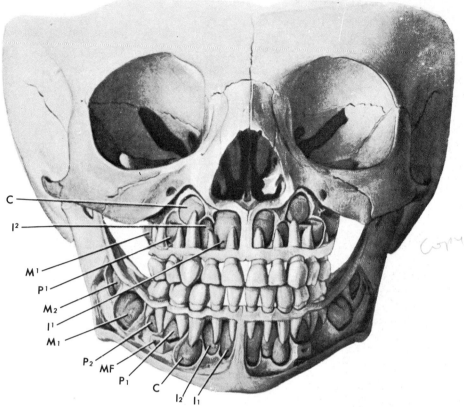

Figure 2–168   Skull of a 4-year-old child. (From Sicher, H.: Oral Anatomy. St. Louis, The C. V. Mosby Co., 1949.)

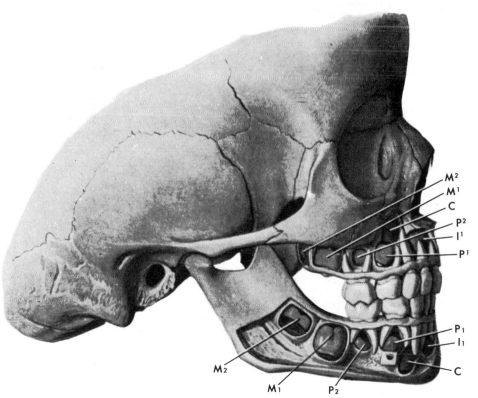

Figure 2–169   Lateral view of skull in previous figure. (From Sicher, H.: Oral Anatomy. St. Louis, The C. V. Mosby Co., 1949.)

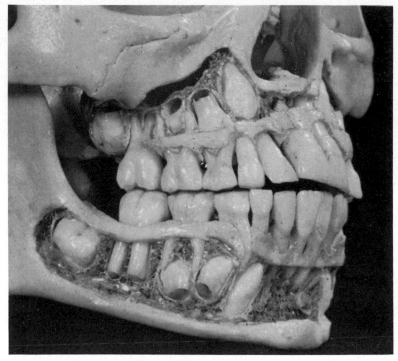

Figure 2–170   Skull of an 8-year-old child. (From Finn, S. B.: Clinical Pedodontics, 1st ed. Philadelphia, W. B. Saunders Co., 1957.)

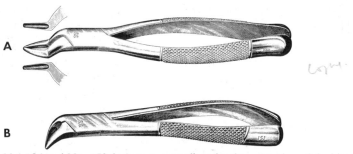

Figure 2–171   *A*, The No. 286 and No. 150 forceps are excellent for the extraction of deciduous maxillary teeth. *B*, The No. 151 forceps is my choice for the extraction of deciduous mandibular teeth.

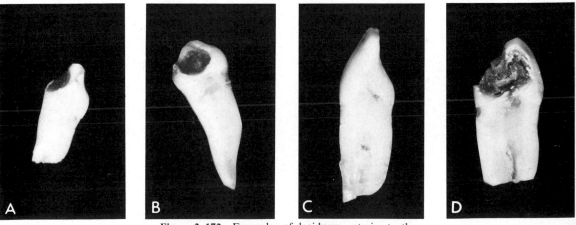

Figure 2–172   Examples of deciduous anterior teeth.

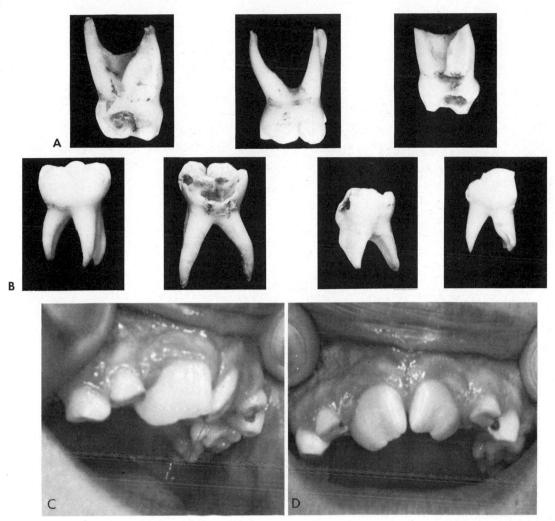

Figure 2–173   *A*, Examples of deciduous maxillary molars. *B*, Examples of deciduous mandibular molars. *C* and *D*, Examples of geminous maxillary central and lateral incisors.

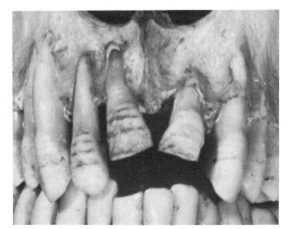

Figure 2–174   Retention of the deciduous maxillary incisors in this unusual case of congenitally missing permanent maxillary central and left lateral incisors. Whether or not the deciduous left lateral incisor was also congenitally absent is not known. The brown transverse streaks on the labial and buccal surfaces of these teeth were the result of an intake of water containing 1 to 7 parts per million (ppm.) of fluorine during their formation.

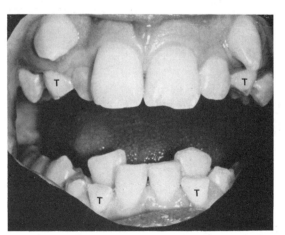

Figure 2–175   Crowding of permanent maxillary and mandibular teeth, possibly due to overretention of deciduous (temporary, *T*) maxillary cuspids and mandibular lateral incisors. It would also appear that there is a tooth-jaw discrepancy. There is no premature loss of the deciduous cuspids. The decision for, and the time of, the elective extraction of deciduous or permanent teeth is one for joint consultation with the orthodontist.

113

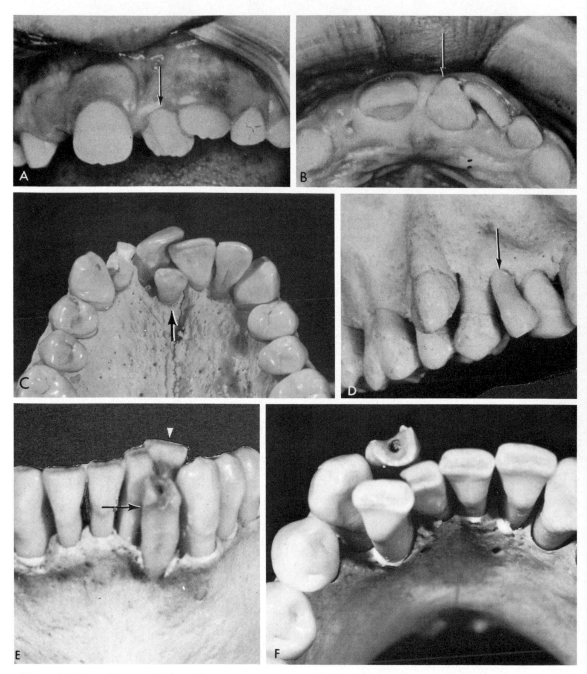

Figure 2–176 *A*, Large, well-formed supernumerary central incisor erupting in the midline and displacing distally and labially the left maxillary central incisor. *B*, This occlusal view of the contact between these teeth indicates the use of Apexo straight elevators driven along the root of the supernumerary tooth to dislodge it from its alveolus. (See Chapter 4, Figure 4–17.) The use of forceps might inadvertently dislodge the partially erupted permanent central incisor. *C*, Mesiodens erupting in the midline of the palate. Removal of this rudimentary tooth should be performed as described in *B* and for the same reason. *D*, Overretention of the deciduous cuspid has resulted in the disturbance of the normal path of eruption for the permanent cuspid. *E* and *F*, Overretention of the deciduous lateral incisor has produced this lingual eruption of the permanent lateral incisor, aided undoubtedly by a tooth-jaw discrepancy.

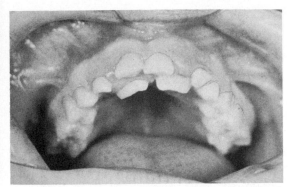

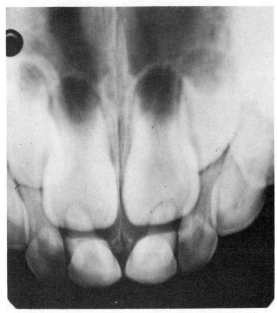

Figure 2-177 The overretention of the primary teeth has resulted in palatal maleruption of the permanent central incisors. (See Figure 2-178.) When primary teeth are retained past the normal time for their loss, they should be radiographed to determine whether there is a reason for the delay. If no reason is found, extraction of the deciduous tooth should be done. (See also Figure 2-179 for an example of delayed eruption due to the presence of a mesiodens.) Other reasons are listed in the text.

Figure 2-178 Radiograph of the case shown in Figure 2-177.

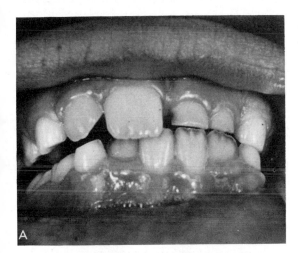

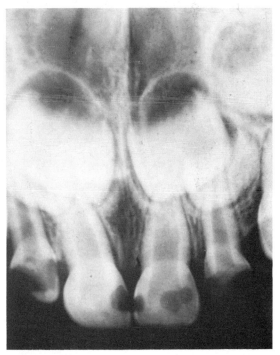

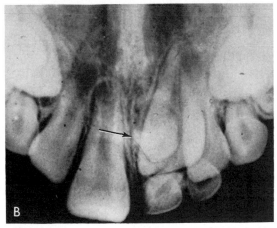

Figure 2-180 The early loss of these four deciduous maxillary incisors, which must be extracted because of advanced caries in this 2-year-old child, will require the placing of a space-maintainer. This case should have orthodontic supervision.

Figure 2-179 A, Seven-year-old child with the deciduous maxillary left central and lateral incisors still in place. B, The reason is revealed in this radiograph. There is a partially formed mesiodens which has interfered with the normal eruption of the permanent central and lateral incisors. Surgical excision of the mesiodens and extraction of the central and lateral deciduous incisors is indicated to permit the eruption of the permanent incisors.

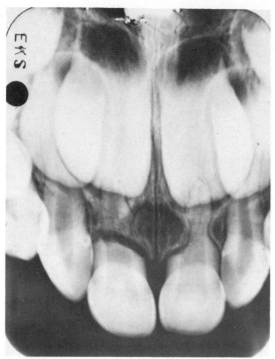

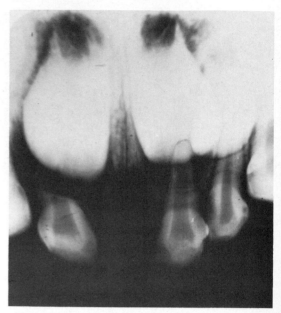

Figure 2–181 A fall severely traumatized the deciduous maxillary central incisors in this 4-year-old child. The left incisor root was fractured about two-thirds of the distance from the apex, and while no union has taken place, it is held in a moderately firm position in its alveolus and is not infected. The right central incisor root apparently was not fractured, but there is an external crescent-shaped area of resorption at the same point on this root at which the fracture occurred on its neighbor's root. This idiopathic resorption was apparently stimulated by the trauma to which it was subjected. There is no sign of resorption of either root as yet. Periodic radiographic examination is required so that these teeth and roots can be surgically excised if these roots do not show signs of resorption at the normal time of eruption for the permanent central incisors.

Figure 2–182 The root of the deciduous left central incisor has resorbed normally as the permanent central incisor has erupted downward. Not so the deciduous right central incisor's root. It is still fully formed, and the permanent central incisor crown has been deflected lingually and slightly distally. The extraction of the right deciduous central incisor is mandatory. The deciduous left central incisor should also be removed, as it is probably loose and ready for removal.

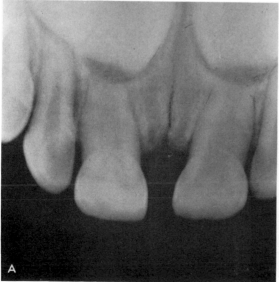
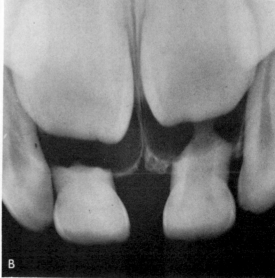

Figure 2–183 There are frequently marked differences in the root resorption rate in deciduous teeth in children of the same age. Note the difference in the rate of root resorption in A and B of the deciduous central incisors in two children, both 6½ years old.

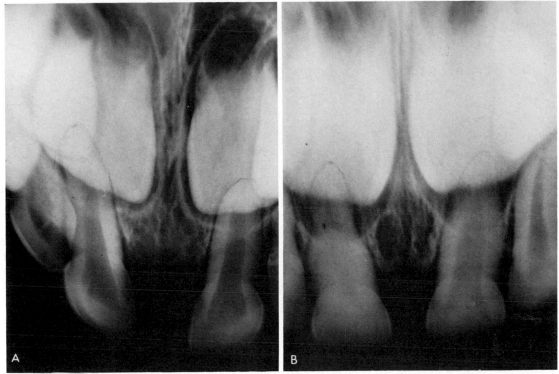

Figure 2–184 *A* and *B,* No evidence of deciduous central incisor root resorption is apparent in either of these 4-year-old children. Evidence is, of course, usually seen at this age. These patients should have radiographic examinations at age 5, and if there is no evidence of root resorption at that age, extractions are recommended.

Figure 2–185 Overretention of the deciduous cuspid in this 12-year-old. This may be due to ankylosis, although such evidence is not radiographically visible. The deciduous cuspid should have been extracted when the patient reached 10 years of age. Radiographically, a dentigerous cyst may be suspected of developing around the permanent cuspid's crown. If so, following the extraction of the deciduous cuspid, the cyst should be marsupialized, not enucleated. See Chapter 12 for the technique. If the normal eruptive force of the cuspid is now missing, the crown should be "lassoed" and moved into place by the orthodontist.

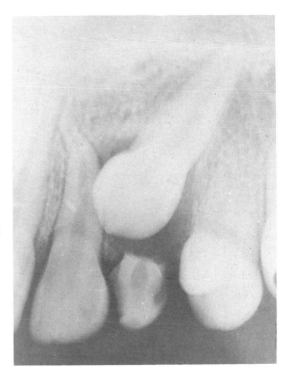

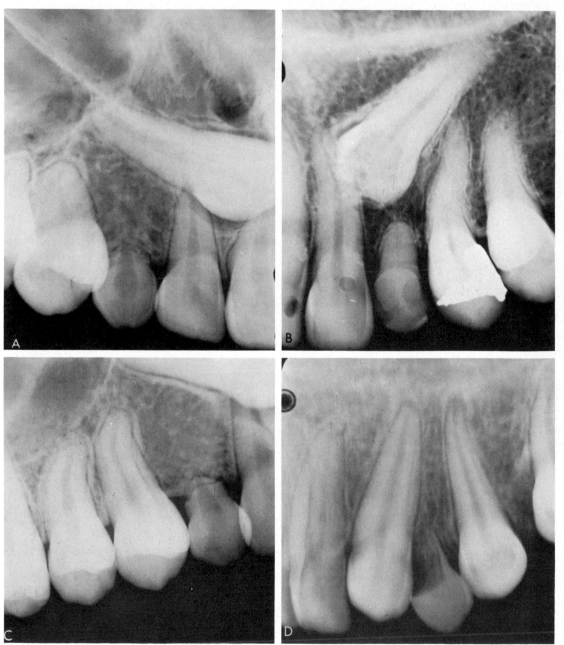

Figure 2–186   *A, B* and *C,* In all three of these cases, patients around the age of 10, the crowns of the permanent cuspids should have been exposed, the deciduous cuspids extracted and the permanent cuspids orthodontically moved into position in the maxillary arch. *D,* The extraction of this ankylosed deciduous cuspid when the patient reached the age of 10 would have permitted the permanent cuspid to erupt in its normal position in the maxillary arch.

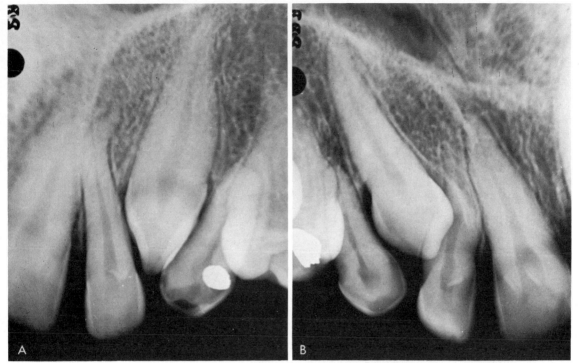

Figure 2–187 Two examples of overretention of deciduous maxillary cuspids that, had they been removed when the patient reached approximately 10 years of age, would have permitted the normal eruption of the maxillary permanent cuspids.

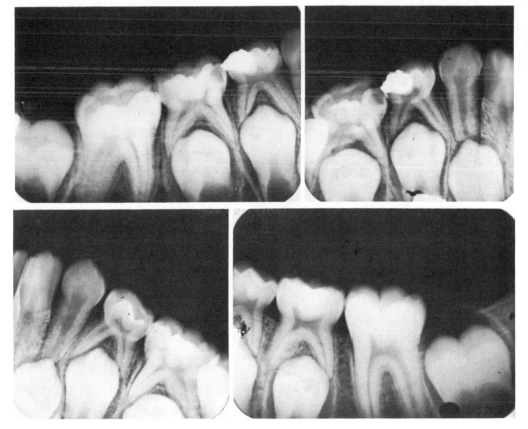

Figure 2–188 Radiographs of an 8-year-old child. The position of the bicuspid crowns high up in the bifurcation of the roots of the deciduous molars, with no radiographic evidence of root resorption in the deciduous molars or cuspids, reveals the possibility of overretention of these teeth. Unless there is positive evidence of resorption within a year, extraction of the deciduous teeth must be considered if the child does not have any of the disorders affecting tooth eruption, such as hormonal, metabolic, developmental or nutritional diseases. (See the cases of cleidocranial dysostosis in Chapter 5, beginning page 366.) This case should be kept under observation.

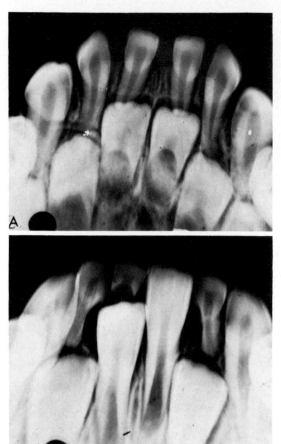

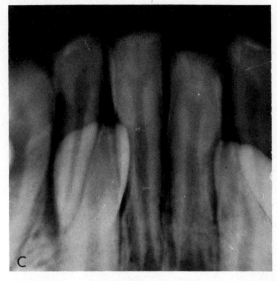

Figure 2–189   *A*, Radiographically, it appears that there is very little, if any, resorption of the deciduous central incisor roots. This is a 4½-year-old child, and the progress of resorption should be checked periodically. *B*, Eruption of the right central incisor is prevented by the right deciduous lateral incisor. It and the enamel cap of the deciduous central incisor should be extracted. *C*, No resorption of the roots of the deciduous lateral incisors is apparent. The crowns of the permanent lateral incisors are erupting lingual to these retained deciduous lateral incisors that should be extracted.

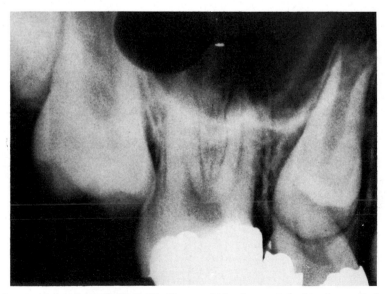

Figure 2–190   This second deciduous molar in this 11-year-old has been retained too long and should be extracted to permit the eruption of the second bicuspid if the eruptive force is still present; if it is not, by traction the bicuspid should be moved into position.

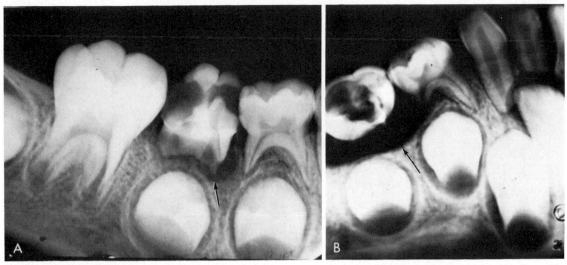

Figure 2–191 *A* and *B*, Deciduous mandibular molars with evidence of periapical pathosis. Extraction is indicated for the second deciduous molar in *A* and both molars in *B*. Space-maintainers are necessary. It is of interest to note the condensing osteitis due to infection beneath the second deciduous molar in *B*. No such defensive activity is present beneath the second deciduous molar in *A*.

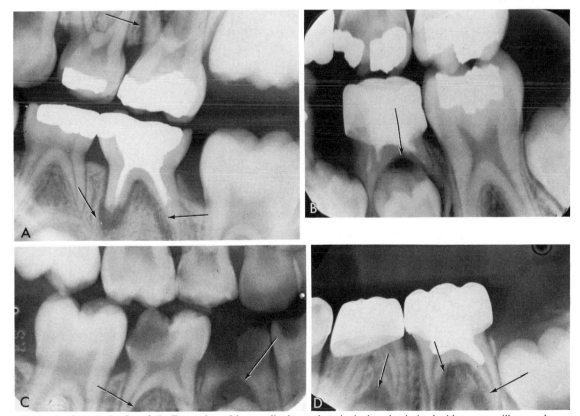

Figure 2–192 *A, B, C* and *D*, Examples of intraradicular and periapical pathosis in deciduous maxillary and mandibular molars. A study of each individual film before extraction will reveal what difficulties may be encountered and how, if possible, they can be avoided or coped with. It should be noted that in cases *B, C* and *D*, where the areas of apical pathosis (acute or chronic inflammatory tissue) are in contact with the succedaneous tooth follicle, curettement is contraindicated following the extraction of the deciduous molars, thereby avoiding damage to or enucleation of the forming tooth in its crypt.

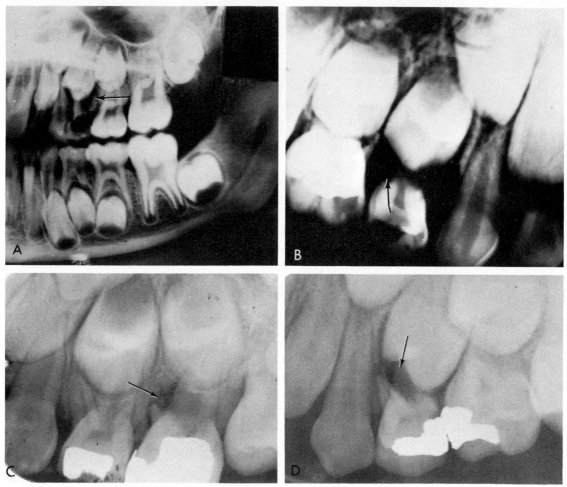

Figure 2–193   *A, B, C* and *D,* Examples of periapical pathosis involving deciduous molars with buccal fistulas. Curettement was contraindicated for the reason stated in the previous legend. Space-maintainers were placed, following the extraction of these teeth.

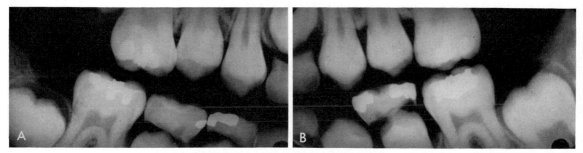

Figure 2–194   It is surprising to learn how long these enamel "caps" sometimes maintain their position, and thus prevent the full eruption of the permanent teeth. These persistent enamel crowns should be promptly removed.

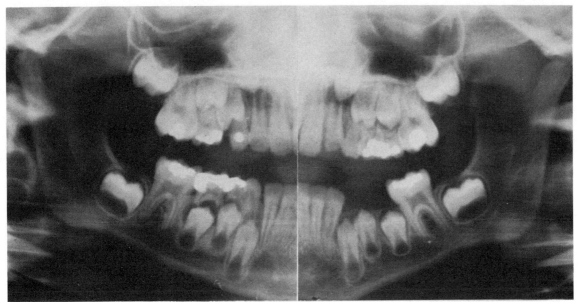

Figure 2–195 Premature loss of the right mandibular III, IV and V deciduous teeth, without placement of space-maintainers, has resulted in the forward drift of the mandibular first permanent molar by a distance of 7 mm., as compared to the same area on the left mandible, where III, IV and V are still in position. It is obvious that repositioning of the right first mandibular permanent molar is necessary to permit the normal eruption of the permanent cuspid and first and second bicuspids.

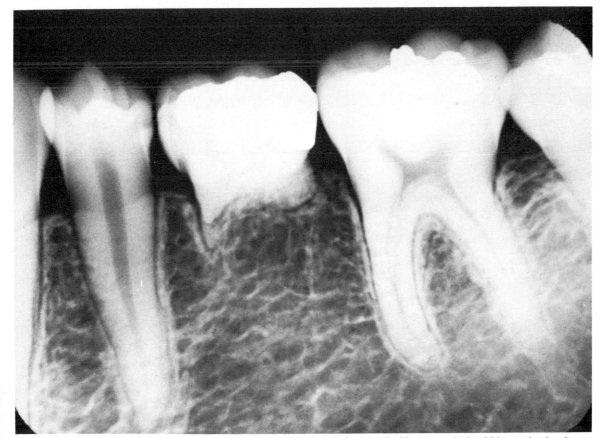

Figure 2–196 Where the succedaneous tooth is congenitally missing, the deciduous tooth should be retained as long as it is not diseased and a normal occlusal plane is maintained.

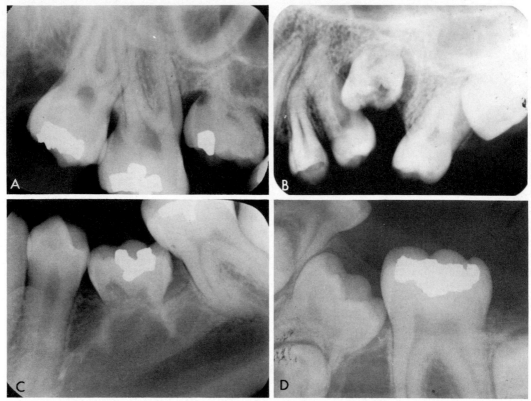

Figure 2–197 Deciduous molars locked beneath the enamel contours of the crowns of the adjacent permanent teeth. In *A*, *B* and *C*, the permanent bicuspids are congenitally absent. In *B* there is evidence of caries in the deciduous crown and a radiolucent area surrounding it. This tooth should be extracted. Whether or not the deciduous molars in radiographs *A* and *C* should be retained is dependent upon whether there are periodontal pockets developing. In both *A* and *C* there is radiographic evidence that interseptal bone is in the early stages of resorption, and so extraction is indicated here to protect the adjacent permanent teeth from periodontoclasia. In *D* the impacted second deciduous molar is preventing the eruption of the permanent bicuspid and should be surgically excised. If there is not sufficient space for the bicuspid, this should be provided by orthodontic treatment.

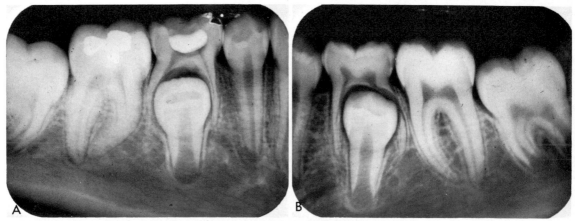

Figure 2–198 *A* and *B*, Overretention of these deciduous second molars is preventing the normal eruption of the permanent bicuspids. The technique for the removal of these teeth is shown in Figure 2–199.

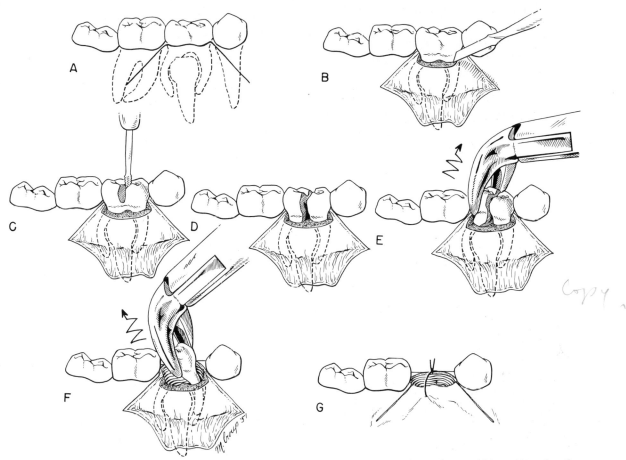

Figure 2–199 Removal of a primary second molar whose roots embrace an unerupted second bicuspid so that the unerupted tooth is not traumatized or extracted. *A*, The flap extends around the neck of the tooth, then onto the buccal mucosa both mesially and distally at a 45-degree angle. *B*, The mucoperiosteal flap is reflected, and removal of the gingival third of cortical bone is effected with mallet and chisel. *C*, Cutting through the crown (buccolingual) with the crosscut fissure bur. *D*, The crown is split through the bifurcation. *E*, Removal of the distal fragment with No. 300 or No. 151 forceps, bringing the fragment mesially. *F*, Removal of the mesial fragment with No. 300 or No. 151 forceps, bringing the fragment distally. *G*, Approximation and suturing of the flap.

Acute infectious stomatitis, acute or chronic Vincent's infection, and herpetic stomatitis are contraindications to extraction of primary teeth until the infection is cured.

2. When the primary teeth interfere with the normal eruption and alignment of their permanent successors. This may be due to (*a*) improper resorption of roots, causing deflection of erupting tooth, found mainly in anteriors, especially lower anteriors; (*b*) irregular resorption of roots of molars, one root being resorbed more slowly than the others: (*c*) prolonged retention. However, in considering the advisability of extraction of primary teeth because of overretention, as Finn states, "One should always keep in mind that age per se is not an acceptable criterion in determining whether a primary tooth should be removed. A primary second molar should not be removed just because a child is 11 or 12 years of age, unless there is a special indication. For some patients the second premolars are ready to erupt at 8 or 9 years of age, while in other cases these same teeth do not show sufficient root development at the age of 12. A primary tooth that is firm and intact in the arch should never be removed unless a complete clinical and roentgenographic evaluation has been made of the entire mouth and especially of the particular area.

"Occlusion, arch development, size of teeth, amount of root, resorption of the primary tooth involved, and state of development of the underlying permanent successor and adjacent teeth, presence or absence of infection—all of these factors must be considered in determining when and how a primary tooth should be removed."

3. When there is a sinus opening through the mucoperiosteal membrane overlying the root.

4. When the roentgenogram reveals evidence of periapical pathosis.

5. When the root is fractured as a result of trauma, with subsequent development of infection.

6. When rudimentary supernumerary teeth or mesiodens are found in the radiographs to be preventing the eruption of the permanent teeth. These should be carefully removed without damaging or dislodging the permanent tooth or teeth.

Note: A primary tooth should not be extracted to make room for any tooth other than its immediate successor. Often a lower primary lateral is removed to make room for a permanent central which is apparently crowded. This should not be done unless so advised by the orthodontist. Eruption problems subsequent to premature removal of deciduous teeth are not infrequent. This is especially true if a space maintainer is not inserted. When a deciduous tooth is prematurely extracted, the patient (and/or his parents) is advised to have the area examined at the age when the permanent successor is supposed to erupt. In cases in which eruption has not occurred, surgical intervention to expose one third of the crown of the permanent tooth is then indicated.

Resorption of Roots in Primary Teeth. Radiographs of primary teeth before extraction will reveal the extent, if any, of resorption of the primary roots. This is particularly true of the anterior primary teeth and mandibular molars, and to a lesser degree the maxillary molars. In the latter the lingual root is "blocked out" to some extent by the permanent tooth crown. If the radiographs reveal that half of the root has been resorbed, then there is no question in the mind of the dentist, when he checks the tooth on removal, whether the root is fractured or resorbed. Without radiographs there is always this question. However, if the root has been fractured, it is smooth and sharply defined as contrasted with the roughened appearance of a resorbed root.

Technique for the Extraction of Primary (Deciduous) Teeth. As has been stated repeatedly, dental radiographs, and a careful study of them, are essential before the extraction of any tooth, and in my opinion, more so before the extraction of any primary tooth, loose or firmly held in the alveolar process.

The relationship of the partially formed permanent tooth crown and its crypt to the primary roots is visualized. Where the primary roots partially encircle the permanent crown, it is necessary to section the crown of the primary molar, and remove the roots individually. This is best done by cutting half way through the crown of the primary molar with a disk or knife-edged stone, and then splitting the crown by the use of a narrow straight elevator placed in this groove, or by the use of crosscut burs.

While posterior primary teeth with resorbed roots are usually uncomplicated extractions, posterior primary teeth whose roots have not resorbed are difficult to extract. Whether they are maxillary or mandibular molars, the roots in either case are quite divergent, so that there must be considerable expansion and compression of the supporting alveolar process to permit the removal of these teeth in one piece. Not infrequently one (or more) of the roots is fractured. It is necessary that these roots be removed without injury to the crypt of the partially formed bicuspid which is contained in the alveolar bone between the roots of the primary molar.

It is necessary to remove primary roots which have fractured for the same reasons that permanent roots are removed. There is the additional reason that the normal eruption of the permanent tooth may be retarded or deflected. Occasionally these roots are the nucleus for the formation of cysts which displace the adjacent permanent teeth. The technique for the removal of primary roots will be contained in Chapter 4.

The so-called "cowhorn" forceps is contraindicated for the extraction of primary molars because of the great possibility of injury to the crypt of the permanent tooth which lies below the bifurcation of the deciduous roots.

The soft tissues about the necks of the primary teeth should be incised and loosened with the periosteal elevator. When the buccal-lingual movements of the primary molar are seen to stretch the mucoperiosteum to the point where a tear is imminent, then a single vertical incision in the mucoperiosteum is indicated, starting at the mesial interproximal space and carried toward the mucobuccal fold at a 45-degree angle for a distance of 0.5 cm.

FORCEPS TECHNIQUE FOR THE EXTRACTION OF PRIMARY (DECIDUOUS) TEETH

While the standard so-called "universal" forceps No. 150 can be used for primary maxillary extractions and the No. 151 for primary mandibular extractions, the forceps No. 300 for primary maxillary extractions and No. 301 for primary mandibular extractions are smaller and can be covered with the hand so as not to frighten the child.

Basic Forces Exerted in the Extraction of Primary Teeth. These forces are as follows:

MAXILLARY AND MANDIBULAR SIX ANTERIORS. Labial pressure, with mesial rotation and removal in the labial direction.

MAXILLARY AND MANDIBULAR MOLARS. Buccal, then lingual, pressure, with the greatest pressure toward the lingual and removal in the lingual direction.

Trauma to Permanent Teeth or Partially Erupted Permanent Teeth. The same rules for the application of forceps apply to the removal of primary teeth as to the extraction of permanent teeth. While in the extraction of permanent teeth the beaks of the forceps are placed well up on the roots of the teeth to be extracted, care must be taken not to place the beaks of the forceps high up on the roots of primary maxillary or mandibular teeth because of the great possibility of removing the partially formed permanent tooth with the primary tooth. Should this inadvertently happen, the partially formed tooth and any surrounding bone should be carefully freed in one piece from the primary roots and replaced in the alveolus. The soft tissues are then sutured over the alveolus to hold the bone and tooth in position.

Curettes should not be used to remove periapical granulomas following primary tooth extraction because of the danger of injury to the permanent tooth bud. Instead postoperative roentgenograms are made six to eight months later to determine whether the granuloma has been replaced by bone or a cyst has developed. The latter is not a frequent occurrence.

Occasionally, because of faulty application of forceps or the injudicious use of elevators, partially formed or partially erupted permanent molars or bicuspids are dislodged from their sockets. These should be immediately replaced, and the patient warned not to chew on that side of his mouth, and to avoid disturbing the replanted tooth as much as possible. Most of these teeth will become reattached, and the root will be completely formed. The chance for successful completion of the roots is directly proportional to the amount of incomplete calcification.

The greater the required calcification for completion of the root, the greater the possibility of successful retention of the tooth and final calcification of the root, because of the increased area of soft tissue of the tooth-forming organ, the pulp, which can again be placed in contact with the blood vessels in the alveolus.

The author has seen several of these cases, one in which the partially formed bicuspid (see Figure 2–200) was out of the patient's mouth for at least 15 minutes before being replaced. In this particular case the root was eventually completely formed of solid dentine with no pulp chamber or root canal.

In lower primary molars with deep central caries the beaks of the forceps should engage the mesial root. When buccal then lingual pressures are applied, the mesial half of the crown and root will most likely be extracted because the crown will fracture through the bifurcation of the roots. Now the beaks are applied to the remaining root and attached coronal portion, and buccal, then lingual pressures applied until this portion of the tooth can be lifted out of the alveolus.

Extensively decayed primary maxillary molars usually fracture at the bifurcation with a loosening of one or more of the roots. The loose roots can be lifted out with a hemostat, while elevators carefully used will be necessary to remove tightly held roots.

Primary teeth decayed to the gum line can usually be removed by the spear-pointed end of a periosteal elevator; if not, then by the use of Apexo elevators.

After the tooth is removed, any sharp edges of bone are removed and a suture is inserted, particularly if a flap has been made or there is excessive bleeding from the socket.

EXTRACTION OF NEONATAL TEETH

At birth occasionally prematurely erupted primary mandibular central incisors and rarely

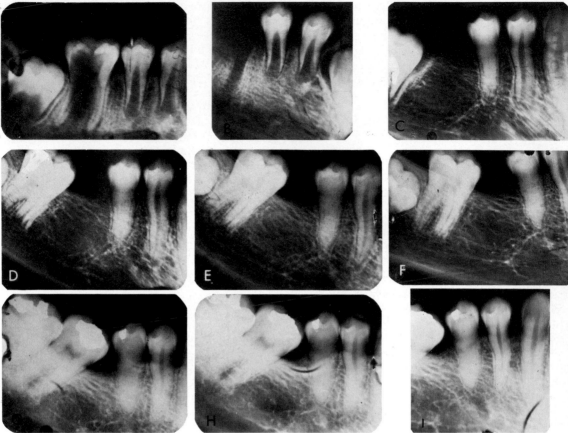

Figure 2-200 Replantation of an accidentally extracted erupted and partially formed mandibular second bicuspid in a 10-year-old. See Case Report No. 3.

other primary teeth are seen. If they are firmly attached to the alveolar ridge and the mother can nurse the baby without her nipples' being traumatized, these teeth are left in place. If the nipples are lacerated by these teeth, then consultation with the pediatrician regarding other methods of feeding is indicated. The alternate to this is the extraction of the tooth or teeth, which should be avoided if at all possible. However, if these prematurely erupted teeth are loose and do not become more firmly fixed within a week, then they should be extracted to avoid the possibility of their becoming dislodged and aspirated. (See also the treatment of eruption cysts in the newborn on page 630.)

While the author has not seen any excessive hemorrhage following the extraction of these loose teeth, Thoma and Goldman warn of this possibility as a result of hypothrombinemia, which may be present during the first 10 days of life, or as a result of the vascular developmental papilla accompanying the incompletely formed tooth.[35]

REPLANTATION OF TEETH

It has been generally agreed that replanted teeth are not retained permanently. They either become infected or resorb. In the case report here, there is *no indication of resorption or infection after nineteen years!* Of course, it was realized that this case was one of the two best indications for replantation: namely, an erupted tooth, with a *partially formed root, in a young patient.*

The replantation of *partly formed unerupted* teeth has been more successful than the replantation of erupted teeth.

Certainly when either unerupted or erupted partially formed teeth are accidentally dislodged from their sockets during the extraction of adjacent teeth, they should be immediately replanted without any treatment.

If a fully formed tooth has been accidentally dislodged, the root canal must be treated and filled. Sometimes this is done before replanting and sometimes later. The tooth should be

Case Report No. 3

REPLANTATION OF AN ACCIDENTALLY EXTRACTED ERUPTED AND PARTIALLY FORMED MANDIBULAR SECOND BICUSPID

The patient, C. C., a boy aged 10, came to the dental clinic for extraction of a carious and abscessed left first mandibular molar.

A dental student inadvertently "popped out" (onto the floor) a fully erupted, partially formed second bicuspid when attempting to extract the carious first molar with an elevator.

After extracting the first molar, I picked up the partially formed second bicuspid (Fig. 2–200A), washed it in sterile normal saline solution, immersed it briefly in 70 per cent alcohol, and replaced it in the alveolus.

There was a blood clot in the alveolus which was displaced by the insertion of the tooth. We felt that this clot had protected the socket from the invasion of bacteria-laden saliva. The tooth was out of its normal environment for 15 minutes.

The patient and his parents were informed about the accident, and instructions were given to the patient to confine himself to a liquid diet for a week, and to avoid all trauma to the replaced bicuspid.

A roentgenogram (Fig. 2–200B) was taken and the patient was discharged.

Recovery was uneventful. Only slight tenderness was present for about a week.

The tooth became reattached, and circulation into the pulp tissue was reestablished. However, as can be seen in the follow-up roentgenograms (Fig. 2–200C to F), which cover 19 years, the root was completed as a solid mass of cementum and dentine *without a pulp chamber.*

There is, of course, no response to the electric pulp tester. The color of the tooth is identical with that of the first bicuspid (Fig. 2–200G to I).

---

splinted in position, and occlusal trauma to the tooth prevented by grinding the occlusion of the opposing tooth. Prophylactic penicillin therapy is recommended. If infection develops, the tooth should be immediately treated.

These teeth should be checked by radiographs periodically. Evidence of resorption of bone or tooth structure is an indication for extraction.

For information on transplantation, see Figures 3–83 and 3–84 and accompanying text, as well as Chapter 23.

BLOOD AND OTHER FLUID LOSS DURING ORAL SURGICAL OPERATIONS

Use of Vasoconstrictors. Pasqual* studied blood loss in 125 patients requiring maxillary and mandibular odontectomy and alveolectomy.

One hundred two patients received thiopental sodium and nitrous oxide and oxygen. Average number of teeth extracted was 19 with an average blood loss of 244.0 cc.

Twenty-three patients received the same type of general anesthesia but with the addition of a local anesthetic containing a vasoconstrictor (epinephrine hydrochloride 1:100,000). Average number of teeth extracted was 17 with an average blood loss of 59.8 cc.

The difference in average blood loss between the two series of patients was found to be 184.2 cc. The number of teeth and duration of surgery are important in blood loss measurement, but blood loss is significantly reduced when vasoconstrictors in local anesthetic solutions are used in conjunction with general anesthesia.

The study concluded that all patients, with the exception of those who exhibit allergic or systemic manifestations to local anesthetic drugs or their vasoconstrictors, should receive, in addition to general anesthesia, a local anesthetic drug with a vasoconstrictor when a maxillary and mandibular odontectomy and alveolectomy is performed.

Fluid Therapy. Meyer,* in a study on blood volume considerations in oral surgery, reported in part as follows:

FULL-MOUTH ODONTECTOMIES. "Thirty-five healthy patients admitted to the hospital in consecutive order for full-mouth odontectomies were selected for this study. Blood volume determination and other related parameters were measured when the patients were admitted to the hospital; measurements were also made after preoperative fasting, immedi-

---

*Pasqual, H. N.: Abridgement of thesis submitted to the Graduate Faculty of the School of Dentistry, University of Pittsburgh, in partial fulfillment of the requirements for the degree of Master of Science.

*Meyer, R. A.: Blood volume considerations in oral surgery. J. Oral Surg., *29*:617–621 (Sept.), 1971.

ately after surgery, 24 hours postoperatively, and 72 hours postoperatively. During surgery, which was done with the patients under general endotracheal anesthesia, gravimetrically measured blood loss was replaced routinely as it occurred with 5 per cent dextrose in water administered intravenously so that effects on blood volume would remain constant. During the operation a third of the patients, randomly selected, received local injections of 1:100,000 epinephrine as a vasoconstrictor for hemostasis; a third received 1:20,000 phenylephrine (Neo-Synephrine), and a third received standard saline solution. For 24 hours postoperatively, a half of the patients received only oral intake as tolerated, simulating conditions at home if they had been treated at the dentist's office and discharged; the remainder of the patients received oral intake plus at least 2000 ml. of fluids administered intravenously."

RESULTS. "The results can be summarized as follows:

1. Intraoperative blood loss was not significantly different regardless of the vasoconstrictor injected. However, blood loss in the postoperative period was significantly less in those patients who received 1:20,000 phenylephrine as a vasoconstrictor.

2. Gravimetrically measured blood loss was about two thirds of the amount of the actual blood loss, as measured by RISA.*

3. Since blood loss during surgery was replaced with intravenous fluids as it occurred, no patient showed cardiovascular instability during surgery. No patient required a blood transfusion, even though losses in excess of 1000 ml. occurred in two patients.

4. Patients who received intravenous fluids to supplement oral intake during the first 24 postoperative hours lost less weight, had lower temperatures, higher intake, higher urine output, less decrease in blood volume, fewer respiratory complications, and no cardiovascular complications when compared to patients who received only oral intake."

CONCLUSIONS. Dr. Meyer concludes, "In the past, full-mouth odontectomies ... often were done in the dental office or as outpatient procedures. Our studies indicate that, because of blood losses, fluid deficits, and difficulty in

maintaining adequate oral hydration, intravenous therapy in a hospital environment is a definite improvement in the standard of care for these patients." I agree.

POSTOPERATIVE CARE

ROUTINE POSTOPERATIVE INSTRUCTIONS TO THE PATIENT

Printed postsurgical instructions, such as those which follow, should be given to every patient.

General Comments. Uneventful postoperative experiences in the past should not lull you with a sense of security from postoperative complications now or in the future.

After the extraction of one or more teeth, or other surgical procedures in the mouth, general and local treatment is necessary to prevent development of infection, or to control infection already present.

Cleanliness of the mouth and teeth, and attention to the following details are absolutely essential to this end. Faithful compliance with these instructions will help prevent postoperative complications, add to your comfort, and hasten recovery. Report promptly any condition which gives you concern.

Bleeding. Keep the gauze sponges held firmly between your jaws and over the operative site for a full half hour after the operation.

Do not use a mouthwash for 6 hours after oral surgery. Vigorous use of a mouthwash may stimulate bleeding if used before the blood clots are formed. If mild bleeding occurs, hold hot salt water in your mouth until it cools to body temperature; then fill your mouth again with hot salt water and repeat the procedure. Do this until 1 pint of hot salt water has been used.

If profuse and continued bleeding occurs, call your dentist. In the meantime, place a warm soaked tea bag over the bleeding area, cover with cotton or gauze, biting firmly for about twenty minutes. If tea is not available, soak a large wad of cotton or clean linen cloth in vinegar, place this over the bleeding area, and bite firmly into this pack, forcing it against the socket. Hold it securely for thirty minutes.

Discoloration. After the surgical procedures in your mouth, the soft tissues have been replaced and sutured in position. These sutures are necessary for good healing and to control postoperative hemorrhage. In some cases there is bleeding in spite of the sutures.

---

* Radio-iodinated serum albumin (^{131}I).

In others, bleeding into the oral cavity is prevented, but the bleeding continues for a short time beneath the tissues, and gives rise to swelling of the soft tissues of the face. This swelling is followed by discoloration. This is a perfectly normal postoperative event, and you should not be worried if this happens in your particular case.

The purplish black discoloration is the same as that seen in bruises of other parts of the body. The purplish black fades into greenish yellow, then yellow and back to normal. The discoloration will spread between the tissue layers as the muscles move and thus distribute the blood elements, which cause the discoloration. Heat in any form, such as heat lamps, electric pads, hot water bottles, and the like, should be applied to the face to aid in the dissipation of this discoloration.

Pain. Surgical operations in the highly sensitive oral cavity can be expected to produce some postoperative pain.

A prescription has been written for you. Have it filled and take the medication as needed for your pain.

Occasionally, severe pains will develop in the jaw, face or ear, from 2 days to 2 weeks after the extraction of teeth. The pain is accompanied by a bad taste in the mouth. In most cases this indicates that the blood clot in the tooth socket has decomposed, exposing the bony walls of the socket. Return for treatment of this socket to control the pain and facilitate healing.

Swelling and Stiffness. Swelling of the facial soft tissues may be due to bleeding beneath the oral tissues extending into the overlying facial tissues. It may also be due to the invasion of the tissues with the fluid and blood elements concerned in tissue healing or in the elimination of infection. To reduce ordinary immediate postoperative swelling, apply an ice cap, or towels wrung out of ice water, to the face briefly and intermittently for the first day only.

The day after operation, apply heat to your face, in any convenient form. At least 4 hours of heat should be applied to the face each day. To prevent stiffness, and to stimulate circulation, chew gum vigorously and as often as possible, so long as stiffness and swelling persist.

Sharp, Bony Projections. During the healing process small, sharp fragments of bone may loosen, and work up through the gum. These are not roots, and often work out themselves. Return for their simple removal.

Oral Hygiene. Rigid cleanliness of the oral cavity, and remaining teeth, if any, is essential. Place 0.3 gm. of oxychlorosene sodium (Kasdenol) in a glass of lukewarm water, and use as a mouthwash four times daily. This will promote healing, and destroy objectionable odors and tastes.

Remove all white film from the gums by means of a cotton applicator, or clean piece of gauze wrapped around a clean finger. The cotton applicator or gauze should be dipped in the solution described above for a mouthwash and rubbed over the gums.

Brush your teeth with a dentifrice, avoiding the operative site.

Diet. Avoid meat and food that is difficult to masticate, for a few days. Eat plenty of fruit, and drink eight to ten glasses of water, fruit juice or other fluids daily.

Supplement your diet at each mealtime by taking two multivitamin capsules immediately after each meal. These capsules contain the vitamins C and B, which are necessary for tissue repair.

Elimination. Maintain your normal time of elimination. If necessary, a mild laxative, such as milk of magnesia, may be taken.

Special Instructions.

....

....

....

....

PHYSIOLOGY OF COLD

Local cold applications produce a diminution of capillary blood flow; the number of open capillaries is decreased, tissue metabolism is reduced, and the normal rate of exchange between blood and the tissues is decreased.

A reactive hyperemia follows the application of cold with a compensatory dilatation of the cutaneous vessels. Cold applications on the skin first cause a contraction of the tissues, producing a blanching effect. This is due to the contraction of the muscular and elastic fibers of the tissues, which press the blood out from the capillaries. This constriction of the blood vessels in return affects the vascularity of the tissues subjacent to the site of application. Cold applications abstract heat from the part and lessen the sensibility of the peripheral nerve endings, thus relieving pain.

Logan Clendening, in his book on hydrotherapy, states: "Cold applications at first produce a transient anemia, later followed by considerable congestion, which is a passive hyperemia." In chilling the tissues, we impede the circulation, inhibit leukocytosis and flow of lymph to the affected part with subsequent diminution of pressure on the nerve fibers and distention of the tissues, and thereby control swelling of the part. By the same physiological process, this may inhibit healing by depriving the injured tissues of increased circulation, which we know from our pathology of inflammation is nature's response to injury and carries all the elements of regeneration and bacterial defense. Hence our applications should be brief and particularly avoided in undernourished cases where there is a diminished blood supply, as in an aged person. Cold aggravates stasis at the site of inflammation; thus prolonged use may lead to necrosis and gangrene.

The effect of cold applications on bacterial incubation is questionable, and cannot be answered scientifically. Staphylococci and streptococci will grow in a suitable environment at temperatures far lower than that to which it would be safe to expose human tissues, and are generally too deep-seated to be influenced by a direct cooling effect. If we did reduce the temperature to the point of inhibiting bacterial growth, we would materially damage the tissues, and this would be a serious factor in the ultimate healing. It is by far the best procedure to follow and maintain the physiological process. It can readily be seen that cold applications have a limited use.

Uses of Cold. Cold is used in order to minimize inflammation in all early cases of trauma in which there is no acute infection; after extraction of a tooth or teeth or after surgical removal of impacted teeth when there is no active infection; in cases of early fractures of the jaws or dislocations of the mandible; and after various surgical treatments of oral tissues, as in the removal of an abnormal frenum or epulis, and so forth. Cold controls bleeding by contracting blood vessels; hence it may prevent ecchymosis and hematoma. Trismus, or false ankylosis, is an inflammation of the muscles of mastication with edema, preventing flexibility. It may be caused by impacted or erupting third molars, intramuscular injections, or any traumatic disturbances, and may be prevented by early cold applications.

If the action of the cold, in cases of swellings for which it has been recommended, has not produced a reduction of the condition after 24 hours, heat should be applied. Cold therapy is most commonly applied in the form of ice bags, cold cloths, or cracked ice in a towel. The application should be intermittent and for periods not longer than 20 minutes, since frostbite may occur, which can lead to necrosis and gangrene. Pain may also be relieved by the evaporation of a cold solution, provided the dressings are not too thick. For this purpose a 60 per cent alcohol solution or equal parts of boric acid solution and alcohol may be applied at frequent intervals. Cold retards chemical and physiological inflammatory processes and delays suppuration, which may or may not be desirable. Applications of cold to early edemas produced by trauma cause vasoconstriction, retard swelling and are analgesic. From the foregoing usages and applications of cold, we can readily see and appreciate that cold therapy has a limited use in oral swellings and has its greatest value if used early and if the application is not too prolonged.

Cold therapy, in oral surgery, has much more limited application than heat and should be used:

1. Immediately after trauma to face or jaws to reduce swelling and minimize the accumulations of tissue fluids and exudates. *However, 24 hours postoperatively, stop the cold applications and start heat to the face or jaws from a luminous source, such as sunlight, a tungsten or carbon filament lamp.* In addition if trismus is present, have the patient start chewing gum.
2. As a postoperative procedure in odontectomy, reduction of fractures and other surgical pursuits in which infection is not a factor.
3. For relief of pain in pulpitis, facial neuralgia and other conditions.

HEAT THERAPY

Inflammation is nature's response to injury and nature's front-line defense to fight bacterial invasion and trauma. The leukocytes of the blood are the important factors in front-line defense, while the macrophages, lymph and inflammatory exudates are the secondary reinforcements.

Application of heat increases vascularity to the part, thus inducing hyperemia, nature's front-line defense. It relaxes tissues, assists absorption, localizes infection, hastens resolution, and will hasten suppuration in the presence of pathogenic infection. Local suppuration cannot be regarded as an evil in septic infection. If an inflammatory necrosis is present, certainly there is no more rapid process of getting rid of the dead soft tissues than suppurative liquefaction and elimination of the pus by surgical incision and drainage.

POSTOPERATIVE VITAMIN THERAPY

After oral surgery there is a period of diminished food intake, which lowers the body's stores of vitamin C and the B complex vitamins. The vitamin deposits of B complex as well as the plasma ascorbic acid level are reduced still further very quickly when the postoperative convalescence is aggravated by the noxious effects of fever, increased metabolism and increased diuresis. Drugs, especially the salicylates which are given for analgesia and hyperpyrexia, increase the excretion of vitamin C. When glucose infusions are given, the rate of elimination of the vitamins by way of the kidney is rapidly increased. It can readily be seen that it is essential to supplement the dietary intake with B complex vitamins and vitamin C to prevent any interference with vital biologic mechanisms or deranged metabolic functions.

Ascorbic acid is essential for the maintenance of connective tissue, bone, teeth and perhaps blood vessels.[6] If vitamin C falls to deficiency levels, wound healing may be retarded, capillary fragility increased, and important detoxication mechanisms weakened.

Thiamine itself is intimately concerned in intermediate carbohydrate metabolism and in biologic oxidation reactions.[6]

When nicotinic acid amide or compounds with similar functions are inadequate to supply the needs of the body, a state of generalized reduction in normal cellular respiration supervenes.[6]

It is the author's practice to prescribe, after oral surgery, 900 mg. of ascorbic acid, 60 mg. of thiamine hydrochloride, 30 mg. of riboflavin, and 900 mg. of niacinamide daily. This is continued, depending on the need, for a week or two.

There are several preparations on the market which contain in one tablet one sixth of the above dose. The patient is instructed to take two such tablets after each meal. When hyperemesis prevents oral intake, the parenteral route is necessary.

ANTI-INFLAMMATORY AGENTS

There has been an observable ebb and flow of interest in the anti-inflammatory effects of antihistamines, steroid agents, and enzymatic debriding compounds on tissues contiguous to the oral cavity. Hinds, in a splendid review of the later stages of the reparative phenomenon, concluded a discussion of anti-inflammatory agents by observing that there was no substitute for careful technique.[21] Snyder's finely tailored and carefully pursued clinical investigation demonstrated no appreciable effects of antihistamines on the inflammatory response following surgery.[33] There is no substitute for precise, accurate surgery for controlling excessive postoperative inflammation and for producing a sound blood clot in dental alveoli.

Alling and Kerr[3] clearly demonstrated that the early viability of the coagulum of dental alveoli was dependent on having a relatively undamaged residual periodontal membrane from which angioblasts and fibroblasts could originate to organize the clot. Alling followed this work by an elaboration of the principles into clinical applications.[2]

POSTOPERATIVE DIET

Modern clinical research has proved that proper food greatly influences the rate and completeness of recovery from burns, injuries, operations and other physiologic disturbances. Because of this fact, patients should be given special diets that emphasize protein foods — meat, milk, eggs, cheese, poultry and fish. This emphasis is made because protein foods promote healing and prevent much loss in weight. Of course, the remainder of the diet consists of vegetables, fruits, and cereals to help supply important vitamins and minerals essential in a well-balanced diet.

REFERENCES

1. Aldus, A. E. M.: Indications for tooth extractions. Ned. Tandartsenbl., *14*:379 (Oct.), 1959.
2. Alling, C. C.: Postextraction osteomyelitic syndrome. Dent. Clin. North Am., 621–636, (Nov.), 1959.
3. Alling, C. C., and Kerr, D. A.: Trauma as a factor causing delayed repair of dental extraction sites. J. Oral Surg., *15*:3–11 (Jan.), 1957.
4. Amler, M. H., Johnson, P. L., and Salman, I.: Histological and histochemical investigation of human alveolar socket healing in undisturbed extraction wounds. J.A.D.A., *61*:32–44 (July), 1960.
5. Behrman, S. J., and Wright, I. S.: Dental surgery dur-

ing continuous anticoagulant therapy. J.A.D.A., *62*:172–180 (Feb.), 1961.

6. Bondy, P. K., and Rosenberg, L. E.: Duncan's Disease of Metabolism: The Genetic and Biochemical Basis of Disease. 7th ed. Philadelphia, W. B. Saunders Co., 1974.

7. Brauer, J. C., Demeritt, W. W., Higley, L. B., Lindhal, R. L., Massler, M., and Schour, I.: Dentistry for Children. New York, McGraw-Hill Book Co., Inc., 1958.

8. Burrell, K. H., and Goepp, R. A.: Abnormal bone repair in jaws, socket sclerosis: a sign of systemic disease. J.A.D.A., *87*:1206–1215 (Nov.), 1973.

9. Cavallo, D. J.: Exodontia after irradiation of the jaws. Report of a case. J.A.D.A., *69*:551 (Nov.), 1964.

10. Collins, L. H., and Crane, M. P.: Internal Medicine in Dental Practice. 5th ed. Philadelphia, Lea & Febiger, 1960.

11. Davidson, Donald: An Analysis of One Thousand Cases of Oral Surgery during Pregnancy. Thesis, University of Pittsburgh School of Dentistry, 1951.

12. De Angella, V.: Selection of teeth for extraction as an adjunct to orthodontic treatment. J.A.D.A., *87*:610–616 (Sept.), 1973.

13. Degnan, J.: Current oral surgical opinion concerning the value of preirradiation exodontia. Oral Surg., *18*:3 (Sept.), 1964.

14. Dodson, W. S.: Irradiation osteomyelitis of the jaws. J. Oral Surg., *20*:467 (Nov.), 1962.

15. Eiseman, B., Spencer, F., and Dachi, S. F.: The role of the dentist in the diagnosis and prevention of cerebrovascular accidents. Oral Surg., *16*:1174 (Oct.), 1963.

16. Fernandez-Herlily, L.: The management of the surgical patient who has had corticosteroid therapy. Surg. Clin. North Am., *45*:589 (June), 1965.

17. Finn, S. B.: Clinical Pedodontics. 4th ed. Philadelphia, W. B. Saunders Co., 1973.

18. Frank, A. L., and Weine, F. S.: Nonsurgical therapy for the perforative defect of internal resorption. J.A.D.A., *87*:863 (Oct.), 1973.

19. Frigoletto, R. L.: Pulp therapy in periodontics. J.A.D.A., *86*:1344–1348 (June), 1973.

20. Grossman, L. I.: Bacteriologic status of periapical tissue in 150 cases of infected pulpless teeth. J. Dent. Res., *38*:101 (Jan.–Feb.), 1959.

21. Hinds, E. C.: Control of postoperative edema. J. Oral Surg., *16*:109–118 (Mar.), 1958.

22. McIntyre, H., Nour-Eldin, F., Israels, M. C. G., and Wilkinson, J. F.: Dental extractions in patients with haemophilia and Christmas disease. Lancet, *7104*:642–646 (Oct.), 1959.

23. Meyer, R. A.: Blood volume considerations in oral surgery. J. Oral Surg., *29*:617 (Sept.), 1971.

24. Neumann, B.: Planned serial extractions in orthodontic treatment. Cesk. Stomatol., *60*:371–381 (Sept.), 1960.

25. Rhymes, R.: Natal teeth. Oral Surg., *18*:541 (Oct.), 1964.

26. Rhymes, R., and Williams, C.: Blood loss following extraction of teeth. J.A.D.A., *69*:347 (Sept.), 1964.

27. Rominger, C. J., Looby, J. and Duncan J.: Role of alveolectomy in the prevention of radionecrosis of the jaws and oral soft tissues; report of case. J. Oral Surg., *20*:72 (Jan.), 1962.

28. Sakellarious, P. L.: Replantation of infected deciduous teeth: A contribution to the problem of their preservation until normal shedding, preliminary report. Oral Surg., *16*:645 (June), 1963.

29. Schmuth, G.: Serial tooth extraction, an orthodontic procedure. Med. Klin., *54*:1833 (Oct.). 1959.

30. Shira, R. B., Hall, R. J., and Guernsey, L. H.: Minor oral surgery during prolonged anticoagulant therapy. J. Oral Surg., *20*:94 (Mar.). 1962.

31. Simpson, H. E.: The reattachment of mucoperiosteal flaps in surgical extraction wounds in macacus rhesus monkeys. Aust. Dent. J., *4*:86–89 (Apr.). 1959.

32. Sleeper, E. L.: Prophylactic dental treatment prior to irradiation of jaws. Alpha Omegan, *44*:101 (Sept.). 1950.

33. Snyder, B. S.: Effect of antihistaminic agents on inflammatory response following surgical trauma. J. Oral Surg., *18*:319–326 (July), 1960.

34. Tainter, M. L., et al.: Alleged hemostatic action of gelatin, coagulen, fibrogen and histidine administered by mouth. J.A.D.A., *26*:420, 1939.

35. Thoma, K. H., and Goldman, H. M.: Oral Pathology, 5th ed. St. Louis, The C. V. Mosby Co., 1960.

36. Wallace, J. R.: Erupted mandibular central incisors in a newborn infant. Oral Surg., *16*:501 (Apr.). 1963.

CHAPTER 3

ORAL SURGERY FOR DENTAL PROSTHESIS

Oral surgery for dental prosthesis includes those surgical operations in the oral cavity which are necessary in order that the artificial denture may rest upon a firm base, free from marked osseous protuberances or undercuts, and devoid of interfering muscle attachments, excess mucoperiosteum, hyperplasias, and fibrous or papillary growths. This surgery includes the removal of both hard and soft tissues. It also includes those oral or extraoral operations which are indicated for the restoration of lost bone.

Whole alveoplasty by definition is: "The surgical alteration of the shape and condition of the alveolar process, in preparation for immediate or future denture contruction."* This term, unfortunately frequently used today, has the additional meaning of including soft tissue plastic surgery designed to correct inadequate ridges by increasing the sulces height on the maxilla and depth on the mandible. These procedures should be called vestibuloplasty, as described by Obwegeser, MacIntosh and others. They list five commonly used procedures for ridge extension in the upper arch. These are (1) the submucosal vestibuloplasty, (2) the secondary epithelialization vestibuloplasty, (3) the alveolar ridge skin grafting vestibuloplasty, (4) the buccal sulcus skin grafting vestibuloplasty (buccal inlay procedure — Dewel uses mucosa from the palate for his labial inlay grafting, as will be described later), and (5) the tuberoplasty. Each of these procedures has its particular indications and limitations.

In previous editions of this book I have discussed and described the use of subperiosteal implants. I have eliminated this material from this edition because I believe that with the

present state of knowledge of both subperiosteal and endosseous implants, they are both doomed to failure.

TYPES OF ORAL OR EXTRAORAL PROSTHETIC SURGICAL PROCEDURES

OPERATIONS IN THE ORAL CAVITY

Operations in the oral cavity are concerned with (1) soft tissue hyperplasias, cartilage-like tissue, fibromatoses, muscles, and fibrous bands which interfere with the placing of a denture and with its retention, and (2) osseous tissue abnormalities of the denture-bearing areas.

Abnormalities of Soft Tissues. The soft tissues that interfere most with the placing of dentures on the maxilla are the low insertion or hypertrophy of the labial frenum, as well as the low attachments or hypertrophy of the depressor septi, incisivi labii superioris, nasalis, alar part, and the buccinator muscles (see Figure 3–5). In addition, there may be interfering bands of fibrous scar tissue present, resulting from trauma or infection of the contiguous soft tissues of the jaws. Hyperplasias in the labial or buccal sulci, on the crest of the ridges or on the hard or soft palate are frequently seen in patients who have worn poorly fitting dentures for many years.

On the mandible, interference with satisfactory denture construction will result from the high attachments or hypertrophy of the lingual frenum and the genioglossus, mentalis, incisivi labii inferioris and buccinator muscles. Hyperplasias and fibrous scar tissue bands similar to those seen on the maxilla may also be present on the mandible.

Abnormalities of Osseous Tissue. Among the abnormalities in this category are those

---

*Dorland's Illustrated Medical Dictionary. 25th ed. Philadelphia, W. B. Saunders Co., 1974.

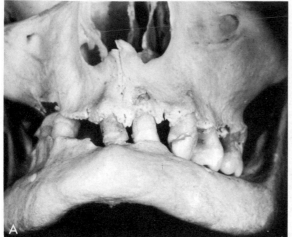

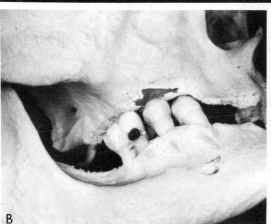

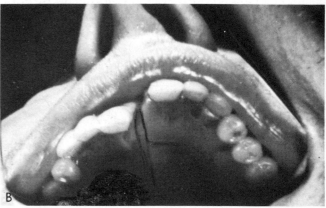

Figure 3–1 In these days of great concern about "balanced occlusion," it is of interest to study the "occlusion" in the three views of this anatomic specimen. One can surmise that this patient did not suffer any of the so-called "malocclusion maladies" one hears so much about today; otherwise he or she would have sought relief.

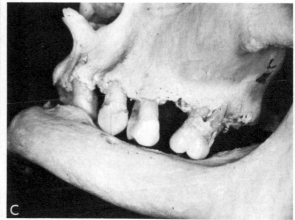

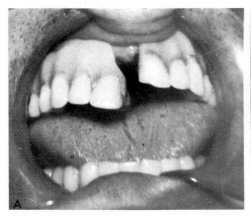

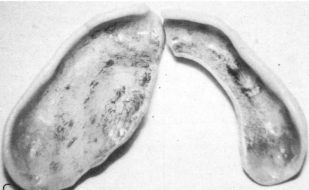

Figure 3–2 This middle-aged male patient had been satisfactorily masticating his food with this broken maxillary denture for 3 years at the time this photograph was taken. We discovered him during the routine dental examinations made of all patients admitted to a government hospital. He had no dental complaints. He proved his ability to eat by chewing peanuts and eating an apple!

This is just another proof of the statement that 90 per cent of the successful use of artificial dentures rests with the patient.

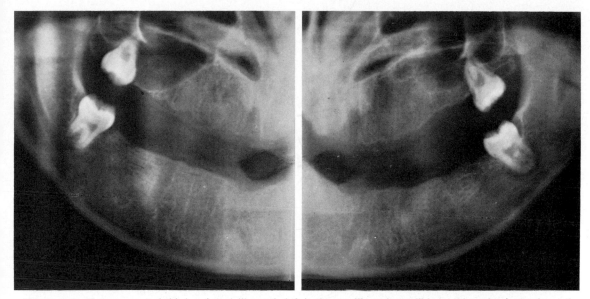

Figure 3–3 Four unerupted third molars deliberately left in the maxilla and mandible by this patient's dentist at the time the remaining teeth were extracted and dentures were made. As they gradually erupted the patient "relieved" the sore spots himself. At present all third molars are erupted and in occlusion. The patient claims that he now can masticate better than ever and has less trouble with the stability of his dentures than before the molars erupted. It was our opinion that there was, at this time, no justification for the extraction of the third molars.

We did suggest a rebasing of the dentures and pointed out that this should be done periodically so that the "occlusion" of the dentures and his third molars would be the same. This was received with skepticism by the patient, as he was "getting along fine" even though there was not the "normal" occlusion that we indicated was necessary. Theoretically, what we recommended was correct, but to the patient, it was not needed.

variations in the height of the alveolar ridge due to the extraction of the maxillary and/or mandibular teeth in small groups or singly at different periods during the patient's lifetime. The time variation between extractions results in greater or less disuse atrophy of the alveolar ridge and, when all the teeth are lost, there is a so-called "roller-coaster ridge" of "hills and valleys."

On examining the edentulous maxilla and

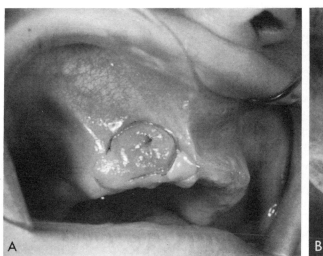
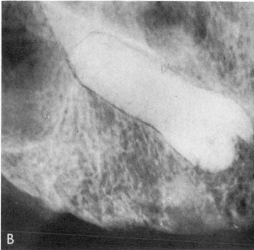

Figure 3–4 *A*, Hyperplastic pyogenic tissue as the result of trauma produced by the denture flange on the soft mucoperiosteal tissue over the hard labial surface of the retained maxillary cuspid. While usually it is the resorption of the alveolar crest that creates the opportunity for the compression and injury of the mucoperiosteal tissue between the tooth crown and the denture, this is an example of how labial resorption can produce the environment for the damage described in this case. Removal of the cuspid (*B*) is mandatory.

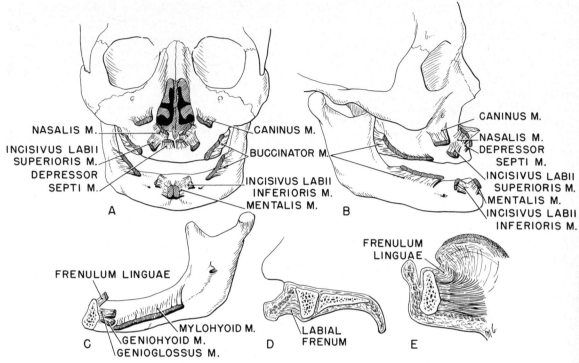

Figure 3–5 Muscle and frenum origins which may interfere with the insertion or stability of artificial dentures.

mandible and finding rounded projections, "hills and valleys" which appear to be osseous structures, keep in mind the possibility that there is contained within the maxillary or mandibular ridge either an unerupted tooth such as an impacted third molar or a cuspid, a cementoma or an intermedullary enostosis. These rounded projections do not resorb as does the surrounding alveolar process; therefore, they stand out prominently on the ridges.

The author has heard some dentists state that they do not believe in the removal of unerupted third molars at the time the remaining erupted teeth are extracted. They claim that the removal of the maxillary unerupted third molars will result in a collapse of the tuberosity, and so they leave the maxillary third molars present with the idea that they will form a good maxillary tuberosity to aid in the retention and support of the maxillary denture. While this reasoning sounds good from a theoretical standpoint, from a practical standpoint, the alveolar bone which has surrounded the maxillary unerupted third molars gradually resorbs under the denture and eventually the

only thing which separates the maxillary third molar from actually contacting the maxillary denture is the thin mucoperiosteal membrane. This very quickly becomes traumatized, inflamed, and infected, and subsequently the patient develops a subperiosteal abscess which can and frequently does extend up into the soft tissues of the cheek, producing cellulitis.

Generalized exostoses that produce deep undercuts on either the maxilla or the mandible, usually in the form of gingival cortical beads extending entirely around the necks of the maxillary or mandibular teeth, require reduction. There may be multiple exostoses or osteomas present on the cortical bone. On the palate there may be the various forms of torus palatinus or, lingual to the maxillary molars, small or large single or multiple osteomas. Prognathism or a marked overbite or overjet may be present in the premaxillary region as a result of the gradual protrusion of the anterior teeth over a prolonged period of time.

On the mandible, in addition to the above-enumerated abnormalities, there may be mandibular tori consisting of single or multiple osseous eminences projecting from the lingual cortical plate, generally in the cuspid and bicuspid regions. Frequently there is a marked sharp lingual projection involved in the second and third molar regions of the mandible; this has been termed the "mandibular balcony." Sharp "saw-toothed" or "knife-edged" ridges on the edentulous or partially edentulous mandible are often found. The genial tubercles, multiple or single, may encroach on the denture-bearing area and have to be removed, with subsequent replacement of the genioglossus and geniohyoid muscles. However, if a patient has been satisfactorily wearing a full lower denture without irritation of the soft tissues, there is no indication for the excision of genial tubercles no matter how large.

Before any surgery is undertaken on the edentulous mandible or maxilla, a complete radiographic examination should be made of both jaws. This is to rule out the possibility of the presence of retained roots, teeth, residual infection, cysts or tumors.

Other surgical procedures which fall into this classification are: (*a*) Surgery necessary for the insertion of immediate dentures either maxillary or mandibular or both (alveoplasty). (*b*) The insertion of experimental devices, with the *patient's informed consent,* to support and retain dentures. (*c*) The transplantation of developing teeth. (*d*) Excision of tissue which prevents the normal eruption or position of teeth.

EXTRAORAL OPERATIONS

Extraoral operations include: (*a*) surgery to correct prognathia or micrognathia of the mandible or maxilla; (*b*) insertion of bone grafts or metal or acrylic implants to replace bone loss due to disease or trauma.

REMOVAL OF LABIAL FRENUM (FRENECTOMY)

REMOVAL OF A HYPERTROPHIED LABIAL FRENUM ATTACHED TO THE CREST OF THE RIDGE PRIOR TO CONSTRUCTION OF A MAXILLARY DENTURE

The following technique is illustrated in Figure 3–7.

As seen in Figure 3–7*A*, there is low attachment of the labial frenum. If local anesthesia is used, infiltrate into the labial frenum at its origin and insertion. Inject slowly, using 0.5 cc. at each point. Wait five minutes for anesthesia.

Raise the lip (Fig. 3–7*B*), and place a hemostat parallel to the labial surface of the alveolar ridge and in contact with the mucosa covering the labial surface of the alveolar process up to the mucolabial fold. Lock the hemostat on the fibers of the frenum. Pull the lip up and out until it is at a right angle to the labial surface of the alveolar process. Place a second hemostat parallel to the lifted and pulled-out lip (at a right angle to the first hemostat) and lock this hemostat over the fibers of the frenum where these fibers enter the lip, extending the beaks of the hemostat to the mucolabial fold.

The tips of the beaks of the two hemostats should now touch each other (Fig. 3–7*C*), and the labial frenum caught between them then forms an inverted V. The assistant holds the hemostats absolutely still—*no traction!*

With a sharp No. 11 Bard-Parker blade cut around the outside surfaces of the two hemostats (Fig. 3–7*D* and *E*), so that when the cut is completed the two hemostats fall away with the tissue of the frenum between them. The lateral margins of the surgical wound are now undermined by means of surgical scissors or a

Figure 3–6 Low insertion of a hypertrophied labial frenum chronically inflamed as the result of trauma from the labial flange of the denture. Treatment indicated is a labial frenectomy. See Figure 3–7.

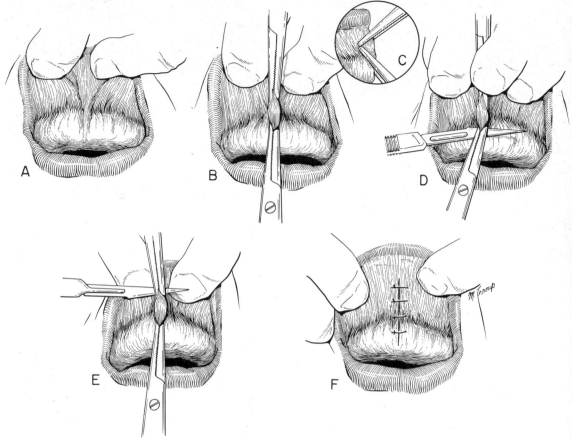

Figure 3–7   Labial frenectomy. Study the text for explanation.

straight hemostat. This will permit a sliding movement of the mucosa so that it can be approximated and sutured without tension. If the cut were made on the inside of the two hemostats, between them, bruised and crushed tissue would be left behind after the hemostats were removed. This damaged tissue would then be subject to sloughing, infection, slow healing, and weak margins through which the suture material could slip and cut, thus failing to hold the edges of the incision together until healing takes place.

For these reasons, always cut outside of the two hemostats.

Place sutures as shown in Figure 3–7F, after the mucosa of the lip has been undermined and freed. When placing sutures on the inside of the lip, be sure that the mucous glands are covered by mucous membrane.

Place several thicknesses of 1-inch iodoform gauze between the labial surface of the alveolar ridge and the lip. Instruct the patient to keep this gauze dressing in place for 2 hours. After the removal of gauze, have the patient rinse his mouth every hour with a mouthwash.

REMOVAL OF LABIAL FRENUM AS AN AID IN ORTHODONTIC TREATMENT OR TO CORRECT DIASTEMA OF THE MAXILLARY CENTRAL INCISORS

Diastemas of the Central Incisors. The labial frenum, which attaches the lip to the alveolar process, usually recedes from its original insertion into the nasopalatine papilla (palatal papilla) by the time the permanent central incisors erupt. When this does not take place, a diastema results between the permanent central incisors. Moyers[42] lists this malposed frenum along with six other causes (Table 3–1) present in 82 patients "who were referred for examination with the *primary complaint of excessive spacing* between the maxillary central incisors."

Because prominent orthodontists have referred to the "few separated central incisors in adults as compared to children," and because

(Text continued on page 146)

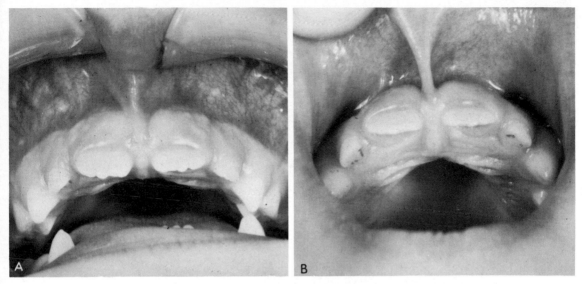

Figure 3–8 *A*, A 6-year-old with a typical broad, thick labial frenum that is inserted through the interproximal tissue and into the nasopalatine papilla. *B*, This is proved by the blanching of these tissues when traction is made on the frenum by pulling the lip up to stretch the frenum.

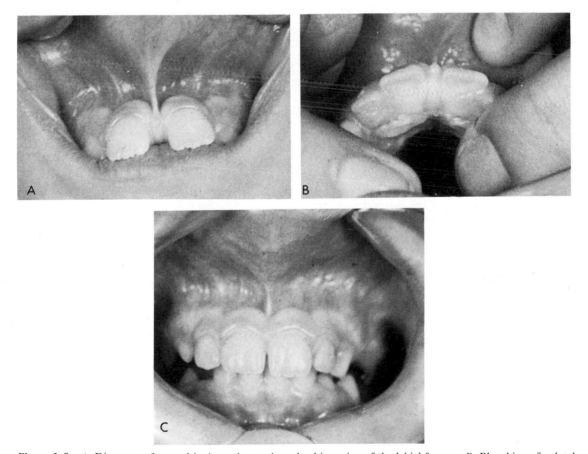

Figure 3–9 *A*, Diastema of central incisors due to the palatal insertion of the labial frenum. *B*, Blanching of palatal tissues when tension is applied to lip, proving that the diastema is due to the labial frenum. *C*, Six months after labial frenectomy the diastema has closed. See Figure 3–10 for the technique to be used in cases of diastema of the permanent central incisors.

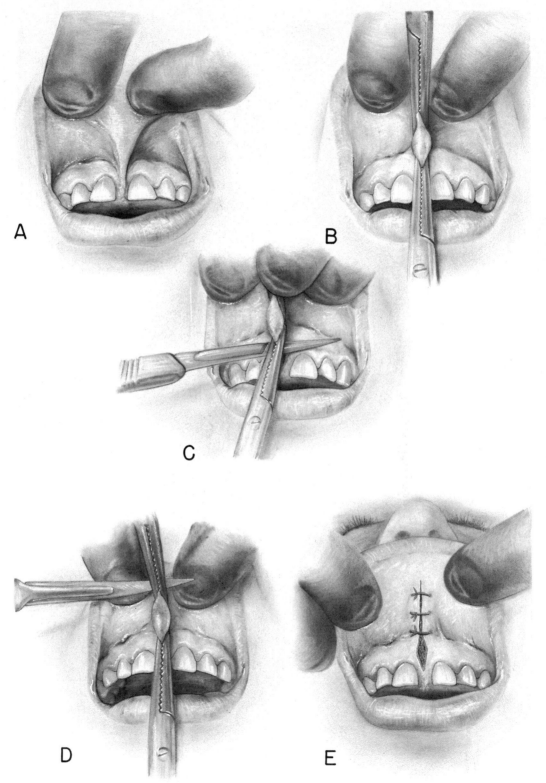

Figure 3–10   Technique of labial frenectomy. Study the text for explanation.

(Figure 3–10 continued on opposite page)

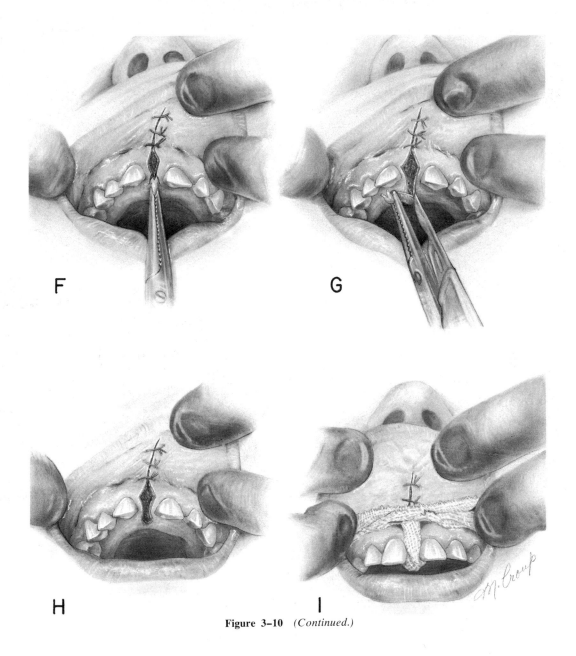

Figure 3–10 *(Continued.)*

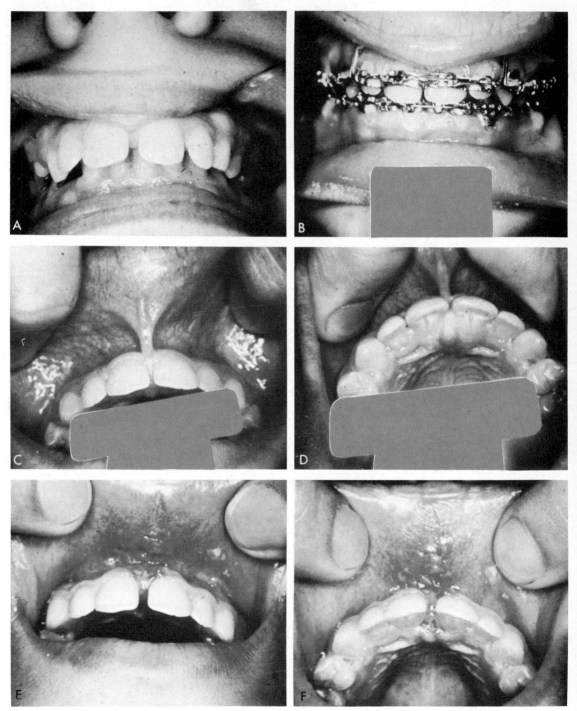

Figure 3–11   *A*, Diastema of the maxillary central incisors in a 14-year-old. *B*, Diastema closed with orthodontic appliance. *C*, Three months after removal of appliance, diastema returned. Twice more the diastema was closed and it reopened. *D*, It is very obvious that the thick, broad malpositioned labial frenum shown in *C* and *D* is the original cause of the diastema, and it will continue to produce the diastema until it is surgically removed. The statement has frequently been made in the orthodontic literature that the process of mechanically closing the maxillary central incisors will crush and destroy the fibers in the labial frenum as they pass between the incisors. I have never seen it happen. *E* and *F*, Two weeks following the surgical excision of the frenum.

(*Figure 3–11 continued on opposite page*)

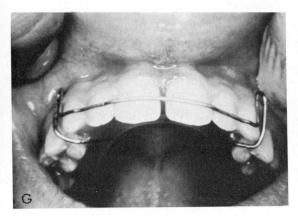

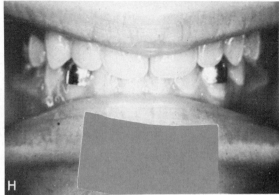

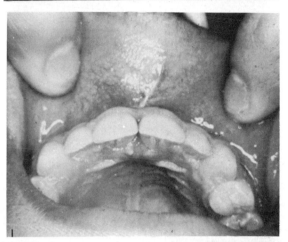

Figure 3–11 (*Continued.*) *G*, The diastema is once more closed mechanically. *H* and *I*, Central incisors now remain in contact. The diastema is closed.

In this patient and older ones presenting with a diastema due to a frenum such as this, it is necessary to excise the frenum and then mechanically close the diastema.

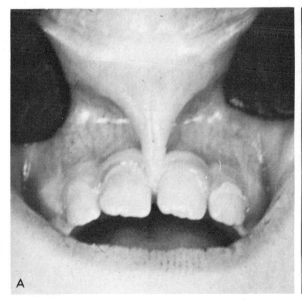

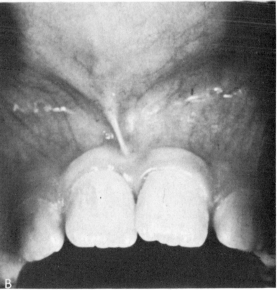

Figure 3–12 *A*, An excellent example of a hypertrophied, broad, thick labial frenum in an 11-year-old whose four maxillary incisors were all fully erupted. Her parents were advised that this "space" would be closed by the eruption of all her "front" teeth. This is by no means a certainty. Furthermore, in our experience and in that of others, if there is interseptal blanching and blanching of nasopalatine papilla when the upper lip is pulled up and out, as illustrated in this figure, surgical excision of the frenum and its extension through the interseptal space is indicated, even though the cuspids have not erupted. A distema due to a frenum such as the one illustrated here, or one even smaller, will not be closed by the eruption of the permanent maxillary cuspids. Figure 3–11 is an example. *B*, Six months after surgical excision of the frenum, the diastema has closed spontaneously. In fact, there is even a slight overlap at the mesial incisal angle.

Table 3-1   *Diastema of the Central Incisors**

CAUSES	NUMBER OF CASES	PER CENT OF CASES
Supernumerary teeth at the midline	3	3.7
Congenitally missing lateral incisors	9	11.0
Unusually small teeth	2	2.4
Malposed labial frenum	20	24.4
Spacing a normal part of the growth process	19	23.2
Incomplete fusion of the median palatine process	27	32.9
Incomplete fusion of the median palatine process plus congenitally missing lateral incisors	2	2.4
		100.0

*From Moyers, R.: Spacing between the maxillary central incisors. Alpha Omegan, 46:80–82, 1952.

statistics on the actual incidence of diastemas in adults have not been available in the literature, such a survey has been made.* In this survey the incidence of diastemas between the maxillary central incisors of 5253 black adults was found to be 9.7 per cent.† The incidence in 8350 white dental students was 15.49 per cent.‡ The lowest incidence was found in East Indians, 5.48 per cent.†

Our surgical clinical experience, supported by that of others, has proved that these "smile-ruining gaps" could have been prevented during their childhood in the 24.4 per cent of the 82 patients found in Moyers's survey. This could have been accomplished by the comparatively simple surgical procedure of excising the abnormal malpositioned labial frenums, together with their interproximal tissue, as described below and illustrated in Figures 3–7, 3–10 and 3–13.

In some cases the diastema closes spontaneously when the lateral incisors erupt, creating medial pressure on the central incisors. If this does not occur and other possible causes of a diastema, such as the presence of supernumerary teeth (mesiodens), malocclusion or tongue pressure, are eliminated, then if tension of the lip and its frenum produces ischemia in the area of the nasopalatine papilla (Fig. 3–9), the frenum, which is usually hypertrophied, and its attachment into the papilla should be carefully excised.

Technique for Excision of a Hypertrophied Labial Frenum.   The technique for frenectomy in a case of diastema is the same as that in fitting a denture, described on pages 139 to 140 and illustrated in Figure 3–7A to E. These steps are again illustrated in Figure 3–10, and beginning with step F, are varied in the following way:

Cut a V-shaped wedge of mucoperiosteum from between the central incisors down to the interseptal bone (Fig. 3–10F and G). Remove this tissue from the interseptal space. Be careful that the necks of the teeth are not exposed.

If the space between the central incisors is great enough, a rectangular piece of mucoperiosteum is removed. In both cases, the tissue should extend 3 mm. behind the linguogingival periphery of the central incisors, *down to the bone,* and also should extend labially for 5 mm. (Fig. 3–10H).

Pack this trench between the central incisors with iodoform gauze into which has been spatulated a thick paste of zinc oxide and eugenol (Fig. 3–10I). Instruct the patient to keep this packing in position for 5 days. This prevents a bridging in of tissue into this space. Place several layers of 1-inch iodoform gauze between the labial surface of the alveolar ridge and the lip. Leave in for 2 hours. Patient is to rinse mouth as described before.

---

*Archer, W. H., and Hayden, C. L.: Incidence of diastema of the central incisors. Int. Assoc. Dent. Res. Abstr., 119, 1970. Paper presented at the International Association for Dental Research, 48th General Meeting, March 16–19, 1970.

†Survey supervised by the author and Cedric L. Haydn at the Port of Spain Community Hospital, Trinidad.

‡The following schools cooperated in this study: University of Alabama, Loma Linda University, University of California, University of Southern California, Georgetown University, Emory University, Loyola University of Chicago, Northwestern University, Indiana University, University of Iowa, University of Louisville, University of Maryland, Tufts University, Creighton University, University of Nebraska, Fairleigh Dickinson University, New Jersey College of Medicine and Dentistry, Columbia University, State University of New York at Buffalo, Ohio State University, Case Western Reserve, University of Oregon, University of Pittsburgh, Meharry Medical College, University of Washington, West Virginia University, University of Puerto Rico, Dalhousie University, University of Toronto, McGill University, University of Montreal.

REPOSITIONING THE ATTACHMENT OF THE DEPRESSOR SEPTI MUSCLE

A large, wide hypertrophied depressor septi muscle that has its origin in the interproximal space between the central incisors and whose fibers fan out widely and are interwoven with the red zone of the orbicularis oris muscle, as

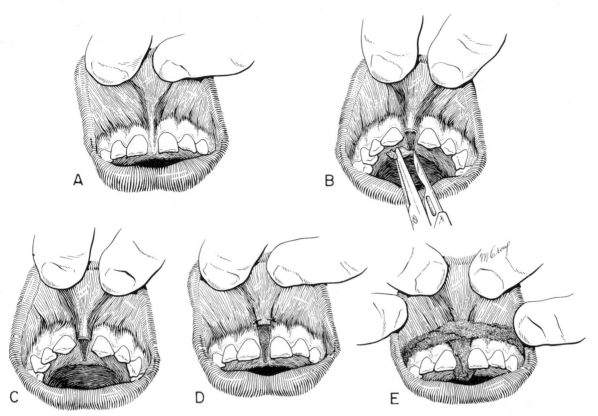

Figure 3-13 Repositioning the origin of the depressor septi muscle. (See text for description of technique.)
Note: See the photographic case report in Chapter 22 (Figure 22-29), which illustrates the surgical technique of osteotomy to close diastemas such as that illustrated in Figure 3-14A in adults.

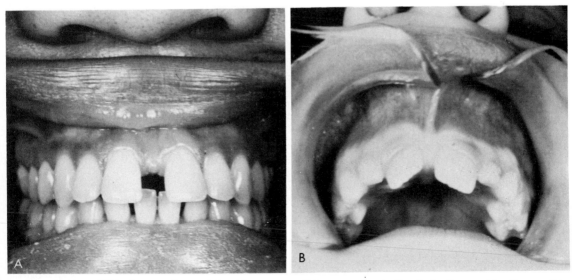

Figure 3-14 *A,* Wide diastema in an adult with a very small frenum under the lip. *B,* An 8-year-old with a small labial frenum inserted into the mucoperiosteal membrane high on the labial surface. Obviously these diastemas were not produced by the frenum.

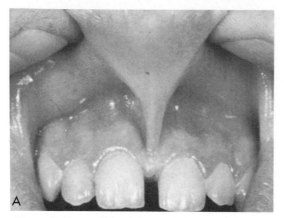

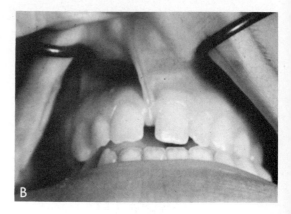

Figure 3–15   *A,* This 18-year-old girl, when a youngster, was told that her front teeth would come together when her "eyeteeth came in." When this prophecy failed to come true, she was referred to have the frenum "clipped." In addition to, and below, the frenum is a large broad depressor septi muscle which should be repositioned as shown in Figure 3–13. However, the diastema will not, at this age, close spontaneously after surgery because the maxillary teeth have all erupted. Surgery will aid the orthodontic procedure now necessary to close this space.

B, A 20-year-old who had been advised in the same manner as *A.*

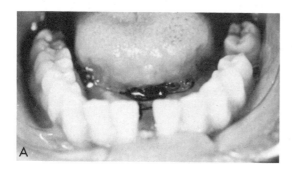

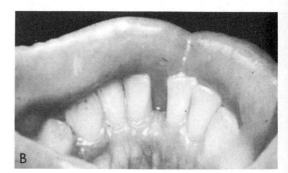

Figure 3–16   *A,* An example of the comparatively rare diastema of the mandibular central incisors. *B,* Lingual view. No lingual frenum.

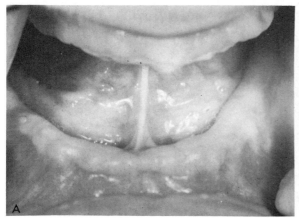

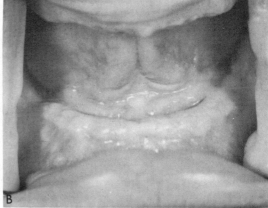

Figure 3–17   *A,* Short, fibrous lingual frenum with its origin near the crest of the alveolar ridge. This obviously would interfere with the seating of the lingual denture flange unless the flange was deeply notched. *B,* Postoperative appearance of the case shown in *A,* showing the free lingual space obtained for the lingual flange of the denture.

is shown in Figure 3–12, should have its alveolar attachments repositioned. The reason a portion of the muscle is not resected (*i.e.*, myotomy performed) is that the contour of the lip may be changed. The technique for repositioning is illustrated in Figure 3–13.

In Figure 3–13*A* is shown the fusion of the muscle fibers with the dense collagenous tissue that extends between the central incisors. This dense collagenous tissue is dissected free from between the central incisors down to the crest of the interseptal osseous tissue from the labial to the lingual side, as shown in Figure 3–13*B*. Vertical cuts are now made alongside the origin of the depressor septi muscle, as shown in Figure 3–13*C*. The origin of this muscle is then sharply dissected away from the labial cortical bone, freed and elevated until the cut edge reaches the labial sulcus. Here it is sutured to the deep periosteum, as shown in Figure 3–13*D*. Strips of iodoform gauze are placed between the central incisors and along the labial sulcus (Figure 3–13*E*) and held in position for at least an hour.

In edentulous cases, in which such a muscle would interfere greatly with satisfactory denture retention and functioning, the muscle is repositioned as described, but it is not necessary to dissect out the dense collagenous tissue across the crest of the ridge.

ANKYLOTOMY (LINGUAL FRENOTOMY) FOR ANKYLOGLOSSIA

Ankyloglossia. Ankyloglossia (tongue-tie) is caused by an abnormally short frenum and/or genioglossus muscle which markedly restricts the range of motion of the tongue. This results in speech defects. Figure 3–20*A* is a drawing of an actual case of ankyloglossia in a girl who had great difficulty in talking.

Edentulous patients with ankyloglossia not only have speech defects but the short frenum or genioglossus muscle has its origin at or near the crest of the mandibular ridge, and this prevents seating and retention of the mandibular denture during speech or mastication.

As indicated above, a short, fibrous frenum alone can produce ankyloglossia. This is demonstrated in Figure 3–17*A* in an edentulous patient. Figure 3–17*B* shows the postoperative result.

Occasionally cases of tongue-tie are the result of both a short lingual frenum and a short genioglossus muscle, as shown in Figure 3–18. In this situation, not only must the frenum be cut but a myotomy of the genioglossus muscle is also necessary to free the tongue.

Technique for Ankylotomy. Anesthesia can be local or general. If local anesthesia is selected, bilateral blocking of the lingual nerve is required. Local infiltration of anesthetic solution distorts the tissues, thus preventing an accurate line of incision. After anesthesia is secured (tip of the tongue is numb), the mouth is propped open and a suture is passed through the midline of the tongue ¼ inch from the tip to hold the tongue up during the operation. The short, fibrous lingual frenum and/or genioglossus muscle is made taut by upward traction on the tongue suture; with sharp, straight scissors it is cut midway between the tip of the tongue and its origin, the lingual surface of the symphysis of the mandible (see Figure 3–20*B*). The cut is directed posteriorly parallel to the floor of the oral cavity for a distance of 1½ to 3 inches, or until the tip of the tongue can touch the lingual surfaces of the maxillary anterior teeth with the mouth open. Cutting the lingual frenum along this line will prevent trauma to the salivary carunculae and submaxillary ducts which are, and should always be, below the cutting edges of the scissors.

If necessary, transect the genioglossus muscle in addition to the lingual frenum.

The lateral edges of the surgical incision are undermined with the scissors. With 000 black silk suture on a curved needle, approximate the cut edges of mucosa in the floor of the mouth and on the under surface of the tongue. Thus, the horizontal incision becomes a vertical one. Use interrupted sutures, ½ inch apart. In Figure 3–20*D* is shown the frenum of the tongue after ankylotomy. Many of these patients still need speech therapy to correct the faulty diction which they have developed.

If ankyloglossia is present in edentulous mouths, exactly the same technique of lingual frenotomy as described above is carried out.

CORRECTING INADEQUATE MAXILLARY AND MANDIBULAR SULCI

There are three factors that may result in the reduction or obliteration of the mandibular or maxillary sulcus: (*a*) resorption of the alveolar process (the most frequent cause); (*b*) abnormally high muscle attachments on the mandible or low on the maxilla; and (*c*) scar tissue resulting from trauma to or infection of the contiguous soft tissues of the jaws.

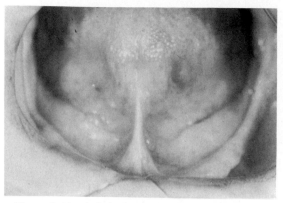

Figure 3–18 Ankyloglossia due to shortness of both lingual frenum and genioglossus muscle.

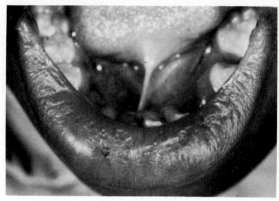

Figure 3–19 Short lingual frenum in a 10-year-old who had a pronounced speech defect.

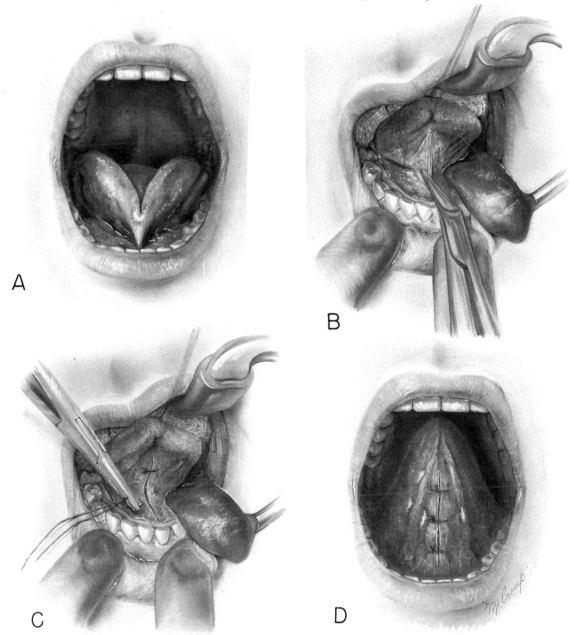

A

B

C

D

Figure 3–20 Ankylotomy for ankyloglossia. *A*, Drawing of a severe tongue-tie in an 18-year-old female which made normal speech impossible. (See text for description of technique.)

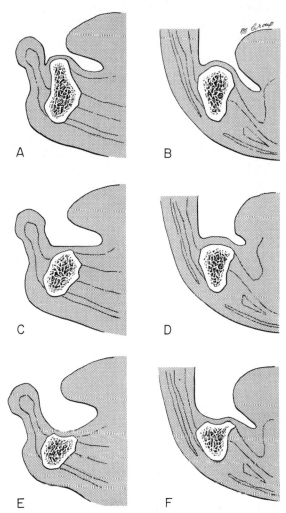

A

B

C

D

E

F

Figure 3–21 Variation in level of mandibular sulcus and condition of alveolar ridge. (See text.)

It can usually be determined by digital examination of the mandible whether or not there is adequate alveolar process remaining, as shown in the cross section of the mandible in the anterior region in Figure 3–21A and the molar region in Figure 3–21B, that will permit a successful sulcus-deepening operation. In Figure 3–21C and D it is obvious that a considerable portion of the alveolar ridge has been resorbed. However, it is possible to deepen somewhat the sulcus both anteriorly and buccally when this much alveolar process remains, though it is impossible to deepen the sulcus in either the anterior region or molar area shown in Figure 3–21E and F. The alveolar process in both of these drawings has been completely resorbed, and we have an atrophied mandible in which the mental foramen is probably on the crest of the ridge in the bicuspid area.

VESTIBULOPLASTY WITH SECONDARY EPITHELIALIZATION

Technique for Deepening the Mandibular Sulcus. On the mandible, the muscles whose origins most frequently interfere with the placing of conventional dentures, or at least the construction of an adequate flange labially and buccally on a lower denture, are, beginning at the midline, the mentalis muscle, the inferior incisor muscle (also known as the incisivus labii inferioris) and the buccinator muscles. It is usually muscles in the anterior region of the mandible that give trouble.

The technique for the removal of these

(*Text continued on page 155*)

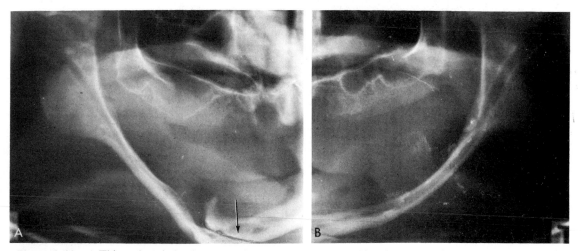

A B

Figure 3–22 *A*, This patient, in her late seventies, "just bumped" her chin. The arrow points to the overriding of the right and left fragments of the fracture. *B*, The corpus of this mandible was nothing but cortical bone with the inferior canal between.

EXCISION OF SHARP RESIDUAL ALVEOLAR BONE, DEEPENING OF THE ANTERIOR MANDIBULAR SULCUS, AND LOWERING OF THE MENTAL INFERIOR NEUROVASCULAR BUNDLES

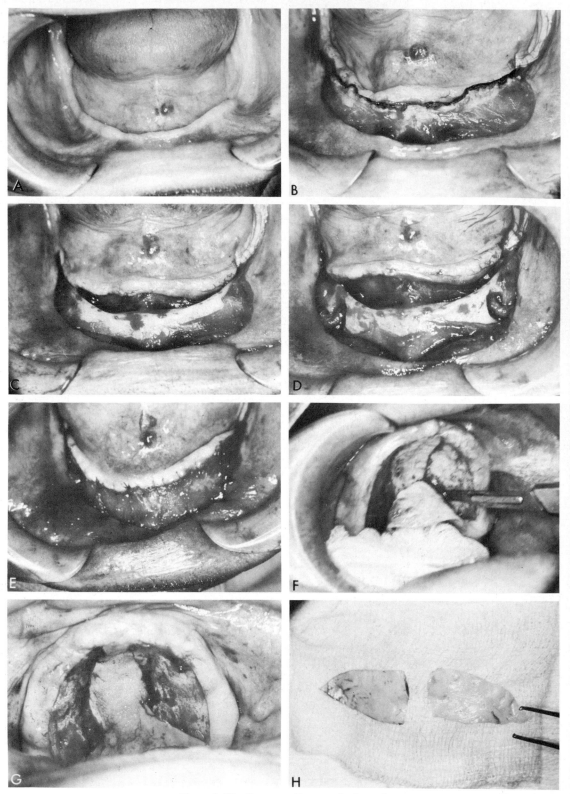

Figure 3–23   *See opposite page for legend.*

(Figure 3–23 continued on opposite page)

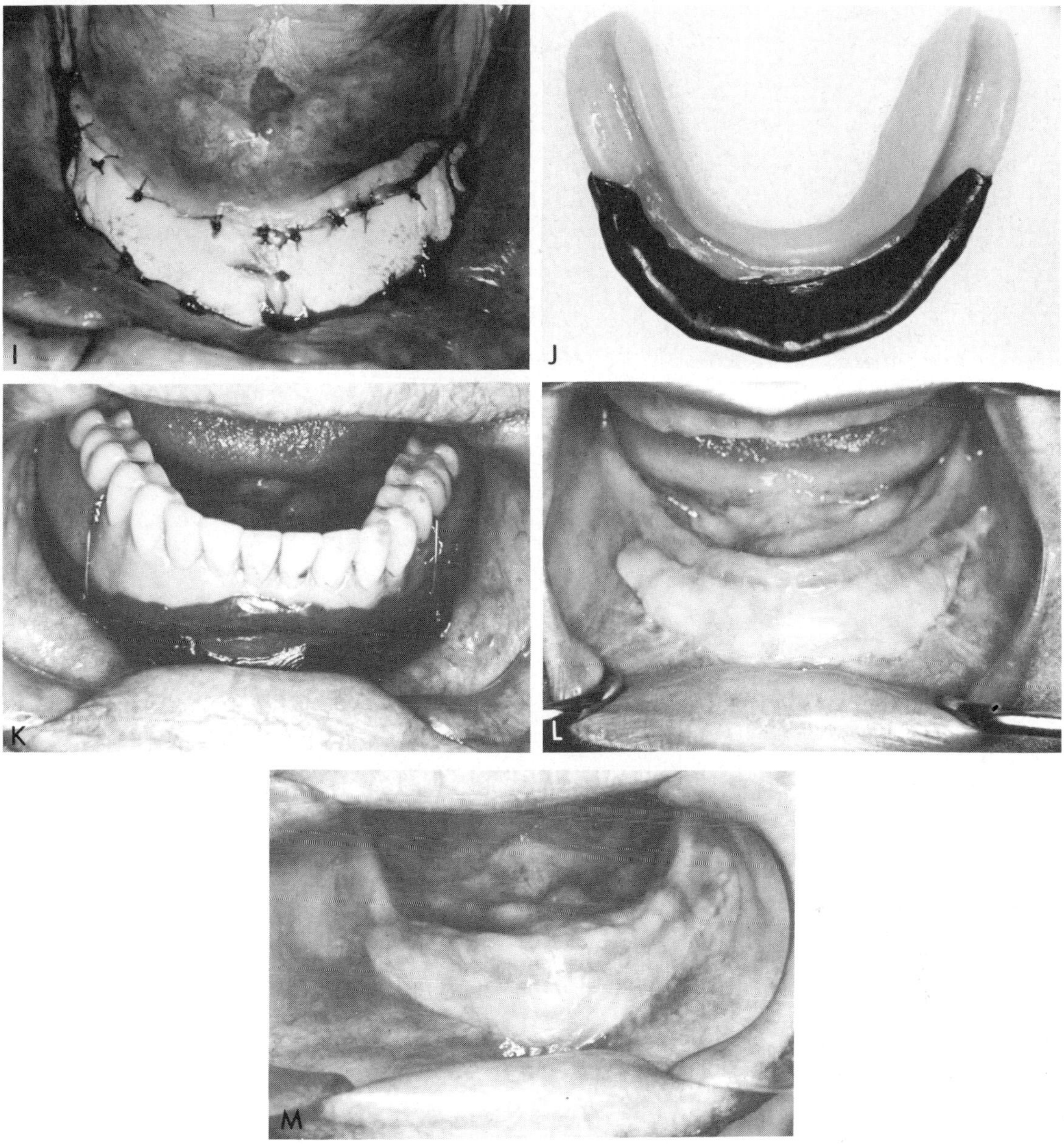

Figure 3–23 (*Continued.*)

Figure 3–23 *A*, This case illustrates extensive loss of the vestibule in the anterior area of the edentulous mandible. In addition, the patient reported intense pain during mastication for which the inner surface of the denture had been relieved in the area of the crest of the ridge.

B, The mucoperiosteal tissue was reflected from the sharp irregular crest of the ridge with extreme difficulty.

C, The thin sharp irregular osseous projections were excised with bone shears and the ridge rounded and smoothed with rotary files and diamond stones.

D, Bilaterally the mental foramens were enlarged laterally and inferiorly to lower the mental neurovascular bundles to prevent the denture flanges creating painful pressure on the mental nerves.

E, The lingual mucoperiosteal tissue is folded down over the crest of the rounded bone and sutured to the periosteum. The labial mucosa is sutured to the periosteum deep in the new sulcus.

F, A mucosal split thickness graft is removed from the palate.

G, The palatal bilateral sites from which the two grafts were secured for the labial inlay technique.

H, The size and shape of the two grafts.

I, Grafts sutured to place.

J, Compound addition to the labial flange of the mandibular denture to hold the grafts against the periosteum without producing pressure necrosis.

K, Mandibular denture held in place by circumferential wires for about a week.

L, Graft 3 weeks later. No denture should be inserted until 4 or 5 weeks later.

M, Four months later. (Photographs courtesy of Dr. Frank Pavel.)

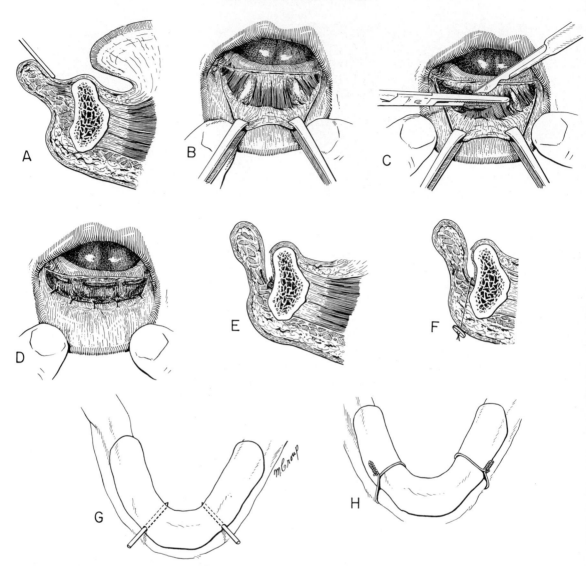

Figure 3–24   Deepening the mandibular sulcus. *A,* As the lip protrudes or is held out, the sulcus is completely obliterated. *B,* An incision has been carried out beginning in the mucobuccal fold in the region of the first molar, curving up toward approximately the crest of the ridge (actually just below the crest of the ridge), along the ridge just above the origin of the muscles enumerated on page 138, across the symphysis to the molar region on the opposite side, and again curved down toward the mucobuccal fold. Special care is exercised to cut only through the mucosa and not through the periosteum. By blunt dissection, the mucous membrane is dissected free from the mentalis muscles in the midline and the right and left inferior incisor muscles for a distance of at least 1.5 to 2.5 cm. The muscles are further bluntly dissected out with a periosteal elevator and hemostats until they stand forth prominently.

C, One beak of a hemostat is then placed beneath the mentalis muscle, the hemostat being held against the labial cortical plate of the symphysis. The hemostat is then closed and, with a No. 15 blade, the origin of the muscle is cut free from the labial cortical plate. Then on the other side of the hemostat the segment of muscle held between the beaks of the hemostat is cut free. The intact periosteum remains attached to the underlying bone. The same procedure is carried out for the right and left inferior incisor muscles. The rest of the muscle retracts into the lip. *D,* The mucosa is sutured into the depth of the sulcus to the periosteum. Ordinarily, this method will suffice for the retention of the mucosa and the maintenance of the increased sulcus. *E,* Cross section, showing the mucosa sutured to the depth of the sulcus and showing the labial cortical plate still covered with periosteum. It is imperative that the periosteum not be disturbed during this procedure. The exposed periosteum will very shortly become epithelialized.

F, Another method for the retention of the mucosa in the depth of the sulcus just created. The incised mucosa is "tied down" to the underlying periosteum by sutures which pass out through the soft tissues overlying the symphysis of the mandible and are tied to buttons. The author prefers the technique shown in *B.*

G, An acrylic splint has been attached to the mandible by means of Roger Anderson pins which have been drilled through the flange of the base plate into the cortex of the mandible. The exposed portions of these pins are covered with soft compound so that the lip is not traumatized by the projecting ends of the pins. *H,* Circumferential wiring of a splint to help in maintenance of the new sulcus and to protect the exposed periosteum.

muscles, or at least a portion of them, and the deepening of the sulcus for those cases in which the alveolar ridge is adequate is shown and described in Figure 3–24.

In Figure 3–25 is shown an example of a thick, broad mentalis muscle which has a high attachment practically on the crest of the edentulous mandible. This muscle can be partially resected (*i.e.*, myotomy performed), as shown in Figure 3–26, and the sulcus simultaneously deepened by following the technique described in the legend of Figure 3–26. This particular situation, in which only the mentalis muscle requires myotomy, is found more frequently than that in which all three muscles (right and left inferior, nasal and mentalis) require operation, as mentioned previously.

Technique for Deepening the Maxillary Sulcus. The labial and buccal sulcus on the maxilla can be materially shortened by the low attachment of the depressor nasal septi muscle in the midline, the nasalis muscle (alar part) next to it on either side, the superior incisor muscle (also known as the incisivus labii superioris) and the buccinator muscle. One or more or all of these muscles may have a very low origin on the alveolar bone, or the level of resorption of the alveolar process has reached the point of origin of the muscles just enumerated. In either event, it becomes necessary to remove these muscle attachments in order to deepen the sulcus so that the denture can have a flange which is adequate to support as well as retain the maxillary denture.

The description has already been given of the removal of the enlarged labial frenum, which is a frequent source of irritation and restriction of denture construction. In addition

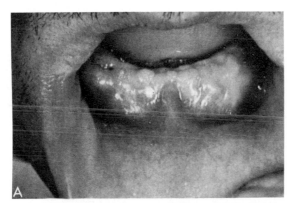

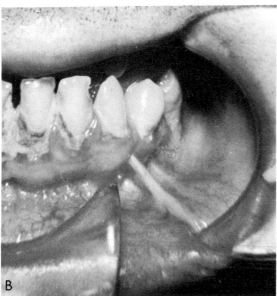

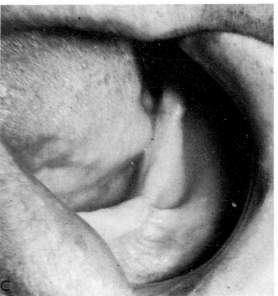

Figure 3–25 *A,* An example of a high mentalis muscle origin. This should be excised as shown in Figure 3–26. *B,* Fibrous bands. *C,* Fibrous bands and muscle insertions that have reduced the sulcus by over 50 per cent.

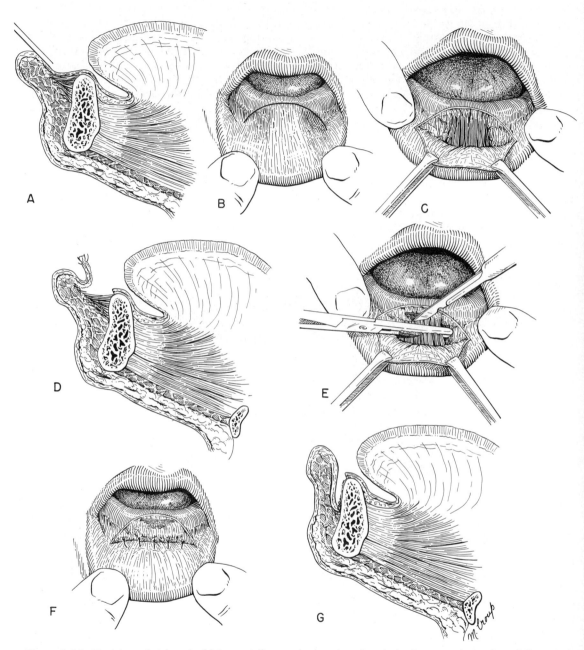

Figure 3–26 Excision of a broad, thick mentalis muscle (myotomy) and simultaneous deepening of the anterior mandibular sulcus.

A, Mentalis muscle origin at the crest of the ridge. *B,* Semicircular incision made just through the mucosa. *C,* Mucosa dissected free from the mentalis muscle and the periosteum covering the symphysis at either side of the muscle origin. *D,* Lateral view. *E,* The muscle bundle is freed from surrounding tissue and grasped at its point of origin. It is cut free and a piece removed by cutting on both sides of the hemostat. The remaining muscle retracts into the lip. *F,* The mucosa is then turned down and sutured to the periosteum in the mucolabial fold. *G,* The new space created by this method is shown here. The exposed periosteum gradually becomes covered with new epithelium. Unfortunately 50 per cent of this additional space is lost in about a year, because of scar contraction.

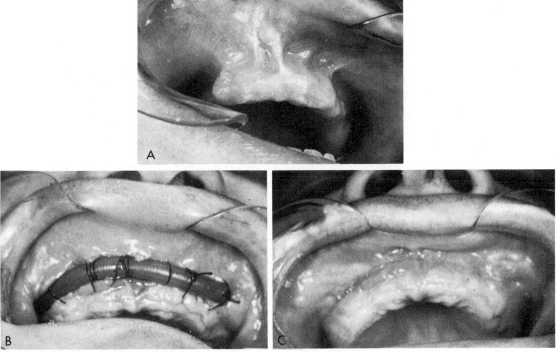

Figure 3-27 *A*, Low origin of multiple muscle bundles. *B*, The mucosa was incised and dissected from the muscle bundles, which were then cut as described in Figure 3–24. Then the edge of the mucosa was sutured to the periosteum and a piece of gum tubing was sutured as shown to maintain the new sulcus. It is not necessary to pass the sutures through the outside of the lip. *C*, End result 10 days later.

to the labial frenum we not infrequently have, as has been mentioned, an enlarged depressor nasal septi muscle. This may be associated, and generally is, with the labial frenum. In other words, there may be a fibrous band attached near the crest of the ridge that consists solely of fibrous tissue, or there may be a fibrous band of labial frenum and just beneath it an enlarged hypertrophied depressor nasal septi muscle. In this particular situation after the frenum has been excised, as has been described and illustrated in Figure 3–7, the muscle is now exposed. By blunt dissection with a hemostat the depressor nasal septi muscle is further exposed and undermined, at which time one beak of the hemostat is placed beneath the muscle and the other on top; the muscle is grasped and severed closely at its attachment to the crest of the maxillary alveolar ridge. It is then dissected upward toward the outer lip and cut free on the other side of the hemostat. The mucosa is undermined on both sides by scissor dissection, and the edges of the incision are brought together and sutured with 000 black silk.

In Figure 3–27*A* is shown an example of low attachments, bilaterally, of the nasalis muscle (alar parts) and the superior incisor muscles. As the lip is elevated, all four of these muscles can be seen to stand out prominently. These muscle bundles were exposed by making a semicircular incision, starting in the mucobuccal fold in the region of the first molar, down to the crest of the ridge just distal to the attachment of the superior incisor muscle, along the crest of the ridge, entirely across the ridge beyond the muscle attachments on the left side of the ridge until the area of the first molar was reached, and then curved up toward the mucobuccal fold. Care was taken in making this incision to cut only through the mucosa, not through the periosteum. The mucosa was next carefully dissected upward from the superior incisor and nasalis muscles on both sides. When the muscles had been clearly exposed, they were freed by blunt dissection with a hemostat, picked up by a hemostat as previously described, and cut free at the point of origin on the alveolar process; then on the other side of the hemostats another cut was made, and this section of the muscle was removed. The same procedure

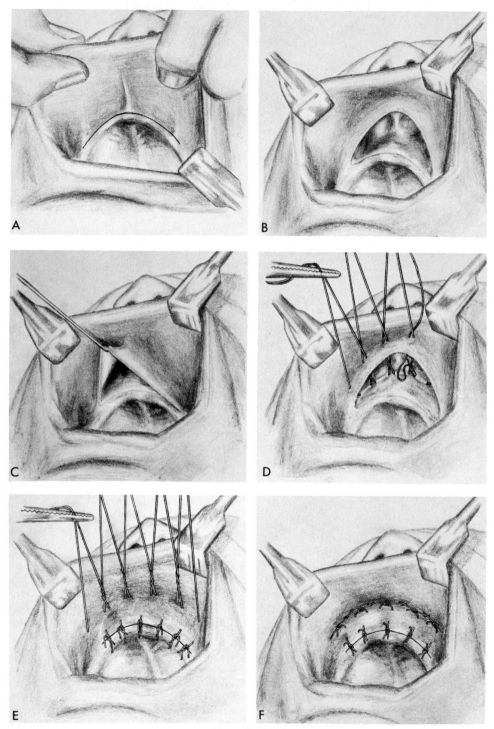

Figure 3–28 (1)

Figure 3–28   Deepening the anterior maxillary sulcus. *1,* Technique used by Wallenius. Study the text for the description of the technique illustrated in these drawings.

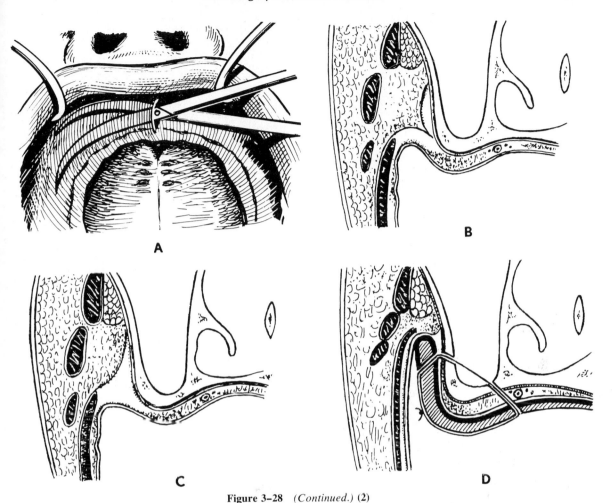

A

B

C

D

Figure 3–28 *(Continued.)* **(2)**

Figure 3–28 *(Continued.)* 2, Obwegeser's technique for submucosal vestibuloplasty. (*1*, From Wallenius, K., and Öwall, B.: Effect of ridge extension on retention and function of dentures. Odontol. Revy, *18*:361–371, 1967. *2*, From Obwegeser, H.: Die submuköse Vestibulumplastik. Dtsch. Zahnaerztl. Z., *14*:696, 1959.)

was carried out for all four of these muscles. The edge of the mucous membrane was then elevated and sutured into the sulcus to the periosteum. The technique is the same as that illustrated for the mandible (Fig. 3–24). As a further retentive device, rubber tubing was sutured over the cut edge of the mucosa in the depth of the sulcus, as shown in Figure 3–27B. Figure 3–27C illustrates the healed area 2 weeks following operation.

It has been revealed, however, that within less than 1 year the denture-bearing area provided at operation in most cases will be reduced by about 50 per cent because of scar contraction. Vestibuloplasty with secondary epithelialization in the labial and buccal sulcus of the mandible and the maxilla should therefore be recommended only when a very wide

denture-supporting area is expected to be gained at the end of operation.

SUBMUCOSAL VESTIBULOPLASTY FOR DEEPENING THE MAXILLARY SULCUS

Many modified methods have been suggested to diminish or exclude relapses due to scar contraction. Transitory forms of reduction of residual ridges, as seen in Figure 3–21A and C for the mandible and corresponding features for the maxilla may thus be treated according to the methods of Wallenius and Öwall,[58] as illustrated in Figure 3–28 (*1A* to *F*). An incision is made along the boundary between the fixed and the mobile mucosa (*A*).

The frontal aspect of the upper jaw is freed from subcutaneous tissue, the periosteum being kept intact. The region toward the canine fossa is laid bare on each side to the desired height. The piriform aperture forms the upper and medial limit of the operative field. The nasal spine can be removed through an incision in the periosteum, which is immediately sutured with fine catgut. The insertions of nasalis, incisivus, depressor septi and possibly caninus muscles can be detached close to the periosteum without damaging the latter. Preparation of the frontal aspect of the maxilla should be carried out to the level envisaged for the future mucobuccal fold (*B*).

A flap consisting entirely of mucous membrane is raised from the inner surface of the lip. Blunt dissection is used to remove subcutaneous tissue to a distance from the wound margin corresponding to the envisaged height of the gingivolabial fold (*C*).

After hemostasis, the first stage in the fixation of the gingivolabial fold is carried out. Mattress sutures are inserted initially to act as stay sutures. Stitches are passed through the flap from the frontal side at a distance from the wound margin determined by the desired height of the gingivolabial fold. By lifting the flap forward and upward the operator can see to insert stitches firmly into the periosteum. The needle is then passed out through the flap again at the same level as before. These sutures should bite into the periosteum slightly above the desired level of the future mucobuccal fold, if possible. Ordinarily five such sutures are inserted, and it should be arranged that they overlap and lie at the anticipated level of the fold (*D*).

The wound edges are now approximated and firmly sutured together, the stitches biting into the periosteum. The stay sutures are interlocked by twisting each once round its neighbor (*E*).

The new mucobuccal fold is now formed by tying the stay sutures under moderate tension. The anchorage of the upper suture line ensures that the mucosa over the entire region lies firmly against the periosteum. The intertwined sutures, biting firmly into the periosteum, provide excellent fixation for the mucobuccal fold at its new level (*F*).

Two of the essentials of this technique are that the denture-bearing area created at the operation be covered by adjacent oral mucosa and that the mucobuccal fold be optimally fixed to the periosteum. The requirements for rapid healing by first intention are satisfied, and scar contraction is negligible. Furthermore, healing proceeds without the operator's

resorting to troublesome splints, tubing or extraoral appliances, and late results have been controlled.

PRONG DENTURES

The construction, by conventional methods, of satisfactory dentures for jaws with severe resorption of the alveolar ridge is difficult or sometimes impossible because of poor denture-supporting tissues. For such cases as that illustrated in Figure 3–21*E* it is impossible to deepen the sulcus, and ridge augmentations by various techniques of grafting bone are far from satisfactory. Consequently, other methods of treatment have been designed in order to secure the retention and the stability of dentures. In the prong denture technique devised by Wallenius and Öwall[59] – see Figure 3–29 (*2*) – extensions from the denture base, fitting to surgically created skin-folded pockets, are planned in such areas as to enable neutralization of forces otherwise displacing the denture – see Figure 3–29 (*3*). In the upper jaw the anchorage should counteract horizontal forces and prevent the denture from falling by gravity. This is achieved by the creation of pockets placed in between the bony floor of the nasal cavity and the nasal mucosa. The denture is effectively retained by its extensions into these pockets and by the upper lip's exerting pressure in a dorsal direction on the denture, which is thereby locked against the underlying bone. Owing to the severe loss in the height of the crest in cases in which this method is indicated, the denture may be inserted horizontally in a ventral-dorsal direction. Even if tubera maxillaris are preserved in an otherwise severely resorbed jaw, the denture can still be inserted horizontally.

The same principle can be applied to the lower jaw. Anchorage in pockets on the labial side of the mandibular body provides satisfactory retention of the denture. The mandibular pockets should be directed as much horizontally as possible, according to the declination of the frontal aspect of the protuberantial area of mandibles with advanced resorption. The muscles of the lower lip and the chin will improve retention of the tips extending from the denture base into the pockets.

Surgery. Via a vestibular approach, the maxilla is bluntly dissected on both sides of the midline to the caudal part of the piriform aperture. The dissection is performed via 1-cm. horizontal incisions through the mucosa high up in the frontal fornix. The access to the

(*Text continued on page 164*)

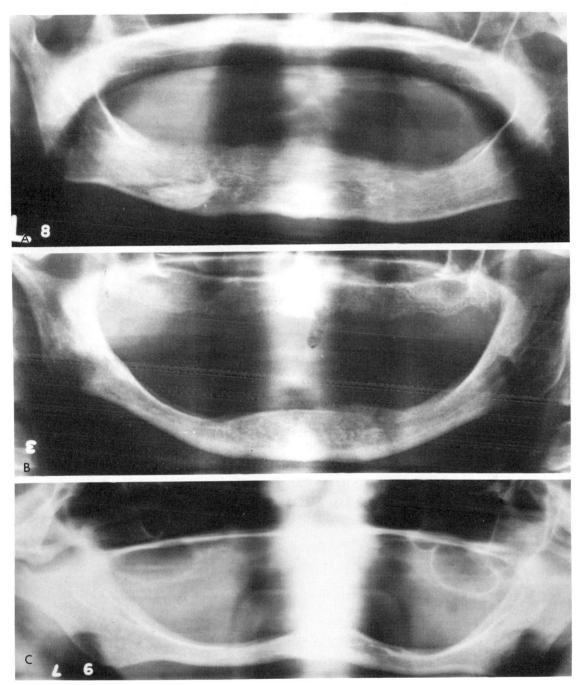

Figure 3–29 (1)

Figure 3–29 *1A, B,* and *C,* These panoramic radiographs illustrate the progressive resorption of the alveolar process in both the maxilla and mandible as age progresses. (Also see Figure 3–22 for a mandible so thin that a very moderate blow fractured it.) There certainly cannot be a deepening of the sulci in these cases on either the maxilla or the mandible. Attempts to augment the height of the maxillary and mandibular ridges, for the most part, have failed. What can be done for these cases? Wallenius[59] suggests "prong dentures." See the accompanying text and illustrations with legends for parts *2* through *7* of Figure 3–29.

(Figure 3–29 continued on following page)

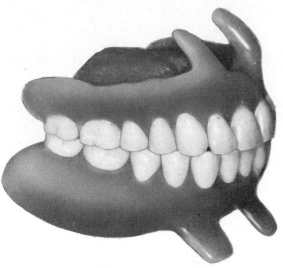

Figure 3–29 *(Continued.)* **(2)**

Figure 3–29 *(Continued.)* *2,* Maxillary and mandibular prong dentures. The prongs fit into skin-folded pockets in the vestibulum of a patient with extreme resorption of the jaws.

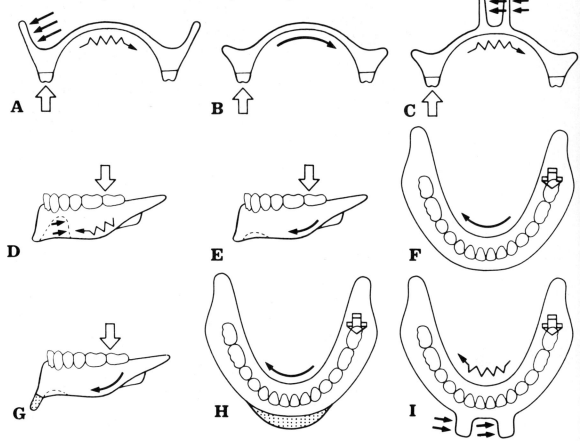

Figure 3–29 *(Continued.)* **(3)**

Figure 3–29 *(Continued.)* *3,* A sketch demonstrating dislocating and stabilizing forces on maxillary and mandibular dentures. *A,* Persisting ridge in maxilla. Denture retained against horizontal dislocation. *B,* Advanced reduction of ridge. Denture not retained against horizontal dislocation. Adhesion seal breaks and denture becomes loose. *C,* Prongs extended from the denture into the nasal cavity counteract horizontal dislocation. *D,* Persisting ridge in mandible. Denture retained against horizontal dislocation. *E* to *F,* Low frontal ridge and sloping lateral ridges. Denture may slide horizontally. Lateral and occlusal views. *G* to *H,* Slight sulcus deepening or an extended horizontal area gained at operation will not retain denture against horizontal dislocation. Lateral and occlusal views. *I,* Prongs extended from the denture into skin-folded pockets keep the denture from horizontal dislocation.

(Figure 3–29 continued on opposite page)

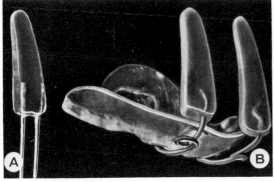

Figure 3–29 *(Continued.)* **(4)**

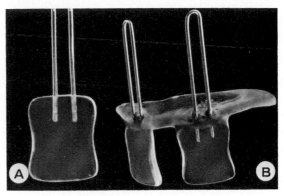

Figure 3–29 *(Continued.)* **(5)**

Figure 3–29 *(Continued.)* *4,* Prong and graft carrier for maxilla. *A,* Prong for maxilla. Standard form: length, 24 mm.; width at base, 5 to 7 mm.; width at tip, 3 to 4 mm. *B,* Graft carrier. Prongs and fixation plate united with steel wires.

5, Prong and graft carrier for mandible. *A,* Prong for mandible. Standard form: length, 15 mm.; width, 13 mm.; thickness, 3 mm. *B,* Graft carrier. Prongs and fixation plate united with cold cure acrylate. Prong direction adjusted by aid of steel handles, which are removed before suturing to the oral mucosa.

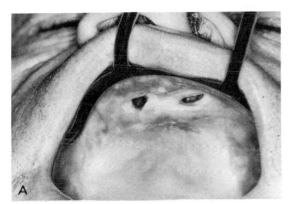

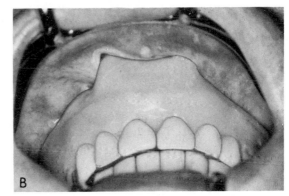

Figure 3–29 *(Continued.)* **(6)**

Figure 3–29 *(Continued.)* *6A,* Extremely resorbed maxilla. In vestibulum, entrances to skin-folded pockets into the piriform aperture are seen. *B,* Same case. Maxillary denture *in situ.* The right skin-folded pocket is somewhat opened because of tension from the lip elevator.

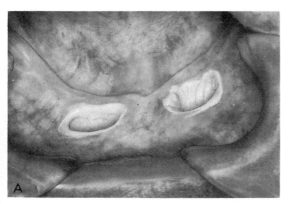

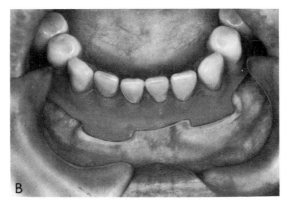

Figure 3–29 *(Continued.)* **(7)**

Figure 3–29 *(Continued.)* *7A,* Skin-folded pockets in the regions of the lower lateral incisors, pointing frontally toward the mandible. *B,* Same case with mandibular prong denture *in situ.*

(2 to 7, From Wallenius, K., and Öwall, B.: A 5-year follow-up study of retention of prong dentures by skin-folded pockets. Int. J. Oral Surg., *1:*26–33, 1972.)

nasal cavity is often sharply cornered, owing to a threshold of compact bone. The edge of this bone may be excised. Dissection is continued onto the bony floor of the nose, the mucosa of which is loosened and lifted from the underlying bone under the control of a nasal speculum. At the bottom of the dissection, a perforation is made into the nasal cavity. In this way tunnels are formed on either side of the nasal septum, and their size, direction and shape are adjusted according to standardized graft carriers that are identical with the prongs of the denture—see Figure 3–29 (4A). The prongs have a handle approximately 3 cm. long, by which it is possible to check manually that they are parallel and that they are properly related to the underlying bony surface before the prongs are united with a fixation plate by cold-cure acrylate. The handles and excess acrylate are then removed. It may sometimes be more expeditious, and easier, to join the prongs to the fixation plate before the operation by means of stainless steel wires. The stainless steel wires are exposed and bent to form loops in order to permit bending and adjusting the prongs in the direction necessary for them to fit into the dissected pockets—see Figure 3–29 (4B). A skin transplant with an area of about 4 by 8 cm. and about 0.5 mm. thick is taken from the inner aspect of the left arm, for example. The graft appliance is lined with the skin so that the rough surface is facing outward and then placed into position. Through holes in the periphery, the plate is sutured to the mucosa and left in position for 10 days, during which time the transplants have taken, and now line the pockets.

In the mandible the pockets are placed along the body between the periosteum and the mental muscle. Incisions about 1 cm. wide are made in the regions of the lateral incisors for blunt dissections of pockets, which then are prepared to receive shovel-shaped prongs of a standard size and form—see Figure 3–29 (5A). In the same way as for the maxilla, the prongs are used separately for manual determination of their direction in relation to the fixation plate or are united preoperatively by stainless steel wires with a fixation plate covering the area frontal to the second bicuspids—see Figure 3–29 (5B).

After the end of the 10 days' fixation period, the prongs and the plate are removed, and prosthetic treatment should be started immediately—see Figure 3–29 (6 and 7).

Prosthetics. During the first postoperative period, which lasts several months, the skin-folded pockets have a tendency to collapse rapidly, and reinsertion of prongs may, after a few hours, already have become difficult. A reserve obturator or a duplicate denture with prongs should be on hand to prevent the pockets from collapsing during the prosthetic treatment.

At the office visit during which the graft appliance is taken out and excess skin is trimmed away, the fixation plate may be cut off to allow the united prongs to be polymerized onto a previously prepared denture or onto an old denture for temporary use.

A reserve obturator may be fabricated directly in an alginate impression of the mucosal surface of either the denture with prongs or the graft appliance. Standard prongs are inserted into the impression, and the obturator is completed in cold-cure acrylate.

The patient should keep the reserve obturator or duplicate denture for use in case of an accident with the denture, and he should be informed of the risk of pocket collapse.

An individual impression tray may also be fabricated by taking an impression of the mucosal surface of the temporary denture and using standard prongs. During the impression the polished standard prongs should not be covered with impression material and should be allowed to stay in the model for polymerization to the definite denture. During prosthetic procedures care must be taken not to change the direction of the prongs, and during laboratory handling the shape of the prongs must not be changed by unnecessary grinding or polishing.

Mouth and Denture Hygiene. The patient should be instructed in oral and denture hygiene. It is recommended that he rinse and aspirate the pockets with some syringe device, *e.g.*, a rubber ear ball. During the first months physiologic saline is used; afterward, tap-water.

HYPERPLASIA OF MUCOPERIOSTEUM OF ALVEOLAR RIDGE CRESTS

Etiology. Alveolar mucoperiosteal hyperplasia is most frequently found in persons who have worn the same set of dentures for many years without having them remade, rebased or relined. It is also seen in patients who had dentures inserted immediately after a maxillary and/or mandibular odontectomy with little or no alveolectomy and who have not had their immediate denture rebased after healing and resorption of the alveolar process has occurred (see Figure 3–31).

Hyperplastic tissue is also frequently seen in patients with a full upper denture and a partial lower denture, and particularly so in those patients who do not wear their partial lower dentures. In these cases, the maxillary anterior ridge is rapidly broken down because of the pounding of the natural anterior mandibular teeth against the anterior portion of the maxillary denture during mastication. The space formerly occupied by alveolar bone is then filled with fibrous hyperplastic mucoperiosteal tissue.

BURNING, PAINFUL RIDGES. In many of these cases of "flabby ridges," at the base of the soft tissue there is a narrow, sharp "saw-toothed," or "knife-edged," alveolar ridge. During mastication the dentures compress the hyperplastic tissue against this thin, sharp edge of bone, producing hyperemia and pain with every bite. The history is sufficient to make the diagnosis, but it can readily be confirmed by removing the dentures and pressing the flabby tissue with your fingers against the ridge. The patient will wince with pain. Furthermore, relieving the inside of the denture over these areas gives only transitory relief, if any. Treatment consists of the reduction of this sharp osseous ridge, as described on page

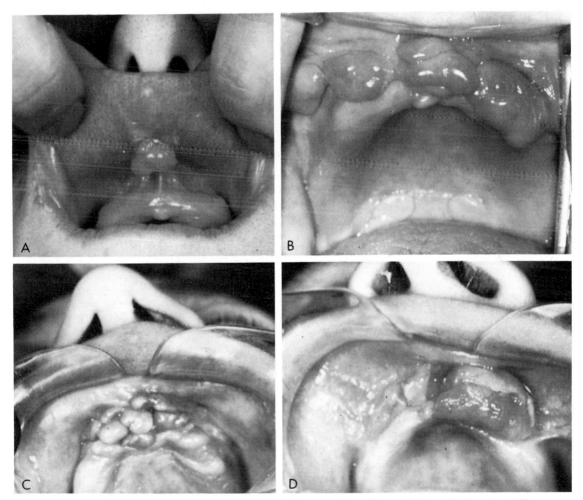

Figure 3–30 Examples of anterior maxillary mucosal and mucoperiosteal hyperplasia. *A*, Pedunculated fibromatous mass arising from the labial mucosa of the lip due to denture trauma. *B*, Multilobular masses of inflammatory hyperplasias arising from the mucosa of the lip and the mucoperiosteum of the crest of the anterior maxillary ridge. Note the flattened bilateral fibropapillomas that have developed along the posterior border of the denture. *C*, Same as *B* but with smaller lobes and not acutely inflamed. *D*, Large unilateral rolls of friable hyperplastic tissue. Treatment: excision as described in the text.

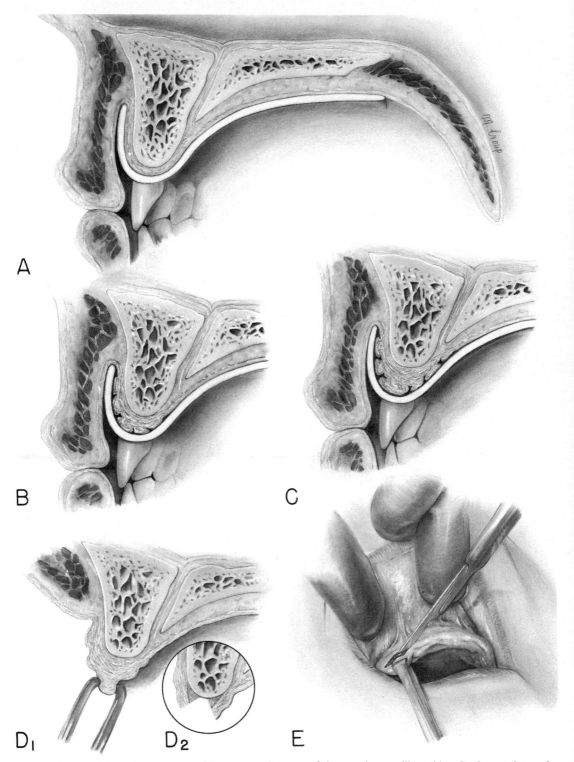

Figure 3–31   Excision of hyperplasia of the mucoperiosteum of the anterior maxillary ridge. Study text for explanation.

(*Figure 3–31 continued on opposite page*)

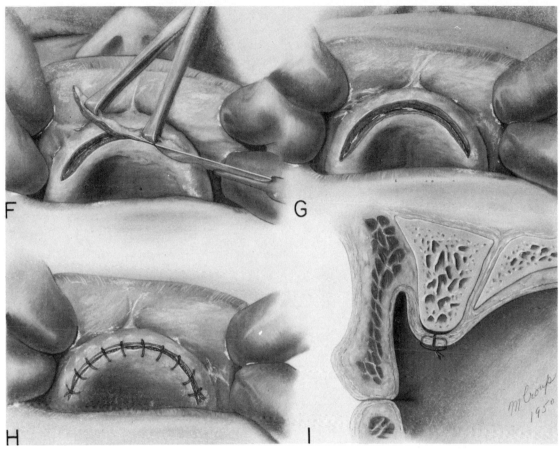

Figure 3–31 (*Continued.*)

190 and illustrated in Figure 3–60. Because mucoperiosteal hyperplasia is almost always present, this and the sharp ridges are excised at the same operation. The patient's lower denture is temporarily relined with a mixture of zinc oxide powder and eugenol.

Technique for Excision of Hyperplastic Tissue from Crests of Maxillary and Mandibular Ridges. In Figure 3–31*A*, *B* and *C* is shown the progressive atrophy of the maxillary alveolar process and subsequent growth of hyperplastic tissue into this area. If local anesthesia is used for this surgical procedure, infiltration in the mucobuccal and mucolabial fold on each side of the median line, plus palatine injections on the maxilla and lingual injections on the mandible, will suffice.

With several Allis tissue forceps, grasp the flabby hyperplastic soft tissue at its crest and hold it up, as shown in Figure 3–31*D*. Next, cut a V-shaped groove through the fibrous

mass down to bone along the crest of the ridge, as illustrated in Figure 3–31D_2, *E* and *F*, and remove this strip of tissue. The labial, buccal and lingual tissues shown in Figure 3–31*G* are slightly loosened with a periosteal elevator and the edges approximated with a continuous lock stitch 000 black silk suture, as shown in Figure 3–31*H*. This assures that the crest of the alveolar ridge will be covered with a reasonably thick cushion of mucoperiosteum, as shown in Figure 3–31*H* and *I*.

Exactly the same procedure is followed for the excision of hyperplastic flabby tissues from the mandibular ridge.

If in addition to the hyperplasia there is present a thin, sharp edge of bone, as previously described, after the mucoperiosteal membrane has been loosened on either side of the groove, the sharp edge of bone is removed according to the technique described and illustrated on page 190, Figure 3–60.

EXCISION OF HYPERPLASIA OF THE CREST OF THE ALVEOLAR RIDGE

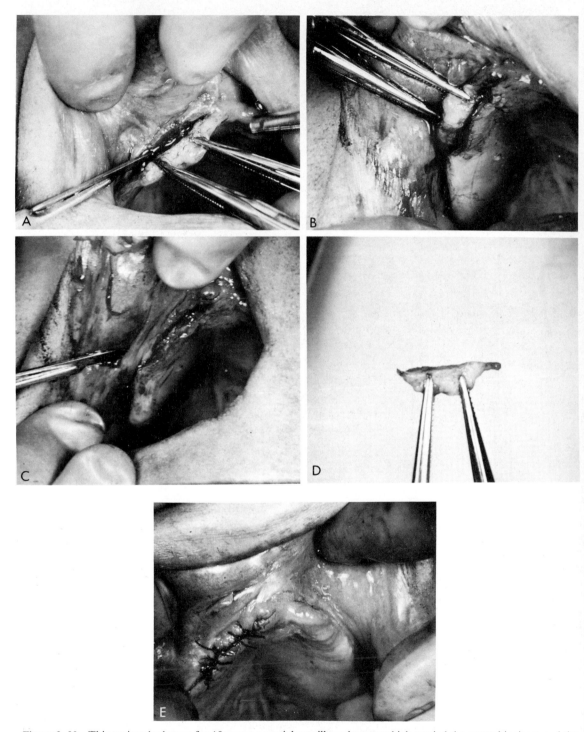

Figure 3–32 This patient had worn for 10 years a partial maxillary denture which carried the central incisors and the molars. She had had her remaining teeth extracted 5 years before this operation and an immediate "temporary" full denture inserted. This denture has never been rebased, and as the alveolar process resorbed in these areas beneath the full denture, the spaces were filled with hyperplastic tissue. This tissue was excised bilaterally, but only the right side is shown in *A* to *E* inclusive. The technique is illustrated and described in the text. See Figure 3–31 and the accompanying text.

HYPERPLASIA OF ORAL VESTIBULAR MUCOSA

Hyperplasia of the oral mucosa may be found in the maxillary or mandibular vestibule; on the inner mucosa of either lip, but usually the upper; and in the floor of the oral cavity. This proliferation of the mucosa is due to (a) mechanical irritation of the vestibular mucosa by an overextended denture flange, and (b) extensive resorption of the alveolar ridge and consequent shifting of the stress of mastication to the denture flanges, which now sink deeper in the soft tissue of the oral vestibule or into the mucosa of the floor of the oral cavity.

The ill-fitting denture moves freely under masticatory stress, producing a traumatic inflammation and the subsequent growth of multiple folds or flat semispherical lobules of fibrous hyperplastic tissue. These folds may be fissured, with a portion of the hyperplastic growth resting inside the denture between the labial or buccal flange and the resorbed alveolar ridge and the other portion draped over the outer surface of the denture flange (see Figure 3–33). They may be confined to the anterior portion of the maxilla or extend from the midline all the way posteriorly to the tuberosity. Occasionally, hyperplastic flaps of tissue are found along the posterior border of the denture where it has been traumatizing the soft palate.

Malignant neoplasms have developed in these hyperplastic growths (see Figures 13–131 to 13–134, pages 825 to 828).

Technique for Removal. Raise the lip. Then lock three or four or more Allis tissue forceps along the base of the hyperplastic mucosa. Holding all the forceps, move the mass to make certain that the forceps do not contain any of the underlying muscle fibers in their beaks. With a No. 9 Dean's scissors, cut between the beaks of the Allis forceps and the lip. Do not pull on the forceps when cutting. Insert sutures along the line of incision. (See the photographic case reports, Figures 3–34 and 3–35, and see the technique illustrated in Chapter 13, page 826, Figure 132A to F inclusive.) Adjustments must now be made in the denture so as to prevent recurrence of the hyperplastic growth.

FIBROMATOSIS OF THE TUBEROSITY (BULBOUS TUBEROSITIES) AND MANDIBULAR THIRD MOLAR AREAS

Fibromatous enlargement of the tuberosities of the edentulous maxilla or of the mandibular third molar areas can and does reduce the intermaxillary space to such an extent that it may be impossible to construct efficient dentures. See Figure 3–37A for the illustration of a unilateral fibromatous tuberosity and Figure 3–37B for the illustration of bilateral fibromatosis of the mandibular third molar areas, which contact the maxillary tuberosity. Even

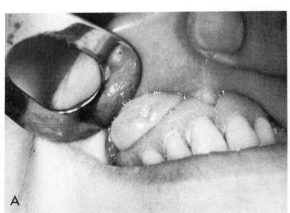
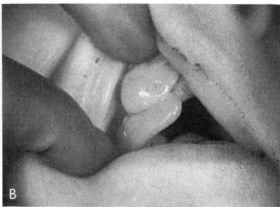

Figure 3–33   *A,* Unilateral bifid semispherical hyperplasia of the vestibular mucosa caused by the mechanical irritation of an overextended labial denture flange and resorption of the alveolar process in this area. *B,* Denture removed, showing bifid growth. The denture flange fits between the two semispherical flattened growths. This patient had worn a partial upper denture for many years and the last teeth she had extracted were in this area. Little or no alveolectomy was performed at the time of extraction. An immediate denture was inserted. Disuse atrophy of this area of the alveolar process created a situation favorable for the development of the hyperplasia seen here.

Photographic Case Report

EXCISION OF HYPERPLASIA OF THE MUCOSA OF THE LIP DUE TO DENTURE TRAUMA

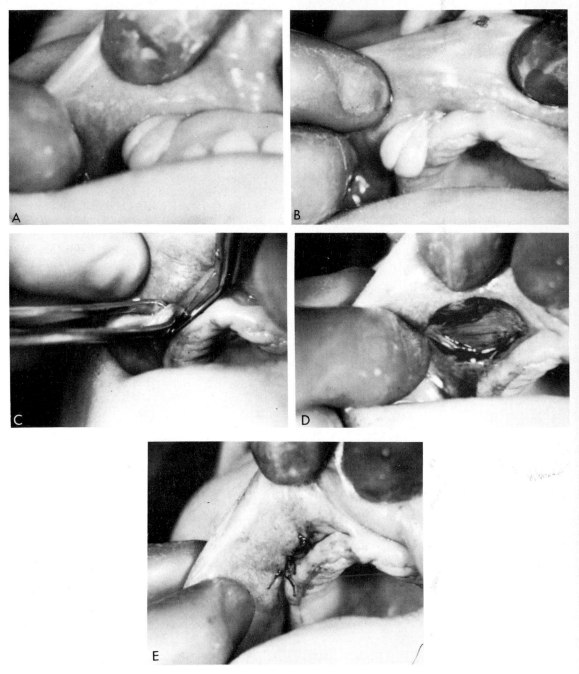

Figure 3–34　The technique for the excision of this unilateral hyperplasia, similar to that shown in Figure 3–33, is described in the text and so is not repeated here.

Photographic Case Report

EXCISION OF A ROLL OF HYPERPLASTIC MUCOSA FROM THE FORNIX OF THE ANTERIOR MAXILLARY VESTIBULE

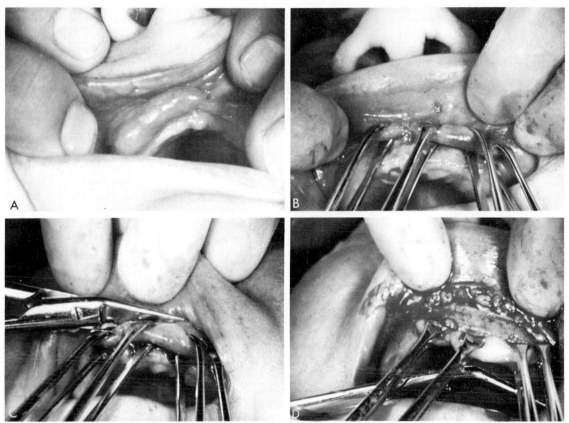

Figure 3–35   The technique illustrated here is described in the text. Suturing is similar to that shown in Figure 3–34E.

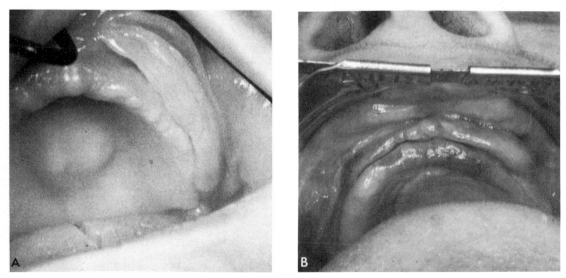

Figure 3–36   *A,* Unilateral maxillary leaf-like multiple folds of hyperplastic vestibular mucosa extending from the midline to the tuberosity as the result of denture flange irritation and resorption.

B, The so-called epulis fissuratum. A roll of hyperplastic tissue whose growth was the result of irritation by the edge of the labial flange of the denture.

if the intermaxillary space is not encroached upon, these fibromatous enlargements have such marked undercuts buccally, and occasionally palatally, as to prevent extension of the buccal denture flange to the vestibule or to prevent adequate palatal seating and sealing of the posterior border of the denture. This means poor denture retention.

Sometimes the tuberosity in partially edentulous cases becomes so large that it interferes with mastication and thus becomes traumatized and inflamed. Because fibromatosis of the tuberosity is such a dense, hard mass it can be mistaken for bone. A radiographic examination should be made of the tuberosities (usually both are affected) before surgery to determine whether the mass is dense, hard, cartilage-like fibrous tissue or if it is an unerupted third molar or bone (see Figure 3–39). While all require surgical reduction, the technique is different for each condition.

However, if the radiograph reveals that the floor of the maxillary sinus proximates the crest of the ridge and tuberosity, surgery to reduce the height or width or to remove undercuts would result in opening the maxillary sinus and so is contraindicated.

Technique for Reduction of the Fibromatosis. The objective in this plastic operation is to reduce the fibromatous enlarged tuberosities or the fibromatous enlarged mandibular third molar soft tissue areas to a size and shape to conform, to a reasonable degree, to the rest of the ridge. A starting point is to estimate the required amount of tissue to be removed to ac-

complish this result. As a rule, if one third of the bulbous mass is excised from the center and the two remaining sides are undermined submucosally, and then brought together and sutured, the desired result will be obtained.

In Figure 3–37 (2A) is an example of a bilateral fibromatous tuberosity. Before actually making the incision through the mass of tissue, one might draw with an indelible pencil the lines of incision on the tuberosity, or over the fibromatous tissue in the mandibular third molar area, to mark accurately the one-third wedge section to be cut out of the center, as shown in Figure 3–37 (2B). Note that the wedge-shaped cuts start at the same point, which is that area on the crest of the ridge which is the junction of normal ridge and beginning fibromatosis, and they end at a point at the most posterior aspect of the tuberosity. This V-shaped incision, made with a No. 15 Bard-Parker blade, is carried through the center of the mass, making certain that the blade contacts bone throughout the entire cut. The wedge-shaped tissue is grasped with an Allis forceps, lifted from its groove and freed at any point at which it is still adherent to the cortical bone.

In Figure 3–37 (2C) are shown the cuts in this cross section; it will be noted here that while it is a wedge-shaped bilateral incision, the lines of cleavage do not meet at the same point on the crest of bone. The distance between these two slanting cuts, at the crest of the bone, is dependent also on the size of the fibromatous tuberosity. The larger the tuberos-

(Text continued on page 176)

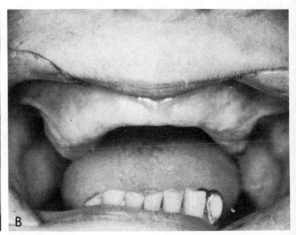

Figure 3–37 (1)

Figure 3–37   *1A,* Fibromatosis of the right maxillary tuberosity. The left tuberosity was reduced in size with the technique illustrated in *2A* to *F.*

B, Bilateral fibromatosis of the mandibular retromolar area. As shown here, it is in contact with the maxilla even in the open-bite relationship of the mandible and maxilla. This will have to be surgically reduced as shown in Figure 3–38.

(Figure 3–37 continued on opposite page)

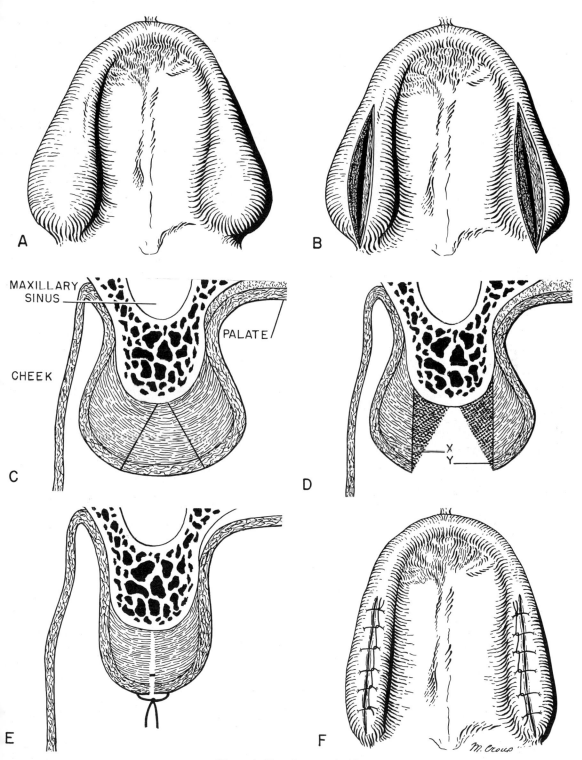

Figure 3–37 *(Continued.)* **(2)**

Figure 3–37 *(Continued.)* 2, Reduction of the fibromatous bilateral enlargement of the tuberosities by a plastic procedure. See text for description of technique.

A, Bulbous tuberosities are in the great percentage of cases made up of dense fibrous tissue. Radiograph before cutting into them.

B, Cut wedges in each tuberosity down to the bone and remove.

C, Cross section enlargement showing wedge to be removed.

D, Wedge is removed. Now the buccal and the lingual portions are undermined by cutting out *X* and *Y*.

E, The two sides are now sutured together.

F, Occlusal view showing reduced tuberosities and continuous sutures.

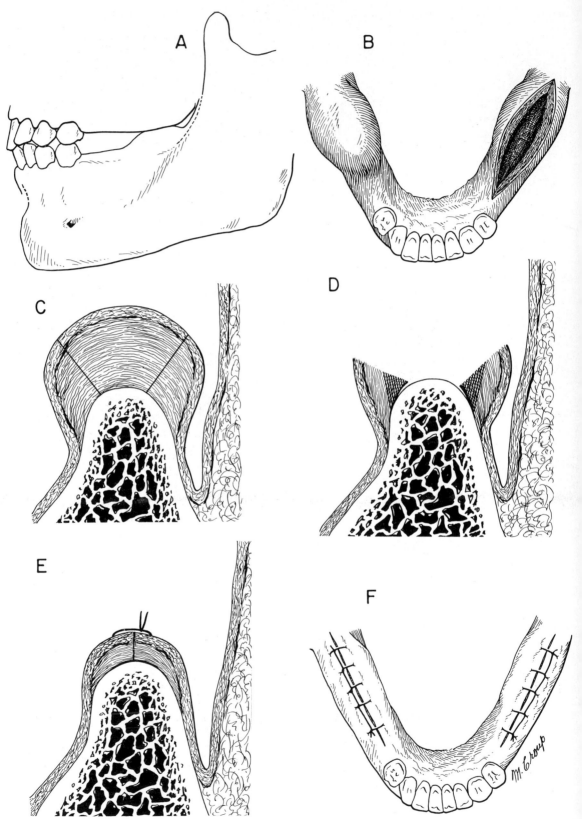

Figure 3–38 Bilateral fibromatous enlargement of the tissue in the retromolar area. The same technique as described in Figure 3–37 (2) is used for reducing this tissue. See the text also.

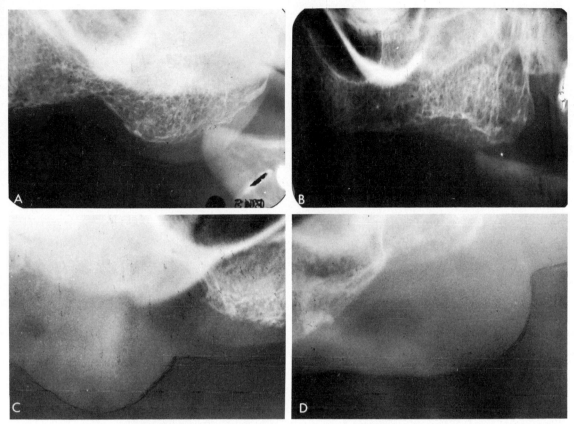

Figure 3–39 *A*, This enlarged tuberosity is cancellous bone. It is reduced by reflecting a large flap buccally and lingually, reducing the size by chisels or bone shears, smoothing with a bone file, replacing the soft tissue, trimming the excess tissue, and suturing. The floor of the maxillary sinus in this case is not proximal to the crest of the tuberosity, so there is no danger of opening the maxillary sinus when reducing the size of this tuberosity.

B, Another example of an enlarged osseous tuberosity.

C and *D*, Enlarged dense, fibrous tuberosities which developed following the loss of excessive bone when the second and third molars were extracted. When necessary, these can be reduced as shown in Figure 3–37 (*2*).

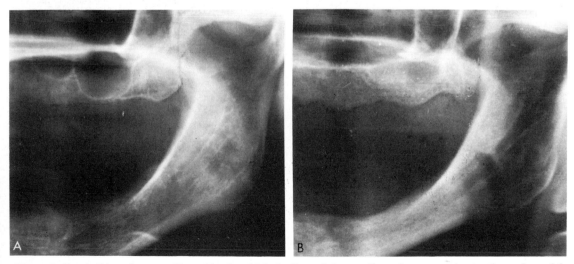

Figure 3–40 *A*, Edentulous maxillary ridge in which the floor of the maxillary sinus approximates the surface of the ridge in the area formerly occupied by the bicuspids and first molar. The sinus does not extend into the normal tuberosity.

B, In this edentulous maxillary ridge there is no approximation of the maxillary sinus to the crest of the ridge throughout its length. If changes were indicated in the shape of this ridge, they could be made without danger of entering the maxillary sinus. This is not true in *A* except in the tuberosity.

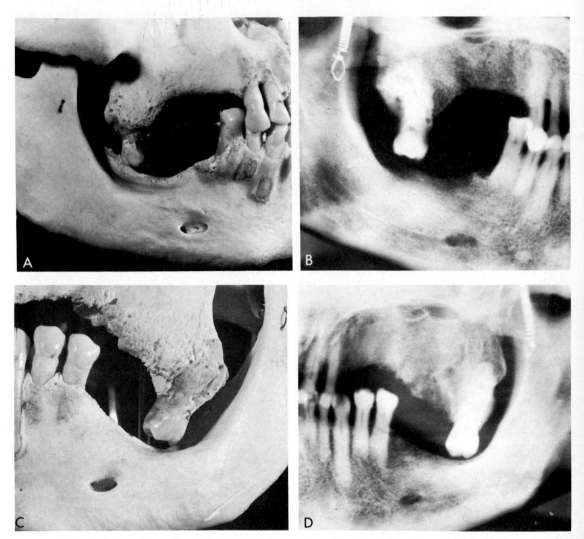

Figure 3-41 *A*, Anatomic specimen of an elongated maxillary tuberosity and its erupted third molar, demonstrating how nature strove to bring this tooth into mastication with its nonpresent mandibular opponent. Note that at least it did reach the mandibular ridge. *B*, Panoramic radiograph shows that the tuberosity is solid bone. The maxillary sinus did not change position.

C, Another example of an elongated tuberosity and its erupted molar. *D*, Again the tuberosity is solid bone.

ity, the greater the wedge and the greater the distance between the cuts at the crest of the osseous ridge.

In Figure 3-37 (*2D*) is illustrated the wedge removed; sections *X* and *Y* are those areas of submucosal fibrous tissue which the operator estimates he must remove in order to approximate the buccal and lingual flaps. The reason that these sections are not removed with the original incisions is that one must remove one or more of these areas until, by trial, it has been determined that the two flaps will meet in the midline without being under tension, as shown in Figure 3-37 (*2E*). Extreme care must be taken in undermining the buccal and lingual flaps to remove sections *X* and *Y*, to avoid getting too close to the covering mucosa,

since this would cut off its blood supply and cause subsequent sloughing of this flap.

Figure 3-37 (*2F*) shows the closure of these cuts by the lock stitch continuous black silk sutures.

FIBROMATOSIS OF THE PALATE

Bilateral fibromatosis of the palate is illustrated in Figures 3-43 and 3-44. These palatally projecting masses of fibrous tissue prevent the construction of a maxillary denture. The technique for their reduction is illustrated in Figure 3-45, in which *A* and *B* reveal the extent of this fibromatous tissue. In Figure 3-

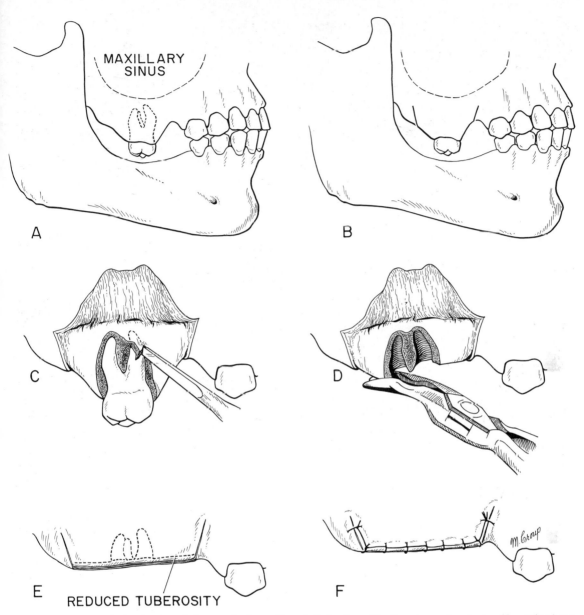

Figure 3–42 Surgical reduction of elongated tuberosities. *A*, Extrusion of tooth and carrying down of investing bone due to long-standing loss of opposing teeth. Radiograph this area to locate the floor of the maxillary sinus before cutting into the tuberosity. *B*, Incise the mucoperiosteum along the crest of the ridge and toward the mucobuccal fold as shown. *C*, Flap is turned back buccally and palatal tissue is loosened, the bone is removed over the buccal roots with a chisel, and the molar extracted. *D*, The tuberosity is now reduced in size and height with a bone shear until approximately the size of the anterior ridge. *E*, The soft tissues are replaced and the excess overlapping portions are removed, half from the buccal and half from the palate. *F*, The edges are approximated with a continuous suture.

45*B*, the cross section shows the marked undercuts which were present in this particular case. The easiest and most exact method for reducing this bulky, dense tissue is illustrated in Figure 3–45*C*. By means of a radiosurgical loop, both fibromatous enlargements are planed down until the desired contour of the palate is reached, as is shown in Figure 3–45*D*. These raw, painful surfaces are protected by placing into the palate an iodoform gauze–wrapped sponge, the palatal surface of which is covered with a thin mix of zinc oxide and eugenol, for the first 72 hours. The sponge is held in place by sutures passed over the

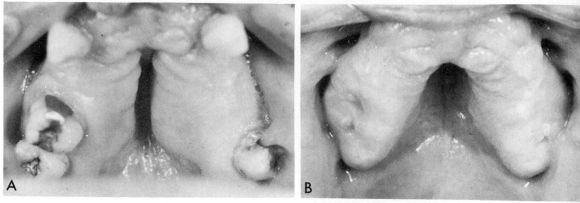

Figure 3–43 *A,* Bilateral fibromatosis of the palate. *B,* Appearance following surgical treatment as shown in Figure 3–45.

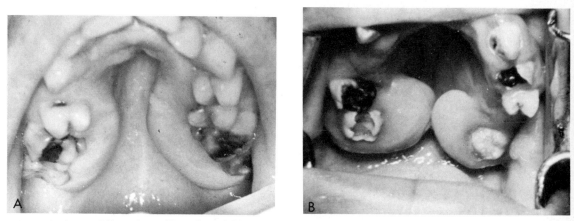

Figure 3–44 *A,* Bilateral maxillary lingual fibromatous growths in the molar regions. *B,* Large bilateral nodular dense sessile fibromas. These are not reduced by undermining but are planed down as described in the text.

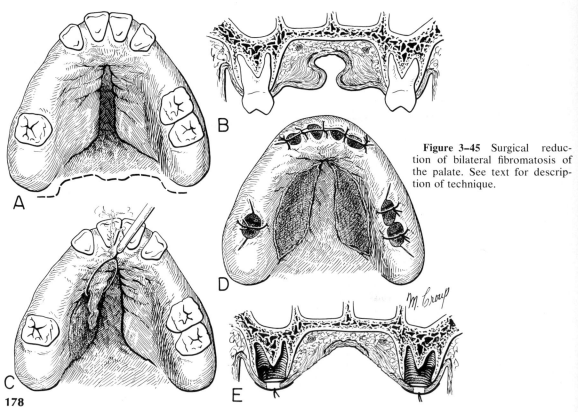

Figure 3–45 Surgical reduction of bilateral fibromatosis of the palate. See text for description of technique.

sponge and through the mucoperiosteal tissue on the right and left alveolar ridges. An impression should be made, if possible, at the time of surgery and a temporary acrylic splint made to cover and protect the palate during the period of epithelialization after the sponge is removed. These drawings were from the practical case shown in Figure 3–43. The few remaining teeth were extracted at the same operation because of advanced periodontoclasia.

VERRUCOUS PAPILLOMATOSIS OF THE PALATE (INFLAMMATORY PAPILLARY HYPERPLASIA OF THE PALATAL SOFT TISSUE)

These small multinodular papillary outgrowths develop under the palatal area as the result of trauma (see Figure 3–46). Some authors label these lesions as precancerous. The author has only seen a carcinoma *in situ* in these lesions. Conservative excision of the epithelium down to the corium is all that is necessary to prevent this possibility.

The electrosurgical excision of these papillary outgrowths seen under dentures is illustrated in Figure 13–15 and described on pages 808 and 809.

REMOVAL OF OSSEOUS STRUCTURES, PROTUBERANCES OR EXCRESCENCES WHICH INTERFERE WITH THE PLACING OF DENTURES

ALVEOPLASTY

Alveoplasty is the surgical contouring of the alveolar process in preparation for the

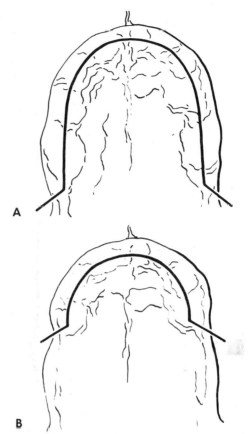

Figure 3–47 Line of incision of the mucoperiosteal flap. *A*, For complete maxillary alveolectomy. *B*, For anterior maxillary alveolectomy.

support of immediate dentures or those which will be inserted a few weeks postoperatively.

ALVEOLECTOMY AND ALVEOLOTOMY

Alveolectomy is the surgical excision of the alveolar process. The only time the complete

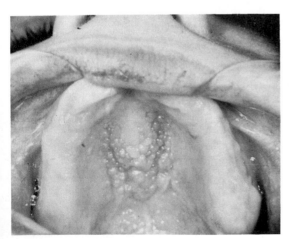

Figure 3–46 Papillary hyperplasia (verrucous papillomatosis) of the palatal mucoperiosteum.

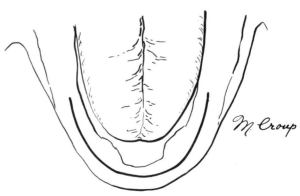

Figure 3–48 Line of incision of the mucoperiosteal flap for torus mandibularis. The incision is carried along the crest of the ridge from the first molar area on the left to the first molar area on the right and reflected lingually.

Photographic Case Report

MAXILLARY ODONTECTOMY AND ALVEOLECTOMY

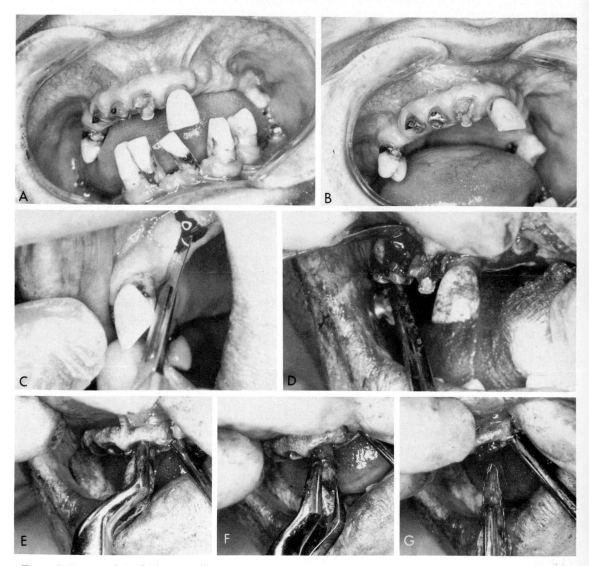

Figure 3–49 *A* and *B*, Carious maxillary roots and advanced loss of alveolar bone around the roots of the three remaining widely separated teeth.

C, Incision through the mucoperiosteal tissue along the crest of the edentulous areas between the isolated teeth and roots.

D, The mucoperiosteal flap is reflected.

E, Central incisor is grasped on the cementum of the neck of the root with a No. 286 forceps.

F, Tooth is rotated mesially.

G, It is lifted out of its alveolus.

(Figure 3–49 continued on opposite page)

removal of the alveolar process (alveolectomy) is indicated is in jaws that will be subjected to radiation during the treatment of a malignant neoplasm (see page 107). Therefore the term alveolectomy as commonly used is incorrect, but usage has made it generally accepted. A partial alveolectomy is all that is ever needed and this solely to prepare the al-

veolar ridges for the reception of dentures. This includes the removal of marked osseous undercuts, wherever present, or sharp cortical plates; reduction of irregularities of the crest of the ridge or elongations; and the removal of exostoses.

While it is recognized that the alveolar process atrophies from disuse after the teeth

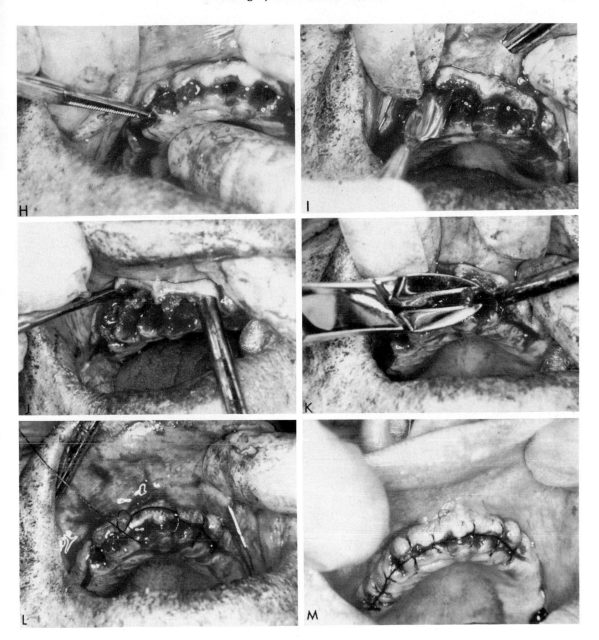

Figure 3–49   *(Continued.)*
H, Large periapical granuloma is grasped with a hemostat and removed *(I).*
J, Flap reflected showing the sharp, irregular alveolar process and cortical bone.
K, Reduction of the bone with a 5C bone shear.
L, Soft tissues trimmed and sutured.
M, Tissues after suturing.

are extracted, nevertheless only the minimum amount of bone necessary to permit the insertion of the denture should be removed. For reasons of esthetics (maxillary prognathism) or to achieve the necessary intermaxillary space, additional alveolar process must occasionally be removed.

Alveolotomy means cutting into the alveolar process. Alveolotomy is done to expose and permit the removal of an embedded tooth, or roots, or to expose a cyst or a tumor, or for an apicoectomy.

Technique for Maxillary and/or Mandibular Partial Alveolectomy.   The various steps in this procedure follow (see also Plate I, page 55, and Figures 3–47, 3–51, 3–59 and 3–60).

If the case is one in which the remaining teeth have just been extracted, the mucoperiosteum should be reflected by the periosteal elevator to a minimum depth of 10 mm. from the gingival line all around the area to be trimmed.

At a point midway between the buccal and lingual surfaces of the last tooth in line (the most distal tooth to be extracted), extend the incision through the buccal mucoperiosteal tissue toward the mucobuccal fold at an angle of 45 degrees for at least 15 mm. Incise across any space where teeth have been extracted previously.

Reflect the mucoperiosteal tissue with a periosteal elevator and hold it back with the index finger of the left hand, or by a broad periosteal elevator, or by a tissue retractor.

Keep the ridges free from blood by suction apparatus throughout the operation.

Place the bone shear or single-edge bone-cutting rongeur with one blade on the crest of the ridge and the other blade beneath the undercut to be removed, starting in the upper or lower central incisor region and proceeding to the distalmost portion of the alveolar ridge.

Free the mucoperiosteal membrane from the crest of the ridge and expose the lingual cortical bone. This procedure will reveal many sharp interseptal osseous projections.

Remove these sharp interseptal osseous projections with end-cutting rongeurs.

Smooth the labial and buccal surfaces of the ridges with the bone file. Hold the bone file in the same position as a straight operative chisel, with the same finger rests, and file small areas in succession with a pulling motion.

Examine the dental radiographs again for periapical radiolucent areas, and where present explore these areas with the curette. Enucleate any soft tissue mass encountered. Explore all tooth sockets with a small bowl curette and remove any spicules of bone or tooth structure or filling material that may have dropped into the socket.

Return the flap to its original position, approximate the ends of the soft tissue, and iron it into position with the moist index finger.

Note the amount of overlapping of the soft tissue. This overlapping has been caused by removal of underlying bone, leaving less bone to be covered by the same tissue.

With scissors, remove that amount of mucoperiosteum which has just previously been seen to overlap.

Iron this soft tissue back into place with the moistened index finger, approximating the cut edges of the mucoperiosteum, and note whether you can feel through the mucoperiosteal tissue any sharp projections remaining labially, buccally or on the alveolar ridge.

If there are any sharp projections of bone, lift the mucoperiosteal tissue and remove them with the bone file or, if large enough, with the bone shear.

Suture the mucoperiosteum back into place so that the soft tissue is held against interseptal bone. I prefer a continuous 000 black silk suture, as illustrated. However, interrupted sutures may be used if desired. (Review the rules for suturing on pages 102 to 106.)

Certain conditions indicate the need for additional sutures. (*a*) Reflect the lips and pull the lip back. If this causes the flap to pull away, the flap needs more suturing at the point at which it pulls away. Other indications are (*b*) continued free bleeding; (*c*) bulging or gaping of the flap.

Note: In placing sutures, the needle is inserted through the labial or buccal mucoperiosteal tissue and then through the lingual soft tissue. The lingual mucoperiosteum is still attached and so will not be elevated by the needle.

Sutures are tied twice the first time and once the second, making a square knot. Study illustrations on suturing and knot-tying.

Objectives of Alveolectomy. Alveolectomy is done (*a*) to correct abnormalities and deformities of alveolar ridges that would interfere with proper adaptation of artificial dentures or other appliances; (*b*) to remove sharp or projecting ridges of the alveolar process; these are sometimes a source of facial neuralgias or localized pain; (*c*) to remove diseased interseptal bone when a gingivectomy is done; diseased interseptal bone is removed with a file; (*d*) to reduce tuberosities so as to obtain clearance for a denture base, or to remove undercuts; (*e*) to correct maxillary prognathism.

OSSEOUS OUTGROWTHS OR EXCRESCENCES

Congenital Abnormalities. These are bulky outgrowths usually found (1) on the maxillary tuberosities; (2) as a projection of the anterior maxillary alveolar process over the lower arch, called *overjet;* (3) as the elongation of the anterior maxillary alveolar process below the normal lip line, called *overbite;* (4) as an osseous outgrowth of the median raphe of the palatine bone known as *torus palatinus* (palatal osteoma), which may vary in size from a slight elevation of 3 mm. to a lobulated mass of 10 to 15 mm. in depth and 40 to 50 mm. in circumference; (5) as osseous excrescences on the lingual surface of the mandible known as *torus mandibularis* (mandibular osteoma) in the region of (*a*) the bicuspids, (*b*) the cuspids, (*c*) the central incisors; these vary from the size of a half pea to that of a half hickory nut; (6) as marked sharp undercuts on the lingual surface of the mandible extending from the molar region posteriorly, or, in some cases, from the cuspid region posteriorly to the third molar; they are called the "lingual balcony" by some authors; (7) as abnormally prominent mylohyoid ridges, also producing undercuts; (8) as prognathism of the maxilla or mandible.

Acquired Abnormalities. These may be the result of:

1. Removal of teeth at different times over a period of years. This results in an irregular rate of disuse atrophy of the alveolar process. In addition the early loss of an occluding tooth or teeth results in the gradual extrusion of the opposing tooth or teeth with its supporting alveolar process (see Figures 3–39 and 13–168*G, H*). See Figure 3–42 for the surgical reduction of elongated alveolar processes at the time of extraction.

2. Peculiar eating habits. Tobacco chewers develop a hyperostosis or a thickening of the cortical bone.

3. Chronic low-grade gingival infections. The buccal or labial cortical plate shows bony protuberances, multiple nodular exostoses (see Figure 2–16).

4. Chronic infections causing destruction of bone, interseptal and intraradicular.

5. Deformity following healed but malunited, poorly aligned fractures of the maxilla or mandible whose malpositions, however, do not warrant refracturing.

6. Deformity following the removal of a large cyst.

7. Osteomas.

CORRECTION OF MAXILLARY PROGNATHISM

A case of maxillary prognathism with marked overbite and overjet* is shown in Figure 3–51. The amount of overgrowth of the maxilla as compared to the mandible is shown in Figure 3–51*A* and *B*. To correct this abnormality, the mucoperiosteal flap is reflected in the manner which has already been described in the section on alveolectomy and is illustrated in Figure 3–51*C*, except that in cases of maxillary prognathism the labial flap is reflected much higher on the cortical bone than in the average case for an alveolectomy. It may be necessary in the reflection of this flap, labially, to excise the origins of the depressor septi muscles, the incisivi labii superioris and the nasalis muscles.

The next step is illustrated in Figure 3–51*D*. By means of a chisel, the labial cortical plate is removed in its entirety from cuspid to cuspid area all the way to the apices of these teeth. Interseptal bone is also reduced for a distance of several millimeters. The teeth now are luxated and removed, and the palatal mucoperiosteal flap is reflected as shown in Figure 3–51*E*. In order to reflect this flap, it is necessary to sever the vessels as they exit from the nasopalatine canal. This can be done and the bleeding controlled by packing a short strip of iodoform gauze into the canal for 3 to 5 minutes. Postoperatively, of course, this area of the palate is numb. However, this should not be alarming because the nasopalatine nerve will grow back into the anterior palatine mucosa tissue within a period of a few months.

(*Text continued on page 187*)

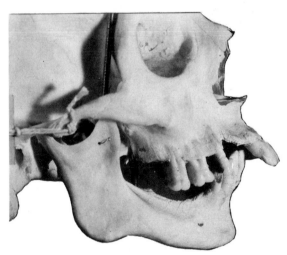

Figure 3–50 In this case the cause for the protrusion of the anterior maxillary process is the long-continued driving force of the lower anteriors during mastication, the full force being exerted on the upper anterior teeth because of the lack of occluding posterior teeth. This is not a true exostosis, but a localized maxillary prognathism mechanically induced.

---

*In the *Glossary of Prosthodontic Terms* (J. Prosthet. Dent., 6 [Mar.], 1956), the Nomenclature Committee of the Academy of Denture Prosthetics indicate a preference for "vertical overlap" instead of "overbite" and for "horizontal overlap" instead of "overjet." The older terminology has been retained here because it appears still to have the widest usage.

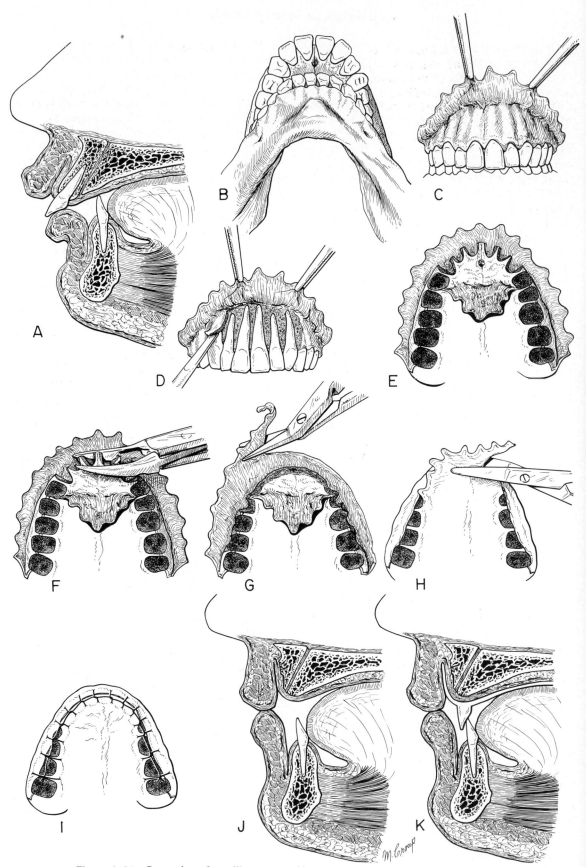

Figure 3–51 Correction of maxillary prognathism. See text for description of technique.

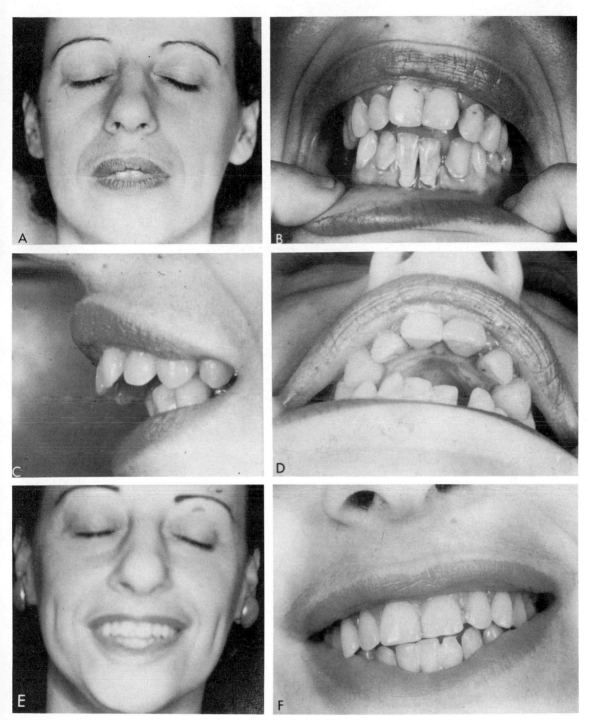

Figure 3–52 Maxillary prognathism. *A,* Note full, protruding maxilla and upper lip which does not cover the upper teeth. *B,* Evidence of periodontal disease. *C* and *D,* Extent of overgrowth and overjet (horizontal overlap). *E* and *F,* Postoperative results after surgical procedure shown in Figure 3–51.

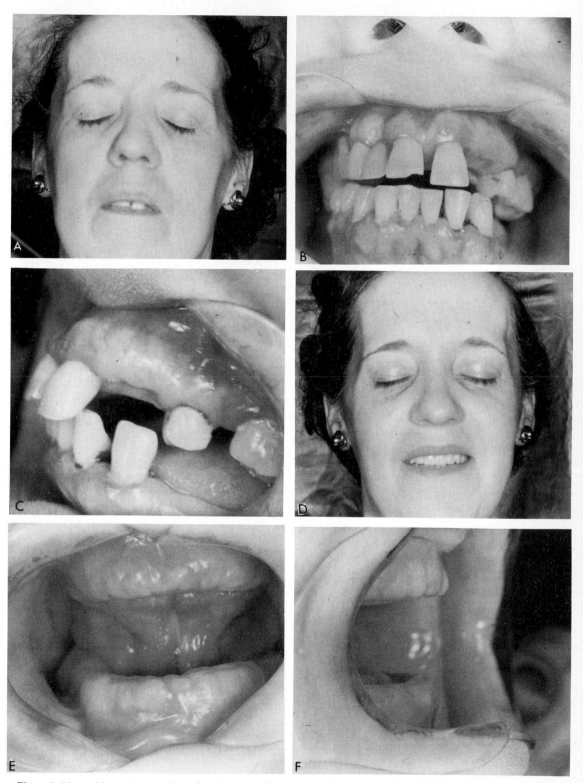

Figure 3–53 *A*, Not only does this patient have maxillary prognathism, but also there has been a marked overgrowth of mandibular anterior alveolar process so that the mandibular anterior teeth might follow the maxillary anterior teeth in an attempt to bring them into occlusion. *B*, Overgrowth of maxillary and mandibular alveolar process; note the multiple nodular exostoses present in both jaws, and the evidence of periodontoclasia. *C*, Profile of anterior maxilla and mandible showing the deep undercuts in both jaws. *D*, Postoperative results after surgery as illustrated in Figure 3–51. *E*, Healed edentulous ridges demonstrating that although quite extensive excision of bone was performed on both jaws, there are still excellent ridges for denture support. *F*, Note the excellent relationship of the ridges to each other, the very slight undercuts and the intermaxillary space.

Additional bone is removed from the anterior maxilla with bone shears, as shown in Figure 3–51*F* until that portion of the maxilla that has protruded beyond the normal contour of the maxilla has been removed. This means, of course, that quite frequently the nasopalatine canal is involved in the line of cutting. However, this should not prevent the removal of bone because, as has been stated, the neurovascular bundle containing arteries, veins and nerves will reestablish itself into the palatal mucosa.

The flaps are now replaced; in Figure 3–51*H* is shown the excision of that portion of the palatal flap which protrudes over the crest of the newly formed ridge. It is well to permit this mucosa to project over the crest of the ridge because it is much thicker than the labial flap and will offer a cushioned base, as it were, for the denture. The labial flap is trimmed in the anterior portion so that the two flaps approximate, and then the entire periphery is sutured, as shown in Figure 3–51*I*, with a continuous lock stitch suture. *J* shows the healed ridge in relation to the mandibular teeth, and in *K* the new denture has been inserted.

LINGUAL "BALCONY": SHARP UNDERCUT INTERNAL OBLIQUE RIDGES

These bilateral ridges may be found at the time of extraction (see Figure 3–54) or in those cases of advanced resorption of the alveolar process. In both cases they should be removed as illustrated in Figure 3–54. Two views of these "balconies" are shown in *A* and *B*, and *D* shows a cross section. *C* illustrates the line of incision to expose the operative side adequately. In *D* the vertical line shows the buccal-lingual position of the incision. In *E*, the mucoperiosteal flap is reflected, exposing the mylohyoid muscle insertion which is cut bilaterally; *F*, the sharp, bony undercut is removed with bone shears and (*H*) smoothed with a file. A chisel or rotary file (*G*) may also be used. The flap is sutured back into place (*I*).

LOCALIZED UNDERCUTS OF ALVEOLAR PROCESS OF MAXILLA OR MANDIBLE

The technique for removal of undercuts is as follows:

Make an incision along the crest of the ridge, starting at a point 10 mm. beyond the undercut on each side; at each end cut toward

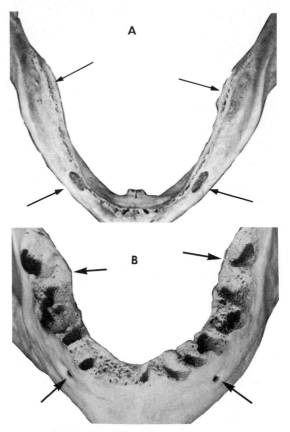

Figure 3–54 Sharp lingual balconies are indicated by upper arrows in both *A* and *B*. Note relationship of mental foramen (lower arrows) to the crest of the ridge.

the mucobuccal fold at a 45-degree angle for 1 cm.

With a periosteal elevator strip the mucoperiosteum from the bone for at least 10 mm. below the undercut.

Using rongeurs, place one blade on the top

(Text continued on page 191)

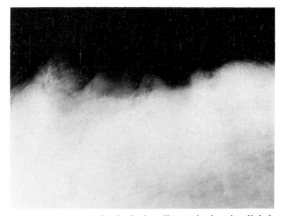

Figure 3–55 *A*, Periapical radiograph that is slightly underexposed will show the sharp, pointed projections of alveolar bone which produce acute pain under dentures and must be excised.

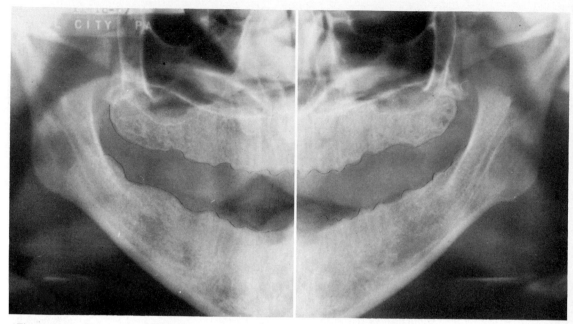

Figure 3-56 Panoramic radiograph revealing alveolar irregularities in both the maxilla and mandible, which require surgery as described and illustrated in previous figures.

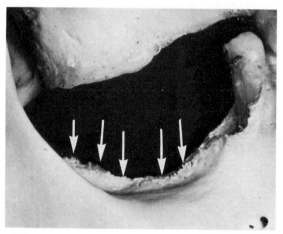

Figure 3-57 Anatomic specimen of the corpus of the mandible, showing a "saw-toothed" osseous ridge, such as was shown in previous radiographs.

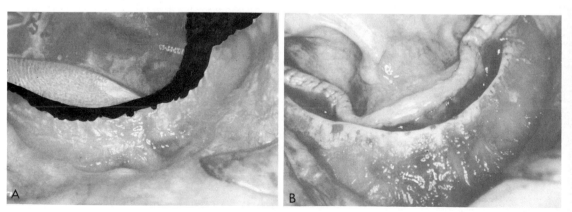

Figure 3-58 *A,* Patient in whom the mucoperiosteal tissue was reflected, a most difficult task in view of the adherence of the tissue to these sharp, thin projections of bone.

B, Ridge following excision of the sharp bone and smoothing of the ridge. (Photographs courtesy of Dr. Frank Pavel.)

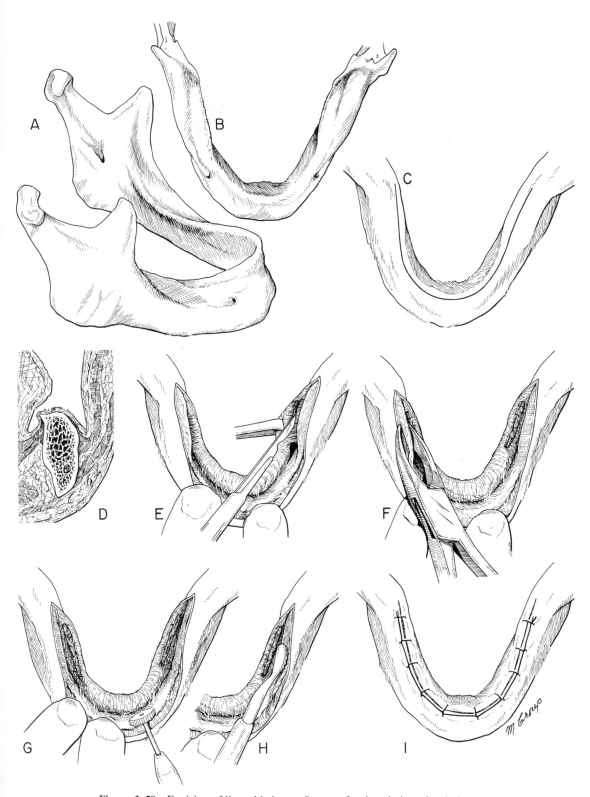

Figure 3–59 Excision of lingual balcony. See text for description of technique.

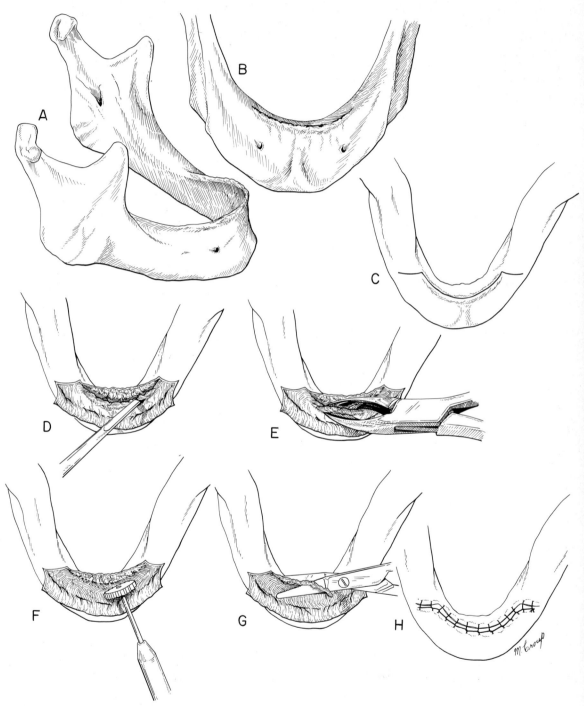

Figure 3–60   Excision of a "saw-toothed" residual mandibular alveolar ridge. See text for a description of the technique.

of the ridge and the other blade under the undercut, and cut off the protruding bone. *Caution: Be careful not to overtrim.* Err in favor of leaving too much bone or tissue in place, rather than too little.

Use a bone file to smooth the exposed bone.

If any sharp points or projections remain on the crest of the ridge, reflect the mucoperiosteum to the lingual side and remove the sharp projections with a bone file; or, if the projections are large, remove with rongeurs.

Replace the soft tissue flap over the ridge and note the degree of overlapping.

Trim away the excess of soft tissue from the edges of the flap until they approximate each other without tension and cover the ridge.

Suture the edges of the flap back into position without tension. (Study the illustrations.)

SHARP "SAW-TOOTHED" OR "KNIFE-EDGED" MANDIBULAR RIDGE

In mandibles the last vestige of the alveolar process is a narrow, sharp, saw-tooth or knife-edge of bone. These are extremely painful, and in many cases even extensive hollowing out of the denture fails to provide relief from the burning pain these patients experience.

In Figure 3–60 is an example of such a case in which just the anterior area is involved (*A* and *B*). *C* shows an outline of the flap. In *D*, the flap is reflected labially and lingually and the ridge is removed with a chisel and mallet or a bone shear (*E*). In *F*, the ridge is smoothed with a rotary bone file. *G* shows excess tissue being cut off. In *H*, flaps are secured with a continuous suture.

REMOVAL OF BONY MAXILLARY TUBEROSITIES

Bony maxillary tuberosities are to be differentiated from hyperplasia of the mucous membrane or cartilaginous maxillary tuberosities (see Figure 3–39).

Precaution: Always radiograph these areas to make sure that the maxillary sinus does not dip down into this tuberosity area.

Make an incision through the mucoperiosteum, starting distal to the tuberosity and cutting anteriorly along the crest of the ridge, using a No. 12 Bard-Parker blade to start the incision.

Then change to a No. 15 Bard-Parker blade and extend the incision 10 mm. beyond the point at which the bone is to be removed, and extend the incision at a 45-degree angle to the mucobuccal fold.

The mucosa overlying these masses is perfectly normal unless it has been traumatized (as the mucosa over the torus palatinus, which may be traumatized by eating). It is therefore necessary, when removing these outgrowths, to take care not to tear the mucous membrane. Make the incision through the entire thickness of soft tissue to the bone, and lay the tissue back with the end of the periosteal elevator.

The flap is now reflected, exposing the undercut.

Remove the bony undercut with bone shears. Place one blade on the crest of the ridge and the other blade beneath the undercut, and cut away the bone forming the undercut.

After the bony undercut has been removed, free the lingual mucosa toward the palate, and reduce the height of the ridge in the tuberosity area with rongeurs and bone shears.

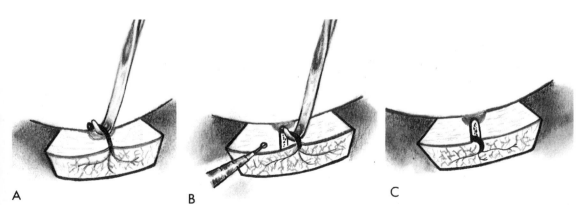

A   **B**   **C**

Figure 3–61 *A,* Mental foramen on the crest of the edentulous mandibular ridge. The neurovascular bundle is elevated with a hook.

B, The bone is carefully cut away beneath the bundle.

C, The neurovascular bundle is lowered into its new position below the edge of the flange of the denture.

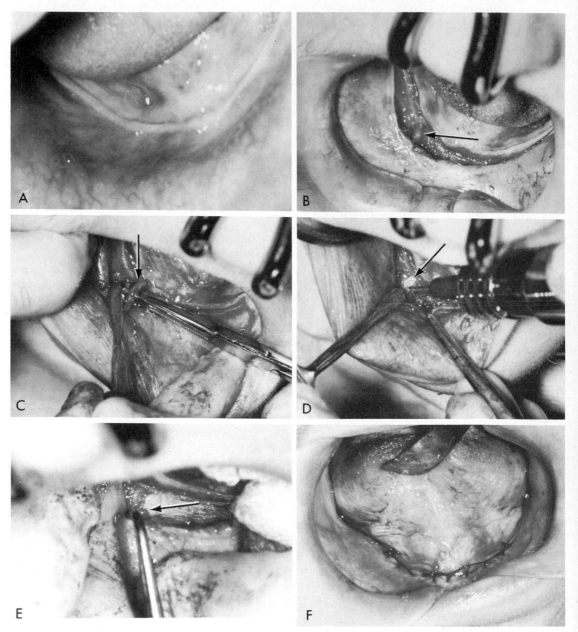

Figure 3–62   *A,* Edentulous mandible with very little remaining alveolar process. This is the so-called "flat floor" of the oral cavity. This patient has worn her dentures with satisfaction and very capable mastication, but now complains of bilateral pain in both mental foramen areas.

B, Mucoperiosteal membrane is incised along the crest of the ridge from the right molar area to the left. The dentist exercises great care *not* to cut the bilateral neurovascular bundles as they exit from the foramina, which now are on the superior surface of the mandible. See arrow and Figure 3–63.

C, The flap is reflected with a periosteal elevator, and the neurovascular bundle is lifted with a closed hemostat slipped beneath it.

D, The bundle is held away from the bone as the foramen is enlarged inferiorly and laterally with a round bur. Care must be used not to cut into the bundle with the bur.

E, Enlarged foramen with the neurovascular bundle at the inferior border. See arrow.

F, Same procedure was carried out on the opposite foramen, and the mucoperiosteal flaps are sutured back into place.

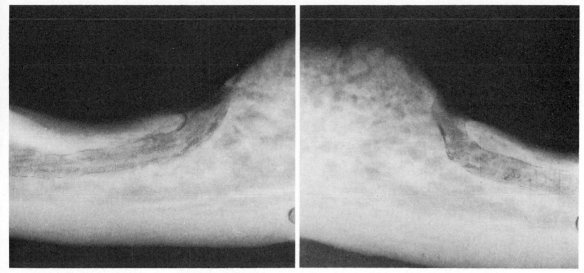

Figure 3–63 Bilateral periapical radiographs of the mental foramen areas, which clearly show the foramina opening onto the crest of the corpus.

Smooth down the ridge with bone files to free the ridge of any sharp margins, or points.

Replace the flap in position over the tuberosity area. There will now be considerable overlapping of this soft tissue flap. With scissors cut away the excess soft tissue so that the ends of the flap approximate without overlapping.

Suture the flap into position without tension.

REDUCTION OF ELONGATED ANTERIOR MAXILLARY RIDGE

Often there is elongation of the anterior maxillary alveolar process below the normal lip line. The problem here is to reduce the height of the anterior maxillary alveolar process.

First make impressions and stone casts of the case, and mount these on an articulator.

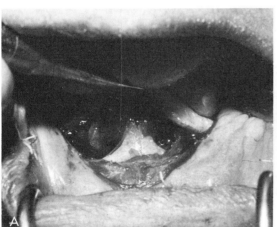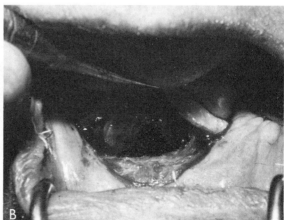

Figure 3–64 *A,* It is rare that enlarged genial tubercles are a source of trouble to patients wearing full lower dentures. In fact, their presence frequently helps to stabilize the denture. In the absence of symptoms, their presence alone is not an indication for their removal. In *A,* however, we see an enlarged genial tubercle in which the overlying mucosa was constantly the site of painful ulceration under the denture, in spite of attempts to relieve the pressure by grinding and polishing the denture where it impinged on the genial tubercles.

B, The superficial fibers of the genioglossus muscles are dissected away, and the osseous tissue is removed with burs. The flap is sutured into place.

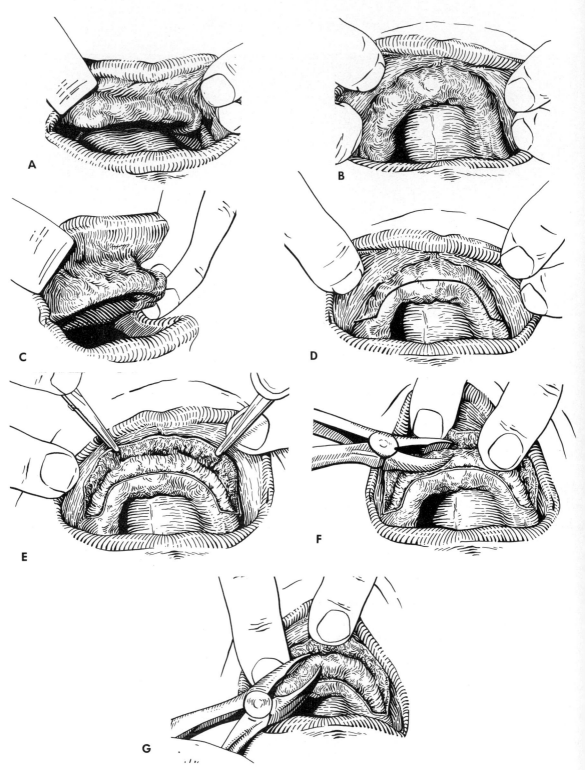

Figure 3–65 Alveolectomy of an irregular and protruding edentulous anterior maxillary alveolar ridge.

A to *C*, Anterior, inferior anterior and right lateral views, respectively. These views show the irregular, markedly undercut and protruding anterior maxillary alveolar ridge.

D, The incision is made along the midpoint of the crest of the ridge, and in both bicuspid areas it is carried toward the mucobuccal fold at a 45-degree angle.

E, The labial mucoperiosteal flap is reflected to the mucolabial fold. The palatal tissue is loosened for a distance of 1 cm.

F, The undercuts are removed with a bone shear by placing one edge beneath the undercut, the other on the crest of the ridge.

G, The length of the ridge is reduced with the bone shear by placing one blade on either side of the ridge.

(Figure 3–65 continued on opposite page)

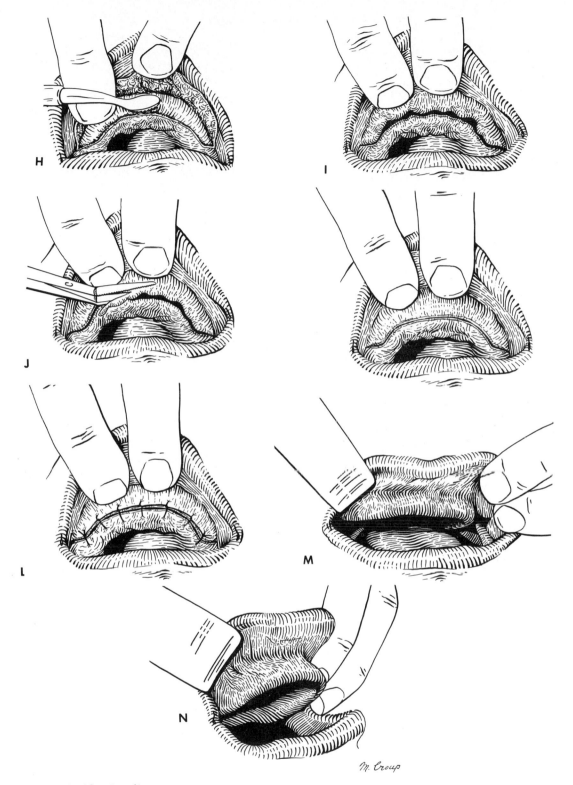

M. Croup

Figure 3–65 (*Continued.*)

H, The ridge is smoothed with a bone file.

I and *J,* The soft tissues are replaced and the excess tissue (*I*) is trimmed from both the labial and palatal flaps (*J*) with a No. 9 Dean's scissors until they meet without tension or excess.

K, Soft tissue in apposition after trimming.

L, Soft tissue flaps approximated with a continuous suture.

M, This anterior view shows that the ridge is smooth.

N, This right lateral view shows that the marked undercut is reduced by half and the height of the ridge reduced one third.

Trim the stone casts to the desired size and shape. This model will guide the operator during surgery.

The technique described below is illustrated in Figure 3–65.

Make the incision along the crest of the maxillary ridge, using a No. 15 Bard-Parker blade to cut the mucoperiosteum until bone is contacted. Extend the incision to include all the area involved, and further extend to a point 10 mm. beyond the area involved on each side. The area involved is usually from cuspid to cuspid.

After extending the incision 10 mm. beyond the area involved on each side, extend the incision toward the mucobuccal fold at a 45-degree angle.

Reflect the mucoperiosteum to the mucobuccal and mucolabial folds, using a periosteal elevator. In reflecting the palatal mucoperiosteum, the nasopalatine foramen may be exposed if it is too close to the crest of the ridge.

It may be necessary to sever the nasopalatine neurovascular bundle and cut away a portion of the nasopalatine canal and surrounding bone to achieve a satisfactory ridge, one which will permit the construction and insertion of a cosmetically and mechanically satisfactory maxillary denture.

Cut away the excess bone, from the upper anterior ridge from bicuspid to bicuspid areas, with rongeurs and bone shears.

Smooth the ridge with bone files.

Replace the mucoperiosteal flap in position.

It will be noted that there is now a considerable overlapping of this flap. With scissors cut away the excess mucoperiosteum from the edges of the flap so that the ends of the flap approximate without overlapping.

Suture the flap into position.

REDUCTION OF OVERJET (HORIZONTAL OVERLAP)

Overjet is the projection anteriorly of the alveolar process of the maxilla over the lower arch.

For the removal of overjet the same technique is used as for the removal of overbite, except that the thickness of the ridge is also reduced. Study Figure 3–65.

REMOVAL OF TORUS PALATINUS (PALATAL OSTEOMA)

A study of the various benign osseous outgrowths along the median palatine suture of the maxilla that are illustrated in Figures 3–66, 3–67, and 13–4 to 13–5 will indicate why it is necessary that these osseous protuberances be removed in order to facilitate the placement of a full or partial maxillary denture. In addition, in cases in which the construction of a denture is not contemplated, these osseous outgrowths are frequently the site of traumatic ulcers resulting from infections of scratches or abrasions as the result of mastication of harsh foods. Frequently, these patients seek surgical relief from these recurrent extremely painful ulcerations; the only relief that can be given, of course, is the

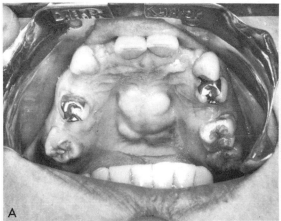 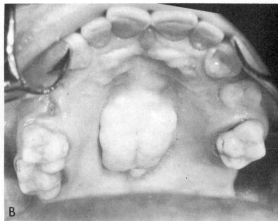

Figure 3–66 Examples of the lobular type of torus palatinus in which there is a marked undercut around the tumor. These are frequently large and may interfere with speech. In some cases there may be food retained beneath the bony ledge, and an area of infection results which may produce a localized osteomyelitis. Certainly they present a problem to the prosthodontist, the best solution to which is surgical removal.

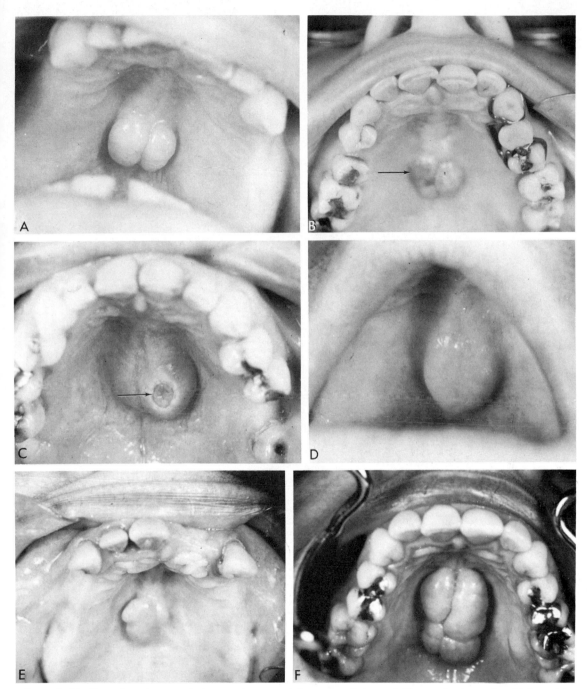

Figure 3–67 Examples of torus palatinus. *A*, Large, nodular torus palatinus. *B*, Traumatic ulcers of multiple nodular torus palatinus as the result of trauma by food during mastication. *C*, Large healing ulcer on a spindle-type torus palatinus, also the result of masticatory trauma. *D*, Large spindle-type torus palatinus. *E*, Nodular torus palatinus. *F*, Large lobular torus palatinus.

Excision of tori is only indicated when these are repeatedly traumatized or if they interfere with the insertion of partial or full dentures that will traumatize the mucosa over the tori.

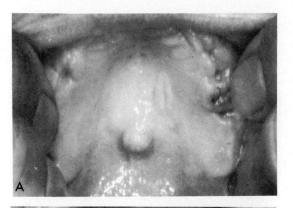

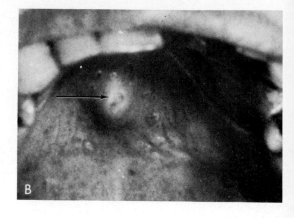

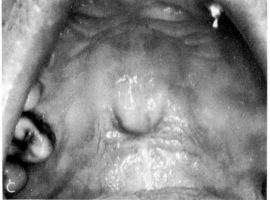

Figure 3–68 *A* and *B*, Small pedicle types of tori. Note the ulceration of the mucosa from food trauma in *B*. This evidence of trauma is an indication for its removal. *C*, A larger multinodular torus.

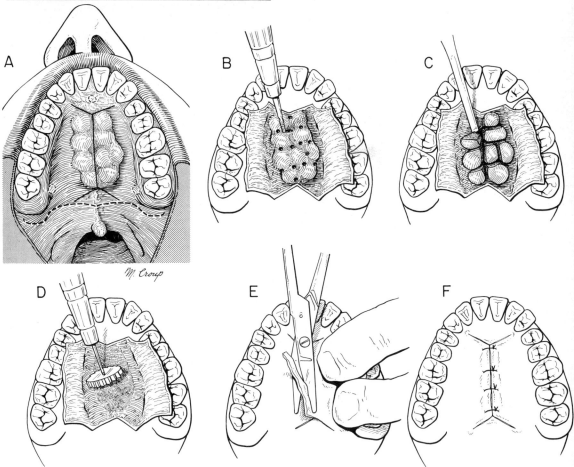

M. Croup

Figure 3–69 Surgical removal of torus palatinus. See text for a description of the technique.

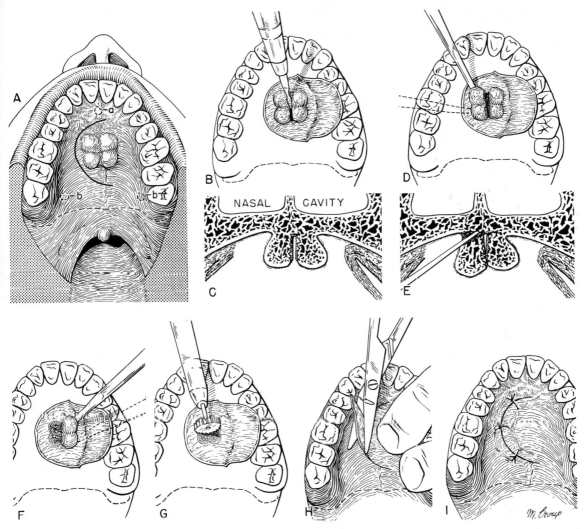

Figure 3–70 Excision of multiple nodular torus palatinus. *A*, Semicircular incision is made. Broken line is edge of hard palate. *a*, Incisive foramen. *b*, Greater palatine foramen. *B* and *C*, Flap is reflected and groove cut through the middle with a crosscut fissure bur. *D* and *E*, One half of torus is removed by cutting through the pedicle base with a chisel. *F*, The remaining half is removed in the same manner. *G*, Palate is smoothed with a small cutting wheel. *H*, The excess mucoperiosteal membrane is trimmed. *I*, Flap is sutured into place with silk sutures.

surgical excision of these bony outgrowths. In a survey, out of 5379 blacks examined 1086 had torus palatinus (or 18.5 per cent).* Out of 1161 whites examined 161 had torus palatinus (or 13.8 per cent).† The reader is referred to pages 196 to 198 for additional information concerning tori palatinus and mandibularis.

Technique for Excision of a Nodular Torus Palatinus. In Figure 3–69*A* is shown a large nodular torus palatinus. In the midline, the dark line shows the incision carried from the anterior end to the posterior end of this bony growth. At either end of this midline incision, lateral incisions are carried right and left for a distance 0.5 cm. beyond the width of the torus. The broken posterior line represents the end of the hard palate. Right and left in the palate the circular broken lines illustrate the greater palatine foramen, which of course must be avoided in making the lateral incision, and, behind the central incisors, the incisive foramen, which is also avoided in making the incision.

In Figure 3–69*B* is illustrated the reflection of the mucoperiosteal membrane from the torus. Reflecting this membrane without tearing it is a very difficult task because it is quite thin. There is a scarcity of fibrous material in

---

*Survey supervised by the author and Cedric L. Haydn at the Port of Spain Community Hospital, Trinidad.

†Dental students examined in the U.S.A.

the tissue; the squamous epithelium is closely adherent to the periosteum, which, in turn, is firmly attached to the various bony nodules. To reflect and elevate this membrane from these rounded bony eminences, to dissect it out from the lines of fusion and depressions without tearing is exceedingly difficult. When the flap has been reflected to the periphery of the osteoma, the mucoperiosteal membrane becomes much thicker and is more readily reflected. Once the flaps are reflected, they can be held back with sutures to the adjacent teeth or with broad periosteal elevators. Then, with a spear-point bur, beginning points are drilled in the lines of fusion in the midline and between the various nodules. These drill-point holes are connected with a crosscut fissure bur.

Next, as shown in Figure 3–69C, the various nodules are removed with a single-bevel chisel. The edge of the chisel is placed against the base of the osteoma (torus) with the bevel approximating the palatine bone. When the chisel is now tapped with the mallet, a planing action results, whereas if the chisel is rotated so that the bevel is away from the palatine bone, striking the chisel may result in penetration of the nasal cavity (see Figure 3–71). The palate is then smoothed and rounded with a rotary file, as shown in Figure 3–69D. The mucoperiosteal membrane is now re-

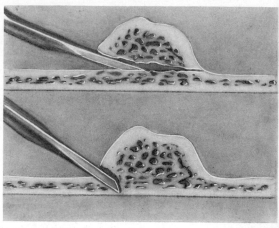

Figure 3–71 To *plane bone* or remove osteomas, the bevel must approximate the cortical plate as shown in the top of this drawing. If the bevel is turned up, as shown in the bottom drawing, the chisel will *penetrate bone*. Additional note: chisels must be razor sharp before using. This means they must be sharpened before every operation.

placed, and it will be found that the flaps are not as large as they were originally because the thin membrane possesses elastic qualities and so the flaps shrink somewhat in size. The excess (overlapping) portions are removed with scissors, as shown in Figure 3–69E, and

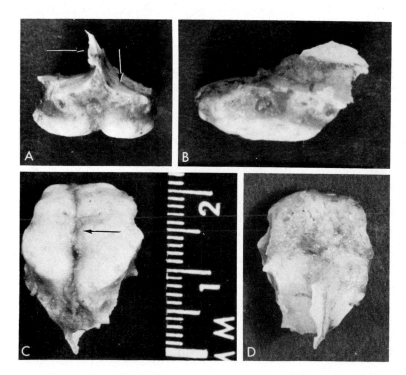

Figure 3–72 *A*, Segmental fracture of the torus palatinus with part of the floor of the nasal cavity (right vertical arrow) and septum (left horizontal arrow). This was the result of an attempt to excise a moderate-sized torus palatinus with a chisel. This would have been successful except for the fact that in this case the palatal process of the maxilla lateral to the torus was very thin. See *A* of Figure 3–73 for a schematic drawing. Also study the text.

B, Lateral view of specimen. *C*, Palatal view. Note midline fissure and seminodular surface. *D*, Nasal side. Note that the osseous union of the torus with the floor of the nasal cavity was cut halfway to the distal end of the torus when the fracture took place.

the flaps are approximated and sutured into place, as shown in Figure 3–69F.

Surgical Sequelae to Be Avoided in Removing a Torus Palatinus. FRACTURE OF THE PALATAL PROCESS AND NASAL FLOOR. Segmental fracture of the entire torus palatinus with the palatal process of the maxilla and of the nasal floor with a portion of the nasal septum. See an example of this in Figure 3–72. A study of the schematic drawing A in Figure 3–73 will show why this happened. Every oral surgeon has successfully removed many of the smaller palatal tori in a few minutes by repeated cuts with a sharp chisel around the base of the torus, thereby separating it from the palatal process of the maxilla. However, if the patient has the anatomic condition shown in A of Figure 3–73, where the palatal process of the maxilla consists only of thin cortical bone separating the oral cavity from the nasal

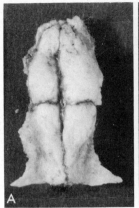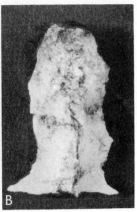

Figure 3–74 Where there is posterior sloping and merging of the torus palatinus and the palatine bone, as shown here, instead of a clear-cut demarcation, a portion of the palatine bone will fracture off with the excised torus, when a chisel alone is used. To avoid this the torus must be divided into sections with a bur and then the individual segments excised with a sharp chisel. Or the entire torus palatinus must be reduced by a bur (see Figure 3–75).

A, Inferior view. B, Superior view (nasal side). Note the smooth area, which is the superior surface of the palatine bone.

cavity, an attempt to cut this tori from the palate with a chisel will produce the segmental fracture shown in Figure 3–72. If the palatal process of the maxilla is as thick as that shown in B of Figure 3–73, then this technique can be carried out.

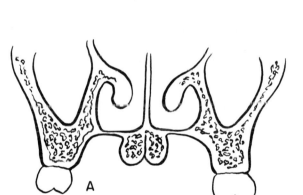

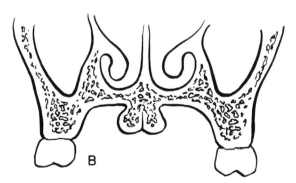

Figure 3–73 A, If an attempt is made to sever the torus palatinus from its base with a chisel alone in the anatomic situation shown here, a segmental fracture of the palate and floor of the nose will result. See example of this in Figure 3–72. B, On the contrary, in this case, in which there is a reasonably thick palatal process on either side of the torus, it can be cut from the palate with a chisel without a segmental fracture.

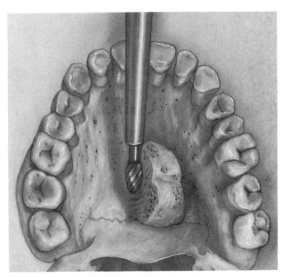

Figure 3–75 Removal of a torus palatinus by means of the ultra-high-speed turbine unit and bur.

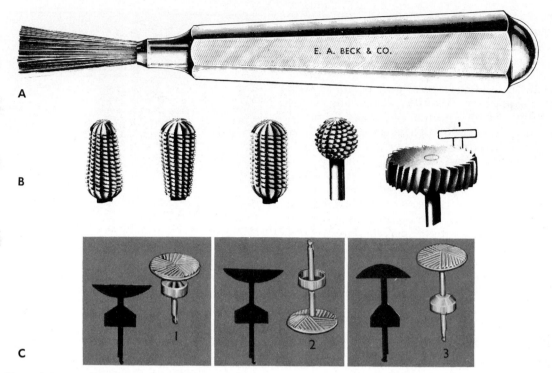

Figure 3–76 *A*, Cleaning brush for saws, files and burs—an *absolute necessity* whenever burs or files are used. All burs quickly clog with bone. The bur then acts as a burnisher and will burn the bone. The bur should be changed as soon as the cutting leaves are filled with bone and replaced with a clean bur. The assistant cleans it and replaces it on the tray.

B, Types of bone burs and a wheel-type rotary file.

C, A very helpful rotary file in three different shapes (note silhouettes). No. 1 file smoothes buccal and labial bone spurs and irregularities during alveolectomy. No. 2 file removes lingual protuberance in region of lower third molar. No. 3 file removes small torus palatinus and torus lingualis.

To determine whether or not the palatal process on either side of the torus is thin, place a diagnostic or transilluminating light against the palatal tissue, first on one side of the torus and then the other, each time looking into the nasal cavity with a nasal speculum. If the palatal process is thin, the nasal cavity will be illuminated. In these cases it is necessary to remove the tori with a bur, or to cut it into segments with a bur and then cut off the small segments with a sharp chisel.

PALATINE BONE FRACTURE. The torus may be almost completely separated from the palatal process of the maxilla and then the last cut with the chisel fractures out with the torus a section of the palatine bone, as shown in Figure 3–74. This results in a marked defect in the junction of the hard and soft palate that

Figure 3–77 *A*, Nodular torus palatinus. *B*, The mucoperiosteum has been stripped from the nodular torus palatinus. *C*, Appearance of the nodular torus palatinus 31 days later. *D*, Immediately after removal of "shell" and underlying tissue. *E*, Outer surface of "shell" after it was exfoliated. *F*, Inner surface of "shell." *G*, One week after removal of "shell." *H*, Two weeks after removal of "shell."

As can be observed from this process, tori arise from the cortical bone from which they receive no nutrition. Stripping the overlying mucoperiosteum *(B)* removes their sole source of nutriment, and they are then decalcified by the action of saprophytic organisms indigenous to the oral cavity. In the usual case this decalcification takes place in 21 days. In edentulous or very clean mouths, the decalcification period is prolonged *(C)*. The outer shell of the torus is exfoliated *(E)*, and there remains a succulent tissue that can be removed with a curette reaching down to cancellous bone *(D)*. This live bone limits the decalcification process, and the area is epithelialized in the normal time, usually 10 to 14 days *(H)*. The responsible organisms are pigmented species of *Neisseria, Micrococcus,* and *Streptococcus mitis.*

Photographic Case Report

DESTRUCTION OF TORUS PALATINUS BY DEPRIVING IT OF ITS BLOOD SUPPLY

Eduard G. Friedrich

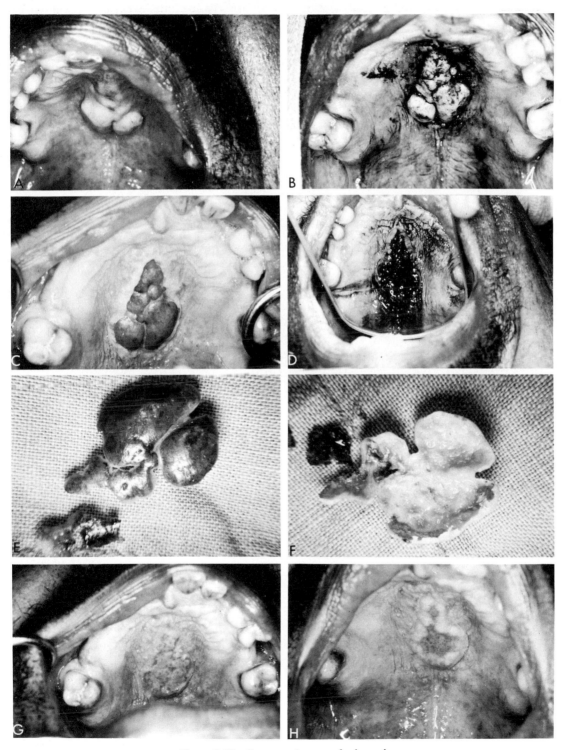

Figure 3–77 *See opposite page for legend.*

makes the construction of a full maxillary denture more difficult. To avoid this, do not try to remove even moderately large tori in their entirety when the posterior border encroaches on the palatine bone. With burs, following the suture lines, cut the tori into small sections and cut these sections off with a sharp chisel.

ʹNasal Bleeding. Do not cut the grooves so deeply as to penetrate into the nasal cavity. Brisk nasal bleeding may result. Seldom does this require nasal packing to control the bleeding, but if the bleeding does not stop within 5 minutes, packing is indicated.

The reader is referred to pages 196 to 203 for additional information and illustrations on osteomas in these areas.

REMOVAL OF POSTERIOR LATERAL PALATAL EXOSTOSES

These multiple exostoses found occasionally in the vicinity of the greater palatine foramen (Figure 3–78) give rise to marked discomfort to patients wearing maxillary dentures. Palpation will reveal their presence beneath the mucoperiosteal membrane. The lines of incision (Figure 3–78A and B) preserve the blood supply to the flap and produce a minimum of hemorrhage. The flap is reflected, and the greater palatine vessels and foramen are exposed (Figure 3–78B). (This is the same type of flap that should be used to remove the lingual root of a molar retained in a ridge, particularly so in those cases in which

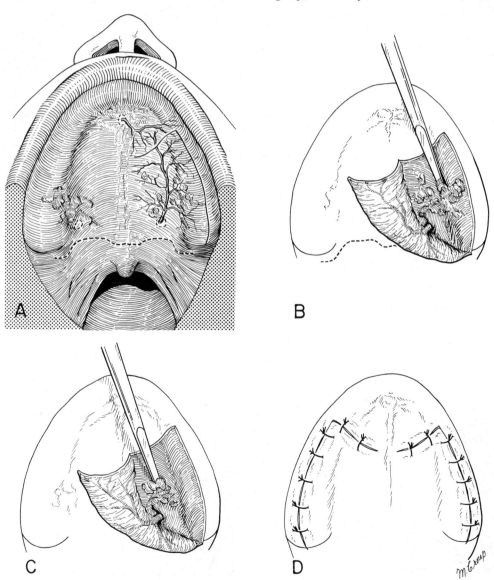

Figure 3–78 Removal of palatal exostoses in the region of the greater palatine foramen. See text for a description of the technique.

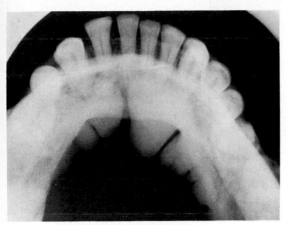

Figure 3–79 Occlusal radiograph of very large multinodular lingual exostoses (tori mandibularis).

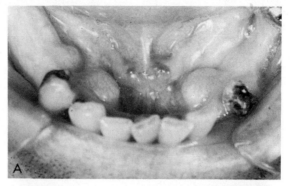

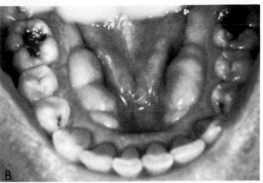

Figure 3–80 Multinodular torus mandibularis.

the floor of the maxillary sinus is buccal to the root tip.) The bony exostoses are planed off with a chisel (Figure 3–78B and C). *Extreme care must be taken to use easy blows of the mallet to prevent cutting the greater palatine artery as it leaves the foramen.* This is a most difficult hemorrhage to control. Flaps are sutured into place with interrupted sutures (Figure 3–78D).

REMOVAL OF TORUS MANDIBULARIS (MANDIBULAR OSTEOMA)

These bony excrescences are found on the lingual surface of the mandible in the region of bicuspids and cuspids. They may vary from the size of a half pea to that of a hickory nut; they may be single or multiple (see Figures 3–80 and 3–81).

Spray the mouth with antiseptic solution, before making the incision.

The following technique is illustrated in Figure 3–82.

Mark the incision along the crest of the mandible from the first molar area on one side of the mandible to the first molar area on the other side.

Reflect the mucoperiosteal flap to 1 cm. below the torus mandibularis on both sides of the mandible. In the anterior region the flap need not be reflected quite this far.

A gauze sponge is now inserted into the operative field between the reflected lingual mu-

(*Text continued on page 209*)

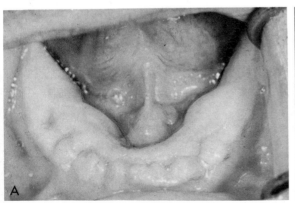

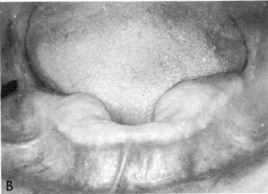

Figure 3–81 Two examples of the broad, sessile type of torus mandibularis.

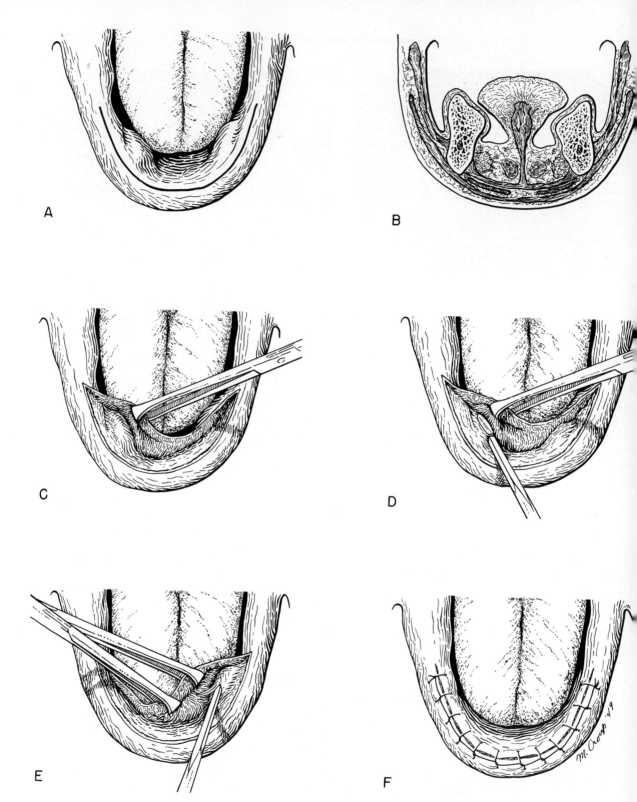

Figure 3–82 Surgical removal of torus mandibularis.
A, Line of incision on the crest of the ridge is shown on occlusal view of an edentulous mandible.
B, Coronal section of the mandible in the bicuspid area.
C, Flap is reflected lingually.
D, Growth of bone on the right side of the mandible is removed with a chisel.
E, Growth of bone on the left side of the mandible is removed with a chisel.
F, Soft tissues are approximated with a continuous suture.

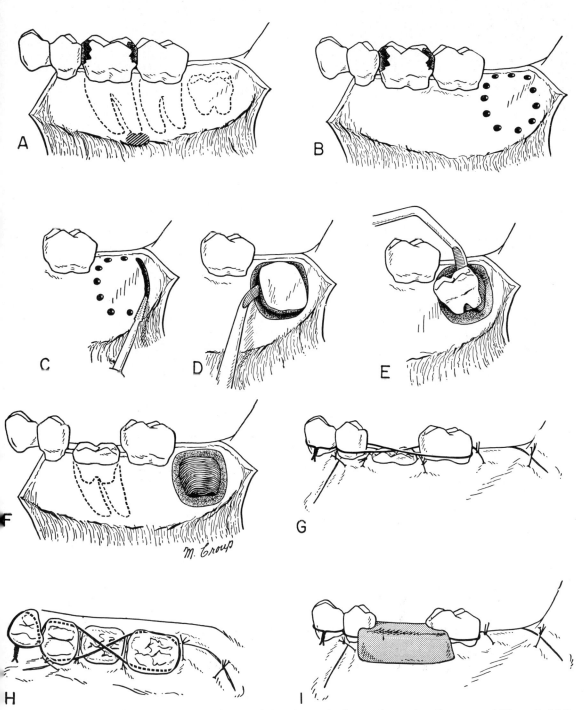

Figure 3–83 Transplantation of a mandibular third molar to the first molar socket. See text and Figure 3–84 for description of technique.

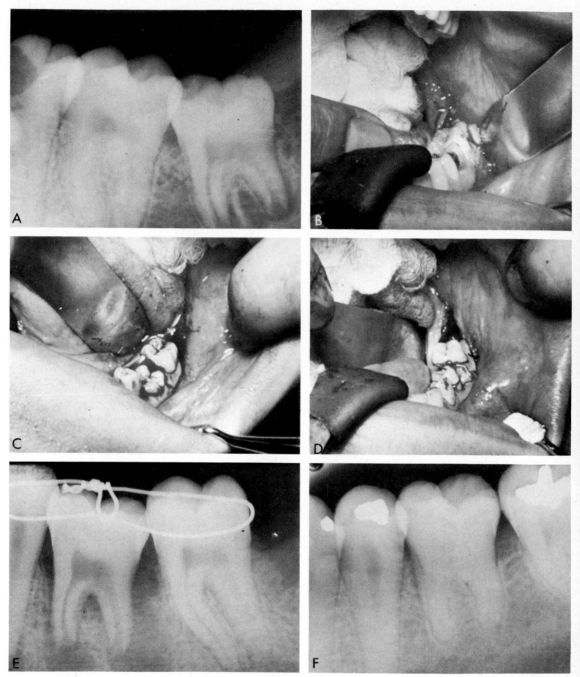

Figure 3–84 Transplantation of a third molar into the socket of a first molar that has just been extracted. *A,* Unerupted third molar before transplantation. *B,* Third molar crown exposed. *C,* Third molar inserted into the second molar's alveolus, from which the second molar has just been extracted. *D,* Third molar held in place by a wire ligature passed around the neck of the first molar, over the occlusal surface of the transplanted molar, and around the neck of the second molar. *E,* Appearance 3 weeks postoperatively. *F,* Appearance 5 years postoperatively. (Courtesy of Frank J. Andren, D.D.S., Parma, Ohio. *A, E* and *F,* From Andren, F. J.: Teens' unerupted third molars used in autogenous transplants. Clin. Dent., *2*(2):1 (Mar.), 1974.)

coperiosteum, the body of the mandible, and the surgical space that lies inferior to the torus (osteoma). This will prevent the loss of the excised bone into the deep structures in the floor of the oral cavity.

Remove the osseous excrescences with a sharp chisel and mallet. The chisel is placed as described for the removal of palatal osteomas. This bone is very dense, like ivory, and cannot be removed with rongeurs.

File smooth with bone files or bone-cutting wheels.

Remove the gauze sponge from the depth of the operative field.

Replace the flap; if edges overlap, remove the excess of the flap with Mayo-type curved scissors until the edges approximate each other.

Insert a continuous suture, or interrupted sutures, to close the line of incision.

TRANSPLANTATION OF DEVELOPING TEETH

The technique and conclusions that follow are excerpts from the articles by Apfel,[4] Hale[30] and Clark,[20] whose articles the reader is referred to for more detailed information on this subject.

The cases reported by these men were mandibular third molar transplants to the first molar bed. For best results the third molar must have developed a bifurcation and roots of 2 or 3 mm. The host area must be free of *acute infection.* Chronic infection is not a contraindication. The third molar must not be too large to fit in the new location.

Technique. Transplantation technique is illustrated in Figure 3–83. *A,* A flap is reflected to expose both operative sites. *B, C* and *D,* The bony crypt of the unerupted third molar is opened widely. *E,* The third molar is elevated from its bed and allowed to remain while the first molar is extracted. *F,* The third molar is transferred to a new site. It should not be wedged into the new socket, but fit freely. *G, H* and *I,* Preferably an acrylic or metal splint should be used to support and protect the tooth for the first 2 to 4 weeks, but a wire matrix covered with a medicated cement as shown here is fairly satisfactory.

REFERENCES

1. Adelson, H.: Orthodontist cites frenectomy dangers. Ill. Dent. J., *30*:40–41 (Jan.), 1961.
2. Adams, C. P.: The relation of spacing of the upper central incisors to abnormal fraenum labii and other features of the dento facial complex. Dent. Rec., *74*:72, 1954.
3. Apfel, H.: Autoplasty of enucleated prefunctional third molars. J. Oral Surg., 8:289, 1950.
4. Apfel, H.: Preliminary work in transplanting the third molar to the first molar position. J.A.D.A., *48*:143, 1954.
5. Backlund, E.: Diastema mediale superioris—frekvens och etiologi. Sven. Tandlak. Tidskr., *57*:273–291 (May), 1964.
6. Baume, L.: Physiological tooth migration and its significance for the development of occlusion. J. Dent. Res., *29*:346, 1960.
7. Bedel, W. R.: Nonsurgical reduction of the labial frenum with and without orthodontic treatment. J.A.D.A., *42*:510–515 (May), 1951.
8. Behrman, S. J.: Implantation: principles, practices and predictions. J. Dent. Med., *10*:116, 1955.
9. Behrman, S. J.: The development of antibiotic resistant organisms; its significance to the dentist. N.Y. State Dent. J., *21*:297, 1955.
10. Behrman, S. J.: The current status of implants in denture prosthesis. Alpha Omegan, *52*:30 (Sept.), 1959.
11. Behrman, S. J.: The implantation of magnets in the jaw to aid denture retention. J. Prosthet. Dent., *10*:807–841, 1960.
12. Behrman, S. J., and Egan, G. F.: The implantation of magnets in the jaw to aid denture retention; an original brief research report. N.Y. State Dent. J., *19*:353, 1953.
13. Bergstrom, K., and Jensen, R.: Diastema mediale och frenulum labii superioris. Sven. Tandlak. Tidskr., 55:59–71, 1962.
14. Bernier, J. L.: Management of Oral Disease, p. 416. St. Louis, The C. V. Mosby Co., 1955.
15. Brauer, J. C., et al.: Dentistry for Children. New York, McGraw Hill Book Co., Inc., 1958.
16. Broadway, R. T., and Gould, D. G.: Surgical requirements of the orthodontists. Br. Dent. J., *108*:189–190, 1960.
17. Byars, L.: Surgical management of the mandible invaded by cancer. Surg. Gynecol. Obstet., *98*:564–570, 1954.
18. Ceremello, P. J.: The superior labial frenum and the midline diastema and their relation to growth and development of the oral structures. Am. J. Orthod., *39*:120–139, 1953.
19. Chapman, H.: Separation of the permanent upper centrals. Trans. Br. Soc. Study Orthod., 249, 1935.
20. Clark, H. B., Tam, J. C., and Mitchell, D. F.: Transplantation of developing teeth. J. Dent. Res., *34*:322, 1955.
21. Conley, J. J.: The use of vitallium prostheses and implants in reconstruction of the mandibular arch. Plast. Reconstr. Surg., 8:150, 1951.
22. Conley, J. J.: Technique of immediate bone grafting in the treatment of benign and malignant tumors of the mandible and a review of 17 consecutive cases. Cancer, 6:568, 1953.
23. Curran, M.: Superior labial frenectomy. J.A.D.A., *41*:419–422, 1950.
24. Dewel, B. F.: Contraindications for surgical resection of the maxillary labial frenum. Dent. Dig., *50*:254, 1944.
25. Dewel, B. F.: The normal and the abnormal labial frenum. I. Clinical differentiation. J.A.D.A., *33*:318, 1946.

26. Dewel, B. F.: The labial frenum, midline diastema, and palatine papilla: A clinical analysis. Dent. Clin. North Am., 175–184. (Mar.), 1966.

27. Felber, P.: Dauerresultate von Selbstregulation des Diastemas der oberen zentralen Inzisiven nach Lippenbandresektion. Schweiz. Mschr. Zahanheilk., *58*:646–647, 1948.

28. Finn, S. B.: Clinical Pedodontics. 4th ed. Philadelphia, W. B. Saunders Co., 1973.

29. Gould, A. W.: An investigation of the inheritance of torus palatinus and torus mandibularis. J. Dent. Res., *43*:159 (Mar.-Apr.), 1964.

30. Hale, M. L.: Autogenous transplants. J.A.D.A., *49*:193–198, 1954.

31. Healy, M. J., *et al.:* The use of acrylic implants in one-stage reconstruction of the mandible. Surg. Gynecol. Obstet., *98*:393–406, 1954.

32. Heskia, J. E., and Deplagn, H.: Les indications chirurgicales au cours des traitements orthodontiques. Rev. Fr. Odontostomatol., *12*:740–752 (May), 1965.

33. Howe, Geoffrey: Surgical preparation of the mandible for prosthesis. J. Oral Surg., *22*:118 (Mar.), 1964.

34. Jacobs, M. H.: The abnormal frenum labii. Dent. Cosmos, *74*:436, 1932.

35. Kelsey, H. E.: When is the frenum labium a problem in orthodontics? Am. J. Orthod., *25*:124–129, 1939.

36. Kruger, G. O.: Oral Surgery, p. 136. St. Louis, The C. V. Mosby Co., 1959.

37. MacIntosh, R. B.: Surgical improvement of the deficient mandibular ridge. J. Mich. Dent. Assoc., *51*:91–94 (Mar.), 1969.

38. Mallett, S. P.: A method of preparing and using stainless steel in oral surgery. Oral Surg., *16*:1160 (Oct.), 1963.

39. Mayer, D. M., and Swanker, W. A.: Anomalies of Infants and Children, p. 173. New York, McGraw Hill Book Co., Inc., 1958.

40. Miller, S. C.: Oral Diagnosis and Treatment. Philadelphia, Blakiston Co., 1952.

41. Moore, C. H.: The incidence of torus palatinus in the newborn. Unpublished Thesis, Department of Oral Surgery, University of Pittsburgh, 1960.

42. Moyers, R.: Spacing between the maxillary central incisors. Alpha Omegan, *46*:80–82, 1952.

43. Obwegeser, H.: Surgical preparation of the maxilla for prosthesis. J. Oral Surg., *22*:127 (Mar.), 1964.

44. Porter, K., and Flanagan, V. D.: Glycogen in papillary hyperplasia of the palate. Oral Surg., *16*:1331 (Nov.), 1963.

45. Robinson, H. B. G.: Neoplasm and "precancerous" lesions of the oral regions. Dent. Clin. North Am., 621–626 (Nov.), 1957.

46. Saltzmann, J. A.: Orthodontic Principles and Prevention. Philadelphia, J. B. Lippincott Co., 1957.

47. Schwartz, A. B., and Abbott, T. R.: The rational treatment of abnormal labial frenum. Am. J. Dis. Child., *52*:1061, 1936.

48. Schwartz, A. B., and Abbott, T. R.: Effect of growth and development on abnormal labial frenum. Am. J. Dis. Child., *71*:248–251, 1946.

49. Small, I. A., *et al.:* Teflon and Silastic for mandibular replacement: experimental studies and reports of cases. J. Oral Surg., *22*:377 (Sept.), 1964.

50. Stones, H. H., and Livingston, E.: Oral and Dental Diseases, p. 210. London, Edward Arnold (Publishers) Ltd., 1962.

51. Tait, C. H.: Medial fraenum of the upper lip and its influence on spacing of upper central incisor teeth. N.Z. Dent. J., *25*:116, 1929.

52. Taylor, J. E.: Clinical observations relating to the normal and abnormal frenum labii superioris. Am. J. Orthod., *25*:646, 1939.

53. Thoma, K. H.: Oral Surgery. 5th ed. St. Louis, The C. V. Mosby Co., 1969.

54. Tuerk, M., and Lubit, E. C.: Ankyloglossia. Plast. Reconstr. Surg., *24*:271–276 (Sept.), 1959.

55. van Du Wast, W. A. M.: Gingival hyperplasia caused by "Dilantin" medication. Acta Med. Scand., *153*:399–405 (Jan.), 1958.

56. Virtanen, I.: Deepening of the whole floor of the mouth for satisfactory prosthetic treatment: a combined submucosal plastic operation. Suom. Hammaslaak. Toim., *56*:115–129 (June), 1960 (in English).

57. Waite, D.: Inflammatory hyperplasia. J. Oral Surg., *19*:210, 1961.

58. Wallenius, K., and Owall, B.: Effect of ridge extension on retention and function of dentures. Odontol. Revy, *18*:361–371, 1967.

59. Wallenius, K., and Öwall, B.: A 5-year follow-up study of retention of prong dentures by skin-folded pockets. Int. J. Oral Surg., *1*:26–33, 1972.

60. Walsh, T. S., Jr.: Buried metallic prosthesis for mandibular defects. Cancer, *7*:1002–1008, 1954.

61. Whitman, C. L., and Rankow, R. M.: Diagnosis and management of ankyloglossia. Am. J. Orthod., *47*:423–428 (June), 1961.

62. Wilson, H. E.: The labial fraenum. Trans. Europ. Orthod. Soc., *36*:34, 1960.

CHAPTER 4

THE USE OF ELEVATORS IN ORAL SURGERY

USE OF ELEVATORS IN EXTRACTION OF TEETH AND REMOVAL OF ROOTS

There is no question in the minds of experienced men that forceps are the best instruments for general use in the removal of teeth; hence it is absolutely necessary to become proficient in the use of forceps before attempting to master the use of elevators.

Each manufacturer has his own particular models of elevators, and the result is a bewildering array of elevators on the market today. Many of them are superfluous. Since only about 10 basic designs exist, it is necessary for the dentist to master the use of only a few of these elevators in order to perform efficient oral surgery.

Indications for Use of Elevators. Elevators are used to reflect mucoperiosteal membranes; to luxate and remove teeth which cannot be engaged by the beaks of forceps, such as impactions and malposed teeth; to remove roots, fractured or carious; to loosen teeth prior to the application of forceps; to split teeth which have had grooves cut in them; and to remove intraradicular bone.

REMOVAL OF TEETH. Elevators are indicated for removing the entire tooth in the following situations: *impactions*—whether maxillary or mandibular—because of the inability of the operator (as a result of the abnormal location or position of these impacted teeth) to use forceps; *malposed teeth,* lingually, buccally or labially crowded teeth, especially maxillary or mandibular bicuspids or lateral incisors so located that it is impossible to apply the forceps without impinging on adjacent teeth, or in the process of luxation, creating pressure on the adjacent teeth; teeth that are extensively *decayed,* in which there is little doubt that the crown will fracture under the pressure of the beaks of the forceps; teeth that

have *tilted* anteriorly, because of the early loss of the proximating or adjacent teeth, making it impossible to place the beaks of the forceps on the tooth to be extracted such that the beaks of the forceps will be parallel to the long axis of the tooth. (See Figure 4–6.)

REMOVAL OF ROOTS. Elevators are indicated for removing roots in the following situations: roots fractured at the gingival line, at midlength or at the apical third; roots left in the alveolus from previous extractions (which may be recent or of several years' standing).

Dangers in the Use of Elevators. Elevators should be used with the utmost caution at all times because of the dangers of damaging or even of extracting adjacent teeth; of fracturing the maxilla or mandible; fracturing the alveolar process; slipping and plunging the point of the instrument into the soft tissue, with a possible perforation of great blood vessels and nerves; penetrating the maxillary antrum or forcing a root or a third molar into the antrum; or forcing the apical third of the root of the lower third molar into the mandibular canal or through the lingual plate of the mandible into the submaxillary or pterygomandibular space, depending upon the position of the impacted third molar in the mandible.

Rules When Using Elevators. The following rules should be observed when using elevators:

1. Never use an adjacent tooth as a fulcrum unless that tooth is to be extracted also.
2. Never use the buccal plate at the gingival line as a fulcrum, except where odontectomy is performed, or in the third molar areas.
3. Never use the lingual plate at the gingival line as a fulcrum.
4. Always use finger guards to protect the patient in case the elevator slips.
5. Be certain that the forces applied by the

211

elevator are under control, and that the elevator tip is exerting pressure in the correct direction.

6. When cutting through interseptal bone, take care not to engage the root of an adjacent tooth, thus inadvertently forcing it from its alveolus.

Parts of an Elevator. All elevators have the following parts: (*a*) *handle* (this may be a continuation of the shank, or at a right angle to it), (*b*) *shank,* (*c*) *blade* (the part which engages the crown or root).

CLASSIFICATION OF ELEVATORS

Elevators are classified according to their use or according to form.

According to Use. The classification of elevators according to their use is as follows:

1. Elevators designed to remove the entire tooth (1L — 1R).
2. Elevators designed to remove roots broken off at the gingival line (30 — 4 — 5).
3. Elevators designed to remove roots broken off halfway to the apex (30 — 4 — 5, or 14L — 14R, or 11L — 11R).
4. Elevators designed to remove the apical third of the root (apical fragment ejectors Nos. 1, 2 and 3).
5. Elevators designed to reflect the mucoperiosteum (periosteal elevators) before forceps or extracting elevators are used. (See pages 37 to 40 in Chapter 2 for technique and Figures 2–20 and 2–21.)

According to Form. Elevators classified

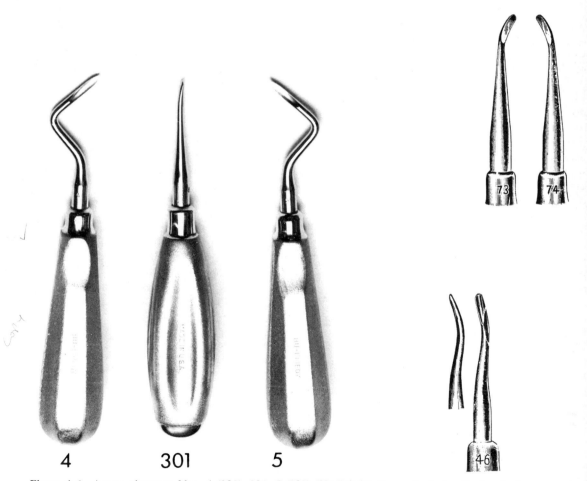

Figure 4–1 Apexo elevators Nos. 4 (302), 301, 5 (303) (Hu-Friedy) are particularly effective in the removal of roots fractured at the gingival line. Apexo elevators Nos. 73 and 74 are excellent instruments for the removal of impacted maxillary third molars, impacted cuspids and some roots. No. 46, a lingual root elevator, is a modified No. 301, particularly good for lingual roots or application to the lingual surface of anterior roots.

Figure 4–2 Winter elevators technique. Elevator No. 11L is used for the removal of the right lower third molar where there is a thick buccal plate to act as a fulcrum. A pathway is made with a spear-point bur between the bifurcation of the roots, and then the point of the No. 11L is forced down into the bifurcation and the handle is rotated buccally, lifting the tooth from its socket.

On the left side of the mandible this instrument is used to cut out the septum and remove distal molar roots that have been fractured. No. 11R is used to remove mesial roots on this side of the mandible.

No. 11R is used for the removal of the left lower third molar where there is a thick buccal plate to act as a fulcrum. The same technique is used as described for No. 11L. These elevators are also useful in helping to remove vertically impacted lower third molars, or for rolling lingually horizontally impacted lower third molars, or for bringing the roots of a horizontally impacted lower third molar forward into the space occupied by the crown which has been severed from the roots and removed.

On the right side of the mandible 11R or 14R is used to cut out the septum and remove distal roots that were fractured. No. 11L or 14L is used to remove mesial roots on this side of the mandible. (See Fig. 4–36C.)

No. 14L is used for the removal of mandibular molar roots from deep sockets, either right or left, when application can be made through an adjoining socket, e.g., where the intervening bone is thin. Primarily this instrument and its mate are valuable for the removal of molar roots. No. 14L is used for the removal of the distal roots of the lower left first, second and third molars, and the mesial roots of the lower right first, second and third molars.

No. 14R is used for the same purpose as No. 14L; note that this instrument, however, is used for the removal of mesial roots of the lower left first, second and third molars and the distal roots of the lower right molars.

Nos. 1L and 1R are indicated for the extraction of mandibular third molars in a normal or approximately normal position. They are also used for vertically impacted mandibular third molars, and to loosen all the mandibular and maxillary teeth by wedging between the necks of adjacent teeth; by using one as a fulcrum its neighbor is moved distally.

This technique of course is only used when all the remaining mandibular or maxillary teeth are extracted. The soft tissue around the necks of all the teeth is incised and reflected so that it is not crushed when the points of these elevators are wedged between the teeth. The anterior-posterior movement of the handle moves the teeth, thus compressing the interseptal bone and loosening the teeth. Forceps are now applied to extract the teeth.

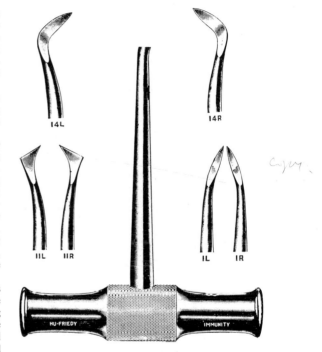

according to their form are as follows:

1. Straight: wedge type (straight apex).
2. Angular: right and left.
3. Cross bar (handle at right angle to shank).

ELEVATORS COMMONLY USED

The following set of elevators is adequate to take care of 90 per cent of all needs for elevators in exodontia. These do not include apical fragment ejectors (see Figure 4–27). This set of elevators includes:*

1. Apexo elevators:
   a. Left Apexo elevator No. 4 (corresponds to 302 of other manufacturers).
   b. Straight Apexo elevator No. 30 (formerly known as No. 81).
   c. Right Apexo elevator No. 5 (corresponds to 303 of other manufacturers).
   d. Miller Apexo elevators Nos. 73 and 74 (see Figure 4–1).
2. Cross bar elevators: Nos. 1L – 1R, 11L – 11R and 14L – 14R (see Figure 4–2).

WORK PRINCIPLES IN USE OF ELEVATORS

The work principle as applied to the use of elevators may be that of the lever, the wedge, the wheel and axle or a combination of two or more of these principles.

Lever Principle as Applied to the Use of Elevators. In using elevators, the work principle most frequently made use of is the lever (Fig. 4–3). The elevator is a lever of the first class. In a lever of the first class the position of the fulcrum is between the effort (E) and the resistance (R). In order to gain a mechanical advantage in a lever of the first class, the effort arm, on one side of the fulcrum, must be longer than the resistance arm, on the other side of the fulcrum.

Wedge Principle as Applied to the Use of Elevators. Some elevators are designed primarily to be used as a wedge (Fig. 4–4); these are called *wedge elevators*. (Apexo elevators

---

Note: Remember that similar instruments are given various numbers by the different manufacturers. Except where noted otherwise, the elevator instrument numbers used in this book are those of Hu-Friedy, Inc.

are wedge elevators.) The wedge elevator is forced between the root of the tooth and the investing bony tissue parallel to the long axis of the root, by hand pressure or by mallet force.

While the wedge principle can be, and is, used as the sole principle in removing teeth, it is most frequently used in conjunction with the lever principle. The wedge in its simplest form, as in a chisel, is a movable inclined plane which overcomes a large resistance at right angles to the applied effort. The effort is applied to the base of the plane, and the resistance has its effect on the slant side. Some wedges are movable double inclined planes. They may also be regarded as two inclined planes placed base to base. The sharper the angle of the wedge, the less effort required to make it overcome a given resistance.

The wedge may be either a single or a double inclined plane. The No. 16 forceps is a double wedge.

Wheel-and-Axle Principle as Applied to the Use of Elevators. The wheel and axle is a simple machine, being really a modified form of the lever. The effort is applied to the circumference of a wheel which turns the axle so as to raise a weight. The effort arm is Rw and the resistance arm is ra (see Figure 4–5).

While the wheel-and-axle principle can be, and is, used as the sole work principle in removing teeth, it is also used in conjunction with the wedge principle, and in some cases with the lever principle.

In Figure 4–6 is illustrated the use of two work principles in the extraction of a mandibular molar. The first work principle is the wedge and the second is the wheel and axle. In Figure 4–6*A* will be seen a situation which is very common, namely, a lower molar which has drifted forward so that it would be impossible to apply forceps to the tooth in such a manner that the beaks of the forceps would parallel the long axis of the tooth. Incorrect application of forceps on a tooth mesially inclined, as shown here, would result most probably in fracturing the crown.

The best technique for extraction in these cases is to make a flap, as shown in Figure 4–6*B*, then use a No. 301 straight Apexo elevator as a wedge, driving it into the space occupied by the periodontal membrane along the mesial aspect of this tooth and using a mallet as the driving force. This wedge driven alongside the tooth accomplishes two things: (1) because of the wedge principle, it has a tendency to elevate the tooth from its socket; (2)

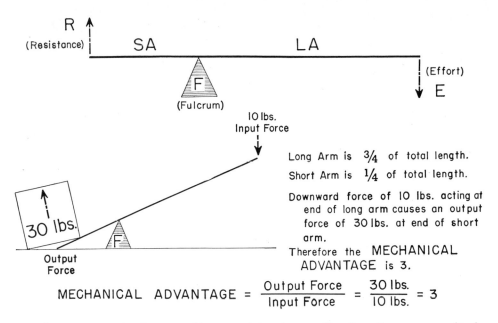

Long Arm is $\frac{3}{4}$ of total length.

Short Arm is $\frac{1}{4}$ of total length.

Downward force of 10 lbs. acting at end of long arm causes an output force of 30 lbs. at end of short arm.

Therefore the MECHANICAL ADVANTAGE is 3.

$$\text{MECHANICAL ADVANTAGE} = \frac{\text{Output Force}}{\text{Input Force}} = \frac{30 \text{ lbs.}}{10 \text{ lbs.}} = 3$$

The lever is the simplest machine used to change the direction or magnitude of a force.

R–Resistance; E–Effort; SA–Short Arm; LA–Long Arm.

Formula of Levers: R × SA = LA × E.

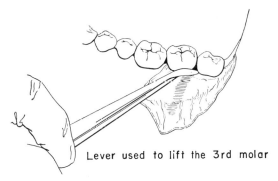

Lever used to lift the 3rd molar

Figure 4–3 Lever work principle as applied to the removal of teeth.

at the same time, it creates a pathway alongside the root. This pathway should be large enough—and if it is not, widen and deepen it with a surgical bur—to accommodate the working point of the cross bar elevator 14R or 11R for the right side or 14L or 11L for the left side. The working point of this elevator is placed deep into the pathway created, and when the handle is rotated, as shown in Figure 4–6C, the heel of the working edge utilizes the crest of the alveolar bone as a fulcrum and the working tip engages the side of the root as shown in Figure 4–6D. As the handle is rotated, the tooth is elevated superiorly and dis-

tally from its socket. The angle of the tooth is such as to facilitate its removal by moving it about the circumference of the circle which its roots would make if they were continued on around. (This is shown very nicely in Figure 4–6D.)

Once the tooth has been removed from its socket, the lingual periosteal membrane is loosened, as shown in Figure 4–6E, so that the collar of bone which projects above the surrounding osseous structure can be removed with the bone-cutting shears, as shown in Figure 4–6E and F. The soft tissue flap is replaced, and the excess tissue, shown in Figure

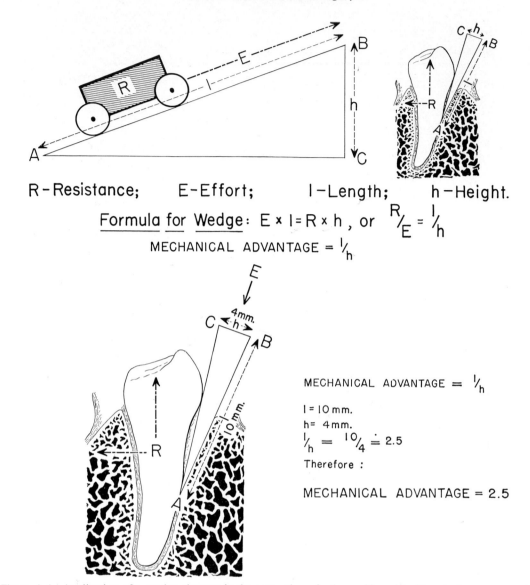

R – Resistance;   E – Effort;   I – Length;   h – Height.

Formula for Wedge: $E \times I = R \times h$, or $\dfrac{R}{E} = \dfrac{I}{h}$

MECHANICAL ADVANTAGE $= \dfrac{I}{h}$

MECHANICAL ADVANTAGE $= \dfrac{I}{h}$

I = 10 mm.
h = 4 mm.

$\dfrac{I}{h} = \dfrac{10}{4} \doteq 2.5$

Therefore :

MECHANICAL ADVANTAGE = 2.5

Figure 4-4 Application of a wedge elevator in the extraction of a lower bicuspid with actual measurements and showing the mechanical advantage. Each pound of pressure applied is multiplied by 2.5.

4–6*G*, is trimmed with scissors; one 000 black silk suture generally suffices to close the wound, as shown in Figure 4–6*H*.

PROTECTION OF THE PATIENT DURING THE USE OF ELEVATORS

As has been described, the elevators produce a great multiplication of force when they are applied to the teeth and jaws by the dentist. Two principles apply in protection of the patient: (1) his jaws must be supported to prevent dislocation of the mandible, and (2) other tissues in the oral cavity must be protected from potential damage, i.e., the accidental slipping and plunging of the point of the elevator into adjacent or distal soft and hard tissues (see Figures 4–7 to 4–14). This is especially necessary when using the wedge-type elevator No. 301, No. 4 or No. 5. Similar protection is essential when using the other elevators.

Protection is best accomplished by (1) careful and continuous control of the *direction* of *force* so that it is directed *into the bone* surrounding the tooth or *against* the tooth being luxated, and (2) surrounding the immediate operative area with the fingers, as shown in the accompanying figures. On the maxilla,

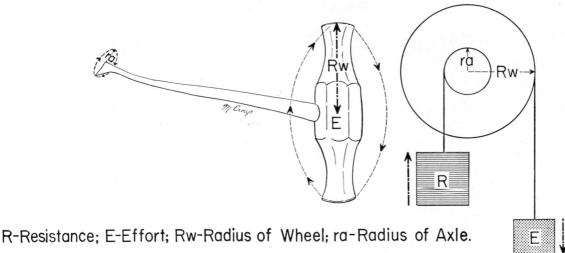

R-Resistance; E-Effort; Rw-Radius of Wheel; ra-Radius of Axle.

Effort x Radius of the Wheel = Resistance x Radius of the Axle

Formula of the Wheel and Axle Work Principle: $\frac{R}{E}$ $\frac{Rw}{ra}$

MECHANICAL ADVANTAGE = $\frac{Rw}{ra}$

MECHANICAL ADVANTAGE $\frac{Rw}{ra}$

Rw = 42 mm.

ra = 9 mm.

$\frac{Rw}{ra} = \frac{42}{9} = 4.6$

Therefore:

MECHANICAL ADVANTAGE = 4.6

Each pound of pressure applied to the crossbar is multiplied 4.6 times.

----BUCCAL PLATE

----LINGUAL PLATE

Figure 4–5 Wheel-and-axle work principle as applied in the use of the No. 11L or 11R cross bar elevators.

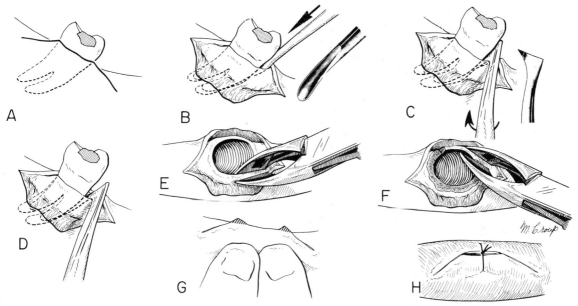

Figure 4–6 Use of the wedge and the wheel-and-axle work principles in extraction of a mesially inclined mandibular molar with no adjacent tooth. See text for a description of this technique.

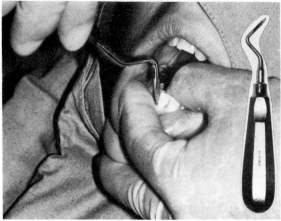

Figure 4–7

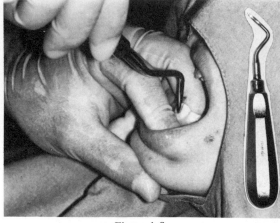

Figure 4–8

Figure 4–7   Study the position of fingers of the left hand as it supports the mandible (the left arm encircles the head) to prevent overstraining the temporomandibular joint or even dislocating it. At the same time, the left thumb and left index finger protect the labial and lingual tissues if the sharp tip of the Apexo elevator slips. These are wedge-type elevators (see Figure 4–4 for the principles involved and also study the text).

Figure 4–8   Protection and support of the mandible's left side during use of the Apexo elevator is achieved by the operator's standing in front of the patient, the left thumb beneath the mandible, the left index finger in the buccal vestibule and the second finger on the lingual side.

grasp the dental arch with the index finger and thumb so that the alveolus containing the root is between them. On the mandible, the first and second fingers should straddle the alveolus and *the thumb should be placed beneath the mandible, supporting it and thus offsetting the downward pressure of the elevator, which might otherwise dislocate the mandible.*

This placing of fingers buccally, labially and lingually affords the operator immediate information concerning whether or not pressure is being created on adjacent teeth which are *not to be extracted.* Adjacent teeth should *never* be used as fulcrums unless they are also to be extracted. This position also means that if the working point of the elevator slips, it will

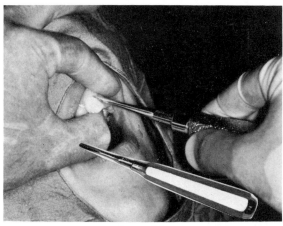

Figure 4–9

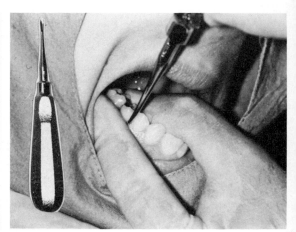

Figure 4–10

Figure 4–9   Protection and support of the anterior maxilla during use of the straight Apexo elevator. The operator stands in front of the patient, the thumb is on the lingual side and the index finger on the labial side. Elevator technique is described in the text and in Figure 4–15.

Figure 4–10   Protection and support of the mandible during use of the straight Apexo elevator. The body of the mandible is supported by the fingers of the left hand, except for the index finger, which is in the buccal vestibule. The thumb is supporting and protecting the lingual tissues and floor of the oral cavity. (Read text.)

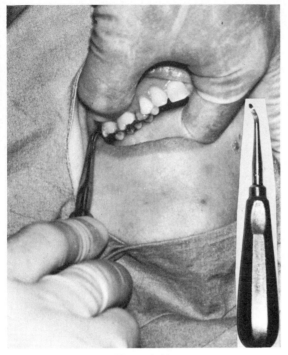

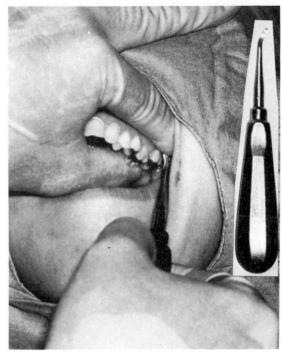

Figure 4-11   Figure 4-12

Figure 4-11 Protection and support during use of right elevator No. 74 in the right maxillary molar region. Note the position of the thumb and index finger.

Figure 4-12 Protection and support during use of left elevator No. 73 in the left maxillary molar region. Study the position of the thumb and index finger.

plunge into the finger of the operator rather than into the patient's surrounding bony tissues, soft tissues, nerves and blood vessels. This is a constant reminder to the operator of possible injury to himself as well as to the pa-

tient. It is far better for the dental surgeon to injure his finger than to run the risk of seriously injuring the patient, with a possible lawsuit ensuing.

To prevent the fracture of the mandible as

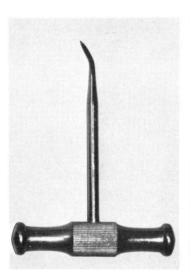

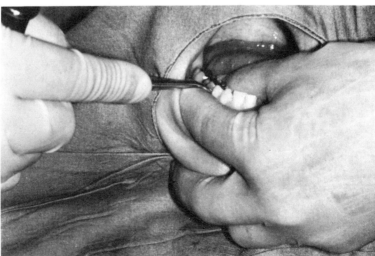

Figure 4-13 Protection and support during use of the 1R cross bar elevator on the right side of the mandible. The operator is at the side of the patient; the left arm encircles the head. Note the support of the mandible with the fingers of the left hand, except for the index finger, which is in the buccal vestibule. The thumb protects the floor of the oral cavity while at the same time supporting the lingual surface of the mandible.

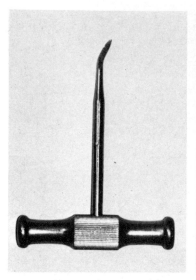
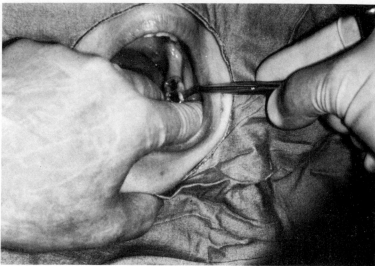

Figure 4–14   Protection and support on the left side of the mandible during use of left elevator No. 71. The operator stands in front of the patient; the operative site is spanned by the index and second fingers, while the thumb supports the jaw.

well as maxillary tuberosities containing teeth, the dentist must estimate just how much pressure can safely be applied before the danger point of fracture is reached. This is obviously not a precise determination, but certainly one can expect that a small mandible on a female patient will not accept the same amount of force without fracturing that a large-boned male patient's mandible would.

SPECIFIC USE OF CERTAIN ELEVATORS

PERIOSTEAL ELEVATOR

Because extracting elevators require a fulcrum to be effective and because the fulcrum is bone in 98 per cent of the cases, before the extracting elevators the dentist must use the periosteal elevator for reflecting the mucoperiosteum away from bone to prevent its being crushed. The full technique for use of the periosteal elevator is described in Chapter 2 (pages 37 to 40).

NO. 301 STRAIGHT APEXO ELEVATOR

The No. 301 straight Apexo elevator (see Figure 4–1) is primarily used on the maxilla, where the upper central or lateral cuspid or bicuspid has fractured at the gingival line.

The straight Apexo elevator is used as a wedge. Place this wedge on the mesiolabial aspect of the tooth in the space occupied by the periodontal membrane. Apply apical pressure, and a slight labiolingual motion; then enter the elevator at the distal side, and repeat; then enter the elevator at the mesial aspect, and repeat. (See drawings of technique in Figure 4–15.) The surgical mallet can be used to drive the elevator along the root, as shown in Figure 4–15B.

There are two main points of entrance, distal and mesial. After having inserted the point of the straight Apexo elevator at each of the two points of entrance (distal and mesial) and with the aforementioned pressures and motions, repeat this whole circuit or procedure until the elevator has penetrated to a depth of 5 mm. at each of the two points of entrance (distal and mesial). After the elevator has penetrated to a depth of 5 mm. at each of the two points of entrance (distal and mesial), use a half rotary motion with apical pressure.

NOS. 4 (302) AND 5 (303) APEXO ELEVATORS (R & L) ON THE MANDIBLE

In these Apexo elevators the blade is at a 45-degree angle to the handle. (The shank is at a 45-degree angle to the handle, and the blade is at a 90-degree angle to the shank.) The principle of their use is the same as that for the straight Apexo elevator; that is, they are used as a wedge. These elevators may be used on all lower teeth where fracture of the root has occurred at the gingival line. The mucoperiosteum is reflected first with the periosteal elevator.

POSITION OF OPERATOR. In the removal of all lower left roots the operator is in front of the patient. The mandible is supported by the thumb, which is placed beneath the mandible, the index finger is in the mucobuccal fold, and the second finger is on the lingual side.

In the removal of all lower right roots the operator stands to the side of the patient. The thumb is on the lingual tissues, the index finger in the mucobuccal fold, and the third, fourth and fifth fingers support the mandible.

Removal of Root Broken at the Gingival Line. Study the illustrations in Figure 4–20.

Insert, with a rotary motion and simultaneous apical pressure, the point of the No. 4 Apexo elevator along the mesial surface of the root in the space occupied by the periodontal membrane, parallel to the long axis of the root (Fig. 4–20A), until a depth of 2 to 3 mm. is gained. If the point fails to penetrate this space with moderate pressure on the handle, drill a starting point with a small, round No. 4 bur alongside the mesial and distal surface of the root.

Next use the No. 5 Apexo elevator and

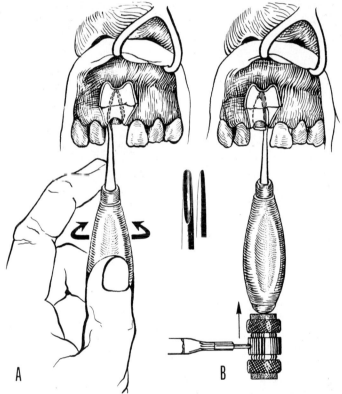

Figure 4–15 Removal of the root of the upper left central incisor fractured at the gingival line, with use of No. 301 (No. 81) straight Apexo elevator. The same technique can be used for the removal of any maxillary single root fractured at the gingival line.

A, Root fractured at the gingival line and the mucoperiosteal flap reflected. The No. 301 Apexo elevator, with concavity always turned toward the root, is wedged into space occupied by periodontal membrane. After forcing the tip alongside the root for approximately 5 mm., rotate the handle. *B,* Now carry out the same procedure on the distal surface. This wedging action, first on the mesial surface and then on the distal, plus the rotation of the blade of the Apexo elevator, lifts the root from the socket. Instead of hand pressure, the tip of the blade of the straight Apexo elevator can be driven alongside the root by the mallet. This is a considerably safer procedure because it eliminates the possibility of the instrument's slipping and being driven into the soft tissues of the face, which is ever present when hand pressure backed up by some of the body weight is used. The instrument might slip when struck by the mallet but the force is expended once the blow has been struck, whereas hand pressure backed up by body weight can be compared to the uncontrolled force exerted by the sudden release of a compressed spring. In using this technique, observe the following points: (*a*) Do not attempt to "pry" the root from the socket. (*b*) Do not create pressure on adjacent teeth. (*c*) After the root is removed, be sure that all loose particles of alveolar plate are removed. (*d*) If this wedging action, first on the mesial surface, then on the distal, back to the mesial, then the distal, and so on, does not result in the root's being freed from the socket, it indicates that the root has a marked curve or is excementosed.

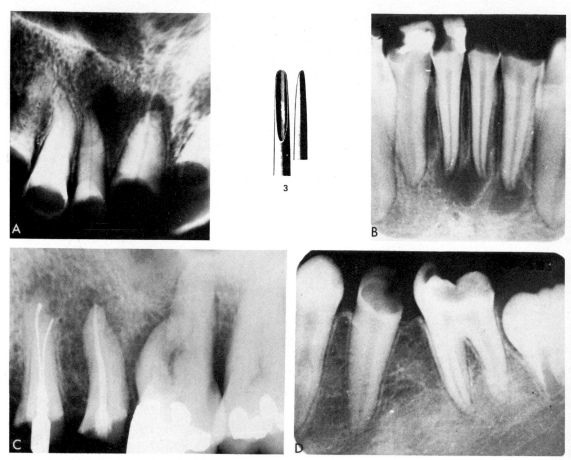

Figure 4–16   In single-rooted teeth with extensive caries of the crowns, as shown in *A, B, C* and *D*, tooth removal can be effected or at least facilitated by the use of a No. 3 elevator which is wedged between the root and its alveolus. While hand pressure can be used, the safest and most effective way is to tap the elevator with a mallet, as previously illustrated, on both the mesial and distal surfaces of the root. Keep the elevator as nearly as possible parallel to the long axis of the root. If this double wedging action does not deliver the tooth, the extraction is completed with the forceps.

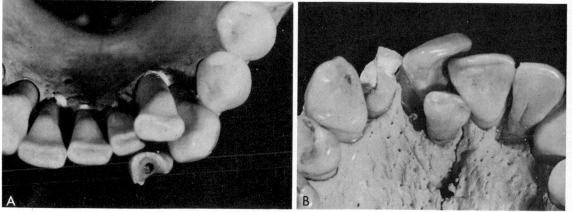

Figure 4–17   *A*, Supernumerary mandibular central incisor. Labial placement makes it rather difficult to grasp this tooth with a forceps. The Apexo elevator wedged alongside the roots of this tooth mesially and distally will effect its removal.

B, Rudimentary supernumerary central incisor erupted on palate. If the crown cannot be grasped with a No. 286 forceps and rotated without impinging on the adjacent teeth, drive with a mallet the straight Apexo elevator alongside the root, first on the mesial surface and then on the distal. This wedging action parallel to the root will effect the delivery of this tooth. (See Figure 4–18.)

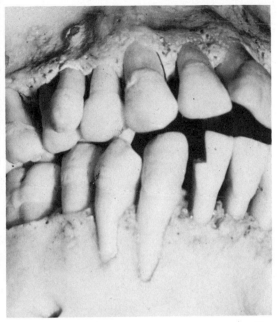

Figure 4–18 Rudimentary supernumerary maxillary cuspid in buccal position to the bicuspids. A straight Apexo elevator inserted parallel to the root will readily remove these teeth. See Figure 4–15 for this technique.

repeat the procedure. Insert the point of the elevator along the distal surface of the root in the space between the tooth root and alveolar bone occupied by the periodontal membrane;

drill a starting point if necessary, and insert parallel to the long axis of the root (Fig. 4–20*B*). Then with a rotary motion and bucco-lingual pressure gradually enlarge the space by compressing the alveolar bone until entrance and a depth of 3 mm. is gained.

Next insert the point of the No. 4 Apexo elevator on the mesial surface of the root, using more and more rotary and apical pressure until a depth of 6 mm. is gained (Fig. 4–20*C*).

Again insert the point of the No. 5 Apexo elevator on the distal surface of the root.

Repeat the foregoing procedure (as was done with the No. 4 Apexo elevator) with the No. 5 Apexo elevator, except that at this time it is done on the distal surface of the root instead of on the mesial surface. Use more and more rotary and apical pressure until a depth of 6 mm. has been gained.

Alternate these procedures using a rotary motion with apical pressure until the root moves out of the alveolus.

If this fails to remove the root, then use the double Apexo elevator technique (Fig. 4–20*D*).

Double Apexo Elevator Technique. Place the No. 4 Apexo elevator in the left hand, and the No. 5 Apexo elevator in the right hand. Then place the points of both elevators in against the root on opposite surfaces and, using both elevators with lever pressure occlu-

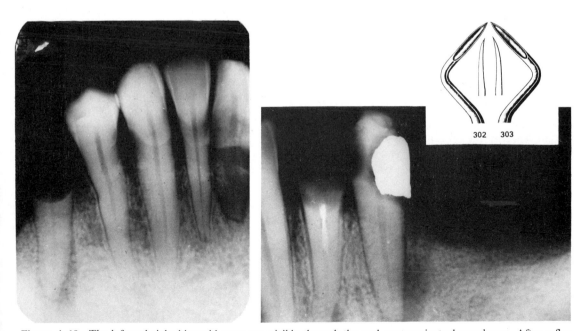

Figure 4–19 The left and right bicuspid roots are visible through the oral mucoperiosteal membrane. After reflection of the soft tissues, the roots can be removed with the Apexo elevators, as shown in Figure 4–20.

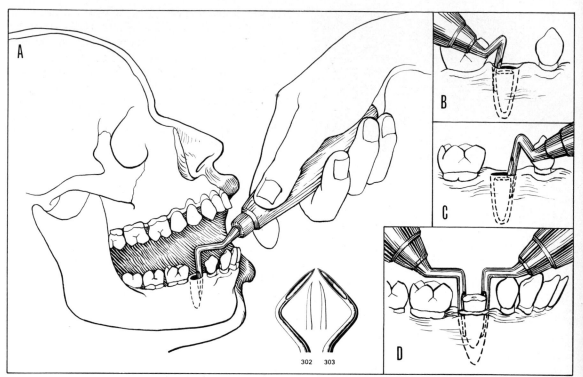

Figure 4–20 Use of Apexo elevators Nos. 302 (4) and 303 (5) as wedges for the removal of a lower bicuspid root fractured at the gingival line.

sally, elevate the root to the surface (Fig. 4–20D).

Double elevators and the preceding technique are used on lower cuspids, lower bicuspids, lower central and lateral incisors and lower molars.

USE OF CROSS BAR ELEVATORS ON THE MANDIBLE

Cross bar elevators are used on the mandible for the following purposes: to remove molar roots fractured at or below the gingival line; to fracture off crown or split roots after a groove has been cut in with a crosscut fissure bur (elevators 14L, 14R); to loosen teeth (elevators 1L, 1R); for the removal of impactions (elevators 73, 74, 1L, 1R, 11L, 11R). For details of the procedure for impacted teeth, see Chapter 5.

Removal of Roots Broken Off Halfway to the Apex. GENERAL RULE. Cases in which the roots are broken off halfway to the apex require the reflection of the mucoperiosteum and the removal of the buccal or labial plate of alveolar bone. This procedure is the so-called open or flap operation, or surgical removal of the root.

OPEN OR FLAP OPERATION (SURGICAL REMOVAL OF ROOT). This is performed for two reasons:

1. To enable the operator to see clearly the field of operation. Never work blindly, or in a pool of blood, when roots are broken off in the alveolus. Such a procedure is not only inefficient but fraught with the danger of further complicating the operation by, for example, (a) displacing roots into the maxillary sinus, (b) displacing them into the mandibular canal, (c) forcing the roots through the lingual cortical plate of the mandible in the lower third molar area into the submandibular space, or (d) forcing them through the cortical plate of the maxilla out into the soft tissues overlying the maxilla.
2. To remove the outer alveolar plate so that the alveolar elevators can function in the same manner as though the root had fractured at the gingival line.

EXCEPTION. The exception to the rule is the so-called blind operation, in which the operator is guided by a well-developed sense of touch, together with the mental visualization of the location of the root tip, in the delicate movements of his instrument.

The blind operation is used in the removal

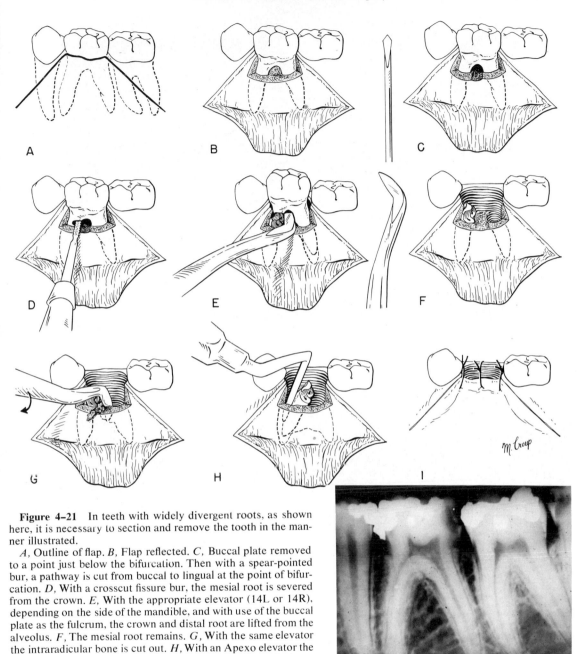

Figure 4–21 In teeth with widely divergent roots, as shown here, it is necessary to section and remove the tooth in the manner illustrated.

A, Outline of flap. *B,* Flap reflected. *C,* Buccal plate removed to a point just below the bifurcation. Then with a spear-pointed bur, a pathway is cut from buccal to lingual at the point of bifurcation. *D,* With a crosscut fissure bur, the mesial root is severed from the crown. *E,* With the appropriate elevator (14L or 14R), depending on the side of the mandible, and with use of the buccal plate as the fulcrum, the crown and distal root are lifted from the alveolus. *F,* The mesial root remains. *G,* With the same elevator the intraradicular bone is cut out. *H,* With an Apexo elevator the mesial root is removed with distal pressure. *I,* The soft tissue flap is returned to its position and sutured.

of posterior apical third fragments located where direct vision, or indirect by means of mirrors, is impossible.

APICAL FRAGMENT EJECTORS

Root Tips Broken Off at the Apical Third. The apical fragment ejectors are miniature elevators shaped just like the straight, right and left Apexo elevators, but smaller. Numbers of apical fragment ejectors are 1, 2 and 3. No. 1 is straight; No. 2 and No. 3 are for mesial and distal application (see Figure 4–27). Apical fragment ejectors are used to remove roots, or parts of roots, fractured at the apical third of the root.

Note: These roots usually fracture on the bias (see Figure 4–28). The thin blade is in-

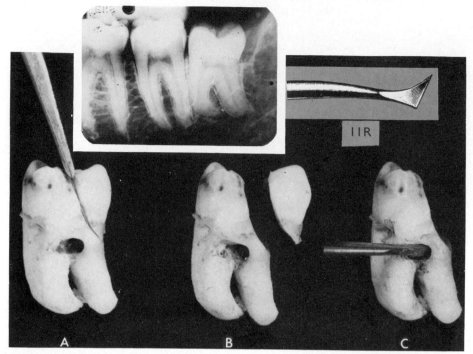

Figure 4–22 Vertically impacted mandibular third molar. *A* and *B,* Distal portion of the crown split off to create distal space. *C,* 11R elevator tip inserted into a purchase point drilled into the neck of the third molar. With use of the cortical bone as a fulcrum the handle of 11R is rotated, moving the tooth superiorly and distally out of the alveolus.

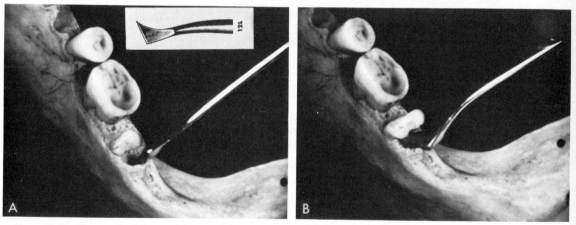

Figure 4–23 Removal of the mesial root of the mandibular second molar fractured at the gingival line. *A,* The tip of the 12L elevator is placed in the distal alveolus. *B,* The handle of the elevator is rotated, cutting through the intraradicular bone, engaging the root and lifting it from the alveolus.

Figure 4–24 Removal of mandibular molar roots fractured at the gingival line or halfway to the apex. Cross bar elevators Nos. 14L or 14R, 11L or 11R are used for the removal of roots from deep sockets.

A, Mesial root of the first molar and the distal root of the second molar have been fractured.

B, A large mucoperiosteal flap is reflected, exposing the buccal cortical plate over both sockets. The thin gingival cortical plate of bone is removed with end-cutting rongeurs until thick cortical bone is reached. If this is not done, the thin bone and overlying soft tissue will be crushed and lacerated, giving rise to much postoperative pain.

C, Place the blade of cross bar elevator No. 14R or 11R in the mesial root socket of the second molar alveolus. Using the junction of the buccal plate with the interseptal bone as a fulcrum, rotate the handle so that the blade cuts through the intraradicular bone.

D, Lift this intraradicular bone from the alveolus. In some cases it will be seen that the bone and root can both be lifted from the tooth socket.

E, If the root remains, replace the blade in the apical region and rotate the handle, again directing the tip of the blade beneath the apex of the distal root.

F, Now lift the distal root from the socket. In using this technique, note the following points: (1) Do not use an adjacent tooth for a fulcrum. To do so will injure this tooth severely or may even extract it. (2) Be careful that the point of the blade only passes beneath the apex in a short arc. If too large an arc is used, you may cut not only beneath the apex, but also through the interseptal bone and lift out the adjacent tooth.

H, I, J and *K* illustrate the technique as described, applied to the mesial root. Note that elevator No. 14L or 11L is used in this case.

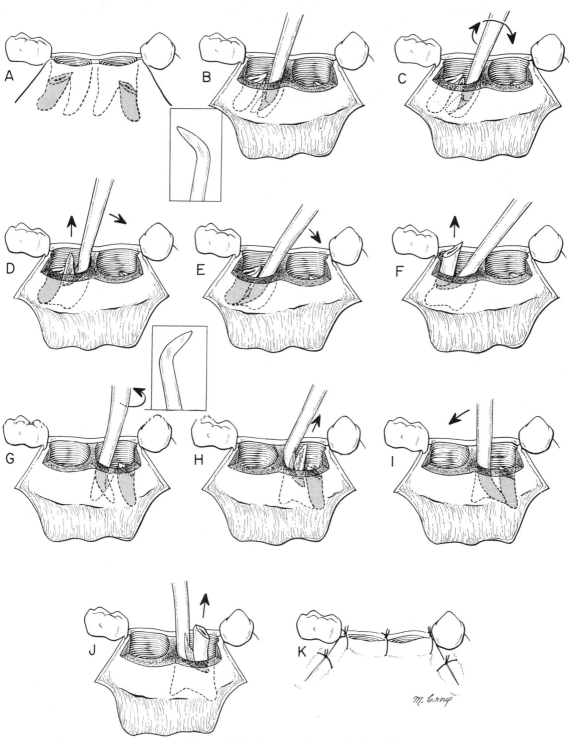

Figure 4–24 *See opposite page for legend.*

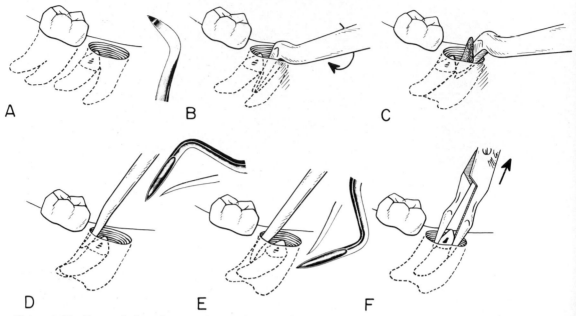

Figure 4–25 Removal of one lower molar root broken off below the gingival line with marked angulation. *A*, Root *in situ*. *B*, Insertion of appropriate elevator (11R, 14R, or 11L or 14L for left side) for removal of intraradicular bone. *C*, Removal of bone. With a straight root or one with mesial inclination in these circumstances, repeating the above maneuver will remove the root (see Figure 4–24). With this type of inclination, however, the possibility of extracting the adjacent tooth because of the force required precludes this technique. *D*, Apexo elevator (4, 5) inserted with blade face reversed in order to create space distally. *E*, Blade face is reversed and root is tilted mesially. *F*, Root grasped with apical fragment forceps.

serted between the root tip flange and the wall of the socket.

PROCEDURE.   The following steps should be observed in the use of apical fragment ejectors for root tips broken off at the apical third:

1. Examine the root of the fractured tooth to determine how much of the root is left in the alveolus.
2. Place the point of the apical fragment ejector into the alveolus, keeping it against, or in contact with, the alveolar wall all the way, with the curvature turned toward the wall until the flange on the fragment is gently contacted. (Study Figure 4–29*A* and *B*.)
3. With the tip of the apical fragment ejector, move the root tip flange from the alveolus toward the center of the socket. Using only a slight pressure, force the tip of the instrument between the flange of the root and the wall of the alveolar bone, thus creating a space between the root tip flange and the wall of bone. Then use the opposite instrument tip to further loosen the root, and create more space (Fig. 4–29*D*). This not only serves to

loosen the root from the alveolus but also creates a space for one sharp beak of the apical fragment forceps. (Study Figure 4–29*A*, *B* and *C*.)

4. Next use the apical fragment forceps to grasp the flange of the root tip, and then gently rock the tip back and forth, and lift the tip from the socket (Fig. 4–29*D*). If the root flange is on the tooth's mesial side, use the No. 2 apical fragment ejector. If on the distal, use the No. 3 apical fragment ejector.

Apical fragment forceps are also called splinter forceps. Apical fragment forceps resemble a hemostat with long, thin, sharp beaks (see Figures 4–27 and 4–30). Study the illustrations in Figures 4–29 and 4–31 to 4–34; they illustrate the removal of the apical third of a maxillary central incisor.

RETAINED ROOTS AND THEIR TREATMENT

Should all dental roots or portions of roots completely invested in the alveolar process be
(*Text continued on page 235*)

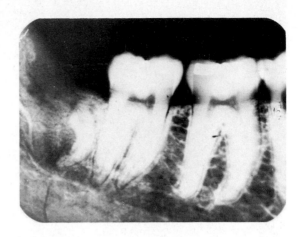

Figure 4–26 This mesial root of a mandibular third molar should be removed by carefully following the technique illustrated in Figure 4–25. Note the relationship of the apices of the second and third molars to the inferior alveolar canal. Obviously care must be taken to avoid injury to the neurovascular bundle contained therein.

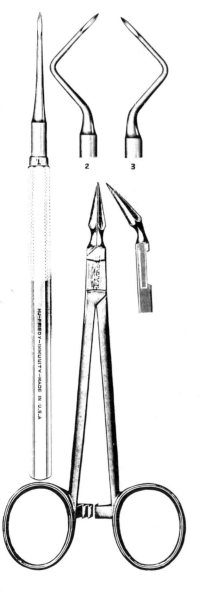

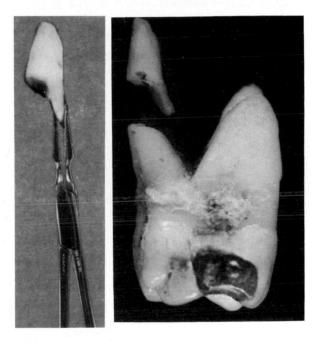

Figure 4–27 Apical fragment ejectors (*left*). These are invaluable instruments for the removal of apical third root fragments, particularly when used in conjunction with the apical fragment root forceps, as described in the text. Also shown are apical fragment fine pointed forceps (*right*).

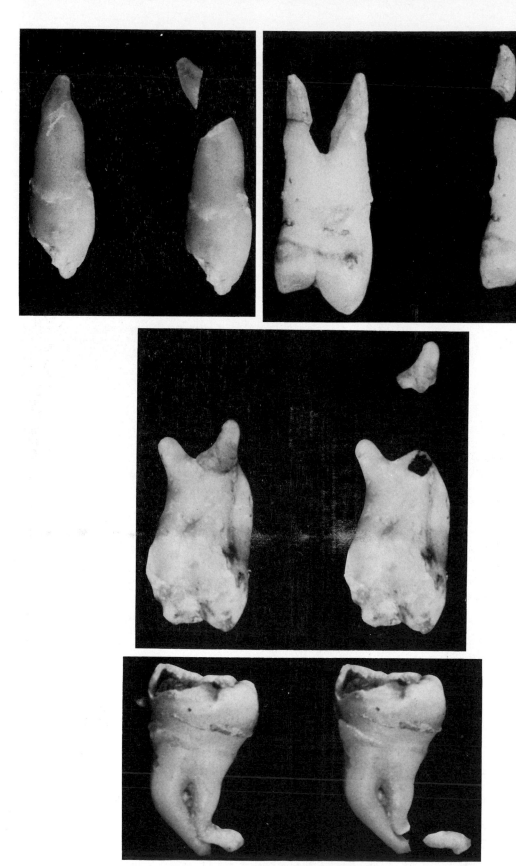

Figure 4–28 Examples of apical root fractures when these teeth were extracted.

(Figure 4–28 continued on opposite page.)

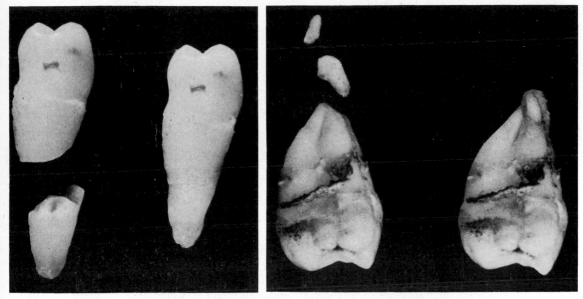

Figure 4–28 *(Continued.)*

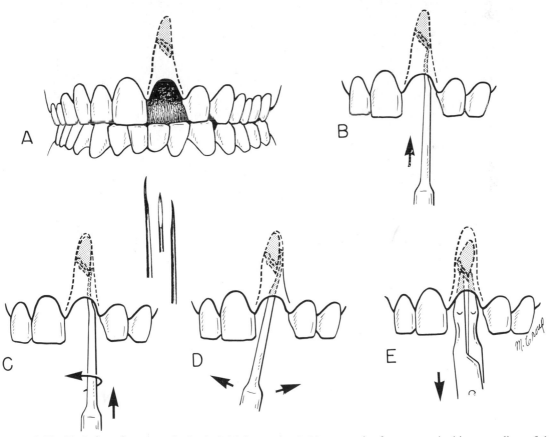

Figure 4–29 Technique for removal of apical third root tip. *A*, Most root tips fracture on the bias regardless of the location of the tooth. *B*, Slide the apical fragment ejector up the alveolus on the same side as the root flange. *C*, Contact the flange and gently work the point between the flange and the alveolus, moving the flange away from the socket wall. *D*, Rotate the tip of the instrument and work it between the flange of the root tip and the alveolus, gradually increasing the space between the root tip and the alveolus. *E*, Slide the apical third root tip forceps up the side of the alveolus and grasp the flange. Rock the tip, and withdraw.

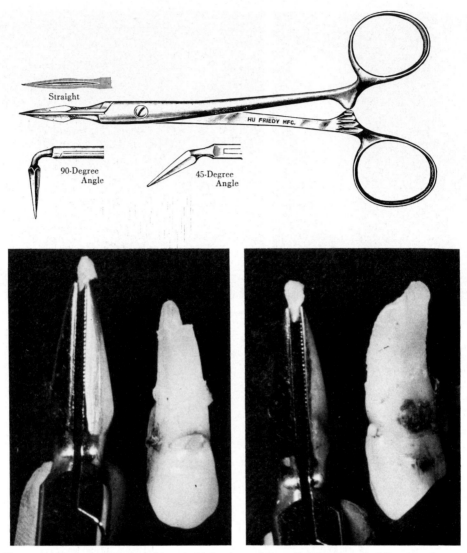

Straight

90-Degree Angle

45-Degree Angle

HU FRIEDY MFG.

Figure 4–30 Study Figures 4–31 to 4–34 for the technique in using the apical fragment forceps.

Figure 4–32 Removal of lower bicuspid root tip, preserving contour of alveolar crest. *A,* Root *in situ.* An incision through the mucoperiosteum is made as outlined. Some operators do not make incisions and flaps but work directly through the soft tissue. This has one disadvantage: In case this technique is not successful the flap for the alveolotomy has a badly traumatized base compromising the blood supply. *B,* Mucoperiosteal flap reflected. C_1, Instrument with marker (disc of rubber dam) attached for measuring root length. C_2, Instrument placed in socket and distance from crest of ridge to fractured tip measured. *D,* Same distance marked on buccal surface. *E,* Sharp elevator inserted through buccal bone with a rotary to-and-fro motion at estimated site of apex. The operator gauges the site of insertion by using the measurement obtained in *D* and adding to it the estimated length of the root tip as seen in a radiograph. *F,* Elevator under root tip dislodges it upward. *G,* Root tip grasped with apical fragment forceps. *H,* Flap sutured.

Warning! Carefully examine the dental radiograph of this area to determine the relationship of the inferior alveolar canal to the apex. If it is close, extreme care must be taken to avoid traumatizing the neurovascular bundle with the sharp, straight apical fragment ejector. If this bundle is traumatized, postoperative anesthesia will persist for a varying period of time, depending on the extent of trauma.

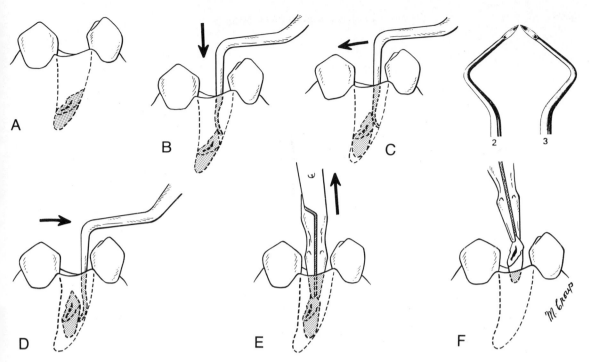

Figure 4–31 Removal of bicuspid apical third root tip fractured on the bias. *A, B,* Slide the tip of the apical fragment ejector down the side of the alveolus against which the flange of the root tip rests. To assure contact with the flange, have the concave surface of the instrument turned toward the alveolus. *C,* After contacting the flange, work the tip of the instrument gently between the alveolus and the root substance until the flange has been moved away from the wall of the alveolus. *D,* The opposite apical fragment ejector is now inserted and the tip of the fragment ejector is worked around the root tip, enlarging the alveolus in this area and loosening the root tip as shown. *E, F,* The root flange is grasped by the apical fragment forceps and removed.

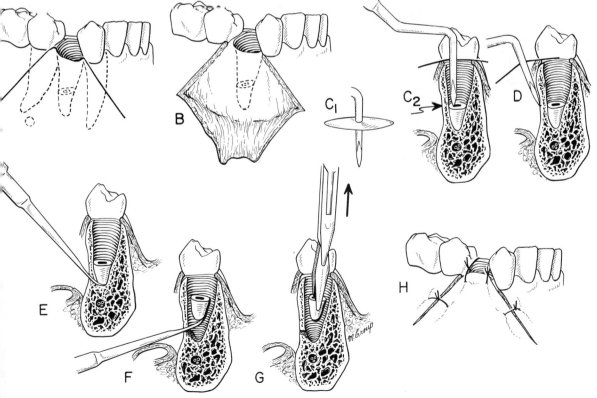

Figure 4–32 *See opposite page for legend.*

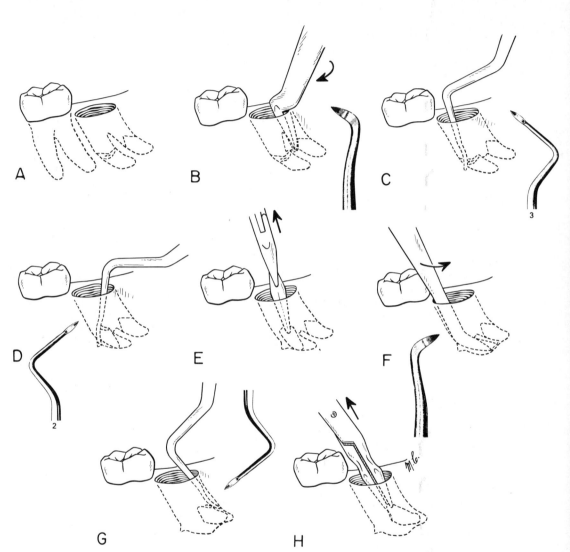

Figure 4–33   Removal of lower molar roots with marked angulation broken off at apical third. *A*, Roots *in situ. B*, Removal of enough intraradicular bone with suitable elevator (11R or 14R; on the left side use 11L or 14L) to create enough space to tilt one root. *C*, Insertion of sharp Apexo elevator (4, 5) with blade reversed in order to gouge a groove in bone mesially. *D*, Elevator blade reversed to engage root in previously created groove and tip it distally. *E*, Root grasped and removed with apical fragment forceps. *F*, Removal of remaining intraradicular bone with elevator. *G*, Mesial tipping of distal root. *H*, Removal with apical fragment forceps.

Warning! Know from your radiographic examination the relationship of the roots to the neurovascular canal. In addition in the lower third molar area, frequently the lingual cortical plate overlying the apices is very thin or absent. This would permit the easy dislodgment of apices by the elevator into the submaxillary space, from which they are extremely difficult to recover.

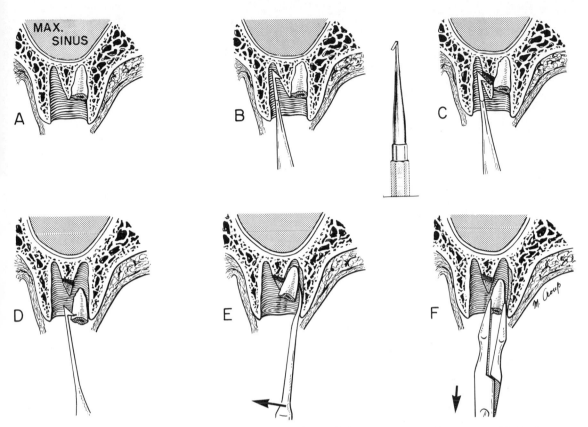

Figure 4–34 Removal of bicuspid or lingual molar root in proximity to antrum. *A,* Root *in situ.* Notice how any apical force, as might occur during wedging actions of elevator, will push the root into the antrum. *B* and *C,* Williams apical pick inserted into adjacent socket and intraradicular bone removed. If this bone is too dense to be removed in this manner, cut it out with a round bone bur. *D,* Williams apical pick reinserted, root engaged and removed with downward pressure. *E* and *F,* If the root cannot be engaged with the hook, drill a pathway along the lingual surface of the root with a small round bur, insert a straight No. 1 apical fragment ejector into this space, and with a wedging action move the root into the center of the socket, where it can be grasped with the apical fragment forceps and removed.

removed? This decision must be made individually on each case. The majority of retained roots are not infected. Retained roots in healed alveolar ridges usually do not have any radiolucent areas either on one surface or surrounding them. Radiolucency (which is determined radiographically) is not automatic proof that this is an infected area, as has been shown by Grossman,* who proved that 85.3 per cent of all nonvital teeth with periapical radiolucent areas were sterile. However, there is no known method to determine preoperatively whether or not this particular radiolucent area represents one of the 15 per cent that are infected, so we recommend removal of all root segments that are associated with a well-cir-

cumscribed radiolucent area. (See Figure 4–35.)

Roots are frequently found in healed ridges beneath bridge pontics. The alveolar bone in these areas is frequently made up of diffuse radiolucent marrow spaces that all too frequently are incorrectly diagnosed as residual infection. These areas represent disuse atrophy of this protected area of bone beneath the bridge pontic. (See Figure 4–37.) Many of these root fragments have been fractured and left in position in the alveolus when teeth with vital pulps were extracted. Kronfeld has rationalized that the pulp in the fragment perhaps remains, normal bone forms around it, and the fractured surface becomes covered with cementum. Some fragments become covered by thick layers of cementum and become rounded or elliptical. (See Figures 4–39 and 4–40.) There is no indication to re-

*Grossman, L. I.: Bacteriologic status of periapical tissue in 150 cases of infected pulpless teeth. J. Dent. Res., *38*:101–104 (Feb.), 1959.

(*Text continued on page 244*)

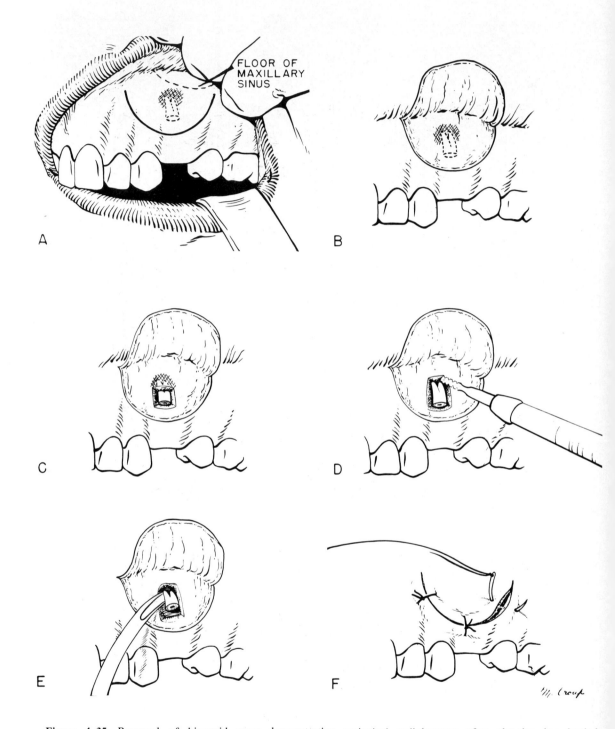

Figure 4–35 Removal of bicuspid apex demonstrating periapical radiolucency after alveolus has healed. *A,* A semicircular incision is made in the mucoperiosteum. *B,* Mucoperiosteal flap is reflected, exposing cortical bone overlying root apex. *C,* Bone is removed over root with chisel. *D,* Groove is cut around tip with bur. *E,* Root apex is lifted from its crypt by elevator No. 73 or No. 74. *F,* Flap is sutured with 00 plain catgut.

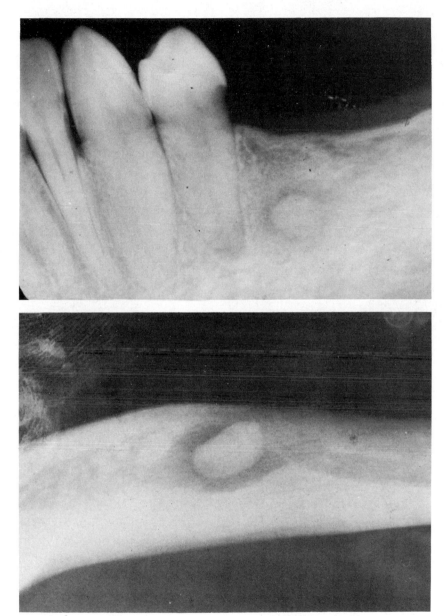

Figure 4–36 Retained roots surrounded by radiolucent areas. These roots should be excised. Study the text for the reasons.

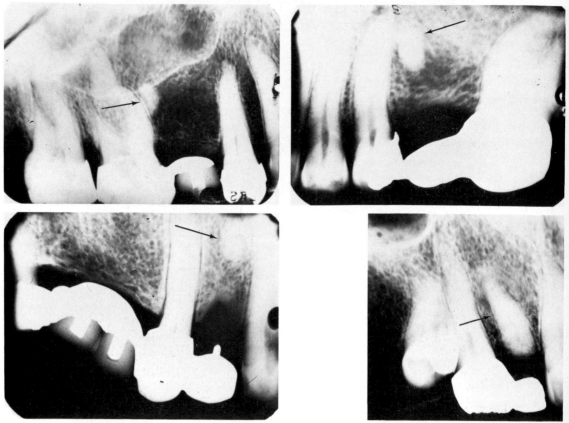

Figure 4–37   These roots should not be removed. Study the text for the reasons.

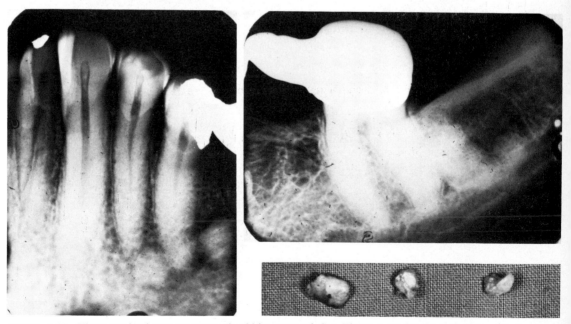

Figure 4–38   These retained root segments should be removed. See Figure 4–39 for the technique of their removal and study the text for the reasons.

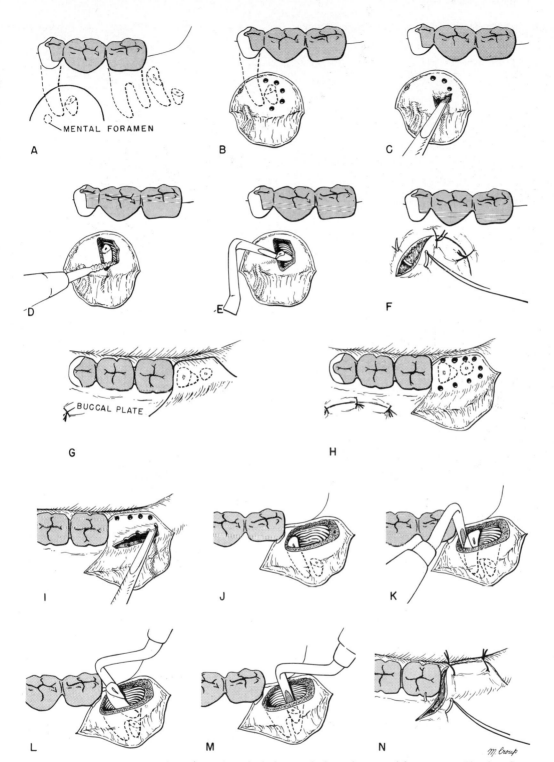

Figure 4–39 *A*, Semicircular incision is made to include vessels from the mental foramen. *B*, Flap is reflected and holes are drilled through cortical plate with a No. 3 Feldman spear-pointed drill. *C*, Cortical plate is removed with a No. 2 Gardner chisel. *D*, Cancellous bone around superior and distal surfaces is cut out with a No. 560 crosscut fissure bur. *E*, With a No. 4 Apexo elevator inserted along mesial surface, the root tip is moved distally and out. *F*, Replace flap with 00 plain catgut suture.

G, Outline of flap to expose bone over third motor roots. *H*, Flap is reflected and holes drilled through cortical bone with No. 3 Feldman spear-pointed drill. *I*, Cortical bone is removed with a No. 2 Gardner chisel. *J*, Cancellous bone around and above roots is cut out with curettes and rongeurs. *K*, With a No. 4 Apexo elevator inserted along the mesial surface, the root is moved distally. *L*, With a No. 5 Apexo elevator, the root is lifted from the socket. *M*, With a No. 5 Apexo elevator inserted along the distal surface, the root tip is moved mesially and occlusally. *N*, Flap is sutured back in place with 00 plain catgut.

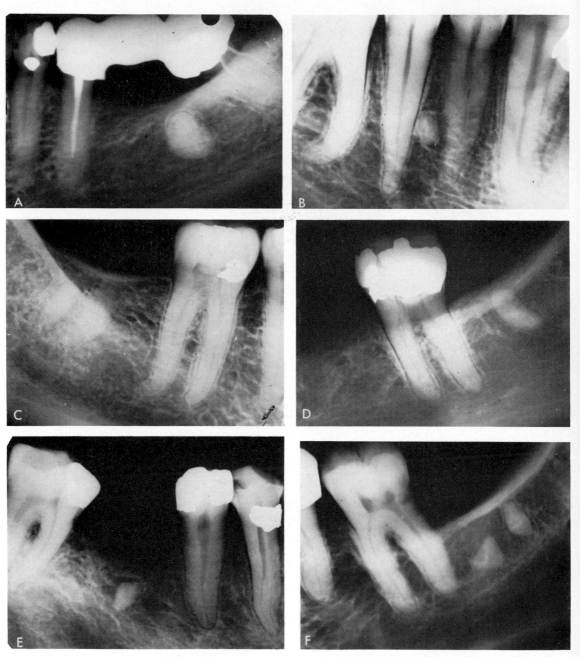

Figure 4–40 See text for a description of these roots. *A, B, C, D* and *F* should not be removed. *E* should be excised.

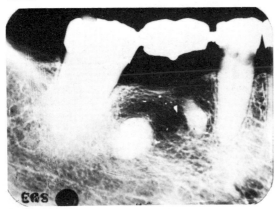

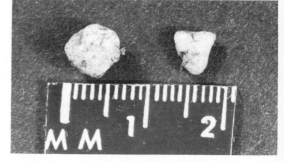

Figure 4–41 Retained roots in which removal is indicated. Note round molding of one of the roots.

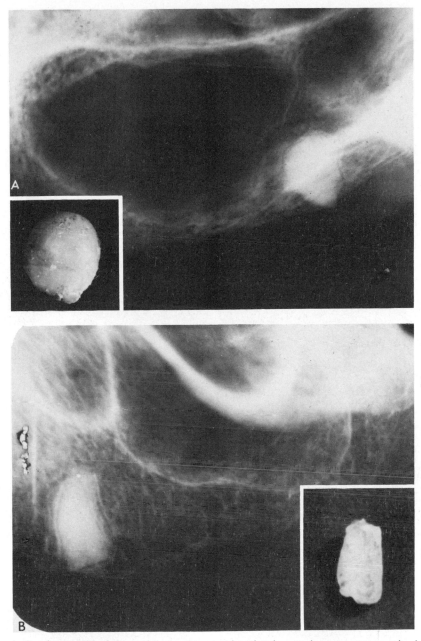

Figure 4–42 *A*, Good example of the molding and contouring that is seen in some roots retained in the bone. *B*, Moderate change in this root which looks to be a mesiobuccal root of a maxillary molar.

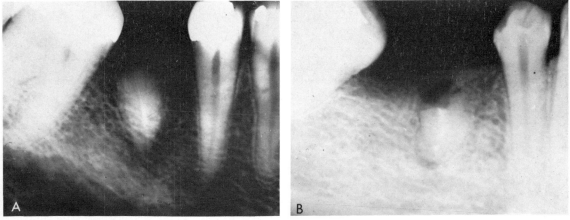

Figure 4–43 *A*, A root? *B*, A root. Area in *A* was explored and a root was found.

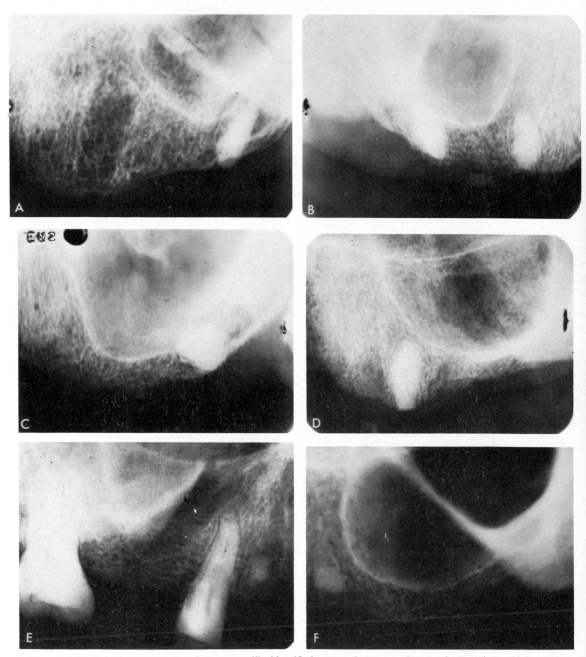

Figure 4–44 Objects in *A, B, C* and *D* are readily identified as root fragments, but not in *E* and *F*, which appear to show sclerotic areas.

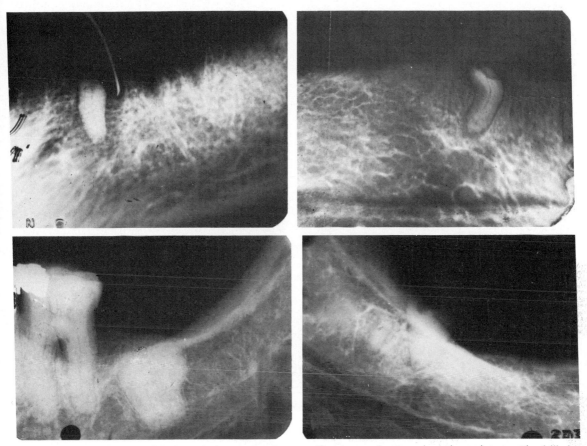

Figure 4–45 Roots just visible through the mucoperiosteum. Use Apexo elevators; insertion points must be drilled.

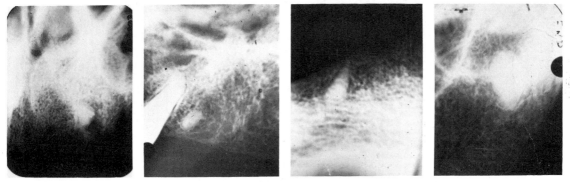

Figure 4–46 Root fragments at or close to the crest of the ridge. These should be removed; study the text.

move the roots illustrated in Figure 4–40, except those in *E*. This root (*E*) has a well-demarcated area of radiolucency around two thirds of its circumference and therefore should be removed.

If the root lies at the crest of the ridge or close to the surface of the alveolar bone, and the patient is wearing dentures, it will be only a matter of time before the surrounding alveolar bone has resorbed, leaving this hard, nonresorbable dental tissue on the surface just beneath the mucoperiosteal membrane. Masticatory action compresses the soft tissue between the denture base and the hard root substance, resulting in pain and inflammation, a breakdown of the soft tissue, invasion of bacteria and infection. Therefore, a root in such a location should be removed. (See Figures 4–42 to 4–46.) In cases in which the root is deeply buried in the bone and radiographically negative, the patient should be informed that he has a retained root (or roots), which is non-symptomatic at this time. At future routine oral examinations, the situation existing at that time should be evaluated, even though the possibility of trouble's developing from the presence of the root (or roots) is remote. In our radiographic survey of dental root material *completely covered with bone,* only 10 per cent revealed evidence of the loss of surrounding osseous tissue. Some authors refer to retained roots as foreign bodies. I do not agree with this designation of root substance in alveolar bone as foreign to its present environment.

REMOVAL OF ROOTS FROM HEALED RIDGES OF THE MAXILLA OR MANDIBLE

The removal of these roots presents the following problems:

1. Localization: If there are remaining teeth adjacent to the retained root, the problem of localization is simplified.
2. Exposure and removal of these roots without damaging the roots of the adjacent teeth.
3. Localization of roots in the edentulous ridge: A careful study of the osteologic landmarks revealed on the dental film is a help in localizing these roots. When additional help is needed, two radiopaque sutures (26 gauge stainless steel wire cable suture) should be passed through the labial or buccal mucoperiosteal membrane 2 cm. apart, in the area in which these roots are located. Occlusal and shift-sketch radiographs are made of this area. For the technique see Chapter 16, page 989. An appropriate mucoperiosteal flap is reflected. The radiopaque sutures are left in the flap until the root is located. This permits replacement of the flap during exploration and further radiographic examination, if necessary, to aid in locating the root.
4. Roots located close to the maxillary sinus or inferior alveolar canal may be forced into these structures during the attempted removal. Extreme care and delicacy in operative manipulations are necessary to prevent such a complication.

LOCALIZATION OF ROOTS APPROXIMATING THE MAXILLARY SINUS AND THEIR REMOVAL

As stated, the localization of roots in edentulous areas in the maxilla or mandible where there are adjacent teeth is a fairly simple matter because from the radiographs of these areas we can measure and locate, with a good degree of accuracy, the position of the remaining root in relationship to the adjacent teeth. There is one situation, however, in which we have an additional factor to be determined, and that is a root located as shown in Figure 4–48, in an area close to a maxillary sinus which dips down around the adjacent teeth (see Figure 4–48*B*). When viewing the radiograph of the area shown in Figure 4–48*B*, the dentist may wonder whether this root is in the maxillary sinus, or is a buccal root (located to the buccal side of the maxillary sinus), or a lingual root (not in the maxillary sinus but to the lingual side of the maxillary sinus). The method for determining whether this root is located buccally or lingually is solved by the shift-sketch radiographic technique described in Chapter 6. In this particular instance, the root was a lingual root.

The technique for the removal of this root is as follows: A flap is made as illustrated in Figure 4–48*A*. As can be seen, an incision is made around the neck of the second molar, along the crest of the maxillary ridge (on the labial side of the teeth), until the midpoint of the distal surface of the second bicuspid is reached, around the second and first bicuspids, and then at a right angle toward the midline of the palate. The reason for making this comparatively large flap is to avoid cutting through the greater palatine artery. The

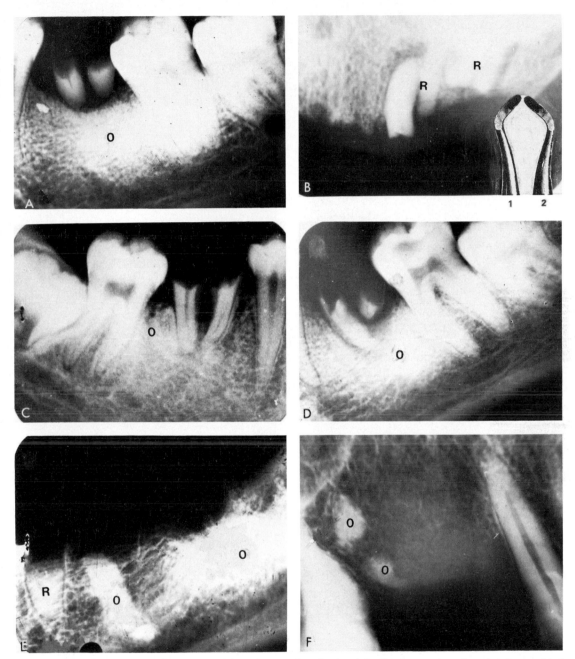

Figure 4–50 Examples of condensing osteitis and osteosclerosis. *A* and *D,* Good examples of condensing osteitis (at *O*), which are actually sclerotic bone formed as a direct result of local infection at the apices of the retained roots. The osteosclerosis shown at *O* in radiograph *C* is the result of trauma (pressure) along the mesial root of the second molar, which has tilted mesially. In radiograph *E* there is a large idiopathic dense area of osteosclerosis in the edentulous molar area, a retained root at *R* and another osteosclerotic area which simulates an elongated root. *F,* Areas marked *O* are small sclerotic areas in bone. The irregular margins are the main point in the differential diagnosis between roots and osteosclerosis.

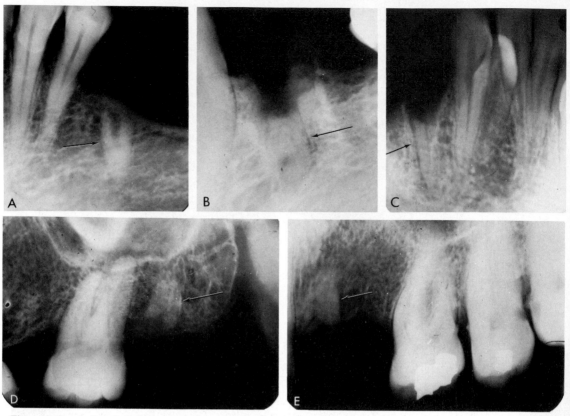

Figure 4–51 *A*, *B* and *C* show large roots in which the lamina dura is clearly discernible in at least one side of each root. This is a valid point when differentiating between a root and sclerotic bone. *D* and *E*, The two areas under examination in these radiographs are not readily identified as roots. I would not advise surgery at this time and would radiograph again in a year. If the radiographs are the same, no further attention is necessary unless symptoms present.

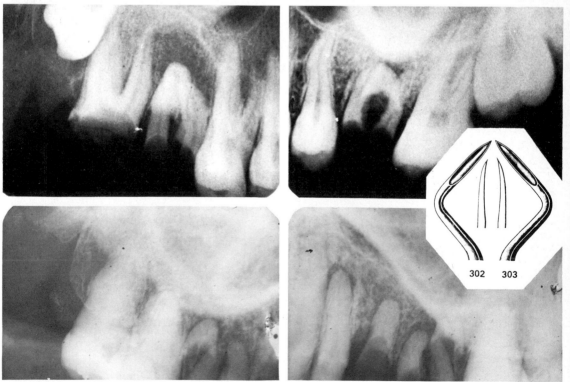

Figure 4–52 Carious roots at and below the gingival line. These are best removed by the Apexo elevators using the technique illustrated in Figure 4–20.

and radiograph a second time. If we see on comparison of the second radiograph with the first that the image of the root has moved mesially (in relation to the wire cable sutures), then the root is in the buccal cortical plate. If it has moved distally, then the root is in the lingual cortical plate. In the case illustrated in this figure, the root is again lingual. The technique for its removal is very similar to that shown in Figure 4–48.

In Figure 4–49A is shown a posteroanterior view of the maxillary sinus, a modified Waters' position, which may be helpful in localizing the buccal-lingual relationship of the root.

In Figure 4–49C is illustrated the incision, starting distal to and then up over the tuber-osity along the crest of the ridge until the vicinity of the maxillary cuspid is reached, and then at right angles toward the palate for exactly the same reason as was stated previously, namely, to avoid cutting the greater palatine artery. The flap is reflected as shown in Figure 4–49D. As can be seen, the greater palatine artery is lifted with the flap and reflected simultaneously. Measuring from the radiopaque sutures that remain in the buccal mucosa, we localize the immediate vicinity of the retained root and expose it by use of the spear-point bur and then enlarge the opening with a crosscut fissure bur, as shown in Figure 4–49D. The root substance is lifted from its crypt (Fig. 4–49E) and the flap sutured into position (Fig. 4–49F).

CHAPTER 5

IMPACTED TEETH

The term "impacted teeth" is often used incorrectly to include unerupted teeth and malposed teeth, when precise distinctions can be made (see Table 5–1). Descriptive terms should be applied intelligently when classifying impacted teeth. It is apparent that in many cases a complete description of the impacted tooth will include one or more of these terms. In many other cases the term "impacted" is not applicable.

CAUSES OF IMPACTED TEETH

The explanation for the occurrence of impacted teeth that appears to be most logical is the gradual evolutionary reduction in the size of the human mandible or maxilla. This results in a mandible or maxilla that is too small to accommodate mandibular or maxillary third molars. In substantiation of this theory, we note the congenital absence of maxillary or mandibular third molars, or the presence of rudimentary third molars in their place. Other teeth are also congenitally absent or malformed, but they are not so frequently found as are the third molars.

Nodine[32] points out that for at least 200 years it has been believed that civilization could be held responsible for the withdrawal or elimination of a stimulus that excites an adequate development of the human jaws, a development that would provide sufficient room for the normal eruption of all the teeth. This lost stimulus is the force demanded for, and the shock attendant upon, the mastication of hard food. The modern diet does not require a decided effort in mastication, and so, according to Nodine and others, this growth stimulus of the jaws is lost, and modern man has impacted teeth.

This theory is strengthened by the facts, brought out by Nodine, that the examinations of the jaws and teeth of ancient Egyptians and modern Bedouins, of Eskimos of the North, and Australian Aborigines of the South, and of the Indians of Mexico, showed that these people *did not have impacted teeth*. Their food, whether animal, fish or vegetable, is simple — simple in variety, and simple in preparation. Its consistency when prepared is such that it requires just as much forceful chewing by the child immediately after weaning as by the adult.

Turner[43] points out that 22 per cent of the Eskimos are missing mandibular third molars and 12 per cent maxillary third molars. North American Indians have 16 per cent of their

Table 5–1 *Impacted, Malposed and Unerupted Teeth*

TERM	DEFINITION	COMMENT
Impacted tooth (See Figures 5–1, 5–2 *B* and *D*, and 5–3*B*)	A tooth which is completely or partially unerupted and is positioned against another tooth, bone, or soft tissue **so that its further eruption is unlikely,** described according to its anatomic position.*	An unerupted tooth in a normal position to erupt in a 12-year-old cannot be considered "unlikely" to erupt and therefore cannot be diagnosed as impacted. The same tooth in a 20-year-old could be considered "unlikely" to erupt and could be diagnosed under this definition as an impaction.
Malposed tooth (See Figures 5–2, 5–3 and 5–4)	A tooth, unerupted or erupted, which is in an abnormal position in the maxilla or mandible.	A malposed tooth cannot be diagnosed as impacted unless it meets the criteria set forth in the definition of an impaction.
Unerupted tooth (See Figure 5–5)	A tooth not having perforated the oral mucosa.*	Many unerupted teeth do meet the requirement for a diagnosis of impaction.

*From Committee on Hospital Oral Surgery Service: Oral Surgery Glossary. Chicago, American Society of Oral Surgeons, 1971.

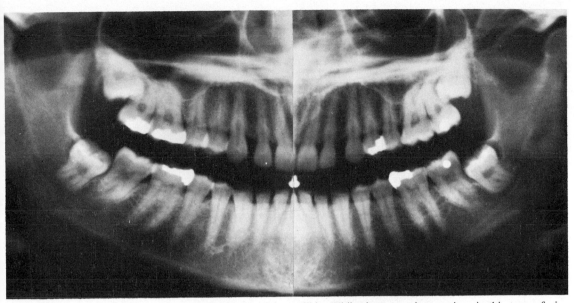

Figure 5–1 Panoramic radiograph of the maxilla and mandible. While there are shortcomings in this type of view (see Chapter 16), there are also advantages. It is essential to have periapical and occlusal as well as bitewing radiographs in addition to the panoramic one, if all the essential information required in diagnosis for oral surgery is to be obtained. I regret that too often only the panoramic view is used to aid in diagnosis.

This panoramic radiograph reveals that the patient has right and left maxillary and mandibular mesioangular third molar impactions. It is of interest to note that the concern, expressed often by some orthodontists and oral surgeons, that mandibular impactions are the cause of crowded, overlapping mandibular teeth, is not proved here. Quite the contrary, because here is a case in which there is spacing between all six mandibular and maxillary anterior teeth.

mandibular third molars and 8 per cent of their maxillary third molars missing, but *no impactions*.

Nodine suggests that "the major basic causes of aberrant or impacted teeth in the adults of Western Europe, Great Britain and

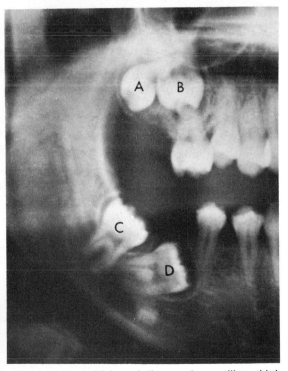

Figure 5–2 *A*, Malposed distoangular maxillary third molar. *B*, Vertically impacted maxillary second molar that appears to be buccal to the first molar. *C*, Malposed mesioangular unerupted mandibular third molar. *D*, Horizontally impacted mandibular second molar. The first mandibular molar is missing. The patient had had teeth extracted but was not certain whether they were deciduous.

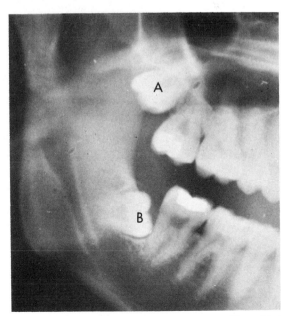

Figure 5–3 *A*, Malposed distoangular maxillary third molar. The occlusal surface was visible in the tuberosity. *B*, Horizontally impacted mandibular third molar.

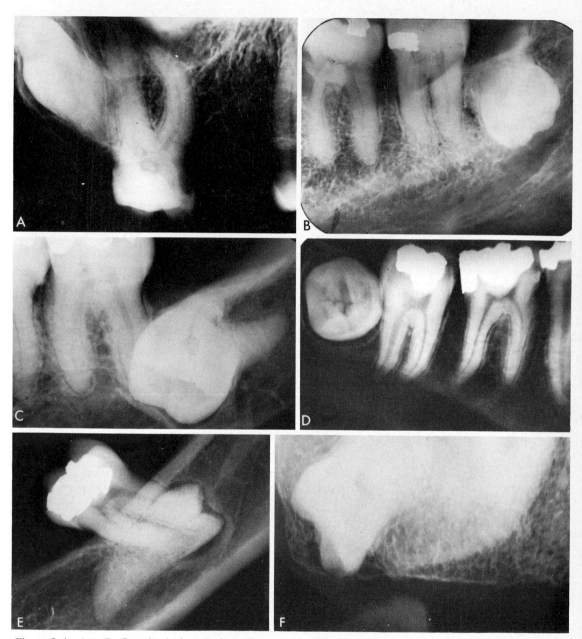

Figure 5–4 *A* to *D*, Completely impacted maxillary and mandibular third molars very oddly malpositioned in the bone. *E*, A horizontally impacted second mandibular bicuspid, probably fused to the molar. Should these symptom-free middle-aged patients have these impacted teeth excised? In my opinion, no. There is further discussion of this matter in the text on pages 258 and 259.

F, Distoangular third molar completely covered with bone in an edentulous maxilla that is symptomless. This 60-year-old patient has been wearing dentures for 10 years. Should this tooth be "prophylactically" removed? The patient was told that this tooth was present when her dentures were made and advised to have this area radiographed and examined periodically, which she has done. The oral tissues were normal. I advised the patient to continue to observe the soft tissues in this area and to continue her periodic radiographic examinations. (See Chapter 3 for further discussion of this subject.)

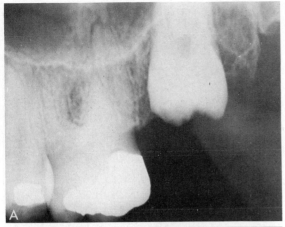

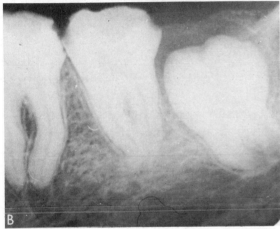

Figure 5-5 *A,* An unerupted maxillary third molar in a normal position to erupt. The crown is still covered with mucoperiosteal tissue. *B,* An unerupted mandibular third molar in a normal position to erupt. In this two-dimensional radiograph there appears to be a thin layer of bone, as well as the covering of mucoperiosteal membrane, over the crown.

Ireland, the United States and Canada" are artificial feeding of babies; the habits of babyhood and childhood; the soft, sweet food of children and youths; and crossbreeding, producing disproportion.

CONGENITALLY MISSING THIRD MOLARS AND SUPERNUMERARY MOLARS

JAMES GUGGENHEIMER, D.D.S., AND
JACK L. PECHERSKY, D.M.D.

Five hundred twenty randomly selected panoramic roentgenograms obtained during the years 1970–71 of a 13- through 16-year-old male and female (American) population were examined. The roentgenograms were reviewed to determine the presence or absence of third molars as well as supernumerary teeth in the region of the third molar. (See Figure 5–6.) Table 5–2 summarizes these findings.

The age range utilized in this study was selected on the basis of unpublished data which demonstrate that a child of age 13 presents some radiographic evidence of third molar calcification. Furthermore, the extraction of third molars would be unlikely prior to age 17 without the patient's knowledge. Third molars determined to be missing were therefore assumed to be congenitally absent.

LOCAL CAUSES OF IMPACTION

Berger[4] lists the following local causes of impaction: irregularity in the position and pressure of an adjacent tooth; the density of the overlying or surrounding bone; long-continued chronic inflammation with resultant increase in density of the overlying mucous membrane; lack of space due to underdeveloped jaws; unduly long retention of the primary teeth; premature loss of the primary teeth; acquired diseases, such as necrosis due to infection or abscesses; and inflammatory changes in the bone due to exanthematous diseases in children.

SYSTEMIC CAUSES OF IMPACTION

Impactions may also be found where no local predisposing conditions are present. In

Table 5-2 *Third Molar Findings in 520 Patients*

CONDITION	NUMBER OF PATIENTS	PER CENT OF TOTAL ($N = 520$)
All four third molars present	432	83.07
Missing one or more third molars	83	15.96
Missing one third molar only	30	5.76
Missing two third molars only	31	5.95
Missing three third molars only	5	0.96
Missing all four third molars	15	2.88
Patients with supernumerary molars (fourth and/or fifth molars)	5	0.96

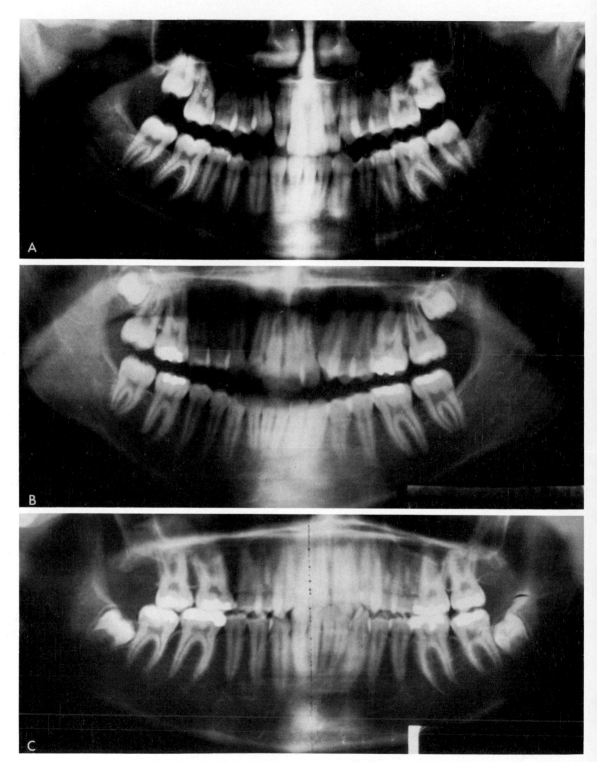

Figure 5–6   *A*, Panoramic radiograph of a 12½-year-old patient who has not had any permanent teeth extracted. Note the congenital absence of all four third molars.

B, Panoramic radiograph of a 14-year-old, with no extractions of any permanent teeth. Note the congenital absence of both mandibular third molars. The crowns of the maxillary third molars are fully formed.

C, Panoramic radiograph of another 14-year-old with congenital absence of the maxillary third molars. The mesial inclination of the fully formed mandibular third molars is not conclusive evidence that these teeth will be impacted. (Courtesy of James Guggenheimer, D.D.S., University of Pittsburgh, School of Dental Medicine.)

these cases there are, according to Berger[4]:

A. Prenatal causes
  1. Heredity
  2. Miscegenation

B. Postnatal causes: all those conditions that may interfere with the development of the child, such as
  1. Rickets
  2. Anemia
  3. Congenital syphilis
  4. Tuberculosis
  5. Endocrine dysfunctions
  6. Malnutrition

C. Rare conditions
  1. Cleidocranial dysostosis (see two case reports, beginning on page 366)
  2. Oxycephaly
  3. Progeria
  4. Achondroplasia
  5. Cleft palate

Cleidocranial dysostosis is a rare congenital condition in which there is defective ossification of the cranial bones, complete or partial absence of the clavicles, delayed exfoliation of the primary teeth, unerupted permanent teeth and rudimentary supernumerary teeth.

Oxycephaly is the so-called "steeple head," in which the top of the head is pointed.

Progeria represents premature old age. It is a form of infantilism, marked by small stature, absence of facial and pubic hair, wrinkled skin, gray hair, and the facial appearance, attitude and manner of old age.

Achondroplasia is a hereditary, congenital disturbance of the skeleton producing a form of dwarfism. In this condition, cartilage fails to develop properly.

Cleft palate is a deformity manifested by a congenital fissure in the midline.

The same local or systemic causes may be the etiologic factors in unerupted or malposed teeth. It has been my observation that impacted teeth occur in the following order of frequency:

1. Maxillary third molars
2. Mandibular third molars
3. Maxillary cuspids
4. Mandibular bicuspids
5. Mandibular cuspids
6. Maxillary bicuspids
7. Maxillary central incisors
8. Maxillary lateral incisors

Maxillary or mandibular first molars are rarely impacted.

COMPLICATIONS ARISING FROM RETAINED IMPACTED TEETH

Impacted, malposed or unerupted teeth should be removed because of the presence of infections; pathologic resorption of adjacent teeth and investing osseous structure such as is seen in cysts and tumors; pain, fractures or other complications.

Infections. Among the complications necessitating the removal of impacted teeth may be listed the following: pericoronal infection, acute or chronic alveolar abscesses, chronic suppurative osteitis, necrosis and osteomyelitis.

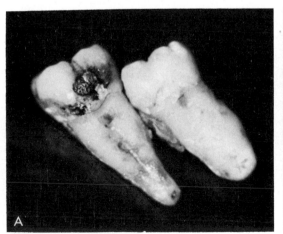 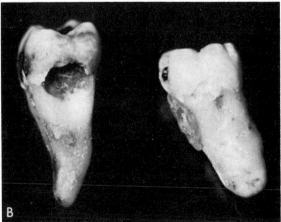

Figure 5–7 *A*, Vertical impaction, position B, of the mandibular third molar. *B*, Distogingival caries in the second molar. Frequent mention is made in the literature of the claimed production of pressure erosion of the tooth, which "impedes the eruption" of the impacted tooth. This I have never seen in enamel. Actually, the incidence of caries is not common in these cases.

Pain. Pain may be referred not only to the areas of distribution of the nerve involved and even to the associated nerve plexus, but also to remote regions. Pain is often referred to the ear.

Pain may be slight and restricted to the immediate area of the impacted tooth, or it may be severe, even excruciating, involving all the lower and upper teeth on the affected side, the ear, the postauricular area, any part of the area supplied by the trigeminal nerve, or even the entire area supplied by this nerve. This includes temporal pain. Pain may be intermit-

tent, constant or periodic. However, the dentist must make a careful assessment of the source of pain. For example, in some cases one must be certain that the pain is due to an impacted third molar and not to caries in the *second molar* (see Figure 5–7).

Pain may be intermittent facial neuralgia, simulating tic douloureux. (Read the case report on facial neuralgia and migraine caused by a vertically impacted mandibular third molar on page 1701.) Tic douloureux is distinctive in that the pain is excruciating, lancinating and sudden as the result of con-

---

Case Report No. 1

CHOROIDITIS CURED BY THE EXCISION OF A PALATALLY IMPACTED UNERUPTED MAXILLARY RUDIMENTARY SUPERNUMERARY CUSPID*

Patient. C. A., a man aged 42, was admitted to the Eye and Ear Hospital.

Chief Complaint. "Blurred vision" of the right eye had begun 2 weeks before and increased in severity over a 3-day period. The patient had received foreign protein and some tablets from his family physician prior to admission. This helped his vision slightly. One day prior to admission the patient claimed that he was able to see only the third line of the eye chart, whereas he had been able to read the eighth line 2 weeks ago. He had noticed a twitch in his right eye for about a year, but never blurred vision before. He did not have pain. He had the feeling that a foreign body was present in his eye and that there was pressure in the eye.

Physical Examination. Findings were essentially negative.

Local Eye Examination. In the right eye the lids, conjunctiva and sclera were all normal; the cornea was clear, the anterior chamber normal, the pupils dilated, the media clear; the optic nerve was well outlined and yellowish in color; the vessels were normal in size and course, with a small white exudate of choroid just above the macular vessel: the macular reflex was absent. The left eye was normal, with no pain, no photophobia, no diplopia. Vision was 20/200 in the right eye, 20/20 in the left eye.

Ears. The patient complained of pain around

the right ear, but no other physical defects in this area.

Laboratory Examination. Within normal limits.

Oral Examination. There was almost a complete complement of teeth in a good state of repair. There was some resorption of gingival soft tissues that was physiologic. There were no gingival pockets, nor could pus be expressed with pressure to the gum tissue. The electric pulp tester indicated that all teeth were vital.

Radiographic Examination. This revealed a rudimentary supernumerary cuspid in the right cuspid area of the palate. (See pages 374 to 386 for examples of mesiodens, supernumerary and rudimentary teeth.)

Hospital Course. No specific treatment was prescribed, and the patient's temperature remained normal.

On the fourth day after admission the patient felt that his vision had improved somewhat. The feeling of intense pressure and the foreign body sensation were still present. It was decided to excise the rudimentary supernumerary cuspid embedded in the osseous tissue of the palate.

Operative Notes. The technique for the excision of this palatal rudimentary cuspid is illustrated and described on pages 329 to 331 and in Figure 5–101.

Postoperative Course. Almost immediately after recovering from the anesthetic, the patient claimed that his vision had improved greatly and that the severe pressure in his eye was relieved. His vision was tested and found to be 20/40 in the right eye and 20/30 in the left eye. His vision continued to improve and on the first postoperative day was 20/20. The patient was discharged 8 days after admission.

---

*Adapted from Archer, W. H., and Fox, L. S.: Choroiditis caused by a palatally impacted unerupted maxillary rudimentary supernumerary cuspid. Oral Surg., 5:861–863 (Sept.), 1952.

CHOROIDITIS TREATED BY SURGICAL REMOVAL OF UNERUPTED IMPACTED MAXILLARY THIRD MOLAR*

PORUS S. TURNER, M.D.S., AND SHREE C. JOSHI, M.S., D.O.M.S.

A man aged 25 reported to the eye surgeon with a chief complaint of progressive loss of sight in his left eye during the last 8 days.

Local Eye Examination. Vision in the right eye was 20/20, and in the left eye, moving body only. Projection was good in both right and left eyes. Externally, the right and left eyes were normal. Pupils were dilated with a mydriatic for examination of the fundus. The fundus of the right eye was normal. In the left eye, the media showed fine vitreous opacities, particularly in the posterior part; a roughly circular yellowish raised area of exudative inflammation with indistinct and fluffy margins at the macular area was seen. The overlying retina also showed mild exudative changes; retinal vessels were normal.

Physical Examination. Findings were negative.

Laboratory Examination. Findings were negative.

Diagnosis. Macular choroiditis.

Medical Treatment. Injections of crystalline penicillin, 100,000 units, procaine penicillin, 300,000 units, and streptomycin, 1 gm., daily for 6 days, were prescribed, as well as betamethasone, 0.5-mg. tablets, one tablet four times a day for 6 days. With the above treatment the patient reported minimal to no improvement.

At this stage he was referred to the dental section for possible septic foci in the mouth.

Oral Examination. Clinical examination revealed a full complement of teeth, with no periodontal pockets. All the teeth were vital.

Radiographic Examination. Examination of the oral cavity showed nothing abnormal except an upper left third molar that was unerupted and impacted mesially against the second molar.

Surgical Treatment. It was decided to extract the impacted third molar in the hope it would have a favorable influence on the choroiditis. It was so decided because of knowledge of a similar ocular condition reported by Archer and Fox (see Case Report No. 1), which had apparently resolved after extraction of an unerupted impacted maxillary cuspid.

Operative Procedure. (The technique used by Dr. Turner is illustrated and described in Figure 5–84.)

Postoperative Notes. No attempt was made to evaluate the condition of the eye immediately after the operation. However, when the patient was seen the next day, he claimed a great improvement in his eyesight—in his own words, "Before the operation I could not see the watch on my hand; now I can actually read the time on it."

Postoperative Course. Vision in the right eye was 20/20, and in the left eye, 20/40. The exudate in the choroid and retina was completely absorbed, and the appearance of the fundus had returned almost to normal, with disappearance of the vitreous opacities. At subsequent examination (after a period of one week) it was noted that the vision in the left eye had further improved to 20/30. To this date the vision in the left eye remains 20/30.

Summary. A case of macular choroiditis of unknown cause with its subsequent resolution after removal of an unerupted impacted maxillary third molar has been presented. The valuable consultation with Dr. W. Harry Archer is gratefully acknowledged.

DISCUSSION

DICK KATZIN, M.D.

The original concept of bacterial metastasis from primary septic foci, such as dental abscesses, periodontoclasia, infected tonsils and inflamed sinuses, to a secondary focus in the uveal tract of the eye is not now generally accepted as the primary factor responsible for choroiditis. Direct infection by a few protozoan, bacterial and viral agents has been implicated as the cause in a significant number of cases. The incidence of cases has shifted over the years from the bulk's being caused by tubercle bacilli and *Treponema pallidum* to the present time, when those are relatively rare and *Toxoplasma gondii* and *Histoplasma capsulatum* represent the largest numbers. Many other cases and recurrences of old cases are thought to be an autoimmune disease or a hypersensitivity to organisms rather than due to direct invasion. Yet in another very large group, probably at least one third of all cases, no cause or even presumed cause can be uncovered. It is into this group that unusual cases of the kind presented in Case Reports 1 and 2 fall, and the relationship between removal of the impacted teeth and the improvement in the ocular inflammation is suggestive and very interesting.

The treatment of choroiditis, therefore, is specific only in those cases in which diagnosis based on clinical appearance of the lesions and supported by serologic testing or, very rarely, histologic examination can point to a specific etiologic agent and thus specific treatment. Other treatment is

---

*Adapted from Turner, P. S., and Joshi, S. C.: Choroiditis treated by surgical removal of unerupted impacted maxillary third molar: Report of a case. J. Oral Surg., *31*:59–60 (Jan.), 1973. Copyright by the American Dental Association. Reprinted by permission.

nonspecific and anti-inflammatory in nature, directed toward preventing the host defenses from damaging the eye and vision severely during the course of the inflammation.

In the two cases presented, no specific explanation is known for the dramatic improvement in the ocular condition after the removal of the impacted teeth.

---

tact with a trigger zone on the face or lip. This differentiates it from other facial neuralgias.

Pain may be due also to caries, or to a tooth whose crown has split alongside a filling but is held in place by its attachment to the gingival tissues and is painful only when the fragment is moved during mastication.

Fractures. The frequency with which fractures of the mandible occur through the areas occupied by impacted teeth proves that these teeth are a weakening factor because of the displacement of bone.

Other Complications. Impacted teeth are malposed bodies, and as such are potential sources of various complications which, while not rare, are encountered less often than those just mentioned. They may be:
1. Ringing, singing or buzzing sound in the ear (tinnitus aurium)
2. Otitis
3. Affections of the eye, such as
   a. Dimness of vision
   b. Blindness
   c. Iritis
   d. Pain simulating that of glaucoma

PROPHYLACTIC REMOVAL OF THIRD MOLARS?

In my opinion there is no more justification for the routine removal of all nonimpacted third molars, partially or completely formed, than there is for routine tonsillectomies, appendectomies or hysterectomies as prophylactic procedures.

THIRD MOLARS AND MALOCCLUSIONS?

In regard to crowding of dentition Laskin states, "Removal of unerupted or impacted third molars is often recommended in patients during or after orthodontic treatment because it has been claimed that these teeth sometimes can produce an anterior force that will cause separation in the contact points and subsequent crowding of the mandibular incisors. Undoubtedly the condition generally develops during the eruption period of the third molar. Whether the two events are related, however, remains unproven. If an anterior force were projected from the improperly

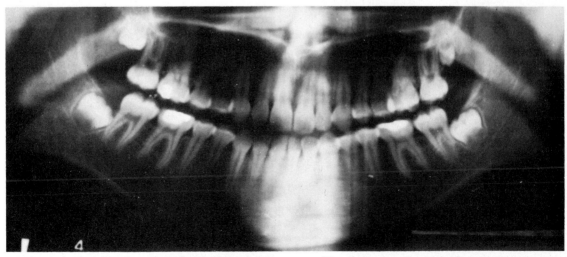

Figure 5–8 Dentition in a 13-year-old. All third molars were arbitrarily "ordered" extracted as a "preventive measure." The removal of these symptomless, partially formed mandibular third molars was, in our opinion, unjustified presumptive prophylactic surgery and was refused. In the mouth of a 13-year-old the position of the third molar crowns shown in these radiographs is common and does not prove that these teeth will become impacted. It is of interest to note the formation of a rudimentary upper left third molar.

erupting molar, it would require a corresponding forward shift of all the posterior teeth in order to be transmitted to the incisors. Moreover, the most likely place for such disruption of the tooth contact to occur would seem to be in the canine region. The fact that the relationship of the upper and lower posterior teeth does not change and the crowding usually affects the incisors tends to dispute the role of the erupting third molar in the etiology of this process. An anterior drift does occur normally, but this drift is due to the force of the occlusion on the mesially inclined teeth rather than to the force of eruption."[29]

On this subject of the third molar and malocclusions Weinstein writes, "In orthodontics, the most controversial role of the third molar is whether it contributes to the development of malocclusion or to relapse or return to irregular alignment, particularly in the anterior dental segment. It has been suggested that the erupting tooth transmits an anterior component of force down the dental arch that results in a breakdown in the continuity of contact areas of the incisors and canines. *Before indicting the third molar and extracting it, the evidence should be examined carefully.*

"The idea that pressure from erupting third molars caused a crowding of anterior teeth usually is based on less than discriminating clinical observations; for example, Waldron's poll of 12 eminent orthodontists. Since several studies, Garn, Lewis and Bonne, Moorrees and co-workers, and Rantanen show third molar crown completion at the age of 13.9, 12 and 15 to 16.5 years, respectively, and in other studies, Garn, Lewis and Bonne, Moorrees, Fanning and Hunt as well as Rantanen give the eruption ages as 16 to 21 or more, 20.5 and 21.8 to 23.3 years, respectively, *it is difficult to relate these* late ages to the observed anterior arch crowding at a much earlier age.

"In the few studies associating third molars with this secondary crowding, Bergstrom and Jensen, in a study of 60 dental students, concluded that these molars appear to exert some influence on the dental arch, whereas Shanley's evaluation of three groups, one with normal erupted third molars, the second with impacted third molars and the third with congenitally missing third molars, *showed no significant differences either in arch length discrepancies or actual inclination of mandibular incisors.*

"Stemm made a longitudinal study of changes in the mandibular arch of 29 individuals from mean age of 15 years 6 months to mean age of 19 years 5 months and divided them into groups with and without third molars. *He concluded that the third molar does not contribute to any irregularity in malalignment or malocclusion that may develop in the remainder of the arch....*

"*Relapse:* The relapse or return to the original irregular alignment of anterior teeth is a constant prick to the ego of the competent orthodontist, and an irritant to the perfection seeking parent. Obviously, there are several variables that singly or in combination might contribute to this after-treatment change in tooth alignment...."

Dr. Weinstein goes on to discuss orthodontic reasons and then concludes, "To put the onus on the last in the dental line—the third molar—demands reliable evidence."* To Dr. Weinstein and many others this has not been done.

Based on my own observations, I am completely in accord with the statements made by these authorities. See Chapter 2, Figures 2–105 and 2–106, for additional information on this subject.

IMPACTED MANDIBULAR THIRD MOLARS

It is necessary for the surgeon to classify mandibular impacted third molars so that he can determine in advance just what difficulties he will encounter in their removal and plan his surgical procedures intelligently. For classification of impacted mandibular third molars, their anatomic position must be determined by a radiographic examination. The radiographs necessary to establish the *true, undistorted anatomic position of the mandibular impacted third molars* are intraoral periapical radiographs, lateral jaw radiographs, bitewing radiographs and occlusal and panoramic radiographs.

CLASSIFICATION OF IMPACTED MANDIBULAR THIRD MOLARS

The following classification, suggested by Pell and Gregory,[33] which includes a portion

---

*Reprinted by permission from Weinstein, S.: Third molar implications in orthodontics. J.A.D.A., *82*:819–823, 1971. Copyright by the American Dental Association.

of George B. Winter's[48] classification, is an excellent one:

A. Relation of the tooth to the ramus of the mandible and the second molar:

Class I: There is a sufficient amount of space between the ramus and the distal side of the second molar for the accommodation of the mesiodistal diameter of the crown of the third molar.

Class II: The space between the ramus and the distal side of the second molar is less than the mesiodistal diameter of the crown of the third molar.

Class III: All or most of the third molar is located within the ramus.

B. Relative depth of the third molar in bone:

Position A: The highest portion of the tooth is on a level with or above the occlusal line.

Position B: The highest portion of the tooth is below the occlusal plane, but above the cervical line of the second molar.

Position C: The highest portion of the tooth is below the cervical line of the second molar.

C. The position of the long axis of the impacted mandibular third molar in relation to the long axis of the second molar (from Winter's classification):

1. Vertical
2. Horizontal
3. Inverted
4. Mesioangular
5. Distoangular
6. Buccoangular
7. Linguoangular

These may also occur simultaneously in
a. Buccal version
b. Lingual version
c. Torsoversion

RADIOGRAPHIC VISUALIZATION OF IMPACTED MANDIBULAR THIRD MOLARS

Periapical Radiographs. It is frequently impossible to visualize completely the impacted third molar on the periapical films because of (1) gagging on the part of the patient, or (2) medial deflection of the film by the soft tissues overlying the ramus. This is particularly true in horizontal Class III cases, in which the impacted third molar is completely imbedded in the ramus, and to a lesser degree in horizontal Class II and I cases of impacted third molars.

Because of the medial deflection of the posterior two thirds of the periapical film, if we are to succeed in securing an image of the impacted third molar on the film it is necessary to direct the central rays at a right angle to the long axis of the film.

Bitewing Radiographs. In Class I and Class II cases of impacted mandibular molars, the only true radiographic visualization of the actual relationship of the crowns of the second and third molars is made by a correctly angled bitewing film. In this case the central ray is directed through the crown of the second molar at a right angle to the film, with a "0" degree vertical angulation.

Occlusal Films. This view reveals the buccal-lingual position of at least the crown of the impacted mandibular third molar. A standard-size occlusal film may be used or a small periapical film can be used. It is placed over the occlusal surfaces of the molar teeth and moved posteriorly until the edge of the film contacts the anterior border of the ramus. The teeth are then closed in occlusion to hold the film in position, the patient's head is tilted posteriorly as far as possible, and the central ray is directed at a right angle to the film through the inferior border of the mandible.

Lateral Radiographic View of the Mandible. A more accurate roentgenogram in Class III horizontal impacted third molars is obtained by a *correctly positioned lateral view* of the mandible—not the *oblique view,* which is frequently mistaken for the true lateral jaw radiograph—or a panoramic radiograph (see Chapters 16, pages 990 to 1012, and 17, page 1028, for specific details on the necessary techniques).

LOCALIZING THE MANDIBULAR CANAL IN RELATION TO THE APICES OF THE LOWER THIRD MOLAR

If the oral surgeon always knew with reasonable certainty the anatomic relationship of the mandibular canal to the roots of impacted mandibular third molars, he could plan his technique so as to avoid that most distressing postoperative complication, anesthesia of the lip.

As a means of locating this canal, Frank suggests that a modification of the "tubeshift" method can be used to determine whether the mandibular canal is medial to, lateral to or below an impacted mandibular third molar.* This technique was first de-

---

*Frank, V. H., D.D.S., Philadelphia, Pa. Personal communication.

MANDIBULAR THIRD MOLARS

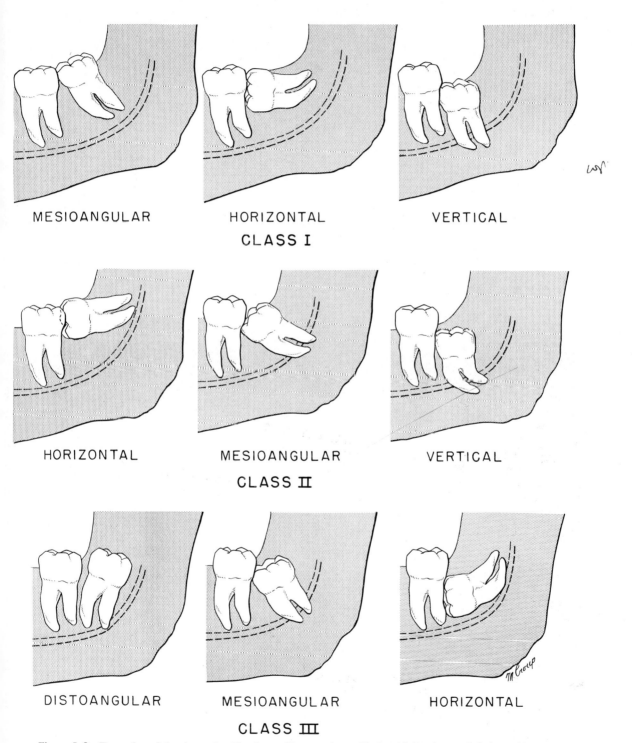

| MESIOANGULAR | HORIZONTAL | VERTICAL |

CLASS I

| HORIZONTAL | MESIOANGULAR | VERTICAL |

CLASS II

| DISTOANGULAR | MESIOANGULAR | HORIZONTAL |

CLASS III

Figure 5–9 Examples of the three classifications of impacted mandibular third molars and their positions.

scribed by Richards.[37] The principle involved is the same as that of the "Clark shift" to localize a maxillary impacted cuspid. Frank's technique follows:

"By placing two films in identical positions in the mouth, when x-raying a lower impacted third molar, and changing the position of the x-ray tube, we can determine whether the canal lies lingually or buccally to the impaction; or in the same plane as the tooth.

"To accomplish this the x-ray angle must be shifted 25 degrees upward and this second film compared to the film taken with the x-ray tube parallel to the occlusal plane of the teeth.

"In the mouth an x-ray taken from 25 degrees below the plane of occlusion will make a distant object move downward in relation to an object in the foreground; i.e., if mandibular canal lies lingual to impaction, it will move downward in relation to the roots of the third molar (see Figure 5–12B). Conversely a canal on the buccal side of roots will appear to move upward on the roots. If the canal remains in the same position, it is directly below the roots, or passes between the roots, or is in a groove in the root substance apically, lingually or buccally.

"There are certain cases in which you may want to take the second film with the x-ray tube pointing downward 25 degrees. This will show the roots of a lingually inclined impacted tooth in greater detail. However, it is more difficult to visualize the mandibular canal.

"Technique for impacted mandibular third molars (see Figure 5–12):

A. An intraoral film is taken in normal position.
  1. Occlusal surfaces of the lower teeth parallel to the floor.
  2. Tube and x-ray parallel to the occlusal surface of the second molar.
  3. This x-ray should be directed so that there is *no* overlap of the contact point between the first and second molars.
B. A second film is then taken. The tube is

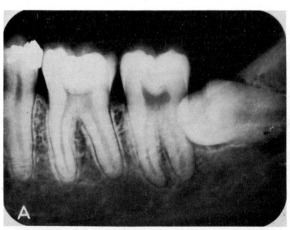
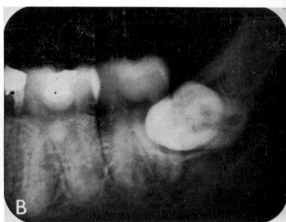
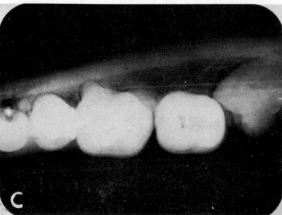

Figure 5–10 Periapical and occlusal radiographs used in studying impacted mandibular teeth before their surgical removal. Localization technique: *A*, Radiograph with the tube in normal position. *B*, When the tube is shifted to the distal side, the third molar image moves mesially, thus proving that the tooth is on the buccal side. *C*, The occlusal view proves the buccal position of the crown.

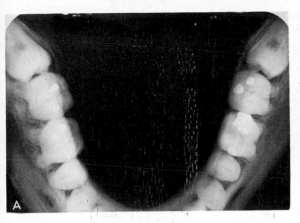

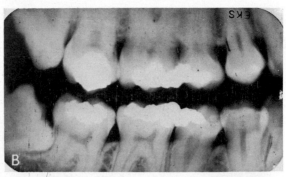

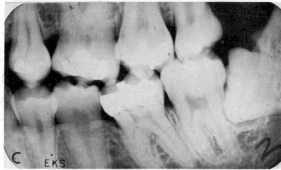

Figure 5-11 *A*, True occlusal radiograph of bilateral horizontally impacted mandibular third molars. This view is of value in determining the thickness of the lingual cortical bone. *B*, and *C*, Right and left bitewing radiographs show the true relationship of the occlusal surface of the crown of the impacted mandibular third molars to the second molars. An extraoral lateral jaw or panoramic radiograph may be necessary to visualize completely the impacted mandibular third molar.

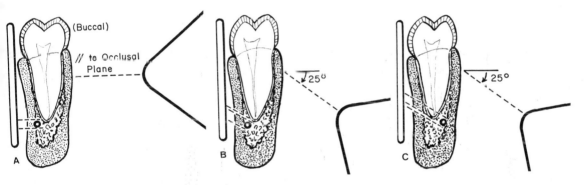

Figure 5-12 See text for a description of the shift-sketch technique illustrated here to localize the roots of the third molar in relation to the mandibular canal.

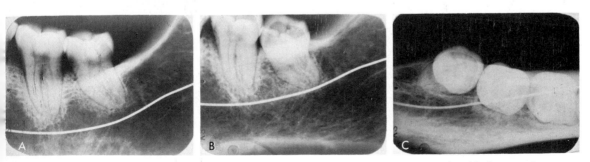

Figure 5-13 *A*, A wire was placed in the mandibular canal, and a roentgenogram was made with the central ray parallel to the occlusal plane. *B*, A second roentgenogram was made, with the central ray now directed at a minus 25-degree angle to the occlusal plane. The canal and its wire appear to have moved up. This indicates that the mandibular canal is on the buccal side of the third molar roots. *C*, This occlusal view proves that the mandibular canal is on the buccal side.

It must be remembered that if the inferior alveolar canal passes *between* the roots of the molar, the shift-sketch method, as described, will *not* show any change in the position of the wire in relation to the third molar roots. This is proof that the actual canal passes through the roots or is in contact with the root or roots. (See text.)

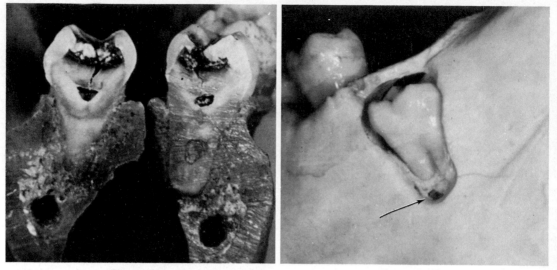

<table>
<tr><td>**Figure 5–14**</td><td>**Figure 5–15**</td></tr>
</table>

Figures 5–14 and 5–15   Two specimens of the mandible prepared to show the relationship of third molar roots to the inferior alveolar canal and its neurovascular bundle.

In Figure 5–14 the canal is below and buccal to the apices of the third molar in a vertical section of the third molar and the mandible.

In Figure 5–15 the lingual cortical plate covering a vertically impacted mandibular third molar has been removed and shows the inferior alveolar canal and its neurovascular bundle passing at an angle between the mesial and distal roots. To prevent severe trauma to this neurovascular bundle when removing this tooth, it would have been necessary to have sectioned the crown and the roots.

directed upward at a 25-degree angle, still at right angles to the first and second molars (see Figure 5–12*B* and *C*). (Both films should be placed in the same position in the mouth, the mesial end of the film positioned at least to the middle of the first molar and the superior edge of the film parallel to the occlusal surfaces of the molars.)

"Localizing the mandibular canal in relation to the roots of a lower third molar impaction is particularly valuable: (*a*) in planning your surgical technique to avoid trauma to

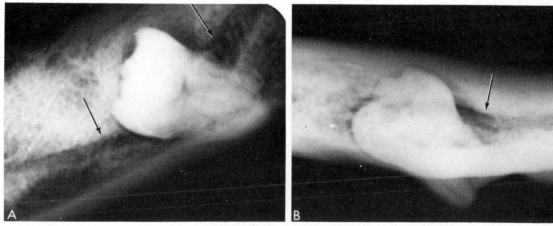

Figure 5–16   This symptomless impacted mandibular third molar was discovered in the radiographic survey of the edentulous mandible of a 48-year-old male when he was having a "complete head-to-toe" physical evaluation. Four items here are of interest: (1) osteosclerotic bone mesial to the crown, (2) a small area of radiolucency superior to the distal surface of the third molar, (3) the inferior alveolar canal, which apparently passes beneath the tooth (*A and B*), and (4) the projection of the roots through the lingual cortical plate.

This fourth condition, incidentally, was discovered during the careful palpation of the soft and hard tissue of the oral cavity, which is an essential part of every oral examination (see Figure 5–35). This possibility was confirmed by the occlusal radiograph, *B*. Our conclusion was that there was no indication for the surgical excision of this impacted tooth. The patient had been wearing complete dentures for over 10 years. The denture did not extend over that area of the mandible in which the third molar was located. The osteosclerosis and osteopetrosis were not due to a pathologic condition.

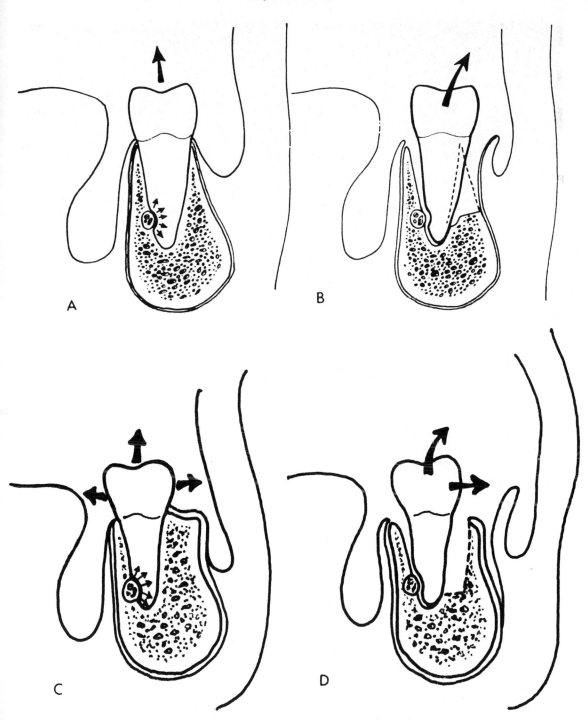

Figure 5–17 As Howe suggests, "The incidence of nerve damage complicating the removal of 'grooved' teeth *(A)* can be reduced by removing the buccal plate and delivering the tooth through the resultant defect *(B)*."

However, as shown in *C* and *D,* in many third mandibular molar areas, the buccal cortical plate is too thick to be removed as Howe has indicated, not only because of the technical difficulty of removing this much dense buccal bone, but mainly because this gross loss of bone would materially weaken the mandible. In these cases I use the technique illustrated in *C* and *D,* in which a groove is created with burs alongside the buccal surface of the roots, and the tooth is moved bucally into this space and removed. Obviously, location of the inferior alveolar canal has been established on the lingual surface prior to this procedure.

(*A* and *B* from, and *C* and *D* modified from, Howe, G. L.: Minor Oral Surgery, Bristol, England, John Wright & Sons, Ltd., 1971.)

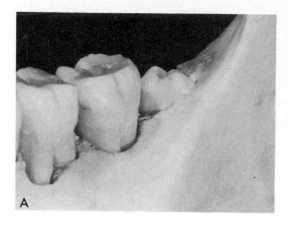

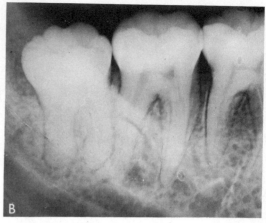

Figure 5–18   *A,* Vertically impacted mandibular third molar with slight distal inclination. *B,* The relationship of the roots of the third molar to the inferior alveolar canal, whether buccal or lingual, is clearly shown in this radiograph. In addition, cancellous bone is locked between the roots buccolingually. To avoid the possibility of injury to the inferior alveolar canal and its contents, and to facilitate the removal of this tooth with a minimum loss of bone and trauma, sectioning of the roots after adequate exposure of the crown is clearly indicated. (See Figures 5–24, 5–25, 5–33 and 5–41.)

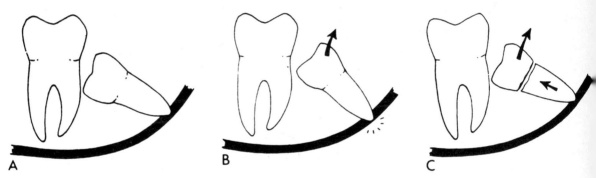

Figure 5–19   *A,* Mesioangular impaction of a notched lower left molar. *B,* Mesial application of force crushes canal contents. *C,* Tooth division minimizes the risk of damage to the canal contents. (From Howe, G. L.: Minor Oral Surgery. Bristol, England, John Wright & Sons, Ltd., 1971.)

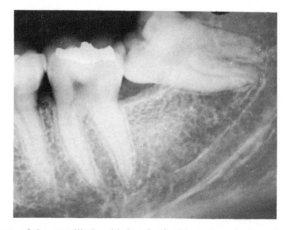

Figure 5–20   While the roots of the mandibular third molar in this case are not as close to the inferior alveolar canal as are those in Figure 5–19, nevertheless injury to the neurovascular bundle could very easily occur. To avoid this, the crown should be split longitudinally and the inferior portion of the crown then cut off with a bur. Following this the roots are moved forward into the space created by the removal of the crown. (See Figure 5–47.)

the mandibular canal and its contents; and (b) when removing root tips lying in close proximity to the canal."*

This should result in fewer cases of anesthesia caused by trauma to the inferior alveolar (mandibular) nerve of the canal.

In all cases in which the mandibular canal approximates the apices of the third molar, the patient should be warned in advance of surgery of the possibility of inadvertent trauma to the inferior alveolar nerve, which would result in numbness (anesthesia) or a burning and tingling sensation (paresthesia) in the lip postoperatively for an unknown period of time. In some cases it is a matter of days; in others, weeks or months; and in some, forever. There is no specific treatment, except surgery in those few cases in which postoperative fibrous bands have "strangled" the neurovascular bundle, or the inferior alveolar canal itself has been occluded. An increase in malpractice suits because of this unfortunate postoperative complication has been noted. Study legends and Figures 5–10 to 5–20 for techniques to help prevent this complication.

SURGICAL TECHNIQUE FOR REMOVAL OF IMPACTED LOWER THIRD MOLARS

The removal of impacted mandibular third molars is a complicated surgical procedure involving soft tissue, muscle and some of the hardest bone in the skeleton. The site of operation is in a restricted area, difficult of access. The field is highly vascular and constantly flooded with saliva, making the continuous use of the suction apparatus a necessity. Strict asepsis must be maintained. The operation must be carefully thought out in advance, with alternate plans of procedure decided upon if the original ones must be changed as the operation proceeds.

Basic Steps in Planning Operative Procedures. Study the radiographs carefully. (1) Determine that your radiographs show exactly the full size, not elongated or shortened, and the actual form of the tooth; also, the number, size and curvature of roots and the proximity of roots or crowns to adjacent teeth or vital structures. (2) Classify the impaction. (3) Study the occlusal views to ascertain buccal-lingual position of the tooth. (4) Carefully note the relationship of the

roots to the inferior alveolar canal. (5) Review the results of the visual and digital examinations of the hard and soft tissues surrounding the operative site.

Assemble all the information gained from the preceding thorough examination, and then plan the operative procedure. If necessary, modify the plan to meet unexpected conditions. In planning: (1) Outline the extent of the soft tissue flaps to be used, keeping in mind the necessity for adequate exposure with maintenance of a good blood supply to the flaps and subsequent support of the soft tissue flaps after operation. When considering the soft tissue flaps, keep in mind the muscles that may be involved, and any foramina and the vessels that may exit from those foramina. (2) Decide whether or not this impaction could be removed by (a) sectioning of the tooth, (b) a combination of some bone removal and the sectioning technique, or (c) solely by the removal of surrounding bone. (3) Estimate the amount of surrounding osseous tissue that must be removed in order to give adequate exposure and create space into which the impaction can be moved en route to its removal. (4) Plan the logical method and choose the best instruments for the removal of this overlying and surrounding bone—whether burs alone, chisels alone or a combination of burs and chisels—or whether a removal of a certain amount of bone plus tooth division may accomplish the desired results. (5) Select the best direction for the removal of the impacted tooth and the instruments necessary to accomplish this result with a minimum of trauma.

Factors Complicating the Removal of Impacted Mandibular Third Molars.

1. Abnormal root curvature.
2. Hypercementosis.
3. Proximity to mandibular canal.
4. Extreme bone density, especially in elderly patients.
5. Follicular space filled with bone, most frequently seen in patients over 25 years of age.
6. Ankylosis. Occasionally the crowns of unerupted teeth in elderly patients are first partially resorbed by osteoclastic activity, and then the eroded surface is filled with bone, owing to the osteoblastic activity. This results in an ankylosis between the tooth and bone that necessitates complete removal of all the bone around the crown of the tooth before it can be luxated, or divided into sections

---

*Frank, V. H., D.D.S., Philadelphia, Pa. Personal communication.

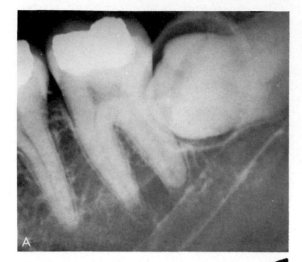

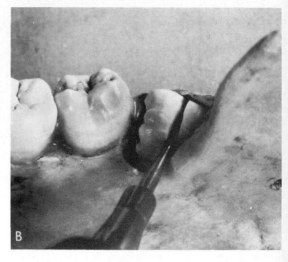

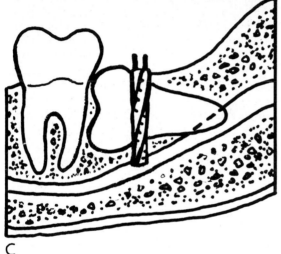

Figure 5–21 *A*, Horizontally impacted Class I, Position B, mandibular third molar. *B*, Sufficient bone from over the crown is removed buccally and superiorly with burs to expose the cementum at the neck of the third molar. *B* and *C*, The crown is then cut off the roots. Special care must be taken in cutting through the inferior surface of the root to assure that the bur does not plunge into the neurovascular bundle in the inferior alveolar canal.

by the bur. The chisel is not effective for splitting these ankylosed teeth.

7. Difficult access to the operative field because of:
   a. Small orbicularis oris muscle.
   b. Inability to open the mouth wide enough.
   c. A large and uncontrollable tongue.

SPECIFIC OPERATIVE TECHNIQUES

Unnecessary Removal of Mandibular or Maxillary Second Molars. Unfortunately, second molars are extracted *unnecessarily all too frequently* to facilitate the removal of impacted third molars. The *only time* the extraction of the second molars is justified in either the mandible or the maxilla is in those *very rare cases* in which the impacted third molar is *below the roots of the mandibular second molar* or *above the roots* of the *maxillary second molar,* and then only when there is a specific pathologic or neurologic reason for removing these third molars that are impacted or fused to second molars. In other cases, unless the second molar is hopelessly decayed or infected, the extraction of the second molar for the purpose of access to the third molar indicates inadequate surgical skill.

The mere presence of these impacted or malpositioned third molars is not an indication for their extraction, with the attendant sacrifice of the second molar. In addition, the potential complications resulting from such a major surgical procedure, such as the involvement of the maxillary sinus, injury to the mandibular neurovascular bundle or fractures of the mandible or the maxilla, are major contraindications to such elective procedures. This same principle applies to all impacted or malposed teeth.

Soft Tissue Flaps. For the removal of impacted mandibular third molars, the incision for the soft tissue flap is started just to the lingual side of the external oblique ridge of the ramus of the mandible at a distance of ¾ inch distally from the lower second molar, and is directed anteriorly until it contacts the midpoint of the distal surface of the second molar.

Continue the incision buccally around the neck of the second molar to the interproximal space between the first and second molars, and then extend it down toward the muco-buccal fold at a 45-degree angle. Reflect the buccal flap carefully with the periosteal elevator, making certain that the periosteum is *stripped back with the oral mucosa* (see Figure 5–22A). An alternate type of flap is shown in Figure 5–22B. Deeply embedded third molars (Position C) require the type of flap shown in Figure 5–22A. Adequate exposure is obtained with the flap shown in Figure 5–22B for impacted mandibular third molars in Positions A and B.

Loosen and turn upward that portion of the mucoperiosteum covering the crown of the impacted tooth. It may be held in this position by means of a broad-blade periosteal elevator. This gives adequate access to the overlying bone.

It is important to keep this incision to the buccal side in order that postoperative infection and trismus may be kept at a minimum. Incisions are not made along the internal oblique ridge of the ramus or the lingual cor-tical plate because of the proximity of the lingual nerve.

To prevent surgical trauma to this nerve, we make our incision from the midpoint of the distal surface of the second molar distally and buccally across the unerupted third molar toward the external oblique ridge, and, if necessary, up along this ridge. Incisions that are carried directly posteriorly shortly pass off the osseous structure because the ramus flares out laterally at this point. It can be seen that an incision starting at the midpoint of the distal surface of the second molar and carried directly posteriorly opens into the ptyergoid mandibular space. It is our technique to disturb the soft tissue to the lingual side of our incision as little as possible. Not only is postoperative trismus reduced, but postoperative trauma to the lingual nerve or submaxillary or parapharyngeal abscesses rarely occur.

The buccal flap should meet these basic requirements: (1) It should provide adequate exposure of the operative site. (2) It should have a wide base to assure a good blood supply to the soft tissues. (3) It should be large enough so that the soft tissue surrounding the operative site is not traumatized during the operation and so that when the flap is replaced, the edges rest on a wide shelf of bone.

Excision of Surrounding Bone. If the impacted tooth is completely covered, remove the bone overlying it by means of bone burs or chisels or both.

BONE BURS. Use sharp burs (preferably spear-point) to start cutting through the dense

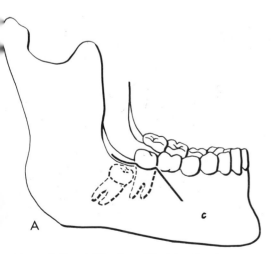
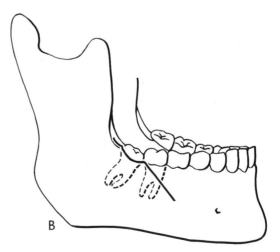

Figure 5–22 *A*, The line of incision for the mucoperiosteal flap shown by the dense black line is that necessary to expose an operative field adequately for the surgical excision of an unerupted impacted mandibular third molar.

B, For a partially erupted impacted mandibular third molar the operative field need not be as large as that shown in *A*. The heavy black line shows the line of incision necessary in these cases.

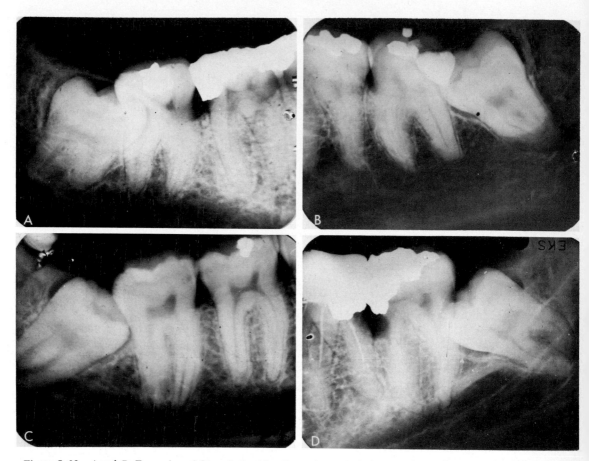

Figure 5–23   *A* and *B*, Examples of Class I, Position B, mesioangularly impacted mandibular third molars. *C*, Class I, Position C, mesioangularly impacted mandibular third molar. *D*, Class III, Position C, mesioangular mandibular third molar impaction. Note that in all four of these impactions there is an intimate relationship with the roots and inferior alveolar canal with its contained neurovascular bundle.

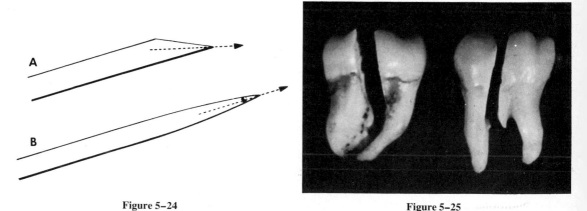

Figure 5–24

Figure 5–25

Figure 5–24   Ends and line of cut of *A*, a chisel, used for removing bone, and *B*, an osteotome, used for splitting teeth. (From Howe, G. L.: Minor Oral Surgery. Bristol, England, John Wright & Sons, Ltd., 1971.)

Figure 5–25   Examples of molars split by a razor-sharp osteotome placed in a buccal groove and struck with a single short, sharp blow from the wrist with the mallet.

cortical plate of bone. When the leaves, or cutting edges, become clogged with the bone chips, clean the bur to avoid overheating and burnishing of the bone, which results in postoperative pain and the death of bone cells. Cut holes in the bone overlying the impacted tooth at a distance of 4 mm. from center to center. Drill down to the impacted tooth with minimum pressure and speed. No drilling is done with bone burs on the side adjacent to the second molar because of the danger of injury to this tooth.

Flush the operative site constantly with sterile water when drilling. Use a suction tip at the same time.

Advantages. Hall has studied the postoperative results from use of the surgical air turbine and burs for removal of bone and has listed the advantages found:

"These were shown to be 50 per cent more effective than other methods commonly employed to remove bone.

"More significant was the pattern of healing. The apposition of new bone to the cut surface and the rate of repair were enhanced when the air turbine unit was used. . . .

"Trauma and postoperative pain were reduced approximately 50 per cent. The lips showed no evidence of abrasion because of the light touch applied, and since the instrument is air-cooled, there is no heat in the handpiece. Since the vibratory range of the instrument exceeds that of sonic perception, minimal trauma is experienced by the patient. Virtually no pain is referred to either the temporomandibular joint or the inferior border of the mandible.

"Postoperative swelling was slightly reduced: most of the edema that occurred could be ascribed to the flap. No edema is attributed to the whisper of air about the surgical bur.

"Postoperative bleeding was relatively the same, but has never created any particular problem.

"The length of time required for surgery is reduced by approximately 60 per cent.

"The small amount of effort required resulted in ease of operation and less fatigue for the surgeon.

"Since the complete unit was autoclavable, sterile conditions were maintained."*

---

*Hall, R. M.: The effect of high speed bone cutting without the use of water coolant. Oral Surg., *20*:150 (Aug.), 1965.

CHISELS. By means of chisels or burs, connect the previously drilled holes and remove the bone overlying the impacted tooth. This method of connecting the previously drilled holes gives the least trauma. Chisels must be *sharp*. Sharpen before using.

Sterilize chisels in a *cold* sterilizing medium, so as not to ruin the cutting edge.

There are two types of chisels: (*a*) the hand pressure chisel — least desirable and most dangerous; (*b*) hand mallet and chisel — satisfactory if you have a trained assistant. Study again the use of the chisel in Chapter 2, pages 32 to 37 and Figures 2–19, 5–24 and 5–25.

After the bone is removed over the impacted tooth, remove that from its height of contour. Sectioning of the crown will facilitate the removal of the tooth and conserve investing bone.

GENERAL RULE REGARDING THE REMOVAL OF BONE. The amount of bone surrounding an impacted, malposed or unerupted tooth that must be removed depends upon the type of impaction, position of the malposed tooth, access to the area in which the tooth is located, and size of the tooth.

Sufficient bone must be removed to allow the tooth to be lifted from its bed without the necessity of heavy pressure. The use of excessive force in an attempt to drive an impacted tooth through the bone is likely to result in a fracture. Never attempt to remove an impacted tooth through a small aperture. If a fracture does not result, there will be excessive trauma, which increases measurably the postoperative complications.

Removal of Impacted Tooth from Its Bed. After the impacted tooth is free (after overlying bone and bone surrounding the height of contour have been removed) sufficient space must be obtained between the height of contour of the impacted tooth and the bone to permit the entrance of an elevator so that the point of the elevator can be placed beneath the crown. In addition, sufficient bone must be removed distal to the impaction to create a space into which the impaction can be moved. The impacted tooth is then lifted from its bed by means of an elevator.

If the impacted tooth is not removed with a moderate amount of pressure, remove the elevator and examine the tooth and its investing bony tissues to determine the reason for its resistance. If insufficient bone has been removed, remove more bone.

If the crown of the impacted tooth is still locked beneath the height of contour of the

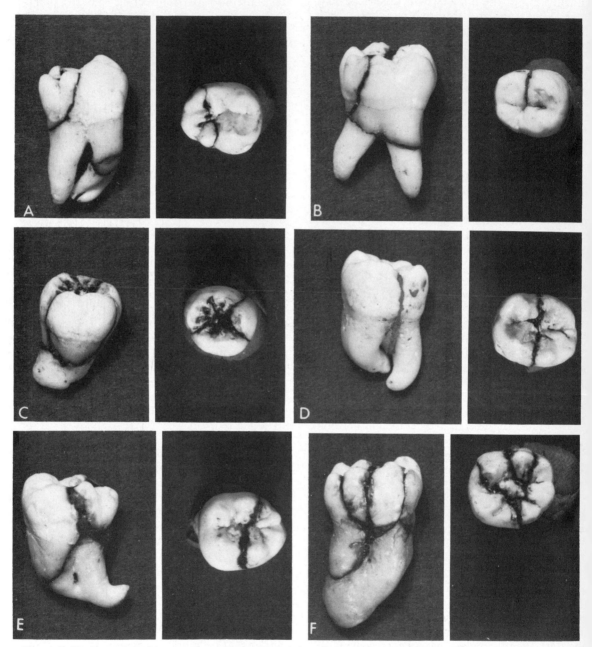

Figure 5–26 Examples of impacted mandibular third molars that were sectioned in order to facilitate their removal and to conserve bone.

Buccal and occlusal views showing the various lines of cleavage when these teeth were split with a chisel. The razor-sharp osteotome (splitting chisel) should be placed in the deepest buccal groove and struck with a short, sharp stroke from the wrist with the mallet.

(Figure 5–26 continued on opposite page)

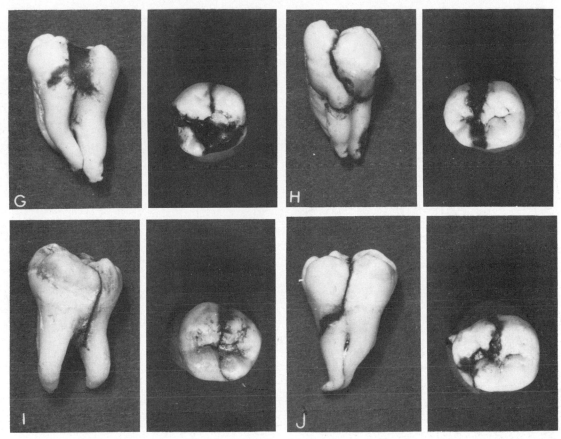

Figure 5 26 *(Continued.)*

second molar, enlarge the space which has been created to the distal side of the third molar, into which the impacted third molar is to be moved. A better method is to section the crown of the third molar.

Do not apply force in the attempted removal of any impacted tooth until all resistance due to dense bone has been removed. This is especially important in lower third molar impactions, because fracture of the mandible may result.

Removal of Residual Tooth Follicle. Because of the potential ability of this tissue to produce an ameloblastoma, it should always be excised following the removal of impacted or unerupted teeth.

Undoubtedly hundreds of thousands of at least segments of these follicles are closed in operative wounds every year, even though conscientious attempts are made to remove them. In spite of this fact, ameloblastomas are not commonly seen. It would appear, therefore, that the "danger" of their develop-

ing is not the hazard that some consider it to be. (See pages 735 to 739 in Chapter 13.)

SPLITTING OR TOOTH DIVISION TECHNIQUE FOR THE REMOVAL OF IMPACTED TEETH

One of the most valuable aids in the removal of many mandibular impacted third molars is the "splitting technique," or the process of reducing the crown into small pieces that are then removed, creating a space into which the remaining portion of the roots can be moved. This is accomplished by chisels or burs and in many cases a combination of both. By this process of destruction of the tooth itself rather than of the surrounding bone, much bone is preserved which otherwise must be regenerated in postoperative healing.

Advantages. Pell and Gregory,[33] pioneers in establishing this technique, list the following advantages, modified by the author's experience, of this method:

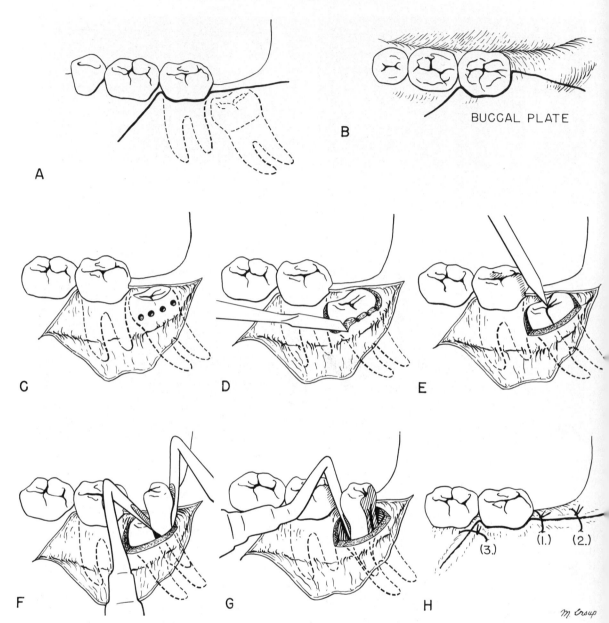

Figure 5–27 Removal of a Class I, Position C, mesioangularly impacted mandibular third molar. *A,* Incision for the required flap. *B,* Occlusal view of the incision for the flap, which is kept out to the buccal side, as shown. To carry the incision straight back would result in the exposure of the lingual structures and cause trismus from the invasion of bacteria into this area. *C,* The flap is turned back and four holes are drilled through the cortical plate with a Feldman spearpoint drill. *D,* With a sharp chisel the buccal and distal bone is removed down to the height of contour. *E,* The crown and roots are split with a sharp bibevel chisel. *F,* The distal root is lifted from its bed by the No. 4 Apexo elevator applied first into the split, with the buccal plate as a fulcrum, and the No. 5 Apexo elevator distally, with the external oblique ridge as a fulcrum, to move the root anteriorly and superiorly. *G,* The mesial root is now moved up into the space created by the removal of the distal root. *H,* Note that only a small amount of bone had to be removed in order to deliver this impacted molar. Only three sutures are needed to close the flap.

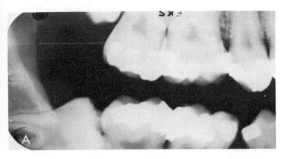

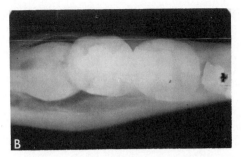

Figure 5–28 *A*, Class II, Position A, horizontally impacted mandibular third molar. *B*, Occlusal view of *A*, taken on a periapical film, which shows that the crown of the third molar is closer to the thin, dense lingual cortical plate than to the thick buccal cortical plate. While it is tempting to remove this thin lingual bone, the too-high incidence of temporary or permanent lingual nerve paresthesia, or complete anesthesia, has usually deterred me from using this technique. Instead, the tooth-splitting technique shown in Figure 5–27 is preferred.

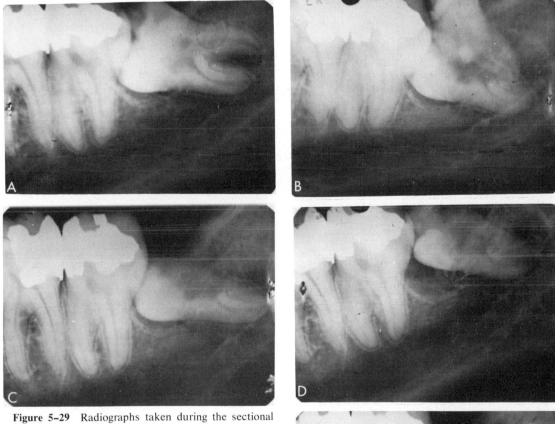

Figure 5–29 Radiographs taken during the sectional removal of the horizontally impacted mandibular third molar. *A*, Periapical film of the impacted molar. See Figure 5–28 for the bitewing film of this case, which reveals the true relationship between the second molar and the occlusal surface of the impacted third molar, and for the occlusal film, which reveals the buccolingual relationship of the impacted third molar.

B, After the soft tissue flap was reflected and a portion of the buccal cortical plate was removed, the tooth was split with a chisel through the bifurcation. *C*, The superior portion of the crown and root (the distal half of the crown and the distal root) have been elevated from the alveolus. *D*, The inferior portion of the crown and root (the mesial half of the crown and the mesial root) were next elevated into the space created by the removal of the distal portion of the crown and the distal root.

E, The impacted tooth has been removed with a minimum loss of investing bone and practically without trauma.

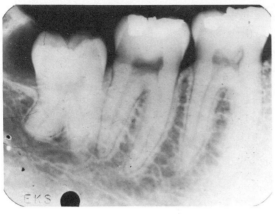

Figure 5–30 Class I, Position B, vertical "impaction," with a distal, well-circumscribed radiolucent area surrounded by a dense, sclerotic line of bone. This simulates a dentigerous cyst. This third molar is labeled as impacted because it is positioned against soft tissue, or in a cyst, and the roots are fully formed. Even if the cyst were marsupialized, thus removing the pressure of the tissue or the cyst fluid against the crown, the possibility that this tooth would fully erupt spontaneously is rather remote. Of course, it could be orthodontically moved up into its place in the arch. This should be done if it could serve a useful purpose.

The field of operation may be kept small. Since little or no work is done posteriorly to the tooth, the incisions are less extensive. This means less postoperative swelling and trismus. However, it is always well to have too much exposure of your operative field rather than too little.

Bone removal is eliminated or considerably reduced.

The operating time is shortened. A single blow of a chisel that splits a tooth will provide space that would require many blows of a chisel or many revolutions of a bur to provide an equal amount of space in bone.

Trismus primarily due to injury to the ligaments of the temporomandibular articulation resulting from forceful elevation of the tooth is eliminated. In this method only small elevators are used.

There is no damage to adjacent teeth and bone. No effort is made to force the impacted tooth past the convexity of the tooth in front, nor is bone subjected to great pressure when it is used as a fulcrum. Subjecting bone to

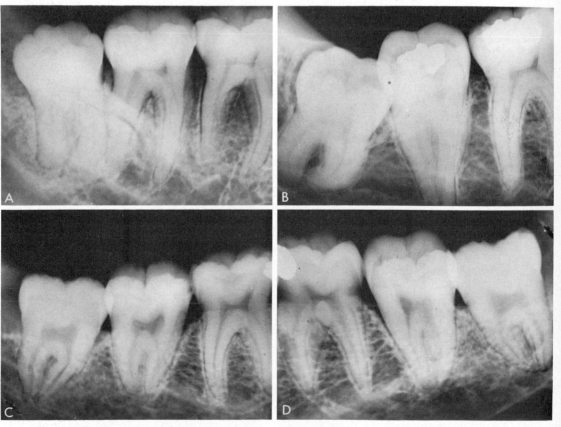

Figure 5–31 Examples of Class I, Positions A and B, vertically impacted mandibular third molars.

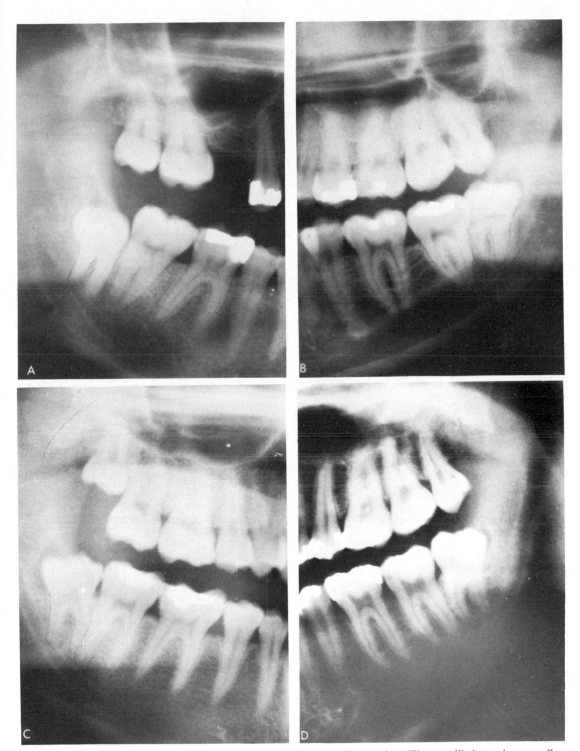

Figure 5–32 Panoramic radiographs showing mandibular and maxillary molars. The mandibular molars are all vertical Class III impactions. *A* is in Position B, while *B*, *C* and *D* are in Position A.

The lack of detail in this type of radiograph compared to that seen in the periapical radiographs is self-evident. However, it is very difficult to get good periapical radiographs in such cases, and at least the complete outline of these teeth is discernible.

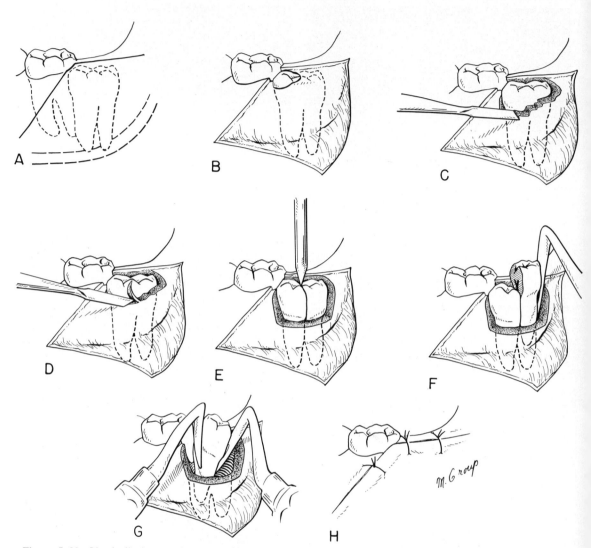

Figure 5–33 Vertically impacted and partially erupted mandibular third molar. Note that the buccal cortical plate and distal bone are above the buccal height of contour of the third molar, which is caught beneath the distal contour of the second molar.

A, Incisions for the mucoperiosteal flap. Note that the distal incision starts at the midpoint of the distal surface of the tooth and is directed distally and buccally to the external oblique ridge. The mesial incision starts at the crest of the mesial interseptal tissue and is directed toward the mucobuccal fold at a 45-degree angle to the gingival line. *B,* Mucoperiosteal flap reflected, giving an adequate exposure of buccal and distal bone. There is no danger of traumatizing this flap during the operation. *C,* A sharp, straight chisel with the bevel turned up is placed well up along the mesiobuccal angle of the third molar and is driven into the buccal cortical plate for several millimeters. *D,* The chisel is now reversed so that the bevel is turned down and the buccal cortical bone, as well as the distal bone, is planed down well below the buccal and distal height of contour of the third molar. *E,* The bibevel splitting chisel is placed in the buccal groove of the third molar. The tooth is split through the bifurcation of the roots by a sharp blow on the chisel with a mallet. *F,* The Apexo elevator is placed in the split, and the tooth segment moved distally; then the elevator is placed distally and the distal half of the third molar is rotated out of the socket. *G,* Adequate space is now provided on the distal side, and into this the mesial half of the crown of the third molar and the mesial root may be moved. An Apexo elevator is forced apically along the mesiobuccal surface of the mesial root, moving this portion of the third molar from beneath the distal contour of the second molar into the space created by the removal of the distal root. It can then be lifted out with two elevators. *H,* Soft tissue flap sutured back into place with 000 black silk.

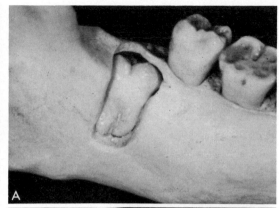

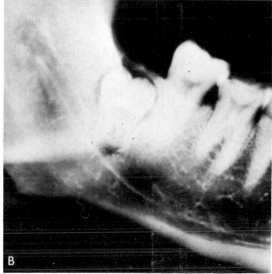

Figure 5–34 *A,* Anatomic specimen in which the thick, dense buccal cortical bone has been removed to reveal the outline of the vertically impacted mandibular Class I molar in Position C. This much bone should *never be excised* to deliver an impacted mandibular molar. (See Figure 5–36 for the correct technique.)

It is very apparent that the inferior alveolar canal is not on the buccal side of the apices of this molar. It was, in fact, located lingually. *B,* Radiograph of this specimen showing the inferior alveolar canal in proximity to the apices of the third molar roots on the lingual side.

excess pressure when it is used as a fulcrum often results in sequestration.

The risk of a jaw fracture is reduced. Most fractures of the mandible result from forced elevations, usually of vertical or mesioangular impactions from which sufficient enveloping bone has not been removed and in which the operator is attempting to drive the tooth forcibly through bone.

Numbness of the lip following the removal of impacted mandibular third molars, the result of heavy leverage that forces the roots of

the tooth against the inferior alveolar nerve, is prevented. (See Figure 5–19.)

Disadvantages. All techniques have their disadvantages. The disadvantages of the chisel-splitting technique are:

Teeth with shallow grooves do not split. Section the crown with a bur.

Teeth in elderly patients are difficult to split. In these cases the crowns are sectioned with a bur.

It is impossible in some cases to place the chisel in line with the long axis of the tooth. This is essential if the tooth is to be split.

Many times the direction of the split results in little advantage because it cannot be controlled.

Patients in general are disturbed by chiseling processes. If the operation is performed under local anesthesia, this is a definite factor to be taken into consideration.

In the preceding instances the alternative is to use a bur.

Technique in Removal of Impacted Third Molars. While it is true that the tooth-splitting technique does in many cases materially reduce the amount of bone that must be removed, it is equally true that the vast majority of lower third molar impactions still require the removal of some portion of the enveloping bone by a bur.

As a general rule the Class I, Position A, mesioangular impacted third molar requires *(Text continued on page 298)*

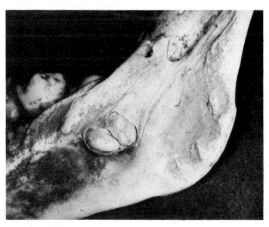

Figure 5–35 Anatomic specimen with a vertically impacted Class I, Position C, third molar whose roots projected through the lingual cortical plate. The inferior alveolar canal is not visible, so it must be on the buccal side of the roots.

This projection of the roots through the lingual cortical plate is unusual and infrequently seen in the customary radiographic examination. Lingual palpation of the soft tissues against the lingual surface of the mandible in this area will reveal situations such as this and should be a part of the oral examination.

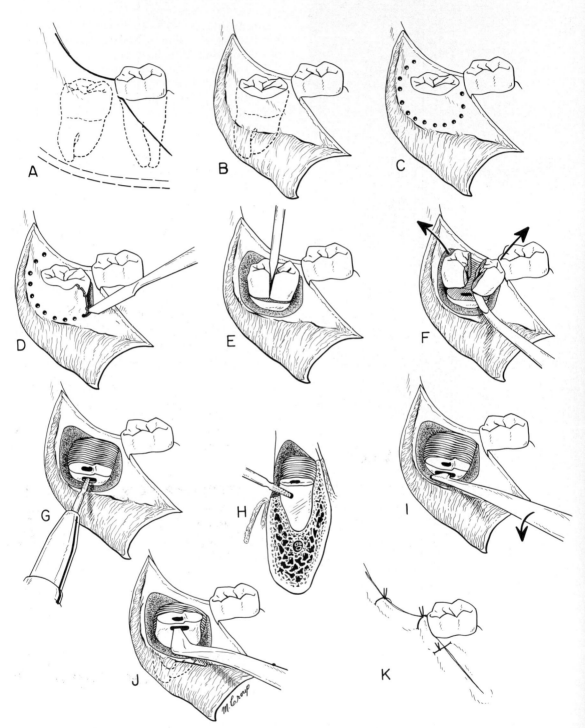

Figure 5–36   Removal of a Class II, Position B, vertically impacted mandibular third molar. *A*, Class II vertically impacted mandibular third molar. *B*, Flap reflected. *C*, Boundary of bone to be removed outlined with spear-point bur holes. *D*, Cortical bone removed to expose crown fully. *E*, An attempt to split the crown and roots has failed and only the crown has split from the roots. *F*, The two halves of the crown are removed. *G* and *H*, A purchase groove is drilled into the root. *I* and *J*, A No. 320 elevator tip is inserted into the groove, and with use of the buccal cortical plate as a fulcrum, the roots are delivered. *K*, Flap sutured.

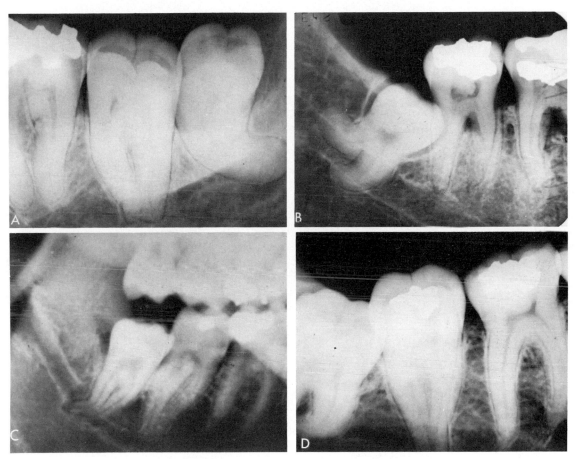

Figure 5–37 Examples of impacted third molars, in which sectioning of the teeth to avoid damage to the neurovascular canal and its neurovascular bundle, containing the artery, vein and nerve, is clearly indicated by the radiographs.

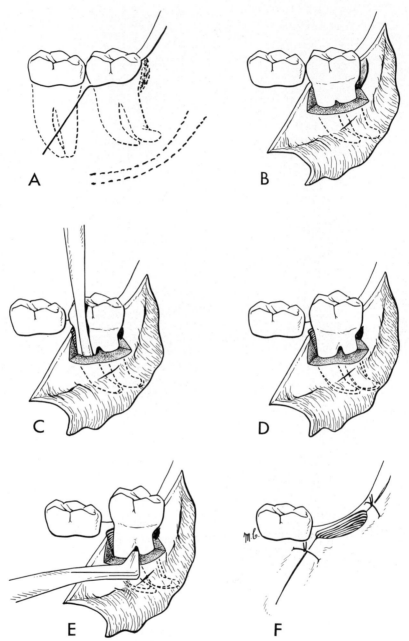

Figure 5–38   Removal of a vertically impacted lower third molar with distal curvature of both roots. In vertical impaction, there is bone over the distal contour of the crown. *A,* Tooth *in situ;* the incision through the mucoperiosteum is diagrammed. *B,* A mucoperiosteal flap is reflected, and bone is removed on the buccal and distal sides. *C,* A straight elevator (81, 1L) is inserted at a mesiobuccal angle, and the tooth is gently luxated distally. This breaks the pericemental attachments of the roots, since the tooth luxates in the same arc as is formed by them. There is practically no vertical component to the force applied, and no attempt is made to remove the tooth with this maneuver. *D,* The pericemental attachments are now severed, and the tooth is slightly elevated in the socket. *E,* With the external oblique ridge as a fulcrum, a suitable elevator (322, 323) is inserted into the bifurcation, and distovertical force is applied. The tooth will move freely out of the socket if there is no distal impediment. Application of this elevator before the maneuver in *C* is performed will result in very little distal component and too much vertical component in the forces applied and will cause fracture of the curved apices. *F,* Incision sutured.

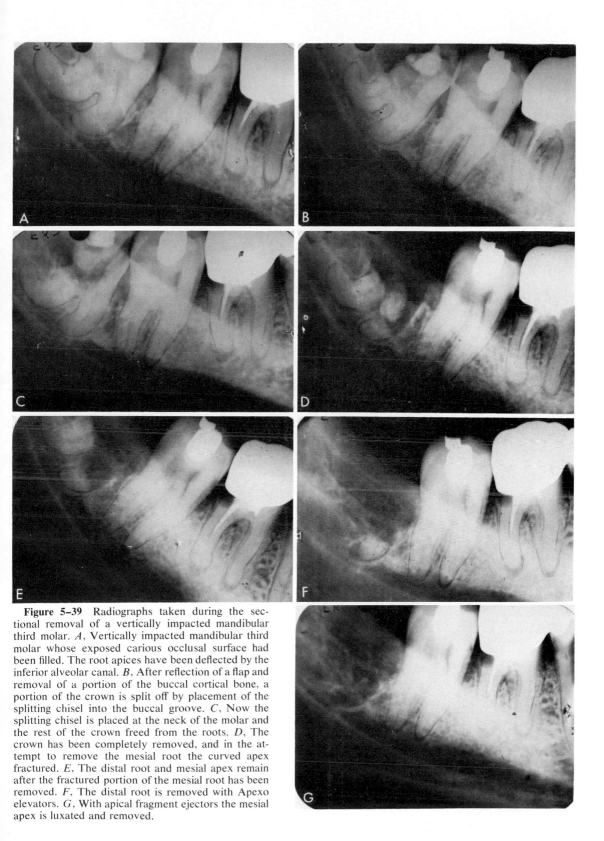

Figure 5–39 Radiographs taken during the sectional removal of a vertically impacted mandibular third molar. *A*, Vertically impacted mandibular third molar whose exposed carious occlusal surface had been filled. The root apices have been deflected by the inferior alveolar canal. *B*, After reflection of a flap and removal of a portion of the buccal cortical bone, a portion of the crown is split off by placement of the splitting chisel into the buccal groove. *C*, Now the splitting chisel is placed at the neck of the molar and the rest of the crown freed from the roots. *D*, The crown has been completely removed, and in the attempt to remove the mesial root the curved apex fractured. *E*, The distal root and mesial apex remain after the fractured portion of the mesial root has been removed. *F*, The distal root is removed with Apexo elevators. *G*, With apical fragment ejectors the mesial apex is luxated and removed.

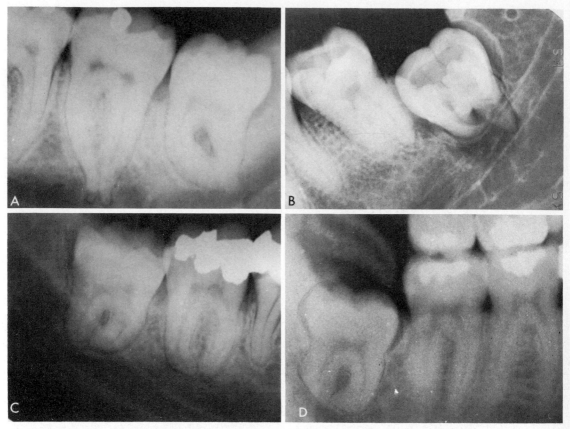

Figure 5–40 Examples of Class I and II vertically impacted mandibular teeth with locked roots. Note relation of roots to the inferior alveolar canal. Technique for the removal of these teeth is shown in Figure 5–41.

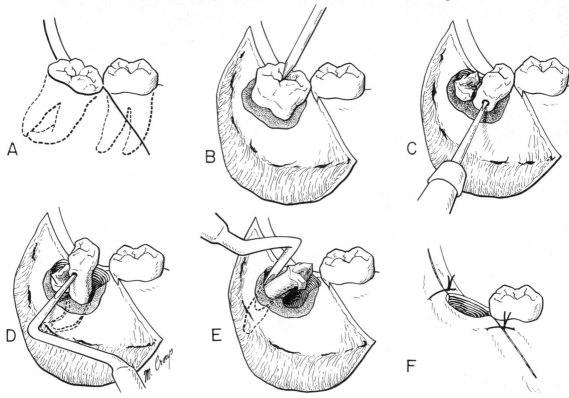

Figure 5–41 *See opposite page for legend.*

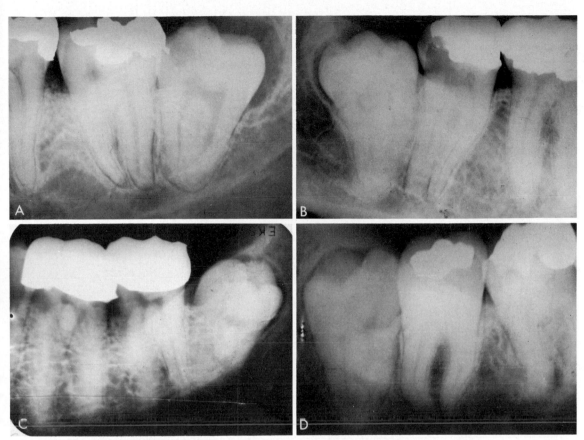

Figure 5–42 Class III vertically and distoangularly impacted mandibular third molars. Radiographically it appears that all these teeth have fused roots. This is a help. To excise these teeth, the operator may follow the technique shown in Figure 5–44, except he does not have to make certain that he splits or cuts the roots apart, since he is removing a tooth with *fused* roots. He does need to split or cut the distal half of the crown off to create distal buccal space into which to elevate the tooth.

Figure 5–41 Removal of a Class I, Position B, mesioangularly impacted mandibular third molar.

A, This case is further complicated by the locking of the intraradicular bone between the roots by the distal right-angled curvature of the apical third of the mesial root, which contacts the distal root. The occlusal surface is visible, and the line of incision in such a case is shown by the heavy black line. *B,* The flap is reflected. The bone has been removed down to the bifurcation by the bur-and-chisel technique already described. The intraradicular bone extending from the buccal to the lingual cortical plates locks this tooth in position. Occasionally, small locked areas of bone are fractured out by the lifting action when elevators are applied to some impactions, but it is always wise to plan to separate these roots and remove each root separately. In this case, a sharp splitting chisel was placed into the buccal groove, parallel to the long axis of the tooth, and a sharp, short blow was struck with a mallet with the hope that the crown would split through the bifurcation of the roots. In this case, the distal half of the crown split off down to the bifurcation. Further separation between the roots is obtained by cutting through the bifurcation from the buccal to the lingual side with a crosscut fissure bur, or the splitting chisel can be placed in the bifurcation and driven between the roots.

C, A purchase point is drilled into the neck of the mesial root, and with the tip of an Apexo elevator this portion of the tooth is raised and moved distally simultaneously, thus unlocking the distal curvature of the apex, as shown in *D.*

E, The same Apexo elevator is now inserted between the distal root and bone along the distal surface with hand pressure, or, if necessary, an entrance point is drilled into the peridental space by a bur and the elevator tip is now inserted into this space. Using the crest of the ridge as a fulcrum, the distal root is moved mesially and out of its socket. *F,* The soft tissue is sutured into place.

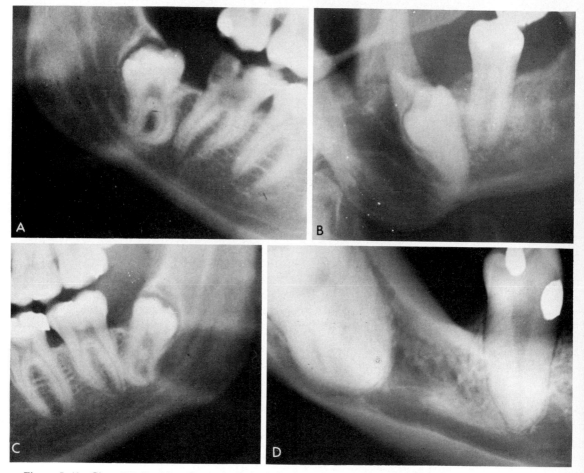

Figure 5–43 Class III, Position C, vertically and distoangularly impacted mandibular third molars. *A* and *C*, Impacted molars with fused roots. Follow the technique shown in Figure 5–44 for their removal. *B* and *D*, Impacted molars with fused roots. See the legend for Figure 5–42 for information on the removal of these teeth.

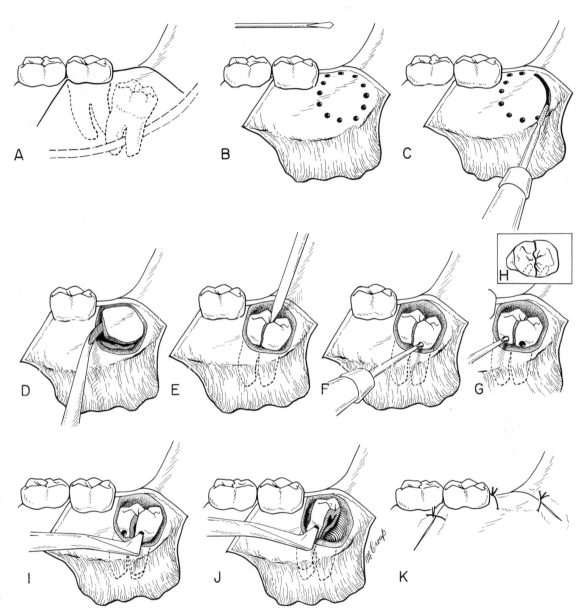

Figure 5–44 Removal of a Class II, Position C, impacted mandibular third molar. *A* to *D*, Exposure of the impacted molar. *E*, The split in this case did separate the crown and roots. If the distal inclination of the third molar will not permit placement of the chisel parallel to the long axis of the tooth, then cut the crown with a bur. *F*, *G* and *H*, Purchase holes are drilled as shown in each half of the tooth at the gingival line. *I* and *J*, A No. 321 elevator is used to remove each segment. *K*, Flap sutured back into place.

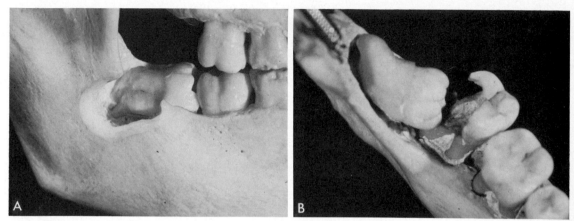

Figure 5–45 *A,* Horizontally impacted mandibular third molar. Note the curvature of the apices and thick buccal cortical bone. This crown has a deep buccal groove, which is ideal for splitting. This tooth should be removed by sectioning of the crown; the roots may then be moved forward into the space created by the removal of the crown. *B,* Horizontally impacted mandibular third molar. Note the extensive destruction of surrounding osseous structure and caries of several molars. The destruction of bone was undoubtedly due to a long-continued (chronic) pericoronitis. It is apparent that if this case had been presented for operation, it would only have been necessary to incise and reflect the overlying soft tissues in order to deliver this third molar.

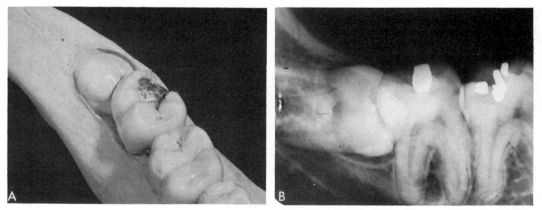

Figure 5–46 *A,* Anatomic specimen showing a Class I, Position B, horizontally impacted mandibular third molar. *B,* Radiograph of another similar case. Note the relationship of the roots to the inferior alveolar canal. See Figure 5–47 for the surgical technique for the excision of these teeth.

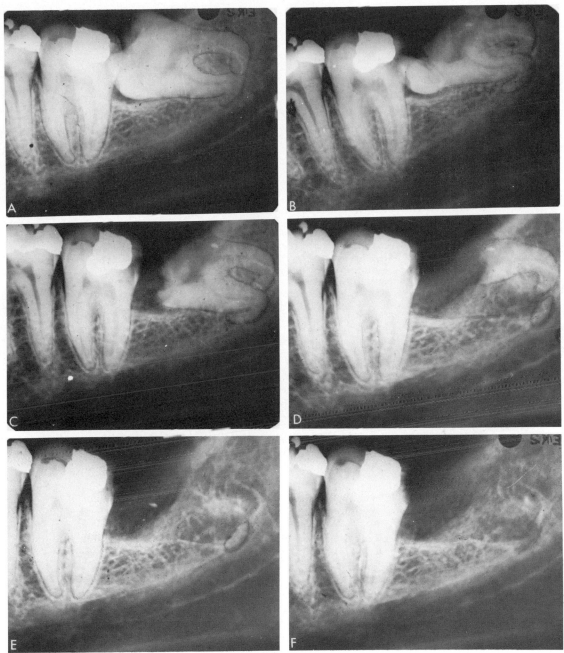

Figure 5–47 *A*, Class I, Position A, horizontally impacted mandibular third molar with sharp mesial curvature of the extreme apical thirds of both roots.

B, After being exposed, two thirds of the crown was split off with an osteotome. *C*, The remaining third of the crown was split off with the osteotome. The bur can also be used for this purpose. *D*, The roots were split with the osteotome. The lower (mesial) root was loose, but during its removal with an elevator the curved apex fractured. *E*, The superior (distal) root was moved down and removed with an Apex elevator. *F*, The small apical fragment was removed with an apical root fragment ejector. (See Chapter 4.)

Figure 5–48   The split-bone technique of Sir William Kelsey Fry. This is a quick, clean technique which has the advantage of reducing the size of the residual blood clot by means of saucerization of the socket. It is only suitable for use in young patients with elastic bone in which the grain is prominent. Although it can be performed under regional anesthesia, endotracheal anesthesia is preferable in most cases. A slight increase in the incidence of transient lingual anesthesia during the postoperative period complicates the use of this technique. (For the purposes of illustration, the soft-tissue retractor has been omitted here.)

After a standard incision has been outlined (A) the soft tissues are reflected to expose the bone enclosing the impacted tooth. A chisel is used to make a vertical "stop cut" at the anterior end of the wound (B). Then with the chisel bevel downward a horizontal cut is made backward from a point just above the lower end of the "stop cut" (C), thus enabling the buccal plate to be removed. A point of application for an elevator is made with the chisel by excising the triangular piece of bone bounded anteriorly by the lower end of the "stop cut" and above by the anterior end of the horizontal cut (D). The distolingual bone is then fractured inward by placement of the cutting edge of a chisel along the dotted line shown in C, with the chisel held at an angle of 45 degrees to the bone surface and pointing in the direction of the second lower premolar on the other side. Provided that the cutting edge of the chisel is kept parallel to the external oblique line, a few light taps with a mallet suffice to separate the lingual plate from the rest of the alveolar bone and to hinge it inward on the soft tissues attached to it (D). Especial care should be taken to ensure that the cutting edge of the chisel is not held parallel to the internal oblique line, for this error in technique may result in extension of the lingual split to the coronoid process. The "peninsula" of bone which then remains distal to the tooth and between the buccal and lingual cuts is excised (E).

A sharp-pointed, fine-bladed straight elevator is then applied to the mesial surface of the tooth and the minimum of force used to displace the tooth upward and backward out of its socket (F). As the tooth moves backward, the fractured lingual plate is displaced from its path of withdrawal, thus facilitating delivery of the tooth. After the tooth has been removed from its socket, the lingual plate is grasped in fine hemostats, and the soft tissues are freed from it by blunt dissection (G).* The fractured lingual plate is then lifted from the wound, thus completing the saucerization of the bony cavity.

After smoothing of the cut bone edges with a bone file, the wound is irrigated with sterile normal saline and closed with sutures. In most cases the solitary suture illustrated in H suffices, and the curved anterior part of the incision comes together, and so the insertion of a suture in this site is seldom required.

(From Howe, G. L.: Minor Oral Surgery. Bristol, England, John Wright & Sons, Ltd., 1971.)

---

*AUTHOR'S NOTE: The removal of this lingual bone frequently exposes the gingival distolingual portion of the root of the second molar. New bone does not replace this lost bone, and so a surgical periodontal pocket is produced. The blunt dissection of this lingual cortical plate, in my opinion, is one of the reasons for "the slight increase" in the postoperative paresthesia or permanent anesthesia seen as a complication in these cases.

We do not remove this bone, and we place two sutures to close the wound, one as described and the second just distal to the neck of the second molar to hold the lingual plate in its normal position during healing.

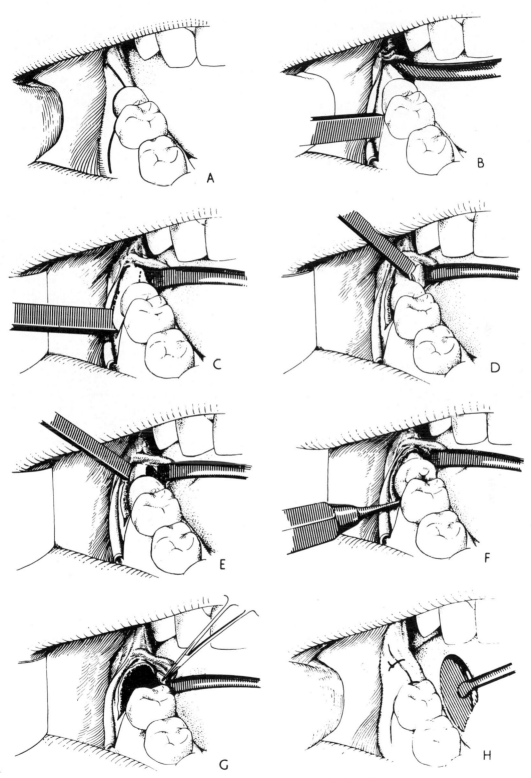

Figure 5–48 *See opposite page for legend.*

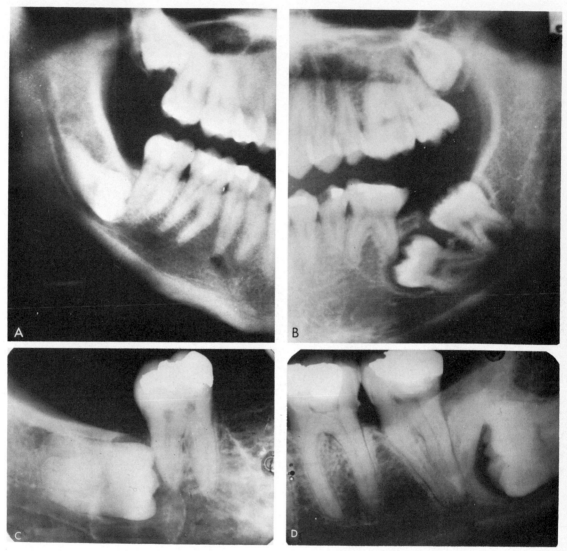

Figure 5–49 *A,* Panoramic radiograph discloses a Position C, mesioangular impaction of the left maxillary third molar and a Class III, Position C, horizontal impaction of the left mandibular third molar parallel to and in approximation with the inferior alveolar canal. (See Figure 5–52 for surgical technique of excision.) *Note:* molars in both *A* and *B* approximate the maxillary sinus. See Figure 5–74 for this nomenclature.

B, A Position C, distovertically impacted right maxillary third molar and two right mandibular molar impactions. The second molar is a Class I, Position C, horizontally impacted tooth with a 3-mm. thick follicle; its roots are proximal to the inferior alveolar canal. The third molar, superior and distal to the second, is a Class II, Position B, mesioangular impaction. This tooth should be the *first* cut out (as illustrated in Figure 5–27). *Then* the *second* molar can be removed (with the technique shown in Figure 5–52).

C, This horizontally impacted Class I, Position C, third molar appears to have a dentigerous cyst around the crown, and it lies parallel to the inferior alveolar canal. Care must be used in the removal of the crown of this tooth in order to avoid severing the neurovascular bundle.

D, Special difficulty will be encountered in exposing the crown of this impacted tooth because of the mesial and superior osteosclerotic bone. Considerable judgment must be exercised in deciding whether or not this tooth should be removed. First, a good lateral jaw or panoramic radiograph should be viewed. Second, are there any symptoms? Third, what is the age of the patient? Fourth, what is the possibility of jaw fracture during or after surgery? A good test is always to ask yourself, "Would I want this tooth removed from my jaw, my wife's or that of a member of my family?"

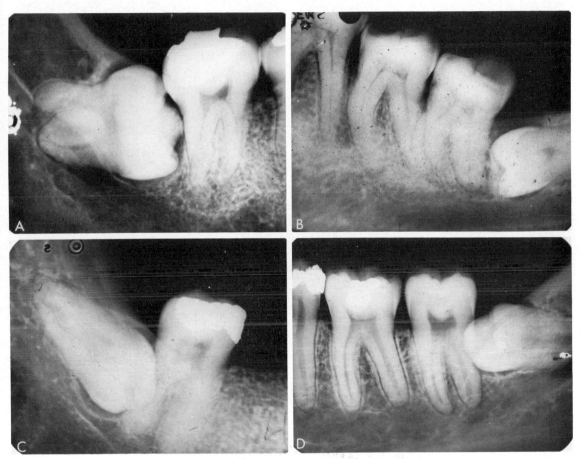

Figure 5–50 Additional examples of horizontally impacted mandibular third molars (*A, C* and *D*), and a fourth molar (*B*). Legends for previous figures have covered the salient points for the treatment of such cases as those illustrated here.

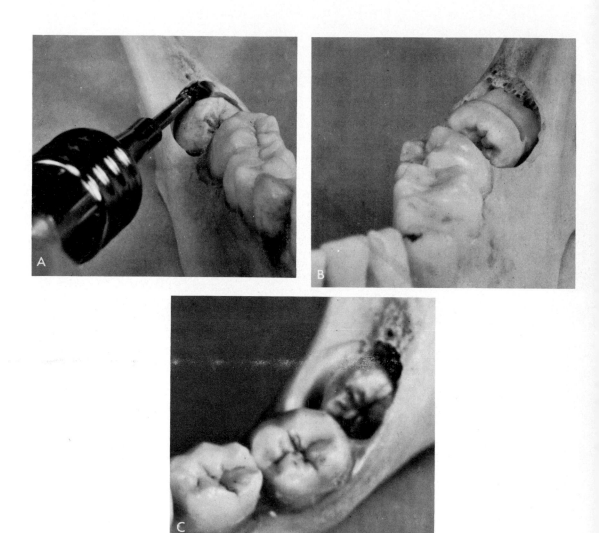

Figure 5–51 Exposure of the crowns of three impacted third molars. These photographs illustrate the point that whenever possible, consistent with the absolute need for adequate exposure, the surgeon should *preserve as much buccal and lingual bone as possible!*

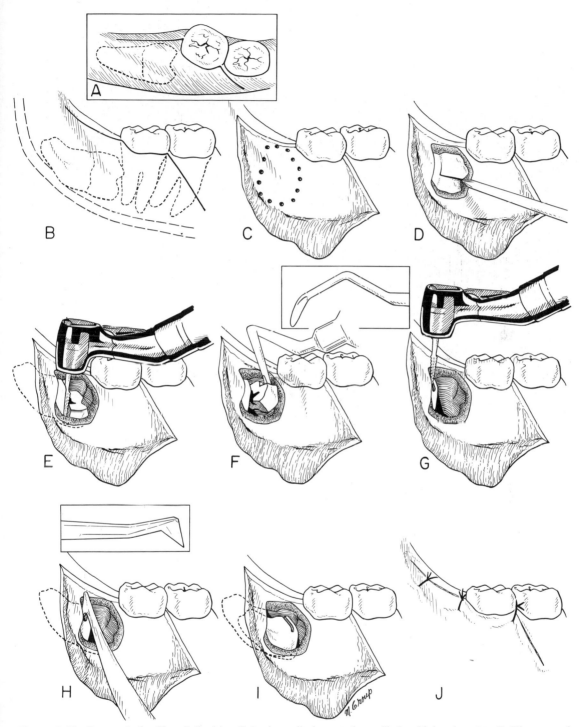

Figure 5–52 Removal of a Class I, Position C, horizontally impacted mandibular third molar. *A* to *D*, The crown is exposed after reflection of a large flap. The crown is split and the superior portion removed. *E* and *F*, The inferior portion of the crown is cut off with a crosscut fissure bur and removed. *G*, Then a purchase groove is cut into the root portion. *H* and *I*, With a No. 320 elevator and use of the cortical bone as a fulcrum, the root portion is moved forward and removed.

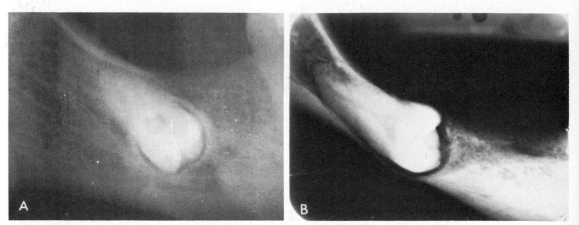

Figure 5–53 *A,* The approach to this impacted tooth can only be determined by good occlusal views. It may be that the crown has penetrated through the lingual cortical bone. If so, it should be removed from a lingual approach.

B, Why this 70-year-old patient had never had a fracture of the mandible is a mystery. Surgical excision of this horizontally impacted third molar was mandated because of traumatic ulceration of the mucosa between the patient's denture and the tooth, and also because of the ease with which a fracture of the mandible could be produced by a minor blow or even excess masticatory pressure (which so far had been limited by persistent pain during mastication). This third molar was removed by sectioning of the crown with burs, then sectioning of the root, in the same manner shown in Figure 5–52. (Study this drawing.) The approach to the tooth was along the superior surface of the mandible; none of the cortical plate was removed. This is a delicate and time-consuming operation because of the hazards of fracture and those of cutting or compressing the neurovascular bundle.

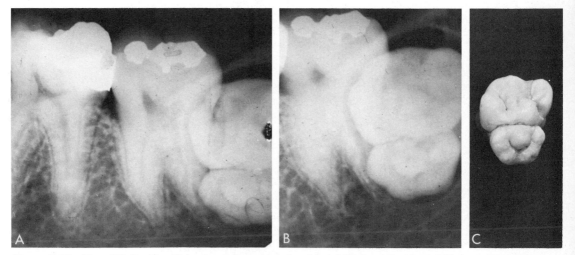

Figure 5–54 Class III, Position C, horizontally impacted and fused third and fourth mandibular molars. These were removed without sacrificing the second molar by adequate exposure through the (fortunately) unusually thin buccal and lingual bone. Sectioning, although planned, was not necessary.

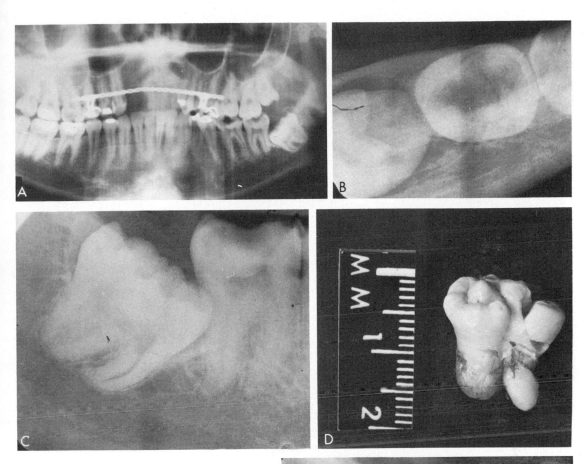

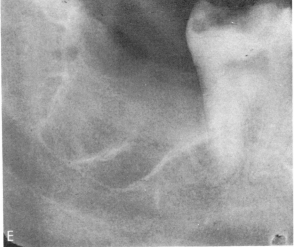

Figure 5–55 *A,* Panoramic radiograph reveals a Class II, Position C, mesioangularly impacted right geminous mandibular third and fourth molar.

B and *C,* Occlusal and periapical radiographs provide information about the buccal-lingual position and the size and shape of the roots and their relationship to the inferior alveolar canal.

D, The crown was fully exposed, and the mesial portion of the crown locked under the distal surface curvature of the second molar was split off into two sections by an osteotome (one slice was lost, as can be noted in the reassembled specimen).

E, A minimum of buccal bone was removed, and the rest of the molar was elevated from its alveolus.

little bone removal. However, in some cases it is necessary to reduce the buccal plate at least at the mesiobuccal corner, in order to expose the mesiobuccal groove. Then the mesial portion of the crown, which is locked beneath the distal convexity of the second molar, can be split free from the roots by means of a sharp splitting chisel that is inserted into this groove and tapped smartly with a mallet.

The greater the depth of the impaction in bone, the more buccal plate that must be removed by planing with chisels at least to the height of contour. In cases in which the buccal bone is very thick (see Figure 5–17C and D), then a groove along the buccal surface to or beyond the height of buccal contour of the impacted tooth can be made with appropriate burs.

EXCISION OF IMPACTED MANDIBULAR MOLARS FROM EDENTULOUS AREAS

Careful radiographic studies must be made of these areas to determine the technique to be used in order to prevent a fracture of the mandible. The radiographs must have a minimum of distortion and include intraoral periapical and occlusal films and an extraoral oblique film. These will reveal the position, size and shape of the embedded tooth and the amount of investing bone.

Technique is dependent primarily on the amount of bone between the inferior border of the mandible and the apex of the tooth to be removed, secondly on the thickness of the buccal and lingual cortical plates. What bone, if any, covers the crown is valueless so far as strength of the mandible is concerned, because it must be removed to gain access to the tooth if the intraoral approach is selected. The extraoral approach will be described later. Technique depends thirdly on the shape of the crown and the number and form of roots, if more than one.

Figure 5–60B shows all that could be visualized of an impacted third molar by an intraoral dental film. An oblique film of the jaw (Fig. 5–60A) reveals considerable bone between the apex of the fused roots and the inferior border of the mandible.

(Text continued on page 305)

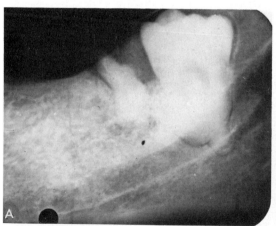

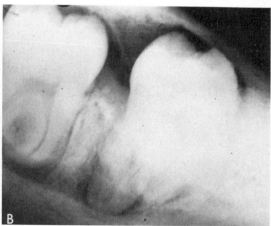

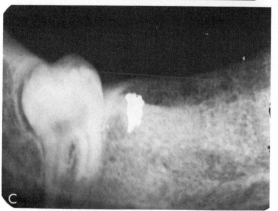

Figure 5–56 Examples of Class I, II and III vertically impacted mandibular third molars in edentulous jaws. Techniques for their excision are shown in Figures 5–57 and 5–60.

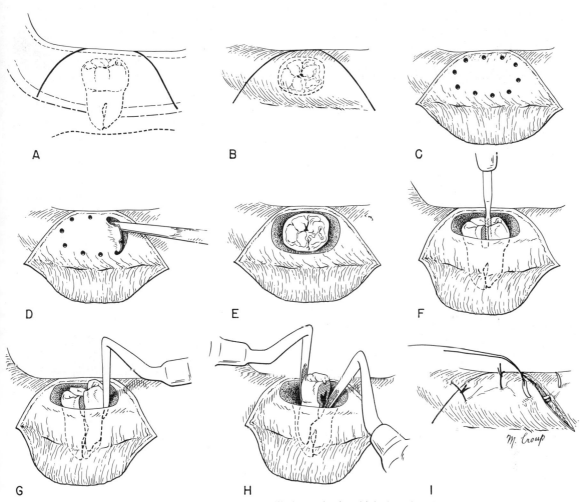

Figure 5–57 Removal of a vertically impacted mandibular molar in which there is only a small amount of bone between the apex and the inferior border of the mandible. In these cases the danger of fracture is great unless a *minimum of bone is removed* and a *maximum retained.*

A, Diagram showing the position of the tooth in the mandible with a heavy line indicating the semicircular flap extending over the crest of the ridge. Note that both mesial and distal portions of the incision extend onto the buccal mucosa. *B,* Occlusal view of the impacted tooth and incision. *C,* Elliptical series of holes made with a spear-point drill through the cortical plate after the periosteum is reflected. *D,* Holes are connected with a hand mallet and chisel and a bur. *E,* View showing the occlusal surface of tooth after a bony window has been removed. Bone has been removed almost down to the height of contour on the buccal and lingual sides.

Note, however, that a deep and wide space has been created in the bone on the mesial and distal surfaces. Bone removed in these areas will *not weaken the mandible.* This permits the sectioned pieces of the crown to be moved into these spaces, partially rotated to free the lingual and buccal surfaces from beneath the cortical plates, and then removed. This can be done with very little force. *F,* Use of the fissure bur to cut through the crown of the tooth (buccolingually) to the bifurcation. *G,* No. 5 Apexo elevator now inserted along the mesial surface. The cortical bone may be used as a fulcrum for moving the mesial segment distally and occlusally. *H,* With both No. 4 and No. 5 Apexo elevators, the distal fragment is moved into the mesial space and out occlusally. *I,* Only a small amount of bone has been removed. The tissue is approximated and sutured into position with interrupted sutures. Note that the needle is passed from movable tissue to fixed tissue.

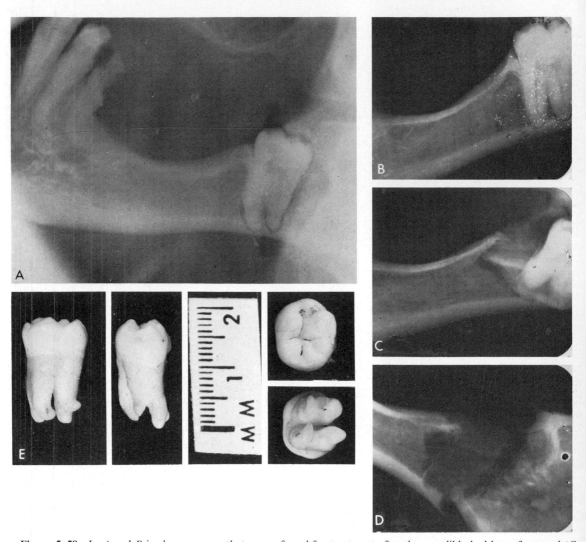

Figure 5–58 In *A* and *B* is shown a case that was referred for treatment after the mandible had been fractured *(C and D)* in an attempt to remove this tooth. The fracture shown in *C* and *D* resulted from an attempt to split the crown and roots with a chisel. Splitting of teeth with an osteotome when the roots approximate the inferior border of the mandible, as shown even in this poor radiograph, is contraindicated for the reason shown here. Treatment of the fracture was further complicated because the large section of mesial and distal bone, plus the lingual cortical plate, all of which were adherent to the molar (as shown in *C*), had been cut away from the tooth *(E)* and discarded.

Following the accident, the ideal treatment would have consisted, first, of the manual replacement of this fragment, which still had the lingual mucoperiosteal tissue attached, and then of immobilization of the three segments of the mandible by means of extraoral skeletal fixation. This not being possible, healing required 16 weeks of fixation. A study of the radiograph shows that a safer technique in such a case is that illustrated in Figure 5–57.

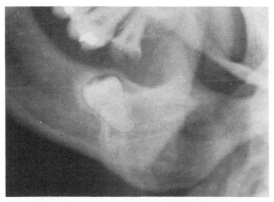

Figure 5–59 Extraoral oblique radiograph of the right body of the mandible, which is essential to show the entire outline of the mesioangularly impacted third molar, which is completely covered with bone (unerupted), and its relationship to the inferior alveolar canal.

300

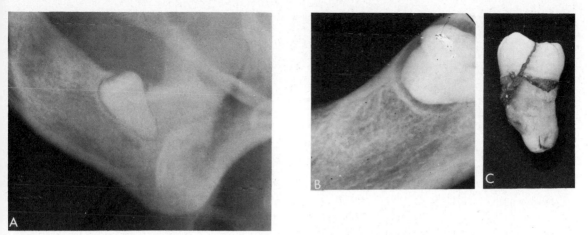

Figure 5–60 *A*, Another case of an impacted mandibular third molar in an edentulous mandible. However, a portion of the crown in this case is exposed on the ridge. *B*, This inadequate periapical radiograph should not be used as the sole diagnostic aid or for surgical guidance. The extraoral oblique right or left view (whichever is indicated), as shown in *A*, or a panoramic radiograph, should be used to supply the additional information not available in this periapical view. *C*, The sectioned tooth reassembled after excision. (See Figure 5–61 for technique.)

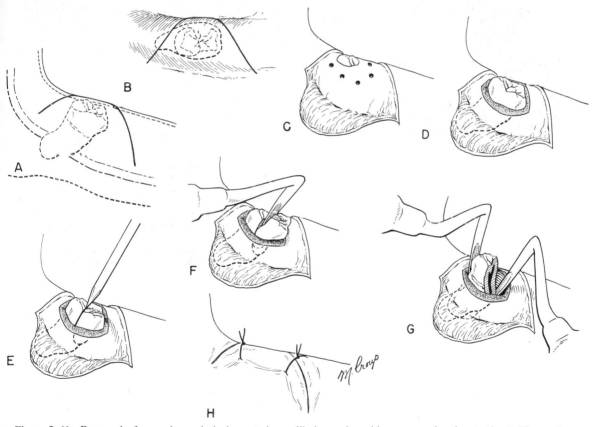

Figure 5–61 Removal of a mesioangularly impacted mandibular molar with no approximating teeth. *A*, The molar and a heavy line indicating the incison for the required flap. *B*, Occlusal view of the impacted tooth and line of incision. This semicircular incision begins and ends on buccal tissues but is carried over the midline of the crest of the ridge to the lingual cortical plate. It is recognized that this violates one of the rules of flap-making, namely, that the continued blood supply to that portion of the flap which is lingual to the midline is cut off. However, in this particular flap circulation is quickly reestablished, and there is little danger of sloughing of the lingual portion of the flap. *C*, Flap is turned back and a semicircular series of holes is drilled with a spear-point bur through the cortical plate. *D*, With a bur and a mallet and chisel the bone is removed down to the height of contour. *E*, After the crown is exposed, it is safe in this particular case to reduce the crown by splitting, because of the dense, heavy buccal plate of bone and the amount of bone between the apex and the inferior border of the mandible. Neither of these factors was present in the case shown in Figure 5–57. *F*, Insertion of No. 4 Apexo elevator into the split and elevation of the mesial crown fragment. *G*, The distal and mesial cortical plates may be used as fulcrums, and then both No. 4 and No. 5 Apexo elevators are inserted, moving the tooth into the mesial space created and out occlusally. *H*, Approximation and suturing of tissues with two interrupted sutures.

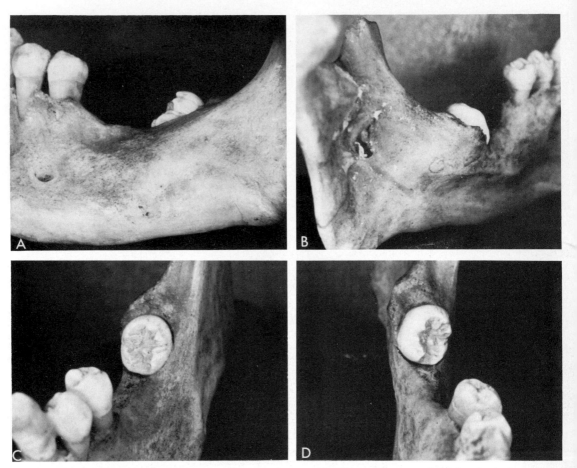

Figure 5–62 Anatomic specimen of a mandible, showing a malposed, partially erupted third molar in four different views. A study of this patient will help the surgeon understand the osseous environment of impacted third molars, such as those shown in Figures 5–59 and 5–60. We become so conditioned to the "picture" revealed by a two-dimensional "shadowgraph" (*i.e.,* radiograph) of a three-dimensional anatomic area that we lose perspective. The surgeon should always pick up an anatomic specimen of the area in which he is going to operate at the same time he is studying his radiographs and planning his operative procedures. To do so will materially aid in preventing preoperative miscalculations revealed only during surgery.

A, Buccal surface. *B,* Lingual surface. *C,* Occlusal view from the buccal side. *D,* Occlusal view from the lingual side. These two views give us very impressive reminders of the great difference in the osseous tissue that is present bucally and lingually.

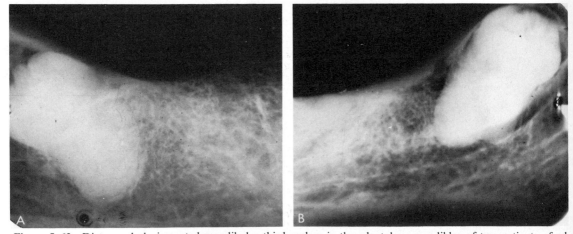

Figure 5–63 Distoangularly impacted mandibular third molars in the edentulous mandibles of two patients of advanced age. *A,* Surgical excision by sectioning of the Class I impacted molar was necessary in this patient because denture pressure of the mucoperiosteal tissue against the enamel surface of the tooth resulted in pressure necrosis of the soft tissue, with localized infection. *B,* This patient's Class III impacted third molar was not in the denture-bearing area and was symptomless. There was no indication for its excision.

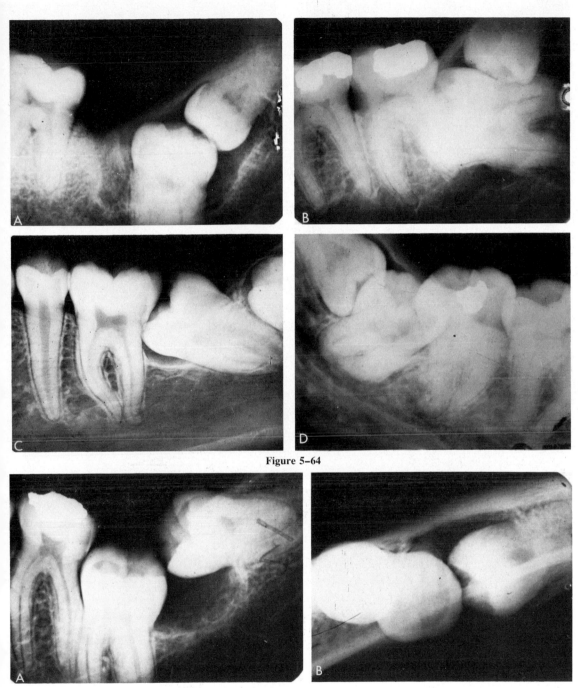

Figure 5–64

Figure 5–65

Figures 5–64 and 5–65 Having studied the various techniques for the excision of single and multiple impacted molars, the reader should be prepared by now to study these and the following examples of mandibular second and third molars and to plan intelligently the sequence of steps necessary to proceed logically with the excision of these teeth at one or two stages.

The experienced, mature surgeon knows when it is in the best interests of the patient to defer the completion of an operation. In my opinion too many multihoured surgical procedures are performed today that could be completed in two operations with a total of fewer hours than the one operation and with reduced debilitation of the patient's vital capacity. One must remember that the nontoxic anesthetic has not been discovered.

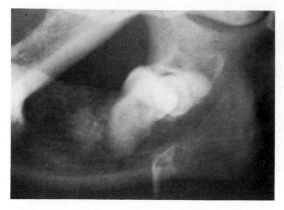

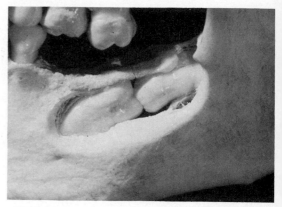

Figure 5–66 Class III distoangularly impacted mandibular third and rudimentary supernumerary fourth molars.

Figure 5–67 A prepared anatomic specimen in which the thick, dense buccal and lateral cortical bone has been cut away to expose the mandibular second and third molars horizontally impacted, occlusal surface to occlusal surface and completely encased in osseous tissue. Obviously this is not the correct surgical approach to expose these teeth for excision. Study Figure 5–72 and its legend for the step-by-step technique for this and similar cases of multiple impactions in the mandible.

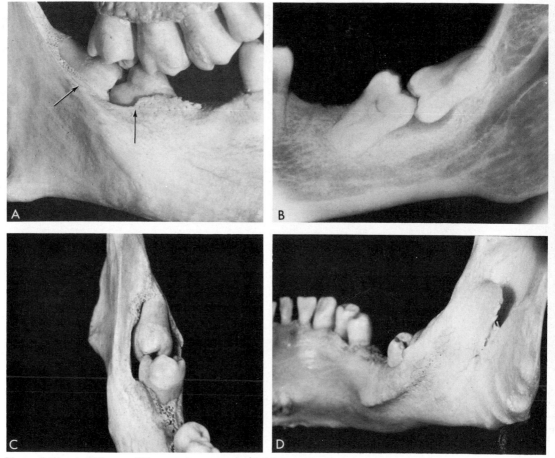

Figure 5–68 *A,* This mandible contains second and third molars impacted occlusal surface to occlusal surface. *B,* Extraoral radiograph. Note the osteosclerotic area beneath these teeth, which was probably the result of defensive osteitis stimulated by apparent chronic infection beneath the crowns. *C,* Occlusal view. Note the partial resorption of the third buccal cortical bone and the thin lingual bone. *D,* Lingual view. Note the thick, prominent internal ridge.

The technique used in this particular case is illustrated in Figure 5–61 and described in this chapter. Figure 5–60C shows the removed tooth reassembled.

Occasionally the second molar is impacted with the third molar, both in horizontal position with their occlusal surfaces in contact with each other. Such a case is illustrated in Figures 5–69 to 5–71.

It is apparent that if a fractured mandible is to be prevented in this case, a minimal amount of bone must be removed. To deliver these through this small opening, the teeth must be sectioned with burs.

The technique for the removal of these

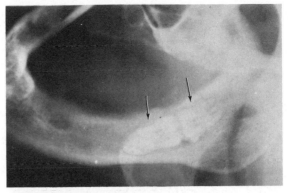

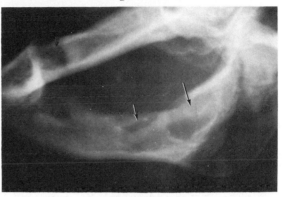

Figure 5–70

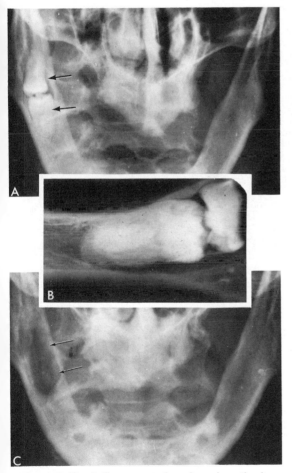

Figure 5–71

Figure 5–70 Oblique extraoral film shows a double-rooted third molar and a single-rooted second molar. It also strikingly reveals the necessity of extreme caution in applying pressure to remove these teeth if a fracture of the mandible is to be prevented.

Figure 5–71 Oblique view gives evidence of the minimal amount of bone removed.

Figure 5–69 *A,* Posteroanterior view gives the buccolingual relationship of these teeth and the thickness of the lingual cortical plate as compared with the thin buccal plate. (See Figure 5–72 for the surgical technique in the removal of these impacted teeth.)

B, Intraoral dental film taken in routine oral radiographic diagnosis revealed this situation. Note the inferior alveolar canal and its relationship to the second and third molars.

C, Postoperative view, showing the minimal amount of bone that was removed.

teeth is illustrated in Figure 5–72. Whether or not both teeth are removed at one sitting depends on the difficulties of each individual case. It is good practice to inform the patient before starting that the operation may be done in two stages. This case was. The postoperative radiographs are shown in Figures 5–69C and 5–71.

OPERCULECTOMY

The newly erupted mandibular third molar may have a dense, fibrous operculum covering two thirds, or less, of its occlusal surface (see Figure 5–73). Frequently, this tissue is the source of much discomfort to the patient because it may be acutely inflamed either as the result of masticatory trauma from the opposing maxillary third molar or because of infection resulting from the growth of bacteria

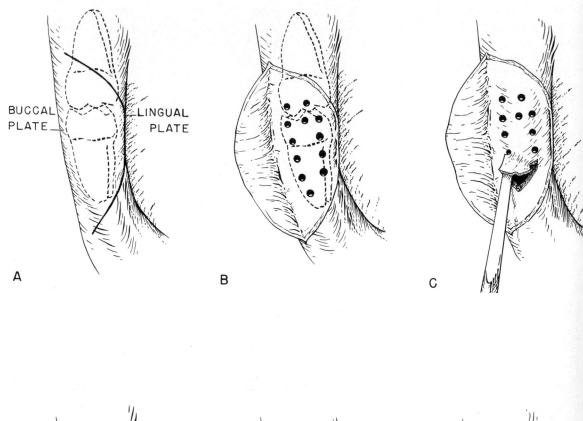

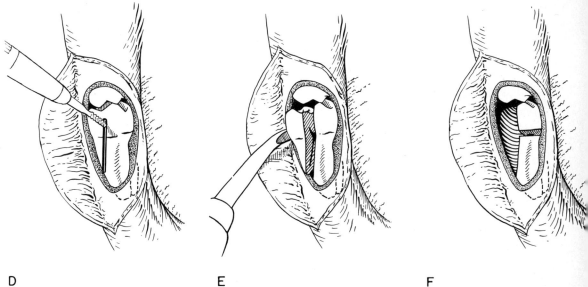

Figure 5–72 Surgical treatment of horizontally impacted second and third mandibular molars.

First stage: A, A semicircular flap is made to expose the bone over the second molar. *B*, Holes are drilled through the cortical bone to the tooth. *C*, Overlying bone is removed with a chisel. *D*, A groove is cut into the tooth with a crosscut fissure bur. *E*, The tooth is split and a segment removed with a No. 73 elevator. *F*, A portion of the crown is cut off with a crosscut fissure bur. *G*, The remainder of the tooth is removed with elevators Nos. 73 and 74. *H*, Soft tissues are sutured with 00 plain catgut.

Second stage: I, After healing of the second molar socket, another semicircular flap is made. *J*, Holes are drilled through the cortical bone over the crown. *K*, The bone is removed with a chisel. *L*, A groove is cut in the gingival line with a crosscut fissure bur. *M*, The crown is split and removed. A groove is cut into the neck of the root. *N*, Roots are moved forward with cross bar elevator No. 322. *O*, The flap is sutured back into place.

(Figure 5–72 continued on opposite page

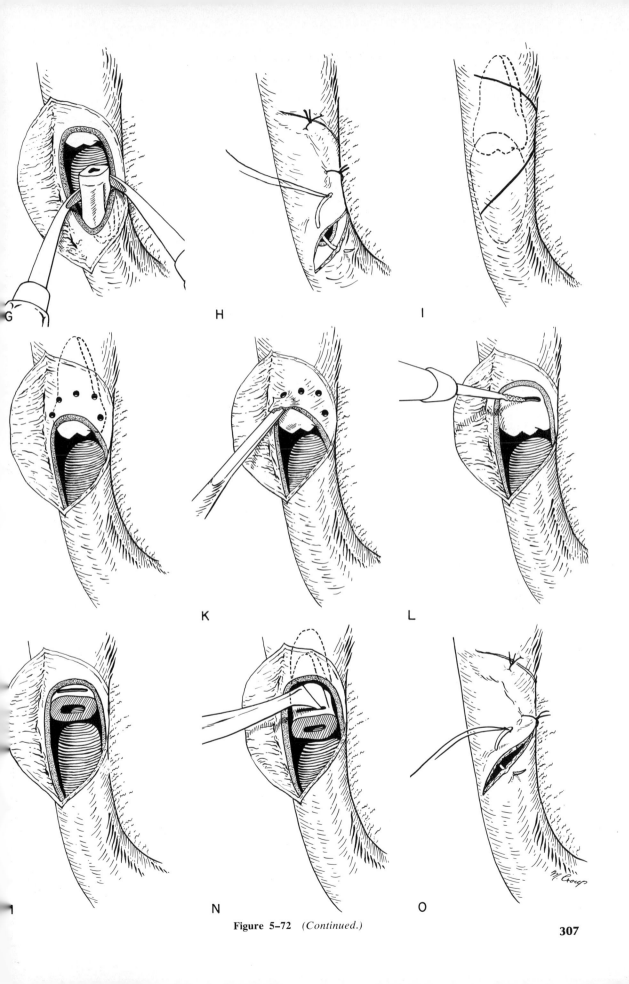

G   H   I

K   L

N   O

Figure 5-72 *(Continued.)*

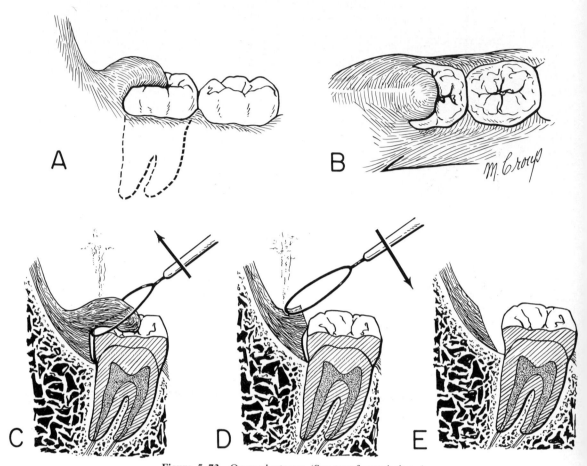

Figure 5-73 Operculectomy. (See text for technique.)

in the ideal incubator that lies beneath this covering and in the crypt distal to the crown. This condition is not, as yet, an acute pericoronitis, which is described on this page.

Operculectomy is indicated, and it is carried out as shown in Figure 5-73A to E. In A and B is shown an operculum covering 50 per cent of the occlusal surface of a fully erupted mandibular third molar. The most efficient method for removing this dense fibrous mucoperiosteal tissue is to use a radiosurgical loop. The loop is placed beneath the lid of tissue as far posteriorly as the wire loop can be inserted—if possible, down around the distal surface of the tooth, as is shown in C. When it has reached this position, the current is turned on and the loop is moved superiorly. This cuts off the bulk of the tissue. Now, it is necessary to plane the tissue distally so as to remove the distal crypt. This is accomplished, as shown in D, by placing the loop on the crest of the tissue approximately ½ cm. distal to the crown and cutting downward so that the tissue is planed downward toward

the gingival line, with the end result shown in E.

IMPACTED OR PARTIALLY ERUPTED THIRD MOLARS WITH PERICORONAL INFECTION

PERICORONITIS

Pericoronitis is caused by two factors. The first is bacterial growth in the ideal incubator that lies below the soft tissue flap covering the crown of the partially or completely unerupted third molar. Beneath the flap there is protection, moisture, warmth, food and darkness. In such an environment bacterial growth flourishes. Frequently the predominant organisms are the fusiform bacillus and spirillum. In some cases of acute pericoronitis the typical necrotic margin of acute Vincent's infection may be observed along the edge of the soft tissue flap. Microscopically the clinical diagnosis is confirmed by the presence of great numbers of fusiform bacilli and spirilla.

The second factor in pericoronitis is traumatic irritation of the mucosa overlying the mandibular third molar by the cusps of the opposing maxillary third molar. With subsequent inflammation, lowered vitality of the tissues and invasion by microorganisms, the irritation may initiate or enhance a case of pericoronitis. Often the upper third molar has not only erupted into position, but, being unopposed by the unerupted or partially erupted lower third molar, it actually has erupted into supraocclusion in an attempt to come into articulation. The soft tissues overlying the lower third molar are therefore traumatized during the masticatory excursions of the mandible.

Symptoms. In acute pericoronitis the soft tissues overlying the partially erupted tooth become red, edematous and extremely painful. The inflammatory process spreads to the adjacent soft tissues, and trismus follows because the overlying soft tissues contain muscle fibers from the buccinator muscle and the superior constrictor muscle of the pharynx. The patient complains of difficulty in eating and swallowing. Frequently the patient has chills, fever, general malaise, constipation, and a foul odor to the breath. The submaxillary and cervical lymph nodes may be indurated and tender.

Treatment. If the exciting factor is the overeruption (elongation) of the maxillary third molar, this tooth should be extracted at the first visit.

The patient should be informed of the necessity for the extraction of the maxillary third molar, plus the additional fact that because of the elongation of the maxillary third molar, the normal contact between the maxillary second and third molars has been lost. Food debris and bacteria accumulate in the interproximal space because of this loss of contact, and eventually the interseptal alveolar bone is broken down between the roots of the second and third molars. If this situation is permitted to continue, the second, as well as the third molar, will be lost. There are, therefore, two valid reasons for the extraction of the maxillary third molar.

The pericoronitis should now be treated. Three methods of treatment of pericoronitis are advocated by various authorities: (1) the conservative method, (2) removal of the tooth, and (3) surgical removal of the overlying flap.

CONSERVATIVE METHOD OF TREATMENT. Irrigate beneath the flap with a quart of warm normal saline solution. This is best accomplished by using a large irrigating can, to which is connected several feet of rubber tubing with a small irrigating tip on the end. The container is suspended several feet above the patient's mouth. A suction apparatus can be used to remove the normal saline solutions from the oral cavity, thus making the irrigation a continuous one, without the necessity of interrupting the process to permit the patient to expectorate.

Hayward irrigates the region below the flap with 1 cc. of iodine lotion. The lotion is prepared as follows: phenol, 5 per cent, 6 cc.; tincture of aconite, 12 cc.; tincture of iodine, 18 cc.; and glycerin, 24 cc.

To irrigate with the medicaments, use a 10 cc. glass syringe and a 20 gauge 3½-inch needle. The needle is annealed by heating 1 inch of the tip in a flame and then bending this end in a gentle curve. The sharp end is ground off with a stone and smoothed and polished with abrasive disks.

This treatment is carried out daily until the acute symptoms subside. Then the third molar is extracted, or, if this tooth can assume a normal position in the arch and serve a useful purpose, the overlying soft tissue flap is removed, preferably with the so-called electrosurgical scalpel.

Instruct the patient to rinse the infected area with a pint of hot normal saline solution every hour.

Prescribe phenoxymethyl penicillin (penicillin V), 250 mg. 4 times daily. If the clinical response is not satisfactory within 48 hours a mixed infection may be suspected. In this case, erythromycin or chloramphenicol should be considered. A culture should be secured as a guide to further management (see Chapter 8, "Antibiotic Therapy").

REMOVAL OF THE TOOTH. While authorities generally agree that removal of the tooth during *acute pericoronitis is contraindicated,* nevertheless there is a wide divergence of opinion.

However, I am not in favor of early surgery in *acute pericoronitis.* Maximum antibiotic therapy and adequate local treatment, as just described, is given the patient (see Chapter 8, "Antibiotic Therapy"). After treatment of the acute disease and the disappearance of the acute symptoms, with the ensuing chronic pericoronitis in which the overlying flap is still inflamed and moderately

BACTEREMIA AND SEPTICEMIA FROM PERICORONITIS

Patient. C. E., a man aged 35, was admitted to the hospital on September 12, at 11:45 A.M., with a complaint of chills and fever.

History. Seven days before admission the patient had had a "toothache" in the right mandibular third molar area, and he visited his dentist. The dentist found an infected tooth (pericoronal infection about a vertically impacted partially erupted mandibular third molar) and would not extract the tooth until the infection subsided. The dentist prescribed penicillin lozenges twice daily for 3 days. The patient had neither chills nor fever during this time.

On September 8 the patient was referred to a physician because of a fever. The physician advised conservative treatment of the tooth. Sulfanilamide was prescribed and the penicillin was stopped. The patient was not satisfied, and he called another physician, who gave him 300,000 units of Crysticillin intramuscularly. Four to five hours after this injection the patient became increasingly ill, with headache, chills and fever.

On September 9 the patient felt better and was given an additional 300,000 units of Crysticillin. During the afternoon and evening of this day he again had a rise in temperature, and marked pain in the right mandibular third molar area. On September 10 he felt well. On September 11 he again had chills and fever and was given another injection of 300,000 units of Crysticillin. On September 12, shortly after admission to this hospital, he suffered chills and fever; his temperature was 102° F.

Physical Examination. Findings in the physical examination of this patient were negative.

Oral Examination. Oral examination revealed a moderate degree of pericoronitis of the mandibular right third molar. There was no trismus or parapharyngeal involvement. There was moderate submaxillary induration and edema of the right side of the face. The tonsils were absent. The tongue was essentially normal.

Impressions. The diagnostic impressions were pericoronitis of the mandibular right third molar, and bacteremia with septicemia.

Therapeutic Treatment. On the day of admission to the hospital the patient was given 300,000 units of penicillin intramuscularly every 3 hours, a hot saline mouthwash hourly, with magnesium sulfate dressings of the right cheek hourly. Forced fluids were ordered. Urinalysis, blood sugar, and nonprotein nitrogen determinations were indicated. Nembutal, 1½ grains at bedtime, and aspirin, 15 grains every 4 hours, were prescribed.

On September 16 penicillin, 300,000 units, was given every 6 hours. A white blood cell and differential count were ordered.

On September 17 penicillin, 300,000 units, was continued every 12 hours. The patient was up and around.

On September 19 the patient was given an enema at night in preparation for operation on the following day.

Operation. On September 20 odontectomy of a vertically impacted lower right third molar was performed.

Postoperative Orders. After the operation, penicillin, 300,000 units every 3 hours, was prescribed. On the first postoperative day, penicillin, 300,000 units every 12 hours, was given. These drugs were discontinued on the second postoperative day, and the patient was discharged on the third postoperative day.

Summary. Table 5–3 presents the findings of the blood counts performed on four different days. Table 5–4 presents the temperature readings.

Conclusion. It is felt that this patient had bacteremia secondary to the pericoronal infection, although this was not conclusively established by blood cultures, which were negative because of the antibiotics. However, the repeated attacks of chills and fever, particularly on September 12 and 13, establish the presence of a blood stream infection.

By September 14, the third day of admission, the bacteremia was well controlled. However, antibiotic therapy was continued, and on September 20, 8 days after admission, the soft tissue that surrounded and partially covered the offending tooth appeared normal and so the impacted tooth was removed. The patient did not have chills or an elevation of temperature, and recovery was uneventful.

Table 5–3 *Blood Picture*

	SEPT. 12	SEPT. 13	SEPT. 14	SEPT. 17
Red blood cells	4,490,000		3,780,000	4,120,000
White blood cells	19,200	19,200	17,200	10,750
Neutrophils	76	81	71	
Lymphocytes	17	13	17	
Monocytes	7	3	6	
Esinophils		5	5	
Basophils			1	

Table 5–4 *Temperature Chart (°F.)*

DATE	8 A.M.	12 M.	4 P.M.	8 P.M.	12 P.M.
9/12		100.8°	102.2°	102.2°	98.4°
9/13	102.2°	100°	100.6°	103°	100°
9/14	99.6°	98°	99°	98.4°	98°
9/15	97°	98°	98.2°	98°	97.8°
9/19	97.6°	98°	98.6°	98.6°	97°
9/20	97°	97.8°	97.8°	98°	98°
9/21	97°	99.4°	99.4°	99.2°	99°
9/22	98°	98.6°	99°	98.4°	98°
9/23	96.4°	98.2°	98.2°	98°	98°

sore, and from beneath which free pus can be expressed by pressure, it is our procedure to incise these flaps widely. If it is a simple impaction, the third molar is removed. If it is a difficult impaction in which considerable bone must be removed, then the flap is incised and the removal of the tooth is deferred until all symptoms have disappeared.

If the *case presents with chronic pericoronitis* and the removal of the third molar is decided upon, the following procedure is carried out:

Prescribe preoperative antibiotic therapy (see Chapter 8).

Irrigate beneath the flap with 1 cc. of the iodine lotion, as has been described.

Under general anesthesia, make an incision through the soft tissue over the middle of the occlusal surface and carry it posteriorly over the distal margin ridge of the crown or its vicinity. The electrosurgical scalpel is an ideal instrument for this operation.

The third molar is removed with a minimum of trauma.

Place a gauze sponge over the socket.

Instruct the patient to rinse his mouth in this region with a pint of hot normal saline solution three times daily.

Give the patient the printed postoperative instructions already prescribed.

SURGICAL REMOVAL OF THE OVERLYING FLAP. It is extremely difficult to remove correctly the thick, dense fibrous tissues overlying the third molars with the usual scalpel or scissors. This tissue is freely movable and slides away beneath the scalpel. In addition, it is next to impossible to secure the correct angulations through the soft tissue around the crown of the third molar with the standard scalpels.

An easier and better way to remove these flaps is by means of the electrosurgical scalpel (see Figure 5–73). The electrosurgical scalpel has the following advantages: (1) It is not necessary to create pressure on the tissue to effect a separation of the tissue. Because of this fact the cuts can be made accurately, since there is no sliding or lateral motion of the soft tissues. (2) The incisions are much less bloody, and so visibility is markedly increased. Further hemostasis can be readily secured by the use of the electrocoagulating blunt electrode. (3) The possibility of dissemination of infection is minimized. The cutting currents are of extremely high frequency, producing a molecular disintegration of the tissues. The lymphatics and capillaries are sealed as they are cut.

IMPACTED MAXILLARY THIRD MOLARS
CLASSIFICATION OF IMPACTED MAXILLARY THIRD MOLARS

For some reason no one has previously classified impacted maxillary third molars. Yet these teeth can and do present variations in anatomic position that materially complicate their removal and increase the possibility of operative or postoperative complications.

A classification of maxillary third molar impactions, based on anatomic position, follows:

A. Relative depth of the impacted maxillary third molar in bone:

Class A: The lowest portion of the crown of the impacted maxillary third molar is on a line with the occlusal plane of the second molar.

Class B: The lowest portion of the crown of the impacted maxillary third molar is between the occlusal plane of the second molar and the cervical line.

Class C: The lowest portion of the crown of the impacted maxillary third molar is at or above the cervical line of the second molar.

B. The position of the long axis of the impacted maxillary third molar in relation to the long axis of the second molar:

1. Vertical
2. Horizontal
3. Mesioangular
4. Distoangular
5. Inverted
6. Buccoangular
7. Linguoangular

These may also occur simultaneously in
a. Buccal version
b. Lingual version
c. Torsoversion

C. Relationship of the impacted maxillary third molar to the maxillary sinus:

1. Sinus approximation (S.A.): no bone, or a thin partition of bone between the impacted maxillary third molar and the maxillary sinus, known as *maxillary sinus approximation.*

2. No sinus approximation (N.S.A.): 2 mm. or more of bone between the impacted maxillary third molar and the maxillary sinus, known as *no maxillary sinus approximation.*

SURGICAL TECHNIQUE FOR REMOVAL OF IMPACTED MAXILLARY THIRD MOLARS

Basic Steps in Planning Operative Procedures. The following steps should be ob-

MAXILLARY THIRD MOLARS

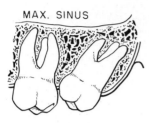 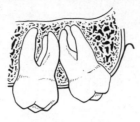 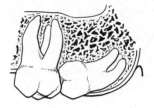

MESIOANGULAR, N.S.A. – DISTOANGULAR, N.S.A. – HORIZONTAL, N.S.A.

CLASS A

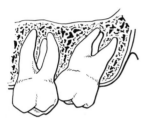 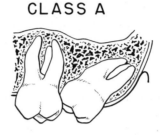 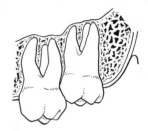

MESIOANGULAR, N.S.A. – HORIZONTAL, N.S.A. – VERTICAL, S.A.

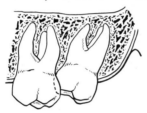 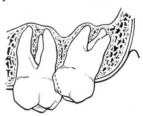

MESIOANGULAR, N.S.A. – MESIOANGULAR, S.A.
(LINGUAL DEFLECTION)   (BUCCAL DEFLECTION)

CLASS B

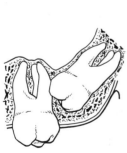 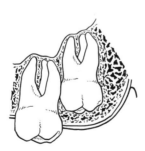 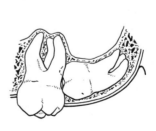

MESIOANG-
ULAR, S.A. – VERTICAL, S.A. – HORIZONTAL, S.A. –
MESIOANG-
ULAR, S.A.

CLASS C

Figure 5–74 Examples of classification of maxillary third molar impactions. See text for details. N.S.A., no (maxillary) sinus approximation; S.A., (maxillary) sinus approximation.

Figure 5–76 Examples of mesioangularly impacted maxillary third molars, all in Position C and approximating the maxillary sinus.

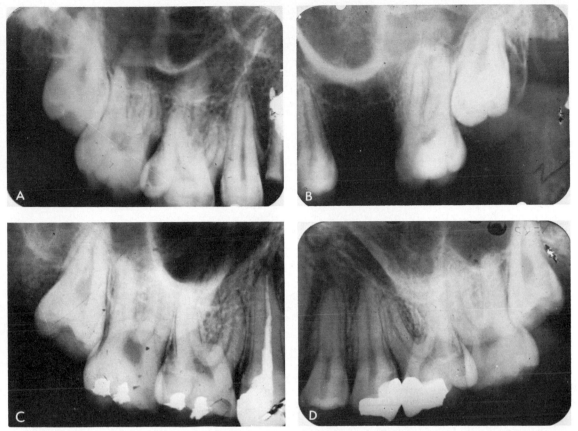

Figure 5–75 Examples of vertically impacted maxillary third molars, all in Position C and approximating the maxillary sinus. (See Figure 5–84 for the technique for excising these impacted teeth.)

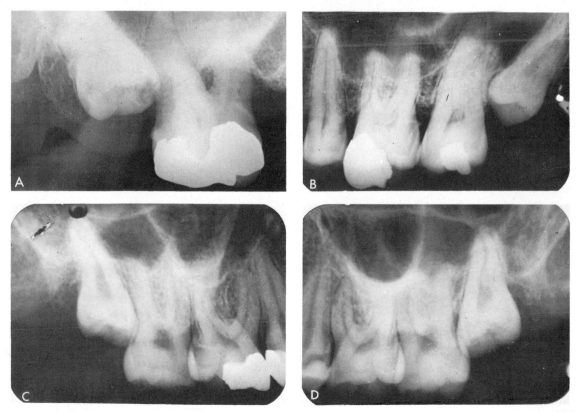

Figure 5–76 *See opposite page for legend.*

313

served in the removal of impacted maxillary third molars:

1. Make a visual and digital examination of the soft tissues, hard tissues and teeth adjacent to and overlying the impacted tooth.
2. Study radiographs of the tooth to be removed, the surrounding anatomic structures and adjacent teeth.
3. Classify the type of impaction (see Figure 5–74).

Factors Complicating the Removal of Impacted Maxillary Third Molars. Factors that will complicate the operative technique for the removal of impacted maxillary third molars include maxillary sinus approximation; the presence of an impacted maxillary third molar partly within or immediately above the roots of the second molar; fusion of the third molar with the roots of the second molar; abnormal root curvature; hypercementosis; proximity to the zygomatic process of the maxilla; extreme bone density, especially in elderly patients; follicular space filled with bone, most frequently seen in elderly patients; difficult access to the operative site because of a small orbicularis oris muscle or an inability to open the mouth wide enough.

Note: It is extremely difficult to secure

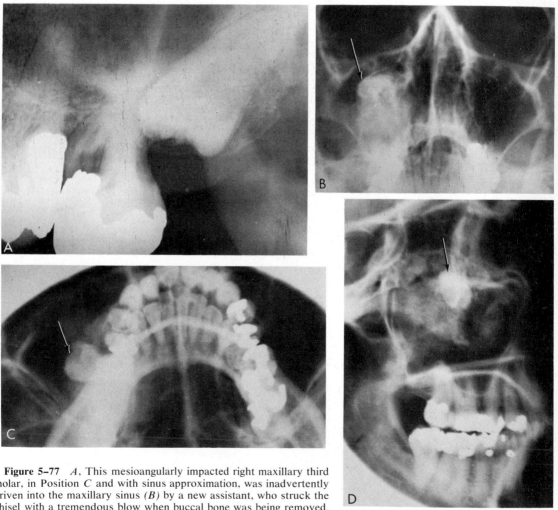

Figure 5–77 *A,* This mesioangularly impacted right maxillary third molar, in Position *C* and with sinus approximation, was inadvertently driven into the maxillary sinus *(B)* by a new assistant, who struck the chisel with a tremendous blow when buccal bone was being removed. Because of the brisk bleeding that followed and because we did not know for certain whether the molar was in the maxillary sinus or the sphenomaxillary fossa, the bleeding was controlled and the wound closed. *B,* The Waters view of the maxillary sinuses the next day revealed the third molar in the right maxillary sinus, two thirds of which was full of blood. Note the difference in the radiolucency in the right and left maxillary sinuses. *C,* A basal radiograph a week later, as well as a true lateral view of the facial bones *(D),* showed that the maxillary sinus was now clear of blood and the third molar still in the same position. It was removed by a Caldwell-Luc operation. Recovery was uneventful.

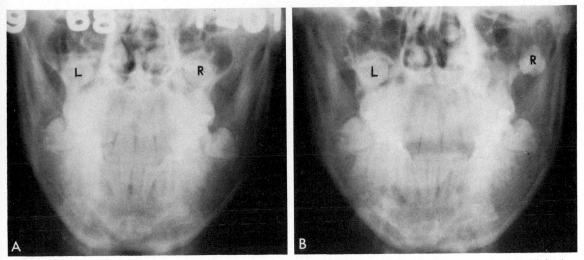

Figure 5–78 *A,* Right and left maxillary third molar crowns in a 14-year-old female whose parents were advised to have all her unerupted partially formed "wisdom" teeth extracted "to prevent future trouble." *B,* When their dentist attempted to remove the right third molar crown, it was unfortunately forced out, and then posteriorly and superiorly into the infratemporal fossa. Crown is marked *R.* (See Figure 5–81*C* and *D.*)

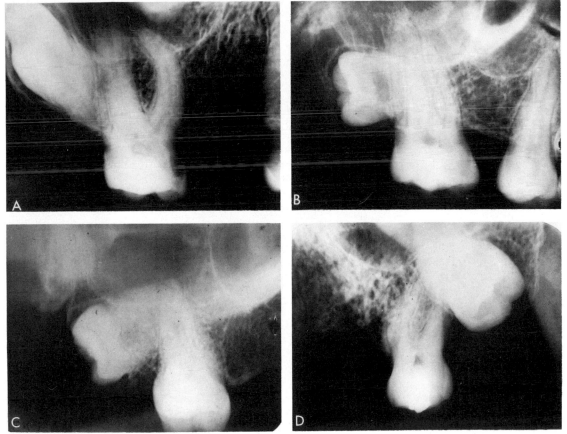

Figure 5–79 (1)

Figure 5–79 *1,* All four of these maxillary third molars—two of which are in distohorizontal positions (*A* and *B*) and two of which are in distoangular positions (*C* and *D*)—appear radiographically to have roots that are fused to those of the maxillary second molars. In my opinion there is no justification for sacrificing these second molars without there being a specific reason for doing so, and in these patients *there was not.* My opposition to the so-called "prophylactic surgical excision of all impacted teeth" has already been noted.

A famous surgeon many years ago emphasized that before performing any surgery the operator should be certain that the patient would not be worse off afterward than he was before. This is certainly doubly true for elective surgery.

(Figure 5–79 continued on following page)

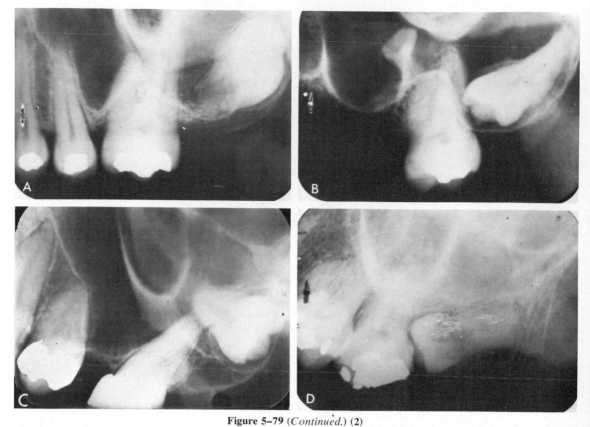

Figure 5–79 *(Continued.)* **(2)**

Figure 5–79 *(Continued.)* 2A to C, The removal of these three malposed, symptomless maxillary third molars would almost certainly result in an opening into the maxillary sinus. While this does not automatically mean that these sinuses would become infected or that an antro-oral fistula would be created, in my opinion the risk contraindicates this elective surgery. *If* these patients become edentulous, and *if* eventually their maxillary dentures traumatize and destroy the mucoperiosteal tissue overlying these teeth, then the risks pointed out above will have to be taken, but not until then. D, This horizontally impacted maxillary third molar has chronic pericoronal infection. Excision is indicated.

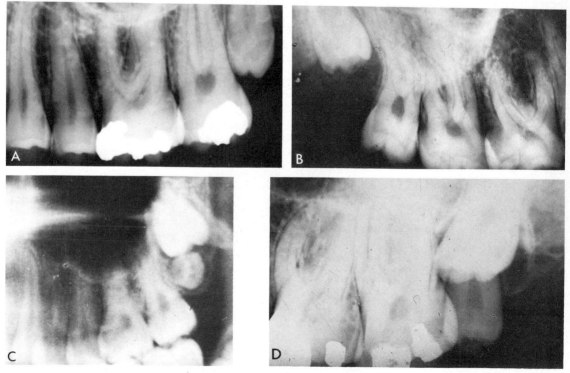

316 **Figure 5–80** *See opposite page for legend.*

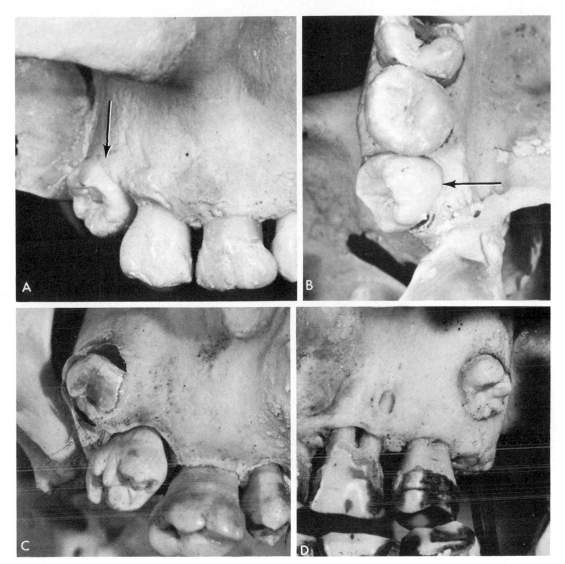

Figure 5–81   *A* and *B*, Anatomic specimens of malpositioned maxillary third molars, complete or partially formed. *C*, Crown of the maxillary third molar in its crypt high in the tuberosity of the maxilla. Note the relationship of this crown to the infratemporal fossa and how easy it would be to displace this tooth into the space, just as shown in Figure 5–78. *D*, Unerupted maxillary third molar in distobuccal version. Molars in this position are always difficult to remove because of their inaccessibility and the ease with which they can be pushed into the infratemporal fossa. Once the molar is exposed by removal of bone over the crown, the appropriate Apexo elevator placed between the buccal cortical plate and the crown will usually permit the easy delivery of this tooth.

direct vision into this area regardless of whether or not the orbicularis oris muscle is small and whether or not the patient can open his mouth wide enough. Actually, better vision is obtained in some cases by having the mouth partially closed, thus permitting greater retraction of the cheek.

Soft Tissue Flap.   For removal of impacted upper third molars, the incision is made starting beyond the tuberosity in the hamular

---

Figure 5–80   *A*, Rudimentary unerupted maxillary third molar. *B*, Rudimentary unerupted maxillary fourth molar. *C* and *D*, Rudimentary maxillary third molars preventing the eruption of the normal maxillary third molars. These rudimentary teeth should be excised to permit the third molars to erupt. The rudimentary third molar in *A* and the rudimentary fourth molar in *B*, *if symptoms warrant removal*, should be excised.

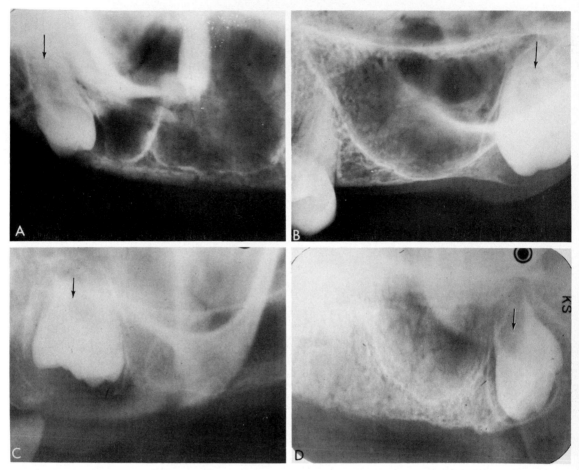

Figure 5–82 *A* to *D,* Unerupted partially formed maxillary third molars. These are not edentulous maxillas, and excision is not indicated. In *A* there is a lingual root of a maxillary molar. The patient's history was negative for sinus disease, as was the radiographic examination. Other periapical views with less elongation were better diagnostic films and were negative for areas of radiolucency. These films were interpreted as indicating that this root was not in the maxillary sinus but in the lingual cortical bone. We did not remove it.

notch with a No. 12 Bard-Parker blade. The mucous membrane overlying the tuberosity is incised from the distalmost portion of the tuberosity forward (anteriorly) until the midpoint of the distal surface of the upper second molar is contacted.

Continue the incision buccally around the neck of the second molar to the interproximal space between the first molar and the second molar, and then toward the mucobuccal fold at a 45-degree angle. Make this last incision with a No. 15 Bard-Parker blade. The muco-periosteal tissue covering the crown of the impacted tooth is loosened and reflected. It may be held out of the way by a broad periosteal elevator. The palatal portion of the mucoperiosteal tissue over the tuberosity is loosened and held by tissue forceps or a suture. This provides adequate access to the bone overlying the impacted tooth.

Removal of Overlying Bone. In an upper third molar impaction, this bone is, as a general rule, not dense, and it can readily be removed with chisels or rongeurs, exposing

Figure 5–84 Excision of a mesioangular impaction of the maxillary third molar. *A,* The incision starts in the pterygopalatine fissure midway between the palatal and buccal surfaces of the tuberosity, up over the tuberosity contacting the midpoint of the distal surface of the second molar, then around the neck of the second molar toward the mucobuccal fold, as illustrated. *B,* The flap is reflected, and the buccal and occlusal bone is carefully removed down to the height of contour with a chisel. *C,* With the buccal cortical plate over the distal root of the second molar as a fulcrum, the No. 74 Miller Apexo elevator is inserted beneath the crown and pressure directed buccally and occlusally, lifting the third molar from its bed.

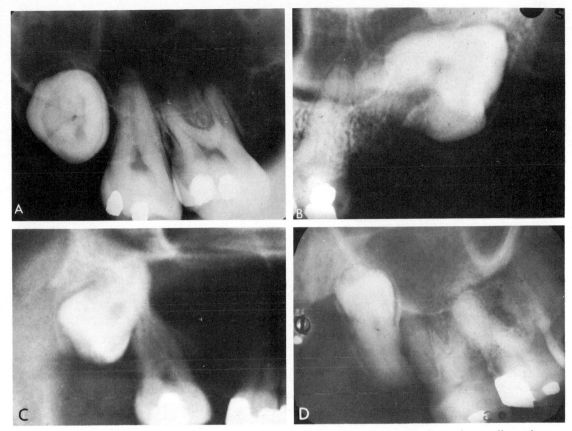

Figure 5–83 The statements made in the legend for Figure 5–79 (*1* and *2*) apply also to these radiographs.

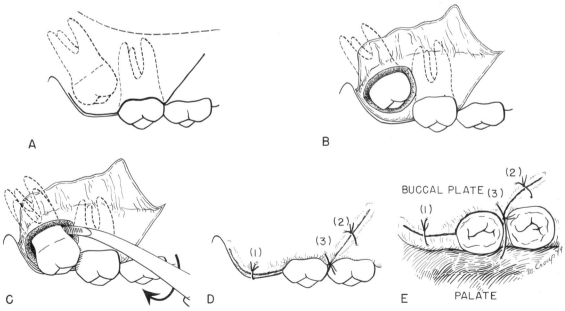

Figure 5–84 *(Continued.)   D,* The flap is replaced and sutured. *(1)* Suture soft tissue back over the tuberosity. *(2)* This is a very difficult place to suture and is not essential if suture *3* can be placed through the interproximal space. *(3)* The interproximal suture is placed from the buccal side to the lingual aspect over the contact point and tied on the buccal side. *E,* The appearance of the occlusal surface of the first and second molars, as well as the palate and buccal aspects of the alveolar ridge.

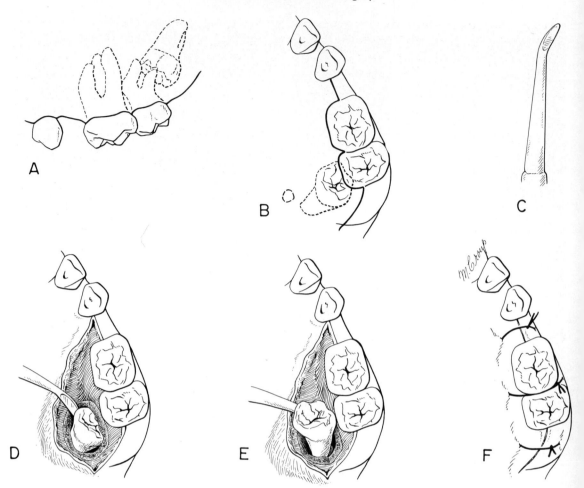

Figure 5–85 Removal of a maxillary third molar that is mesioangularly impacted in the palate. In this case the impacted third molar appeared to be fused to the second molar. However, it was possible to identify the roots of the second molar, which seemed to be superimposed over the crown of the third molar. In view of the fact that it was impossible to palpate the crown of the third molar buccally, it was felt that this crown and the main body of the tooth must be in a palatal position. The shift-sketch technique confirmed this possibility.

In *A* and *B* will be seen the line of incision for the exposure of the osseous structure overlying this tooth, namely, up over the tuberosity, around the lingual neck of the second molar and the first molar and across the space present in this case between the first bicuspid and the first molar. *D* shows the reflection of the flap; of course, the reason the flap was made in this manner was to prevent cutting through the anterior palatine artery. The overlying osseous structure was removed with bursi, and with the elevator, the crown was lifted from its crypt and the tooth delivered, as shown in *E*. Sutures were placed as shown in *F*, and the flap was closed.

Note: Extreme care must be taken to avoid cutting the anterior palatine artery at its exit from the posterior palatine foramen.

the crown of the impacted tooth. In this operation extreme care must be exercised not to drive the tooth inadvertently into the maxillary sinus or the pterygomaxillary space. Because of this danger, the sectioning technique is not applicable to, nor is it necessary for, maxillary third molar removal.

After the overlying bone has been removed, exposing the crown of the impacted tooth, remove sufficient bone to expose the crown's height of contour.

Removal of Impacted Upper Third Molar.
After the impacted tooth is exposed and the overlying bone and bone surrounding the height of contour have been removed, sufficient space must be obtained between the height of contour of the impacted tooth and the bone to permit the entrance of an elevator, so that the point of the elevator can be placed beneath the crown, near the gingival line, at the mesiobuccal angle.

The appropriate elevator is inserted above

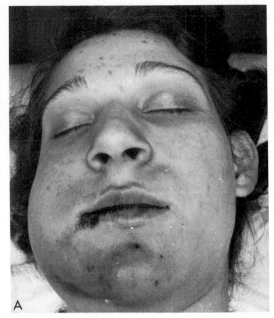

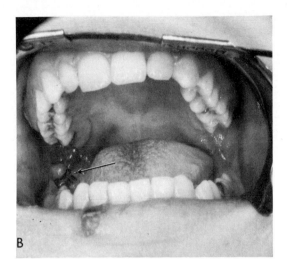

Figure 5–86 *A,* Appearance of an 18-year-old patient 24 hours after the removal of a Class I, Position C, vertically impacted mandibular third molar and a similarly classified maxillary third molar. Note the very early signs of ecchymosis in the skin of the buccal and submandibular region and the trauma to the lip. *B,* Bleeding was brisk during surgery but was controlled by the sutures when the patient was removed from the operating room. During the night the pressure beneath the flap was sufficient to tear out the sutures and open the flaps, as can be seen.

This patient had been scheduled for removal of four impacted third molars (all were similar in location). The difficulty encountered in the removal of the right two was sufficient to defer the excision of the other two until the patient had fully recovered. To do so was in the best interests of the patient. One should never "bulldoze" ahead on cases which turn out to be more difficult than expected. In fact, it is our policy to tell all patients scheduled for the excision of four impacted molars that we *may find* it necessary to divide the operation into two for the reasons previously stated.

the height of contour (the Miller elevators Nos. 73, for upper left, and 74, for upper right, are most useful in this operation). By using the buccal plate as a fulcrum, the tooth is then elevated buccally and distally from the alveolus.

Extreme care must be exercised in the placing of the elevator to make certain that it

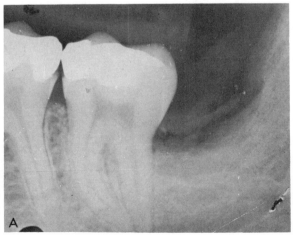

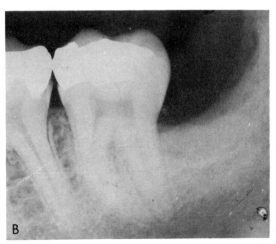

Figure 5–87 Sequestrum of a portion of the buccal cortical bone weeks following the excision of an impacted mandibular molar. This pressure necrosis was produced by repeated excessive pressures from the various elevators that, quite rightly, had made use of this bone as the fulcrum point. Here again, one must exercise "judgment" as to how much pressure is not "too much" pressure. As previously stated, one should create adequate space into which the tooth can be moved without more than *moderate pressures* with elevators by sectioning the crowns—and, if necessary, the roots—by burs or osteotomes.

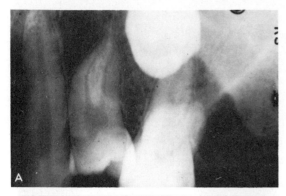

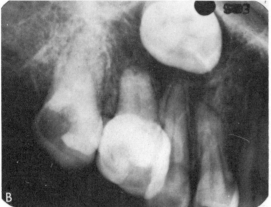

Figure 5–88 Impacted maxillary first molars are rarely seen. Two examples are illustrated here.

is above the height of contour and that pressure is to the distal and buccal sides. This is to prevent the impacted tooth from being forced into the maxillary sinus (see Figure 5–77) or into the pterygomaxillary space (see Figure 5–78).

If the tooth is forced into the maxillary sinus, it will necessitate the surgeon's opening into the maxillary sinus above the bicuspid area to remove the tooth.

Note the following points: The most important thing in the removal of impacted teeth is adequate exposure, which means removal of the overlying and surrounding bone well past the height of contour of the crown of the impacted tooth. There must be room sufficient to pass an elevator point up between the height of contour of the tooth and the surrounding bone, so that the tip of the elevator can get above the crown of the tooth.

IMPACTED MAXILLARY CUSPIDS

The removal of a deeply embedded, horizontal, palatally impacted cuspid, in close relationship to the maxillary sinus, or nasal cavity, or both, is one of the most difficult

surgical procedures in the oral cavity. In fact, the average palatally impacted cuspid presents many more difficulties than the average mandibular third molar impaction. The "average" case is the least difficult of each type of impaction.

ETIOLOGIC FACTORS

Several etiologic factors in addition to those thought to cause most impacted teeth

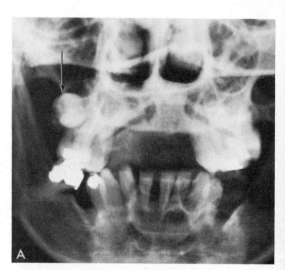

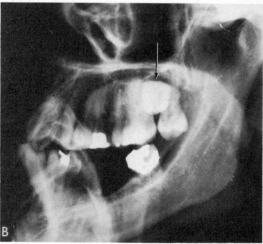

Figure 5–89 *A,* Posteroanterior radiograph of the maxilla and mandible reveals the impacted left maxillary second molar. *A* digital examination of this patient had revealed this buccal bulge, and radiographic examination confirmed our suspicion that this was a very rare impaction of the second molar.

In the very few cases I have seen (in 48 years) of impacted maxillary second molars, all the crowns have been in the buccal position. With bicuspids, the crowns are usually on the lingual side. *B,* True lateral head radiograph reveals that the second molar is located between the roots of the first and third molars. The technique for the excision of this tooth is shown in Figure 5–90.

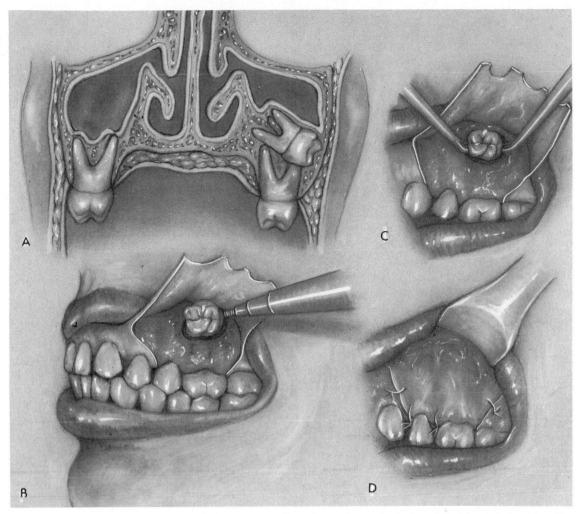

Figure 5-90 Excision of a transversely impacted maxillary first molar. *A*, Sagittal section shows relationship of impaction to the teeth and to the floor of the maxillary sinus. *B*, Large mucoperiosteal flap reflected. Note lines of incision. This produces a clearly visible field and adequate bone support when the flap is replaced and sutured. Also shown is the exposure of the crown by removal of the overlying cortical bone with round and crosscut burs. Note that space around the anterior, inferior and distal surfaces of the crown has been created with a crosscut fissure bur. No superior bone has been removed because of the proximity of the maxillary sinus. Care must also be taken to avoid trauma to the roots of adjacent teeth. It may be necessary to section the crown of the impacted tooth to avoid trauma to adjacent roots. This can be determined when the crown is exposed. *C*, With Miller elevators, and use of the buccal cortical plate as a fulcrum, the tooth is luxated and removed; or, the crown can be grasped with a No. 150 or No. 286 forceps, luxated and removed. *D*, Mucoperiosteal flap replaced and sutured. Ties are on the buccal side.

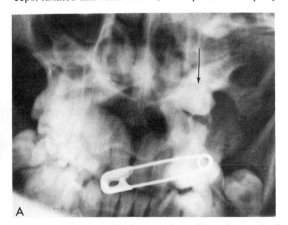
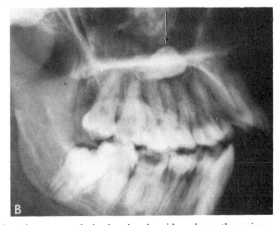

Figure 5-91 *A*, This impacted maxillary first molar is positioned transversely in the alveolar ridge above the apices of the molar and bicuspid roots, with the crown in the buccal bone. *B*, This true lateral head radiograph reveals the horizontal position of this molar. The technique for excision is shown in Figure 5-90. (The pin in *A* is from the drape.)

have been suggested for impaction of maxillary cuspids. A summary of Dewel's[13] discussion of these factors follows.

The hard palatal bone offers more resistance than does alveolar bone on the ridge to the eruption of the cuspid that is misplaced lingually.

The mucoperiosteal tissue covering the anterior third of the palate, being subjected to repeated stress and pressure during mastication, becomes very dense, thick and resistant. It is attached more firmly to the osseous structure than is any other soft tissue membrane in the oral cavity.

Eruption of teeth is dependent, to some extent, on an associated increase in apical development. This aid to the eruption of cuspids is minimized because this root is normally more fully formed at the time eruption is due than is that of any of the other permanent teeth.

The greater the distance a tooth must travel from its point of development to normal occlusion, the greater the possibility of deflection from its normal course and of resultant impaction. The cuspid has the greatest distance of all the teeth to travel before reaching full occlusion. It is equally true that the shorter the distance a tooth must travel from its point of development to full occlusion, the less the possibility of impaction. First permanent molars have the shortest distance to travel and are *rarely* impacted.

During development, the crown of the permanent cuspid lies immediately lingual to the long apex of the primary cuspid root. Any change in the position or condition of the primary cuspid because of caries or premature loss of the primary molar is reflected along its full length to the end of its root, and may thereby easily cause a deviation in the position and direction of growth of the permanent cuspid tooth bud.

Delayed resorption of the primary cuspid root can affect eruption of the permanent cuspid.

The cuspids are the last of the permanent teeth to erupt; hence they are vulnerable for a long period of time to any unfavorable environmental influences.

The cuspids erupt between teeth already in occlusion and are competing for space with the also currently erupting second molars.

The cuspid is preceded by a primary cuspid whose mesiodistal diameter is much less than that of the permanent cuspid.

Because of these factors, the cuspid is the third most frequently impacted tooth.

The great majority of these cases are found in female patients, probably because the bones of the skull and the maxilla and mandible in the female are, on the average, smaller than those in the male.

POSITIONS OF IMPACTED CUSPIDS

Rohrer[38] has shown that impacted cuspids occur in the maxilla 20 times more frequently than in the mandible. Why this is true when the same etiologic factors are present, no one has been able to explain.

In the maxilla malposed cuspids are found three times as frequently on the palatal side of the arch as on the labial or buccal side. In the maxilla they are almost always rotated upon their longitudinal axis and are usually in an oblique position. Frequently impacted maxillary cuspids are found in a horizontal position.

Impacted mandibular cuspids are rarely found in a horizontal position or on the lingual side of the dental ridge, being located most often in the labial surface of the mandible.

Aberrant maxillary and mandibular cuspids have been found between the first and second bicuspids, in the nose, in the maxillary sinus, in the orbit, in the lip, under the tongue and under the chin.

LOCALIZING IMPACTED MAXILLARY CUSPIDS

It is imperative that the position of impacted cuspids be carefully determined prior to operation. This is best decided by a complete radiographic examination. To establish whether they are in the palatal process or the labial process, the radiographic shift-sketch technique is used. This is illustrated and described in Chapter 16, "Oral and Panoramic Radiographs and Localization." (See Figures 16–4 and 16–6 for sectional roentgenograms showing a palatally impacted cuspid and its relationship to adjacent maxillary teeth and the maxillary sinus. See Figures 16–9 and 16–10 to 16–13 inclusive for localization technique.)

These radiographs must be studied and correctly interpreted. Unfortunately, seldom, if ever, do they reveal the marked apical curvature that is present so frequently. The radiograph may suggest that the root of the palatally located cuspid passes through the alveolar process, ending in the labial cortical bone (see Figure 5–109). Unfortunately, even the occlusal view is often of little value in proving or disproving this possibility. It then must finally be decided when the crown and a portion of the root are exposed at the operation for removal.

There are, however, some clinical clues that can be investigated: There may be a distinct bulge seen on the palate; by palpation a bulge might be felt on the buccal aspect of the maxilla.

Labial impactions in which the cuspid crown is in contact with the apical third of the lateral incisor root will cause deflections of the apical portion of the root lingually and of the crown labially. However, horizontal palatal cuspid impactions in which the cuspid crown is in contact with the gingival or middle third of the lateral incisor root also move the lateral incisor crown labially. Movement of the lateral incisor crown can be used as a guide only by carefully checking with all of the other diagnostic aids.

Impacted maxillary cuspids are most frequently found in the following positions: (a) in the palate, with the crown located to the lingual side of the upper lateral incisor and the root extending posteriorly in the palate parallel to the bicuspid roots; (b) with the crown to the lingual side of the maxillary central incisor and the root extending posteriorly in the palate parallel to the bicuspid roots, or between the bicuspid roots and extending through to the buccal surface; (c) with the crown of the impacted tooth on the palatal area and the body of the root on the buccal surface of the maxilla; (d) with the crown of the impacted tooth on the buccal surface of the maxilla, and the root extending to the lingual side of the bicuspid roots on the palate; (e) with the entire tooth lying in the buccal cortical plate; (f) in an edentulous mouth; (g) bilaterally impacted either in the palatal process or labial cortical plate of the maxilla.

CLASSIFICATION OF IMPACTED MAXILLARY CUSPIDS

Impacted maxillary cuspids are classified as follows:

Class I: Impacted cuspids located in the palate.
1. Horizontal.
2. Vertical.
3. Semivertical.
Class II: Impacted cuspids located in the labial or buccal surface of the maxilla.
1. Horizontal.
2. Vertical.
3. Semivertical.
Class III: Impacted cuspids located in both the palatal process and labial or buccal maxillary bone; e.g., the crown is on the palate and the root passes through between the roots of the adjacent teeth in the alveolar process, ending in a sharp angle on the labial or buccal surface of the maxilla.
Class IV: Impacted cuspids located in the alveolar process, usually vertically between the incisor and first bicuspid.
Class V: Impacted cuspids located in an edentulous maxilla.

CONTRAINDICATION TO THE REMOVAL OF IMPACTED CUSPIDS

When the cuspid can be brought into normal position either by surgical positioning or by a combination of surgery and orthodontia at an early age, it should not be removed. See photographic case reports (Figs. 5–112 to 5–126) of this combined technique. Figures 5–112 to 5–117 show two labially semivertically impacted maxillary cuspids (Class II) brought into place in the dental arch, and Figures 5–120 to 5–123 show bilateral palatally impacted cuspids (Class I) that were similarly treated.

TECHNIQUE FOR SURGICAL REMOVAL OF PALATALLY IMPACTED CUSPIDS

Plan operative procedure with the following steps: (a) carefully study radiographs to ascertain the position and relationship of the cuspid to other teeth and to the maxillary sinus; (b) classify the impaction; (c) plan the type of soft tissue flap; (d) decide whether sectioning of the tooth will facilitate its removal and at the same time conserve bone.

Factors Complicating the Removal of Impacted Maxillary Cuspids. Because of the usual proximity of the crown and root of impacted cuspids to the adjacent teeth (central

MAXILLARY CUSPIDS

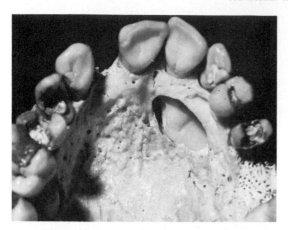

Figure 5–92 Horizontally and palatally impacted maxillary cuspid. The dentigerous cyst about the crown of this tooth materially aids in its removal, since surrounding bone has been destroyed, thus reducing the amount of bone that must be removed to expose the crown. In a case like this one, use the technique shown in Figure 5–101 to remove a cuspid from the palatal process of the maxilla.

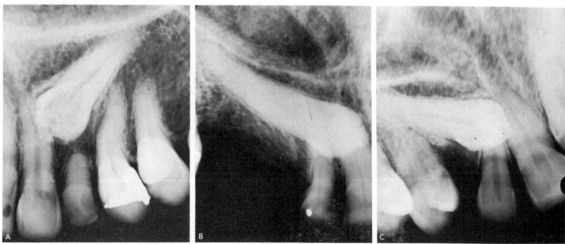

Figure 5–93 Examples of palatally impacted maxillary cuspids.

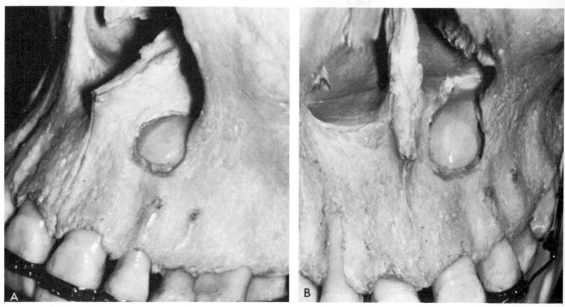

Figure 5–94 Anatomic specimen with a grossly malposed maxillary cuspid just beneath the osseous floor of the nasal cavity.

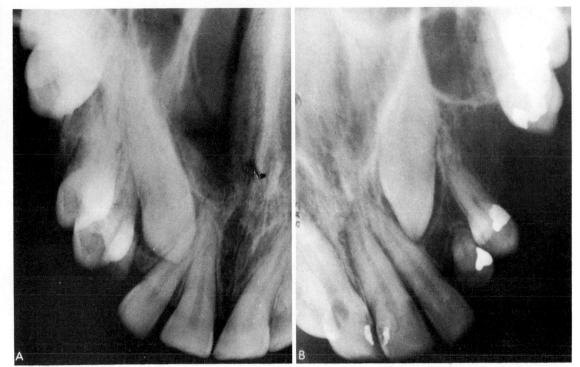

Figure 5–95 *A,* Impacted maxillary cuspid deflected during eruption by the carious deciduous root. *B,* While the deciduous cuspid is also still present in this case, it is hard to blame the impaction on it because of the bone intervening between its apex and the permanent cuspid, lying impacted against the lateral incisor.

and lateral incisors and bicuspids), there is a greater danger of injury to adjacent teeth and vital structures in the area of surgery.

In the greater percentage of these impactions, the root portion is separated from the maxillary sinus and nasal cavity by a thin partition of bone, and in some cases solely by the ciliated epithelial lining of the maxillary sinus. For this reason, the possibility of forcing the cuspid root into the maxillary sinus during the sectional removal of an impacted cuspid is always present. Not infrequently openings of various sizes into the maxillary sinus are created. Rigid asepsis should be followed; otherwise, an acute infection of the maxillary sinus may ensue. With strict

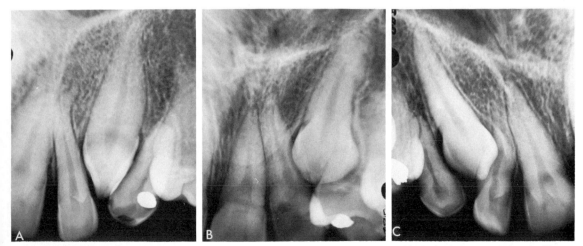

Figure 5–96 *A* and *C,* Vertically impacted partially erupted maxillary cuspids lodged between the deciduous cuspids and the permanent lateral incisors. *B,* Cuspid vertically impacted between the lateral incisor and first bicuspid.

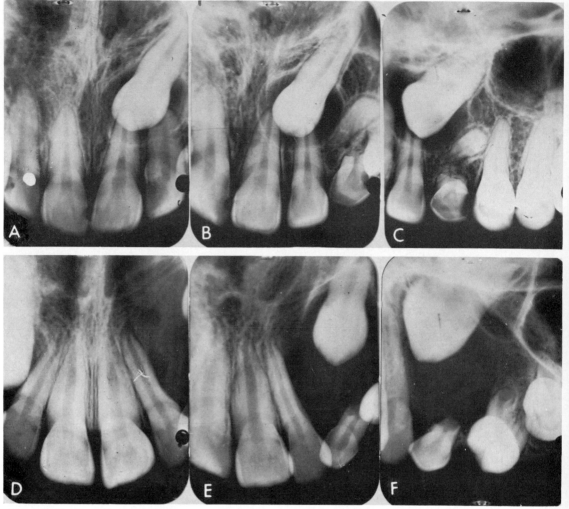

Figure 5–97   Examples of dentigerous cysts involving maxillary impacted cuspids. *A* to *C,* Views of a beginning dentigerous cyst. Note the rudimentary cuspid. *D* to *F,* Vertically impacted maxillary cuspid and dentigerous cyst. Note the deflection of the lateral incisor root.

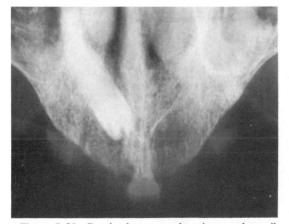

Figure 5–98   Retained symptomless impacted maxillary cuspid in an edentulous maxilla. This patient, who is in her late fifties, has been wearing dentures for 18 years without any knowledge of the presence of this impaction. In my opinion there is not any reason for the excision of this tooth.

asepsis these accidental perforations of the membrane of the maxillary sinus do not result in infection. When the thick, dense palatal mucoperiosteal tissue is sutured back into place and held in contact with the palatal process for several hours by gauze pressure packs in the palatal arch, healing takes place without complications.

Most impacted cuspid roots have a pronounced curvature at the apical third, in some cases almost a right angle.

Occasionally the crown is in the palate and the root is above the apices of the bicuspids (Class III) or even on the buccal surface of the maxilla. If the latter is true, follow the technique described and illustrated in Figure 5–109.

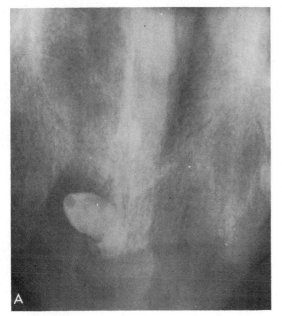 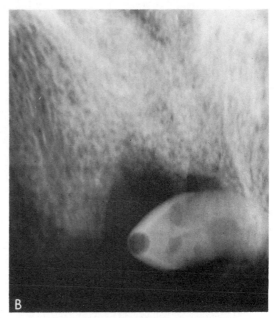

Figure 5–99 *A* and *B*, Rudimentary impacted cuspid at the crest of the ridge in this edentulous maxilla. The patient has ulceration of the mucoperiosteum over the crown, and there is chronic discharge of pus. Radiolucency around the carious crown indicates loss of bone. Excision of this tooth is certainly indicated.

REMOVAL OF IMPACTED CUSPIDS IN CLASS I POSITION

Use a No. 12 Bard-Parker (BP) blade to incise the tissues around the necks of the teeth, beginning on the lingual side of the maxillary central incisor and extending to the distal edge of the second bicuspid.

With a No. 15 Bard-Parker blade, beginning at the crest of the interdental papilla on the lingual side, between the maxillary central incisors, carry the incision straight back along the center of the palate for 1½ inches. This incision traverses the nasopalatine (incisive) canal and results in minor bleeding that is controlled by pressure with a sponge for a few minutes. If this doesn't control the bleeding, pack a short strip of iodoform gauze into the canal. Reflect the mucoperiosteum from

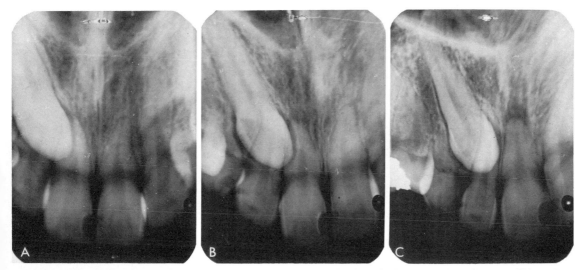

Figure 5–100 Shift-sketch radiography (see Chapter 16) for localization of this impacted maxillary cuspid. *A*, Central incisor view. *B*, The x-ray tube was moved distally, and another radiograph was made for the lateral incisor. Note how the crown of the cuspid has moved distally also. *C*, The x-ray tube was again moved distally and another radiograph of the cuspid region made. Note how the crown of the impacted cuspid has moved further distally. This proves that the cuspid is located in the palate.

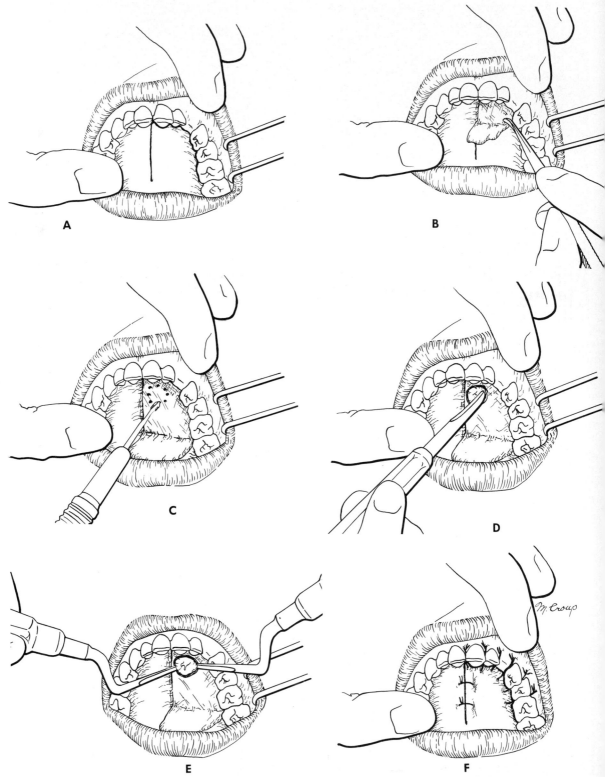

Figure 5–101 Removal of a palatally impacted maxillary cuspid. *A,* The incision is made. *B,* The mucoperiosteum is reflected. *C,* Holes are drilled around the crown of the impacted tooth. *D,* The opening is enlarged with a crosscut surgical bur. *E,* The tooth is elevated from the socket with No. 73 and No. 74 elevators. *F,* The flap is sutured back into place.

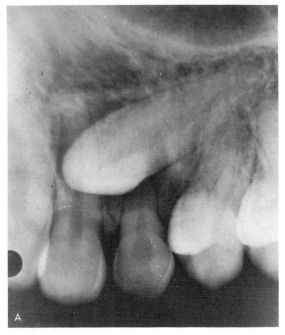

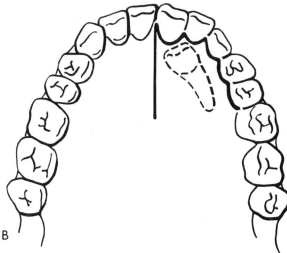

Figure 5-102   *A*, Palatally impacted maxillary cuspid. Note the retained deciduous cuspid. *B*, Outline of the flap to expose the operative field.

the hard palate by means of the periosteal elevator until the overlying osseous structure is completely exposed. At this point, a bulge in the bone may be seen, or a portion of the crown of the impacted cuspid may be visible.

Take a spear-pointed drill, or bone bur, and drill holes in the palatal bone 3 mm. apart around the crown of the impacted tooth, being careful not to damage the roots of the adjacent teeth.

By means of a bur or a chisel and a mallet, connect the drilled holes around the crown of the impacted tooth in the palatal process, and remove the bone overlying the crown. Enlarge the size of the opening with burs so that the complete crown may be seen.

The exception to this rule is those cases in which a portion of the crown of the impacted tooth is in contact with the roots of the upper central or lateral incisors or bicuspids. If the roots of these teeth are exposed, they will be damaged. In these cases, *enlarge the opening on the opposite side of the crown* by means of bone burs or cut the crown from the root (see Figure 5-107).

After the crown of the palatally impacted cuspid has been completely exposed, place a No. 73 and No. 74 Miller Apexo elevator on each side of the crown, and with a double lifting action, attempt to lift the impacted tooth from its crypt in the palate. Extreme care must be exercised to prevent injury to the adjacent teeth.

If this does not remove the impacted tooth, enlarge the opening and repeat the procedure, using the two elevators in the same way (see Figure 5-101).

If the impacted tooth is still not removed, grasp the crown with a No. 286 forceps, and with a rotary motion attempt to remove the cuspid. The use of the No. 286 forceps is particularly advantageous when there is a hook on the root of the impacted tooth. Using elevators would probably fracture this type of root.

Clean out all debris, remove any spicules of bone, and trim smooth the edges of the bony crypt. Remove the tooth follicle, if present, and *suture the flap back into position.*

Then pack gauze over the mucoperiosteal flap (palatal packing) to the level of the occlusal surface. Cut a tongue blade to fit the distance between the buccal surfaces of the right and left maxillary bicuspids and round the cut end. (The other end is already rounded.) Place this over the palatal packing and instruct the patient to bite on it. If the patient is asleep, silk sutures are passed around the contact points of the bicuspids on both sides of the arch, over the palatal packing, and tied. Keep this palatal packing in place 4 hours.

ALTERNATE TECHNIQUES FOR REMOVAL OF CLASS I IMPACTED CUSPIDS

This technique is indicated when the tip of the cuspid crown is in contact with the roots of the central and lateral incisors. (Study Figure 5-103.)

(Text continued on page 335)

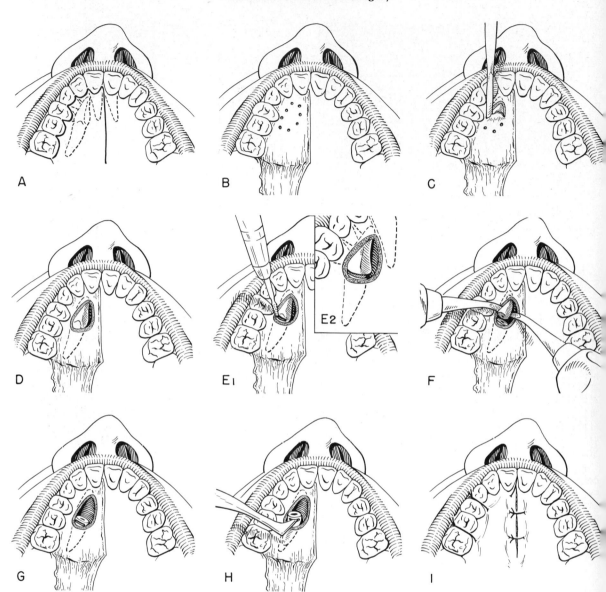

Figure 5–103 Sectional removal of an unerupted cuspid in the palate. This method of excision is necessary when the crown of a palatally impacted maxillary cuspid is in contact with the roots of the central and lateral incisors. *A*, Incision for the palatal flap. *B*, The flap is reflected, and holes are drilled through the bone. *C*, Some bone overlying the crown of the cuspid is removed with a chisel. *D*, To prevent exposure of adjacent roots, the crown of the cuspid is not entirely exposed. *E*, A groove is cut into the tooth with a wide crosscut fissure bur. *F*, The crown is lifted from the socket with elevators. *G*, More root surface is exposed, and another groove is made. *H*, Root is removed with a No. 323 Barry elevator. *I*, Palatal flap is sutured into place.

Figure 5–106 Single flap for exposure of bilaterally impacted cuspids. This is used when the cuspids are close to the midline because if tissue is left in the midline, as in the double flap technique, it is traumatized and usually sloughs. Blood is supplied to this flap via the anterior palatine arteries. *A*, Flap outlined. *B*, Mucoperiosteal covering of the palatal process reflected posteriorly and holes drilled in bone prior to exposure of the crowns by the removal of these segments of bone with crosscut fissure burs.

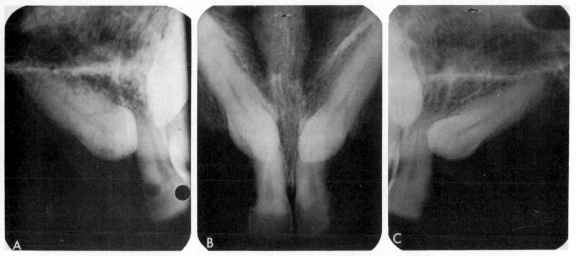

Figure 5–104 Bilateral palatally impacted maxillary cuspids.

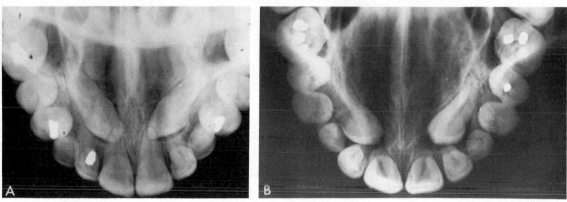

Figure 5–105 *A,* Bilateral palatally impacted maxillary cuspids whose crowns are in contact with the roots of the central incisors. The crowns of the cuspids must be sectioned as shown in Figure 5–103. Note the retained deciduous cuspids, which should not be extracted. *B,* Bilateral palatally impacted cuspids whose crowns are not in contact with the roots of the central incisors but are close to those of the lateral incisors. Note also that there are radiolucent areas about both cuspid crowns caused by possible developing dentigerous cysts. The loss of investing bone around the cuspid crowns will facilitate the removal of these teeth. After the crowns are exposed it may be found that little, if any, additional bone must be removed to deliver these teeth. See Figure 5–103. Note the retained deciduous cuspids, which should not be removed.

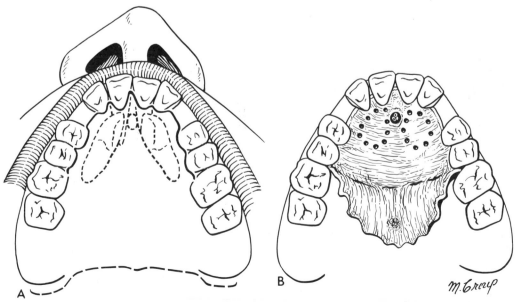

Figure 5–106 *See opposite page for legend.*

Photographic Case Report

EXCISION OF BILATERAL PALATALLY IMPACTED MAXILLARY CUSPIDS

Paul M. Burbank, D.M.D.

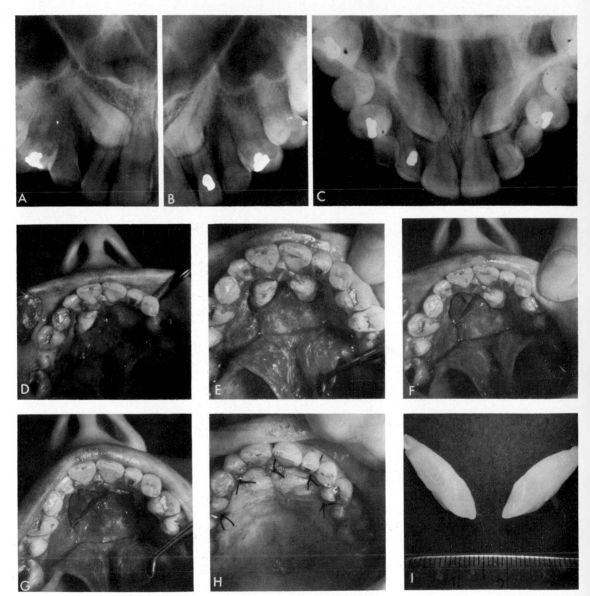

Figure 5–107   Bilateral impacted maxillary cuspids in 32-year-old female. *A* to *C*, Preoperative periapical and occlusal radiographs. *D*, Flap retracted and right cuspid exposed. *E*, Both impacted cuspids exposed. *F*, Right cuspid extracted. *G*, Both cuspids removed and area debrided. *H*, Palatal flap repositioned and sutured. *I*, Extracted impacted maxillary cuspids.

After the crown of the impacted cuspid is partially exposed, cut off the crown with a large crosscut fissure bur. This loss of tooth structure permits the crown to be moved back from under the bony ledge that surrounds the necks of the incisors and facilitates the removal of the crown.

Drill a slot into the root of the impacted tooth with a bur. Then insert the point of an Apexo elevator into this slot and move the root forward, using the cortical bone of the palate as a fulcrum.

Complete the preparation of the crypt, replace the flap, and insert the palatal packing as described above.

REMOVAL OF IMPACTED CUSPIDS IN CLASS II POSITION

The technique for this operation is illustrated and described in Figure 5-108.

REMOVAL OF IMPACTED CUSPIDS IN CLASS III POSITION

The steps for this operation are illustrated and described in Figure 5-109. The cuspid crown is in the palatal bone and the root is on the buccal side of the maxilla.

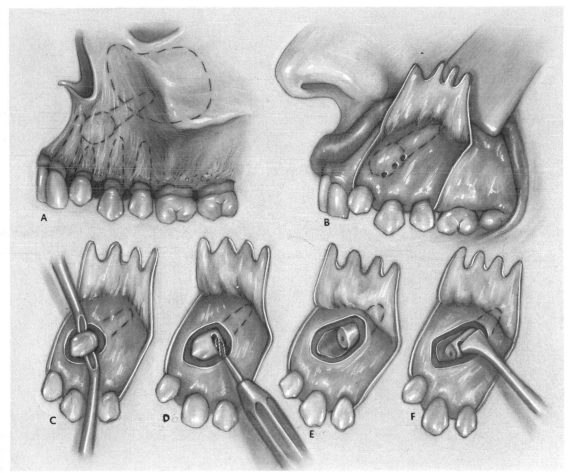

Figure 5-108 Removal of a labially impacted maxillary cuspid. *A,* Note the relationship to the nasal cavity, maxillary sinus and roots of the maxillary teeth. The primary cuspid is still in place. *B,* With a Feldman drill and crosscut burs, expose the crown. *C,* Using the cortical plate as a fulcrum, insert the No. 73 and No. 74 Miller Apexo elevators beneath the crown and lift the tooth from its bed. *D,* If the bone overlying the root is too thick and dense to permit delivery of the tooth by the above technique, then cut halfway through the crown with a crosscut fissure bur, fracture the crown from the root and remove the crown. *E,* With the chisel expose several millimeters more of the root surface. *F,* Cut a groove into the root. Place the tip of the No. 11R elevator into this groove and, using the cortical plate as a fulcrum, move the root into the space created by the removal of the crown.

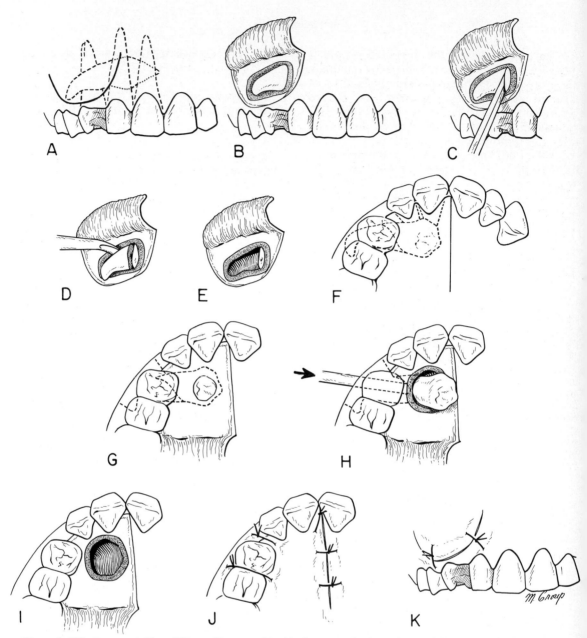

Figure 5–109 Impacted Class III maxillary cuspid with the crown in the palate and the root on the labial surface.

A, A semicircular labial flap is made over the root.

B, The root is exposed by removal of bone with burs and chisels.

C, The root is severed with a sharp chisel or cut off with a crosscut fissure bur. If a chisel is used, the blow is directed upward to prevent traumatizing the roots of the adjacent teeth.

D and *E,* The root is elevated from its bed.

F, G and *H,* A palatal flap is outlined, cut and reflected, and bone overlying the crown is removed to expose the periphery completely.

H and *I,* A blunt instrument is placed in contact with the root end of the crown through the buccal crypt and tapped with a mallet, driving the crown out of its crypt.

J and *K,* The flaps are replaced and sutured.

REMOVAL OF IMPACTED CUSPIDS IN CLASS III WHEN THE CROWN IS ON THE LABIAL SIDE AND THE ROOT EXTENDS INTO THE PALATE

If the crown of the impacted cuspid is on the labial surface of the maxilla, with the root extending to the lingual side of the bicuspid roots on the palate, the procedure that follows is used.

The incision for the flap is made around the necks of the teeth, and then to the mucobuccal fold at a 45-degree angle. Reflect the mucoperiosteum with a periosteal elevator (see *B* and *C* of Figure 5–108).

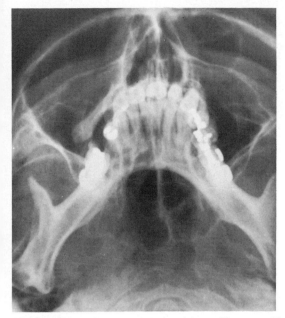

Figure 5–110 Unerupted malposed maxillary cuspid located in the anterior and lateral wall of the maxillary sinus. This tooth was removed by exposure of the cortical bone in this area with a large semicircular incision, removal of the bone covering the crown, grasping the crown with a forceps and rotation of the tooth until it was free. The maxillary sinus was not disturbed. An elevator could not be used because the surrounding bone was too thin to act as a fulcrum.

Remove the labial and buccal plate over the area with bone burs and chisels. Drill holes as described before, but be careful to control the depth of penetration to avoid injury to the roots of the teeth and to the maxillary sinus (see *C* and *D* of Figure 5–108).

Next attempt to *engage the crown with No. 286 forceps. The tooth is rotated mesially and distally, and toward the labial side,* and then is *removed from its bed.*

If this attempt is unsuccessful, cut off the crown, reflect a palatal flap, remove bone over the root and push the root out with a blunt instrument passed through the labial opening.

Clean out all debris, remove any sharp spicules of bone, and smooth the periphery of the labial and palatal osseous openings. Remove the tooth follicle, if present, and suture the flaps back into position; use black silk suture. Pack palate with gauze as described. Keep the gauze packing in place for 4 hours.

REMOVAL OF IMPACTED CUSPID IN AN EDENTULOUS MOUTH

The incision for the palatally impacted cuspid is along the crest of the ridge and back

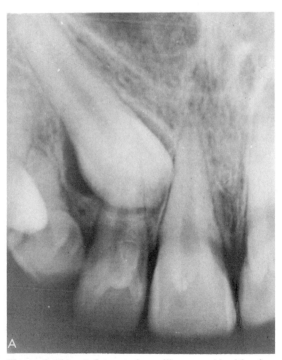

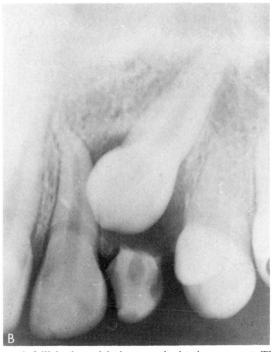

Figure 5–111 *A,* Impacted maxillary cuspid with a large tooth follicle that might be an early dentigerous cyst. The deciduous cuspid, which has a fully formed root, should be retained. *B,* A small dentigerous cyst appears to be developing around the crown of this impacted cuspid. The deciduous cuspid crown will not serve any useful purpose and should be extracted.

Photographic Case Report

BILATERAL LABIALLY IMPACTED MAXILLARY CUSPIDS, THE SURGICAL EXPOSURE OF THEIR CROWNS, AND THEIR SUBSEQUENT MOVEMENT INTO THE DENTAL ARCH BY THE ORTHODONTIST*

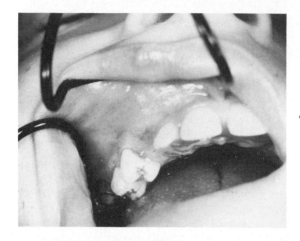

Figure 5–112 In this patient both maxillary cuspids were located labial to the arch.

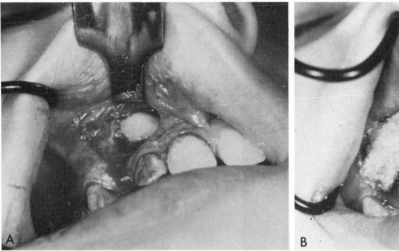

Figure 5–113 *A*, The crowns were exposed by excising the mucoperiosteal membrane and osseous structure covering the crowns. The opening must be a large one; otherwise, the tissue will grow back over the crown. *B*, Medicated cement mixed with cotton fibers is packed into each cavity.

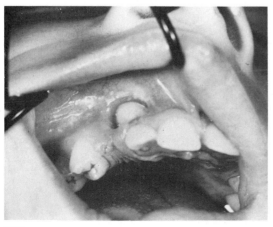

Figure 5–114 Soft tissue healed around the exposed crown.

---

*This case was carried to successful conclusion as the result of skilled orthodontic treatment by Dr. Joseph L. Polk of Pittsburgh.

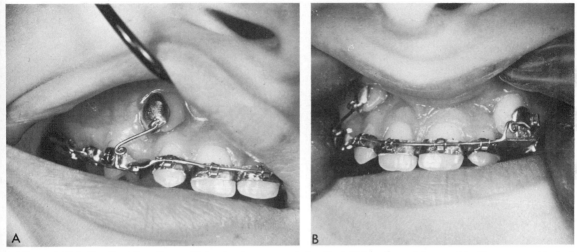

Figure 5–115 Small gold castings with hooks were cemented to the labial surface of the cuspids. These were attached to the orthodontic appliance.

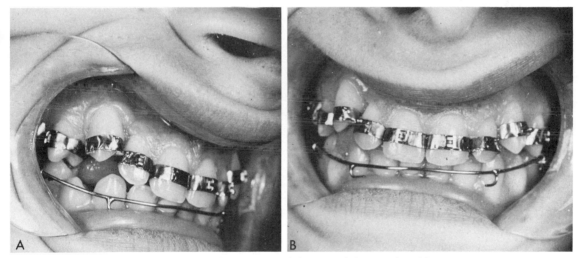

Figure 5–116 Cuspids moved almost to their normal position.

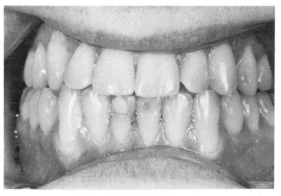

Figure 5–117 End result.

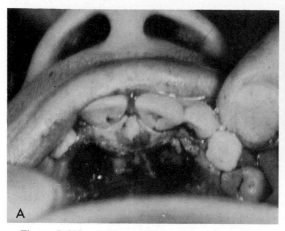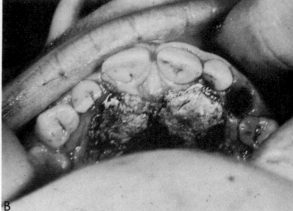

Figure 5–118 *A,* The maxillary permanent cuspids were impacted vertically in the palate. The overlying soft and osseous tissue is excised so that the complete contour of the crown is exposed. *B,* Spaces filled with medicated cement.

along the center of the palate for 1½ inches. The technique of exposure and removal is the same as already described. However, there is not the danger of exposure of the roots or trauma to adjacent teeth.

REMOVAL OF BILATERALLY IMPACTED CUSPIDS IN THE PALATE

The question of whether to remove one or both of these impacted teeth at one time depends on the difficulty of the case. In uncomplicated bilateral impactions in young, healthy adults, both teeth can be removed at one time. In difficult impactions, the teeth should probably be removed at different

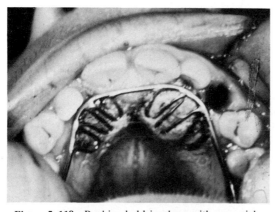

Figure 5–119 Packing held in place with a special appliance. The dressings are changed until the periphery of the opening epithelializes. In some cases the cuspids will now erupt (see Figures 5–120 to 5–123). In either case, the orthodontist now proceeds with his treatment.

times. Techniques have already been described.

The question of the type of palatal flap arises in these cases. A single bilateral flap is reflected, cutting the nasopalatine (incisive) neurovascular bundle where it enters the flap. The nerve and blood supply will be reestablished in the flap in a few weeks' time. The collateral blood supply is adequate to maintain the vitality of the flap (see Figure 5–106).

It is especially important to insert and maintain a palatal packing in these cases, as previously described!

SURGICAL PROCEDURES AS AN AID IN ORTHODONTIC TREATMENT

Surgical procedures may be undertaken to expose the crown of an impacted or unerupted tooth in the hope that it will erupt spontaneously, so that it can then be brought into alignment by orthodontic means.

Locate the unerupted tooth, using periapical radiographs, the shift-sketch x-ray technique and occlusal views.

Administer premedication, especially if the patient is a child.

Secure anesthesia, general or local.

Exposure of Palatally Located Unerupted Cuspids. Excise the soft and hard tissue over the area of the crown, past the height of contour of the crown (Fig. 5–118*A*). With the radiosurgical coagulation tip control the bleeding.

In children the bone is not too dense. Use bone burs to remove the overlying bone

(*Text continued on page 346*)

Photographic Case Report

BILATERAL PALATALLY IMPACTED CUSPIDS SURGICALLY EXPOSED AND MOVED INTO THE DENTAL ARCH BY ORTHODONTIC TREATMENT

B. F. DEWEL, D.D.S.

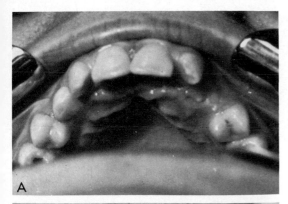

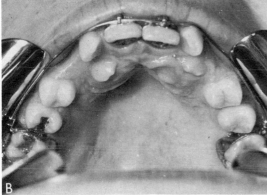

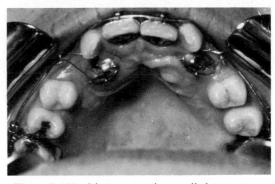

Figure 5–121 Ligature traction applied to cast caps was used to carry the cuspids buccally, after which rotation was accomplished by standard orthodontic procedures.

Figure 5–120 *A,* This is the first of a series of photographs illustrating the orthodontic correction of a palatally impacted right cuspid. It shows the case as it originally appeared before treatment. *B,* Surgical removal of the mucoperiosteum and palatal bone structure overlying the cuspid was accomplished 5 months prior to this photograph. The tooth erupted with no assistance other than operation.

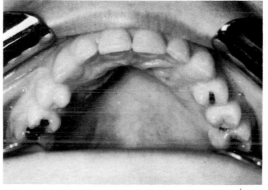

Figure 5–122 Normal arch form and tooth position are illustrated in this photograph taken 2 months after the removal of all appliances. The case was self-retentive.

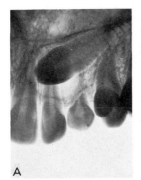
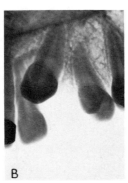
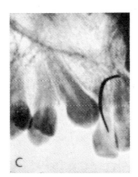
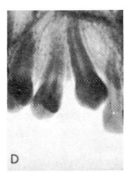

Figure 5–123 *A* and *B,* Intraoral roentgenograms provided partial evidence of the position of the impacted right cuspid. Stereoroentgenograms were not necessary in this case. *A,* Before operation; *B,* 5 months later.

C and *D,* The left cuspid improved its position only a little during the 5 months that the right cuspid made such marked progress. End-to-end occlusion with the lower cuspid prevented this tooth from further eruption. *C,* Beginning of treatment; *D,* 5 months later.

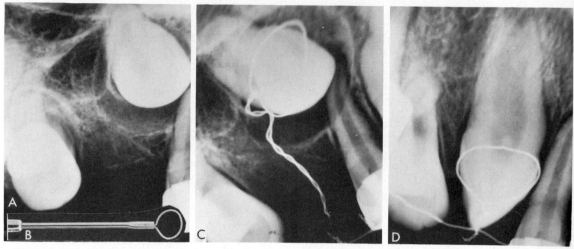

Figure 5–124 *A,* Impacted unerupted cuspid whose crown was exposed labially and "lassoed" with a wire ligature. *B* shows the wire loop ligature held in the tubular tip of the ligature cartridge. The loop is preformed to fit the impacted tooth and "pigtailed" in place by rotation of the instrument. *C* and *D,* The orthodontist then moves the cuspid into its place in the dental arch.

(*A, C* and *D,* Courtesy of Dr. Italo H. A. Gandelman. *B,* Courtesy of SRS Company, Napa, Calif.)

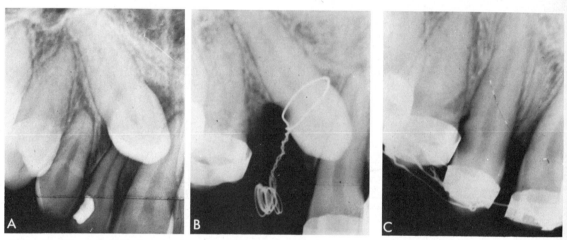

Figure 5–125 *A,* Labially impacted maxillary cuspid. The nonvital lateral incisor and the deciduous cuspid were extracted. *B,* During the removal of bone from around the crown the root at the neck of the cuspid was inadvertently cut into by the bur. *C,* Cuspid moved into place. (Courtesy of Dr. Italo H. A. Gandelman.)

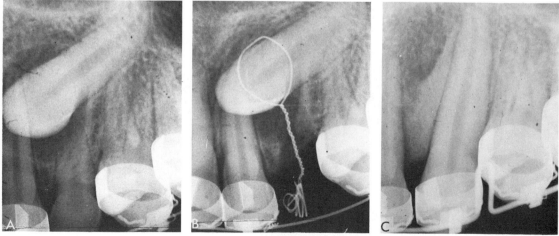

Figure 5–126 *See opposite page for legend.*

MANDIBULAR CUSPIDS

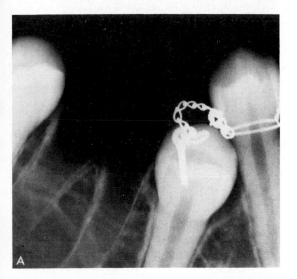

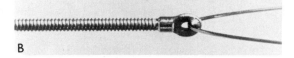

Figure 5–127   This assembly is used for impacted and malposed teeth and minor tooth movement. Anchors for elastic bands, chain links and ligature wires are included. (Courtesy of Whaledent, Inc., New York.)

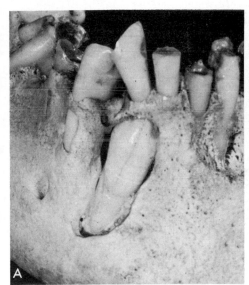
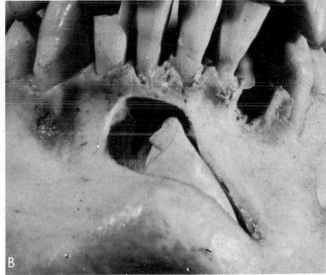

Figure 5–128   Anatomic specimens of unerupted impacted mandibular cuspids in the symphysis of the mandible. *A,* Vertical labial impaction of a cuspid. *B,* Semihorizontal labial impaction of a cuspid in the symphysis of the mandible. (*Note:* In dry specimens, such as these, the teeth become so dry that the crowns spontaneously split off, as shown.)

Because of the dense cortical bone found in the symphysis, these teeth are not easily elevated from their malpositions. After exposure of the crown by the reflection of a flap, and the removal of overlying bone, it can be decided whether or not the removal of the crown will facilitate the extraction of this tooth. (See Figure 5–131 for technique of removal.)

Figure 5–126   Another example of a case in which a labially impacted cuspid crown was exposed, the deciduous cuspid was extracted, and the orthodontist then moved the cuspid into its position in the arch. (Courtesy of Dr. Italo H. A. Gandelman.)

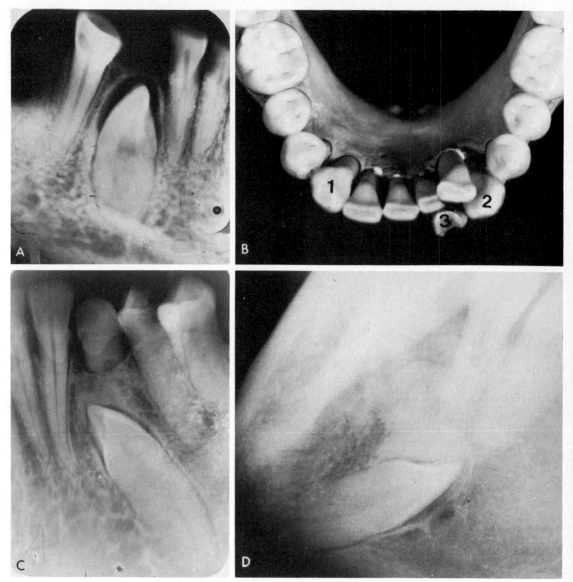

Figure 5–129 *A*, Vertically unerupted mandibular cuspid with what appears to be a small dentigerous cyst surrounding the crown. This patient, age 65, was unaware that he had this symptomless condition in his jaw. Marsupialization was proposed, not with any expectation that the cuspid would erupt but to prevent enlargement of the cyst. Patient refused but promised to have periodic examinations. We never saw him again.

B, Anatomic specimen. *1* indicates the right mandibular cuspid, fully erupted and in normal position and occlusion. *2* is the left mandibular cuspid, impacted beneath the mandibular left lateral incisor and first bicuspid. This situation was precipitated by the retention of the deciduous left lateral incisor (*3*), which is still crowded labially into the arch. In a young patient the deciduous lateral incisor would be extracted and the patient referred to an orthodontist.

C, Vertically impacted mandibular cuspid. It is not often that one sees a case in which the primary cuspid is still in position in the mandible of an adult.

D, Impacted mandibular cuspid at the inferior border of the mandible. Note the area of osteosclerosis superior to the crown. In both cases *C* and *D*, the patients were in their late fifties and the cuspids symptomless, so surgery was not advised. Periodic examination was recommended and followed by both patients for many years and removal was never indicated.

Figure 5–131 Excision of a vertically impacted mandibular cuspid. *A*, Outline of mucoperiosteal flap. *B*, Holes are drilled through the labial cortical bone around the crown. *C*, The crown is fully exposed. *D*, An attempt is made to luxate and remove the cuspid with elevators. *E*, If the crown is locked, cut a groove and snap the crown off at the gingival line. *F*, Expose more of the root and make another groove. *G*, Remove the root. *H*, Suture the flap back into place.

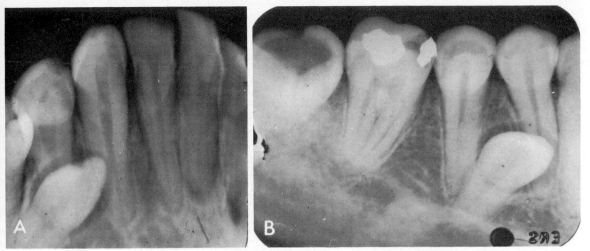

Figure 5–130 Impacted supernumerary mandibular cuspid with a small developing dentigerous cyst. These two roentgenograms illustrate the shift-sketch method of localization. *A* is the first roentgenogram taken. *B* is the second. Observe the change in the position of the supernumerary cuspid crown from *A* to *B*. In *A* it appears as though the supernumerary cuspid crown partially overlaps the erupted cuspid root. In *B* the x-ray tube has been moved distally and the supernumerary crown has moved away from the cuspid root. The rule is: if the unerupted tooth moves in the *same direction as* the x-ray tube, the unerupted tooth is to the *lingual* side. This supernumerary impacted cuspid is in the lingual area of the mandible.

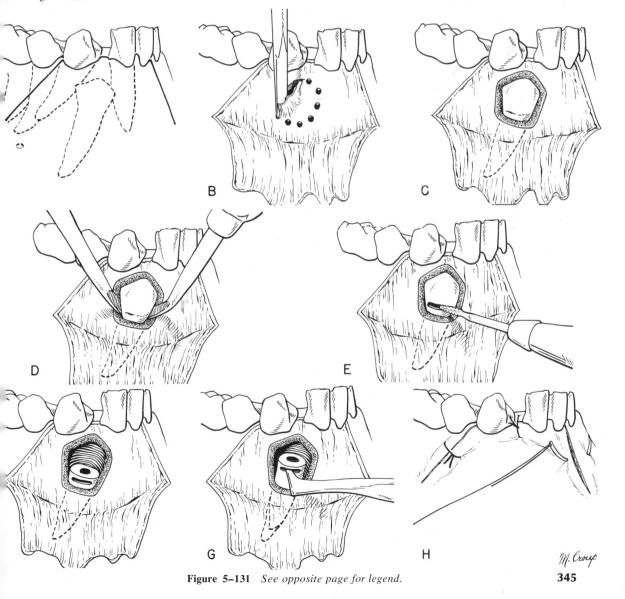

Figure 5–131 *See opposite page for legend.*

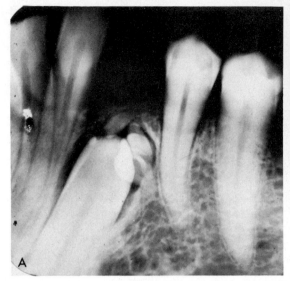
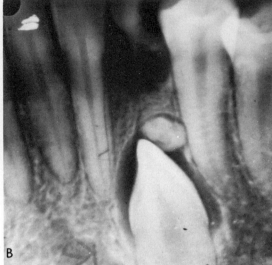

Figure 5–132 *A* and *B*, The eruption of these mandibular cuspids has been prevented by the presence of compound odontomas in the tooth follicles, as can easily be seen in these radiographs. The crowns should be exposed and the odontomas excised. Because this wasn't done when the normal eruption force was present for both of these cuspids, they will have to be moved up into place by the combined help of the orthodontist and the oral surgeon.

down to the crown of the tooth and past its height of contour.

Fill the cavity with a medicated cement consisting of zinc oxide, eugenol and powdered rosin. Incorporate asbestos fibers or cotton fibers into the mass of cement until it is thick; then pack this mass of cement around, under and over the tooth (Fig. 5–118*B*).

Cover the area with burlew dry foil; burnish into place; leave in place for 4 to 5 days. If difficulty is encountered in keeping these dressings in place, an appliance such as is shown in Figure 5–119 can be used.

IMPACTED MANDIBULAR CUSPIDS

Impacted mandibular cuspids are usually vertically impacted and are found close to the labial surface (Fig. 5–128*A*). Occasionally they are located beneath the apices of the mandibular incisors, lying transversely at a 45-degree angle to the lower border of the mandible (Fig. 5–128*B*). Rarely are they found in a horizontal position or on the lingual side of the dental arch. However, in Figure 5–129*D* a radiograph is shown of a semi-horizontally impacted mandibular cuspid beneath the apices of the bicuspids. Also in this figure are radiographs of vertical cuspid impactions and a mandibular cuspid dentigerous cyst. The labial or lingual positions of these teeth must be determined by the occlusal x-ray film.

Technique for Removal of Mandibular Cuspids. A technique for the excision of labially impacted mandibular cuspids, as shown in Figure 5–132, follows.

In all mandibular cuspid impactions make incisions for a large flap. Reflect the flap and cut the muscle origins that are located in the operative area.

Drill holes through the labial cortical plate of bone around the crown with spear-point burs. Be careful not to cut the roots of the adjacent teeth. Remove the cortical bone with a chisel or crosscut fissure burs.

Expose the crown completely, using bone burs. This process is known as "windowing" the cortex.

Try to luxate and remove the cuspid with elevators No. 73 and No. 74 placed beneath the crown and using the labial cortical bone as a fulcrum.

If the crown is locked, cut a groove and snap the crown off at the gingival line.

Expose more of the root and make another groove.

Remove the root with a No. 11L or No. 11R cross bar elevator, using the buccal cortical bone as a fulcrum and the wheel-and-axle work principle to lift the root.

Suture the flap into place with 000 black silk in an atraumatic needle.

Photographic Case Report

DENTIGEROUS CYST ABOUT THE CROWN OF AN UNERUPTED IMPACTED LEFT MANDIBULAR PERMANENT CUSPID IN A 12-YEAR-OLD BOY

Paul M. Burbank, D.M.D.

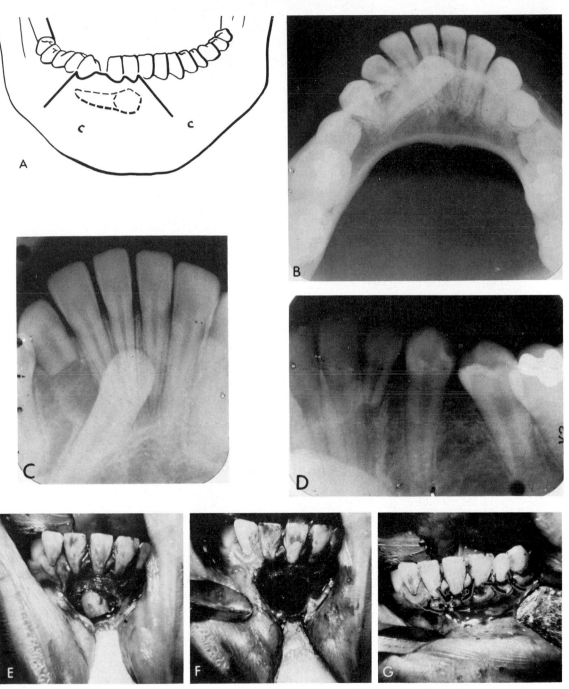

Figure 5–133 *A,* Outline for the mucoperiosteal flap. *B* to *D,* Periapical and occlusal views of the impacted cuspid. *E,* The mucoperiosteal flap has been reflected, the overlying thin cortical bone removed and the cuspid crown exposed. The crown has been cut from the root at the gingival line with a crosscut fissure bur. This permits its removal without necessitating the removal of gingival cortical bone from around the necks of the permanent central incisors. *F,* The cuspid crown has been extracted, the cuspid root has been moved up into the space thus created and removed, and the cystic sac has been enucleated. *G,* The mucoperiosteal flap is replaced and sutured into position with 000 silk in atraumatic needles. These are passed through the crests of the interdental soft tissues. This technique is illustrated diagrammatically in Figure 5–131.

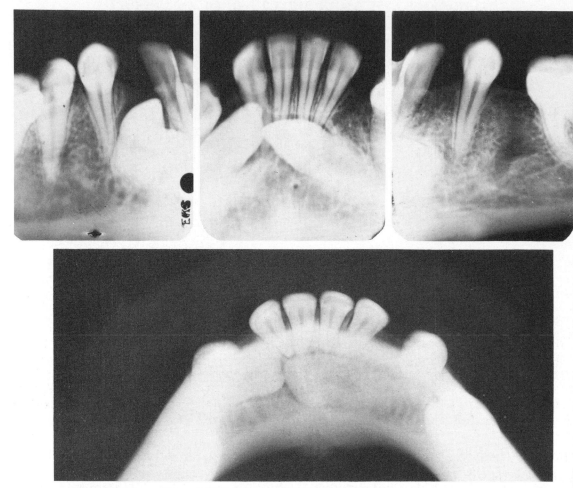

Figure 5–134   Bilaterally impacted mandibular cuspids.

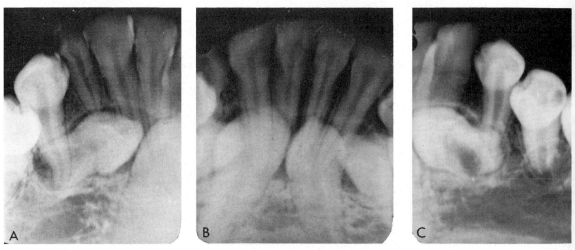

Figure 5–135   Bilateral vertically impacted mandibular cuspids whose crowns are in contact in the midline of the symphysis of the mandible labial to the central and lateral incisors. In addition, there are right and left supernumerary rudimentary partially formed cuspids.

This is a case that required consultation with the orthodontist to decide whether it would be feasible to remove the supernumerary teeth and then move the cuspids into these areas, as well as to expand the arch. It was agreed that this could and should be done.

MANDIBULAR BICUSPIDS

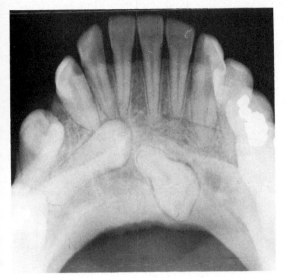

Figure 5-136 The symphysis of the mandible is an unusual location for bilateral mandibular first bicuspids.

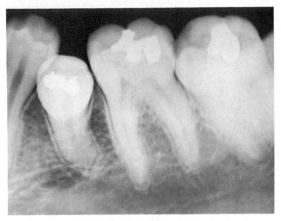

Figure 5-137 Vertically impacted mandibular second bicuspid.

IMPACTED MANDIBULAR BICUSPIDS

Impacted mandibular bicuspids (premolars) are usually found in the vertical or near vertical position, and more frequently with a lingual inclination than with a buccal one (Figs. 5-137 and 5-138). Impacted supernu-

merary mandibular bicuspids are frequently found. Of all the supernumerary teeth that may develop in various areas in the dental arches, the supernumerary mandibular bicuspid most nearly exactly duplicates the normally erupted bicuspids. They rarely present the rudimentary forms found elsewhere in the arches.

(Text continued on page 357)

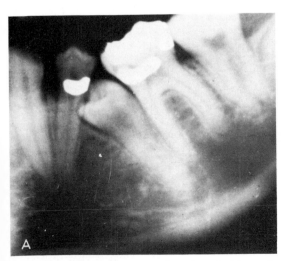

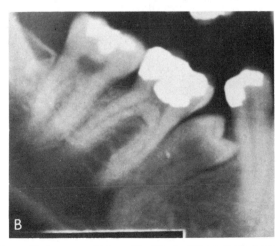

Figure 5-138 Further examples of vertical impactions of mandibular second bicuspids. Most of these teeth have a lingual inclination. See Figure 5-139 for excisional technique.

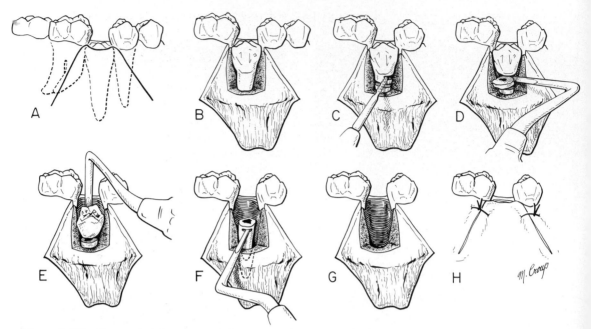

Figure 5–139   Figures 5–137 and 5–138 demonstrate impacted mandibular second bicuspids whose eruption was prevented by the partial closure of the space in the dental arch. This was caused by forward movement of the first molar, and so only a portion of the occlusal surface of the bicuspid was visible.

Vertically impacted bicuspids such as this are removed after a flap is made, as illustrated in *A*. The flap is reflected *(B)*, and the buccal cortical bone is removed from around the crown and the gingival third of the root *(B and C)*. Additional space is created with burs, mesially and distally, beneath the height of contour of the crown, so that after a segment of the root has been removed by cutting through it with a crosscut fissure bur *(C)*, and removing a section *(D)*, the crown can then drop down into the space created by the removal of this section and be moved out buccally with an Apexo elevator *(E)*. A purchase point is then drilled into the root *(F)*; an Apexo elevator is placed into the purchase point, and with the buccal bone serving as a fulcrum, the remaining portion of the root is elevated from the alveolus. The flap is replaced and sutured into position *(H)*.

If these vertically impacted teeth are on the buccal side of the arch, their removal is a relatively uncomplicated process, the technique being that described in Figure 5–131 for mandibular cuspid labial impactions. If, however, as happens occasionally, the bicuspid is in lingual position, then the technique illustrated in Figure 5–148 is used.

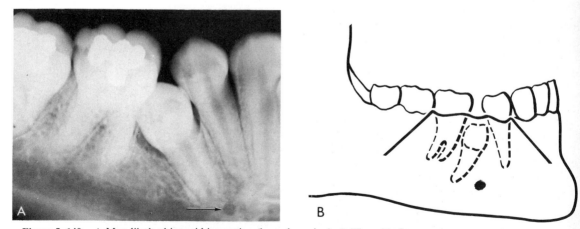

Figure 5–140   *A*, Mandibular bicuspid impaction (buccal version). *B*, The wide flap necessary to expose the operative site and to protect the neurovascular bundle which exits into this flap.

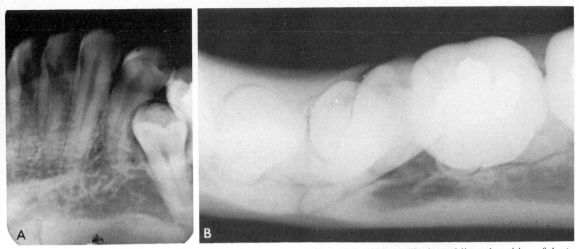

Figure 5–141 *A,* Lingual vertical impaction of a second mandibular bicuspid. *B,* The buccal-lingual position of these teeth can be demonstrated by an occlusal view, which is mandatory in these cases.

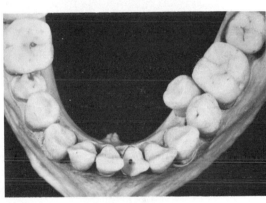

Figure 5–142 Anatomic specimen of a lingually malposed, fully erupted mandibular second bicuspid. This tooth is not impacted.

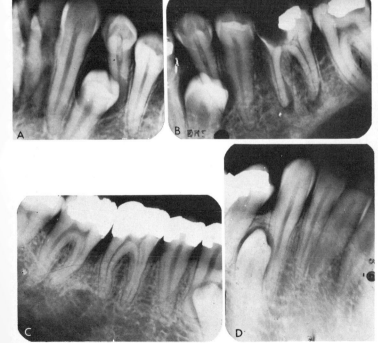

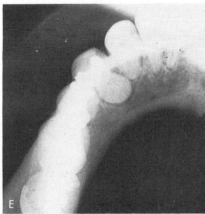

Figure 5–143 These lingual vertically impacted supernumerary bicuspids were removed with the technique shown in Figure 5–148.

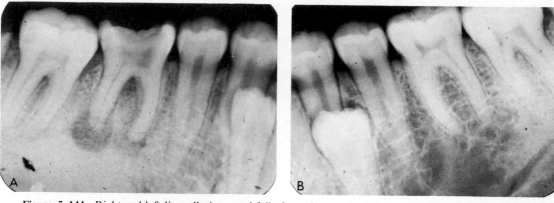

Figure 5-144 Right and left lingually impacted fully formed normal supernumerary mandibular bicuspids.

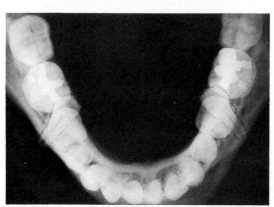

Figure 5-145 Occlusal radiograph of the impacted supernumerary mandibular bicuspids in a transverse vertical position in the jaw, with the crowns projecting lingually and the roots projecting into the buccal cortical bone.

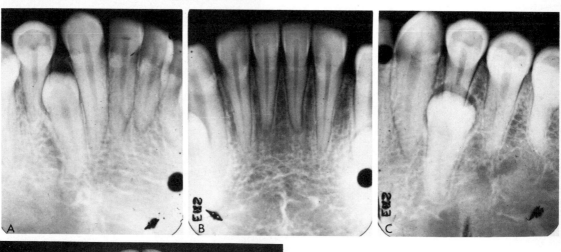

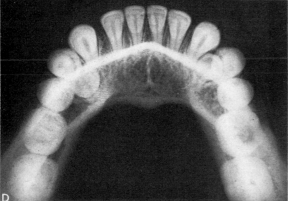

Figure 5-146 A to C, Lingual bilateral supernumerary fully formed vertically impacted mandibular bicuspids. D, Occlusal view confirms the complete containment of these teeth in the lingual bone.

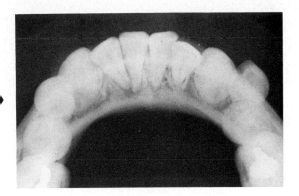

Figure 5–147 Occlusal radiograph of a buccal vertically impacted mandibular bicuspid. These are not seen as frequently as are the lingually positioned bicuspids.

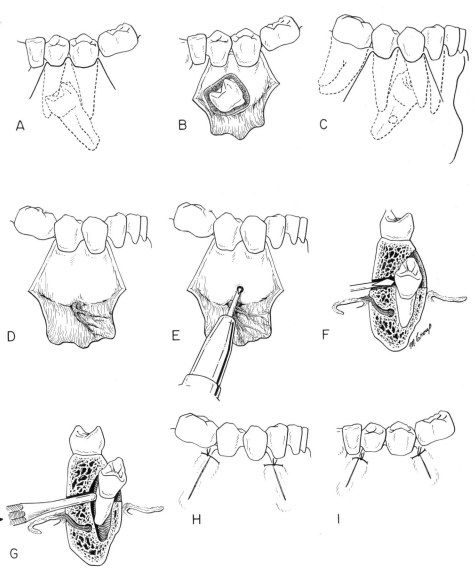

Figure 5–148 Surgical excision of a lingual vertically impacted mandibular first bicuspid. *A* and *B*, Lingual flap reflected and covering bone removed. *C* and *D*, Buccal flap incised and reflected. *E* and *F*, With a large spear-point bur a pathway is drilled upward from the buccal side toward the lingual side, contacting the crown of the impacted tooth. *G*, A blunt instrument is passed through the hole, contacting the crown, and then tapped with a mallet, driving the impacted tooth up and out of its crypt. *H* and *I*, Buccal and lingual flaps are sutured back into place.

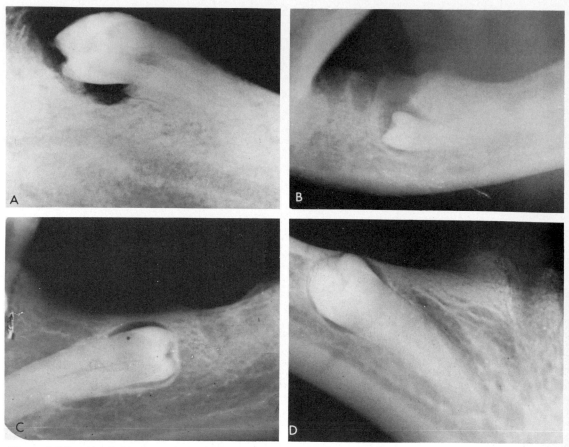

Figure 5–149 *A* to *D*, Horizontally impacted mandibular bicuspids in edentulous areas of the mandible. There isn't any question about the necessity of removing *A*, *C* and *D* because of the certainty of traumatic irritation from dentures. In *B* the radiolucency around the crown requires further investigation to confirm the need to excise it. Is there a fistula draining this area? Was there a recent extraction or multiple extractions, as the alveolus-like areas of radiolucency would indicate? If there is infection, then surgery is indicated, but to avoid destroying the alveolar ridge, occlusal views should be taken to determine whether or not a buccal or lingual approach should be made to excise this tooth. Perhaps even an extraoral exposure would be indicated.

Figure 5–150   Examples of horizontally impacted mandibular bicuspids. See Figure 5–153 for excisional technique.

Figure 5–151   Bilateral impacted mandibular first and second bicuspids in a 10-year-old child.

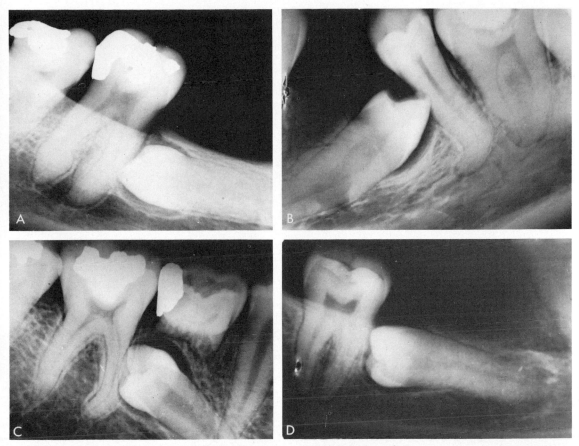

Figure 5–150 *See opposite page for legend.*

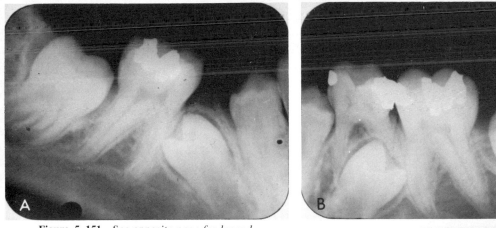

Figure 5–151 *See opposite page for legend.*

Figure 5–152 Horizontal impaction of a mandibular second bicuspid. See Figure 5–153 for operative technique.

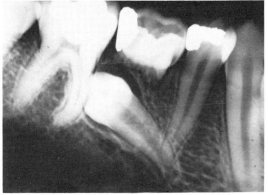

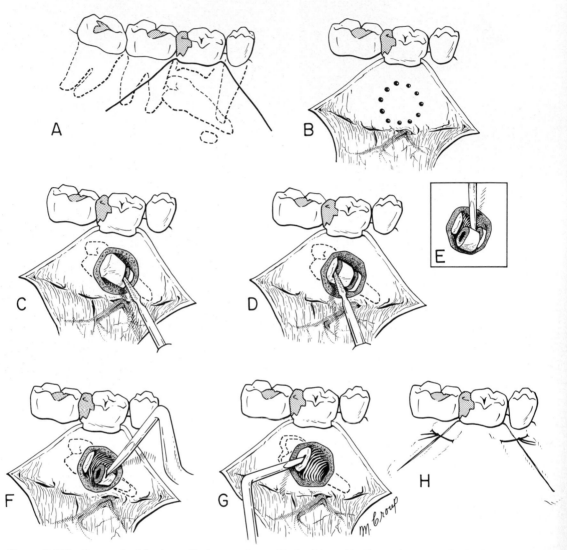

Figure 5–153   Removal of horizontally impacted mandibular bicuspid. Shown is a completely formed left mandibular second bicuspid with the crown engaging the mesial root of the first molar. Rarely is it possible to move a fully formed tooth surgically so that normal eruption might eventually take place. The teeth that respond best to surgical movement with subsequent normal eruption are those whose roots are not completely formed. Possibly those teeth whose roots are half formed offer the best potentialities for continued development and eventual eruption into a normal position in the arch after surgical repositioning.

It was desirable, in the case illustrated here, to remove the bicuspid without encroaching upon or damaging the primary molar, the first molar or the first bicuspid. This was accomplished with the technique that follows.

A flap with a wide base is made, as illustrated in *A,* to avoid the mental foramen. The flap is reflected *(B),* and it will be seen that the vessels that exit from the mental foramen are contained within the reflected flap. An opening is made through the cortex by drilling a series of holes through the cortex with a spear-point surgical bur. These holes are then connected with a crosscut fissure bur, and this segment of cortical plate is removed. From around that portion of the root that is exposed, as shown in *C,* additional bone is removed superiorly and inferiorly with small round burs. Then, with a crosscut fissure bur, as shown in *C* and *D,* a segment of the root is cut through and removed, as shown in *E.* The root is moved forward after a purchase point has been drilled into it, as shown in *F,* by means of the Apexo elevator, with the cortical plate serving as a fulcrum. The crown is next engaged; the Apexo elevator tip is placed into a purchase point drilled into the substance of the crown, and with the buccal cortical plate serving as the fulcrum, the crown is moved backward into the space that has been created and is removed from the crypt *(G).* The flap is now replaced and sutured into position *(H).*

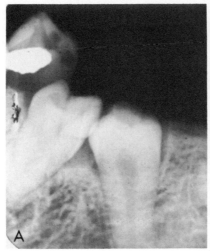

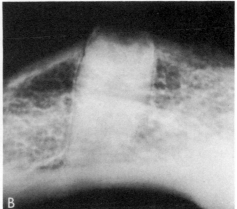

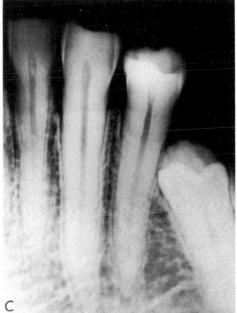

Figure 5–154 Examples of vertical impactions of mandibular bicuspids.

EXTRAORAL REMOVAL OF IMPACTED TEETH

Occasionally the malposition of the unerupted tooth is such that the extraoral approach is indicated for its removal. Such a case is illustrated in Figures 5–155 and 5–156. This patient had had swelling and pain in this area, for which an intraoral incision for drainage had been made some weeks prior to the admission of the patient to the hospital for removal of the tooth and enucleation of the cyst. There was no swelling at this time. The operation was performed under general anesthesia.

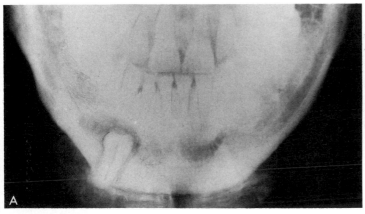

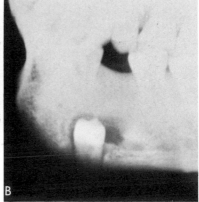

Figure 5–155 Impacted mandibular bicuspid with a dentigerous cyst at the lower border of the mandible. See Figure 5–156 for the technique for removing this bicuspid and the cyst.

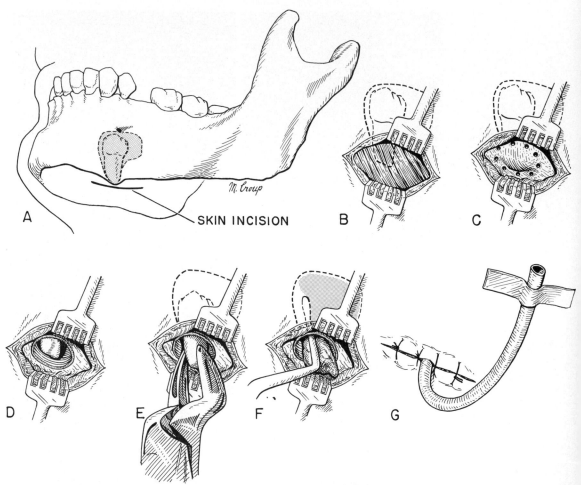

SKIN INCISION

A   B   C   D   E   F   G

Figure 5–156 *A*, Unerupted mandibular second bicuspid with a dentigerous cyst. See radiographs of this case in Figure 5–155. *B*, Incision through the skin exposing the triangularis and platysma muscle bundles. *C*, Muscle incised through to the inferior border of the mandible, revealing the periosteum, which was incised and reflected, exposing the buccal cortical bone and inferior border of the mandible. A series of holes was drilled through the cortical bone around the periphery of the cyst. *D*, The section of cortical bone was removed with a chisel and crosscut fissure burs, and a window was cut out of the cyst, exposing the apex of the bicuspid. *E*, The root was grasped with a No. 286 forceps and the tooth removed. Care must be taken to make sure that the circumference of the opening through the cortical plate is a little larger than the largest diameter of the crown. *F*, The remaining portion of the cyst is now enucleated. *G*, Insertion of a rubber catheter into the surgical wound prior to closing. This tube permits irrigation with penicillin in normal saline solution.

IMPACTED MAXILLARY BICUSPIDS

These are comparatively rare. Two cases are illustrated here in Figures 5–157 and 5–158. A dentigerous cyst enveloping the crown of a palatally located maxillary bicuspid is exceedingly rare (Fig. 5–159). Localization of an embedded maxillary bicuspid is very difficult. Many are contained within the alveolar ridge. However, an occlusal radiograph should always be taken to aid in locali-

zation, and the shift-sketch technique should be used.

REMOVAL OF IMPACTED MAXILLARY BICUSPIDS

The technique for removing impacted maxillary bicuspids is dependent on the location, the formation of the tooth, its relationship to the adjacent teeth, the maxillary sinus, and
(*Text continued on page 364*)

MAXILLARY BICUSPIDS

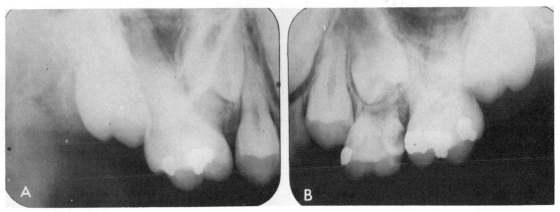

Figure 5–157 Impacted maxillary right first and second bicuspids and left second bicuspid in an 11-year-old. Note the congenital absence of the maxillary third molars.

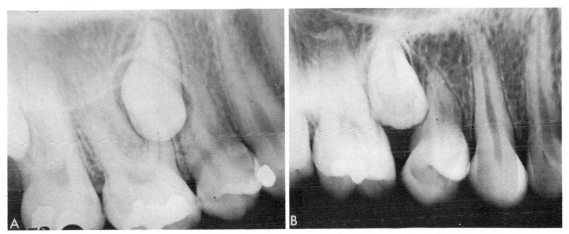

Figure 5–158 *A,* Vertical impaction of the maxillary second bicuspid on the buccal side of the arch. Note the well-circumscribed radiolucent area about the crown. The well-defined osteosclerotic border around the radiolucent area is strongly suggestive of a dentigerous cyst. *B,* An impacted maxillary second bicuspid with the crown on the buccal side of the alveolar ridge and the roots in the palate.

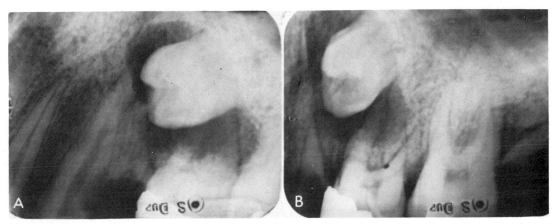

Figure 5–159 A dentigerous cyst containing a malpositioned maxillary bicuspid. On the basis of the shift-sketch roentgenographic technique this tooth is closer to the buccal than to the lingual side of the alveolar ridge.

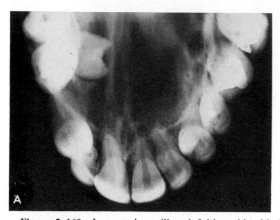

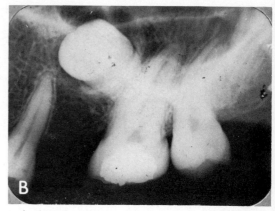

Figure 5–160   Impacted maxillary left bicuspid, with the crown in the palatal bone and the root in the buccal cortical plate.

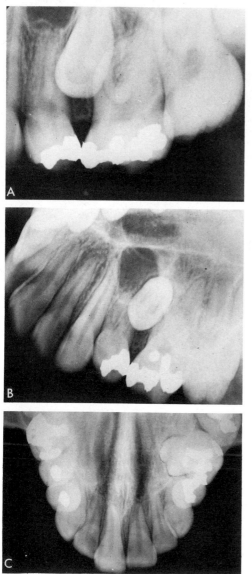

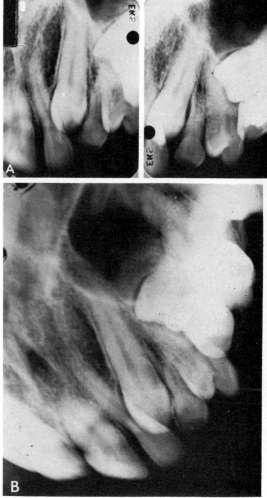

Figure 5–161   *A* to *C,* Series of radiographs of one impacted maxillary second bicuspid.

Figure 5–162   Palatally impacted maxillary cuspid and bicuspid.

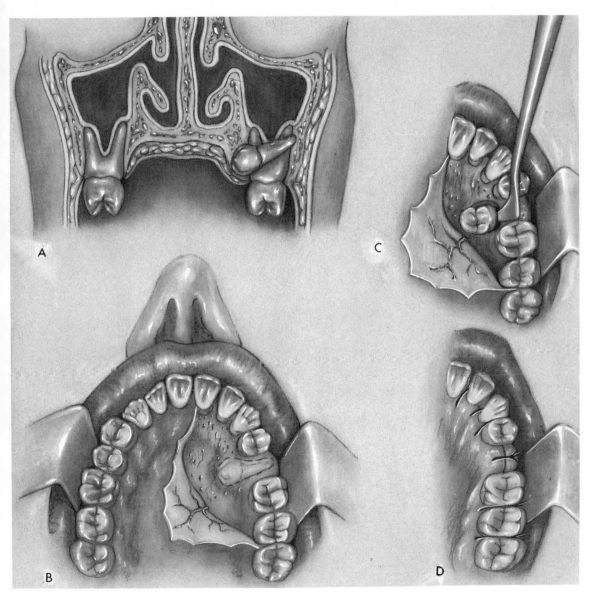

Figure 5–163 Surgical excision of a maxillary left bicuspid with crown in palatal bone and root in the buccal cortical plate. *A,* Sagittal section showing the position of the impacted malposed second bicuspid and its anatomic relationship to the maxillary sinus. *B,* This is one of the few areas in the oral cavity in which a so-called "envelope flap" will provide adequate access. Note that the posterior palatine vessels are elevated with the flap. This type of flap is necessary in this area to avoid the danger of cutting across the anterior palatine vessels, with subsequent hemorrhage. *C,* The crown of the bicuspid is exposed, and a purchase point or groove is cut into the neck. A No. 11L elevator tip is inserted into the groove, and with the crest of the alveolar ridge as a fulcrum, the tooth is removed. If adequate exposure of the crown will permit, the beaks of a No. 286 forceps can grasp the crown, and with careful luxation the tooth can be loosened and removed. *D,* Flap replaced and sutured with 000 silk.

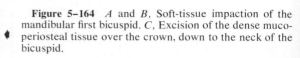

Figure 5–164 *A* and *B*, Soft-tissue impaction of the mandibular first bicuspid. *C*, Excision of the dense mucoperiosteal tissue over the crown, down to the neck of the bicuspid.

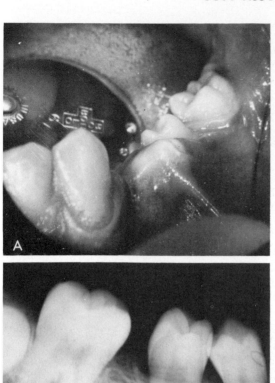

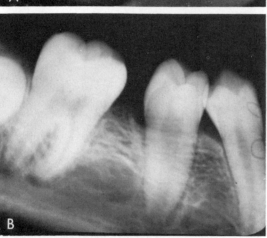

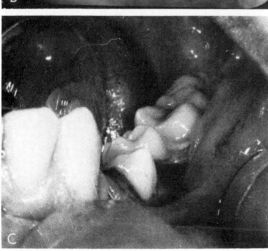

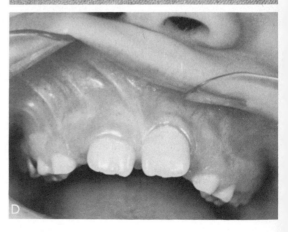

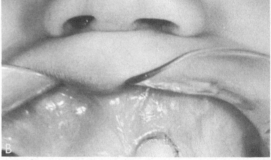

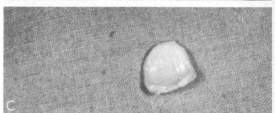

Figure 5–165 *A*, Soft-tissue impaction of the maxillary left central incisor. *B*, and *C*, Excision of dense cartilage-like tissue, completely exposing the labial surface and the incisal edge of the tooth. Note that the excised tissue *(C)* retains its rigid contour even after its removal. *D*, The central incisor was fully erupted within three weeks. See Figure 5–169 for technique.

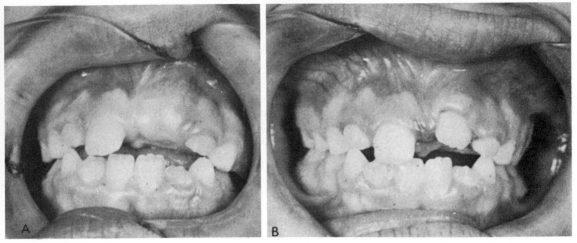

Figure 5–166 *A,* A soft-tissue impaction of the maxillary left central incisor. *B,* The thick fibrous tissue over the unerupted crown was removed, exposing the labial and incisal surfaces. The tooth began to erupt almost immediately, as shown here a week later. See Figure 5–169 for this technique.

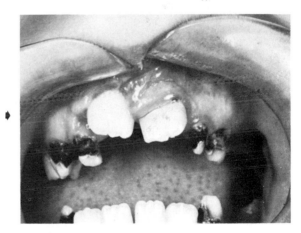

Figure 5–167 A postoperative view of a case similar to that in Figure 5–166 2 weeks after the labial surface and the incisal edge of the maxillary right central incisor were exposed by the technique shown in Figure 5–169.

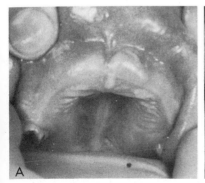
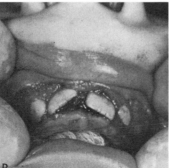
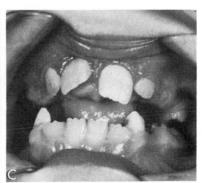

Figure 5–168 *A,* Fibromatosis of the maxilla that has prevented the eruption of the permanent teeth in this 9-year-old boy. *B,* Teeth exposed widely. *C,* Three weeks postoperatively.

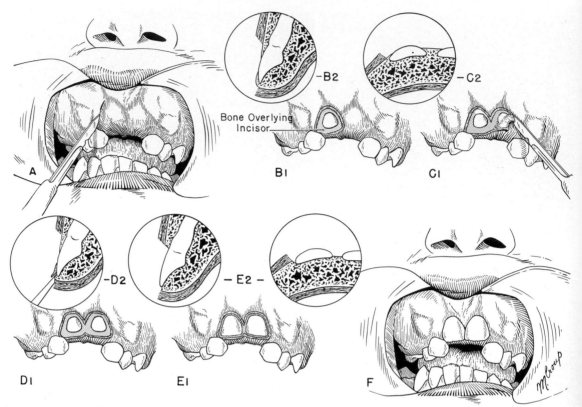

Figure 5–169　Fibrous tissue excision and osteotomy to allow the eruption of impacted unerupted maxillary central incisors. Drawings made of an actual patient.

A, Diagram showing the initial incision with a No. 15 blade. Note the two swellings marking the attempts of the central incisors to erupt. *B1*, Incision completed around the periphery of the right bulbous area, revealing the underlying retaining cortical plate and a portion of the labial surface of the crown. *B2*, Cross section showing the position of the tooth in the alveolus and the amount of eruption that has so far occurred. Note the thickness of the fibrous tissue. *C1*, Completing the left peripheral incision. *C2*, Horizontal section through the alveolus showing the thickness of the fibrous tissue and the amount of osseous retention. *D1*, Excision of tissue overlying both incisors completed. Note how the periphery was followed in both cases and the bevel of the incision. *D2*, Removal of the bone with the chisel. Note that the bevel of the chisel faces the bone to obtain a shaving action rather than deep gouging. *E1*, Complete labial surfaces of both crowns exposed to height of contour. *E2*, Cross and horizontal sections showing the labial and incisal surfaces now free of retaining fibrous and osseous structure. *F*, Postoperative view showing the central incisors now prepared to complete their eruption into normal position.

the nasal cavity, and whether it is involved in a cyst. If the bicuspid is located buccally, or is in the alveolar process midway between the buccal and lingual surfaces, a large buccal flap is reflected and overlying osseous tissue is removed with burs and chisels to expose the crown. The tooth may have to be sectioned in order to facilitate its removal.

If the bicuspid is mostly in the palatal process of the maxilla, a large palatal flap is reflected starting at the gingival line of the lateral incisor and continuing distally around the necks of all the posterior teeth on that side until the mesial-lingual angle of the second molar is reached. If the full thickness of the mucoperiosteal tissue is now reflected, this creates what is called an "envelope flap," which gives inadequate exposure to the operative site, so an incision is made from the lingual side of the lateral incisor to the midline of the palate. This then permits the palatal flap to be reflected and eliminates working in a trough, as one is forced to do if he uses the "envelope flap." When freeing the full thickness of the mucoperiosteal (that is, including the periosteum) covering the palatal process, we lift with the flap its contained anterior palatine artery, vein and nerve. This

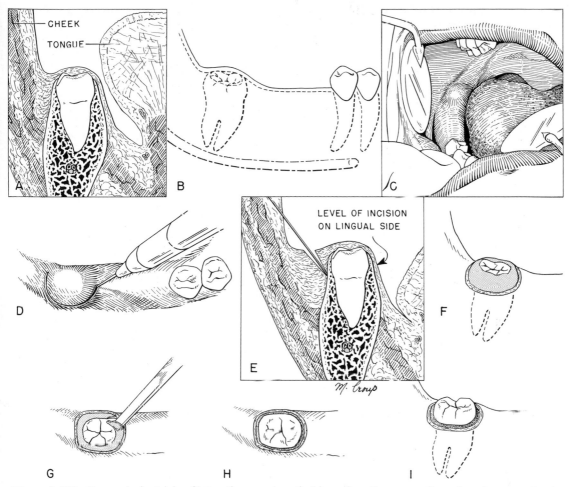

Figure 5-170   Removal of retaining fibrous tissue and cortical bone from the crown of a molar whose eruption has been prevented, in order to allow the eruption of that tooth.

A and B, Sections showing the heavy restraining band of fibrous tissue, and accompanying alveolar bone, extending onto the occlusal surface of the unerupted molar. *C,* Intraoral view showing the bulge caused by the retained tooth. *D,* Buccal portion of incision of fibrous tissue made with a radiosurgical knife. It is difficult to cut this tissue because it compresses and waves under the pressure of the scalpel blade. For this reason, as well as the excess bleeding that accompanies this operation, the radiosurgical knife is the ideal method to remove this dense, highly vascular tissue. *E,* Radiosurgical knife held at approximately 45 degrees and incision made into fibrous tissue down to the area of the gingival line of the retained crown. *F,* Removal of fibrous tissue around the height of contour, revealing a portion of the occlusal surface of the tooth and the encasing cortical bone. *G,* Removal of cortical bone with mallet and chisel. *H,* Occlusal surface of retained molar exposed. *I,* Crown of molar exposed with both fibrous tissue and alveolar bone removed down to below the height of contour.

avoids trauma to this important neurovascular bundle, and the danger of a most difficult-to-control hemorrhage.

Once the operative site is adequately exposed, then the same technique may be used for exposure and removal of the bicuspid as is used for the excision of palatally impacted cuspids. Admittedly, however, access is much more difficult. In addition, care must be taken not to involve the nasal cavity or the maxillary sinus. Small openings may be created and are of no concern because when

the palatal flap is returned and sutured into place, healing will normally follow.

SOFT-TISSUE IMPACTIONS

Fibromatosis Preventing the Eruption of Teeth.   The eruption of teeth can be, and often is, prevented by dense fibrous tissue. This is frequently observed in cases of delayed eruption of the permanent central incisors, in which early loss of primary teeth with subsequent masticatory trauma to the ridge results in fibromatosis. Mandibular third molars for which the approximating teeth have been lost sometimes slowly attempt to erupt, carrying with the crown the alveolar process and dense, fibrous mucoperiosteal membrane that is found in this region. Many times fibers of the buccinator muscle are contained in this tissue.

To expose these teeth adequately the technique that is illustrated in Figures 5–169 and 5–170 should be followed. The most frequent error in these cases is *inadequate exposure!*

Case Report No. 4

CLEIDOCRANIAL DYSOSTOSIS

L. D., aged 16 years, was referred with the complaint that he still had his maxillary anterior "baby teeth," and so was self-conscious about his appearance (Fig. 5–171).

General Appearance. The body had the typically enlarged skull with a bulging forehead (Fig. 5–172) from the hydrocephalic pressure that expanded the cranial vault, inasmuch as the fontanelles and sutures had remained open. When he removed his shirt it was apparent that there was defective development of the clavicles. However, he could not quite bring his shoulders together (Fig. 5–173).

Oral Examination. In the anterior maxilla were four widely separated primary incisors and cuspids that were abraded halfway to the gingival line. In the left maxilla a bicuspid was present, and the first and second permanent molars. In the right maxilla the space usually occupied by the perma-

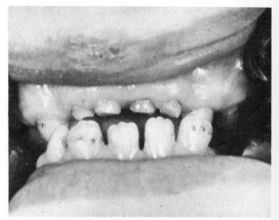

Figure 5–171 Retained abraded deciduous maxillary six anterior teeth in patient aged 16 with cleidocranial dysostosis (see page 374).

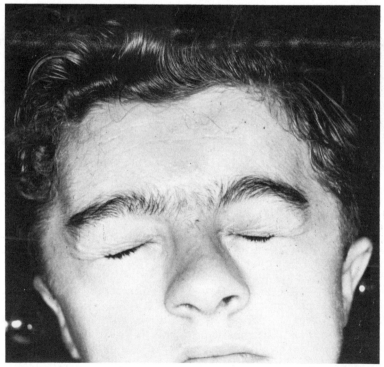

Figure 5–172 Large head, out of proportion to the bones of the face, with a bulging forehead and prominent cranial bosses.

nent bicuspid was edentulous, and the first and second molars were present.

The permanent mandibular incisors were in place. The right primary cuspid was present, the right primary molars were missing, and the bicuspids were not visible. The right mandibular first and second permanent molars were in position. The left mandibular primary and permanent cuspid and primary molars were missing. The permanent bicuspids were not visible. The mandibular first and second molars on this side were present.

Report on Dental Roentgenograms. See Figure 5–174 and the legend for this report.

Impression. In view of the arrested dental development, the overlong retention of the primary teeth, the delay in the eruption of the permanent teeth, the large number of supernumerary teeth, the large skull, and the defective development of the clavicles, a tentative diagnosis of cleidocranial dysostosis was made.

Hospital Admission Notes. This 16-year-old white boy was admitted to the hospital for study and for tonsillectomy and adenoidectomy because of frequent sore throat.

Physical Examination. The patient had prominence of the clavicles in the outer thirds and spine of the scapulae, but with a normal range of motion of shoulders. It was thought that there was some bilateral congenital abnormality of the shoulder girdle. In addition, there was a large, triangular, flattened skull with teleorism, which could have been a rachitic skull or possibly a hydrocephalus.

Funnel chest was present. The tonsils were ragged and hypertrophied. There were six upper primary teeth.

Laboratory Data. Three urinalyses were essentially negative. Blood cholesterol was 125 mg. per 100 cc. The blood count was as follows: hemoglobin, 15 gm.; red blood cells, 4,650,000; white blood cells, 7600, with 71 per cent polymorphonuclears and 24 per cent lymphocytes. The bleeding time was 1 minute and 30 seconds; the coagulation time 4 minutes and 40 seconds. A Kahn test was negative. Tuberculin tests, 1:10,000 and 1:1000 were negative. The basal metabolic rate was plus 19.

Roentgen Examination. For the details of this examination see the legends under Figures 5–175 to 5–178.

Treatment. The patient was hospitalized for additional studies and for the removal of his diseased tonsils. It was also decided to remove the upper primary anterior teeth at the same time and remove some of the osseous structure overlying the permanent teeth. It was thought that this procedure, plus thyroid medication, might stimulate the eruption of these teeth. If not, then a partial maxillary denture would answer his complaint about his appearance.

These procedures were carried out. Six months later, there was no sign that the permanent teeth had moved. Although the patient's basal metabolic rate was plus 19, he was put on ¼ grain of thyroid daily.

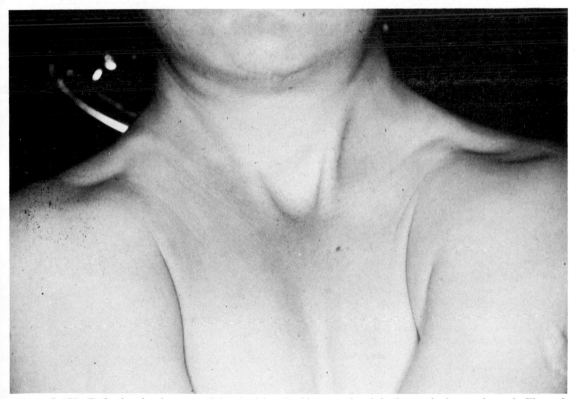

Figure 5–173 Defective development of the clavicles. In this case a break in the continuity, as shown in Figure 5–175, permits near approximation of the shoulders.

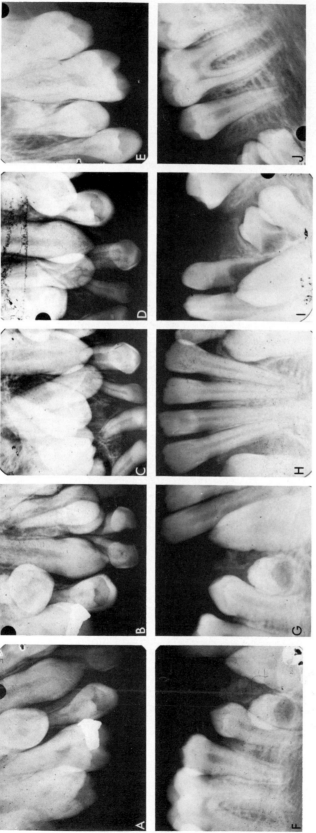

Figure 5–174 The six maxillary primary anterior teeth are still in position, with no resorption of their roots, except the apical third of the left central and lateral incisors. In the maxilla above the apices of these teeth are the four permanent incisors and two supernumerary malformed teeth.

In the upper left bicuspid and molar area the first bicuspid has erupted, and the second bicuspid is unerupted and locked between the roots of the first bicuspid and the first molar. The second molar has also erupted. There are two unerupted rudimentary third molars in the left tuberosity.

In the upper right bicuspid area the primary molars have been lost, but the permanent bicuspids, although formed and in position, have not erupted. There is a supernumerary bicuspid crown in the process of formation between the second bicuspid and first molar roots. The upper right first and second molars have erupted.

In the mandible all four permanent incisors have erupted. The permanent cuspids have not erupted. The primary lower right cuspid is still in position with one half of its root resorbed. The bicuspids on the lower right are unerupted. In the body of the mandible on the mesial side of the first bicuspid and overlapping its crown is a partially formed supernumerary bicuspid crown. The second bicuspid crown is just below the mucosa. The second and third molars in the right side have erupted. There is a partially formed lower third molar. On the lower left the identical situation found on the lower right is present.

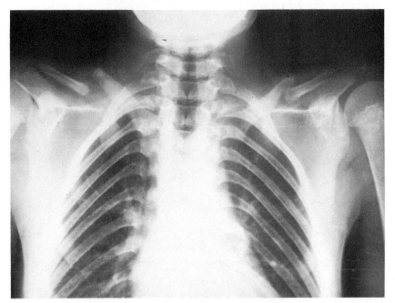

Figure 5–175 Note the break in the continuity of the clavicles through the middle thirds, with well-rounded apposing ends.

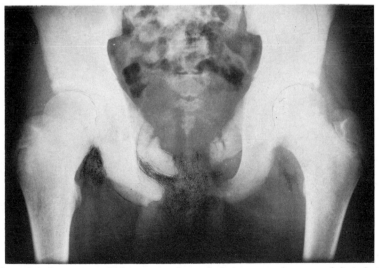

Figure 5–176 The pelvic bones are widely separated anteriorly because of osseous defects in the pubes consisting of complete absence of the vertical rami.

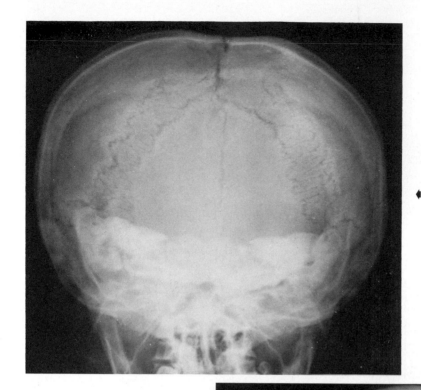

Figure 5–177 The skull is of the brachycephalic type with broad transverse diameter and flattened vertex. The cranial sutures are prominent, the sagittal suture appearing a little wider than usual. The bones of the face are small in comparison to the size of the cranium.

Figure 5–178 The lateral view shows definite evidence of platybasia.

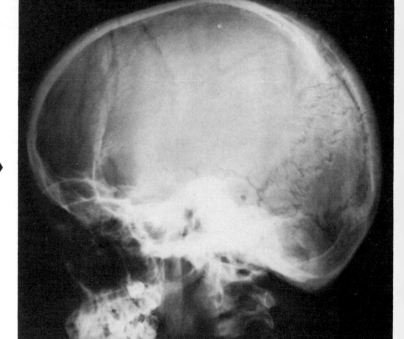

Case Report No. 5

CLEIDOCRANIAL DYSOSTOSIS

E. M., a man aged 42 years, presumably edentulous, was referred because of inflammation of the oral mucosa of the mandible beneath an artificial denture. Oral radiographs revealed the presence of unerupted malformed teeth in both the maxilla and the mandible. This, plus the typical skull forma-

tion, led to a suspicion of cleidocranial dysostosis that was confirmed by radiographic findings of the skull, clavicle and pelvis (Fig. 5–179).

Roentgen Examination Report. For the details of this examination see the legends accompanying Figures 5–181 to 5–183.

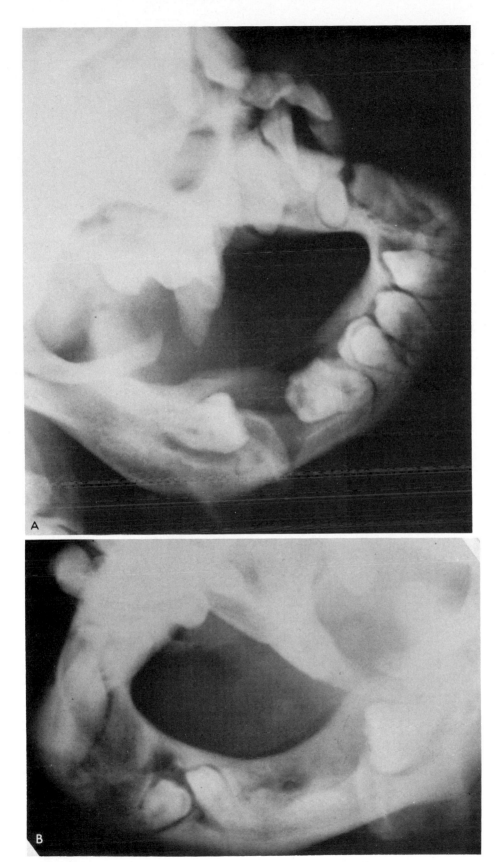

Figure 5–179   Another example of cleidocranial dysostosis (see Case Report No. 5). *A*, Impacted unerupted mandibular cuspids, bicuspids, molars and supernumerary rudimentary teeth. Note the large dentigerous cyst involving the molars. *B*, Impacted unerupted mandibular bicuspids and a third molar in the right side of the mandible.

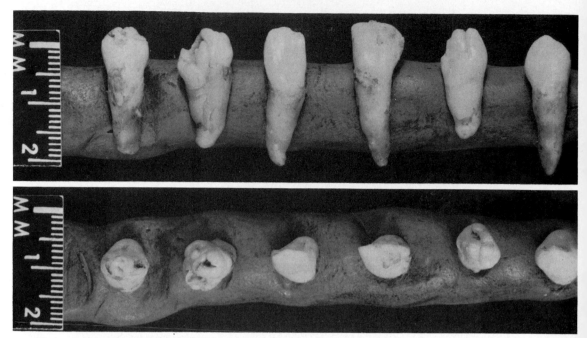

Figure 5–180   Some of the malformed maxillary and mandibular teeth that were removed from this patient.

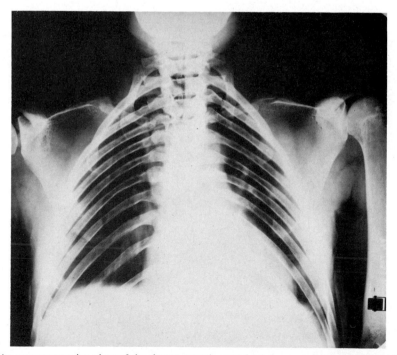

Figure 5–181   An anteroposterior view of the thorax reveals complete absence of the outer half of each clavicle, the distal end of the inner half being well rounded. A slight compound scoliosis is present. The posterior ribs present unusual obliquity from behind and above downward and anteriorly.

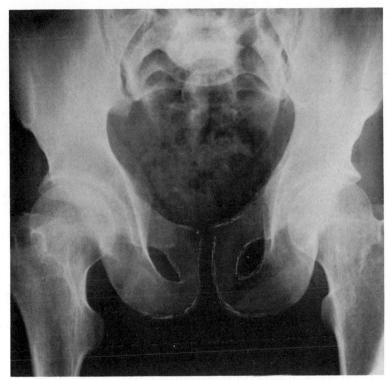

Figure 5–182 The pelvis is narrow, the transtrochanteric film measurement being 26 cm. The sacroiliac joints are wide. The pubes at the symphysis are more widely separated than normal, film measurements being 9 mm. A large osseous defect involves the upper two fifths of the opposing margins of each pubis at the symphysis. There is slight inward protrusion of either acetabulum.

Figure 5–183 The terminal phalanges of the toes present conical configuration without terminal tufting. There is a prominent concave impression at the base of the proximal phalanx of each great toe. Less marked concavities are noted in the bases of the proximal phalanges of the other toes. The proximal epiphyses of the first metatarsal bones are un-united.

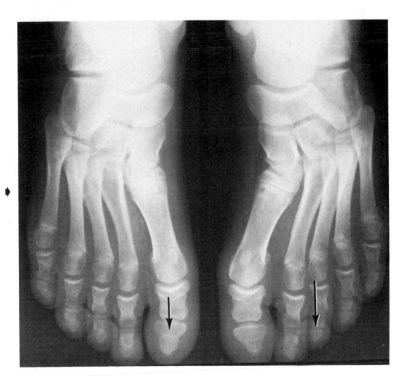

SUPERNUMERARIES, RUDIMENTARIES, MESIODENTES AND DENTES IN DENTE

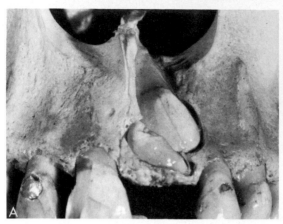 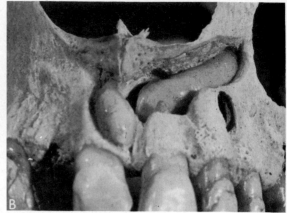

Figure 5–184 *A,* Labially impacted maxillary central incisor and rudimentary supernumerary central incisor. In this case the rudimentary supernumerary tooth prevented the normal eruption of the left central incisor. After reflection of a labial flap, the bone overlying the supernumerary tooth is removed and the supernumerary lifted from its bed. If this procedure is performed early enough in life, the central incisor will erupt by itself. If not, then the permanent central incisor should be adequately exposed and moved into position by orthodontic appliances. *B,* Horizontally and palatally impacted maxillary cuspid. The dentigerous cyst about the crown of this tooth materially aids in the removal of this cuspid, as explained earlier. In a case like this use the technique shown in Figure 5–101 to remove this cuspid from the palatal process of the maxilla.

RETAINED AND UNERUPTED TEETH IN CLEIDOCRANIAL DYSOSTOSIS*

Cleidocranial dysostosis is a rare hereditary disease. It is characterized by (1) delayed and incomplete ossification of the calvarium, (2) hypoplasia or absence of the clavicles, and (3) delayed and defective dentition. There is a delay in the exfoliation of primary teeth because of a delay or failure in the eruption of permanent teeth. There are also many supernumerary teeth in both the maxilla and mandible. (4) A bulging forehead, with prominent cranial bosses that are clinically evident, is found. The head is large, usually brachycephalic, out of proportion to the bones of the face. (5) A poorly developed maxilla makes the mandible appear prominent. There is incomplete ossification of the bones of the skull. Our second patient (E. M., Case Report No. 5) had failure of fusion of the anterior and posterior portions of the zygomatic arch bilaterally, a finding that we had not previously seen reported. (6) Delayed ossification of fontanelles is another finding. The individual bones of the head frequent y fail to unite, with the formation of

accessory centers of ossification occurring, and this creates the appearance of a large number of wormian bones between the chief cranial bones. (7) It is transmitted genetically by either parent to either sons or daughters as an autosomal dominant trait.

RUDIMENTARY SUPERNUMERARY TEETH (MESIODENTES)

While these anomalies can be and are found in any region of the jaws, they are most frequently seen in the maxillary incisor region at or near the median line. Most of them are impacted, although occasionally they are able to erupt in or near the arch.

The technique for their removal is determined by their size, shape and location and is the same as for the removal of any impacted tooth in that area.

The eruption of permanent teeth is sometimes prevented by the presence of supernumerary teeth. An unusual example of this is presented in Case Report No. 6, in which double dens in dente in bilateral rudimentary supernumerary central incisors was found.

Composite odontomas also prevent the eruption of teeth, but this will be discussed in Chapter 13.

*Archer, W. H., and Henderson, S. G.: Cleidocranial dysostosis. Oral Surg., 4:1201 (Oct.), 1951.

(*Text continued on page 384*)

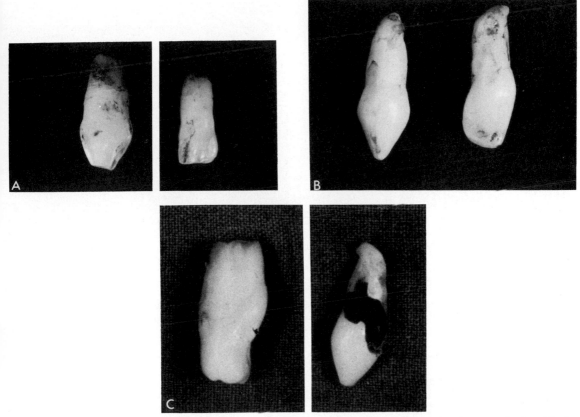

Figure 5–185 *A, B & C,* Examples of peg-shaped mesiodentes and rudimentary-shaped incisors usually found in the anterior maxilla. While the mesiodentes are found in the midline between the central incisors (hence the name), they *are not* a frequent cause for diastema of the maxillary central incisors, as has been frequently stated. They are also located in proximity to other maxillary anterior teeth.

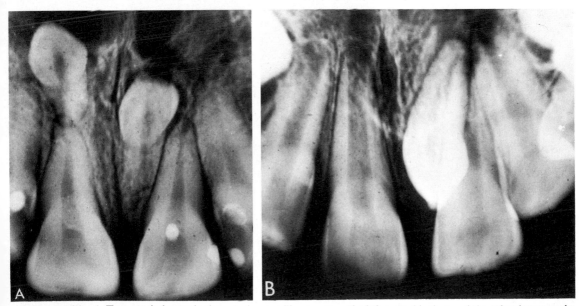

Figure 5–186 *A,* Two mesiodentes in the anterior maxilla, one over the left central incisor and the other between the central incisors which have a diastema. However, note the space also between the central and lateral incisors. *B,* Mesiodens between the maxillary central incisors. Again, note also the space between the central and lateral incisor. The presence of the mesiodens cannot be blamed for the diastema.

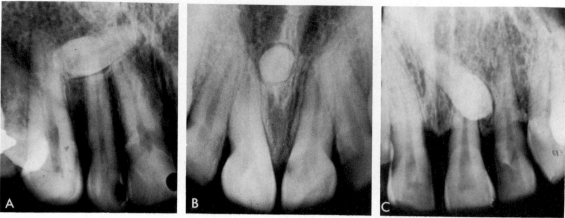

Figure 5–187 Three patients whose radiographs revealed the presence of mesiodentes in their anterior maxillas. Note, as previously stated, that in *A* and *C* the mesiodentes are not between the maxillary incisors but over the spaces of the incisors. *B*, This mesiodens is between the central incisors and at a right angle to the long axis of the incisors.

Note spaces between all maxillary incisors in *A*, *B* and *C*. There is not any relationship between the mesiodentes and these diastemas.

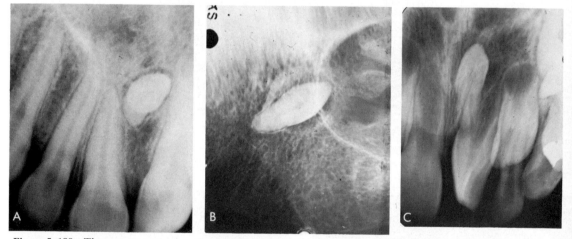

Figure 5–188 Three more examples of mesiodentes. *A*, Again located between the apices of the maxillary central incisors, this mesiodens is at a 60-degree angle to their long axis. *B*, Mesiodens in an edentulous maxilla. The comparatively large radiolucent area about its crown is strongly suggestive of a dentigerous cyst. *C*, An inverted mesiodens (also called a rudimentary supernumerary central incisor) which has impeded the normal eruption of, and deflected the course of, the permanent central incisor.

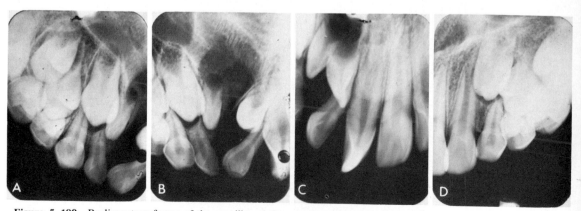

Figure 5–189 Rudimentary forms of the maxillary left central and lateral permanent incisors in a dentigerous cyst.

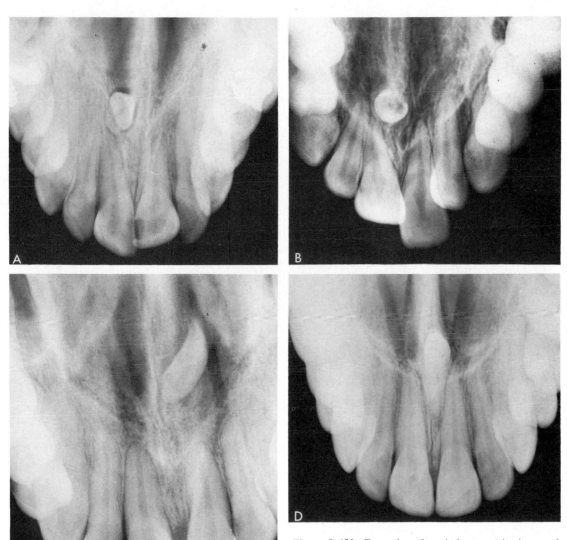

Figure 5–190 Examples of mesiodentes. *A* is close to the floor of the nasal cavity, probably right at the entrance to the nostril. In *B* the radiolucent area in the crown suggests internal resorption. *C* has an unusual curvature of the root. Note the absence of diastema in any of these patients, even in *D*.

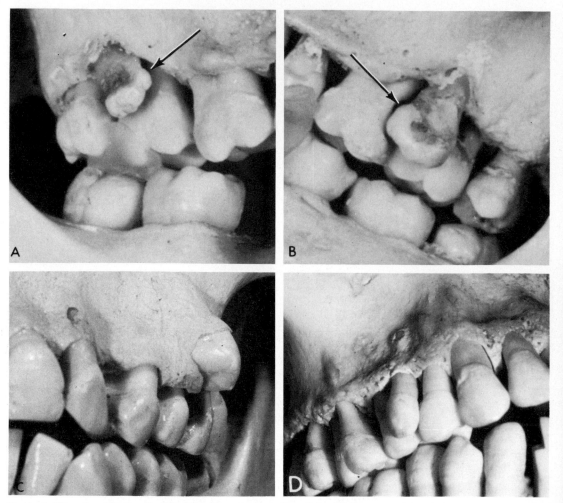

Figure 5–191 *A* and *B*, Poorly formed rudimentary maxillary left and right second molars in eruption buccal to the first and second molars. *C,* Cuspid transposed over the root of the maxillary second bicuspid. *D,* Rudimentary maxillary cuspid situated buccally between the crowns of the maxillary bicuspids.

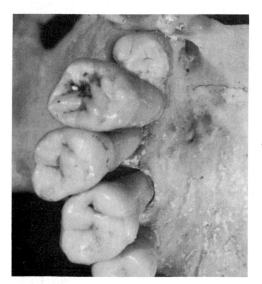

Figure 5–192 Vertically impacted rudimentary supernumerary maxillary third molar. Again the main difficulty in removing this tooth is gaining access to it. Of course, care must be taken to avoid forcing this tooth into the maxillary sinus or into the pterygomaxillary space.

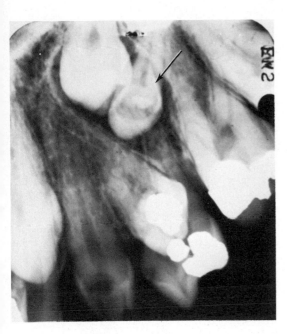

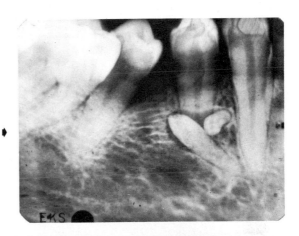

Figure 5–193 Rudimentary supernumerary maxillary bicuspid blocking the eruption of the maxillary first bicuspid.

Figure 5–194 A cystic odontoma composed of typical large and small mesiodentes within what appears to be a cyst. These rudimentary peg-shaped tooth structures are usually seen only in the maxilla.

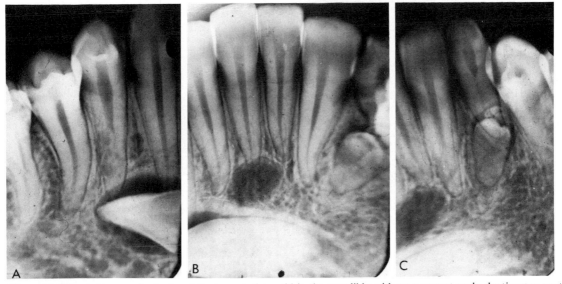

Figure 5–195 *A,* Crown of a horizontally impacted cuspid in the mandible with an apparent early dentigerous cyst developing. *B,* A radiolucent area that appears, inasmuch as the tooth is vital, to be a soft cementoma (cementifying fibroma) on the apex of the mandibular left central incisor. *C,* A small odontoma consisting of two rudimentary tooth forms in the cuspid area.

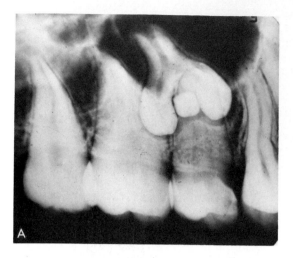

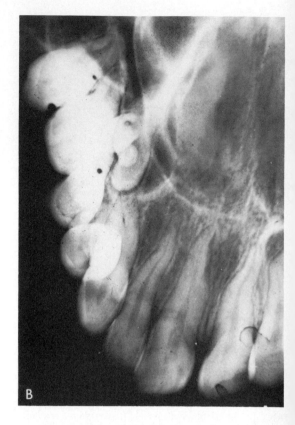

Figure 5-196   Periapical and occlusal radiographs reveal a bizarre odontoma in the right maxillary molar region.

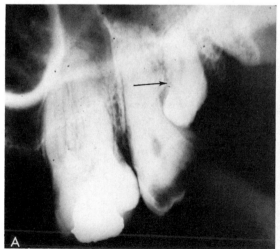

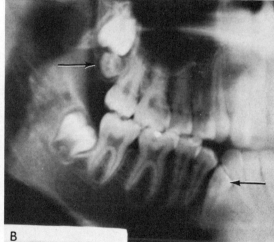

Figure 5-197   *A*, Vertically impacted rudimentary maxillary fourth molar. *B*, Rudimentary partially formed maxillary third molar blocking the eruption of the normally forming maxillary third molar.
The supernumerary third molar should be extracted to permit the normal third molar to erupt.

Figure 5-198   *A*, Supernumerary mandibular first bicuspid fully erupted between the cuspid and first bicuspid. *B*, Partially formed crown of a supernumerary bicuspid located between the apical thirds of the second bicuspid and first molar roots. This should be excised. *C*, Partially formed peg-shaped tooth (mesiodens) impacted in the mandibular area normally occupied by the first bicuspid. This should be excised.

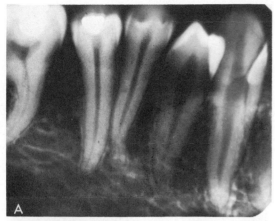

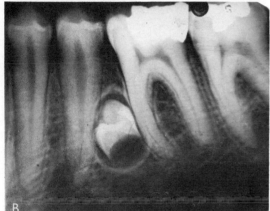

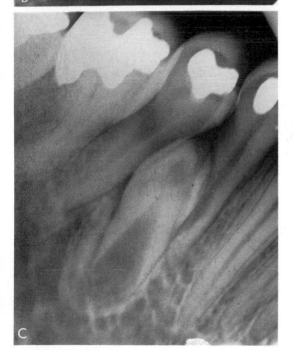

Figure 5–198 *See opposite page for legend.*

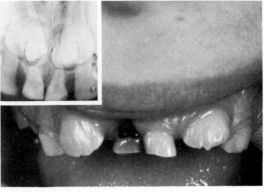

Figure 5–199 Overretention of the maxillary deciduous central incisors. *Inset:* Radiograph reveals that the permanent maxillary incisors are prevented from erupting by the presence of partially formed rudimentary supernumerary teeth, which must be excised to permit the fully formed permanent central incisors to erupt, if the eruptive force has not been dissipated. If it has, they will now have to be moved into place by the orthodontist.

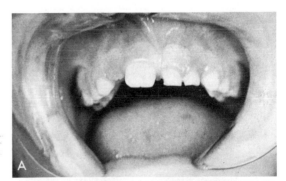

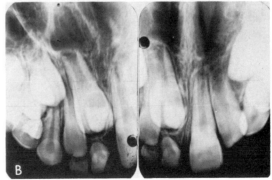

Figure 5–200 *A,* Overretention of the left primary maxillary central and lateral incisors. *B,* The cause, a partially formed rudimentary supernumerary incisor, which is preventing the permanent central incisor from erupting normally.

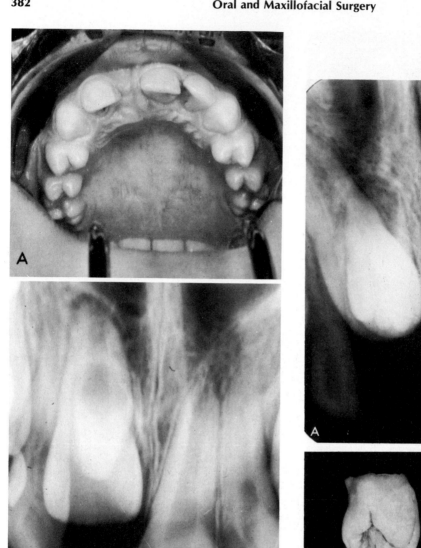

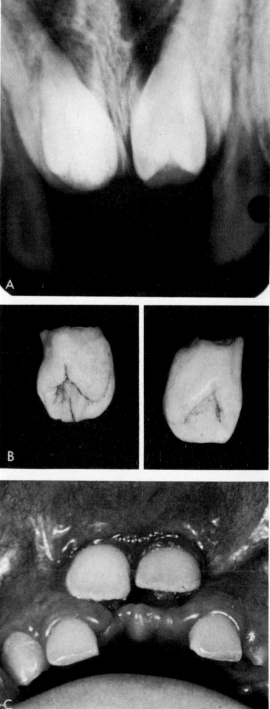

Figure 5–201 *A* and *B*, Another example in which the normal eruption of a permanent maxillary incisor was prevented by the presence of a partially formed rudimentary supernumerary tooth. The patient's dentist had removed the deciduous tooth because he knew it was overretained, but he had not radiographed the area to determine why the permanent central incisor did not erupt. A second dentist did so.

Figure 5–202 *A*, Two fully formed permanent maxillary central incisors whose eruption has been prevented by the partially formed supernumerary rudimentary incisors *(B)*, which were excised from the lingual side of the arch. *C*, At the same time, the labial and incisal surfaces of the permanent teeth were fully uncovered by removal not only of the dense mucoperiosteum but also of the labial and incisal bone. This view is 1 week after surgery.

Photographic Case Report

DELAYED ERUPTION OF PERMANENT MAXILLARY CENTRAL INCISORS DUE TO RUDIMENTARY SUPERNUMERARY TEETH: SURGICAL TREATMENT

PAUL M. BURBANK, D.M.D.

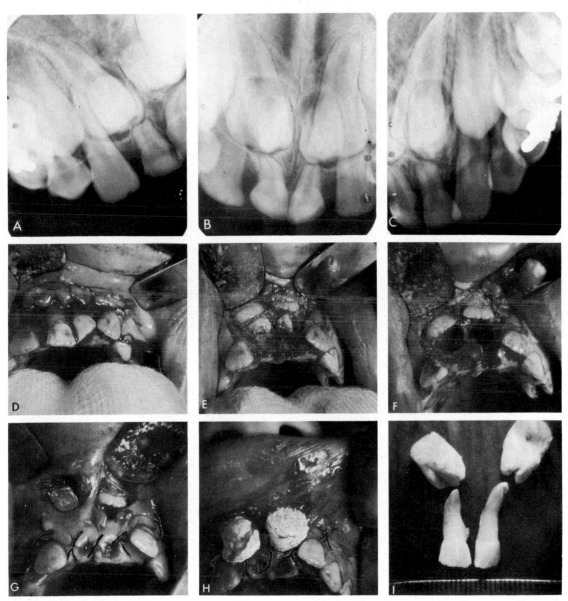

Figure 5–203 Delayed eruption of maxillary permanent central incisors in a 10-year-old boy. *Treatment:* Extraction of retained primary incisors and bilateral supernumerary teeth to allow eruption of the permanent central incisors.

A to *C*, Preoperative periapical radiographs. *D*, Beginning of the operation. *E*, Supernumerary teeth and permanent central incisors exposed. *F*, After the extraction of the primary and supernumerary teeth. *G*, Flap repositioned and sutured; permanent central incisors exposed. *H*, Periodontal pack placed on the permanent incisors to maintain gingival openings. *I*, Extracted primary and supernumerary teeth.

Case Report No. 6

UNERUPTED MAXILLARY BILATERAL RUDIMENTARY SUPERNUMERARY CENTRAL INCISORS PREVENTING THE ERUPTION OF THE MAXILLARY CENTRAL INCISORS

Chief Complaint. Delayed eruption of permanent maxillary central incisors.

Past History. About 1½ years ago, this 9-year-old child was referred to an oral surgeon for the extraction of carious primary teeth. Nine teeth were extracted. No radiographs were taken. It was felt that after their removal the permanent maxillary central and lateral incisors would erupt. The right and left maxillary second incisors did. To determine the cause for the delayed eruption of the maxillary central incisors, radiographs were taken (Fig. 5–205). These revealed two rudimentary supernumerary teeth in the maxillary anterior region, lying in the normal path of eruption of the permanent maxillary central incisors. The patient was admitted to the hospital for excision of the supernumerary teeth.

Physical Examination. Findings in the general physical examination were negative and noncontributory.

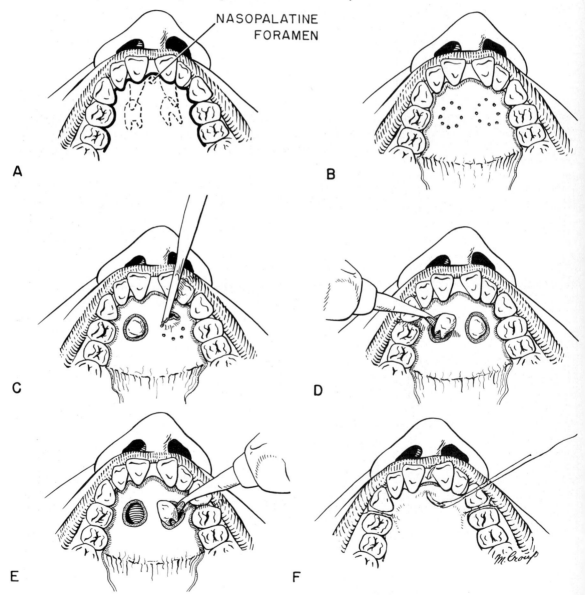

Figure 5–204 Removal of two supernumerary rudimentary incisors in the palate. *A,* Incision for the palatal flap. *B,* The flap is reflected, and holes are drilled through the palatine bone. *C,* Overlying and surrounding bone is removed with a chisel or bur. *D,* The right tooth is elevated from its crypt with a No. 73 Miller elevator. *E,* The left tooth is elevated from its crypt with a No. 74 Miller elevator. *F,* The flap is sutured back into place.

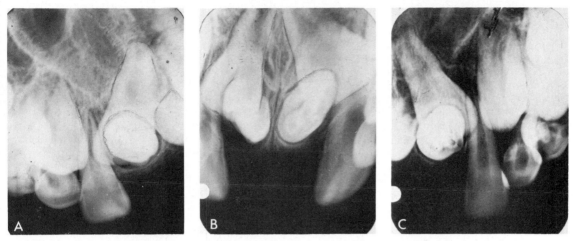

Figure 5–205 Bilateral rudimentary supernumerary maxillary teeth preventing the eruption of the permanent central incisors. On removal it was discovered that there were partially formed bilateral dentes in dente. (See Figure 5–206.)

Laboratory Examination. Results of all laboratory studies were essentially normal.

Preoperative Diagnosis and Treatment. The patient was found to have bilateral rudimentary supernumerary teeth. He was scheduled for surgical removal of these teeth, with routine preoperative orders.

Operation Record. Under Avertin-ether anesthesia the face and mucous membrane were prepared with tincture of Merthiolate, and the lips

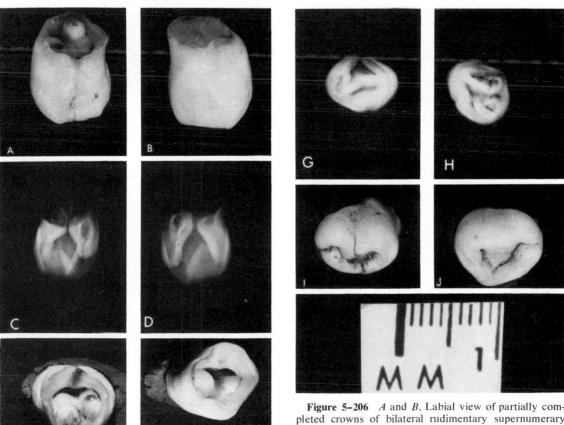

Figure 5–206 *A* and *B*, Labial view of partially completed crowns of bilateral rudimentary supernumerary maxillary incisors. Each crown contains a double dens in dente. *C* and *D*, Labial radiographs of *A* and *B*, which clearly reveal the two dentes in dente in each crown. *E* and *F*, This photograph looking into the completely calcified crowns shows the two miniature crowns of the dentes in dente contained in each of the supernumerary crowns. *G* and *H*, Longitudinal radiographs outline the type of calcification in the dens. *I* and *J*, Photograph of the "incised edges" which are blunt and blend into the fissured lingual cingulum.

coated with petrolatum. A Molt mouth prop was inserted in the mouth, and the jaws were separated. The tongue was grasped by gauze held between the fingers, and brought forward, exposing the tip, which was scrubbed dorsally and ventrally with tincture of Merthiolate. A curved needle with 0 plain catgut was passed through the midline of the tongue ½ inch from the tip and brought forward for a distance of 6 inches. The needle was cut from the suture; a knot was tied in the ends of the four strands; a hemostat was clamped on this knot and held to the cover sheet by a towel clip. A loose oropharyngeal partition was then placed.

An incision was made along the crest of the ridge from the right cuspid to the left cuspid region, and thence at a 45-degree angle to the mucobuccal fold. A mucoperiosteal flap was reflected labially, and overlying bone was removed with a chisel and mallet. Two rudimentary teeth were then exposed. These were removed by means of elevators. On examination these were found to contain partially formed rudimentary teeth within themselves, indicative of dens in dente (Fig. 5–206). The wound was debrided with curettes and the process trimmed with rongeurs and bone files. Crystalline sulfanilamide was sprinkled into the cavity. The tissues were approximated and sutured with 000 catgut.

The patient was removed from the operating room in good condition.

Postoperative Course. The patient had an uneventful postoperative course. Radiographs taken of the rudimentary teeth after extraction demonstrated the outline of the invagination process. The reverse relationship of enamel and dentine in a dens was clearly outlined in the radiographs. A careful study of the radiographs revealed not one but two areas of enamel invagination in each rudimentary tooth (Fig. 5–206).

Summary. A case of double dens in dente in bilateral rudimentary supernumerary central incisors has been presented. As demonstrated by radiographic evidence, this case may also be classified as a mesiodens.

DOUBLE DENS IN DENTE IN BILATERAL RUDIMENTARY SUPERNUMERARY CENTRAL INCISORS (MESIODENTES)

Dens in dente has been the subject of a number of articles in the dental literature. Conflicting theories relevant to its etiology have been propounded. Basically, two theories have been developed.

The cause of dens in dente, according to Kronfeld,[28] is an invagination during the developmental stage of the tooth. The growth of the tooth germ is regarded as centrifugal, and the dens is the result of localized retardation during the growth process followed by ingrowth of tooth tissue and its subsequent enclosure.

Swanson and McCarthy,[42] who published the first case of a bilateral dens in dente, advance a second theory. They "believe these malformations to be caused by a proliferation of the cells of the enamel organ into the dental papilla." This proliferation occurs during the stage of differentiation of the developing tooth germ at the inner enamel epithelium.

Supernumerary teeth are common in the maxillary incisor region. Those developing between the two central incisors are called mesiodentes, occurring singly or in pairs.

Case Report No. 6 illustrates a double dens in dente in bilateral rudimentary supernumerary central incisors. Their position in the maxilla may justify their placement in the category of bilateral mesiodentes. A search of the literature reveals that no such case has been previously reported.

COMPLICATIONS DURING OR AFTER THE REMOVAL OF IMPACTED, MALPOSED OR RUDIMENTARY TEETH

Among the many complications that may occur during or after the removal of impacted teeth the following may be mentioned:

1. Exposure of the inferior alveolar canal.
2. Severance of the inferior alveolar nerve, or injury to or compression of this nerve, resulting in prolonged numbness or paresthesia of the lip.
3. Acute trismus, severe and incapacitating so far as mastication is concerned.
4. Fracture of roots. Maxillary third molar roots may be forced into the maxillary sinus. Mandibular third molar roots may be dislodged through the thin or nonexistent lingual cortical bone into the submandibular space. If the mandibular canal is in contact with the apices of the mandibular third molar, a small fractured apex can be pushed into this canal when attempts are made to remove it unless extreme care is exercised.
5. Disruption of blood supply due to injury to, or compression of, the inferior alveolar artery and vein. Interruption of the blood supply to a palatal flap for

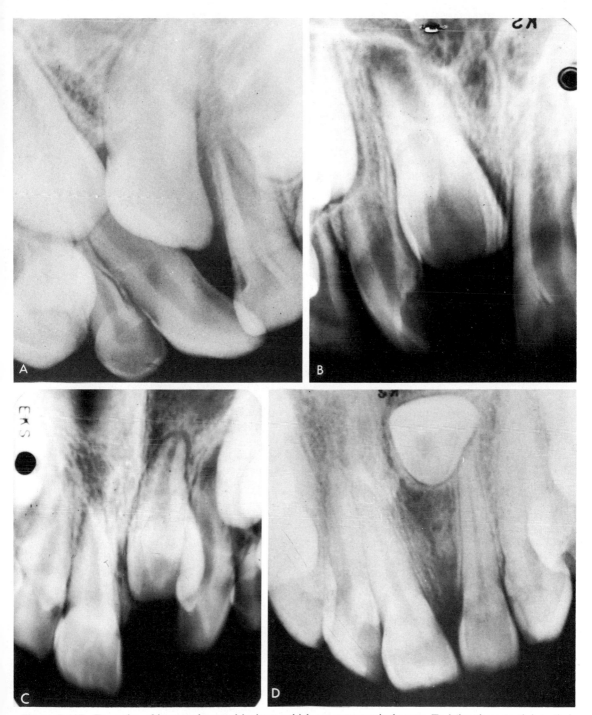

Figure 5–207 Examples of impacted central incisors, which are comparatively rare. To bring these teeth into their normal position in the arch presents a combined oral surgery and orthodontic problem.

too long a time may result in necrosis of the flap.

6. Fracture of a large section of alveolar process.

7. Traumatization or dislodgement of adjacent teeth. This may cause a loss of vitality in these teeth and resultant periapical infection.

8. Discoloration of the soft tissues overlying and below the mandible, below the

eye, in the cheek or in the lower lip, depending on the operative site. This is due to ecchymosis as a result of post-operative bleeding.

9. Injury to the lips, cheeks or mucous membrane from the use of instruments.
10. Opening into the maxillary sinus.
11. Forcing a tooth into the maxillary sinus.
12. Forcing an upper third molar into the pterygomaxillary fossa.
13. Opening into the nasal cavity.
14. Loss of a large section of alveolar process postoperatively, due to necrosis and sloughing because of improper planning of the technique to be used in the removal of the impacted tooth. This is due usually to overtraumatization of the investing bone by excess elevator pressure, dull chisels, burning the bone with rapidly turning burs, or using dull burs.
15. Fracture of the mandible or the maxilla.
16. Extensive laceration and/or traumatization of the soft tissues.
17. Extensive exposure of the roots of adjacent teeth, which may eventually result in the premature loss of those teeth.
18. Forcing an apex through the lingual plate of the mandible into the sublingual space, or into the maxillary sinus, or into the inferior alveolar canal.
19. Pain. This may be the normal amount of postoperative pain associated with normal surgical trauma, or it may be the severe pain of alveolalgia (so-called dry socket).

During operation under local anesthesia on the mandible, if pressure is created by the roots or by the instruments on the inferior alveolar nerve, the patient experiences pain. This is true in spite of the fact that the patient may have profound numbness of the lip, and he has been observed repeatedly even when the anesthetic used was 4 per cent procaine hydrochloride with 1:50,000 epinephrine. Likewise, when pulps are exposed as a result of the splitting or sectional technique, the pulpal tissue is painful when contacted by instruments or the suction tip. Pain as a result of contact with or the compression of the inferior alveolar nerve, or an exposed pulp, is the rule rather than the exception.

NUMBER OF IMPACTED TEETH TO BE REMOVED AT ONE TIME

How many impacted teeth should be removed in one operation will depend upon the difficulty of the operative procedures necessary to excise them, as well as upon the age and physical condition of the patient. As a rule, four very difficult impacted teeth should be divided into at least two operations.

POSTOPERATIVE TREATMENT FOR SURGICAL REMOVAL OF IMPACTED, MALPOSED OR RUDIMENTARY TEETH

After an impacted tooth has been removed, carefully suction out the sockets and explore them with a small-bowled curette for any remnants of tooth structure or bone. This is particularly important when the tooth-sectioning technique has been used.

If remnants of the dental follicle are present, excise this semisac carefully from the surrounding soft tissue in order to prevent the formation of a cyst.

Smooth the periphery of the alveolus with a round surgical bur to remove any sharp or ragged edges. If the buccal plate has been excessively traumatized by compression when it was used as a fulcrum for the shank of an elevator used to remove the impaction, this area should be removed with the chisel or bur to prevent subsequent sequestration (see Figure 25–102).

Suture the soft tissue flap into place over the socket.

If there is excessive bleeding, apply firm pressure with a sponge over the socket for 5 minutes.

Give the patient a supply of gauze sponges, and instruct him to keep one in place over the socket by biting on it. If one sponge does not produce *firm pressure* against the soft tissues when he bites on the sponge, then *two sponges* should be used. As it becomes soggy, he should replace it with a fresh one. This should be continued for at least 1 hour or until the bleeding stops. Continued pressure, as described, will control most bleeding in the oral cavity. See the discussion of hemorrhage, pages 1560 to 1579 in Chapter 25, "Complications Associated with Oral Surgery."

Prescribe basic vitamins. One tablet, taken $1/2$ hour after each meal, will supply the patient with a daily total of 30 mg. of thiamine hydrochloride (vitamin B$_1$); 15 mg. of riboflavin (vitamin B$_2$); 450 mg. of niacinamide; and 450 mg. of ascorbic acid (vitamin C). As a rule a 10-day supply is prescribed.

If the impaction was a mandibular third molar, instruct the patient to chew gum vigorously and constantly beginning 1 hour after the operation.

Prescribe alternate hot and cold applications 1 hour each until bedtime. Advise after that heat in any form as often as possible.

Prescribe medication to control pain, if necessary.

Warn the patient of the possibility of swelling and ecchymosis postoperatively and why.

If there is a possibility that the mandibular canal and its contents might have been traumatized, explain this to to the patient and tell him that he may have transitory numbness of the lip.

Give the patient an appointment to return the next day.

Irrigate the oral cavity the next day and clean the operative area gently with an antiseptic solution.

Remove the sutures 3 days postoperatively.

If pain develops in the socket, the alveolalgia (so-called "dry socket") must be treated as described in Chapter 25.

Always give the patient a list of printed instructions.

REFERENCES

1. Archer, W. H., and Fox, L. S.: Choroiditis caused by a palatally impacted unerupted maxillary rudimentary supernumerary cuspid. Oral Surg., 5:861–863 (Sept.), 1952.
2. Archer, W. H., and Henderson, S. G.: Cleidocranial dysostosis. Oral Surg., 4:1201 (Oct.), 1951.
3. Bean, L. R., and King, D. R.: Pericoronitis: nature and etiology. J.A.D.A., 83:1074–1077 (Nov.), 1971.
4. Berger, A.: The Principles and Technique of Oral Surgery. Brooklyn, Dental Items of Interest Publishing Co., Inc., 1930.
5. Bergstrom, K., and Jensen, R.: Responsibility of the third molar for secondary crowding. Dent. Abstr., 6:544 (Sept.), 1961.
6. Bjork, A.: The Face in Profile, pp. 64, 126, 172. Lund, Berlingska Boktryckeriet, 1947.
7. Bjork, A., Jensen, E., and Palling, M.: Mandibular growth and third molar impaction. Acta Odontol. Scand., 14:231 (Nov.), 1956.
8. Brothwell, D. R.: Dental anthropology, pp. 182–187. In Symposium of the Society for the Study of Human Biology. Vol 5. New York, The Macmillan Co., 1963.
9. Chipman, M. R.: Second and third molars: their role in orthodontic therapy. Am. J. Orthod., 47:498 (July), 1961.
10. Clark, C. A.: A method of ascertaining the relative position of unerupted teeth by means of film radiographs. Odont. Sec. Roy. Soc. Med. Proc., 3:85, 1909–1910.
11. Committee on Hospital Oral Surgery Service: Oral Surgery Glossary. Chicago, American Society of Oral Surgeons, 1971.
12. Dachi, S. F., and Howell, F. V.: A survey of 3874 full mouth radiographs. II. A study of impacted teeth. Oral Surg., 14:1165 (Oct.), 1961.
13. Dewell, B. F.: Clinical diagnosis and treatment of palatally impacted cuspids. Dent. Dig., 51:492 (Sept.), 1945.
14. Dingman, R. O., and Hayward, J. R.: Oral surgery in general practice. J.A.D.A., 35:607 (Nov.), 1947.
15. Duke-Elder, S., and Perkins, E. S.: System of Ophthalmology. Vol. IX. London, Henry Kimpton, 1965.
16. Faubion, B. H.: Effect of extraction of premolars on eruption of mandibular third molars. J.A.D.A., 76:316 (Feb.), 1968.
17. Frank, V. H.: Paresthesia: evaluation of 16 cases. J. Oral Surg., 17:27 (Nov.), 1959.
18. Frank, V. H., D.D.S., Philadelphia, Pa. Personal communication.
19. Garn, S. M., Lewis, A. B., and Bonne, B.: Third molar formation and its developmental course. Angle Orthod., 32:270 (Oct.), 1962.
20. Garn, S. M., Lewis, A. B., and Kerewsky, R. S.: Third molar agenesis and size reduction of remaining teeth. Nature (Lond.), 200:488 (Nov. 2), 1963.
21. Hall, R. M.: The effect of high speed bone cutting without the use of water coolant. Oral Surg., 20:150 (Aug.), 1965.
22. Howe, G. L., and Poyton, H. G.: The inferior dental nerve and extraction of mandibular third molars. Brit. Dent. J., 109:355–363 (Nov.), 1960.
23. Keene, H. J.: Third molar agenesis, spacing and crowding of teeth, and tooth size in caries-resistant naval recruits. Am. J. Orthod., 50:445 (June), 1964.
24. Kim, Y. H.: Treatment of an unusually impacted permanent maxillary central incisor. J.A.D.A., 69:596 (Nov.), 1964.
25. Kitchin, P. C.: Dens in dente. J. Dent. Res., 15:17, 1935.
26. Kitchin, P. C.: Dens in dente. Oral Surg., 2:1181, 1949.
27. Knapp, A. A.: Healing of eye diseases by cure of oral foci. Oral Surg., 5:799–808, 1952.
28. Kronfeld, R.: Dens in dente. J. Dent. Res., 14:49, 1934.
29. Laskin, D. M.: Evaluation of the third molar problem. J.A.D.A., 82:824–828 (Apr.), 1971.
30. Moorrees, C. F. A., Fanning, E. A., and Hunt, E. E., Jr.: Age variation of formation stages for ten permanent teeth. J. Dent. Res., 42:1490 (Nov.-Dec.), 1963.
31. Muller, E. M.: Transplantation of impacted teeth. J.A.D.A., 69:449 (Oct.), 1964.
32. Nodine, A. M.: Aberrant teeth, their history, causes and treatment. Dent. Items Interest, 65:894–910 (Sept.), 1943.

33. Pell, G. J., and Gregory, G.: Report on a ten year study of a tooth division technique for the removal of impacted teeth. Am. J. Orthod. Oral Surg., 28:660 (Nov.), 1942.

34. Picton, D. C. A.: Tilting movements of teeth during biting. Arch. Oral Biol., 7:151 (Mar.-Apr.), 1962.

35. Rantanen, A. V.: The age of eruption of third molar teeth. Helsinki, Tingman, 1967.

36. Reitan, K.: Tissue rearrangement during retention of orthodontically rotated teeth. Angle Orthod., 29:105 (Apr.), 1959.

37. Richards, A. H.: Roentgenographic localization of the mandibular canal. J. Oral Surg., 10:325 (Oct.), 1952.

38. Roher, A.: Displaced and impacted canines, a radiographic research. Int. J. Orthod. Oral Surg. Radiol., 15:1003, 1929.

39. Shanley, L. S.: Influence of mandibular third molars on mandibular anterior teeth. Am. J. Orthod., 48:786 (Oct.), 1962.

40. Sheneman, J.: Third molar teeth and their effect upon the lower anterior teeth. A study of 49 orthodontic cases 5 years after band removal. Am. J. Orthod., 55:196 (Feb.), 1969.

41. Stemm, R. M.: Influence of the third molar on the position of the remaining teeth in the mandibular dental arch. M.S.D. thesis, University of Nebraska, 1961.

42. Swanson, W. F., and McCarthy, F. M., Jr.: Bilateral dens in dente. J. Dent. Res., 26:167, 1947.

43. Turner, C. G., Department of Anthroplogy, Arizona State University, Tempe, Arizona. Personal communication.

44. Turner, P. S., and Joshi, S. C.: Choroiditis treated by surgical removal of unerupted impacted maxillary third molar: Report of a case. J. Oral Surg., 31:59–60 (Jan.), 1973.

45. Verunac, J. J., and Lindsay, J. S.: Treatment of persistent paresthesia after third molar odontectomy; report of case. J.A.D.A., 83:364–366 (Aug.), 1971.

46. Waldron, R.: Question of influence of erupting or impacted third molars on occlusion of treated and untreated cases. Int. J. Orthod., 23:221 (Mar.), 1937.

47. Weinstein, S.: Third molar implications in orthodontics. J.A.D.A., 82:819–823 (Apr.), 1971.

48. Winter, G. B.: Impacted Mandibular Third Molar. St. Louis, American Medical Book Co., 1926.

49. Woods, A. C.: Endogenous Inflammation of the Uveal Tract. Baltimore, The Williams & Wilkins Co., 1961.

CHAPTER **6**

SURGICAL ENDODONTICS

ANDREW E. MICHANOWICZ, B.S., D.D.S.

W. HARRY ARCHER, B.S., M.A., D.D.S.

Apicoectomy, also called root resection and root amputation, is the ablation (cutting off) of the apical portion of a tooth, and the curettement of all periapical necrotic and inflammatory tissue. When the apical portion of the root is not perforated, or resorbed extensively, then curettement of the periapical area without the cutting of the root end is performed in conjunction with filing the surface of the apex smooth. This procedure is known as an *apical curettage*. It serves advantageously in that root length is preserved.

In the past an apicoectomy was considered by many to be the treatment for endodontic failures, and as a result, repeated apicoectomies were performed on some roots until there was little or no root left. Studies have shown that the most common failure of endodontically treated teeth is an improper seal of the apex of the tooth. The repeated apicoectomies did not remove the source of the failures, and the apicoectomy failed, although the surgeon in some cases proved fortunate in removing sufficient root structure, to a point at which the seal was adequate. Apical curettage or apicoectomy or both in conjunction with an adequate root canal filling serves as a useful procedure where access to the apex cannot be gained via the crown of the tooth. Successful repair following root resection and a good root canal seal has been reported as high as 99 per cent.

INDICATIONS FOR APICAL SURGERY

Apical surgery is indicated in the following cases:

1. Teeth in which the operator can gain

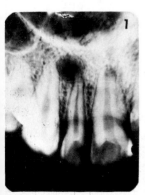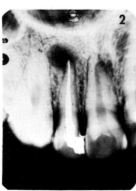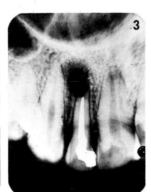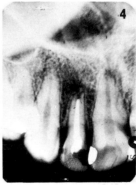

Figure 6–1 By use of the technique illustrated in Figure 6–2 and described on page 393, this nonvital left maxillary lateral incisor was treated (*1*), the root canal filled (*2*) and an apicoectomy performed (*3*). Two years after the surgery (*4*).

access to the apices with reasonable ease and not invade such anatomic structures as the maxillary sinus or the inferior alveolar canal—and for which the patients cannot travel or return for repeated endodontic treatments. Valuable time and effort in such cases can be conserved with immediate endodontic treatment and surgery.

2. Teeth in which root canals cannot be negotiated through the crown portion of the root (because of calcification, post crowns, and so forth). In such cases an apical seal must be placed in the canal following the apicoectomy. Gutta percha, when possible, is the filling of choice, and second is a seal of amalgam.

3. Teeth in which the apical portion of the root (usually severely curved) has been perforated or cannot be negotiated.

4. Teeth in which there is a gouging out of cementum at the apex, and the canal cannot be reshaped and cleansed properly.

5. Teeth in which surgical cleanliness and a negative culture cannot be attained during endodontic treatment.

6. Teeth in young patients that are the etiologic factor in the production of radicular cysts, or that may have been devitalized by the extension of the cyst. The loss of bone, which appears radiographically to involve the apex of the tooth, may not in fact do so. The loss of bone may be buccal or lingual to the apex of the tooth. Remember, radiographs are only two-dimensional and do not reveal depth. In a study, completed by Michanowicz and associates,[11] of teeth in which the radiolucent area appeared to circumscribe two or more teeth, only one tooth was nonvital in 88.6 per cent of cases. A root which radiographically appears to be within the cyst may be to either the buccal or the lingual side. It is absolutely imperative, therefore, before any operative procedures are undertaken, that all teeth which radiographically appear to be involved in a cyst be carefully checked for vitality. (For additional discussion of the subject, study Chapter 11.)

7. Teeth with radiolucent areas that continue to drain in the canal. Some authors claim that conservative endodontic therapy is successful in about 96 per cent of these cases.

8. In teeth that previously have been endodontically treated and filled properly, but whose radiolucent area is nevertheless increasing in size. The tooth should first be checked for traumatic occlusion and the radiograph scrutinized for possible leakage of the root canal. If a leak is suspected, the root canal filling should be removed and the canal retreated prior to the surgery. If no cause for the increasing area of radiolucency can be discovered, this is most likely a radicular cyst.

9. In teeth in which a broken instrument has passed beyond the canal and become an irritant in the periapical tissues.

10. Gross overfilling of the root canal, resulting in irritation of the periapical tissue.

CONTRAINDICATIONS TO APICOECTOMY

Apicoectomy is contraindicated in the following cases:

1. When the general health of patients would be jeopardized—especially those patients who have active systemic diseases, such as rheumatic fever, or who are suffering at present from active rheumatism, nephritis, leukemia, diabetes, syphilis, anemia, cardiac disease or thyrotoxicosis.

2. In teeth with deep periodontal pockets and excessive mobility.

3. In inaccessible teeth and apices.

4. In teeth in which it would be necessary to remove too much root structure, and the crown–root ratio would be so altered that the tooth would exfoliate itself as a result of the trauma.

5. When traumatic occlusion could not be corrected.

6. In teeth that have been treated previously by several apicoectomies, and the root canals are not properly filled.

PROCEDURE FOR APICAL SURGERY

There are three accepted procedures for apicoectomy. The first includes root filling and immediate root resection or curettage. In the second, root filling is followed several days or weeks later by apicoectomy or curettage. The third involves root amputation or curettage on teeth with root canal fillings that are found by subsequent examination to have developed a periapical radiolucent area, or on teeth whose radiolucent area has increased in size with or without a draining sinus. In these cases the operator should attempt to obtain the preoperative radiographs to determine the cause. If the root canal seal is inadequate, then the root filling should be removed and the canal cleansed and refilled prior to the apical surgery.

ROOT RESECTION TECHNIQUE

Premedicate with 1½ grains of pentobarbital or secobarbital if local anesthesia is to be used. If general anesthesia is used, see premedication recommendations on pages 23 and 24.

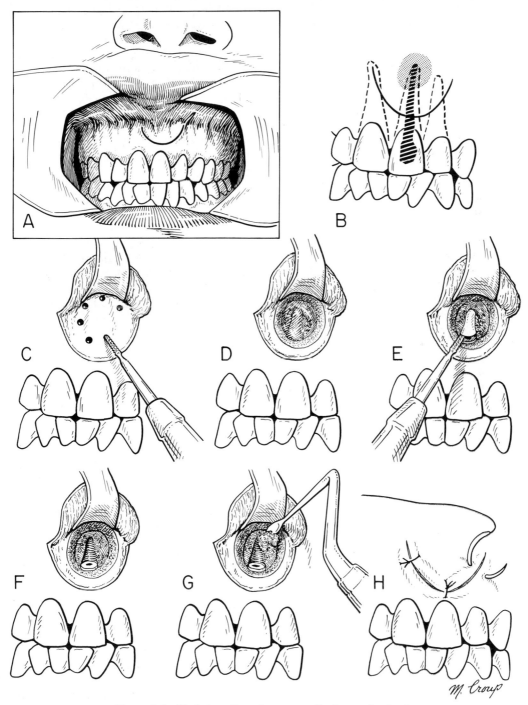

Figure 6–2   Technique for apicoectomy. Study text for details.

Take several good radiographs from various angles, showing length of root, pathologic area and proximity of root to roots of other teeth and to maxillary sinus.

Spray the mouth well with a good antiseptic solution.

Anesthetize the tooth and investing tissues if local anesthesia is to be used. Local anesthesia is best adapted to this purpose.

Isolate the area of operation and scrub with a germicidal solution.

Place the gauze pack, and use the suction tip to keep the area free from saliva and blood.

Make a semilunar incision, beginning in the region of the apex of the mesial tooth and extending down to a point two thirds of the distance between the apex of the root and the gingival line of the infected tooth and extending back up to the apex of the distal tooth (Fig. 6–2A and B).

Retract the flap upward and hold it by a small retractor (Fig. 6–2C).

Remove the bone plate with bone chisels or surgical bur (Fig. 6–2C). Extreme care must be taken not to expose or cut into the roots of adjacent teeth (Fig. 6–2D).

Cut off the apex of the root with a fissure bur. Do not cut off more than one third of the root (Fig. 6–2E and F).

Remove with a curette the surrounding pathologic tissue (Fig. 6–2G).

Round off the end of the cut root and bone margins.

Suture the flap back in place (Fig. 6–2H).

ROOT FILLING AND IMMEDIATE ROOT RESECTION

In this procedure, the preparation, sterilization and filling of the root canal is followed immediately by the apical surgery.

Secure the necessary anesthesia. Inject approximately 2 cc. of a 2 per cent local anesthetic solution with a vasoconstrictor labially and 0.5 cc. lingually into the incisive foramen if the operation is to be performed on an *upper* anterior tooth. In the case of a *lower* tooth, the inferior alveolar and lingual (mandibular) injection is given if an anterior tooth is to be operated upon, or if a bicuspid is to be resected, an injection is given on the same side of the mouth as the tooth, in addition to infiltration in the region of the root apex.

Cleanse the tooth and the interproximal spaces of those teeth to be included in the placement of the rubber dam.

Place the rubber dam in position, using the one-hole technique and clamping the tooth. The No. 9 Ivory dam is preferable for maxillary anterior teeth and No. 211 S.S. White for mandibular anterior teeth.

Swab the tooth and the rubber dam with an antiseptic agent.

Prepare the access into the pulp chamber. *Note:* Remove all decay before opening the chamber. Begin with a sterile No. 2 round bur (diamond or carbide) and *penetrate* the roof of the pulp chamber. Remove the entire roof of the chamber with a short draw-cut occlusal stroke, progressing with the No. 4 and No. 6 round burs to extend the pulp chamber to the peripheral outlines of the pulp horns. The cutting is performed with the shank side of the round bur.

Remove the contents of the pulp chamber with a large, sterile round bur or a spoon excavator.

Control hemorrhage by flooding the chamber with sodium hypochlorite. Absorb excess solution with suction or sterile gauze.

Insert a No. 1 file into the canal until the instrument encounters resistance; the instrument will usually bind at the dentocemental junction, which is approximately 1½ mm. from the apex of the fully formed tooth.

Take a radiograph of the tooth with the file in position, and develop the film.

Grasp the file with a hemostat forceps at the incisal edge or the tip of the buccal cusp and remove it from the canal.

Record in mm. the length of the file that was inserted into the canal.

Read the radiograph and, if necessary, make any minor adjustments in the length recorded. Set stops on all root canal instruments to the corrected length and enlarge the canal. For rapid and efficient cutting, reamers are preferable. The canal is reamed to the radiographic apex.

Irrigate the canal with alternate solutions of hydrogen peroxide and sodium hypochlorite. During the subsequent enlargement of the canal, irrigate the canal only with chlorinated soda.

Do not dry the canal after the use of each subsequent instrument. Instead, irrigate the canal with hypochlorite solution after each one. The canal should be enlarged until a complete surface layer of dentin is removed from the apical third of the tooth.

Irrigate the canal alternately again with hydrogen peroxide and sodium hypochlorite, the final solution being sodium hypochlorite, until no further effervescence is evident.

Dry the root canal with sterile absorbent points cut to the approximate length of the tooth.

Select a diagnostic cone the approximate size of the last reamer used.

Insert the gutta percha cone into the canal so that the cone will bind in the apical third and protrude approximately 1 or 2 mm. beyond the apex of the tooth. Take a radiograph of the tooth to check the fit of the gutta percha cone; then remove it from the canal.

With a small reamer or a lentula, coat the walls of the canal with Grossman's root canal cement. Place a small amount of cement on the tip of the reamer and insert it into the canal. Withdraw the reamer with lateral pressure in a counterclockwise direction, simultaneously placing the cement on the canal walls.

Cover the gutta percha cone with cement and carry it into position in the canal. Withdraw the cone 1 or 2 mm., and reinsert it several times in a slight pumping motion before seating it finally.

Laterally condense the root filling with additional cones, with alternate use of spreaders and with the aid of root canal pluggers (e.g., Starlite 11-D root canal spreader and Starlite No. 8 plugger). The spreader will condense the filling laterally and permit the insertion of additional cones; the plugger will slightly force the gutta percha filling apically to insure an apical seal. When the canal is tightly filled, make a radiograph of the tooth.

Check the radiograph to make certain that the filling extends slightly beyond the apex.

Cut off the excess gutta percha that is protruding through the coronal portion of the tooth (using a No. 2 Ladmore burnisher and/or F. P. Tarno No. 3).

Remove the excess gutta percha 1 to 1½ mm. below the visible crown with a large (No. 10) gutta percha plugger.

Wipe the inside of the chamber with chloroform.

Place a pledget of cotton moistened with sodium peroxyborate monohydrate and water in the coronal portion of the tooth and irrigate with sodium hypochlorite.

Again place a pledget of cotton moistened with sodium peroxyborate monohydrate and water in the coronal portion of the tooth, and seal with gutta percha and cavit, for approximately one week. At that time remove, irrigate and place a translucent restoration.

Remove the rubber dam and instrument tray.

PROCEDURE FOR PERIAPICAL SURGERY

Have the patient rinse with an oral germicidal solution, *e.g.,* oxychlorosene sodium (Kasdenol).

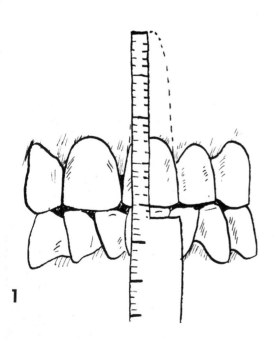
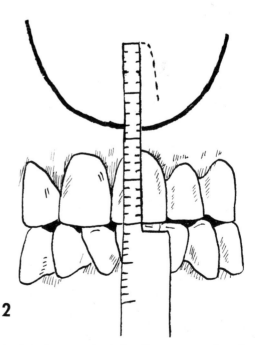

Figure 6–3 Place a surgical ruler on the labial surface of the tooth to its approximate length, as measured on the radiograph (*1*). Outline the incision for the curved flap so that the periapical area is in the center of the half circle (*2*).

If general anesthesia is used, also inject periapically a local anesthetic solution containing 1:50,000 epinephrine.

Wall off the patient's throat by having the patient close his teeth firmly, and pack bilateral oral vestibules with 4-in. by 4-in. gauze sponges.

Cover the patient's eyes with a mask.

Apply surgeon's gloves and cap.

Swab the tissue with nitromersol (Metaphen).

Place a surgical ruler on the labial surface of the tooth to its approximate length and with the dull end of the periosteal elevator, scribe the apex on the tissue; also outline the incision of the flap with the periosteal elevator (Fig. 6–3).

With a No. 15 Bard-Parker scalpel, make a semilunar incision extending from the tip of the apex on the adjacent tooth to that of the one on the opposite side of the tooth involved (Figs. 6–3 and 6–4). When extensive destruction of the cortical plate is present, and to prevent postsurgical dehiscence, a vertical incision is preferable (Fig. 6–4).

Reflect the tissue with a periosteal elevator, gradually raising the flap from one end of the incision to the other. (With most radiolucent areas, the labial plate will be partially eroded, exposing the root of the involved tooth.) Raise the flap labially and place the tissue retractor carefully into position, so that the flap is not turned under, and retract gently but firmly.

With either a No. 6 rounded bur or small rongeurs, gently remove some of the eroded labial plate. Probe the cavity of the lesion gently with a No. 85 right-angle Misdom

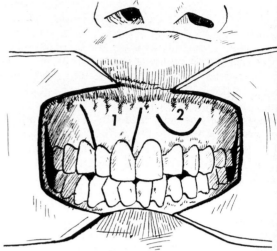

Figure 6–4 In a case of extensive loss of osseous tissue, such as is illustrated in Figure 6–5, the lines of incision for the flap should be vertical (*1*). For comparatively small areas of periapical loss of osseous tissue, semilunar flaps (*2*) are indicated. These would be appropriate for such cases as are illustrated in Figures 6–1, 6–6 and 6–7.

Frank curette to determine the extent of the lesion in all directions and the amount of alveolar bone involved.

Insert a sterile No. 6 round bur into the opening of the labial plate, and with a brush draw-cut stroke, outline a labial window in the cavity of the lesion. Remove sufficient labial plate until the entire labial margins of the cavity are exposed.

Begin to detach the lesion by inserting the edge of the curette between the granuloma-

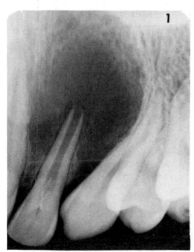
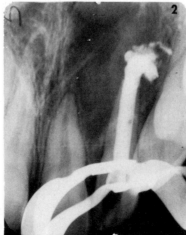
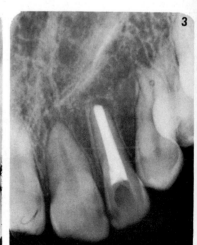

Figure 6–5 An extensive area of destruction of osseous tissue as a result of the traumatic devitalization of the pulp (*1*). Root canal filled (*2*). Two years after a minimal apicoectomy (*3*).

Figure 6–6 Unfortunately, there were not any follow-up radiographs after the initial treatment and root canal filling of this left mandibular central incisor. The radiograph several years later (*1*) shows the extension of bone loss, and on vitality testing, no response from the mandibular right central incisor was demonstrated. A loosely fitted silvercone was removed, and both teeth were treated and filled with gutta percha. The radiograph taken 10 years after periapical curettage (*2*) shows osseous repair.

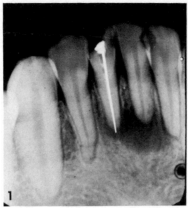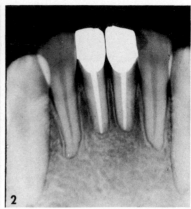

tous tissue and the bony socket, with the concavity of the bowl turned away from the center of the concavity.

When the entire lesion is peeled toward the center of the cavity, so that only the extreme attachment of the lesion remains, turn the bowl of the curette so that the concavity is facing the center of the bony crypt and insert the bowl between the pathologic tissue and the cavity. Peel the entire sac free from its remaining attachment.

Remove the excess gutta percha extruding from the apex with the curette.

Often the lesion extends linguoincisally on the palatal side of the root, and remnants of the lesion cannot adequately be removed. With a No. 558 crosscut fissure bur, remove approximately 2 to 3 mm. of root apex to gain proper access to this area. Make the cut so that the labial portion of the root is slightly lower than the lingual aspect. Remove the resected root tip with a curette.

Irrigate the cavity with oxychlorosene sodium (Kasdenol) solution.

Take a radiograph of the tooth.

When the labial plate is not perforated, the anatomic position of the apex must be determined. Place a sterile ruler on the tooth parallel with the long axis of the root, and determine the location of the apical extent of the root according to the known length of the tooth (using the radiograph). Scribe the labial plate with the dull point of the periosteal elevator where the ruler ends. Approximately 2 mm. from the scribed point or apex, an opening is made in the labial plate with a No. 6 round bur. With a draw-cut brush-away stroke, and air turbine, the labial plate is removed gradually from this starting point to approximately 3 to 4 mm. toward the crown on the mesial and distal aspect of the root end. If a turbine is available, several small openings are made with a fissure bur, and the labial plate may be removed with a chisel.

Irrigate the cavity with oxychlorosene sodium (Kasdenol) solution.

In the cavity place gelfoam, cut to the approximate shape of the cavity.

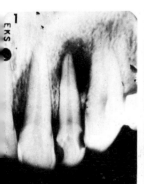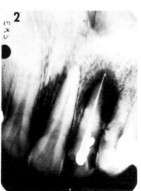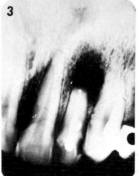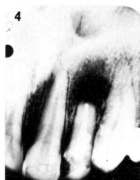

Figure 6–7 This case was one in which both the labial and lingual cortical plates were perforated (*1* through *3*). The radiograph taken 8 years later (*4*) shows a radiolucent area, which is a common result of nonossification in areas when both these plates have been lost. The area is filled with dense fibrous tissue and should not be interpreted as a diseased area. See also Figure 12–23 on page 540. To prove this diagnosis, anesthetize the area and pass the needle of the syringe through this area from the labial to the lingual side. No further treatment is indicated or necessary.

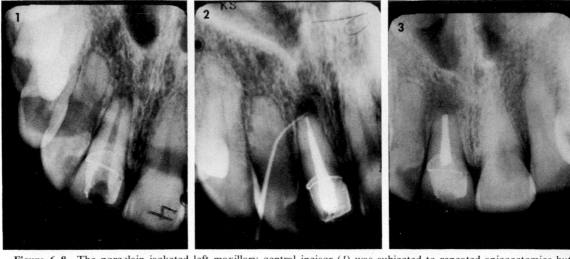

Figure 6–8 The porcelain jacketed left maxillary central incisor (*1*) was subjected to repeated apicoectomies but continued to have a labial draining fistula. A gutta percha point was inserted into the fistula (*2*). The result 10 years after retreatment and apical curettage is shown in *3*.

Suture the flap with single sutures.

Have instruments taken out of the operating room.

Remove packing and mask.

Have the patient rinse with an antiseptic mouthwash of oxychlorosene sodium (Kasdenol) solution.

Give the patient oral and written postoperative instructions.

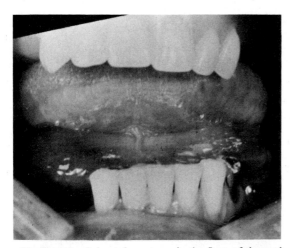

Figure 6–9 A large hematoma in the floor of the oral cavity that formed rapidly as the lower left first bicuspid root was being reamed. Obviously, the reamer passed through the lingual cortical plate and perforated a large blood vessel. Fortunately, the swelling was self-limiting and did not encroach on the larynx. If it had continued, it might have threatened to block the airway, necessitating a tracheostomy. This was a most unusual endodontic complication. It took approximately 10 days for the hematoma to be resorbed. Treatment was hot packs and mouth washes.

POSTOPERATIVE TREATMENT

POSTOPERATIVE INSTRUCTIONS

The patient should be given the same postoperative instructions as described in Chapter 2. A typical set of printed instructions which may be reviewed with the patient are as follows:

1. DO NOT RAISE THE LIP TO LOOK AT THE SUTURES.
2. Place an icepack on the outside of the face, 20 minutes out of every 1½ hours for the first day of the surgery.
3. Beginning with the second day, place ½ teaspoon of table salt in a glass of warm water and rinse three times daily (preferably after meals).
4. Do not chew any hard foods with the tooth for 1 week.
5. Do not brush in the area of the surgery for 1 week; however, brush the remaining teeth as usual.
6. A soft diet is suggested for the first 4 days.

POSTOPERATIVE COMPLICATIONS

If the adjacent teeth become painful, the possibility of trauma to the roots of these teeth during the operation must be considered. A careful study of the postoperative radiographs may help to prove or disprove this contingency diagnosis. It may be that local suppuration has developed. If so, the cavity should be opened and irrigated, and a small ¼-in. iodo-form drain inserted into the bony crypt.

If swelling accompanied by temperature and general malaise persists for 3 days or longer, there is undoubtedly a subperiosteal abscess developing. Treat this as described in Chapter 10. However, it is rarely necessary to extract this tooth. Hot wet dressings applied to the face continuously, hot normal saline mouthwash in the operative area hourly and antibiotics prescribed as discussed in Chapter 8 will often abort these infections. If not, the wound should be reopened and adequate drainage be established when localization of pus has occurred.

These apical areas should be examined by radiograph periodically for several years to make certain that the radiolucent area about the apex diminishes and osseous or fibrous repair takes place.

An apical scar noted as a small radiolucent area some distance away from the root apex may result when both the labial and lingual plates have been perforated.

Case Report No. 1

TREATMENT OF BILATERAL MAXILLARY CENTRAL INCISORS WITH FRACTURED ROOTS*

JERROLD I. WASSERMAN, D.D.S., AND MATTHEW J. HERTZ, D.D.S.

Severe trauma that fractures a fully formed tooth root, with separation of root segments, usually results in pulpal necrosis. In such instances the recommended course of treatment is root canal therapy and, if necessary, removal of the apically fractured section of the tooth if sufficient structure remains for tooth retention.

A 12-year-old patient was seen on an emergency basis, having just received a severe blow to the upper anterior teeth. Clinically, both central incisors were pushed lingually and had class 3 mobility.† Radiographic examination (Fig. 6–10) showed that each tooth had root fractures with a 1-mm. space between root segments. The right central incisor had an apical one-third fracture and the left central incisor had a mid-root fracture.

The teeth were anesthetized, and manual repositioning was attempted. Close adaptation was not possible, although better alignment of the fractured sections was achieved. A full upper acrylic resin splint was constructed (Fig. 6–11), and oral penicillin was prescribed for five days.

The upper splint was constructed by adapting quick-setting acrylic resin around the patient's total arch and having the patient close his mouth in centric occlusion to achieve a semblance of proper occlusion. Cold water was used to help dissipate the heat of setting.

The initial treatment goal was stabilization of the teeth, to be followed by root canal therapy. The prognosis for the left central incisor was considered quite poor, because of the limited amount of bony support for the exposed crown section and its severe degree of mobility.

The splint was worn for 7 weeks. During this period the patient was observed weekly for signs of infection and pain. Radiographs were taken at 2-week intervals (Fig. 6–12). Healing proceeded uneventfully.

After the seventh week the splint was removed (Fig. 6–13). The right central incisor appeared quite firm, but the left central incisor still had class 2 mobility. Upon testing, both teeth surprisingly proved vital. The patient was cautioned not to place much stress on his anterior teeth and was advised to return in 1 month. The gingival tissue had receded about 2 mm. from the normal position around both teeth (Fig. 6–14).

Examination 1 month later revealed two firm central incisors with healthy, normal gingival contours, and radiographs revealed no pathologic signs (Figs. 6–15 and 6–16). The patient had no discomfort, not even while masticating.

The healing properties of a young, healthy child should not be underestimated. Apparently, fibrous union of the fractured root sections occurred during the immobilization period. The blood supply in this area is sufficient to nurture repair in this type of injury.

While no further course of treatment is contemplated, the patient has of course been advised to return at 6-month intervals for follow-up examination.

The last examination was 15 months after the splints had been applied, and both teeth were still vital upon testing.

*Reprinted from Wasserman, J. I., and Hertz, M. J.: Case report/ Treatment of fractured incisors. Dent. Surv., 49:46–47 (June), 1973.

†AUTHOR'S NOTE: Mobility is graded as follows: 1 indicates movement of a tooth that is greater than normal but less than 1 mm. 2 indicates that a tooth can be moved 1 mm. in any direction. 3 indicates movement more than 1 mm. in any direction. If a tooth can be *rotated* or *depressed* in its socket, it is also considered class 3.

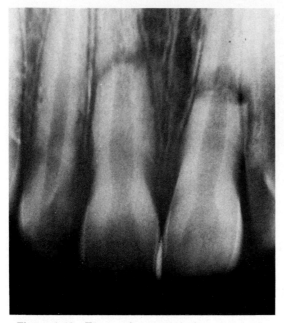

Figure 6–10 Fractured central incisors. (See Case Report No. 1.)

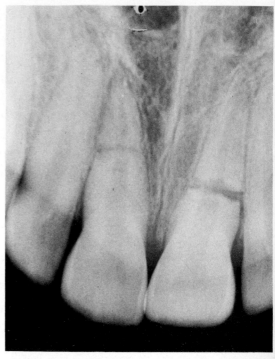

Figure 6–12 Radiograph taken during wearing of the splint.

APICAL FENESTRATION

Severe intraosseous inflammation and edema before, during and after root canal treatment may be relieved by apical fenestration. This procedure is a form of trephination resulting in decompression of the edema. Chestner and associates[3] have suggested the following: A semilunar flap should be cut and reflected, and a 3- to 5-in. diameter trough should be cut with fine chisels or burs perpendicularly through the overlying bone to reach

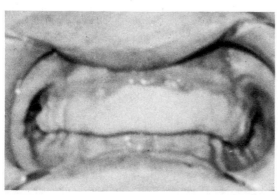

Figure 6–11 Acrylic resin splint.

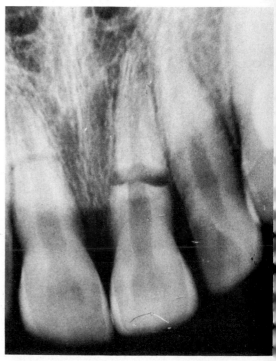

Figure 6–13 Radiograph taken immediately after splint removal.

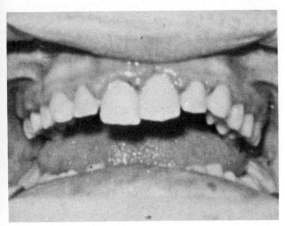

Figure 6–14 Photograph taken immediately after splint removal. Note gingival recession.

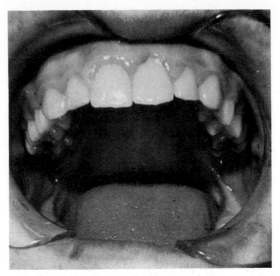

Figure 6–16 Photograph taken 1 month after splint removal. Note healthy gingiva.

the region involved. Neither the root of the tooth nor its apex should be damaged. A rubber dam drain is inserted into the fenestration and secured by suturing into the oral mucosa. The drain should be left in place until root canal therapy is completed, and it is removed 1 or 2 days following the filling of the canal. In patients who are treated for recalcitrant pain, the drain is removed after the discomfort

ceases. Antibiotic therapy is advisable postoperatively.

In a study of posttreatment endodontic pain, Clem[4] has shown that 25 per cent of the patients experience an increase of pain to a moderate level some time during the course of endodontic treatment. When the pain increases and persists to an intolerable level and the pressure cannot be relieved by intracanal methods, apical fenestration becomes the treatment of choice.

ROOT FRACTURES

Root fractures may require surgical intervention and removal of the apical fractured segment. However, it is recommended only after an alternant has failed to stabilize the tooth and preserve the root. Michanowicz[11] suggests that a root fracture should be reduced under a local anesthetic and the tooth ligated for 6 weeks afterward.

Acute symptoms that develop following reduction may necessitate the removal of the pulp solely in the coronal segment or in both the coronal and the apical segments.

The apical segment is surgically removed when a union fails to occur and the apical segment becomes a focus of inflammation. Should the crown–root ratio be affected by removing the apical segment, an endosseous splint is advisable.

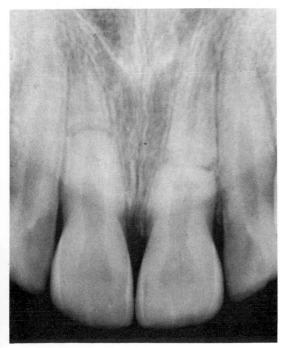

Figure 6–15 Radiograph taken 1 month after splint removal.

Case Report No. 2

REPLANTATION OF AVULSED TEETH*

HARRY BLECHMAN, D.D.S.

Replantation of avulsed teeth—despite an unfavorable long-term prognosis—can be an expedient procedure in children for cosmetic and psychological reasons, and certainly when artificial replacement is not feasible.

Avulsion resulting from athletic injuries and other accidents is common in youngsters. If the practitioner is able to reinsert the tooth in its socket shortly after the accident, it will be retained and will function for up to 10 years.

In a case of this type, the person who telephones before bringing the patient to the office should be instructed to keep the tooth moist by wrapping it in a clean, wet handkerchief or towel. Timing is obviously critical. If the tooth can be replanted in its socket within 30 minutes after the accident,

reattachment of the periodontal ligament and pulp survival are likely, without the occurrence of ankylosis.

Otherwise—as most cases usually present more than ½ hours after the accident—wash the avulsed tooth in a saline solution, scrape off the contaminated periodontal ligament, extirpate the pulpal tissue, conventionally cleanse the root canal, and fill it with a gutta percha cone and sealer. After heat-sealing the apex of the tooth, carefully debride the socket—removing the blood clot—before replantation. The tooth is stabilized in the socket by means of an acrylic splint, which is left in place 2 to 3 weeks, and systemic antibiotics are administered.

Root resorption of the replanted tooth generally begins within a few months, probably because of absence of the periodontal ligament, and the rate of resorption dictates how long the tooth will function before being exfoliated. See Figures 6–17 to 6–22 and their legends.

*Adapted from Blechman, H. *In*: Replantation is urged in youngsters: Avulsed teeth resume function. Clin. Dent., *1*(3):8 (Mar.-Apr.), 1973, by permission of Eli Lilly and Company.

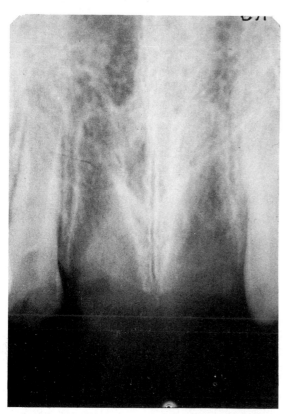

Figure 6–17　Missing (avulsed) upper central incisors. (See Case Report No. 2.)

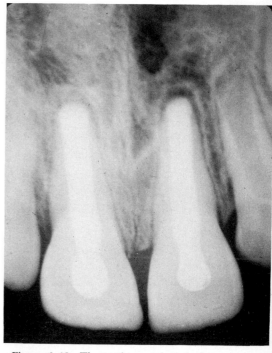

Figure 6–18　The teeth as replanted after root canals were filled with gutta percha.

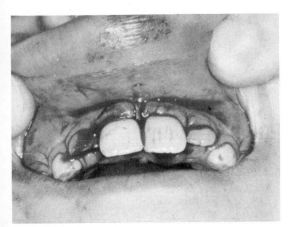

Figure 6–19 The central incisors immediately after replantation.

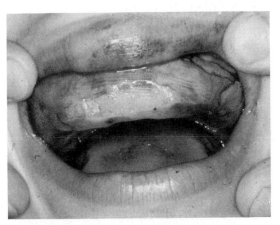

Figure 6–20 A plastic splint in place over the upper arch (to stabilize the replanted teeth).

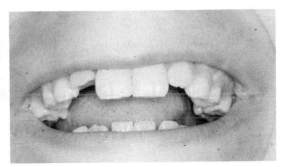

Figure 6–21 Smiling patient at 2-week postoperative interval, following removal of splint.

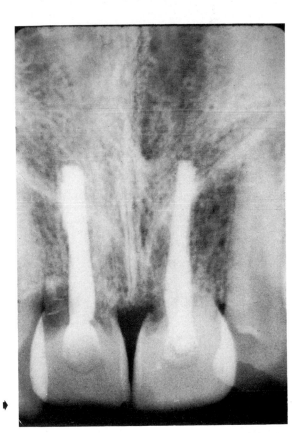

Figure 6–22 The same teeth 7 years later (roots of the replanted central incisors have been totally resorbed, although the teeth—with apparent support from gutta percha points—continue to function).

REFERENCES

1. Baurmash, H., and Mandel, L.: Root and amalgam. N.Y. State Dent. J., *29*:297–306 (Aug.-Sept.), 1963.

2. Blechman, H. *In:* Replantation is urged in youngsters: Avulsed teeth resume function. Clin. Dent., *1*(3):8 (Mar.-Apr.), 1973.

3. Chestner, S. B., Friedman, J., Heyman, R. A., and Selman, A. J.: Apical fenestration: Solution to recalcitrant pain in root canal therapy. J.A.D.A., *77*:846–848 (Oct.), 1968.

4. Clem, W. H.: Posttreatment endodontic pain. J.A.D.A., *81*:1166–1170 (Nov.), 1970.

5. Grossman, L. I.: Endodontic Practice. 7th ed. Philadelphia, Lea & Febiger, 1970.

6. Hamilton, R. E.: Endodontic therapy and immediate root resection employing zinc oxide and eugenol as a filling material. Texas Dent. J., *81*:11–13 (Jan.), 1963.

7. Hiatt, W. H.: Periodontal pocket elimination by combined endodontic periodontic therapy. Periodontics, *1*:152–159 (July-Aug.), 1963.

8. James, G. A.: Simplified techniques in surgical periapical treatment. Dent. Clin. N. Am., 375–382 (July), 1963.

9. Luebke, R. G., et al.: Indications and contraindications for endodontic surgery. Oral Surg., *18*:97–113 (July), 1964.

10. Maurice, C. G.: An annotated glossary of terms used in endodontics. Oral Surg., *25*(3):491–512 (Mar.), 1968.

11. Michanowicz, A. E., Michanowicz, J. P., and Abou-Rass, M.: Cementogenic repair of root fractures. J.A.D.A., *82*:569–578 (Mar.), 1971.

12. Shamblin, J. F.: Root canal therapy and adjunctive periapical surgery for the G. P. J. Philip. Dent. Assoc., *16*:14–17 (July), 1963.

13. Siedler, B.: Indications and contraindications for pulp capping and pulpotomy, regular endodontic therapy, and periapical surgery. Dent. Clin. N. Am., 305–319 (July), 1963.

14. Susser, I. W.: Technique for apicoectomy of anterior teeth. R. Can. Dent. Corps Q., *2*:18–20 (Apr.), 16–17 (July), 1961.

15. Wasserman, J. I., and Hertz, M. J.: Case report/Treatment of fractured incisors. Dent. Surv., *49*:46–47 (June), 1973.

CHAPTER 7

ORAL SURGERY FOR THE CHILD PATIENT

A. D. MACALISTER, E.D., D.D.S.(N.Z.)

INTRODUCTION

Oral surgery for the child patient may already occupy a large proportion of our time, and it is possible that with the necessary and increasing cooperation between orthodontist, pedodontist, general practitioner and oral surgeon this commitment will increase.

Basically, there is no difference between surgery performed upon a young patient and that performed on an older person. The principles will always be the same, but there will be differences in general management. Pediatric surgery is no place for "snap judgment," nor should there be any tendency to think that small patients produce only small problems.

The complete problem must be evaluated in accordance with the physiologic age and individual findings in the particular child.[6] To this end I am sure we can all recall occasions when our judgments were hasty—perhaps because we considered the present problem in the light of a slightly similar case. Perhaps technically, the causes were similar; however, the patients were very different. This in turn led to a complete breakdown of rapport among child, parent and operator. Further, technical difficulties brought about by hasty assessment were increased by the deterioration of patient cooperation.

Many of the texts on pedodontia stress that local anesthesia is the method of choice for minor oral surgery. I, too, believe this up to a point. However, the very young and the proven unmanageable child are definitely candidates for general anesthesia. On the other hand, children of the 8- to 15-year-old age group are in general very good patients.

PREMEDICATION

If the choice is made to operate under local anesthesia, I would hasten to stress the importance of adequate sedation in all cases. The basic principle of premedication for these patients is administration of a drug which will have a rapid action and an effect of short duration. With the wide range of drugs now available it is not too difficult to find a drug or combination of drugs which fulfill these requirements. In most cases dosage by mouth is satisfactory. When more rapid sedation is required, it may be accomplished by the intravenous or intramuscular route. For many years, the barbiturates have formed the basis of outpatient premedication, and from the proven results, they will continue to be first choice. It is true that, infrequently, barbiturates used alone bring about a hyperactive condition in some children. This has been explained as an idiosyncratic reaction to the drug. Perhaps I am fortunate that in my experience this set of circumstances has been rare. In recent years synergistic combinations of drugs have produced the near-perfect oral premedication. For instance, butobarbitone, in combination with codeine or promethazine, has provided a useful range of sedative activity. Combinations of these drugs have been used successfully on many patients of all ages. Further, improvements are found in the "cocktail-type" premedication. I have used such mixtures for a number of years for small children, those with behavior problems and handicapped children. One of my favorite combination is: perphenazine (8 mg.) (Trilafon), pentobarbitone (50 mg.) (Nembutal) and pethidine (75 mg.) (Demerol), and this combination of drugs is given 1¼ hours before operation. The actual dosages are calculated according to an age/weight formula. A further advantage is that these preparations may be given to the child by the parent in the home environment. By the time of the scheduled appointment the effect is maximal. More recently, the widespread use of intravenous diazepam used alone or in combination with methohexital has been widely acclaimed and could well take the place of full anesthesia in a variety of cases.

ANESTHESIA

Many operators have impatiently rejected topical anesthesia as being ineffective. I am sure the main reasons for this are that the material has been applied to a wet mucosa and that insufficient time has been allowed for its effective action. Personally, I would favor the ointment preparations, as I find these more readily controlled than the spray type. Local anesthetics should be injected slowly through a tense mucosal surface.

When preference and facilities indicate general anesthesia, intranasal nitrous oxide and oxygen with the supplement of Fluothane or Penthrane is still an excellent medium for minor surgery which calls for a short anesthetic only. The routine use of a soft latex nasopharyngeal tube aids considerably in the management of these patients. With the now established general acceptance and employment of intravenous drugs, either alone or as an induction for a continuing intranasal anesthetic, there are a number of proven techniques available to skilled operators. Thiopentone, methohexital and more recently propanidid are all in general use. Techniques for the use of these demand adequate facilities and staff, which must always include a trained anesthetist. Even more so than when operating on adult patients, I consider surgery for the child patient no place for the operator-anesthetist.

PARTICULAR MEDICAL PROBLEMS

Rheumatic and Congenital Heart Disease. We know that individuals with rheumatic or congenital heart disease are susceptible to the lodgment of bloodborne bacteria on damaged valves or other parts of the endocardium, causing a bacterial endocarditis. A bacteremia, however transitory, is a potential threat to such patients. It is now widely acknowledged that in order to have an effective prophylaxis at the time of surgery, and for the critical 6- to 8-hour postoperative period, there should be a high blood level of antibiotic at the time of operation. The drug of choice is penicillin, but some physicians have put forward a strong case for the routine use of erythromycin under certain circumstances.[13] It must be emphasized that penicillin or sulfonamides already employed in dosages for long-term prophylaxis against the Group A beta hemolytic streptococcus in susceptible rheumatic children are inadequate for the prevention of endocarditis following an oral procedure. Under these conditions a different drug must be used.

Erythromycin is a good drug to have as an alternative, especially when the patient is presently on a long-term prophylactic dose of penicillin for renal or rheumatic disease. By choice I would always recommend the initial high dosage of the prophylactic drug to be given by parenteral injection within 30 minutes of operation. This can be followed by a 4-day course of an oral preparation. At all times when using antibiotics, and especially so for these purposes, it is better to overtreat than to "play" with the material in token doses and risk development of drug-resistant organisms.

Hemorrhagic Diseases. Oral surgical procedures for patients suffering from hemorrhagic diseases are not the major hazard of a few years ago. With the full cooperation of oral surgeon, physician and hematologist, along with the hospitalization of the patient, this serious problem may now be capably coped with.

PARTICULAR SURGICAL PROBLEMS

IMPACTED TEETH

In the preoperative assessment of particular surgical problems, I would emphasize careful clinical examination, employing palpation, visual comparison and even measurement, all of which are needed to obtain a full and accurate diagnosis. Radiographs must be adequate and cover the full operative field, especially in more than one plane. The panoramic (Panorex), periapical and vertex-occlusal films all have their place in the diagnosis and assessment of pediatric oral surgery.

Operative Considerations. In the age groups we are concerned with, bone has a high organic content, which makes it more pliable with less likelihood of fracture. We may therefore employ this property during the elevation of unerupted teeth, when one may count on a certain amount of compression of the bone. Rather than exploit this property of the bone or employ gross removal of bone to clear an impacted or unerupted tooth in a young patient I would always recommend the sensible use of tooth sectioning techniques. This is far less traumatic, and it does not demand extensive bone removal.

Maxillary Teeth. For many years the impacted maxillary cuspid has provided a high percentage of surgery in the younger age groups. However, in the last decade this situation has markedly changed with the furthering of exposure, ligation and replacement techniques now supported by most orthodontists. The numbers now presenting for removal are low. I do not propose to discuss the details of all the removal techniques, but would mention that on frequent occasions approaches from both labial and palatal sides have been of great value in the conservation of bone, time and temper. This is especially so when the dentist is faced with the mid-alveolar placement of this tooth. More than in any other situation the critical principle for removal of the impacted cuspid is the clearance of the greatest diameter of the crown. At times, because of access, this is not easy to achieve. Once again, sectioning is really the only adequate method for dealing with this difficult task.

Supernumerary Teeth. The problem of supernumerary teeth properly belongs to patients in the 6- to 8-year-old age group. The failure of eruption of central incisors, a large diastema between the teeth, or marked rotation of recently erupted incisors frequently draws attention to the abnormality. An unpublished survey of 6- to 8-year-old children in New Zealand revealed the incidence of midline supernumerary teeth to be 2 to 3 per cent. The size of the mouth, limited access, and recently erupted incisor teeth can all contribute to the difficulties and hazards of this particular problem.

Upper Bicuspids. Removal of upper second bicuspids may prove to be either simple (if the tooth is displaced to the palatal side) or most difficult (when the tooth is impacted high in the mid alveolus beneath the crown of the first molar).

Mandibular Teeth. Probably the most common problem in the mandible is the second bicuspid. Impaction of this tooth is almost inevitably the result of early loss of the second deciduous molar followed by the forward drift of the first permanent molar to overlie the developing tooth bud. This is a true impaction, the tooth being prevented from eruption into its normal position by both the dense bone of the mandible and the presence of the overlying teeth. Access may be difficult even from the buccal aspect. However, when the tooth is seen in an occlusal film to be displaced to the lingual side of the mandible, it is more expedient to approach it from this side. Because of the proximity of adjacent tooth crowns and roots, sectioning of the crowns is the safest and most practical way of treating the problem, and in this precise situation, the dental engine (handpiece) is found to be the instrument of choice. Further, the conscious patient in this younger age group is much more familiar with the sensation of the dental engine than with the jarring blows from a mallet and chisel. The vulnerable anatomic structure in this region is the mental foramen, but if its position is identified when the flap is first raised, the contents of this foramen may be respected and not inadvertently damaged by enthusiastic retraction.

SOFT-TISSUE LESIONS

Frenectomy. In the past, frenectomy held pride of place as perhaps being the most popular of soft-tissue operations in the younger patient. Many a labial and lingual frenum was snipped by midwife, family doctor and dental surgeon. Popularity for this surgery has declined, both because the true nature of the problem has been realized and because of evidence that in many cases the apparent abnormality resolves at a later age. Nevertheless, there are cases which do require surgical attention.

Retention Cysts. Mucous cysts of the cheek and lips are not uncommon in this group of patients. They are best eliminated because of the nuisance they constitute. Clean excision is the treatment of choice. Small sublingual ranulae are not infrequently seen, and if left untreated they may cause some embarrassment to the child. The most convenient solution to this problem is to tie a soft stainless steel suture through the cyst wall and leave it long enough to allow the perforations to epithelialize.

CYSTS

Cysts of both jaws are a relatively common finding in the younger age groups. The commonest is the dentigerous cyst related to the noneruption or impeded eruption of permanent teeth. In most cases, where there is room for the tooth to come into its normal position it is not necessary to remove the involved tooth. Clearance of the crown and saucerization of the cavity by packing are all that is required.

Hemorrhagic Cysts. The majority of cases of hemorrhagic cysts are in the younger age groups. All the cases I have treated to date have been young girls in their early teens. An excellent review by Howe[3, 4] has recently given us a clear exposition of this peculiar entity. The true cause is still hazy, but we may all enjoy the success of the dramatic resolution of this condition following the minimal operative intervention, namely, opening the area and then closing it up.

Multiple Cysts. The more uncommon syndromes which manifest multiple cysts of the primordial (keratinizing) or dentigerous type are likely to be discovered almost by accident. When first seen by a general practitioner, one of the many cases I have seen was diagnosed as an acute abscess requiring drainage. Definitive treatment of this entity demands the complete stripping out of the cyst lining. Even with apparent total surgical excision the recurrence rate is high.

Radicular Cysts. A well-established radicular cyst in the young age groups is not common. Instead, it is more customary for the predisposing circumstances to react more acutely rather than tend toward cyst formation.

Bone Dystrophies. Fibrous dysplasia is a disease of childhood which may involve many bones. In the jaws, the classic clinical signs include migration of teeth, deformity and malocclusion. Radiographic examination shows single or multiple areas which have the classic appearance described as similar to "ground glass" or "orange peel."

Symptomatic surgical excision is the recommended treatment. It is sad to reflect on some of the gross surgical assaults made a couple of decades ago on some very small and harmless areas of fibrous dysplasia in the jaws of young children.

Odontomas. Tumors of calcified tooth-forming tissues may first be discovered when attention is drawn to the nonappearance of a permanent tooth. Early removal is indicated. The compound type presents few problems, as it is usual to find a well-defined soft-tissue sac around the mass. On the other hand, the complex type, of irregular and unyielding shape, requires extensive bone removal for the clearance of its greatest diameter.

FRACTURES

Fractures in children have for some time received scant recognition or even acknowledgment by many clinicians, as something almost to be avoided. It is true that they are not a common occurrence; nevertheless, they do occur and could well increase with the incidence of automobile accidents. Two of the most dramatic facial injuries I have seen in children have been part of the "battered baby syndrome." These cases not only presented with technical difficulties but also had far-reaching psychological and management problems associated with them.

In spite of the difficulties of access and the mixed dentition, with its distribution of teeth unfavorably shaped for splinting, we at least can take comfort from one outstanding attribute of the young: the healing potential of young bone as compared with that of the older age groups. Further, we should always observe the cardinal principle applicable to the treatment of all traumatic injuries of the face and jaws, *i.e., the employment of the simplest procedure which will give a satisfactory end result.* In other words, the simpler the treatment the better.

The most common sites of fracture are the symphysis and subcondylar region. Rowe declares, *"It is time to state unequivocally that there is no indication for open reduction and transosseous wiring in the case of condylar fractures in children unless there is a mechanical interference with mandibular movement. A conservative policy offers the best chance of obtaining a morphologically and functionally acceptable condyle."*[12] This has been substantiated clinically by Blevins and Gores,[1] Rakower and associates,[10] Kaplan and Mark,[5] MacLennan and Simpson,[8] and Rowe and Killey,[11] and demonstrated in animal research by Walker.[14]

Fixation of Fractures in Children. We are fortunate that with the healing potential of young bone the time of immobilization is minimal. The use of splints frequently provides some difficulties, especially in regard to the retention of these splints, but circumferential wires may be used to advantage to reinforce their stability. The use of rubber bands for intermaxillary fixation can further reduce the forces of determined mouth-opening movements that would tend to dislodge splints when circumferential wires were not used. There are some operators who favor pins for intermaxillary fixation, using a malar pin connected by a rod to a mandibular pin. It is generally felt that, where possible, the use of external fixation in young patients should be avoided.* External apparatus is always at risk of being bumped or dislodged, and particularly so in the case of a boisterous youngster. Further, with other definitive means of fixation (splints with circumferential wires or direct wiring techniques) available, the minimum length of time in the hospital is required.

POSTOPERATIVE PHASE

Orr[5] has pointed out that postoperative difficulties in the child are few and that swelling and pain are found to be less than in the older age groups. The prime reason for this is that we are, in general, dealing with young, healthy subjects with a good response to injury, a good blood supply to the soft tissue and a resilient and vascular bone that is not likely to have its blood supply damaged.

To improve postoperative comfort even more, I would stress the importance of well-designed mucoperiosteal flaps. Further, I recommend the use of fine nonabsorbable sutures, which keep the wound edges in position for the required period and which do not tend to become a focus of irritation as sometimes occurs with catgut.

Detailed instructions for the patient, along with explanations of possible complications and the oral hygiene procedures to be followed, all go toward making this phase of the treatment much easier for all. Judicious use of analgesics and hypnotics may further improve the situation. As with any procedure in oral surgery, the patient will remember the experience by how he feels after the operation.

---

*There are, however, fracture cases in children in which the pins are the best and least traumatic form of fixation. See Chapter 18, pages 1189, 1191–1193, and 1195 to 1198.

CONCLUSION

In conclusion I would first stress that the basic principles of good surgery must be even more strictly adhered to when dealing with these younger patients. Secondly, minor oral surgery for young patients presents a real challenge to our skill, judgment and knowledge of patient management, and especially so when the work has to be done under local anesthesia. Finally, the successful completion of surgery for a young patient provides far more of the indefinable rewards than that for many of our older patients.

To me, a grateful parent—with a happy child who has surmounted his fears and worries once a surgical task has been successfully accomplished without any upset—is one of the pleasures of following the specialty.

REFERENCES

1. Blevins, C., and Gores, R. J.: Fractures of the mandibular condyloid process: Results of conservative treatment in 140 patients. J. Oral Surg., *19*: 392 (Sept.), 1961.
2. Boyne, P. J.: Osseous repair and mandibular growth after subcondylar fractures. J. Oral Surg., *25*:300 (July), 1967.
3. Howe, L.: "Haemorrhagic cysts" of the mandible I. Br. J. Oral Surg., *2*:55–76 (Jul.), 1965.
4. Howe, G. L.: "Haemorrhagic cysts" of the mandible II. Br. J. Oral Surg., *3*:77–90 (Nov.), 1965.
5. Kaplan, S. I., and Mark, H. L.: Bilateral fractures of the mandibular condyles and fractures of the symphysis menti in an 18-month-old child. Oral Surg., *15*:136 (Feb.), 1962.
6. Kelsten, L. B.: Paedodontics for the General Practitioner. Chapter 22, p. 307. London, Henry Kimpton, 1956.
7. Macalister, A. D.: Drugs, disease and dentists. N.Z. Med. J., *66*:615–619 (Sept.), 1967.
8. MacLennan, W. D., and Simpson, W.: Treatment of fractured mandibular condylar processes in children. Br. J. Plast. Surg., *18*:423 (Oct.), 1965.
9. Orr, J. A.: The surgical treatment of dental anomalies in children. Br. Dent. J., *106*:53–61 (Jan.), 1959.
10. Rakower, W., Protzell, A., and Rosencrans, M.: Treatment of displaced condylar fractures in children: Report of cases. J. Oral Surg., *19*:517 (Nov.), 1961.
11. Rowe, N. L., and Killey, H. C.: Fractures of the facial skeleton. 2nd ed. Edinburgh, E. & S. Livingstone, Ltd., 1968.
12. Rowe, N. L.: Fractures of the facial skeleton in children. J. Oral Surg., *26*:505 (Aug.), 1968.
13. Tozer, R. A., Boutflower, S., and Gillespie, W. A.: Antibiotics for prevention of bacterial endocarditis during dental treatment. Lancet, *1*:686, 1966.
14. Walker, R. V.: Traumatic mandibular condylar fracture dislocations. Effect on growth in macaca rhesus monkeys. Am. J. Surg., *100*:850 (Dec.), 1960.

CHAPTER 8

ANTIBIOTIC THERAPY

SIDNEY S. SPATZ, B.S., D.D.S.

HAROLD J. ZUBROW, A.B., D.D.S.

An antibiotic is "a chemical substance produced by a microorganism which has the capacity, in dilute solutions, to inhibit the growth of or to kill other microorganisms."[4]

Antibiotic therapy is an integral part of dental practice. In order to use these agents effectively, the practitioner must be cognizant of the basic principles governing this type of therapy.

Diagnosis. An accurate clinical diagnosis will enable the practitioner to hazard an intelligent guess about the kind of organism involved in the condition to be treated. Laboratory studies are helpful, but the treatment of acute cases must be instituted immediately. In these cases, the antibiotic of choice would be one that is usually effective against the pathogens of the oral cavity.

Choice of Antibiotic Agent. The ideal antibiotic, of course, would be one that would act against all pathogens, leave nonpathogens and normal cells unchanged, and be effective in minimal concentrations with no local or systemic side effects. At the present time, no such agent exists, so we are compelled to observe certain reasonable therapeutic principles in order to achieve the best results with the antibiotics now available. After determination of the probable pathogen, either by laboratory methods or by clinical judgment, the antibiotic regimen is instituted. Since most pathogens in the oral cavity are grampositive, our drug of choice will probably include one of the following: (*a*) penicillin, if not contraindicated by a history of allergy or

specific sensitivity to the agent, (*b*) erythromycin or (*c*) tetracycline. The spectrum of these agents is such that they will probably be effective against most pathogens found in the oral cavity.

Dosage. The proper dosage is one that will produce a therapeutic level of the antibiotic in the blood plasma and serum, and also at the site of the disease process. If the pathogen is susceptible to the antibiotic being used, the average recommended daily dose will be adequate in most cases.

Duration of Treatment. Since many of the antibiotic agents are bacteriostatic, and many kill bacteria only during the stage of active multiplication, therapy must be continued for a reasonable time after the clinical course seems to improve. In most conditions encountered in dental practice, administration of the drug should be continued for at least 48 hours following the subsidence of the acute phase, or following surgical procedures in which it was used prophylactically. If therapy is discontinued prematurely, the residue of viable organisms that the body defense has not overcome may again become active and reestablish the disease state.

Administration. The drug should be administered in such a manner as to provide a sustained therapeutic level at the area under treatment. Systemic therapy is generally preferable except in very superficial infections that have caused no constitutional symptoms. In these cases, topical therapy may be considered, provided the antibiotics used locally are not ever likely to be used systemically. Bacitracin, polymyxin, and neomycin fall into this category.

Mechanism of Action. The exact mechanism of action for many of the antibiotics in common use is unknown. The principal mechanisms recognized follow.

PROTEIN COAGULATION. This mode of action is common to the protoplasmic poisons such as phenol, alcohol, etc.

DISRUPTION OF CELL MEMBRANE. Alteration of the permeability of the cell membrane by an antibiotic agent may prevent the cell from securing certain of the organic compounds necessary for reproduction.

COMPETITIVE ACTION. Certain of the sulfonamides will replace compounds essential for cell reproduction.

Emergence of Resistant Strains. The majority of drug-resistant strains are the result of mutation, which occurs independently of the use of antibiotics. Antibiotic therapy does, however, allow the resistant strains to live, while the susceptible organisms are killed. First-step mutants are of low resistance to most of the commonly used antibiotic drugs. The second-step mutants, which are descended from the first-step organisms, are of only slightly increased resistance. The notable exception to this is observed with streptomycin, in association with which organisms at all levels of resistance, and even of drug dependence, arise simultaneously. The emergence of resistant strains can be minimized by the following precautions:

1. Use a large enough dose to inhibit the growth of the organism and first-step mutants.
2. Continue the therapy for a long enough period of time to reduce substantially the number of viable organisms. Most antibiotics should never be prescribed for less than a 72-hour period.
3. Combined therapy. In certain instances, the use of two drugs with synergistic or additive action may delay the emergence of resistant strains, provided that the agents used do not display cross resistance.

Reasons for Failure of Treatment. When a clinical infection fails to respond as expected to surgical or pharmacologic management, or both, several factors should be considered.

DIAGNOSIS. It is true that most bacterial infections in the oral cavity are gram-positive. Occasionally, a patient will be seen with a gram-negative infection, or with a resistant staphylococcal infection that presents a therapeutic challenge.

SURGICAL DRAINAGE. Antibiotic therapy alone will not effect a cure if surgical drainage is indicated and has not been performed.

PATIENT COOPERATION. In cases in which the antibiotic is prescribed orally for an ambulatory patient, one cannot be certain that the patient is actually taking the medication as directed.

INADEQUATE DOSAGE. The patient may be on a satisfactory dosage regime, but the antibiotic level at the site of infection may not be adequate. In such cases, normal dosage schedules may have to be augmented.

ANTIBIOTICS IN COMMON USE

PENICILLIN

Penicillin compounds may be generally divided into two groups.

Naturally Occurring Penicillins. Among these, penicillin G and penicillin V are the most commonly employed.

Semisynthetic Penicillins. In this category are some compounds that are not inactivated by staphylococcal penicillinase. These are used in the management of "resistant" staphylococcal infections. In this group are oxacillin, methicillin and phenethicillin. Phenethicillin has a spectrum quite similar to penicillin V and can be used in the same clinical situations. Oxacillin and methicillin have relatively narrow ranges of antibacterial activity but are effective against staphylococci resistant to the other types of penicillin.

Profile. SPECTRUM. Naturally occurring penicillin compounds are effective against most gram-positive cocci, some gram-negative *Neisseria,* and some spirochetes, including those found in Vincent's infection.

The semisynthetic compounds are effective against many strains of penicillinase-producing staphylococci, and their use generally should be confined to this area.

ACTION. Bactericidal or bacteriostatic, depending on the concentration. Effective only against organisms that are actively reproducing.

DOSAGE. The average adult dosage is 600,000 to 1,200,000 units daily. When necessary, much larger doses may be given with little danger of toxicity. The average adult dosage of phenoxymethyl penicillin (penicillin

V) is 125 to 250 mg. four times daily. This dosage also applies to the semisynthetic penicillins.

ADMINISTRATION. Penicillin may be administered orally, intramuscularly or intravenously. Adequate blood levels can be achieved with penicillin V via the oral route. For most patients who are not critically ill, this is probably the most desirable method of administration.

PRECAUTIONS. Penicillin is the antibiotic most frequently involved in untoward reactions. These are primarily allergic in nature and may range in severity from a mild rash to generalized respiratory and vasomotor collapse. The following precautions should be exercised:

1. Do not give penicillin to a patient who has an allergic history or one who has ever reacted unfavorably to the drug. Patients with a history of asthma, hay fever or other allergy are more apt to have a sensitivity reaction to penicillin. Patients who have had repeated fungal infections may have cross sensitivity to penicillin.
2. Be prepared to treat the patient quickly and properly in the event of an anaphylactoid response (see Management of Allergic Emergencies, page 417).
3. Penicillinase, injectable, may be used to neutralize penicillin. This must be used with care since some severe allergic response has been reported to penicillinase itself. Theoretically, penicillinase will have no neutralizing effect on those semisynthetic penicillin compounds which are not inactivated by penicillinase.

BIOSYNTHETIC PENICILLINS

The use of 6-aminopenicillanic acid as a building block has permitted the development of many synthetic penicillin compounds which have therapeutic properties that differ from the natural penicillins. Some examples follow.

Methicillin. This agent is effective against penicillinase-producing staphylococci.

Ampicillin. Ampicillin is active against both gram-positive and gram-negative organisms, including *E. coli*.

Carbenacillin. Active against *Pseudomonas*, these agents have very specific usage indications and should not be substituted for the natural penicillins.

CLINDAMYCIN AND LINCOMYCIN

Lincomycin (Lincocin) and a derivative, clindamycin (Cleocin), are effective against many anaerobic organisms that are penicillin-resistant, but there is evidence of severe complications from them. For this reason and in order to prevent the development of resistant organisms, their use should be reserved for emergencies.

STREPTOMYCIN

SPECTRUM. Streptomycin is effective against the tubercle bacillus and many gram-negative organisms.

ACTION. It is considered bactericidal.

DOSAGE. The average adult dose is 1 to 2 gm. daily, in divided doses.

ADMINISTRATION. This drug is most effective when given intramuscularly.

PRECAUTIONS. There are few indications for streptomycin therapy in dental practice except in the treatment of a tuberculous lesion, and in combination with penicillin in the treatment of subacute bacterial endocarditis caused by *Streptococcus viridans*. The drug is toxic to the auditory mechanism, and organisms develop resistance to it at all levels at a very rapid rate. Streptomycin has been used in conjunction with penicillin to treat certain mixed infections. However, since the advent of the newer antibiotics, this is no longer necessary except in rare instances.

TETRACYCLINE DERIVATIVES

SPECTRUM. Effective against gram-positive and gram-negative organisms, as well as the rickettsiae and certain of the large viruses, these drugs are commonly referred to as "broad-spectrum antibiotics."

ACTION. The action of these drugs is generally regarded as bacteriostatic.

DOSAGE. The average adult dose is 250 mg. every 6 hours. The children's dose may be calculated as 4 to 5 mg. per pound of body weight, divided into four equal doses in a 24-hour period.

ADMINISTRATION. The primary route of administration is oral. Under compelling circumstances, the drugs may be used intravenously. Tetracycline is to be preferred to oxytetracycline or chlortetracycline, since it is a more stable compound.

PRECAUTIONS. The tetracycline derivatives eliminate much of the normal intestinal flora. This destroys the delicate bacterial balance and sometimes permits an overgrowth of resistant staphylococci. The resulting staphylococcic enteritis can be serious, and a small number of cases have terminated fatally. If severe gastrointestinal disturbance occurs after the third day of therapy, discontinue the drug at once. The absorption of the vitamin B complex is also affected, and it is wise to supplement the vitamin intake during tetracycline therapy. Tetracycline should not be prescribed for pregnant women, since it stains the teeth of the unborn child.

Note: Chlortetracycline (Aureomycin) and oxytetracycline (Terramycin) are similar in action to tetracycline (Achromycin, Panmycin, Tetracyn and others). Tetracycline is the drug of choice in this group.

ERYTHROMYCIN

SPECTRUM. Effective against gram-positive organisms, this drug has essentially the same spectrum as penicillin and may be useful against some penicillin-resistant staphylococci.

ACTION. Erythromycin is bacteriostatic in the usual dosage. Large doses may produce bactericidal activity.

DOSAGE. The average adult dose is 250 mg. every 6 hours.

ADMINISTRATION. The primary method of administration is oral.

PRECAUTIONS. Some cases of gastrointestinal disturbance have been observed, but these occur very rarely.

CHLORAMPHENICOL (CHLOROMYCETIN)

Chloromycetin is a broad-spectrum antibiotic, but it has been shown to produce aplastic anemia and should therefore *not be used*.

BACITRACIN

SPECTRUM. Effective against gram-positive organisms.

ACTION. Bactericidal.

DOSAGE. The usual dose is 500 units per gram of soluble base.

ADMINISTRATION. The route of choice is topical. The drug may also be administered intramuscularly.

PRECAUTIONS. Systemic administration can cause renal damage.

NEOMYCIN

SPECTRUM. Effective against gram-positive and gram-negative organisms.

ACTION. Bactericidal.

DOSAGE. The usual dose is 5 mg. per gram of soluble base.

ADMINISTRATION. The route of choice is topical. The drug may also be administered orally and intramuscularly.

PRECAUTIONS. Systemic administration may cause renal damage and possible damage to the eighth nerve.

POLYMYXIN B

SPECTRUM. Effective against gram-negative organisms and bacilli.

ACTION. Bactericidal.

DOSAGE. The usual dose is 0.1 to 0.25 per cent in aqueous solution.

ADMINISTRATION. The route of choice is topical. The drug may also be administered intramuscularly and orally.

PRECAUTIONS. Systemic administration may cause renal damage and damage to the nervous system.

KANAMYCIN

SPECTRUM. Effective against many forms of staphylococci that may be resistant to other agents.

DOSAGE. Daily dosage should not exceed 2.0 gm. given in two to four divided doses.

ADMINISTRATION. The drug should be given intramuscularly. It may be given orally in preparation for surgery of the gastrointestinal tract.

PRECAUTIONS. The drug is nephrotoxic, and may also cause deafness because of its toxic effect on the eighth nerve.

These newer antibiotics seem to be active against many strains of resistant staphylococci. Their chief field of usefulness is in this area. They are not recommended for treatment of the more common conditions caused by susceptible organisms.

COMBINED THERAPY

Many claims of synergistic activity have been made for commercially prepared combinations of antibiotic drugs. Much investigation is needed in this area, and "combinations" are not recommended for routine use. Combined therapy should be used when the situation clearly demands it and when antibiotic sensitivity studies confirm the need.

ANTIBIOTIC PROPHYLAXIS

There are certain situations in which the clinical indication for antibiotic prophylaxis is quite clear. However, in the great number of situations in which the indication is less clear, the liabilities incurred by the use of antibiotics must be carefully weighed against the hoped-for advantages. In many cases it may be better judgment to wait for the earliest sign of postsurgical complication before initiating antibiotic therapy, thereby giving the patient's own defense mechanism every opportunity to function normally.

Zallen and Strader state, "The question as to whether to use antibiotics preoperatively when performing extraoral surgery for mandibular prognathism is often debated. A study was made of 76 patients who were operated on for prognathism over a 33-month period. The results showed that antibiotics are not indicated when extraoral approaches are used, provided there is a careful preoperative preparation of the surgical site and postoperative management of the wounds."[12]

Goldberg evaluated 118 cases of oral and oral cutaneous lacerations with and without the use of prophylactic doses of antibiotics. His conclusions were "that antibiotics have little value in the prevention of infection in minor oral lip wounds." In oral cutaneous wounds "prophylactic use of antibiotics . . . could seem justified." In spite of this statement, he concluded, "the routine use of these agents (antibiotics) is discouraged, however, because their potential toxicity may outweigh the benefit. . . ."[7]

Although the list of possible prophylactic uses for antibiotics is rather large, it should be noted that these are possible uses, and we do not recommend that antibiotics be used routinely. Specific recommendations follow.

Prevention of Subacute Bacterial Endocarditis Following Oral Surgery. Bacterial endocarditis is a disease due to bacterial infection of the valvular and mural endocardium. This entity is of particular interest to the dental practitioner because dental extraction and other oral surgical procedures often cause a transitory bacteremia. A transient bacteremia can also be initiated by scaling and gingival curettage. This is of little consequence in the patient with no pathologic cardiac condition. However, in patients with damaged heart valves, or with roughening of the endocardium, this bacteremia may be the beginning of an ominous chain of events.

Any patient with valvular heart disease, no matter how minimal, is in danger of contracting endocarditis every time bacteremia occurs. Any operation in an infected field, especially tooth extraction, tonsillectomy, and instrumentation of the genitourinary tract, presents a real hazard. Also, many patients who have had rheumatic fever suffer chronic deforming valvular disease of the heart. These facts indicate clearly that each patient should be questioned prior to dental treatment concerning a history of rheumatic fever, congenital heart disease, or the presence of a heart murmur. Patients presenting a history of rheumatic fever, with or without clinical evidence of valvular damage, should receive antibiotic prophylaxis pre- and postoperatively.

Factors Influencing Postextraction Bacteremia. Many studies have been conducted in an attempt to evaluate the factors that influence the incidence of postextraction bacteremia. In their series of investigations, Okell and Elliot, and Glaser and co-workers, obtained the data presented in Table 8–1.

Several important facts must be considered in evolving a satisfactory prophylactic antibiotic regimen for these patients:

1. Antibiotic therapy will reduce the incidence of bacteremia following oral surgery, but it will not eliminate it. We must therefore assume that the bacteremia does occur, and continue administration of antibiotics for at least 72 hours postoperatively.

2. Oral sepsis tends to increase markedly the incidence and severity of postextraction bacteremia.

3. In about 95 per cent of the cases of subacute bacterial endocarditis, the causative organism is a nonhemolytic streptococcus. *Streptococcus viridans* is the causative organism in about 80 per cent of these cases.

4. The *in vitro* inhibitory level of *Str. viridans* is 0.15 unit of penicillin per cubic centimeter of blood serum. The *in vivo* inhibitory level must be from 2 to 30 times this amount.

Table 8–1 *Incidence of Bacteremia Following Dental Extractions*

INVESTIGATORS	GINGIVAL CONDITION	INCIDENCE OF BACTEREMIA	
		%	
Okell and Elliott[11]	Marked pyorrhea (multiple extractions)	75	
	Moderate pyorrhea (multiple extractions)	70	
	Normal (2 or more extractions)	43	
		Control Group	*Penicillin Group*
		%	*%*
Glaser *et al.*[5]	Normal	57.2	45.4
	Abnormal	78.9	41.4
	Gingivitis	75.0	46.2
	Mild pyorrhea	66.6	12.5
	Severe pyorrhea	100.0	62.5
	Single extractions	62.5	26.9
	Two or more extractions	70.8	71.4
	Causative Organisms		
	Hemolytic streptococci	81.5	
	Alpha hemolytic streptococci		29.4
	Nonhemolytic streptococci	7.4	58.8

TREATMENT GOALS. In the management of the oral surgery patient with increased susceptibility to subacute bacterial endocarditis, we should strive to accomplish the following:

1. Combat the local gingival infections, as in patients having gingivitis, periodontal disease, or other forms of oral sepsis.
2. Reduce the incidence and severity of bacteremia occurring during treatment.
3. Provide an adequate antibiotic level for at least 72 hours postoperatively.

ANTIBIOTIC REGIMEN. A suggested antibiotic regimen for this group of patients is as follows.

Local. First, local preparation of the mouth should be effected with an agent to reduce the bacterial population, *e.g.,* 0.3 gm. of oxychlorosene (Kasdenol) in 8 oz. of H_2O used as a mouthwash three times daily.

Jones and associates, in an excellent study "to determine whether a simple, topical, antiseptic lavage of the oral cavity and gingival sulcus would significantly reduce the incidence of postextraction bacteremias" summarized their findings:

"1. Blood specimens of 201 patients were tested to determine the effects of preextraction treatment with an oral antiseptic on the incidence of postextraction bacteremia.

"2. Bacteriologic evaluation of pre- and postoperative blood samples revealed a 72.7 per cent reduction in the number of postextraction bacteremias in patients receiving a simple preoperative treatment consisting of an oral rinse and gingival sulcus irrigation with a phenolated mouthwash solution [1 to 4 per cent phenol, sodium phenolate, sodium borate, menthol, thymol and glycerin].

"3. Alpha hemolytic streptococci, normal inhabitants of the human oral cavity, were responsible for 88.5 per cent of all positive blood cultures.

"4. The results of this study indicate that use of an antiseptic mouthwash in the manner described can significantly reduce the incidence of postextraction bacteremia and is of value as an additional method of protecting patients from these transitory bacteremias. It is recommended that this system of preoperative treatment be adopted as a regular part of all exodontia procedures.

"It must be emphasized that this treatment is not intended to replace prophylactic antibiotic coverage in patients who have cardiovascular abnormalities. However, antiseptic mouthwash lavage provides these patients with additional protection from the transitory bacteremias associated with exodontia."[10]

Another excellent procedure is to paint the gingival tissues with providone-iodine (Betadine) around the teeth to be extracted 10 minutes before incising. This permits the destruction of bacteria in these areas.

Bartlett and Howell made a study to "determine whether vancomycin, applied to the teeth and gingivae, would reduce the incidence of bacteremias following the scaling and extraction of teeth." They concluded that "the results of the study do not warrant the adoption of vancomycin in clinical practice as a substitute for the accepted regime of systemic antibiotics."[1]

Systemic. *Penicillin* should be used if the patient susceptible to subacute bacterial endocarditis is *not allergic* to penicillin and *not on rheumatic fever prophylaxis.* Penicillin should be administered:

1. One hour prior to the procedure:
   either (a) by injection—
            aqueous penicillin, 600,000 units
            procaine penicillin, 600,000 units
     or   (b) by mouth—
            potassium penicillin V, 500 mg.
2. Following the procedure (four times a day the day of the procedure and the next 2 days):
   by mouth—
            potassium penicillin V, 250 mg.

Erythromycin should be used if the patient *is allergic* to penicillin, or *is on rheumatic fever prophylaxis.* Administration of erythromycin is dependent upon the patient's body weight:

1. Two hours prior to the procedure:
   a. Over   25 kg.: by mouth—
                  erythromycin, 500 mg.
   b. Under 25 kg.: by mouth—
                  erythromycin, 20 mg./kg.
2. Following the procedure (four times a day the day of the procedure and the next 2 days):
   a. Over   25 kg.: by mouth—
                  erythromycin, 250 mg.
   b. Under 25 kg.: by mouth—
                  erythromycin, 10 mg./kg.

These recommendations are the same as those of the American Heart Association and the American Dental Association.

The Diabetic Patient. Most oral surgical procedures will be performed on the diabetic patient only when he is under control. In controlled diabetic patients the incidence of postsurgical complications seems no higher than in nondiabetic patients, so that diabetes per se need not be considered as an indication for antibiotic prophylaxis.

Hematologic Abnormalities. Patients having a blood dyscrasia or other hematologic abnormality will often be treated by a hematologist in conjunction with the oral surgeon. Antibiotic therapy is not used routinely in these cases, but if leukopenia exists, antibiotics may be necessary to combat secondary infection.

Multiple Extractions and Alveolectomy. There is no indication for the routine administration of antibiotics in cases of multiple extractions and alveolectomy, provided each case is evaluated according to the criteria which follow.

GENERAL PHYSICAL CONDITION OF THE PATIENT. The patient who is debilitated or chronically ill and who has a history of greater than normal susceptibility to bacterial infection may benefit from antibiotic prophylaxis.

GINGIVAL SEPSIS. Multiple extractions should not be performed in the presence of acute gingival sepsis. Chronically inflamed tissues seem to heal satisfactorily in the post-extraction period without antibiotics.

NUMBER OF TEETH TO BE REMOVED. The number of teeth being removed at one time need not in itself be an indication for antibiotic prophylaxis.

INVOLVEMENT OF ADJACENT ANATOMIC SPACES DURING ORAL SURGERY. When the surgical procedure is such that adjacent structures or anatomic spaces (*i.e.,* maxillary sinus, submandibular space, infratemporal space) are involved, the prophylactic use of antibiotics is justified in an effort to prevent the establishment of an infection.

THE THERAPEUTIC USE OF ANTIBIOTICS IN DENTAL PRACTICE

Antibiotics may be used therapeutically with success when the following conditions are fulfilled:

1. The disease entity is microbial in origin.
2. The pathogen involved is sensitive to one of the antibiotics in doses that can be readily tolerated.
3. The antibiotic is brought into contact with the diseased area or with the disease-producing organisms.

Several specific cases in which antibiotics may be used therapeutically in dental practice follow.

Acute Vincent's Infection. In cases of Vincent's infection with constitutional symptoms such as malaise, cervical adenopathy, temperature elevation and sore throat, the systemic use of antibiotics is indicated to control the acute phase as quickly as possible. Therapy should also be continued during the period when the initial prophylactic procedures are performed. Penicillin is the antibiotic of choice, and one injection of aqueous procaine penicillin, 600,000 units daily for 4 days, is generally adequate. If there are no systemic manifestations, local therapy may be carried out without antibiotic therapy in many instances.

Acute Pericoronitis. Pericoronitis most frequently occurs around unerupted or partly erupted mandibular third molars. The causative organisms are often those of Vincent's infection, which can multiply readily under the soft tissue flap. Occasionally, pericoronitis will be seen in conjunction with a sore throat, in which case the organism involved will most probably be one of the streptococci. In either case, the acute phase of this condition can be controlled with systemic antibiotic therapy in addition to adequate local measures.

Penicillin is the drug of choice, and the average daily dosage is adequate. If the clinical response is not satisfactory within 48 hours, a mixed infection may be suspected. In this case, erythromycin or tetracycline should be considered. A culture should be secured as a guide to further management.

The occurrence of pericoronitis gives evidence of lowered resistance to infection in the immediate local area, as well as a pathogenic oral bacterial flora. Any surgical procedure in these areas should be accompanied by antibiotics, even though the acute phase has undoubtedly subsided.

Acute Infections. In the management of acute infections of dental origin, therapy of maximum intensity must be used from the outset. Many cases of cellulitis are mixed infections.

Penicillin, erythromycin or tetracycline is usually the drug of choice, coupled with judicious surgical intervention. Treatment may be simplified in cases in which it is possible to secure cultures and perform antibiotic sensitivity tests. If the patient does not respond to therapy within 72 hours, a change to another antibiotic may be wise. Antibiotic sensitivity tests assume a role of greater importance in these instances.

Osteomyelitis. In acute osteomyelitis, antibiotic therapy should be started immediately. The causative organism is usually *Staphylococcus aureus*. Therefore,

1. Administer aqueous procaine penicillin, 600,000 units every 12 hours, if no history of sensitivity is elicited.
2. Secure culture for predominant organism and antibiotic sensitivity.
3. If the clinical course is not markedly improved in 72 hours, change the antibiotic regimen in conformity with the sensitivity studies, which should be available by that time.
4. In patients allergic to penicillin, erythromycin is a good second choice.

PROGNOSIS OF THERAPY

The prognosis of therapy is determined by (1) local condition at the site of the pathologic process, and (2) the general condition of the patient: (a) temperature elevation, (b) leukocyte count and (c) erythrocyte sedimentation rate.

If there is no improvement after 72 hours of antibiotic therapy, a change of drugs may be indicated. This may be guided by laboratory sensitivity studies.

THE MANAGEMENT OF ALLERGIC EMERGENCIES

It is true that penicillin offers the greatest liability as far as allergic response is concerned. It must also be borne in mind, however, that allergic emergencies can arise with the administration of many different drugs.

Allergic responses may range in severity from a mild rash to the life-threatening anaphylactoid reaction.

Support of Vital Functions.
1. Clear airway and institute respiratory support and consider cricothyrotomy if necessary.
2. Support the cardiovascular system and arrest the anaphylaxis by the injection of epinephrine, 0.5 cc. of a 1:1000 aqueous solution into the most accessible vascular site. The floor of the mouth is satisfactory, if access can be gained quickly.
3. Continued support of the cardiovascular system can be provided by the use of such vasopressor agents as mephentermine and metaraminol.
4. Corticosteroids can be used, but only after the primary steps have been completed.

SUMMARY

The indiscriminate use of antibiotics is certainly no greater in dentistry than in any other area of the health professions. However, this is not reason enough to excuse a very poor and potentially dangerous practice. The mushrooming cloud of resistant organisms and sensitivity reactions is surely a by-product of this type of usage. The routine use of these agents in all dental procedures is to be condemned. However, when indicated, failure to make use of these agents with good judgment and with proper scientific logic is also to be condemned.

There is, however, little doubt that the antibiotics together with good surgical judgment, as well as greater consideration for the patient's entire physiology, have contributed much to the improvement of the practice of oral surgery.

REFERENCES

1. Bartlett, R. C., and Howell, R. M.: Topical vancomycin as a deterrent to bacteremias following dental procedures. Oral Surg., 35:780–788 (June), 1973.
2. Beeson, P. B., and McDermott, W. (Eds.): Textbook of Medicine. 14th ed. Philadelphia, W. B. Saunders Co., 1975.
3. Conn, H. F. (Ed.): Current Therapy 1975. Philadelphia, W. B. Saunders Co., 1975.
4. Dorland's Illustrated Dictionary. 25th ed. Philadelphia, W. B. Saunders Co., 1974.
5. Glaser, R. J., Dankner, A., Mathes, S. B., and Harford, C.: Effect of penicillin on the bacteremia following dental extraction. Am. J. Med., 4:55–65, 1948.
6. Goldberg, M. H.: Gram-negative bacteremia after dental extraction. J. Oral Surg., 26:180–181 (Mar.), 1968.
7. Goldberg, M. H.: Antibiotics and oral and oral-cutaneous lacerations. J. Oral Surg., 23:117–122 (Mar.), 1965.
8. Gross, A., Bhaskar, S. N., and Cutright, D. E.: A study of bacteremia following wound lavage. Oral Surg., 31:720–722 (May), 1971.
9. Hurwitz, G. A., Speck, W. T., and Keller, G. B.: Absence of bacteremia in children after prophylaxis. Oral Surg., 32:891–893 (Dec.), 1971.
10. Jones, J. C., Cutcher, J. L., Goldberg, J. R., and Lilly, G. E.: Control of bacteremia associated with extraction of teeth. Oral Surg., 30:454–459 (Oct.), 1970.
11. Okell, C. C., and Elliott, S. D.: Bacteremia and oral sepsis, with special reference to the etiology of subacute bacterial endocarditis. Lancet, 2:869, 1935.
12. Zallen, R. D., and Strader, R. J.: The use of prophylactic antibiotics in extraoral procedures for mandibular prognathism. J. Oral Surg., 29:178–179 (Mar.), 1971.

CHAPTER 9

ORAL SURGERY IN THE HOSPITAL

The amount of oral surgery being performed in hospitals for patients who are admitted solely for that purpose is increasing rapidly. It is now recognized that extensive surgery in the oral cavity, such as is necessary for multiple maxillary and mandibular extractions, with the subsequent alveolectomy, the surgical eradication of cysts, tumors and impacted teeth, the open or closed reduction of fractures of facial bones, the correction of malformations of the jaws, and so on, is just as major a surgery as any other operation involving the head and neck or nose and throat. Particularly is this true when the operation is to be performed under general anesthesia. Prolonged oral surgery under general anesthesia should be performed in a hospital, where the patient can receive appropriate preanesthetic, preoperative and postoperative treatment. Also, there are immediately available those safeguards and services concomitant with modern hospital care. It is inconceivable that any dental (or medical) office would be equipped with the individual specialists and specialized equipment to maintain the life of the patient as would the well-designed hospital environment.

In addition, with the present increase in longevity and the prolongation of life by modern medical means, more and more patients are seen who, because of age and other physical impairments, must be classified as very poor office risks for any type of surgery. An apprehensive elderly diabetic with arteriosclerosis and coronary artery disease, on anticoagulant therapy, is safer in the hospital for what might be considered a minor surgical procedure, such as the extraction of one or two teeth, with local anesthesia, whereas the same procedure on a young person in good health is more likely to be done in the office. Evaluation of the patient's ability to withstand the contemplated surgery (age, physical status, emotional status, and so forth), as well as severity and duration of the procedure itself, must be made when deciding where to perform the operation.

PRESURGICAL EVALUATION AND CLASSIFICATION OF THE PATIENT

Assessment of Physical Status (P.S.). The American Society of Anesthesiologists (A.S.A.) has classified patients into a number of grades according to their general physical condition and "risk." There were originally seven grades, but the classification has been amended by the House of Delegates of the Society as follows:

1. A normal, healthy patient.
2. A patient with a mild systemic disease.
3. A patient with a severe systemic disease that limits activity but is not incapacitating.
4. A patient with an incapacitating systemic disease that is a constant threat to life.
5. A moribund patient not expected to survive 24 hours with or without an operation.

In the event of emergency operation, the number should be preceded with an E. An attempt may be made to put patients into their proper grade for purposes of comparison and assessment of risk. The student of dentistry and the practitioners of dentistry must bear in mind that the foregoing are general classifications and should be considered as such. Many patients, especially those in the older age group (55 years and more), will show overlapping physical status, as P.S. 1 and 2, P.S. 2 and 3, and so forth. Those who fall in the A.S.A. 3 and 4 category will rarely, if ever, be seen outside of the hospital environment. It is paramount that the oral surgeon be familiar with all phases of these patients.

419

ADMISSION OF PATIENTS

GENERAL CONCEPTS

Appointment of the oral surgeon, or other health care professional, to the medical staff is a privilege granted to the applicant by the governing body of the hospital after considering recommendations made by the medical staff through established mechanisms. The medical staff must define in its by-laws the requirement for admission to staff membership and for the delineation and retention of clinical privileges.

In some hospitals, the oral surgery section is a division of the general surgical service (with the same status as urology, gynecology, etc.), and admissions are made directly to the general dentist's or oral surgeon's service. In these cases *the prime responsibility (legal and moral) for the patient's management rests with the dentist or oral surgeon.* The regulations of the Joint Commission on Accreditation of Hospitals (J.C.A.H.) require that dental patients receive the same basic medical appraisal as patients admitted to other services. A physician member of the medical staff must be responsible for the care of *any medical problems* during the hospitalization of dental patients. It is not the intent of the J.C.A.H. that a physician need be in attendance of hospitalized dental patients unless a medical problem is present on admission or arises, but it is the dentist's obligation to request consultation with an appropriate physician when medical problems occur.

In some hospitals, an oral surgeon qualified in physical diagnosis will do the complete history and physical, and this may be acceptable to the medical staff; in other hospitals this same history and physical will be countersigned by a physician member of the medical staff; in still other hospitals, a physician member of the staff or licensed intern or resident physician will do the necessary history and physical. However, whether there is one or are even more consultants, the dentist must realize that if he is the person whose name is on the chart, *he is the responsible doctor.* It is his duty to see the patient regularly, and he must be aware of everything that is going on with respect to that patient, not only of what is happening in the mouth.

For example, if a patient develops anuria postoperatively or develops an elevated postoperative temperature, he should know what to do. This does not mean that he should treat the patient for these conditions if they are beyond his scope of responsibility, but it is his obligation to be able to recognize trouble and to see that the patient is treated properly. If the dentist is not competent to evaluate the patient's postoperative course and see that the indicated medical treatment is carried out, he should not accept the responsibility for admissions directly to his own service. In these cases, the admissions may be handled as medical and dental admissions.

In smaller hospitals and in hospitals in which there is no dental service, admissions are generally made by the patient's physician to his own service. In these cases, the dentist serves as a consultant, and here the prime responsibility for the patient's medical evaluation rests with the physician. This does not absolve the dentist from his duties to see the patient pre- and postoperatively, but the burden of responsibility has passed from his shoulders to the physician's with respect to nondental complications and so forth.

If a dentist has his own service, he should be competent enough to obtain an adequate medical history and evaluate the pertinent findings. Despite the fact that a consultant physician may have done the history and physical examination, it should be repeated because additional important information often comes to light which the patient has glossed over the first time. How to take a history is covered later in this chapter — the ability to evaluate this history depends on the knowledge and training of the examiner.

SPECIFIC MECHANICS OF ADMISSION

The majority of hospitals require that surgical patients be admitted 24 hours before operation or at least spend the night prior to surgery in the hospital. This will provide adequate time for physical evaluation, laboratory procedures and proper preoperative sedation.

The patient enters the hospital and should be seen as soon as possible after admission by the dental intern or resident if there is one available. If not, the dentist should see the patient himself. Although there are many varieties of chart systems in hospital practice, they all conform to one basic standard. A history and physical examination must be written which, in this case, will include the dental examination in the physical or on the consultation sheet. Depending on local practice (as explained previously), this may be divided between physician (or medical resident) and dentist (or dental intern or resident). An ad-

Liver disease (these patients are often "bleeders")

Kidney disease	Tonsillitis
Blood disease	Scarlet fever
Measles	Diphtheria
Mumps	Influenza
Diabetes	Pleurisy
Whooping cough	Pneumonia
Chickenpox	Tuberculosis

Allergies (especially to penicillin and narcotics): also inquire about possible sensitivities to barbiturates, aspirin, adhesive tape, iodine, mercury, etc.—in other words, anything they might come in contact with to which people are often sensitive. It is a good idea to note these allergies in red ink prominently on the front of the chart or chart holder so that a night intern or nurse (who is not going to read a whole chart if he or she is in a hurry) will not inadvertently prescribe or use an allergenic agent.

Syphilis	Rheumatic fever
Gonorrhea	Asthma
Typhoid fever	Arthritis
Malaria	

Patients who have endocardial damage (e.g., from rheumatic heart disease) or who have had valvular heart surgery should receive adequate dosages of antibiotics before and after surgery.

Bleeding tendencies. This factor is *very important,* and the reader is referred to pages 1560 to 1579, Chapter 25, for careful study.

History of having received steroid (cortisone) therapy. This has become a major surgical hazard, since patients who have been on steroid therapy prior to surgery may have adrenal insufficiency and be unable to respond to operative or anesthetic stress, or both. Numbers of these patients have very quietly died postoperatively from the most innocuous surgical procedures. Any patient who has received steroids in the past year (and patients must be questioned most carefully, since many are unaware of the nature of their medication) must be individually evaluated regarding the necessity of placing him again on prophylactic steroid therapy prior to surgery, *during it and postoperatively.* Any history of

treatment for arthritis, rheumatism, allergies, uveitis, iritis, skin diseases or similar disorders by unknown systemic medication should be pursued by calling the prescribing physician or pharmacist, if possible, to make sure exactly what the medication is.

Previous operations and anesthetics: Record any untoward reactions, and so on.

Injuries: Injuries necessitating medical treatment and any complications.

Past oral operations: Note any reactions to local anesthetics, bleeding tendencies, alveolalgia (so-called "dry sockets"), swelling, trismus or delayed healing.

Age.

Systemic Review. The patient is questioned about each system, as indicated, in order to uncover any pathologic condition unknown to him.

General: Night sweats, fever, tremors, weight changes, nutrition.

Skin: Warm, moist or dry, presence of lesions, eruptions, cyanosis, jaundice, multiple petechiae, sores, needle tracks, scars, coloration, etc. (Because of the rapid rise of the so-called drug culture the dentist should be acutely aware, in both the office and hospital, of the signs and symptoms of the drug abuser.)

Head: Headache, syncope, trauma.

Eyes: Diplopia, photophobia, lacrimation.

Ears: Deafness, discharge, tinnitus, dizziness.

Nose: Epistaxis, colds, obstruction, drips, sinusitis.

Throat: Soreness, hoarseness, dysphagia.

Respiratory: Hemoptysis, dyspnea, chest pains, sputum, asthma, orthopnea.

Cardiovascular: Pain, palpitation, tachycardia, vertigo, edema, faintness.

Musculoskeletal: Weakness, joint pain, paresthesia, varicosities.

Gastrointestinal: Appetite, pain, nausea, vomiting, belching, flatulence, constipation, diarrhea, bloody or mucous stools, hernia, hemorrhoids, melena.

Genitourinary: Sores, frequency, burning, incontinence, nocturia, hematuria, water consumption.

Female Reproductive: Periods (frequency, type, duration), abortions.

Nervous: Headaches, convulsions, paralysis, emotions, personality.

Family History. This is taken in order to discover any predisposition in the family toward inheritable diseases or diseases in which inheritance seems to be an important factor, e.g., allergies or diabetes. Record information concerning parents, siblings and children as to whether they are alive and well (abbreviated a. & w.) or if dead, year, ages at death, and causes.

Social Habits. Note occupations, habits, use of drugs, alcohol, tobacco, coffee, sleeping habits, and so on. Pin the patient down as to a definite quantity of various substances used in a given period of time; do not accept a generality such as "an occasional drink." When discussing drugs, a question such as, "Are you now, or have you recently, been taking any medicine or drugs?" will usually elicit most relevant information. Another excellent catch-all question is, "Are you now, or have you recently, been going to the doctor for anything?"

Summary and Impressions. At this point the examiner should have a good general idea of the patient's medical background, and from this information can draw certain conclusions. The final diagnosis may not be obvious but, insofar as the general condition is concerned, certain impressions have been obtained from the history. These impressions may be confirmed or denied by the physical examination and laboratory reports, but the clues appearing in the history should be pursued by ordering the necessary laboratory tests and informing the medical consultant of any significant points recorded.

The impressions are numbered consecutively, starting with the most likely positive diagnosis and ending with the most remote diagnosis consistent with the history.

In recording diagnoses and operations the *Standard Nomenclature of Diseases and Operations* should be consulted. Hospitals keep records of diagnoses and operations by code number rather than name, so the correct terminology must be used so that the medical records department can correctly encode it.

PHYSICAL EXAMINATION

This is the next part of the chart to be filled out by the examiner. If this is the joint responsibility of a medical consultant and the oral surgeon, the dentist fills out an oral examination and gives his conclusions, and the medical consultant follows this with the rest of the physical examination and conclusions. The latter may appear on the regular chart or the special consultation sheet in the chart, according to local hospital practice. It must be emphasized that the use of the term "negative" or "normal" is to be condemned, and some specific comment should be made about each part examined.

The oral and maxillofacial portion of the examination should include the following:

Teeth. Record, diagrammatically, which teeth are present in the mouth and any information concerning caries, mobility, periodontoclasia, or other pathologic condition that is present. The occlusion should be checked for any abnormalities. If dental radiographs are available, this information should also be recorded. If radiographs are taken at the hospital the radiologist's report will contain this information. However, the dentist should always diagnose the oral radiographs also. In the radiographs impacted teeth, cysts, tumors, and so on, should be noted. If necessary, pulp tests, transillumination and percussion should be performed and recorded here.

Mucosa and Gingiva. The presence of inflammatory changes, enlargements or malformations should be noted.

Palate, Pharynx, Lips, Cheeks, Floor of Oral Cavity, Sublingual Tissues. Change in color, inflammation, enlargements, and so on, are noted. Do not hesitate to palpate these tissues bimanually if possible.

Tongue. Any changes in size, papillary color and size, mobility are noted. Grasp tip of tongue with a towel and bring it well forward out of the mouth, then carefully examine sides and base for ulcerations or tumor formation.

Breath and Oral Hygiene.

Lymph Nodes. Bilateral bimanual palpation of neck nodes is performed.

Temporomandibular Joint. Both temporomandibular joints are palpated for evidence of subluxation, pain, cracking and so on. Deviation on opening the mouth is also noted.

Face (Where Applicable). Any abnormalities in appearance and contour (especially following trauma) should be noted. Pupillary size and level, palpable defects and paresthesias are also noted.

Following this examination, one or more conclusions are drawn concerning the findings of the oral examination: *e.g.,* severe periodontoclasia, extensive dental caries, deep tumor of the tongue, or other diagnoses. These are also numbered consecutively like the impressions in the history, with the most important conclusion listed first and the least important last.

EXAMPLES OF HISTORY AND PHYSICAL EXAMINATION

HISTORY

Chief Complaint. Swelling of neck and inability to swallow.

History of Present Illness. Two days ago (April 17, 1975) the patient visited her dentist and had lower left first bicuspid extracted because of persistent toothache of several days' duration. She had no noticeable swelling at the time of extraction. Yesterday morning she awakened with marked swelling of the floor of the mouth and neck and saw her dentist, who gave her 600,000 units repository penicillin intramuscularly. She has gotten progressively worse despite the penicillin, and this morning had great difficulty in even swallowing her saliva. She has had repeated chills followed by hot flashes and has had moderately severe pain. Her dentist saw her this morning and took her temperature, which was 103° F. He referred her to the hospital for admission and oral surgery consultation.

Past Medical History. *Medical:* Denies liver, heart, kidney disease, rheumatic fever, influenza, pleurisy, pneumonia, tuberculosis, allergies, lues, gonorrhea, typhoid, asthma, arthritis, bleeding tendencies. Usual childhood diseases: measles, 1954; whooping cough, 1957; chickenpox, 1958; mumps, 1961.

Previous operations and anesthesia: No history of untoward reactions. T & A — ether (?), 1960. Appendectomy — Pentothal, 1970.

Injuries: No injuries.

Past oral operation: Three extractions under local anesthesia with no complications or anesthetic reactions.

Systemic Review. *General:* No history of night sweats, recent weight changes or tremors. Since present illness there has been a high fever.

Skin: No history of cyanosis or jaundice. Prickly heat in summer.

Head: No history of trauma or syncope. Has had severe headache for past two days over entire head.

Eyes: No history of diplopia, photophobia or lacrimations.

Ears: No history of deafness, discharge, tinnitus, dizziness.

Nose: No epistaxis, obstruction, postnasal drips, sinusitis. Two or three colds every winter.

Throat: No hoarseness. Dysphagia and pain following onset of present illness but not prior to it.

Respiratory: No history of hemoptysis, pain, asthma. Occasional dyspnea following exertion. Orthopnea since yesterday due to swelling of neck.

Cardiovascular: No tachycardia, vertigo, ankle edema, faintness or pain.

Musculoskeletal: No history of weakness, paresthesia, varicosities. In past three years has had occasional episodes of sore, swollen stiff joints. Never seen by a physician during these episodes and has never been checked by physicians since 1970.

Gastrointestinal: No history of nausea, vomiting, diarrhea, flatulence, melena, blood in stools, hemorrhoids, or pain in abdomen. Usually chronically constipated.

Genitourinary: No burning incontinence or hematuria. In past several years nocturia has developed (2–3 times per night), and there has been an increase in water consumption (8–10 glasses daily).

Female Reproductive: Regular periods with no difficulty. Not menstruating now.

Nervous: No history of convulsions or paralysis. Infrequent headaches. No excessive nervousness.

Family History. Mother a & w; father died, 1961, cancer of lung. 2 brothers, a & w, 1 sister, a & w. Married — no children. Age 25.

Social Habits. Housewife, denies use of barbiturates or other drugs, moderate use of alcohol ("at parties only"). Smokes one-half pack of cigarettes daily. No coffee or tea.

Summary and Impressions. This patient has apparently developed an infection of the neck as a result of the extension of dental infection. However, there appear to be one or more modifying factors.

Impressions: 1. Cellulitis of neck due to
2. Possible penicillin-resistant organisms?
3. Possible diabetes?
4. Possible rheumatic fever history?

Signature — D.D.S.

PHYSICAL EXAMINATION

April 19, 1975: A well-nourished, well-developed, white female in moderately severe distress due to inability to swallow and orthopnea.

Teeth. $\overline{4}$ missing. $\overline{4}$ socket healing normally $\overline{7/45}$ with no discharge. No visible caries. Teeth are in a good state of repair with large numbers of amalgam fillings. No periodontoclasia or mobility demonstrable.

Mucosa and Gingiva. In the   345 area there is marked elevation of the lingual mucosa with infection. No other malformations noted. Gingival tissues not hyperplastic or inflamed other than in lower left bicuspid area.

Palate, Pharynx, Lips, Sublingual Tissues, Neck. There is a marked swelling of the left side of the neck in both the submaxillary and submental spaces. It is not indurated but moderately firm to the touch and has passed the soft, doughy stage. The depression under the inferior border of the mandible has been completely obliterated by the swelling. There is a superficial, irregular erythema about 2 inches in diameter over the anterior pole of the submaxillary gland. Bimanual palpation does not elicit fluctuation. There is also a moderate-sized swelling in the floor of the mouth on the left side. That is firm and nonfluctuant. The lips are dry and cracked and the palate is dry but not inflamed.

Tongue. Elevated and deviated to the right. No tremors or masses. Papillae appear normal under thick coating of debris.

Breath and Oral Hygiene. Poor oral hygiene and foul breath.

Lymph Nodes. Submaxillary and submental nodes on left are not palpable due to swelling. No other enlargement or tenderness noted.

Temporomandibular Joint. Palpation not satisfactory because of some degree of trismus present. No tenderness on pressure.

    Impression: 1. Submaxillary and submental cellulitis not as yet fluctuant?
                     Signature — — —

At this point the consulting physician or attending oral surgeon should complete the remainder of the general physical examination and give his impressions. From then on it is the duty of the oral surgeon to proceed with the necessary orders and treatment.

LABORATORY STUDIES

Laboratory studies that are routinely done prior to surgery serve two main purposes. By their proper interpretation the dental surgeon is helped in arriving at a correct clinical diagnosis, and he is able to resolve complicated situations that can make surgery a hazard.

A full-mouth series of dental radiographs can be supplemented by occlusal and bitewing radiographs as well as extraoral views. These radiographs will help to relate the dental problem to the other vital structures of the head and neck.

Blood studies as well as urinalyses are routinely performed for all patients who are admitted to the hospital for surgery. These tests may at times uncover a hidden systemic medical disease that automatically transfers the patient from the class of a *"good surgical risk"* (see earlier Assessment of Physical Status) to one in which any surgical procedure, however minor in nature, would jeopardize his life. For example, a patient with a chief complaint of "loose decayed teeth" who excretes great quantities of sugar in the urine

would definitely warrant a thorough medical evaluation before the surgeon could proceed with reasonable safety.

Included in the blood studies should be a complete blood count (CBC), which provides a reasonable estimate of the patient's circulating red blood cells (RBC) as well as his white blood cells (WBC). The hemoglobin (Hb) and hematocrit (HCT) give a fair indication of the oxygen-carrying capacity of the blood as well as an index of the patient's red blood cell volume. The hematocrit is a laboratory test in which the volume of packed red blood cells is expressed in percentages after the whole blood has been centrifuged.

In patients over 40 years of age an electrocardiogram and chest film are mandatory.

Urine is analyzed for its total volume output, concentration, specific gravity, and presence of abnormal organic and inorganic elements. Of special importance is the presence of abnormally large quantities of sugar and albumin in otherwise normal urine. Their presence is so often the first sign of pre-existent systemic disease.

For normal laboratory values, see tables just inside the front and back covers of *Conn's Current Therapy*.[1]

PREOPERATIVE CHECK-UP BY SURGEON

The morning of operation, the oral surgeon examines the chart to ascertain whether the laboratory and physical findings are normal. He visits the patient, preferably before the preoperative medication has been administered.

If the laboratory findings, history and physical examination are not normal, then the operation should be cancelled and medical treatment carried out until the patient's physical condition will permit surgery with a minimum of risk.

If everything is found to be normal, the oral surgeon proceeds to the operating room, and there checks the instrument set-up to make certain that it and the other equipment, such as the headlight, suction apparatus, and the rest, are ready.

OPERATING ROOM ROUTINE

The dental surgeon should prepare himself for surgical procedures in the operating room in the same manner as the general surgeon prepares himself for his work. Although it is impossible to sterilize the oral cavity, which encompasses the field of operation in most dental cases, the ritual of sterile technique is of great value in minimizing the possibility of introducing pathogenic organisms into the surgical wound. In addition, many features of the technique serve to provide comfort and protection for the oral surgeon.

Aseptic surgical technique briefly consists of the following:

Operating Room. Thorough sterilization of instruments, drapes, gloves, sponges, sutures, and anything else that may come in contact with the field of operation directly or indirectly, e.g., the table covers upon which sterile instruments are placed; setting up sterile tables and instrument trays.

Dressing of Operator and Assistants. The operator and each assistant, after removing street clothes, put on clean cotton scrub suits consisting of trousers and shirts. Cotton clothing does not produce the sparks from static electricity that may develop when nylon or woolen clothing is worn. Static electric sparks have been responsible for tragic explosions in operating rooms. Clean scrub suits, in addition to eliminating dust-laden clothes from the operating room, provide for the comfort of the operator, and conserve his clothes as well.

The operator next dons a pair of shoes or disposable conductive boots. Today a well-equipped hospital has special conductive operating room floors to prevent explosions, and all personnel must wear conductive-soled shoes or special conductive boots that fit over street shoes. These prevent static electricity from accumulating on the operator, which can produce a spark when he approaches a grounded circuit.

Although these practices are still adhered to, including in the construction of all new hospitals, the wide acceptance of the halogenated inhalation compounds has reduced the explosive hazard to zero. The reader should remain aware that these new compounds present their own particular problems and that we are still not in possession of the "ideal inhalation anesthetic."

Next the participants don clean caps and masks. The surgeon puts on a headlight and adjusts the light beam. If he dosen't wear glasses, he puts on a pair of shatter-resistant glasses to protect his eyes from flying debris.

PREPARATION OF HANDS AND ARMS FOR OPERATION

Preparation. Adjust the scrub cap to cover the hair completely, and adjust the mask to cover the nose and mouth. Roll the sleeves well above the elbows. Remove all jewelry and watch. The nails should be short and smooth.

Procedure. Regulate the water in the scrub sink to a desirable temperature. Wash the hands and forearms thoroughly, and cleanse the fingernails with an orangewood stick. Scrub brushes are now supplied in sterile containers or in individual sterile packages impregnated with germicidal concentrate and containing a plastic nail cleaner.

Begin by scrubbing the palm of the hand, using parallel strokes. Scrub the palm in three sections: from the little finger to the thumb scrub all four surfaces of each finger; then close the hand and scrub the knuckles; then scrub the arms to the elbows, using longitudinal strokes and scrubbing in five sections. While scrubbing the hand, be sure to scrub the interdigital spaces thoroughly; while scrubbing the back of each finger, scrub from hand to wrist, using longitudinal strokes. After scrubbing one hand and arm, repeat the procedure on the other hand and arm. Repeat this scrub on each hand and arm. Then rinse the hands and arms, thoroughly draining them from fingertip to elbow. Rinse the brush. Turn off the water with the brush and discard the brush. Walk into the operating room, holding the hands up, and the scrub nurse provides a sterile towel.

Gowns and Gloves. The hands and arms are dried with the sterile towel, and each member of the surgical team puts on a sterile gown. The hands are dusted by the scrub nurse with sterile talcum powder prior to putting on sterile gloves. Strict aseptic technique requires that gloves be put on without touching the outer surface with the hands. From this point the operator and all sterile personnel must be aware that any area below the operative field is to be considered contaminated and is not to be touched.

PREPARATION OF THE PATIENT

The patient is first anesthetized.

The technique used in preparing the patient's face and neck depends upon whether the procedure is to be intraoral or extraoral.

Preparation for Extraoral Procedure. All work is done from a specially prepared sterile table containing only the armamentarium needed for the preparation of the patient. This consists of (*a*) a cleansing solution to remove the surface oil and dirt from the skin (commonly used are germicidal solutions, followed by a washing of sterile water and alcohol; the latter is allowed to dry by evaporation); (*b*) an antiseptic or germicidal agent, such as tinted benzalkonium chloride (Zephiran), thimerosal (Merthiolate) or iodine (the last is much less frequently used); (*c*) sterile stainless steel cups or basins containing the solutions; (*d*) large sterile sponges; (*e*) sponge holders.

The sponges are folded in squares measuring approximately 1½ inches on the side, and grasped with the sponge holder. The cleansing solution is first vigorously applied to the operative site in such a fashion that extension of the cleansed area for a great distance under the drapes is assured. This will preclude contamination with movement of the drapes. The cleansing is repeated several times, never redipping the used sponge in either the cleansing or antiseptic solutions. Then, using folded sponges again, the cleansed area is painted with one of the tinted antiseptic agents. A tinted vehicle is preferred, the better to demarcate the operative site.

The table, its equipment and gloves are now regarded as being contaminated and are

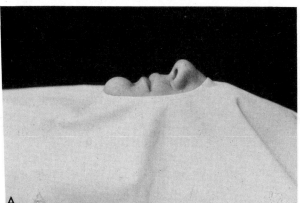
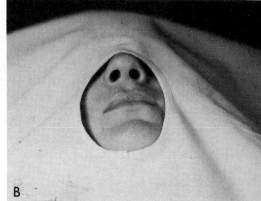

Figure 9–1

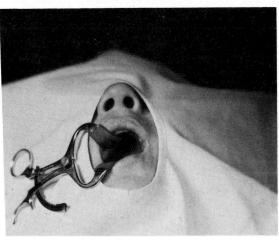
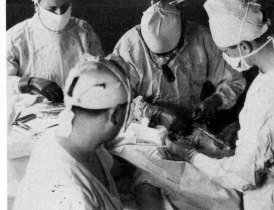

Figure 9–2   Figure 9–3

Figure 9–1 *A,* "T and A" sterile drape over the patient's head and face. *B,* Exposed skin prepared with germicide and the lips coated with petrolatum.

Figure 9–2 Mouth prop placed and the jaws opened.

Figure 9–3 Operating team placing the suture in the tongue in those cases in which endotracheal anesthesia is not used.

discarded. The first assistant need not scrub again, but merely change his gown and gloves. The patient is then draped.

Preparation for Intraoral Procedure. For this preparation the first assistant may wear gown and gloves, and work from the Mayo table. Using large sponges folded into 1½-inch squares, a tinted antiseptic germicidal agent is widely applied to the area around the mouth extending below the chin to the neck and up to the nose, and including both cheeks.

If the solution used is a tincture, the area should be dried with sterile dry sponges, so as to avoid a chemical burn by having a drape which has become wet with the tincture in prolonged contact with the skin. The sponge holder is then discarded; sterile petrolatum is then applied to the lips and commissures of the mouth to keep these areas well lubricated, thereby preventing drying and cracking. The applicator is also discarded. The first assistant need not regown or reglove.

After the patient is thus prepared and draped, the operator, using his tongue retractor and good lighting, should examine the oral cavity and the full aspects of the oropharynx, thoroughly suctioning any collected mucous and blood following nasal intubation and carefully checking for any teeth, tooth fragments or calculus fragments that may have been displaced by laryngoscopy. Despite the fact that modern endotracheal tubes have an inflatable cuff that is expanded against the laryngeal cords to prevent the passage of secretions or foreign material to the bronchial tree, the wise operator will place a moistened pharyngeal gauze pack. Probably the safest is the large one-piece vaginal pack that can be placed in an accordian fold, with the excess easily being cut away.

SURGICAL TEAM

The surgical team consists of the operator and the assistants, the anesthetist, the scrub nurse, and the circulating nurse.

The *operator* is in a sense the captain of the team. He assumes the responsibility, and his instructions are to be respected by other members of the team.

The *assistants'* duties are to (1) keep the mouth and the operative field free of blood, mucus, saliva and debris, by continuous and judicious use of the suction apparatus; (2) do any retraction that is necessary to expose the field properly; (3) cut sutures, use the mallet, keep an eye on the oropharyngeal partition, and notify the surgeon if it requires changing or adjustment; (4) call the operator's attention to anything the operator might overlook.

The *anesthetist's* duties consist in maintaining a suitable level of anesthesia, constantly observing the patient's condition, and advising the operator of any untoward reaction of the patient. The anesthetist should inform the operator of any obstruction of the airway caused by the surgical manipulation, so that the operator and the assistant may take immediate steps to remove or correct any cause of obstruction.

The *scrub nurse's* duties consist in seeing that the sterile instruments, drapes, and supplies are available and properly arranged on the tables. He or she should hand instruments, sponges and sutures to the operator at his request. The nurse should keep the instruments properly arranged during the operation and sometimes may be required to assist in retraction.

The *circulating nurse* ties the surgeon's and the assistant's gowns in the back. This person also adjusts the overhead operating light and table. If additional supplies, instruments, or equipment are needed, this nurse brings them.

INSTRUMENTARIUM FOR ORAL SURGERY

Sterile Instrument Supply Table. The table is set up by the instrument or scrub nurse. It contains the sterile supplies and all the instruments that may be used in oral surgery. Since the table contains sufficient instruments and supplies for several operations, it is not to be contaminated during the operation in progress; it should be covered with a sterile drape. Instruments and supplies that are needed are transferred to the Mayo stand with a sterile instrument forceps. Thus, when a series of cases are operated in sequence, there is no need for delay because of lack of sterile equipment for the succeeding case.

The table should contain, as illustrated in Figure 9–4, the following:

Back Row:
  Sterile drapes.
  Hemostats.
  Metal pan for sterile water to clear suction tip and wash sutures.
  Medicine glasses for antiseptic for preparing face and oral cavity.

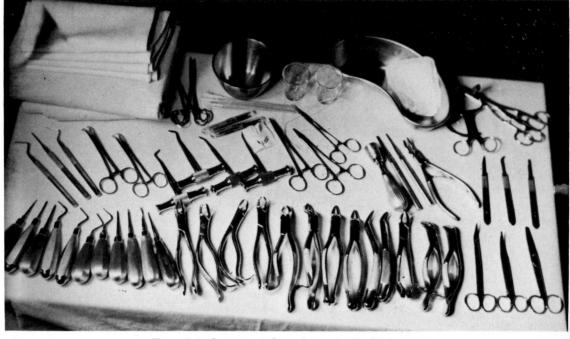

Figure 9–4 Instruments for oral surgery. (See list in text.)

Applicators.

Emesis basin for specimens and teeth.

Molt mouth gag.

Sponge holder (sponges in emesis basin).

Middle Row:

Apical fragment ejectors Nos. 1, 2, 3.

Towel clips.

Cross bar elevators Nos. 322, 323, 370, 371.

Suture.

Needle holder (6-inch) and appropriate needles.

Mallet and chisels (universal and bibevel).

Rongeurs.

Bone files (not shown).

Scalpels (Bard-Parker handle No. 3; blades Nos. 11, 12, 15).

Front Row:

Apexo elevators Nos. 4 (302), 5 (303), 81 (301); Miller elevators Nos. 71, 72, 73, 74.

Forceps (Nos. 286, 150, 10H, 24, 10, 99A, 16, 151, 103).

Dean's scissors Nos. 9, 12 (not shown); 5-inch straight and curved scissors.

Not shown:

Allis forceps.

Apical fragment forceps.

T & A suction tip.

Cogswell suction tip.

Curettes, assorted sizes.

Periosteal elevator.

Retractors (Austin and T & A).

Surgitome, with an assortment of surgical burs.

For the removal of cysts and cystic tumors of the oral cavity that are approached intraorally: iodoform gauze (1/4-inch or 1/2-inch) should be on the main supply table.

For extraoral incision and drainage of abscesses: a large, curved Kelly hemostat (used for blunt dissection) and iodoform gauze or Penrose drains (for drainage) are placed on the main supply table.

For the excision of both peripheral and central tumors: the use of electrosurgery is often indicated, and the appropriate tips must be present, should dissection, fulguration or coagulation be indicated. Iodoform gauze may also be necessary to pack residual cavities and should be on the main supply table.

For the treatment of fractures requiring intermaxillary fixation the following must be added to the main supply table:

1. Arch bars—Jelenko, Winter, Erich, etc., according to the operator's preference.

2. Stainless wire of 24 to 26 gauge to fasten arch bars to teeth or use for Stout-type wiring.

3. Rubber bands (already made or cut from rubber tubing) for intermaxillary fixation.

4. Flat-nose pliers.

5. Wire cutter.

6. No. 1 suture (18-inch) or some other heavy suture-type material to be used by placing around intermaxillary elastics if fracture is reduced and fixed while patient is still anesthetized. This can be fastened to the cheek,

and if the patient develops postoperative vomiting the elastics can be removed with one pull on the cord and aspiration of the vomitus can be prevented.

7. Suitable plastic instrument for holding wire down below the cingulum during tightening.

For the treatment of fractures requiring extraoral fixation or open reduction add:

Roger Anderson pins.

Roger Anderson connecting bars—assorted lengths.

Roger Anderson single and double connector links.

Small wrench.   ⎫ For tightening con-
Socket handle wrench. ⎬ nection and links.

Pin vise for removing pins.

Pin cutter.

Dye (*e.g.,* methylene blue) for outlining fracture.

Electric or hand drill for insertion of pins.

Manipulating handles for fractures.

Stader pin guide.

Stader connecting rods.

Stader wrenches.

Thoma clamp.

Sherman plate and bone screws.

Clip-on screw driver.

Sherman screw bits for drill.

000 catgut for closure of subcutaneous tissues in open reductions.

0000 Dermalon for skin closure in open reductions.

24 or 26 gauge wire for interosseous wiring.

No. 557 for drilling holes for interosseous wiring.

Mayo Table.   This table is placed over the operating table, above the patient, within easy reach of the surgeon and the scrub nurse. On it are placed the instruments the surgeon is using. A minimum number of instruments are kept here; those not in use are removed by the scrub nurse, who turns them over to the circulating nurse for sterilization. When they are sterilized, they are returned to the sterile supply table.

Figure 9–5 illustrates the table as it is set up for a complete maxillary odontectomy and alveolectomy.

Surgical Air Turbine.   This instrument

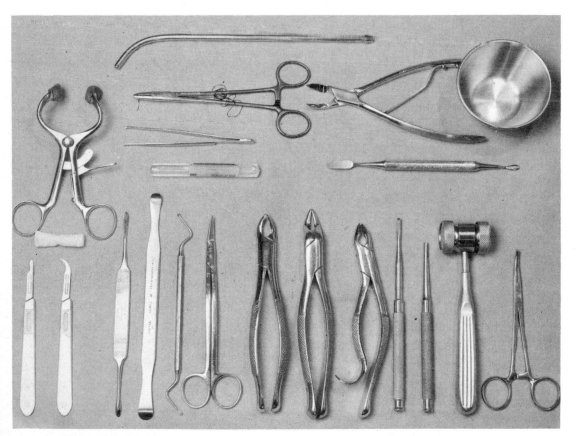

Figure 9–5   Instrument tray set-up for a complete maxillary odontectomy and alveolectomy.

with appropriate burs is standing by, or the dental engine with a sterile arm, cord and handpiece and an assortment of bone burs is made ready for use at each operation.

When the operator has completed the maxillary odontectomy and alveolectomy, the forceps appearing in Figure 9–5 are replaced by the mandibular forceps and the table is set up as shown in Figure 9–6.

IMMEDIATE POSTOPERATIVE TREATMENT

When the operation is completed, a thorough examination is made to see that the oropharyngeal partition is removed and the pharynx is clear of blood clots. The mouth is suctioned, and fresh sterile pressure packs are placed, with an airway inserted if necessary. The drapes, anesthetic armamentarium, and all instruments are removed from the operative area. The patient is transferred from the table to a recovery carriage or his bed, usually being placed on his side or abdomen. The purpose of this position is to try to

prevent any swallowing or aspiration of blood or mucus. The patient is covered with warm blankets and removed to the recovery room or to his own room. Here he is constantly watched, especially for symptoms of shock, respiratory embarrassment and excessive bleeding.

The patient's vital signs, including pulse, respiration rate and blood pressure, are checked every 15 minutes until he has fully reacted, and after that every 30 minutes until he is up and around. Following recovery, providing that no untoward events have occurred, the check for vital signs can return to the routine of four times a day. In the elderly and chronically ill patients, fluid intake and output should be monitored. An emesis basin is kept next to the patient's face so that he may expectorate at any time.

A tank of oxygen and a suction machine are at the patient's bedside, in readiness for immediate use. The patient should never be permitted to become cyanotic. If such should occur, a patent airway should be established, all packs should be removed, the mouth

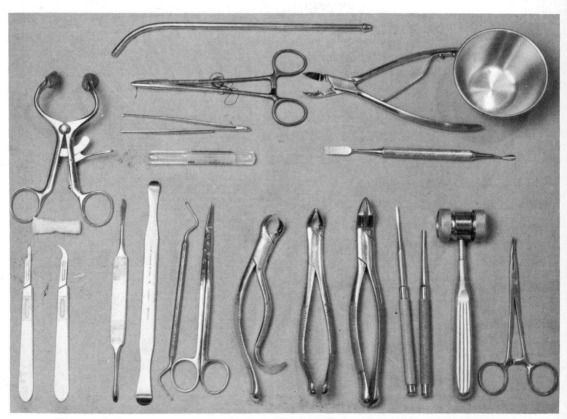

Figure 9–6   Instrument tray set-up for a complete mandibular odontectomy and alveolectomy.

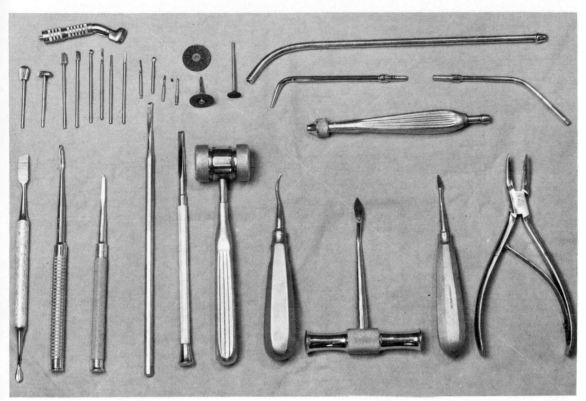

Figure 9–7 Instrument tray set-up for (1) radectomy (root excision by windowing the cortex in an edentulous maxilla or mandible); (2) excision of torus palatinus or mandibularis; (3) excision of exotoses; (4) alveolectomy of edentulous jaws; (5) excision of unerupted teeth from edentulous ridges plus additional appropriate forceps or elevators.

should be suctioned, and oxygen should be applied with a mask. Respirations and pulse rates should be periodically observed until the patient is normal.

Ice packs are applied intermittently for periods not longer than 20 minutes to the operative areas immediately. This reduces the amount of postoperative edema considerably.

If intravenous fluids were started in the operating room, they are permitted to finish unless the patient is reacting too violently. If the needle cannot be kept in the vein, it may be reinserted later when the patient is not too violent (but a well-inserted and well-taped needle in the back of the hand or an Intracath is difficult to dislodge, whereas a needle in the antecubital fossa is almost impossible to retain). How much fluid a patient should receive intravenously depends on how soon oral ingestion can be started. Average patients require 2500 cc. of fluid daily, but more than 1000 cc. intravenously is rarely indicated. It is preferable to use 5 per cent glucose in water rather than saline because

for 24 or more hours postoperatively the kidney tends to excrete less than normal amounts of sodium ion, and saline solutions only add to the sodium excess in the circulation.

Occasionally a patient will become restless and even violent when emerging from anesthesia. Meperidine, 50 to 100 mg., may be given intramuscularly in order to relax the patient. However, respiratory depression of varying degrees may occur even with small amounts of meperidine because of synergistic action with the residual anesthetic. The patient should be carefully observed for this. Sides are placed on the bed, and, if necessary, the patient is placed in restraints. These hold the arms, legs, and even the body of the patient. This might prevent the patient's doing harm to himself and to his attendants.

Drinking and eating are permitted and even encouraged as soon as the patient is able. Approximately 8 hours postoperatively, mouth rinses are started and continued for several days.

Postoperative Orders. It must be remembered that surgery cancels all presurgical orders. Therefore, new postoperative orders must be written for the patient. A representative set of orders might appear as follows:

POSTOPERATIVE ORDERS

1. Remove sponges when patient reacts. Insert sponges as required for bleeding and instruct patient to bite firmly on the sponges.
2. For pain, every 3 hours when required, 10 grains ASA with 1/4 grain codeine orally or meperidine, 75 mg. intramuscularly.
3. Ice packs to face for first 24 hours, 30 minutes each hour, followed by heat tomorrow (hot water bottles or Thermolite).
4. Dental soft diet (nonchewing), force fluids.
5. Multivitamin capsules.*
6. Mouthwash, 0.3 gm. oxychlorosene sodium (Kasdenol) in 8 oz. of H_2O. Use three times a day, beginning 8 hours after surgery.
7. Semi-Fowler position (elevation of head of bed) and out of bed when fully reacted (early ambulation is usually desirable).
8. Special orders as surgeon desires or as are indicated for the specific case.

The patient should be visited daily and progress notes recorded until he is discharged.

DEHYDRATION FEVER

Each cell of the body lives an aquatic existence, and the water surrounding it is, both physically and biologically, an ideal medium for conducting away from the cell excess heat generated in the course of cellular metabolism. Inadequate intake of water, common after oral surgery, results in faulty cooling and is the cause of the "dehydration fever." Unless the oral surgeon is aware of this common cause of postoperative fever, it is often overlooked.

To prevent this, as well as to facilitate the elimination of bacterial products, we routinely order postoperatively about 2500 cc. of fluid daily. If necessary, the intravenous route is taken, using 1000 cc. of a 5 per cent glucose solution in water. However, it is far better physiologically to "force fluids" via the gastrointestinal tract in the form of juices,

ginger ale, or just plain water since there is less likelihood of overloading the cardiovascular system.

Sodium chloride in intravenous solutions is treated with ever-increasing care and respect. In cases uncomplicated by nephritis, heart failure, diabetes mellitus, cirrhosis of the liver, anemia, diarrhea or vomiting, it is safe to give 500 cc. of physiologic saline daily. However, when complications are present, the fluid, electrolyte and acid-base requirements are far more complex, and the medical consultant should decide what is indicated.

It is a good plan, when you suspect that the patient is not getting 2500 cc. of fluids daily, to write orders for the recording of fluid intake and fluid output.*

---

*To meet special conditions of fluid balance for the patient, the oral surgeon should become knowledgeable about certain of the long-chain molecular solutions, such as lactated Ringer's and lactated Ringer's in 5 per cent dextrose and water, as well as the high-molecular dextrans.

Table 9–1 *Dental Soft Diet**
(Carbohydrate, 300 gm.; protein, 78 gm.; fat, 105 gm.; calories, 2500)

BREAKFAST
  Fruit juice—100 gm.
  Cooked cereal
  Soft cooked egg
  Cream—2 oz.
  Milk—8 oz.
  Coffee—sugar

10 A.M.
  Fruit nectar—200 gm.

NOON MEAL
  Cream soup
  Eggnog
  Fruit juice—200 gm.
  Jello or vanilla ice cream
  Tea or coffee
  Cream—sugar

3 P.M.
  Milkshake

EVENING MEAL
  Fruit juice
  Cooked cereal
  Soft cooked egg
  Custard
  Tea or coffee
  Cream—sugar

8 P.M.
  Pep cocktail

---

*There are also composite liquid diets that can supplement a full meal in one glass, if needed.

---

*Order enough multivitamin capsules to give the patient daily 900 mg. of ascorbic acid, 60 mg. of thiamine hydrochloride, 30 mg. of riboflavin and 900 mg. of niacinamide.

Table 9–2   *Full Liquid Diet*

The full liquid diet supplies nourishment in a simple and easily digested form and consists of foods that are liquid or that liquefy at body temperature. This diet is to be used immediately postoperatively following full mouth extractions or for patients with treated or untreated fractured jaws.

FOODS TO INCLUDE DAILY	QUANTITY	DESCRIPTION
Milk	1 quart	As a beverage; in soup or cereal gruel.
Cereals	1 serving	Strained cereal waters and gruels.
Eggs	1 to 2	Custards; raw in beverages.
Fats	As tolerated	Butter; fortified margarine; cream in prepared foods.
Fruit juices*	1 pint	Strained juice.
Potato	1 serving	Mashed.
Vegetables	1 to 2 tablespoons	Strained vegetable juices; strained vegetables in a meat stock or in cream soup.
Soups	1 to 2 servings	Clear broth; strained cream soups.
Beverages	As desired	Coffee, tea, cocoa, carbonated beverages, cereal beverages.
Sweets	As tolerated	Honey, sugar, plain sugar candy.
Desserts	2 servings	Soft or baked custard; plain ice cream; rennet desserts; sherbets; water ices; gelatin.
Miscellaneous	As tolerated	Salt

*Tomato and grape juice are avoided because of the psychological effect upon the patient in case of vomiting.

DIET

Three Diet Orders for Dental Patients.

REGULAR DIET. This is to be ordered not only before surgery but also after surgery for those patients who have had only a very limited amount of work done in the oral cavity or for extraoral operations.

DENTAL SOFT DIET (NONCHEWING). This would be ordered for the majority of dental patients following surgery. It would contain about 2500 calories and would provide three meals and three nourishments for a total of six feedings. Certainly most of the patients should be able to take the majority of these items. (Details of this diet are given in Table 9–1). With the increasing incidence of diabetes mellitus, the oral surgeon should also be aware that A.D.A. liquid diets of varying caloric levels, as 1200 calories or 1500 calories, are available from the hospital dietitian.

The dentist should make sure that the dietary department understands what a dental soft diet really means. To the average dietitian, "soft diet" means *easy to digest*, not *easy to chew*. In some hospitals, to avoid confusion, the word "soft" has been eliminated and the terms "dental diet" or "nonchewing diet" have been substituted.

The order for the dental soft diet is to be marked as such on the ward diet slip, or ordered as a routine diet from the diet kitchen or general kitchen.

Table 9–3   *Sample Liquid Meal Pattern**
(Carbohydrates, 215 gm.; protein, 70 gm.; fat, 70 gm.; calories, 1655)

BREAKFAST
1/2 cup strained fruit juice (orange)
1/2 cup strained cereal gruel (oatmeal)
1 cup milk, whole
1 tablespoon sugar
Beverage (tea or coffee)

MIDMORNING
1/2 cup strained fruit juice (grapefruit)

LUNCH
3/4 cup soup (broth)
1/2 cup dessert (soft custard)
1 cup milk, whole
2 teaspoons sugar
Beverage (tea or coffee)

MIDAFTERNOON
Hi-pro†

DINNER
1/2 cup juice (nectar)
3/4 cup strained soup (cream)
1/2 cup dessert (sherbet)
1 cup milk, whole
2 teaspoons sugar
Beverage (tea or coffee)

BEDTIME
Hi-pro†

*Compiled by the Department of Biochemistry and Nutrition, Graduate School of Public Health, University of Pittsburgh.
†Hi-pro supplement: 6 ounces homogenized milk
1 tablespoon skim milk powder
1 tablespoon chocolate syrup

Table 9–4   *Common Abbreviations and Terms Used in Prescription Writing and Hospital Work*

TERM	LATIN OR GREEK	TRANSLATION
a.c.	ante cibum	before eating
bene	bene	well
b.i.d.	bis in die	twice a day
BMR		basal metabolism rate
BOR		before time of operation
B.P.		blood pressure
Ca		cancer
C.		Centigrade
CBC		complete blood count
C.C.		chief complaint
cc.		cubic centimeter
Det.	detur	let be given
dil.	dilue	dilute
D.T.D.	dentur tales doses	let such doses be given
EENT		eye, ear, nose and throat
EKG		electrocardiogram
elix.	elixir	an elixir
e.m.p.	ex modo prescripto	as directed
enem.	enema	an enema
ENT		ear, nose, and throat
et.	et	and
f., ft.	fac, fiat, fiant	make (thou)
F.		Fahrenheit
F.H.		family history
garg.	gargarisma	gargle
gm.	gramma	gram
gr.	granum	grain
gu.	gutta(e)	drop(s)
h.	hora	hour
Hbg.		hemoglobin
hypo		by hypodermic
H.P.I.		history of present illness
h.s.	hora somni	at bedtime
in d.	in dies	from day to day
kg.	kilogram	a thousand grams
L.	liter	a liter
liq.	liquor	a solution
lues		syphilis

DENTAL LIQUID DIET. This is to be ordered in the majority of instances for the patient who has had a fractured jaw. The basis for making this diet would be a dental soft diet, as outlined in Table 9–1, but when there is need for a dental liquid diet the oral surgeon will order "dental liquid diet," which will be an automatic signal to the dietary department that a dietitian is to interview the doctor to find out exactly what type of food the patient can eat.

DENTAL CONSULTATION IN THE HOSPITAL

Consultations in the hospital are requested for many reasons, such as pain in the face, facial swelling, difficulty in mastication, bleeding in the oral cavity, headaches, tumors in the oral cavity, ulcerations or a potential source of chronic infection. The oral surgeon is often asked, "Are the teeth infected?" The question should read: "Is there a source of infection in the oral cavity?" Too frequently chronic periodontal infection is overlooked in the search for infection.

The types of oral lesions, and conditions that may act both as primary and secondary sources of infection, are numerous.

Infection may be found in the edentulous mouth as well as where a full complement of teeth is present. The following conditions are regarded as potential areas of infection: periapical destruction, periodontal disease, pulpitis, alveolar resorption, pericoronal infection, gingival pockets, subacute residual infection which occasionally is found in the edentulous mouth, infected cysts.

Basically, all reports on the oral cavity should include at least the following: a report of dental x-ray examination using fourteen

Table 9–4 *(Continued)*

TERM	LATIN OR GREEK	TRANSLATION
M.	misce	mix (thou)
mcg.		microgram
mg.		milligram(s)
ml.		milliliter
N.B.	nota bene	note well
N.F.		National Formulary
non rep.	non repetatur	do not repeat
n.s.q.		not sufficient quantity
N.S.S.		normal saline solution
o.d.	omne die	once a day
o.m.	omne mane	each morning
o.n.	omne nocte	each night
OPD		out-patient department
p.c.	post cibum	after eating
placebo	"I will please"	medication given to please patient
p.o.	per os	by mouth
p.r.n.	pro re nata	when required
q.h.	quaque hora	every hour
q. 2h	quaque secunda hora	every 2 hours
q. 3h	quaque tertia hora	every 3 hours
q. 4h	quaque quarta hora	every 4 hours
q.i.d.	quarter in die	4 times a day
qs	quantum sufficit.	a sufficient quantity
RBC		red blood count
S.H.		social habits
S.O.S.	si opus set	if necessary
ss	semis	a half
Stat.	statim	at once
tab.	tablet	a tablet
Tbsp		tablespoon
t.i.d.	ter in die	3 times a day
T.P.R.		temperature, pulse, respiration
Tsp.		teaspoon
Tr., tinct.	tinctus	tincture
u.		units
USP		United States Pharmacopeia
WBC		white blood count

regular films and two bitewing films,* a vitality test of all teeth; a transillumination of alveolar ridges; a report on periodontal tissues, and the depth of pockets; smears in cases of acute and chronic gingival infections; a report on the mucous membrane; a report on the tongue.

The examiner should first examine the patient's mouth carefully and note any gross abnormalities. Secondly, the radiographs should be checked and the vitality test performed. Transillumination may then be done to aid in diagnosis. The results of these procedures should be tabulated, and an attempt made to correlate the information. Areas of rarefaction in the bony structures should be investigated.

Abnormally low vitality readings must be considered, since these may be indicative of a degenerative, liquefactive process of the dental pulp.

This information should then be summarized under the heading Conclusions. This is to be followed by specific advice as to suggested treatments or operation under the heading Recommendations.

REFERENCES

1. Conn, H. J. (Ed.): Conn's Current Therapy 1975. Philadelphia, W. B. Saunders Co., 1975.
2. Douglas, B. L., and Casey, G. J.: A Guide to Hospital Dental Procedure. Chicago, Illinois, Council on Hospital Dental Service, American Dental Association, 1964.

*The panographic films are now commonly used, but the author wishes to emphasize that so far these are all of limited diagnostic value.

CHAPTER 10

ORAL, FACE AND NECK INFECTIONS

GENERAL CLINICAL COMMENTS ON HEAD AND NECK INFECTIONS

The greatest number of infections in and about the mandible and maxilla are odontogenic in origin. Trauma (with or without fracture) and infections from needle puncture cause a small percentage of infections and a tiny percentage results from bizarre etiologic factors, *e.g.*, the infected antrum. For all practical purposes most infections originate within the bone of the mandible and maxilla from odontogenic sources: periapical or periodontal infection, cysts, root fragments, residual infection, pericoronal pockets, etc.

The clinical treatment of infections is both a science and an art. The surgeon will use all scientific facilities available: radiographs, blood counts, vitality tests, temperature readings, cultures, etc. However, the art in treating infections consists in the ability of the surgeon to evaluate *the infection in relation to the patient*. This sounds like a simple statement, but most cases of mismanagement of infection occur because the surgeon forgets that he is dealing with *three* variables: (1) the cause of the infection (bacterial, fungal or viral), (2) the anatomic location, and (3) the ability of the patient to combat infection. It is the interrelationships among these three variables that makes evaluation and treatment difficult. All abscessed central incisors cannot be treated in the same manner merely because they are central incisors—the other factors must also be considered. Antibiotic therapy may be indicated in one case and not in another. Knowledge of what to do and when to do it is based on the knowledge of basic surgical principles and anatomy, reinforced with experience.

THE CAUSE OF INFECTION

Generally speaking, most bacterial infections with which we are dealing are not due to one particular organism. Most infections are due to mixtures of the same organisms that make up the normal oral flora. However, if the patient has been on antibiotic therapy, a resistant strain (of *Staphylococcus* particularly) may survive and produce an aggressive, highly resistant infection that is almost one pure strain. Hemolytic-type organisms will generally spread faster than the nonhemolytic strains, and if they are antibiotic-resistant, the result may be a rapidly spreading infection that is difficult to control.

Fungal infections (*e.g.*, those due to *Actinomyces*), on the other hand, are notorious for their very slow propagation rate. It is almost as if one were watching a bacterial infection in slow motion. They are difficult to diagnose in the early stages, and biopsies and other diagnostic tests may be necessary. Fortunately, they are not common.

There is virtually nothing in the literature about viral infections of odontogenic origin, yet on the basis of other known facts there is no reason to assume that these do not exist. In all likelihood, they are not recognized because they are complicated early in their course by secondary bacterial infections and, like most viral infections, "burn themselves out" in a few days. One may speculate, however, that the dreaded Ludwig's angina (see page 484), in which there is a rapidly spreading nonsuppurative cellulitis of the floor of the mouth and neck, is in reality a viral cellulitis.

THE ANATOMIC LOCATION

When infection occurs in the medulla of the maxilla or mandible it will take the line of least resistance as it spreads. In rare cases it will traverse the medullary bone, producing thrombosis of the arterioles and a resultant osteomyelitis. More commonly it erodes the cortex and spreads into the soft tissues. At this point, the surgeon must recognize that he

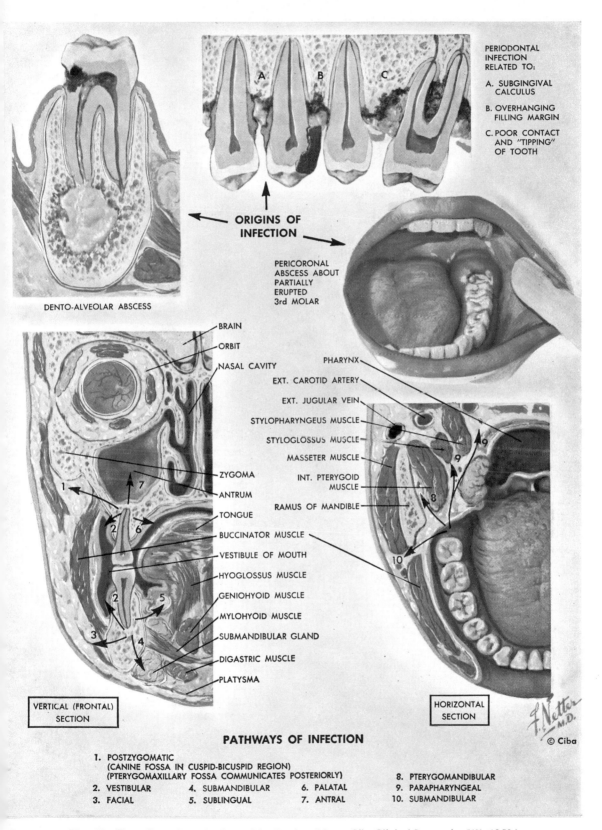

PERIODONTAL
INFECTION
RELATED TO:

A. SUBGINGIVAL
   CALCULUS

B. OVERHANGING
   FILLING MARGIN

C. POOR CONTACT
   AND "TIPPING"
   OF TOOTH

ORIGINS OF
INFECTION

PERICORONAL
ABSCESS ABOUT
PARTIALLY
ERUPTED
3rd MOLAR

DENTO-ALVEOLAR ABSCESS

BRAIN
ORBIT
NASAL CAVITY

PHARYNX
EXT. CAROTID ARTERY
EXT. JUGULAR VEIN
STYLOPHARYNGEUS MUSCLE
STYLOGLOSSUS MUSCLE
MASSETER MUSCLE
INT. PTERYGOID
MUSCLE
RAMUS OF MANDIBLE

ZYGOMA
ANTRUM
TONGUE
BUCCINATOR MUSCLE
VESTIBULE OF MOUTH
HYOGLOSSUS MUSCLE
GENIOHYOID MUSCLE
MYLOHYOID MUSCLE
SUBMANDIBULAR GLAND
DIGASTRIC MUSCLE
PLATYSMA

VERTICAL (FRONTAL)
SECTION

HORIZONTAL
SECTION

F. Netter
M.D.
© Ciba

PATHWAYS OF INFECTION

1. POSTZYGOMATIC
   (CANINE FOSSA IN CUSPID-BICUSPID REGION)
   (PTERYGOMAXILLARY FOSSA COMMUNICATES POSTERIORLY)

2. VESTIBULAR   4. SUBMANDIBULAR   6. PALATAL   8. PTERYGOMANDIBULAR
3. FACIAL   5. SUBLINGUAL   7. ANTRAL   9. PARAPHARYNGEAL
                                                                      10. SUBMANDIBULAR

Plate II   (From Stern, L.: Infections of the Teeth and Jaws. Ciba Clinical Symposia, 5(3), 1953.)

is dealing not with one but with *two* infections in different stages of development. The intrabony pus has spilled into the soft tissues, and the soft tissue infection is at this point developing into a cellulitis. Clinically, it is soft and doughy to the touch. The fate of this infection depends on the anatomic soft tissue pocket into which it has spilled and its delineating muscles and fascia (see description of various spaces later in this chapter).

The other limiting factor is the response of the patient's resistance elements. When the body can "wall off" the infection, its progress is stopped. The fate of this infection is either (1) resolution, *i.e.,* healing without pus formation, (2) fluctuation, *i.e.,* progressing until anatomically and physiologically it is walled off and undergoes central necrosis with pus formation, or (3) extension, *i.e.,* spreading into other soft-tissue spaces or the blood stream.

When the usual acute periapical abscess perforates the cortex, the apical lesion has reached the stage at which intrabony pus is usually present but the soft tissues have not yet undergone necrosis. If this infection progresses, the soft tissues will become more and more indurated until they become brawny, and then a small area of central softening can be palpated. This represents the central necrosis due to bacterial propagation and loss of blood supply. This is the time for the incision and drainage. If the tooth can be safely extracted when the soft tissues are still soft and doughy to the touch, the source of infection is removed and the soft tissues will usually not progress to suppuration but the infection will undergo resolution. At the intermediate stage, judgment about whether or not to do an incision and drainage is difficult, but when there is a firm, brawny swelling, there is no doubt that suppuration will occur. Extraction of the tooth at this stage but failure to treat the soft tissue infection will result in later difficulties.

Antibiotic therapy may complicate this picture and delay the appearance of suppuration beyond the normally expected time. It must be remembered that the blood must carry the antibiotics to the infection, and the area of brawny edema is so densely packed with fluid elements that a very poor blood supply exists. If just enough antibiotic gets into this area to slow down bacterial growth, fluctuation may be a long time in coming. (See the following section for the rationale in antibiotic therapy.) If incision and drainage is necessary, the site for incision is determined by

the anatomic location of the infection. A thorough knowledge of the fascial spaces of the head and neck is a prerequisite.

Anatomically, infections of the oral cavity, face and neck are located in the (1) periapical area, (2) pericemental pocket, (3) upper lips, (4) palate, (5) canine fossa, (6) subperiosteal area, maxilla or mandible, (7) sublingual area, (8) mental and submental areas, (9) buccal space, (10) submandibular space, (11) pterygomandibular space, (12) parapharyngeal space, (13) zygomaticotemporal space, (14) carotid sheath, and (15) areas in the fascial planes anterior to the sternocleidomastoid muscle.

ABILITY OF THE PATIENT TO RESIST INFECTION

The rate of spread of infection is contingent not only upon the type of infection but also upon the patient's ability to resist. This factor resides in the globulin fraction of the plasma and probably in the gamma globulin fraction. The actual biochemistry of "general resistance" is probably related to the individual's ability to synthesize adequate amounts of specific immunoglobulin rapidly to meet sudden demands created by a specific antigen.* There are individuals who cannot do this, and in these patients soft tissue infections are not "walled off" as rapidly and tend to spread further than in the others. Because they are not "walled off," they spread into the blood stream and produce the fever, chills, leukocytosis and elevated sedimentation rate associated with acute general infections and septicemia. These are patients with agammaglobulinemia or hypogammaglobulinemia (not as rare as was formerly believed), blood dyscrasias, uncontrolled diabetes, malignant diseases, nutritional disorders, endocrine disturbances and any other disease-producing metabolic abnormalities. Electrophoresis of blood albumins and globulins will reveal a striking deficiency of immunoglobulins in these patients.

In these patients, no surgical procedures are indicated that will break down any of the few poor physiologic barriers to infection that have been created, for fear of producing a

---

*This is probably mediated in turn by the endocrine system (pituitary-adrenal axis) in the "stress response" of Selye, which also effects the leukocytosis, elevated temperature, etc.

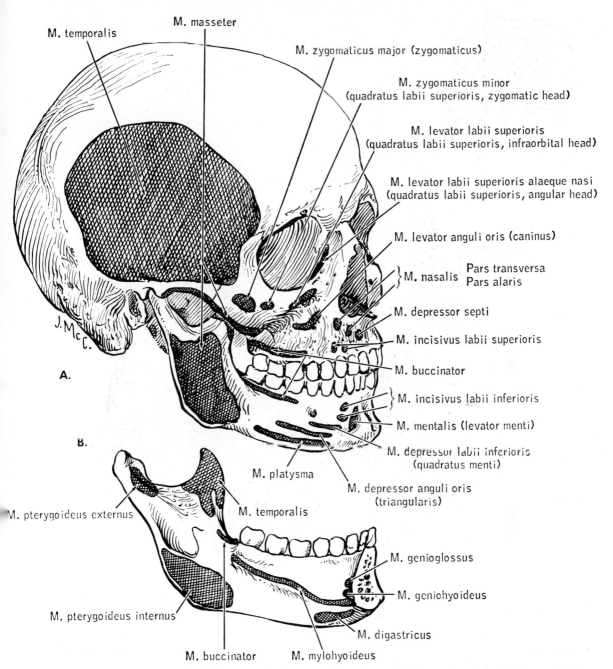

M. temporalis

M. masseter

M. zygomaticus major (zygomaticus)

M. zygomaticus minor
(quadratus labii superioris, zygomatic head)

M. levator labii superioris
(quadratus labii superioris, infraorbital head)

M. levator labii superioris alaeque nasi
(quadratus labii superioris, angular head)

M. levator anguli oris (caninus)

} M. nasalis Pars transversa
              Pars alaris

M. depressor septi

M. incisivus labii superioris

M. buccinator

} M. incisivus labii inferioris

M. mentalis (levator menti)

M. depressor labii inferioris
(quadratus menti)

M. depressor anguli oris
(triangularis)

A.

B.

M. platysma

M. pterygoideus externus

M. temporalis

M. pterygoideus internus

M. genioglossus

M. geniohyoideus

M. digastricus

M. buccinator   M. mylohyoideus

Figure 10–1 *A* and *B*, Skull and mandible, showing the areas of attachment of the muscles of mastication and facial expression. (From Tiecke, R. W. [Ed.]: Oral Pathology. New York, McGraw-Hill Book Co., Inc., 1965. Used by permission of McGraw-Hill Book Company.)

(*Figure 10–1 continued on following page.*)

general septicemia. It is more advisable to approach the problem by building up resistance to the infection by use of antibiotics and other systemic therapy as medically indicated for the specific deficiency present. Following this, surgery can be performed, since the patient will be able to handle the systemic bacteremia that will follow the surgery.

The rationale of antibiotic therapy in the treatment of these infections can be drawn from the above comments. It must be remembered that the drugs do not cure, they only help the body to destroy the infection. When the body has adequately walled off an abscess (as evidenced by a low white count and very little fever), antibiotics are useless as treatment and are only indicated prior to incision

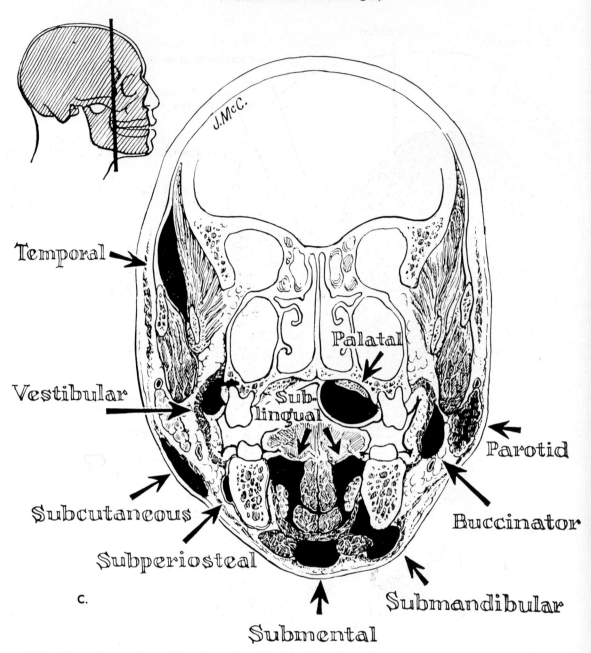

J.McC.

Temporal

Palatal

Vestibular

Sub-
lingual

Parotid

Subcutaneous

Buccinator

Subperiosteal

C.

Submandibular

Submental

Figure 10–1 *(Continued)*   *C,* Frontal section of the head showing various abscesses. (From Tiecke, R. W. [Ed.]: Oral Pathology. New York, McGraw-Hill Book Co., Inc., 1965; after Kampmier and Jones. Used by permission of McGraw-Hill Book Company.)

(Figure 10–1 continued on opposite page.)

and drainage or other surgery to cover the bacteremia that will result from the surgical manipulation. However, an elevated temperature and white count is an indication that a constant or recurring bacteremia (or toxemia) is occurring which the body cannot control itself; therefore, antibiotic therapy is indicated. The best general rule to follow is to use antibiotics (1) if the body does not seem to be able to control the infection, as indicated by

the various tests and observations listed above, and (2) for prophylaxis when a surgically produced bacteremia is expected.

It must also be kept in mind that some organisms are resistant to some antibiotics. Always make a culture and some sensitivity test if possible, so that a refractory infection can be intelligently treated.

The last factor in patient resistance to be considered is hydration. Since oral infection

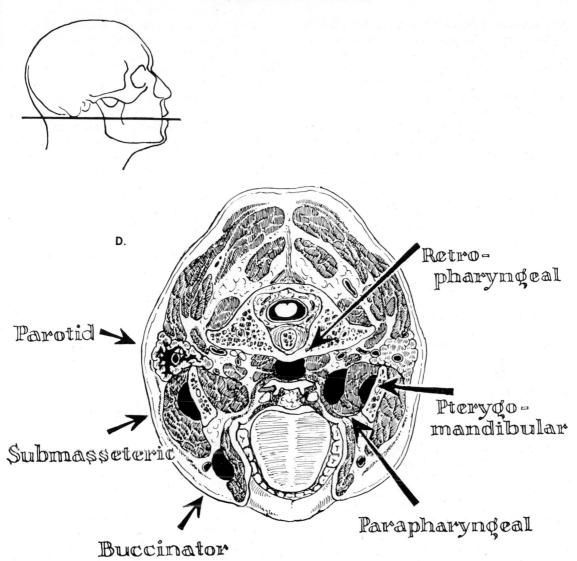

D.

Parotid

Retro-
pharyngeal

Submasseteric

Pterygo-
mandibular

Buccinator

Parapharyngeal

Figure 10–1 *(Continued)* D, Horizontal section of the head at the level of the commissure of the lips showing various abscesses. (From Tiecke, R. W. [Ed.]: Oral Pathology. New York, McGraw-Hill Book Co., Inc., 1965; after Eycleshymer and Schoemaker. Used by permission of McGraw-Hill Book Company.)

will often result in cessation of ingestion of food (and liquids) and the resultant fever produces excessive loss of body fluid via perspiration, a fluid deficit results. This is further intensified by the pathologic renal and circulatory condition that occurs in the presence of infection. There is a shift of fluid to the extravascular spaces,* and with the decrease in circulating volume produced by this shift plus loss of fluid plus lack of replacement there is a decrease in urine production because of the

lack of availability of water to spare in the blood. The increased metabolic activity produces excess nitrogenous waste, and the resultant oliguria (decreased urine production) causes retention of nonprotein nitrogen as well as chloride ion because of the decreased water available for dilution of the urine. Thus a markedly concentrated urine is produced (*i.e.*, high specific gravity) in small volume. In the blood the metabolic products and chloride ions pile up. This will progress until a severe electrolyte imbalance and possible acidosis occur. Ketosis is always present, and there will be ketone bodies in the urine. Dehydration is usually easily recognized clinically

_____

*This is also mediated by the pituitary-adrenal axis.

and, while oral fluids are preferable, 1000 to 2000 cc. of 5 per cent glucose in water can safely be given to most patients in a slow intravenous drip. This will often dramatically transform a toxic, acutely sick patient into a much better looking individual with a much lower temperature.

The correction of dehydration and possible acidosis in patients with cardiac or metabolic diseases should not be attempted by those who are not well versed in fluid balance, since in these patients it is very easy to overload the system with fluids, and more than one patient has died from pulmonary edema due to overaggressive treatment of dehydration.

INFLAMMATION

A basic understanding of the dynamics of inflammation is an obvious prerequisite in the intelligent treatment of infections. The specific details of this fundamental pathologic process will not be recited here since they more properly belong in a course in pathology, but a brief recapitulation may help refresh the memory and serve as a useful reference.

Any irritant—thermal, radioactive, mechanical, bacterial, etc.—provokes a typical tissue response that is designed to eliminate the irritant and restore normalcy. The basic biochemical mechanism is the production of a polypeptide (leukotaxine), which initiates a series of events, starting with vasodilatation of the capillaries, diapedesis of white cell elements and then exudation of certain of the protein fractions of the blood (albumin, globulin, fibrinogen) into the injured area. The net effect is twofold: (a) isolation and fixation of the foreign antigen in the affected area and (b) destruction or removal of the antigenic agent. The exact biochemical mechanism involves a vast complex of interrelated events, both local effects and systemic effects on the bone marrow (leukocytosis) and temperature regulation centers. From a practical standpoint, however, that is, for clinical considerations, it is sufficient to say that when bacteria are introduced into tissues there is an outpouring of fluid and cells into the tissues, producing edema of the affected area. (The only substances capable of blocking this reaction are cortisone and its related compounds.) The sequence of events that follow is determined by the irritant—in this case the organism—and the host's resistance. Staphylo-

cocci, for example, provoke a severe coagulation effect on the capillary exudate, which seals the lymphatics and produces localization of the organism in the affected area. Streptococci, on the other hand, provoke little or no coagulation of the plasma exudate (especially hemolytic streptococci), and consequently the lymphatics remain open and generalized systemic dissemination of the bacteria occurs. This means that the systemic effects of a streptococcal infection—leukocytosis, malaise, elevated temperature, and so forth—will be more severe than in a staphylococcal infection, whereas in the latter there will be a more massive local reaction.

Once the infection is walled off locally, phagocytosis may be adequate to eliminate the organism and tissues destroyed by the elaboration of another substance always present—necrosin. In other cases surgical intervention may be required to eliminate the necrotic tissues (pus). A detailed description of head and neck infections and their surgical treatment appears later in this chapter.*

HEAT AND COLD THERAPY, DRUG THERAPY

Since inflammation, in the presence of infection, is a defense mechanism to eliminate a foreign body, it serves a useful purpose. Rational therapy should therefore be employed to help nature do its job. In a healthy person several modalities are available.

Drugs. Antibiotics are used primarily to control systemic dissemination anticipated from surgical interference. Steroids may be indicated if edema becomes life-threatening, but the routine use of steroids is extremely hazardous because of the effects on the dynamics of inflammation. Large doses of antibiotics must accompany the use of steroids. The use of antihistamines to control edema is controversial and probably useless.

Cold. Whereas ice packs are indicated for postsurgical trauma in which infection is not present, they have no use in the treatment of an acute cellulitis, since they inhibit the physiologic defense mechanism.

Heat. (See also Heat Therapy, following Physiology of Heat.) The use of heat in the

*The author acknowledges the many contributions of Daniel J. Holland, D.M.D., in the preparation of this material.

presence of an acute cellulitis is debatable if the patient does not have a therapeutic blood level of some active antibiotic. There is no doubt that heat will increase local circulation and increase fluid and cellular diathesis, but so much edema may be so rapidly produced as to provoke an ischemic necrosis. However, once a good therapeutic antibiotic blood level is reached, heat in the form of thermal lamps, hydrocollator packs, heating pads, hot moist packs, hot water bottles, and so forth, both intraorally and extraorally is most beneficial because, in effect, this brings the antibiotic into the affected area in higher concentrations. With the antibiotics available today—even in oral doses—extremely high blood levels can be reached rapidly so that heat therapy can be started very early in treatment.

Physiology of Heat

The penetrating depth of heat applied in the form of poultices, compresses or hot water bottles is not great—about 1 mm.—and the heating of the tissues is by conduction. This is in contrast to the greater penetrating depth of luminous sources of heat, such as sunlight and tungsten and carbon filament lamps. The rate at which changes of temperature penetrate the tissues is slow in either method (conduction or radiation). When one attempts to raise the temperature of the tissues beyond 98.6° F. (37° C.), heat is quickly dissipated by the tissues through the action of circulatory reflexes. That is why such large quantities of heat energy are required to alter the tissue temperature to any depth.

Local exposure to heat results in stimulation of the vasomotor reflexes. The *number of open capillaries is increased; tissue metabolism is accelerated; and the rate of exchange between blood and tissues is increased.* Heat causes dilatation of the smooth muscle cells in the walls of the peripheral vessels, producing peripheral vasodilatation and a rise in capillary blood pressure. As the capillaries relax and enlarge, the area of the capillary wall available for fluid exchange is increased. Hence more lymph, more plasma, and more tissue fluid are attracted to the part—diapedesis is enhanced, and the local defense mechanisms are augmented.

With the increase in local circulation rate, the rate of edema formation is increased. Warmth increases the lymphatic capillary network and lymph formation, which in turn *accelerates lymphatic drainage.* The activities of the leukocytes in phagocytosis are stimulated. Both factors are paramount in the battle against infection. *If the infection is markedly pathogenic and is inclined toward formation of pus and localization, either intraorally or extraorally, heat will hasten the process.* Conversely, if the infection is inclined toward resolution rather than localization, then heat will hasten the resolution. There is no substantiation for the theory that heat will produce localization of an infection which, without applications of heat, might otherwise resolve.

Dentists have been prone to avoid prescribing heat for obvious dental infections with secondary cellulitis and have recommended cold. Ice bags never prevent infection, and they generally prolong the duration of the infection by inhibiting the natural tissue defense and combat mechanisms.

Heat Therapy

Application. Intraoral heat is probably best administered in the form of hot irrigations of normal saline solution (120° to 125° F.) or mouthwashes every 2 hours.

Applying heat to the face from luminous or nonluminous sources is most effective. According to Kovács, the advantages of heat radiation over methods of conductive heating (hot-water bottles, poultices, etc.) are: "(1) that its action extends to a greater depth; (2) that there is no pressure over the parts; and (3) that the parts may be kept under constant observation without difficulty. Thus signs of undue heating can be discovered immediately."

TECHNIQUE OF LOCAL RADIANT HEAT APPLICATION. "The patient should be placed in a comfortable, relaxed position and the radiation from the generator directed over the part to be treated, at a distance from which it feels comfortable. The distance will average from 2 to 3 feet, according to the sensitivity of the parts, the intensity of the radiation and the type of reflector.... Exposure is continued for ½ to 1 hour. The routine employment of a time clock for exact measurement of the time of treatment serves as a protection for patient and dentist. Too long exposure, if not too intense, usually does not produce harmful effects in local treatments; in some acute painful conditions it may be helpful to apply infrared radiation for as long as 1 to 2 hours at a time. Dentists and technicians often err by using heat radiation for too short a period to be effective."*

The author prefers the use of continuous heat by the application of wet, hot towels over the swollen area and adjacent tissues and then directing the heat radiation lamp on the wet towel. This procedure maintains heat in the wet dressing until it is partially dry, when it is removed, soaked in hot water and reapplied to the face. The heat lamp is then repositioned.

DANGERS AND PRECAUTIONS.   As Kovács explains, "Exposure to infrared or visible radiation results normally in an erythemal response consisting of individual dark red spots or a confluent network of these, and occurs according to the distance from the lamp, the wattage of the bulb, and the type of reflector, and the sensitivity of the patient. Excess radiation or hypersensitivity or other causes may produce, after the initial erythema, wheal formation, local edema and eventually blistering. Sometimes these blisters only develop overnight. Excess radiation in normal patients always gives rise to a varying degree of burning sensation. Especial precautions are imperative in patients whose skin sensation is impaired, in those with scars on the skin after burns or other injuries which have destroyed part of the normal skin or its nerve endings, and in patients with peripheral nerve injuries.

"If at any time during treatment the patient complains of unpleasant burning over the entire area or over one spot, the heat lamp should be moved a few inches farther away; this process may have to be repeated until the patient feels entirely comfortable. Patients who receive treatment for the first time often think that a severe burning sensation is part of the treatment; such indiscreet patients may become blistered and, therefore, special watchfulness is always indicated when treatment is applied for the first time.

"Anesthetic areas in patients with peripheral nerve injuries and over scars are especially prone to blister, so that in these cases heat generators should be kept at a distance of at least one and a half times the usual space and even then one should always look out for signs of possible blistering."*

Uses.   Specifically, heat is used in all cases of phlegmons or cellulitis resulting from al-

veolar abscess, tooth extraction, and so on in which drainage is not good and infection extends into the surrounding tissues, because it localizes the condition. Localization is an important factor for incision and drainage of purulent fluids. Heat is indispensable in the treatment of osteomyelitis, in which incision and drainage are of utmost importance. Heat is used in all types of edema or inflammatory exudate of the maxilla and mandible that are potential cases of deep cellular infections.

With the advent of penicillin and other chemotherapeutics, heat has become no less important in the treatment of infections. Hot applications inducing increased circulation and fluid exudation serve to carry more of the circulating penicillin to the infected area.

OUTLINE OF SPECIFIC TREATMENT OF INFECTIONS

DENTOALVEOLAR ABSCESS WITH NO SWELLING OF THE FACE

Symptoms.   When a dentoalveolar abscess has formed but the patient's face is not swollen, the following symptoms will probably be present:
1. Tooth feels long.
2. Tooth is extremely sensitive to touch.
3. Excruciating pain.
4. Lamina dura shows break on x-ray (make sure that this tooth is really abscessed and not just in traumatic occlusion).

Treatment.   If endodontia is contraindicated extract the tooth if the patient's condition is physiologically satisfactory. General anesthesia is usually required since local anesthesia is usually only about 70 to 90 per cent effective. No apical curettage is indicated.

DENTOALVEOLAR ABSCESS WITH EARLY SWELLING OF THE FACE

Symptoms.   Patients with a dentoalveolar abscess that has caused early swelling of the face will present with the following symptoms:
1. Patient had a severe toothache that subsided as soon as swelling started.
2. Tissues where abscess has perforated are soft and doughy to the touch.
3. Pain is not as severe as in prior 24 hours.

Treatment.   Extract the tooth if the pa-

---

*Reprinted with permission from Kovács, R.: Electrotherapy and Light Therapy. 6th ed. Philadelphia, Lea & Febiger, 1949.

tient's systemic condition is physiologically satisfactory. Local anesthesia is usually effective, but an effort should be made to circumvent the area of swelling (*i.e.,* tissue infection). With antibiotics today we are less concerned about injecting into infected areas, but the lowered pH (*i.e.,* acidity) in infected areas reduces the efficacy of local anesthetics and usually some form of block anesthesia must be used to anesthetize the nerve outside of the area of swelling. Supportive antibiotic therapy for the next 4 to 5 days should be prescribed.

Discussion. There is a difference of opinion as to treatment. In general, the medical practitioner and the general surgeon hold the view that when swelling is present, teeth should not be extracted, whereas oral surgeons agree almost unanimously that swelling per se is not a contraindication to extraction. It is easy to see why the medical profession as a group hold their view: it is because they see only those cases in which extreme complications have occurred following extractions when swelling was present. They never see the thousands of patients, with swelling of the facial tissues, who are daily having teeth extracted and are given therapeutic doses of antibiotics and vitamins with prompt recovery resulting.

The infection is aborted in the great percentage of cases by extraction of the abscessed tooth. As soon as infection develops in the periapical space, the body immediately builds up a defense wall around this area. As the microorganisms multiply, the cells break down and pus forms. The pressure in the periapical space builds up, resulting in the throbbing pain, and finally the pus breaks out of its bony chamber into the soft tissue and the patient experiences immediate relief from pain. He reports that the pain has stopped but that his jaw has swelled up. Examinations reveal not only swelling of the face but also, in many cases, subperiosteal swelling. The facial swelling is soft at this stage.

Swelling is the result of the body's local reaction to the irritation of the pathogenic microorganisms which have poured out into the soft tissues; these tissues become inflamed, and eventually all the characteristics of inflammation appear: (*a*) calor (heat); (*b*) rubor (redness); and (*c*), as the tissues become tense and indurated, dolor (pain).

If extraction is carried out at this early stage (24 to 48 hours) *of swelling, as a rule adequate drainage is established, through the alveolus,* and what bacteria and their products have spilled out into the tissue planes of the face will quickly fall prey to the first line of defense, phagocytosis, and the humoral defense factors and antibiotics present in the blood plasma in the tissues. However, if extraction is delayed and the defenses of the host are inadequate, the infection travels through the tissue planes to deeper structures, and particularly so if the dentist instructs the patient to apply ice bags or cold wet cloths to the face until the swelling goes down. It is these patients who will eventually show extensive cellulitis with edema and induration, general malaise and high temperature.

Extraction of the offending tooth at this stage will not abort the infection, nor will it make the patient's condition worse. The dentist who expects that the swelling will disappear immediately in these cases will be disappointed.

DENTOALVEOLAR ABSCESS WITH ABSCESS FORMATION IN ONE OF THE FASCIAL SPACES OF THE HEAD AND NECK

Once infection has passed from the alveolar bone into one of the fascial spaces of the head and neck and has progressed beyond the soft, doughy stage into the firm, brawny type of infection, surgical intervention is usually required to remove the tooth as well as the pus in the soft tissues. It must always be remembered that, in effect, we must treat two infections and that antibiotic therapy alone will not cure an abscess in one of the larger fascial spaces, even though the offending tooth has been extracted. Failure to drain the soft tissue abscess will ultimately result in fistulas of the face (see section following) or a re-exacerbation of the abscess.

In abscesses involving the fascial spaces of the head and neck it is imperative that the surgeon identify the space involved and thus, with his surgical knowledge, correctly drain the space with the proper approach. The exact timing of this procedure is an art unto itself because, as any experienced oral surgeon knows, palpation is very unreliable in determining the presence of "laudable pus" in these deep lesions. The general surgeon almost invariably procrastinates much too long in these cases because of his unfamiliarity with the pathologic process (see Figure 10–34).

The spaces involved are: canine and buccal

in the maxilla, and sublingual, submental, submandibular, pterygomandibular (masticator), parapharyngeal and zygomaticotemporal in the mandible.

DENTOALVEOLAR ABSCESS, OR RESIDUAL INFECTION IN A FACIAL BONE, WITHOUT FACIAL SWELLING BUT WITH A SKIN FISTULA

Diagnosis. Any persistent fistula of the face should be suspected of having a dental origin. The author has seen fistulas in areas apparently remote from the teeth (e.g., lateral to the eyebrow; see Figure 10–73) that are the termini of the long fistulous tracts from teeth. Residual chronic infection in a facial bone is always a possibility. The use of a probe, radiopaque dye, gutta percha point, and so on, may be necessary to determine the origin of the abscess.

Treatment. Extraction or treatment of the infected tooth or excision of the residual area of infection in the bone is indicated. This is followed by a cessation of drainage and a "drying up" of the tissues at the orifice of the fistulous tract, which is usually surrounded by pyogenic granulation tissue. See Chronic Skin Fistula and Figures 10–60 to 10–72.

PROPAGATION OF DENTAL INFECTION

The reader is referred to the excellent chapter entitled "The Propagation of Dental Infections" in Sicher and DuBrul's book *Oral Anatomy* for a complete discussion of this important subject. A few pertinent excerpts from this book are quoted or paraphrased in the discussions of maxillary and mandibular abscesses that follow.*

Excluding the hematogenous spread, that is, the spread of bacteria by blood vessels, there are three possibilities for the spread of dental infections:

1. By the invasion of bacteria into lymph vessels, resulting in metastatic inflammation of the regional and more remote lymph glands.
2. By the involvement of the veins that are affected by thrombosis and that then form, by continued clotting of the contained blood, a wide-open roadway for the invasion of bacteria.
3. The most frequent, the spread of infection by continuity (see Plate II).

---

*Reproduced with permission from Sicher, H., and DuBrul, E. L.: Oral Anatomy. 5th ed., 1970; copyrighted by The C. V. Mosby Co., St. Louis.

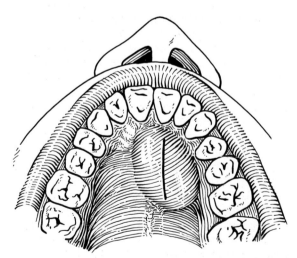

Figure 10–2 Incision for a palatal subperiosteal abscess which may have its origin in any of the six maxillary anterior teeth. In this location probably one of the left anterior teeth is the offender. Keep the incision along the medial border of the swelling. This avoids the anterior palatine artery.

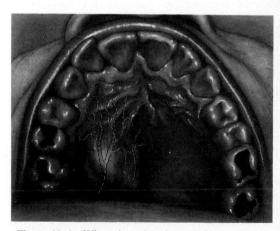

Figure 10–3 When the subperiosteal abscess is in the posterior palatal region, care must be taken when making an incision for drainage to avoid the greater palatine artery; otherwise, a most difficult-to-control hemorrhage may result. The incision should be made along the median border of the swelling, as shown in this drawing.

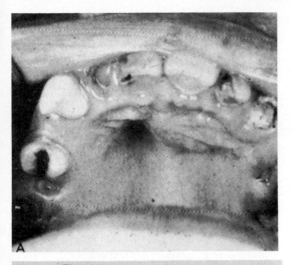

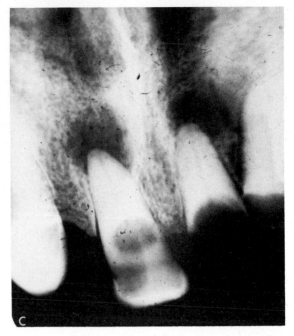

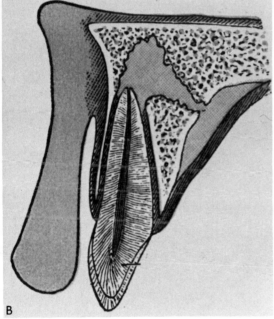

Figure 10-4 *A*, Palatal subperiosteal abscess. *B*, Pathway from the periapical pathosis to the palate, where the pressure of the pus elevates the thick mucoperiosteal tissue. *C*, Radiographs of these anterior teeth reveal periapical radiolucent areas.

(*A*, From Laskin, D. M.: Anatomic considerations in diagnosis and treatment of odontogenic infections. J.A.D.A., *69*:308 [Sept.], 1964. Copyright by the American Dental Association. Reprinted by permission. *B*, From Black, G. V.: A Work on Special Dental Pathology. Chicago, Medico-Dental Publishing Co., 1920.)

DENTOALVEOLAR INFECTIONS OF THE MAXILLA

Maxillary Anterior Teeth

The loose, fat-containing connective tissue of the lips and cheeks is continuous, but it is partially partitioned by the muscles of facial expression that arise from the osseous tissue (see Plate II and Figure 10-36) and end in the skin. These muscles play a role in directing the spread of infection. For this reason dental abscesses that have penetrated the cortical bone do not always localize in the vestibule but often move through the subcutaneous connective tissue to the skin. The reason that periapical abscesses of the maxillary incisors, cuspids and bicuspids usually do localize in their vestibules is that the muscles arising in the region of these teeth are either so small (nasal and upper incisal muscles) or so far away (canine) from the apices that they have little influence on the spread of the infection, so that it moves readily toward the fornix of the vestibule.

In the maxilla a small localized subperiosteal infection may be located in the palate (Figs. 10-2 to 10-8) or on the labial-buccal *(Text continued on page 457)*

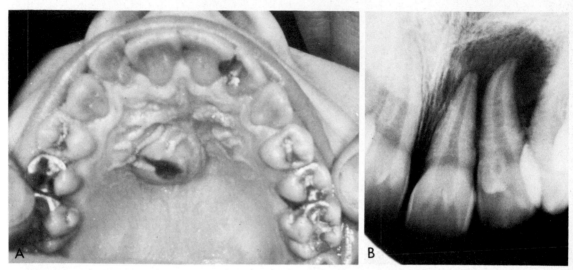

Figure 10-5   *A,* Another example of a subperiosteal abscess, but one located somewhat further back in the midline of the palate than the case shown in Figure 10–4. This was incised and drained. Root canal therapy was then performed and the canal was filled. *B,* Periapical radiograph taken before incision and drainage.

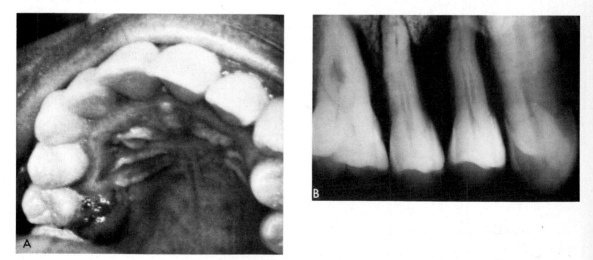

Figure 10-6   *A,* Palatal gingival acute inflammation and subperiosteal infection, with early necrosis of the muco-periosteal tissue. *B,* Periapical radiograph showing extensive loss of tissue from periodontal disease, with soft tissue involvement, as shown in *A.*

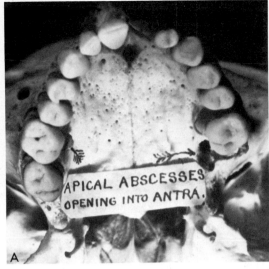

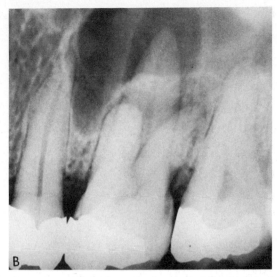

Figure 10–7 *A,* Palatal view of this maxillary anatomic specimen shows bilateral antral subperiosteal fistulas into the maxillary sinuses. *B,* This periapical radiograph of a maxillary molar reveals a well-circumscribed radiolucent area extending around the lingual root of the first molar. This area could represent such a fistula as shown in *A.*

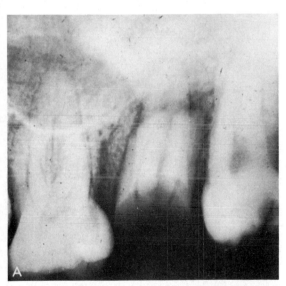

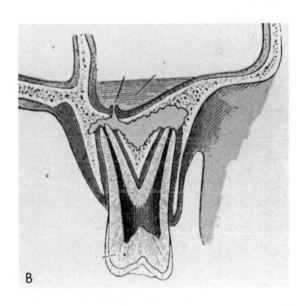

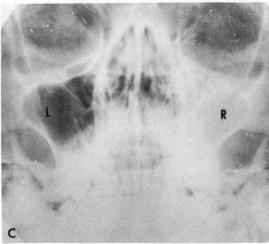

Figure 10–8 *A,* Periapical radiograph showing maxillary molar with apical pathosis. *B,* Drawing showing how the thin space between the apices of the tooth and the floor of the maxillary sinus can be penetrated and infected. *C,* Posteroanterior radiograph taken with the nose and chin in contact with the film holder (Waters' position), which suggests (by the opacity in the area of the right maxillary sinus) the presence of sinusitis. The clinical symptoms, as described in this chapter, confirmed the diagnosis.

(*B,* From Black, G. V.: A Work on Special Dental Pathology. Chicago, Medico-Dental Publishing Co., 1920.)

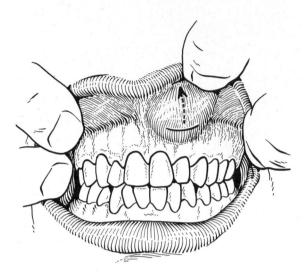

Figure 10–9 Incision to drain a localized subperiosteal abscess that originated from a periapical abscess of the central or lateral incisor. Arrow indicates the direction of the hemostat to separate the deeper structures.

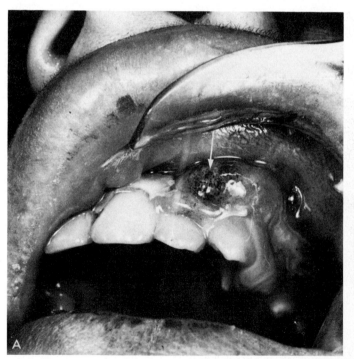
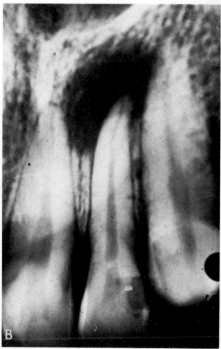

Figure 10–10 *A*, Localized subperiosteal abscess formed by the infected lateral incisor. Note the mottled black and gray dotted area (see arrow). This area of the raised mucoperiosteal membrane is becoming necrotic because the pressure of the pus against this thinned membrane has cut off the blood supply. If this abscess is not promptly incised and drained (see Figure 10–9), the tissue will rupture spontaneously and the abscess will drain by itself. Incising the tissue to establish drainage results in much quicker and better healing, for in spontaneous rupture, a large area of necrotic tissue first has to be sloughed off and then new mucoperiosteal tissue must cover the exposed bone by secondary intention. (See also Figure 10–11.) *B*, Periapical radiograph of offending tooth.

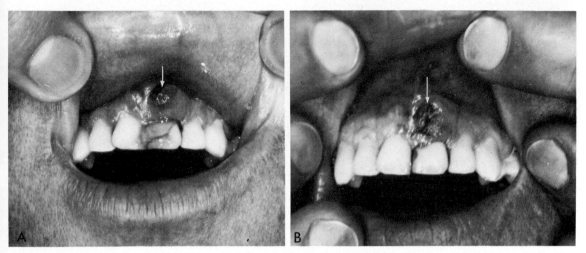

Figure 10–11 *A,* Here we see again (at arrow) the same necrotic process taking place as described in the legend for Figure 10–10. In this case thick pus can be seen escaping from the gingival attachment of the mucoperiosteal membrane, but as shown in *B,* the necrotic process was irreversible and this entire section of the labial mucoperiosteal flap had been destroyed. This subperiosteal abscess required incision and drainage before the pressure necrosis of the soft tissue began to heal. (See Figure 10–9.) The same applies to extraoral abscesses.

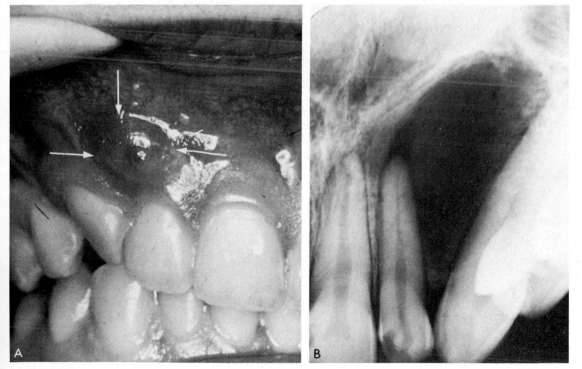

Figure 10–12 *A,* Well-circumscribed maxillary anterior subperiosteal abscess (parulis). *B,* Radiograph shows a large area of diffuse radiolucency.

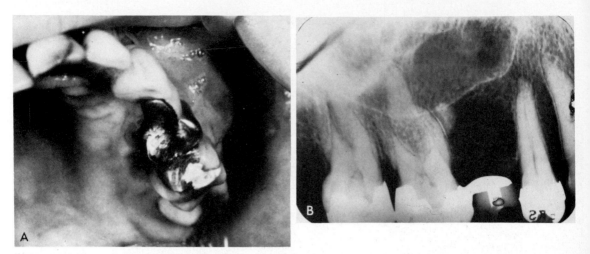

Figure 10–13 *A,* Subperiosteal abscess beneath bridge pontics are not rare. The usual cause is the long-continued slight pressure against the mucoperiosteal membrane, producing chronically inflamed tissue whose resistance to the invasion of oral bacteria becomes lowered. A subperiosteal abscess then develops. However, as is shown in radiograph *B,* in this case, there is a retained root and loss of osseous tissue beneath the pontic is due to residual infection.

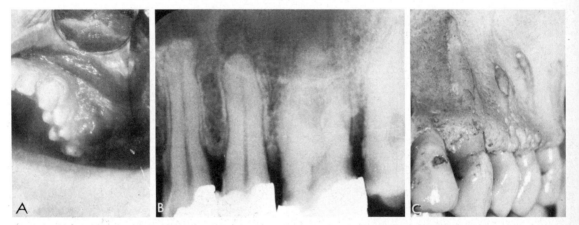

Figure 10–14 *A,* Subperiosteal abscess. *B,* Origin of the abscess. *C,* Dry skull indicates the thin cortical bone, or absence of osseous tissue, over the apices of maxillary cuspids and bicuspids frequently observed in this area.

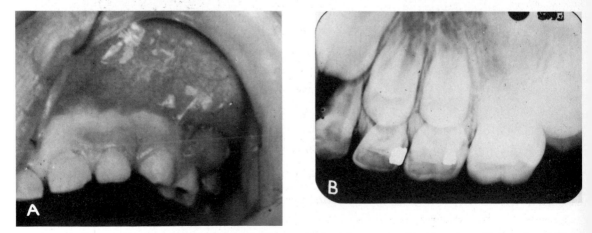

Figure 10–15 *A,* Subperiosteal abscess from a carious and infected temporary (deciduous) maxillary molar. *B,* Non-vital infected temporary second maxillary molar.

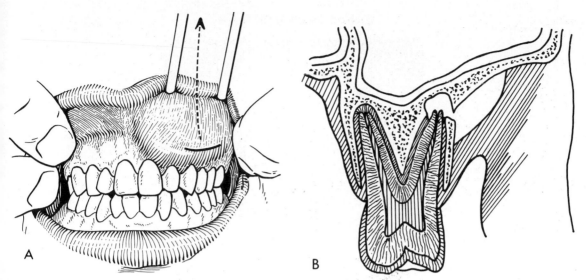

Figure 10–16 *A,* Incision for drainage of a large localized abscess of the left side of the upper face which may have started from any periapical infection from the central incisor to and including the maxillary molars. The arrow indicates the direction of the hemostat in separating the deeper structures. *B,* While the usual route for the penetration of pus is through the buccal cortical plate of bone, we do occasionally see a fistula or subperiosteal abscess on the palatal side of the alveolar ridge.

(*B,* From Black, G. V.: A Work on Special Dental Pathology. Chicago, Medico-Dental Publishing Co., 1920.)

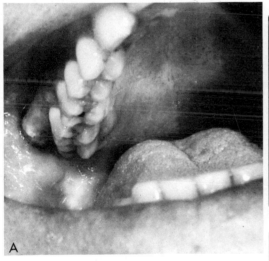

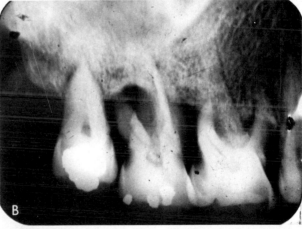

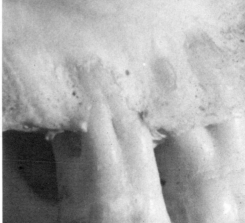

Figure 10–17 *A,* Subperiosteal abscess originating from a periodontal pocket that has stripped the mucoperiosteal membrane from the buccal cortical plate, but has not dissected upward into the soft tissues of the upper face. *B,* Radiograph reveals extent of periodontal pathosis. *C,* Maxillary anatomical specimen which demonstrates the extent of destruction of the supporting alveolar bone around the maxillary molar roots due to advanced periodontal disease.

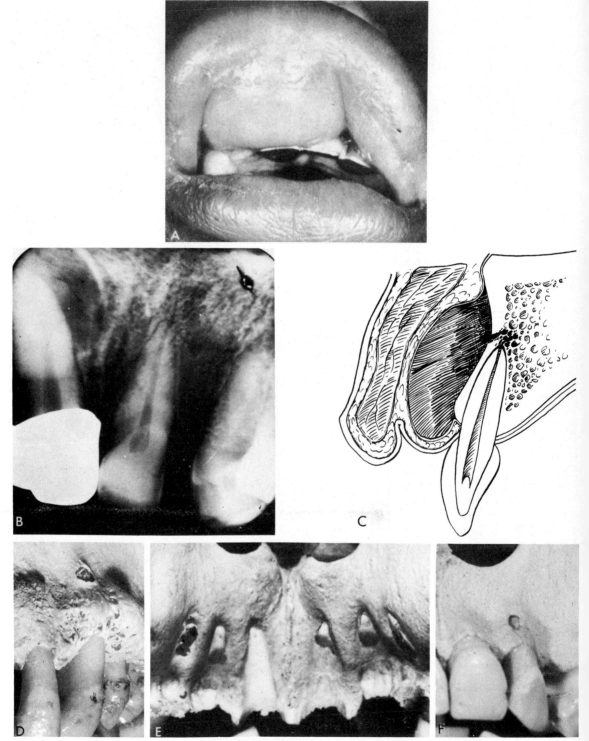

Figure 10–18 *A,* Subperiosteal abscess arising from the right maxillary central incisor. Despite the great size, infection is still contained intraorally by muscle and fascial barriers.

B, Radiograph with large radiolucent area, suggesting an infection that could produce such an abscess.

C, This drawing shows the close relationship of the apices of the maxillary anterior teeth to the labial cortical plate as compared to the palatal cortical plate, and also how the pressure of the pus has stripped the mucoperiosteal membrane away from the labial bone down to its attachment with the periodontal ligaments of these teeth.

D to F, A series of photographs of dry skulls, showing fistulas through this thin cortical bone over the apices of the six maxillary anterior teeth.

(*A,* From Laskin, D. M.: Anatomic considerations in diagnosis and treatment of odontogenic infections. J.A.D.A., 69:308 [Sept.], 1964. Copyright by the American Dental Association. Reprinted by permission.)

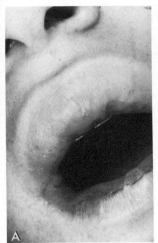
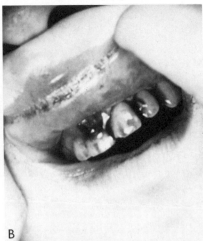
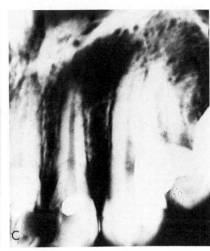

Figure 10-19 *A*, Diffuse cellulitis of the lip from an acute exacerbation of a chronically infected maxillary left lateral incisor. *B*, Within 72 hours the labial periosteum was stripped free to the gingival line, and had broken through the gingival attachment and begun to drain. *C*, Note the diffuse radiolucent area about the apex of the lateral incisor, indicating a prolonged chronic infection.

side of the maxillary ridge (Figs. 10-9 to 10-15). These infections, if not treated properly, may become enlarged (Figs. 10-16 and 10-17) and, as explained earlier in the chapter, spread into contiguous soft tissues.

Lip. When a maxillary anterior tooth is abscessed, the infection may penetrate the labial plate, causing swelling of the lip (Figs. 10-18 and 10-19).

Canine Fossa. If the infection breaks through the labial cortical plate superiorly, the infection can enter the canine fossa (Figs. 10-20 to 10-22). The canine fossa is located in the depressed anterior osseous wall of the maxillary sinus below the infraorbital ridge. It can vary from a shallow concavity to an abnormally deep well. In obese individuals, in whom there is a large amount of fat in the subcutaneous tissue, the canine fossa is not easily located. The canine muscle arises high in the canine fossa just below the infraorbital foramen in an almost horizontal line above the cuspid. A periapical abscess of the cuspid usually breaks through the alveolar cortical plate below the origin of the canine muscle and spreads into the submucous connective tissue of the vestibular fornix.

An exception to this usual area of localiza-tion is in those cases in which the cuspid root is very long and its apex is above the origin of the canine muscle but below the origin of the quadratus muscle. A periapical abscess in such a case most likely will spill into the loose connective tissue in the space between these muscles, containing the branches of the infraorbital nerve and blood vessels. If this happens, the infection may finally spread anteriorly through the gap between the angular and infraorbital heads of the quadratus muscle and thus emerge under the skin just below the inner corner of the eye, or escape posteriorly between the infraorbital head and zygomatic head of the quadratus muscle, emerging under the skin just below the outer corner of the eye (see Figure 10-32).

Maxillary Bicuspids

The same mucle, the canine, having its origin far from the apices of the maxillary bicuspids, permits the localization of periapical abscesses first in the vestibule over these apices.

Buccal Abscess. As illustrated in Figures 10-23 to 10-28, a maxillary as well as man-*(Text continued on page 460)*

Case Report No. 1

MAXILLARY VESTIBULAR AND CANINE FOSSA ABSCESS OF ODONTOGENIC ORIGIN

A 24-year-old man was perfectly well until 6 days before admission, when he awoke with a soft swelling of his upper lip. An ice pack was applied, but the swelling increased and the upper lip became hard and painful. Four days before admission he saw his dentist, who recommended applications of heat. The lip became red, the swelling extended into the right canine fossa, and the labial mucosa became puffy and obliterated the sulcus (see Figure 10–20).

On admission, the temperature was 101.5° F., the white blood cell count was 18,700, and findings for the urine were negative. The upper lip was massively swollen, hard, tender and red. Intraorally, the maxillary right first incisor (which was fitted with a Davis crown) was acutely tender to the touch, and somewhat loose, and the labial gingival tissue was edematous and fluctuant. The radiographs showed a large, well-defined area of bone destruction about the apex of the right lateral central incisor.

The patient was admitted to the hospital ward; hot wet dressings were started; hot mouth irrigations were begun; and penicillin, 600,000 units every 12 hours, was injected intramuscularly. On the day of admission, the lateral incisor was extracted under general anesthesia, and satisfactory drainage was established.

The intraoral and extraoral heat were continued postoperatively, and the next day the lip swelling had markedly diminished. The temperature was 100.2° F., the white blood cell count 12,000. The pus continued to drain through the socket, and the patient was discharged on the third hospital day, with instructions to continue intraoral heat.

Comment.   This was a case of marked cellulitis of the lip of dental origin, with streptococci the causative organisms. Heat helped to localize the infection and to aid drainage established by the removal of the tooth.

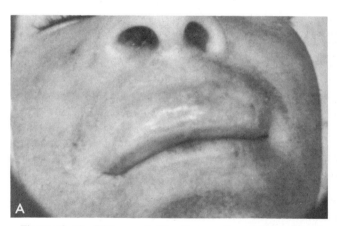
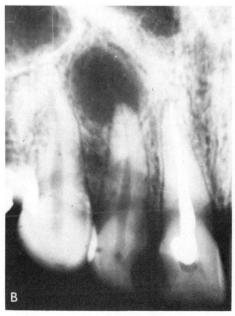

Figure 10–20 Diffuse cellulitis of upper lip extending into the right canine fossa from acute alveolar abscess of the maxillary right lateral incisor (see Case Report No. 1).

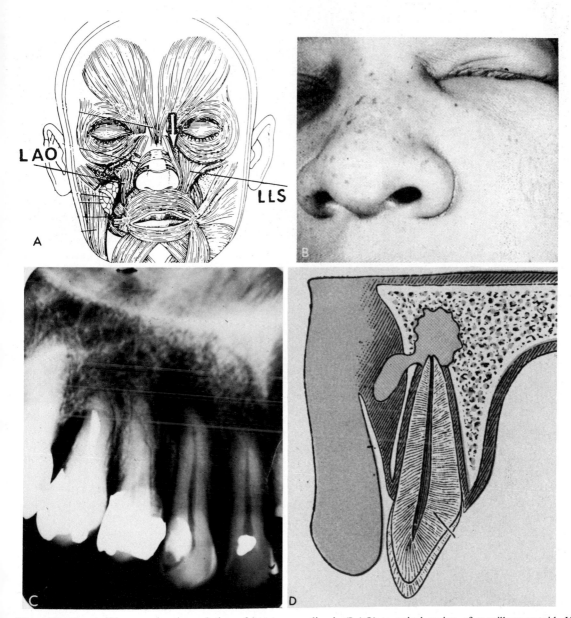

Figure 10–21 *A,* Diagram showing relation of levator anguli oris (LAO) to apical region of maxillary cuspid. If infection perforates bone above attachment of this muscle, it localizes beneath levator labii superioris (LLS) in canine space. Access to skin is afforded through the gap (arrow) between these muscles. *B,* Clinical appearance of the canine space abscess.

C, Periapical radiograph shows a circumscribed area of radiolucency, the probable source of the acute abscess. *D,* This drawing illustrates how the acute abscess has penetrated the labial cortical plate of bone and periosteum and has "spilled out" into the soft tissue in the canine space.

(*A* and *B,* From Laskin, D. M.: Anatomic considerations in diagnosis and treatment of odontogenic infections. J.A.D.A., *69:*308 [Sept.], 1964. Copyright by American Dental Association. Reprinted by permission; *A,* modified from Sicher, *D,* From Black, G. V.: A Work on Special Dental Pathology. Chicago, Medico-Dental Publishing Co., 1920.)

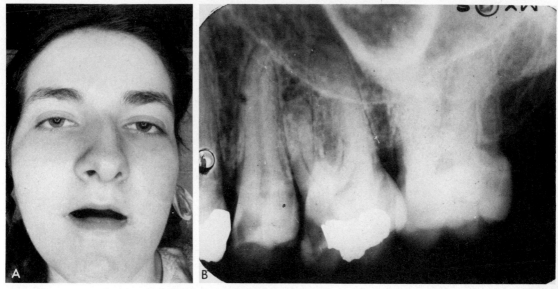

Figure 10–22 Acute maxillary abscess from an infected first molar. The swelling is confined to the upper half of the face. The patient has a typical toxic appearance. Note also the distortion of the right naris due to the swelling. Intraoral incision and drainage were established in the canine fossa region.

dibular bicuspid or molar may be the source of an infection in the buccal space. Discussion of the anatomic relations of this space is included with that of other mandibular spaces, beginning on page 469.

Maxillary Molars

As Sicher points out, "In the region of the maxillary molars it is the attachment of the buccinator muscle to the alveolar process which plays a decisive role for the path of a dental abscess after it has perforated the outer compact layer of the bone. Ordinarily, the line of origin of the buccinator muscle is, in the adult, beyond the level of the root apices of the molars, so that a molar abscess involves the submucous connective tissue, while its spread to the skin is blocked by the buccinator muscle and its fasciae. In persons with relatively long roots, or in young persons in whom the height of the jaws has not yet been attained and in whom the teeth have

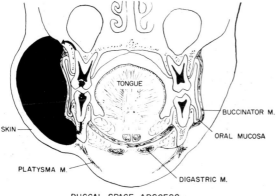

BUCCAL SPACE ABSCESS

Figure 10–23 Diagrammatic representation of buccal space abscess. Although periorbital area is not involved directly, impaired venous and lymphatic drainage often results in great edema of this region. (From Laskin, D. M.: Anatomic considerations in diagnosis and treatment of odontogenic infections. J.A.D.A., 69:308 [Sept.], 1964. Copyright by the American Dental Association. Reprinted by permission.)

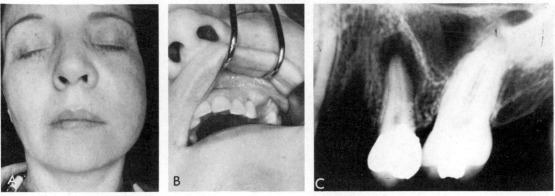

Figure 10–24 *A*, An area of residual infection in the left second bicuspid area broke through into the soft tissues of the upper cheek. Note the distention of the mucoperiosteal tissues and the mucobuccal fold. *B*, Buccal abscess. The infection has spread from the maxilla between the mucosa and the buccinator muscle to the inferior border of the mandible. *C*, Radiograph with well-circumscribed periapical radiolucency.

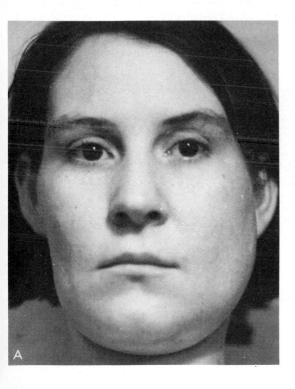

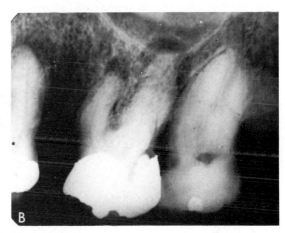

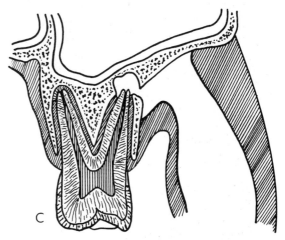

Figure 10–25 *A*, Buccal abscess which originated from the periapical pathosis shown in *B*. In this patient the infection from the buccal roots broke through the thin cortical bone over the apices above the insertion of the buccinator muscle, stripping away the mucoperiosteal membrane, as shown in *C* and Figure 10–23. From this position the pus moved laterally and inferiorly between the buccinator muscle and the skin to the lower border of the mandible and beyond. (*C*, Modified from Black, G. V.: A Work on Special Dental Pathology. Chicago, Medico-Dental Publishing Co., 1920.)

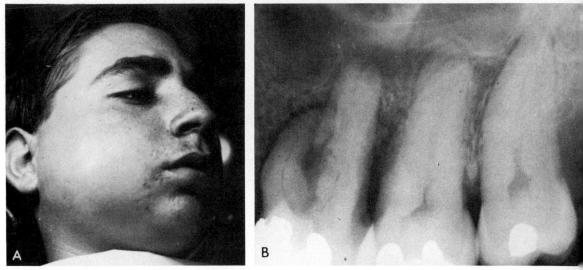

Figure 10–26 This buccal abscess has spread beneath the mandible into the submandibular space. Treatment, incision and drainage obviously should have been instituted before this extension occurred.

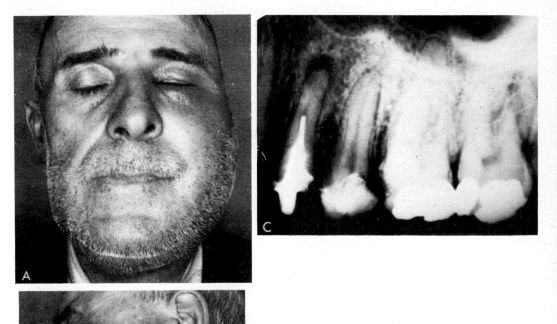

Figure 10–27 Another example of a buccal abscess

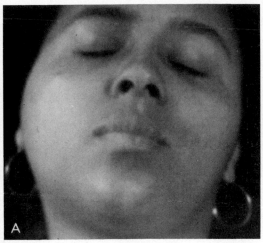
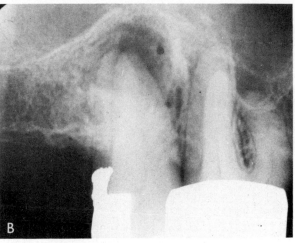

Figure 10-28 *A,* An example of a cellulitis of the face due to a buccal abscess from the infected maxillary second bicuspid. *B,* The buccal fistula was above the insertion of the buccinator muscle, which frequently extends over the bicuspid apices.

not yet sufficiently erupted from the body of the maxilla or mandible, the apices of the molars may reach beyond the line of origin of the buccinator muscle. An abscess perforating the outer plate of the alveolar process is then barred from the submucous connective

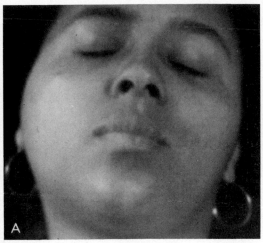

Figure 10-29 Postoperative cellulitis and maxillary abscess with extension into the pterygoid maxillary space following extraction of maxillary molars. Intraoral drainage was established by an incision into the pterygoid maxillary space, as shown in Figure 10-53.

tissue in the vestibule by the buccinator muscle and spreads in the subcutaneous tissue toward the skin."[30]

Differential Diagnosis for Maxillary Abscesses

Acute Maxillary Sinusitis of Dental Origin. The symptoms of acute maxillary sinusitis of dental origin (Fig. 10-30) are severe pain; chills and fever; swelling of the cheek and lower eyelid; marked soreness in any remaining maxillary teeth on that side (the teeth feel elongated); profuse, thick, foul purulent discharge from one side of the nose. The foul odor of the pus is due to the putrefactive and saprophytic organisms from the mouth. The patient has a heavy sense of fullness on the affected side of his face. When stepping off curbs or down steps, he is conscious of movement of the pus in the infected antrum. If the patient stoops and then straightens up, he is momentarily dizzy. The patient feels and looks toxic.

Not all these symptoms need be present in order to make a diagnosis of acute maxillary sinusitis.

Acute Maxillary Sinusitis and Acute Postoperative Maxillary Soft Tissue Infection. When there is considerable swelling as a result of edema in the soft tissues overlying the maxillary sinus, the posteroanterior radiograph of the maxillary sinuses cannot be relied on to determine whether the antrum is

(*Text continued on page 468*)

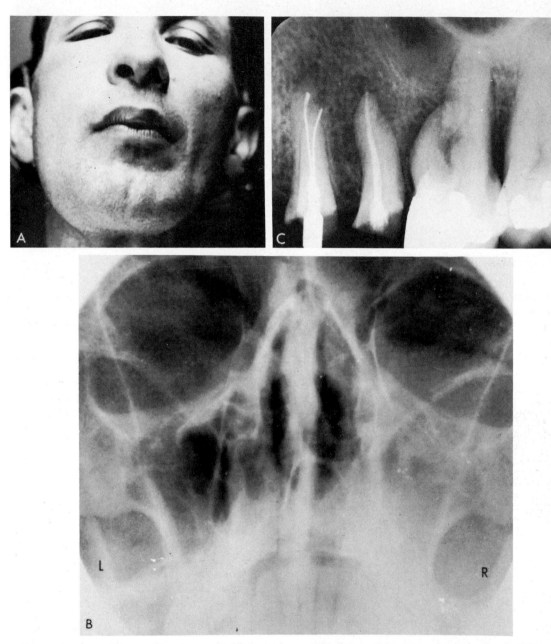

Figure 10–30 *A*, This maxillary facial swelling was incorrectly diagnosed by the patient's family physician as the extension of an acute maxillary sinusitis. He made this diagnosis because of the opacity he saw in his radiograph (*B*) of the patient's right maxillary sinus. His irrigations of this sinus were nonproductive. *C*, Periapical radiographs of the right maxillary teeth revealed the cause of the infection.

(*Figure 10–30 continued on opposite page*)

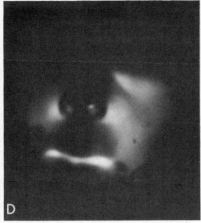

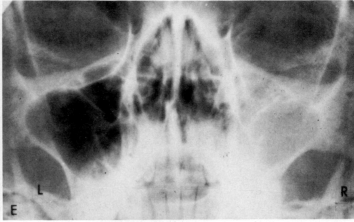

Figure 10–30 (*Continued.*)

D and *E*, Differential diagnosis (see also text). *D*, An example of the use of the transillumination lamp in the diagnosis of maxillary sinusitis. Note the lack of penetration of light (opacity) on the affected right side of the face as compared to translucency of the left healthy side. *E*, An x-ray view in the Waters-Waldron position of a chronic sinusitis involving the right maxillary, ethmoid, and frontal sinuses. There is a fluid level visible in the involved maxillary sinus.

F, The source of the infection was the carious roots of the maxillary second molar.

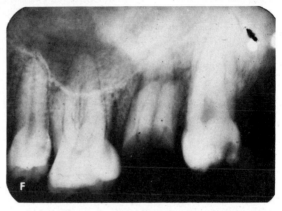

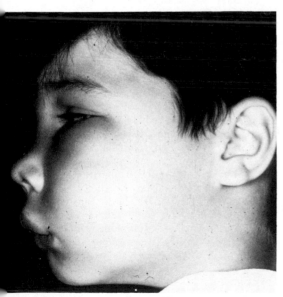

Figure 10–31 Maxillary abscess involving the lip and left side of the face from a periapical abscess of the left lateral incisor of 7 days' duration. Intraoral incision and drainage and extraction of the lateral incisor was performed. This case illustrates the extent to which infection can spread from maxillary anterior teeth.

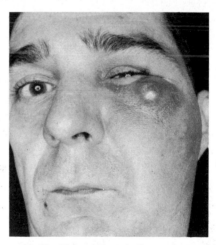

Figure 10–32 This patient had an acute periapical abscess of the first maxillary molar which resulted in extensive edema of the left upper half of his face. He was advised that "nothing could be done until the swelling went down." About a week after the initial swelling, the patient stated that "something broke" in his mouth, and he had a lot of foul-smelling yellow pus in his mouth. The swelling subsided rapidly, and a week later his dentist extracted the offending molar. Several days later the present swelling developed. This was a residual subcutaneous abscess which had developed at the origin of the infraorbital head of the quadratus muscle. Extraoral incision and drainage were done.

465

ACUTE ALVEOLAR ABSCESS OF THE MAXILLARY FIRST MOLAR WITH SECONDARY CELLULITIS OF THE FACE

A 15-year-old boy came to the out-patient dental clinic with a chief complaint of pain and swelling of the right side of the face.

Present Illness. Four days before admission, the patient had had a sharp toothache in the right maxillary cuspid region.

Three days before admission, the right side of the face began to swell; ice packs were applied, but the swelling progressively increased.

On the day before admission, the right eye was closed by the cellulitis, and the patient had malaise and some slight headache, but no cough, nausea or vomiting.

Physical Examination. There was diffuse cellulitis on the right side of the face, with periorbital edema and closure of the eyelids. The cheek tissue was semifluctuant, reddened and tender to the touch (see Figure 10–33*A*).

The maxillary right cuspid and first bicuspid (Fig. 10–33*B*) were deeply carious, sensitive to percussion, mobile, and slightly elongated. There was fluctuant edema of the surrounding buccal and palatal mucosa.

The patient's temperature was 101° F. (rectal); a white blood count showed 15,500 cells per cubic millimeter; findings in the urine examination were negative.

Diagnosis. The case was diagnosed as acute alveolar abscess of the maxillary right cuspid and first bicuspid, with secondary cellulitis of the face. The patient was admitted to a hospital ward.

Treatment. Penicillin therapy was given, hot wet dressings were applied to the right face continuously; hot saline (120° F.) mouth irrigations were administered every 3 hours; and fluid intake was forced.

The offending teeth were removed under nitrous oxide anesthesia (with administration of morphine, 8 mg., and atropine, 0.3 mg., ½ hour before). A free flow of pus was obtained from the tooth socket, the culture of which revealed abundant alpha hemolytic streptococci and some beta hemolytic streptococci.

Two days later the facial swelling had markedly reduced, the temperature was normal, the white blood cell count was lowered to 10,000, and the patient continued to have copious drainage from the tooth socket. He was discharged on the fifth hospital day.

Comment. This was an obvious severe maxillary alveolar abscess with cellulitis, for which ice packs were contraindicated. A regimen of intraoral and extraoral heat and penicillin, plus drainage by the extraction of the infected teeth, brought rapid recovery.

ACUTE MAXILLARY ABSCESS FOLLOWING THE EXTRACTION OF THE FIRST DECIDUOUS MOLAR

An 8-year-old girl came to the out-patient dental clinic with a chief complaint of pain and swelling following a tooth extraction.

Present Illness. Five days before admission to the hospital, the patient had had a toothache in the right maxillary deciduous molar region. The dentist had extracted the right first deciduous molar under ethyl chloride anesthesia. Twenty-four hours later the patient had experienced pain and swelling. She returned to her dentist, who gave her a pill and advised that ice bags be applied to her face, but the condition grew worse. Four days later the dentist extracted the superior right second deciduous molar and lower right first permanent molar. That night the condition grew much worse; the temperature rose to 105° F., and the swelling became more extensive.

Physical Examination. There was diffuse swelling of the right side of the face extending into the temporal region, and evidence of the left side's becoming involved; also, periorbital edema, closure of the right eyelid, and partial closure of the left eyelid. The cheek tissue was semifluctuant, reddened, shiny, and very tender to the touch. The temperature was 105° F. (see Figure 10–34*B*).

Diagnosis. This was established as acute alveolar abscess with extensive secondary cellulitis of the face and head. The patient was admitted to the hospital ward.

Treatment. Hot compresses (towels) were applied constantly by the nurse assigned to the case. The swelling increased in the region of the trachea, and asphyxia was feared. The otolaryngologist was alerted to be prepared to do an emergency tracheotomy. Forty-eight hours later, under nitrous oxide and oxygen anesthesia, drainage was obtained by a submandibular incision. Hot, moist applications and intraoral irrigations were continued. Twenty-four hours later the temperature began dropping, and the swelling was markedly reduced. Three days later incision of a temporal abscess was done. Her condition rapidly improved, and the patient was discharged on the twelfth day.

Comment. In this severe maxillary alveolar abscess with cellulitis and acute infection, ice bags were contraindicated, for they apparently produced stasis. The moist heat applications localized and aided nature's front-line defense (hyperemia to combat the infection. This case, treated before sulfanilamide drugs and penicillin were in use, shows the efficacy of hot, moist applications.

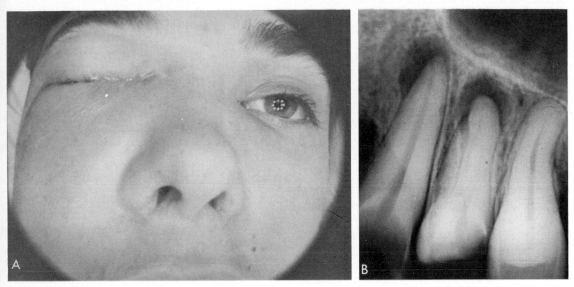

Figure 10-33 *A*, Acute alveolar abscess of maxillary right cuspid and first bicuspid with facial cellulitis resulting in periorbital edema (see Case Report No. 2). *B*, Periapical pathosis.

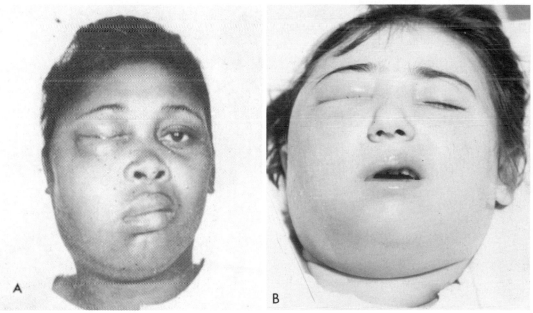

Figure 10-34 *A*, Infection involving submandibular, buccal, pterygomandibular and pretemporal spaces (so-called "pan-facial" abscess). The patient, who had diabetes, had failed to maintain insulin therapy after the extraction of the maxillary right third molar, and diabetes became uncontrolled. This illustrates the interrelationship between anatomic and physiologic factors in the regulation of infectious processes.

B, Acute cellulitis of the face following the extraction of deciduous teeth. Twenty-four hours after hospitalization. (See Case Report No. 3.)

(*A*, From Laskin, D. M.: Anatomic considerations in diagnosis and treatment of odontogenic infections. J.A.D.A., 69:308 [Sept.], 1964. Copyright by the American Dental Association. Reprinted by permission.)

infected, because the fluid in the facial tissues will offer the same resistance to the passage of the x-rays, as *would fluid in the antrum.* Hence, *radiographically the shadows on the film in either case are the same!* If the patient has profuse foul drainage *from the nose,* the antrum is infected. If this discharge is not present, in order to rule out the antrum, the rhinologist should be consulted.

Extension of Localized Maxillary Abscesses

If an anterior central or lateral incisor is abscessed, and the purulent material has penetrated the labial cortical bone, the upper lip will swell to two or three times its normal size. The infection can extend into the cheek, as described earlier.

Abscesses of the maxillary cuspids, bicuspids and molars cause a marked swelling of the cheek that extends up to the eye. Frequently the eye is closed because of the edema that extends into the lid (Figs. 10–31 to 10–33).

Eventually the cellulitis involves the whole side of the face, extending posteriorly to and around the external ear and temporal region and forehead (Figs. 10–34 and 10–35). Simultaneously, there is extension posteriorly behind the maxilla into the buccal and other masticator spaces. There is always a possibility of thrombosis of the pterygoid plexus of veins, with subsequent extension to the cavernous sinus or internal jugular vein. Here there is also the possibility of a blood stream infection by way of the internal jugular vein. Gold and Sager reported a "case of pansinusitis, orbital cellulitis and blindness as sequelae of delayed treatment of a dental abscess." The patient received "neither timely nor correct initial treatment."

Cavernous sinus thrombophlebitis with general septicemia and death, associated with infection of the face, particularly the upper half, is described on pages 510 to 514.

DENTOALVEOLAR INFECTIONS OF THE MANDIBLE

Mandibular Anterior Teeth

Periapical abscesses of the mandibular anterior incisors and cuspids, the apices of which are above the origin of the inferior incisive and mental muscles, when the infection has penetrated the labial bone, will localize in

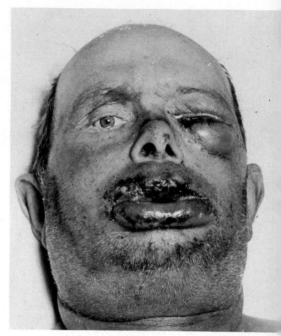

Figure 10–35 This infection of odontogenic origin started in the left canine fossa. Procrastination on the part of a general surgeon resulted in the spread of the infection illustrated here in spite of massive antibiotic therapy. Early intraoral drainage through the fornix of the vestibule in the canine region with adequate antibiotic coverage would have quickly brought this infection under control.

the labial sulcus. If these roots are large, the perforation of the labial plate may be below the origin of these muscles and therefore the infection will be directed along a pathway toward the skin in front of or below the bony chin. If periapical infection of any of the mandibular six anterior teeth perforates the lingual surface of bone, it will involve the sublingual space above the mylohyoid muscle, which has its origin close to the lower border of the mandible.

A small localized subperiosteal infection in the mandible (Figs. 10–38 and 10–39), if not treated early and adequately, may extend into contiguous soft tissues of the mandible.

Mandibular Bicuspids

Diseased mandibular bicuspids (premolars) rarely cause cutaneous abscesses because the muscles in the area of these teeth, namely the depressor anguli oris, the triangular and the quadrate muscles, arise near the lower border of the mandible, below the apices of the bicuspids. When a periapical abscess perforates the labial cortical bone and discharges into the loose connective tissue between the muscles and mandible, it localizes first in the vestibule, where it is readily visible and accessible.

Lingual perforation of the cortical plate will result in infection in the sublingual space above the mylohyoid muscle.

Mandibular Molars

Periapical infection of the first and second mandibular molars can perforate the buccal or lingual bony plate. If on the buccal side, an abscess of the sulcus will result unless the roots are very long and thus below the insertion of the buccinator muscle. In such an event the subcutaneous connective tissue is involved. If on the lingual side, the point of lingual discharge of the abscess may be below, or above, the mylohyoid muscle. If below, there is an abscess in the submandibular space; if above, in the sublingual space. Periapical infections of mandibular third molars routinely perforate the lingual cortical bone, discharging pus into the submandibular space. The infection may spread backward into the parapharyngeal space and downward into the connective tissue of the neck.

Moreover, Sicher explains, "The buccinator muscle also plays a role in the spread of pericoronal abscesses of the lower mandibular third molar. These abscesses involve frequently the submucous connective tissue at the buccal side of the tooth. Here, at the root of the cheek where its mobility is restricted, the vestibule is shallow and the amount of loose connective tissue at the fornix is small. The abscess, therefore, is not very conspicuous before it involves more voluminous layers of loose connective tissue. The origin of the buccinator muscle at the oblique line directs the spreading abscess forward and downward and it becomes more and more voluminous and pronounced when it reaches the level of the second or first molar. Such infections may seem to originate from a second or first molar, and only the knowledge of the peculiar anatomic relations can prevent a faulty diagnosis."[30]

Anatomic Spaces

Infection may invade the loose connective tissue that separates muscles from each other and may spread from one space to others.

Because of this possibility the terms intermuscular and interfascial "spaces" are commonly used. Sicher insists that the term "spaces" should be strictly reserved for those regions (spaces) that are filled with loose, sometimes fat-containing, connective tissue.[30] Therefore, according to Sicher, an interfascial area does not qualify as a "space."

Masticatory Fat Pad Spaces. Three masticatory spaces can be differentiated. "They communicate with each other and with the parapharyngeal space but are at least partly separated from each other, so that infection may, for a time, be confined to either one of the compartments."

BUCCAL SPACE. "This loose, fat-filled area is located between the buccinator and masseter muscles. It connects posteriorly with the pterygomandibular space, and superiorly with the zygomaticotemporal space." (See Figures 10–23 to 10–28.)

PTERYGOMANDIBULAR SPACE. "This space is bounded laterally by the medial surface of the mandibular ramus, medially by the medial (internal) pterygoid muscle, and above by the lateral (external) pterygoid muscle. The pterygomandibular extension of the fat pad, surrounding the lingual nerve and inferior alveolar nerve and the lower alveolar blood vessels, reaches backward to the anterior surface of the deep part of the parotid gland, which is contained in the retromandibular fossa. The masticatory fat pad also sends a rather thin process upward between the lateral and medial pterygoid muscles and finally connects, through the pterygopalatine gap, at the anterior border of the pterygoid process, with the fat in the pterygopalatine space."[30]

Hall and Morris reviewed 20 cases of infection of the pterygomandibular space and found that they most commonly resulted from extraction of a lower molar tooth.[15] Abscesses within this space may apparently "point" (see Figure 10–44) at the anterior aspect of the masseter muscle, either into the cheek or the mouth, or they may "point" posteriorly beneath the parotid gland (see Figures 10–40 to 10–42).

ZYGOMATICOTEMPORAL SPACE (RETROZYGOMATIC) (INFRATEMPORAL). This has been called the retrozygomatic space because it is partially situated behind the zygomatic bone. This, however, does not indicate the relationship to the temporal muscle and is therefore not clearly descriptive. This space lies directly behind the maxilla and zygomatic bones and medial to the insertion of the tem-

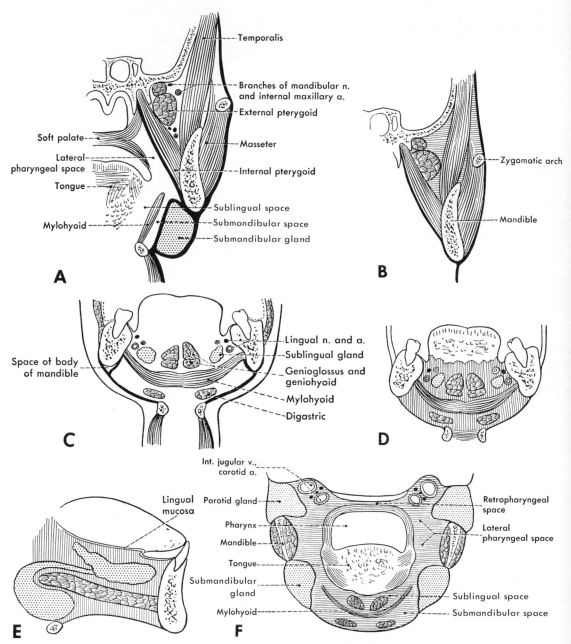

Figure 10–36 Study the text for the various spaces and anatomical structures involved, as illustrated above and described on pages 469 to 474. The external and internal pterygoids are also called lateral and medial pterygoids, respectively. (Modified from Hollinshead, W. H.: Anatomy for Surgeons. Vol. I, Head and Neck. New York, Hoeber, 1954.)

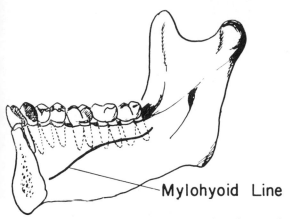

Mylohyoid Line

Figure 10–37 Diagram illustrating relation of roots of mandibular bicuspids and molars to lingual attachment of mylohyoid muscle. Teeth whose periapical infection penetrates the lingual cortical bone *above* the attachment of the mylohyoid muscle to the internal oblique ridge, illustrated above, produce sublingual abscesses. Those that penetrate *below* insertion of the mylohyoid muscle produce submandibular or pterygomandibular abscesses.

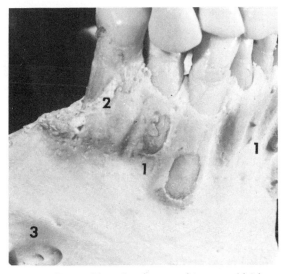

Figure 10–39 Note the absence of (or very thin) bone along the roots near and at the apices of these mandibular teeth (*1*). This obviously facilitates the ease with which a subperiosteal abscess could raise the periosteum and develop into a diffuse infection.

This dry skull is also of interest because of the double-rooted mandibular second bicuspid (*2*) and the distal, markedly inferior position of the mental foramen (*3*), which is usually between and below the apices of the bicuspids.

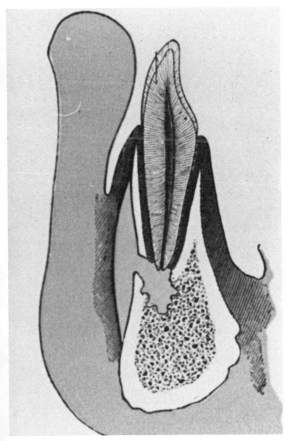

Figure 10–38 Illustrated here is the penetration of the labial cortical bone but not the periosteum, so a subperiosteal abscess has formed. (From Black, G. V.: A Work on Special Dental Pathology. Chicago, Medico-Dental Publishing Co., 1920.)

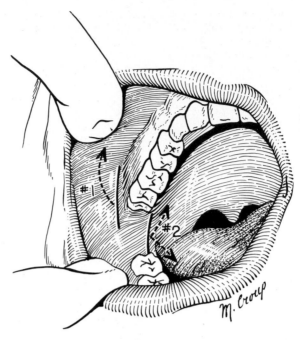

Figure 10-40 This incision medial to the anterior border of the ramus is to drain an abscess of the pterygomandibular space. The posterior part of the buccal space is also opened by this incision through the mucosa and buccinator muscle. A curved hemostat passed laterally and anteriorly through this incision will drain the buccal space. The zygomaticotemporal space is reached through the same incision by passing the hemostat upward along the exposed tendon of the temporal muscle. The parapharyngeal space can be opened by passing the hemostat along the medial surface of the internal pterygoid muscle. This incision will frequently drain these spaces long before there is extraoral pointing, thereby reducing the danger of excessive dissemination of the infection. It is true that drainage is not facilitated by gravity, but drainage tubes can and should be inserted into the spaces, and irrigation with penicillin and saline solutions will accomplish the dual purpose of bactericidal action and forced drainage. Or counterincisions can be made extraorally against the tip of the hemostat in each of these spaces.

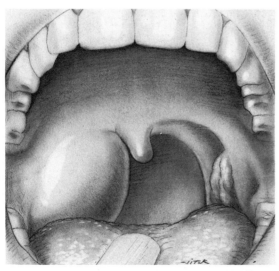

Figure 10-41 Clinical appearance of patient with pterygomandibular space abscess. Such patients generally have difficulty in swallowing and considerable trismus.

poral muscle and is filled with fat that extends upward from the buccal space. The pterygomandibular space is directly below and is considered by some as a part of the zygomaticotemporal space.

Infections of the maxillary teeth that drain through the cortical bone above the buccinator muscle many times spread into the zygomaticotemporal space and on to other spaces.

Parapharyngeal Space. Hollinshead prefers to call this the lateral pharyngeal space.[17] This space has been variously termed the parapharyngeal, peripharyngeal, pharyngomaxillary, pterygopharyngeal, pterygomandibular, and pharyngomasticator space. It extends laterally about the pharynx, and these lateral portions are continuous with the retropharyngeal space (see Figure 10-36A).

Sicher states, "The parapharyngeal space (lateral pharyngeal space) extends upward between the lateral wall of the pharynx and the medial surface of the internal pterygoid muscle. Behind the medial (internal) pterygoid muscle the parapharyngeal space widens considerably and reaches lateral to the styloid process with its muscles and to the deep surface of the parotid gland. The pterygomandibular space therefore communicates with the parapharyngeal space around the anterior and posterior borders of the internal pterygoid muscle."[30]

Incisions for Drainage of Infections of Intermuscular Spaces. As Sicher explains, "Infections may involve one or all of these compartments. They can be opened and explored from one key point." (See Figure 10–43.) "If a vertical incision is made in the most posterior part of the oral vestibule between the posterior ends of the upper and lower alveolar processes, lateral and parallel to the pterygomandibular fold, and if mucous membrane and the buccinator muscle are split, the posterior part of the buccal space is opened and the tendons of the temporal muscle arc exposed. A curved hemostat can be introduced in various directions through the incision. Anteriorly and laterally it enters the buccal space, posteriorly it passes into the pterygomandibular space medial to the temporal tendon. If the hemostat is guided upward along the exposed tendon of the temporal muscle, one can explore the zygomaticotemporal space. The parapharyngeal space is finally accessible from the same incision if the instrument is introduced along the inner surface of the medial pterygoid muscle whose anterior border, easily recognized, serves as a landmark.

Under the guidance of the introduced instrument counterincisions can be made in the temporal region, in the cheek, and below the mandibular angle to secure adequate drainage of zygomaticotemporal, buccal, and parapharyngeal abscesses."[30]

Submandibular Space. Hollinshead states, "The anterior element of the parapharyngeal space is conveniently referred to as the submandibular space (Fig. 10–36). It actually consists of a group of spaces that, however, either communicate with each other or can be made to do so with relatively little pressure by pus. The submandibular space as a whole is limited above by the mucous membrane of the tongue, while its floor is the anterior or superficial layer of deep fascia as it extends from the hyoid bone to the mandible. Its inferior extent is the attachment of the fascia to the hyoid."[17]

Some of the subdivisions of the submandib-ular space are fairly obvious: the mylohyoid muscle, stretching across the floor of the mouth, divides the submandibular space into a portion above this muscle, the sublingual, and a portion below, the submental. The submandibular gland, which lies partly above and partly below the posterior portion of the mylohyoid, enables these two subdivisions to communicate with each other. As has been mentioned, infection may spread from the submandibular space backward into the parapharyngeal space.

SPACE OF THE SUBMANDIBULAR GLAND. "The capsule of the submandibular gland is usually described as enclosing a space, the submandibular space (or, less confusingly, the space of the submandibular gland) but again this description is apt to be misleading: the submandibular gland does not lie loosely within its sheath, so that this latter can be opened and the gland easily shelled out; rather it and its associated lymph nodes arc embedded in this fascia, and the septa of the gland are continuous with the capsule; essentially, therefore, the 'submandibular space' is the substance of the gland and nodes (Fig. 10–36A)."[17]

Submental Space. This space lies between the mylohyoid muscle and the platysma. It contains the anterior bellies of the digastric muscles and the submental lymph nodes in between.

SUBMENTAL CELLULITIS. A periapical infection of the mandibular incisors, cuspids or bicuspids that perforates the lingual bone below the origin of the mylohyoid muscle produces a submental abscess that may extend to the submandibular space.

Surgical Treatment. A transverse incision is made in the skin below the symphysis of the mandible. A hemostat is inserted into the submental space for blunt dissection upward and backward. A drain is inserted.

Sublingual Space. The sublingual space is bounded above by the mucous membrane, medially by the geniohyoid and genioglossus muscles, laterally and below by the mylohyoid muscle.

SUBLINGUAL SPACE CELLULITIS. According to Sicher, "Sublingual space cellulitis involves primarily the connective tissue which surrounds the sublingual gland, Wharton's duct, and the neighboring structures." (See Figures 10–54 to 10–56.) "Such an infection may, however, invade the loose connective tissue which separates the individual muscles from each other.

"The intermuscular connective tissue in

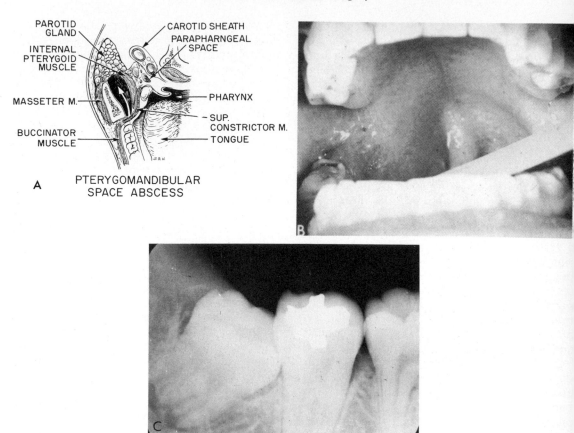

Figure 10–42 *A*, Diagrammatic representation of spread of infection into pterygomandibular space from mesio-angularly impacted mandibular third molar. Note proximity of parapharyngeal space. *B* and *D* to *F*, Clinical appearance of patient with pterygomandibular space abscess. Such patients generally have difficulty in swallowing and considerable trismus. Opening in this patient was achieved by use of extraoral block of third division of trigeminal nerve to relieve pain. *C*, Radiograph of a mesioangularly impacted third molar. (From Laskin, D. M.: Anatomic considerations in diagnosis and treatment of odontogenic infections. J.A.D.A., *69*:308 [Sept.], 1964. Copyright by the American Dental Association. Reprinted by permission.)

the sublingual region is characterized by continuing across the midline from one side to the other (see Figure 10–36*F*). The connective tissue between the mylohyoid and geniohyoid muscles, as well as that separating the geniohyoid and genioglossus muscles, is not interrupted at the midline. Right and left muscles are separated in the midsagittal plane by a thin layer of loose connective tissue. Sublingual cellulitis may therefore spread across the midline and involve two distinct levels of connective tissue, the lower being below and the upper being above the geniohyoid muscles. In the midline itself the cellulitis will involve the tissue between the right and left geniohyoid and the right and left genioglossus muscles and will therefore cause a swelling of the body and base of the tongue itself."[30]

Sublingual cellulitis is confined anteriorly and laterally by the mandible, posteriorly at the midline by the body of the hyoid bone.

Surgical Treatment. If the abscess has raised the mucosa in the floor of the mouth (Figs. 10–54 and 10–55), it should be drained by an incision in the lingual sulcus, ½ inch from the lingual cortical bone, so as to avoid injury to the sublingual gland, the lingual nerve or the submandibular duct (Fig. 10–56). Free-flowing pus is usually released. If not, then a hemostat should be passed beneath the gland posteriorly and anteriorly to locate pus. Finally, a drain should be inserted.

EXTENSION OF SUBLINGUAL SPACE INFECTION. Lateral to the hyoid bone, which is the posterior border of the sublingual space, the infection may spread distally and then

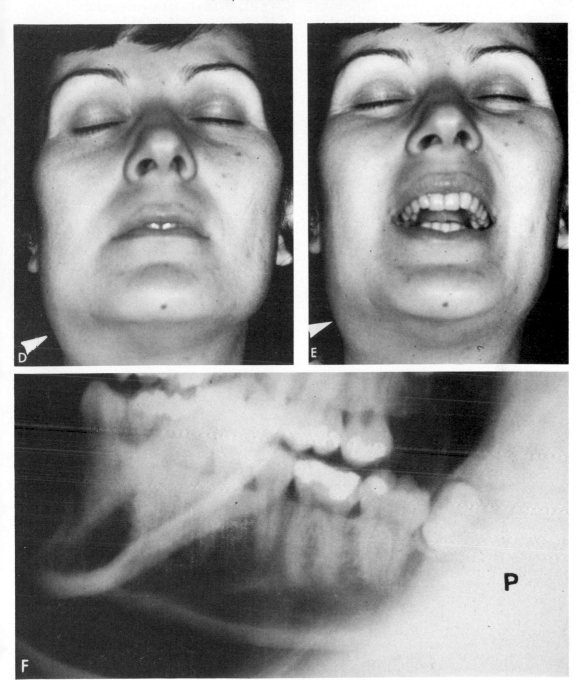

Figure 10–42 (*Continued.*)

pass the posterior border of the mylohyoid muscle. If this happens, the sublingual cellulitis passes the boundary between the submandibular niche and the parapharyngeal space and may spread in the latter downward along the neck. The sublingual cellulitis then ends as a descending cervical cellulitis or (pseudo–) Ludwig's angina. See page 484 for

a description of the criteria for a "true" Ludwig's angina.

"Usually a sublingual cellulitis is not confined to one side, and the best way of opening the infected spaces is a midline incision from the chin to the hyoid bone. The incision of the skin may be made transversely. After reflecting skin and subcutaneous tissue, the

(*Text continued on page 484*)

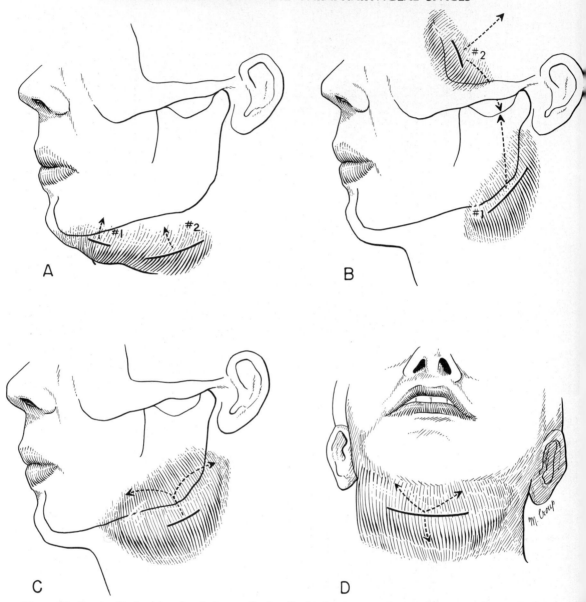

Figure 10–43 *A*, #1, Incision for drainage of a localized subcutaneous abscess. These are frequently seen as a result of an orally compounded fracture of the mandible through the mental foramen or periapical infection from a mandibular bicuspid that has penetrated the cortical plate of the mandible.

#2, Incision for drainage of a localized abscess of the submandibular space or for a subcutaneous abscess. Again, these often follow fractures of the mandible through the mandibular third molar, impacted or otherwise, or from periapical infection of the mandibular second or third molar. This is also the point of drainage of a buccal abscess which has extended below the inferior border of the mandible, as shown in Figure 9–16 *A*.

B, #1, Incision for drainage of an abscess of the parotid space. These abscesses are not common. Parotitis can result from an oral infection.

#2, Incision for drainage of a zygomaticotemporal abscess originating from dentoalveolar infection.

C, Incision for drainage of a submandibular abscess which has spread into the parapharyngeal space. Arrows show the direction which the hemostat must take to separate the deeper structures and assure adequate drainage. It is not necessary to wait for "pointing" of these abscesses before incising for drainage. A soft spot approximately the size of a nickel is frequently found in or near the center of the brawny indurated mass. This is the point to incise for drainage. This spot has the same feeling to the fingertips as a soft spot in a cantaloupe.

D, Incision for the draining of the submental space. Abscesses in this area generally include the bilateral submandibular spaces, and, as is shown by the arrows, the hemostat should, when separating the deeper structure, expose both these spaces. These infections simulate Ludwig's infection.

476

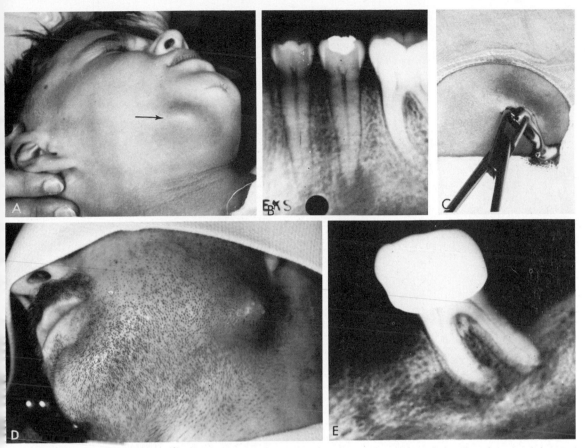

Figure 10–44 *A*, The "pointing" of a submental, submandibular abscess (see arrow). Palpation of the hard, brawny mass of tissue surrounding the area of infection will reveal, in most cases, a comparatively "soft spot" much like that felt in a ripe melon which has been injured in one area. This soft area in the tissue mass indicates that pus has broken through the muscle barrier in that area and is now subcutaneous. Now is the time to incise and drain the abscess through this soft area. To delay will mean that necrosis of the skin will develop. (See Figure 10–73.) It must be remembered that there are exceptions to this "soft spot," or "pointing," and if such does not develop and it appears that the abscess has "localized," or there is "laudable pus," then drainage should be instituted. Study the text for more information on this subject.

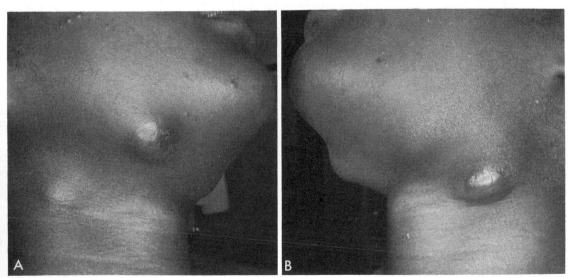

Figure 10–45 Tuberculous lymphadenitis, as shown in this case, can simulate a submandibular abscess. However, the fact that there were similar swellings on both sides of the neck which were soft and fluctuant, and that along the anterior border of the sternocleidomastoid muscle was a hard node, made us suspect the possibility of tuberculous lymphadenitis with chronic abscesses. Diagnosis was confirmed by excision of one of the nodes.

477

Photographic Case Report
INCISION AND DRAINAGE OF A SUBMANDIBULAR AND SUBLINGUAL ABSCESS

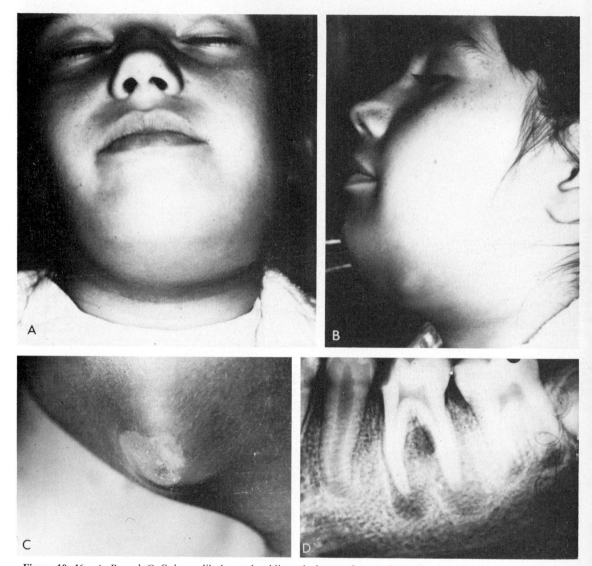

Figure 10–46 *A, B,* and *C,* Submandibular and sublingual abscess from a dentoalveolar abscess of the mandibular left first molar of 8 days' duration. Note in *C* that extraoral spontaneous rupture and drainage are just a matter of hours. *D,* Radiograph showing the mandibular first molar with the periapical pathosis responsible for the facial cellulitis.

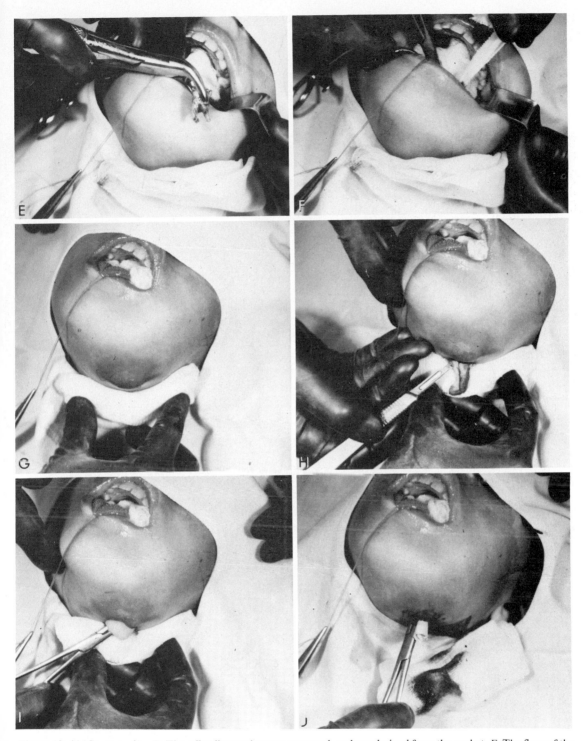

Figure 10–46 (*Continued.*) *E,* The offending molar was extracted, and pus drained from the socket. *F,* The floor of the mouth was elevated, and although swelling subsided when the tooth was extracted, the lingual mucoperiosteal membrane was reflected and an iodoform drain was inserted into the sublingual space. Preoperatively and postoperatively the patient was given 400,000 units of penicillin intramuscularly every 12 hours.

G, Under general anesthesia, the patient is prepared for incision and drainage.

H, Incision was made through the skin, and pus squirted out.

I, Deeper structures are gently opened, allowing thick yellow pus to escape from the submental and submaxillary regions.

J, A rubber cigarette drain is inserted into the submandibular region.

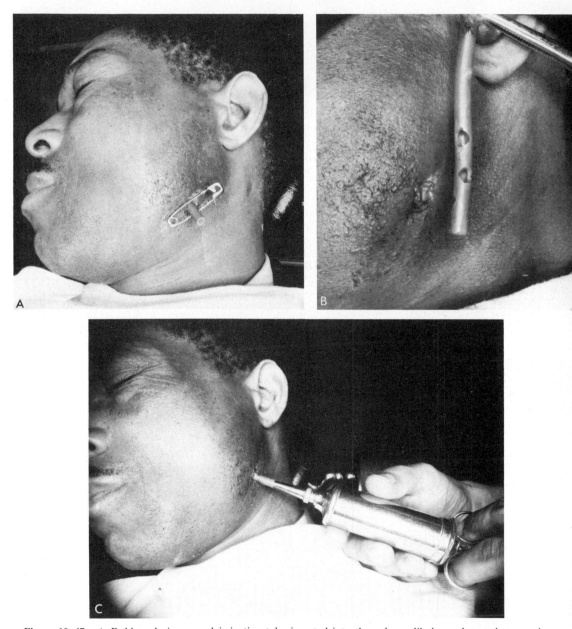

Figure 10–47 *A,* Rubber drainage and irrigation tube inserted into the submandibular and parapharyngeal spaces. This case was a diffuse postextraction cellulitis with submandibular and parapharyngeal abscess, *B,* Openings are cut into the sides of the rubber tube to facilitate drainage and irrigation. *C,* Spaces are irrigated with penicillin solution, 100,000 units in normal saline solution, twice daily.

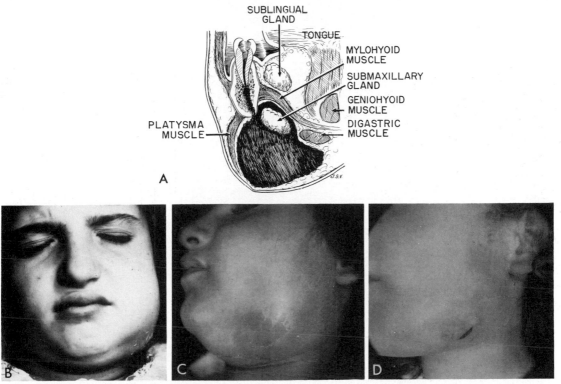

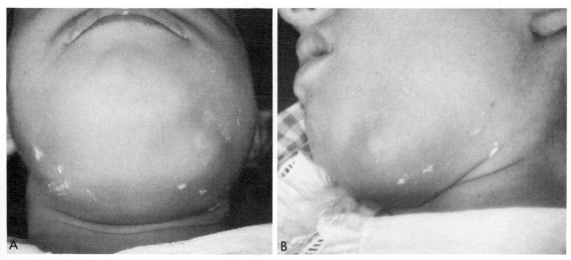

Figure 10–48 *A*, Diagrammatic representation of a submandibular abscess. Note that the pus-filled space is beneath the mylohyoid muscle. This abscess usually enters the submental area as well, and if not treated by incision and drainage, with antibiotic coverage, can become bilateral, simulating Ludwig's angina (See Figure 10–51).

B, *C* and *D* illustrate a typical 9-day-old abscess confined to the submandibular space which was incised and drained. The cause, an extensively decayed first molar, was extracted. Note that the incision should *not be much over an inch,* if any.

Figure 10–49 *A*, Submandibular abscess over a week old. This originated from a periapical abscess of the first mandibular molar. Treatment was immediate extraoral incision and drainage, extraction of the tooth and antibiotic therapy. *B*, Note how the infection has spread to the opposite side and the swelling simulates that seen in the so-called Ludwig's angina. (See Figure 10–58.)

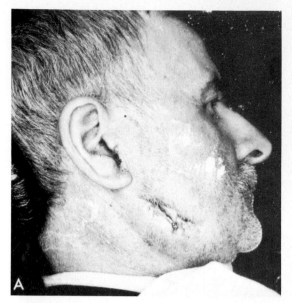

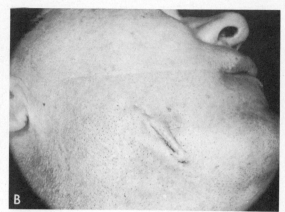

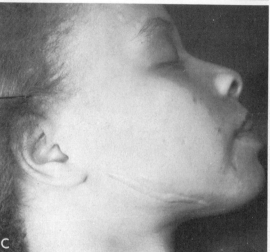

Figure 10–50   *A* to *C*, Examples of postincisional and drainage scars with keloid formation. As has been pointed out, it is not necessary to make incisions this way; one inch long suffices for the majority of cases.

C, Keloid formation in the two lines of incision for drainage of a submandibular abscess. The patient stated that her physician had made the short and shallow incision but failed to obtain any pus. Several days later a general surgeon made the long and deep incision, obtaining a free flow of pus. Both were in error; the short incision was too high and too shallow; the long incision was unnecessarily long and also too high. New growth formations are common in incision lines in blacks.

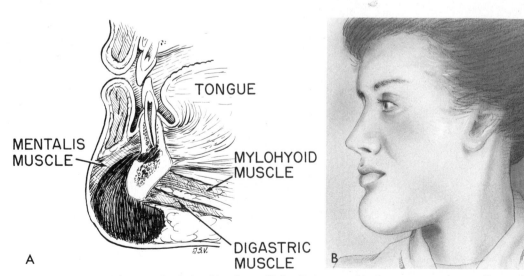

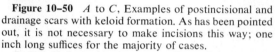

Figure 10–51   *A,* Diagram of relationship of mandibular incisors to alveolar process and mentalis muscle. Infection has extended beneath mentalis muscle into submental space. *B,* Clinical appearance of patient with submental space abscess. (Modified from Laskin, D. M.: Anatomic considerations in diagnosis and treatment of odontogenic infections. J.A.D.A., *69*:308 [Sept.], 1964. Copyright by the American Dental Association. Reprinted by permission.)

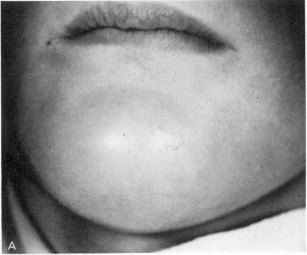

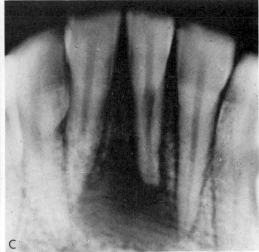

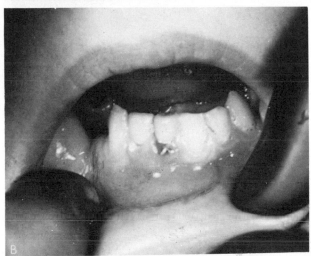

Figure 10–52 *A,* Cellulitis of the soft tissues above and below the mentalis muscle. *B,* Periapical radiograph reveals source of infection. A blow to this tooth during its formative period, at about the eighth year, destroyed the vitality of the pulp. *C,* Approximately 5 years later an acute abscess developed, forming a subperiosteal abscess (parulis), as illustrated in Figure 10–38, with extension into the soft tissues of the chin, an elevation of the mucoperiosteal tissues and beginning drainage at the gingival line.

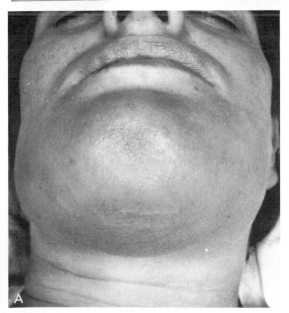

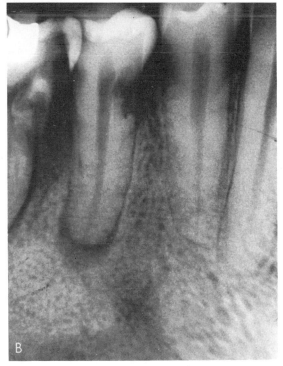

Figure 10–53 *A,* Submental abscess now extending into the submandibular space. Other examples will follow. *B,* This is an example of periapical pathosis which could produce a submental abscess.

483

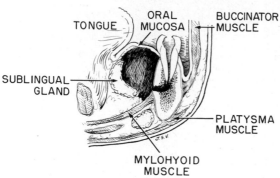

Figure 10–54 Diagram showing development of sublingual space abscess from mandibular first molar. Note that the lingual cortical plate was penetrated above the insertion of the mylohyoid muscle insertion. (Modified from Laskin, D. M.: Anatomic considerations in diagnosis and treatment of odontogenic infections. J.A.D.A., 69:308 [Sept.], 1964. Copyright by the American Dental Association. Reprinted by permission.)

mylohyoid muscle is incised in the midline and then the entire complicated stock of intermuscular connective tissue is accessible. It is especially important to remember that the connective tissue and thus the cellulitis extends laterally below and above the geniohyoid muscles."[30]

Extension of Localized Mandibular Abscesses

The infection in acutely abscessed mandibular incisors, cuspids, bicuspids and molars may spread from the adjacent space to the sublingual, submental, submandibular, pterygomandibular and related spaces. The tissues become tense, shiny, hard, and board-

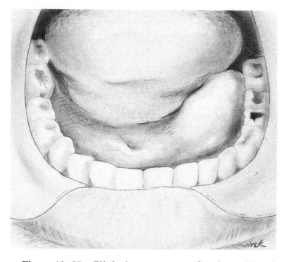

Figure 10–55 Clinical appearance of patient with sublingual space abscess. Spread of infection through loose connective tissue in floor of mouth often results in bilateral swelling and elevation of tongue.

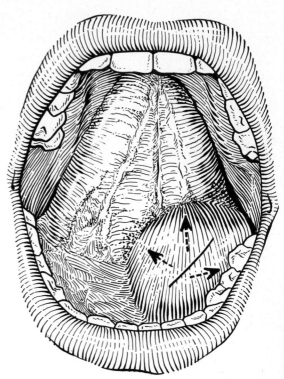

Figure 10–56 Incision for drainage of a sublingual abscess which may originate from any anterior or bicuspid tooth on that side of the mandible. The only requisite is that the infection has broken through above the mylohyoid muscle. Care must be taken not to cut through Wharton's duct. This can be readily avoided by keeping within ½ inch of the lingual cortical plate when making the incision.

like. There is trismus because the masseter, buccinator and internal pterygoid muscles are involved.

The floor of the mouth is swollen, as is the base of the tongue. This causes the tongue to swell and crowd upward against the palate and back into the pharynx. There is considerable difficulty in masticating and swallowing, and still more when the infection spreads posteriorly into the pharynx, with the formation of a parapharyngeal abscess.

The patient is quite apparently toxic and ill. There is a marked rise in temperature, often preceded by chills, and the patient complains of headache and malaise.

Ludwig's Angina. "Ludwig's angina" is loosely applied by many to any case in which bilateral sublingual, submental or submandibular edema is present. Ludwig set down in 1836 the following criteria:

1. The insignificant inflammation of the throat itself, which, even if present early in the disease, fades away soon.

(*Text continued on page 489*)

Case Report No. 4

LUDWIG'S ANGINA FOLLOWING EXTRACTION OF A LOWER THIRD MOLAR

Eight days before admission to the hospital this patient had had a "difficult" lower right third molar extracted. The patient reported that the dentist had a "lot of trouble getting the tooth out." Immediately after the extraction the patient's jaw began to swell. In the next 4 days the swelling quickly spread down his neck, along the side of the jaw, around his chin and along the left side of his neck. Simultaneously, the tissues in the floor of his mouth became swollen, pushing his tongue up and above the occlusal plane of his lower teeth and forcing him to hold his jaws open. Saliva drooled out of his mouth (Fig. 10–57).

The patient had great difficulty in swallowing and breathing, because of the edema of the neck and submandibular regions; undoubtedly, dyspnea was also due to paralaryngeal and perhaps laryngeal edema. He had difficulty in speaking. He had noticed a brownish fluid in his mouth for 24 hours prior to admission. The otolaryngologist was alerted for a possible emergency tracheotomy.

Examination. There was a bilateral massive brawny indurated edema of the tissues of the submandibular region and neck. The skin was tense and did not pit on pressure. There were no soft areas that might indicate suppuration and localiza-

tion. The skin had a cyanotic tint, possibly due to anoxemia, but more likely to sulfathiazole, which the patient had been taking prior to admission. He was not sure how much he had taken. He had stopped because he could not swallow. His temperature was 100° F., pulse 96.

Oral Examination. The tongue was pushed upward and was dry and coated. The mucosa in the floor of the mouth had been raised upward in a dark, reddish roll. The mouth would not open more than ¾ inch, so that the suspected intraoral drainage point could not be located.

Treatment. Hot, wet magnesium sulfate dressings were applied continuously to the neck and jaw. The patient was kept in a semireclining position. One thousand cc. of 5 per cent glucose in normal saline solution were administered intravenously twice a day. Sulfathiazole, 5 gm., was administered in 500 cc. of normal saline solution.

(*Note:* This was a preantibiotic case. Today patients would receive 600,000 units of penicillin intramuscularly twice daily and 250 mg. of tetracycline every 6 hours.)

Progress Notes. On the second day of admission the patient's condition was improved. He could breathe much more easily and did not have

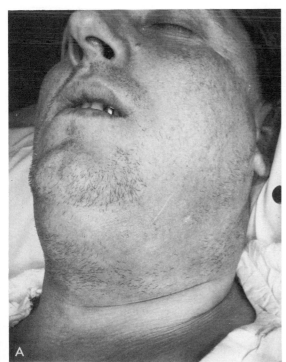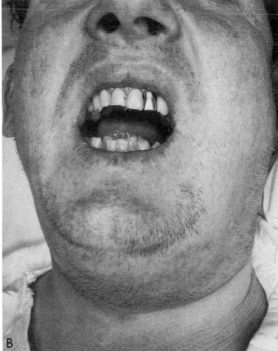

Figure 10–57 Ludwig's angina following tooth extraction. *A,* Bilateral submandibular induration on admission to the hospital. *B,* Edema of the floor of the mouth which pushed up the tongue. (See case report No. 4.)

quite so much difficulty in swallowing. The cyanosis was gone.

On the third day of admission forced fluids by mouth, 3000 cc. daily, were prescribed, along with sulfathiazole, 15 grains four times a day, and potassium citrate, 10 grains four times a day. The swelling was not so indurated; the patient could swallow much more easily and had no trouble breathing.

On the fourth day of admission sulfathiazole, 15 grains, and potassium citrate, 10 grains, three times a day were prescribed. The swelling was decreasing in size slowly.

By the seventh day the swelling and trismus were greatly reduced, and the patient was discharged.

Discussion. This was an atypical case in which the temperature and pulse rate never went as high as one would expect when the extent of the infection is considered. The highest temperature was 101° F. and the highest pulse rate was 96.

While this may have been a case in which the efficacy of sulfathiazole was demonstrated, I personally believe that recovery was undoubtedly due also to spontaneous intraoral drainage. Certainly the sulfathiazole blood level was never anywhere near those that are recommended as being effective (4 to 6 mg. per 100 cc. of blood).

Recovery was prompt in this case, avoiding the necessity of the radical inverted T type of incision recommended by some in these cases.

Case Report No. 5

BILATERAL SUBMANDIBULAR CELLULITIS (PSEUDO–LUDWIG'S ANGINA) ARISING FROM DENTURE TRAUMA

A 45-year-old edentulous man presented himself at the dental school on January 3 for treatment of a large bilateral swelling of the submental region. The floor of the mouth was elevated, and he had difficulty in swallowing and breathing. He was admitted to the Eye and Ear Hospital. The otolaryngologist was alerted for a possible emergency tracheotomy.

History. On December 27 the patient had noticed some spots on his lower gum from traumatic injury due to lower dentures. The lower anterior jaw began to swell and became painful, with pain radiating to the right ear and parietal region. The next day there was continued swelling accompanied by pain. On January 1 he expectorated a great amount of yellowish-red, foul-smelling thick fluid. The swelling decreased considerably, and there was no pain. Later that day the swelling started to increase again, accompanied by pain. This continued through the night and the next day. He had difficulty in swallowing and breathing.

Admission Note. Upon admission the patient's temperature was 102° F., his respiration slightly rapid, and the pulse normal. Penicillin, 600,000 units immediately and every 8 hours intramuscularly, was ordered. Hot, wet magnesium sulfate dressings were applied to the jaw and the neck. Infrared light administered for ½ hour three times daily was ordered. The lower jaw was swollen to twice its normal size (see Figure 10–58).

Physical Examination. The findings were essentially negative, except for adenopathy in the neck and those already noted.

Laboratory Reports. The blood count was as follows: erythrocytes, 4,230,000 per cubic millimeter; leukocytes, 15,700 per cubic millimeter; hemoglobin, 75 per cent. The differential count showed 85 per cent polymorphonuclear leuko-cytes, 12 per cent lymphocytes, and 3 per cent mononuclear leukocytes. The blood coagulation time was 3¾ minutes, the bleeding time 1½ minutes. Wassermann and Kahn tests were both plus 4.

The urine had a specific gravity of 1.023 and had a trace of albumin.

Course. The next day the swelling extended from the lower lip bilaterally over the symphysis and posteriorly toward the angle of the jaw. It had displaced downward the geniohyoid and mylohyoid muscles of the floor of the mouth from their normal positions. The swelling involved the neck and the angles of the mandible. There was tenderness as far down as the clavicles. The tongue, mucous membrane, and genioglossus were forced up into the mouth. In the mucolingual folds on both sides of the mandible in the region of the molars, there was a small sinus opening, around which were small quantities of thick, light yellow pus.

On January 4, by means first of a probe and then of a hemostat, blunt dissection of the muscle planes of both the right and left sides of the mandible was accomplished through the sinus openings. As a result, large quantities of blood-tinted pus drained into the mouth.

Because of the success of this treatment, it was thought that perhaps extraoral incision and drainage could be avoided. That afternoon, however, the swelling had not decreased, the temperature had risen from 99.2° at 9 A.M. to 101.6° F. at 4:00 P.M., and it was decided to incise and drain extraorally the next morning.

The patient continuously applied hot, wet magnesium sulfate dressings to his neck and to the jaw and used hot normal saline solution as a mouthwash.

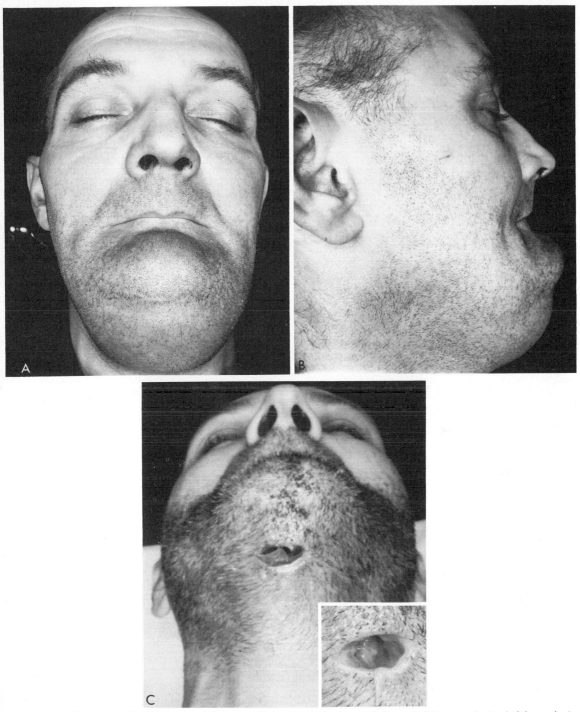

Figure 10–58   *A* and *B*, Bilateral sublingual, submental and submandibular cellulitis (pseudo–Ludwig's angina). Rubber tissue drain. *Inset*, Thick yellow pus drained from the incision for several weeks. (See Case Report No. 5.)

During the night there was evidently spontaneous intraoral drainage, for the temperature at 8 A.M. on January 5 was 97° F., and the patient could now swallow and breathe without difficulty.

Operative Notes. Under Pentothal anesthesia, the face and mucous membrane were prepared with tincture of Merthiolate, and the lips coated with petrolatum. The tongue was grasped by gauze held between the fingers, and brought forward, exposing the tip, which was scrubbed dorsally and ventrally with tincture of Merthiolate. A curved needle threaded with 00 plain catgut 18 inches in length was passed through the midline of the tongue, $\frac{1}{2}$ inch from the tip, and brought forward for a distance of 6 inches. The needle was cut from the suture; a knot was tied in the ends of the four strands; a hemostat was clamped on this knot, and held to the cover sheet by a towel clip. (*Note:* Today intubation would be employed, or if this were deemed too traumatic, then a tracheostomy would be indicated under local anesthesia and general anesthesia administered by this route.)

At the onset of the anesthetic, marked laryngeal spasm occurred. The anesthetic was deepened, but the vocal cords did not relax. A metal airway placed into the pharynx and an increase in the nasal oxygen did not alleviate the rapidly increasing anoxemia. All respiratory efforts ceased. The patient was markedly cyanotic. Manual artificial resuscitation was instituted until the E. & J. resuscitator was applied. After the lungs were inflated and deflated a dozen times, the skin became pink and respirations were resumed.

The skin was prepared by scrubbing with tincture of green soap and then tincture of Merthiolate.

A horizontal incision was made through the skin 8 cm. below the center of the symphysis of the mandible, extending right and left for a distance of 8 cm. The subcutaneous connective tissue was incised down to the fascia covering the platysma muscle. This was incised, and free pus flowed from the wound. The muscle fibers of the platysma were separated by blunt dissection with the hemostat, and the opening thus made was enlarged by separating the beaks of the hemostat, and then withdrawing the hemostat. More pus was found beneath the platysma, and by means of the index finger this muscle was separated from the digastric muscle and the mylohyoid muscle on both sides of the neck, and the submaxillary space was opened. Again by blunt dissection with the hemostat, the mylohyoid muscle fibers were separated and the opening into the sublingual area was enlarged.

A rubber gauze drain 1½ inches wide and 4 inches long was inserted into the sublingual space. Two iodoform gauze drains were inserted on either side between the platysma and mylohyoid and the anterior belly of the digastric muscles.

At the conclusion of the operation, oxygen under pressure was administered, using the E. & J. resuscitator. The respiratory difficulty remained, probably because of the weight of the inflammatory mass on the trachea. An attempt was made to relieve the obstruction by raising the head; this resulted in renewed cyanosis, which was relieved by the means already described. After the application of oxygen for 5 minutes, the patient was taken to his room, where he was placed in bed on his side. A portable suction apparatus was used to clear his mouth and pharynx of the accumulated saliva and pus from the open sinus tracts. A nasal catheter was placed and 100 per cent oxygen was administered by this means. Two cubic centimeters of Coramine (pyridine-3-carboxylic acid diethylamide) were injected intravenously. The patient began to improve and was fully recovered in an hour and a half.

During the operation a specimen of the pus on a sterile cotton swab was taken for culture, and the bacteriologist's report was as follows: Apparently a pure culture of gram-positive cocci in clusters, morphologically resembling *Staphylococcus aureus.*

The medical consultant instituted antisyphilitic treatment.

Postoperative Course. On the first postoperative day the patient's temperature was 98° F.; he was comfortable, and the swelling had decreased considerably. Hot, wet magnesium sulfate dressings and saline mouthwashes were continued.

On the second postoperative day the patient's temperature was 98° F.; the swelling had diminished still more, and the patient inquired about leaving the hospital. Dressings and mouthwash were continued.

On the third postoperative day the drains were removed, and the cavity was irrigated with Dakin's solution through the incision by means of an antrum irrigator joined to a metal syringe. Three rubber drains were placed in the cavity and covered with a dressing.

The drains were again removed, the cavity irrigated with Dakin's solution, and three new drains placed and secured with a safety pin. A dressing was placed, and the patient was discharged after making an appointment to be seen at the dental school in several days.

On the tenth postoperative day, edema and induration had practically disappeared. Free pus was still draining from the extraoral incision; the cavity was irrigated with Dakin's solution; new rubber tissue drains were inserted. The patient was still under antisyphilitic treatment.

On the thirteenth postoperative day the drains were removed, and a small amount of pus drained from the wound; the cavity was irrigated with Dakin's solution. Slight swelling and induration were still present.

On the nineteenth postoperative day the drains were removed. There was no pus; the wound was irrigated with Dakin's solution. No drains were placed in the wound, which was two-thirds closed.

On the twenty-fifth postoperative day the wound was practically closed; there was slight seepage of serum.

By February 21 the wound was completely healed; there was no edema or induration.

2. The peculiar wooden hardness of the swelling, which does not pit on pressure, as in ordinary edema.
3. The hard swelling under the tongue, forming a callus ring within the inner border of the mandible, reddish or bluish in color.
4. The well-defined border of this ⁕hard edema and induration in the neck, which is surrounded by uninvolved healthy connective tissue.
5. The slight involvement or, more often, the lack of involvement of the glands, although the surrounding cellular tissue is involved.

Two types have been described: (1) a septic nonsuppurative inflammatory edema, in which it is impossible to obtain adequate drainage; (2) a septic suppurative type, in which adequate drainage can be obtained, and in which the prognosis is more favorable.

Ludwig's angina is an acute, rapid, diffuse, septic, inflammatory, indurated (with wooden hardness) bilateral cellulitis of the floor of the mouth and neck. The distortion of the tissues of the oral cavity forces the enlarged tongue upward against the palate and backward into the hypopharynx, embarrassing respiration.

The pharynx and larynx may also become involved, thus further restricting respiration and making speech more difficult. It is reported that the majority of deaths from this condition are the result of respiratory obstruction rather than sepsis. Early tracheostomy should be performed, if respiratory embarrassment persists, to prevent asphyxiation or pulmonary complications.

The infection is usually mixed. Culture studies have demonstrated a multiplicity of organisms. These include hemolytic and nonhemolytic streptococci, staphylococci, pneumococci, *Escherichia coli,* and Vincent's organisms.

Treatment. Johnson and associates reported a case of Ludwig's angina in which an emergency tracheotomy was performed, and because of the suspected mixed infection over a period of 10 days, they administered the following antibiotics: "Pencillin G, 4,000,000 units every 12 hours, and streptomycin, 1 gm. every 12 hours, were given intramuscularly; and Staphcillin (2,6-dimethoxyphenylpenicillin sodium), 900 mg. every 4 hours, and tetracycline, 500 mg. every 12 hours, were given intravenously." Treatment was given over a 10-day period, with the total amount of penicillin 58,000,000 units; Staph-

cillin, 53.1 gm.; streptomycin 9.0 gm.; and tetracycline 3.5 gm. They conclude "that establishment of an adequate airway by tracheotomy early in the course of the disease is mandatory. Control of sepsis can then be obtained by intensive antibiotic therapy. There is little rationale for the use of submandibular surgical incision or 'decompression' of the phlegmon unless suppuration, which is a rare finding, supervenes."[18]

MANAGEMENT OF ACUTE INFECTIONS IN THE FACE AND NECK WITH CELLULITIS

Neck infections generally follow infections that originate in the mandible or its contiguous tissues. Infections of the upper face usually come from the maxilla (Figs. 10–30 to 10–34), and of the lower face, from the mandible (Figs. 10–48 to 10–56). There are exceptions to this general observation. An infection of the maxilla, for example, can spread into the buccal or zygomaticotemporal space, or the pterygomandibular, which communicates with the parapharyngeal space, and dissect downward along the fascia of the carotid sheath into the neck and eventually into the chest.

Any patient with extensive brawny edema and induration (see Figure 10–80 and Case Report No. 9) of the soft tissues of the face, neck or floor of the oral cavity, with a temperature of over 100° F. as a result of oral infection, should be hospitalized immediately. Study Death from Dentoalveolar Infection, starting on page 510.

Signs and Symptoms. The signs and symptoms of acute infections in the face and neck are swelling, painful swallowing, trismus, fever, increase in pulse rate associated with increase in temperature, leukocytosis, pain and difficulty in breathing.

TREATMENT

Antibacterial Treatment. The reader is referred to Chapter 8 for a complete discussion of antibiotic therapy.

Local Treatment. The object is to increase the circulation in the area in order to expedite fluctuation or resolution.

Hot dressings are used continuously. Radiation and heat from infrared lamps, such as Biolite or Thermolite, may be given. Hot saline mouthwashes are also useful.

General Therapy. Many of these patients are dehydrated because of their inability to swallow or because of fever, or both. Fever increases vitamin requirements. This is especially true of the B complex and C vitamins. Liquid and soft diets, which are, as a rule, necessarily prescribed in these cases, are usually inadequate in these vitamins. Vitamin supplementation is thus necessary during the illness and convalescence to compensate for the increased metabolic demands imposed by the stress of infection or injury.[27] If patients cannot swallow, 1000 cc. of 5 per cent glucose solution should be given by continuous intravenous drip. To this can be added: 1 gm. of Ceratin (ascorbic acid); 4 cc. of Betalin compound (nicotinamide, 150 mg.; thiamine chloride, 10 mg.; riboflavin, 4 mg.; pantothenic acid, 5 mg.; pyridoxine hydrochloride, 10 mg.).

As soon as the patient is able to swallow, therapeutic doses of multivitamins should be given daily, with a high carbohydrate diet. The vitamin reserve is quickly depleted during infections, so that it is essential that they be replaced to aid in combating the infection and eventually in repairing damaged tissue.

Surgical Treatment. The source of the infection must be located, if still present, and removed. Figures 10–60 to 10–72 illustrate the end results of cases of acute cellulitis of odontogenic origin in which failure to locate and remove the source of infection produced chronic fistulas.

Incision and drainage should be done as soon as fluctuation occurs. The incision may be made intraorally or extraorally as indicated. However, if brawny, massive induration, which pits on pressure, presents in 5 to 7 days with an elevation of temperature in spite of antibiotic treatment, and if there is no fluctuation, then that space in which it is felt that there should be localization of pus should be surgically explored. To delay is to risk dissemination of infection into the carotid sheath, particularly if there is a parapharyngeal infection. Infection of the carotid sheath may result in thrombosis of the internal jugular vein, or erosion of the internal carotid artery. The latter would result in a fatal hemorrhage.

Septicemia is indicated by a positive blood culture, chills and sweats, and temperature spiking (rapid rises and falls in temperature).

Occasionally this rapid variation in temperature over a 24-hour period is due to spontaneous intraoral drainage accompanied by a dramatic drop in temperature. As the pressure in the abscess is now low, the escape valve closes and the abscess fills again, accompanied by a rise in temperature until the pressure permits a reopening of the point of spontaneous drainage, and the cycle is repeated.

ROUTINE ORDERS FOR DENTAL PATIENTS WITH ACUTE INFECTIONS OF THE FACE OR NECK, ON ADMISSION TO THE HOSPITAL

The patient should have a complete physical examination and history taken. There should be a complete red blood cell count and a differential white blood cell count.

A Kahn test should be done, and radiographs should be taken. The patient should receive 600,000 units of aqueous procaine penicillin twice daily. (See Chapter 8.) Hot, wet magnesium sulfate dressings should be applied continuously to the swollen area. An infrared lamp should be applied to the face for 20 minutes out of each hour, repeating the procedure every 2 hours throughout the day. Or continuous heat is prescribed, as described on page 131. Force fluids to 3000 cc.

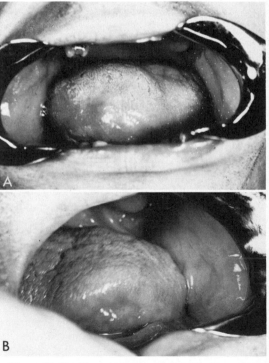

Figure 10–59 Two cases of cellulitis of tongue. Study the text for details.

daily. Measure the patient's fluid intake and output. For the relief of pain, codeine sulfate, 1 grain, and acetylsalicylic acid, 10 grains, may be prescribed by mouth. Place 0.3 gram of oxychlorosene sodium (Kasdenol) in a glass of lukewarm water and use as a mouthwash four times daily.

If a specimen is available, antibiotic sensitivity tests should be performed. If this is not possible, the therapy must be determined by the clinical course alone. If a favorable re-sponse is not obtained within 48 hours, the current therapy should be discontinued and a new regimen established, perhaps utilizing the broad-spectrum antibiotics. The clinician must be constantly aware that antibiotics are capable of masking the symptoms of toxicity. Consequently, freedom from temperature elevation following antibiotic therapy can be regarded as a favorable prognostic sign only if accompanied by evidence of general clinical improvement.

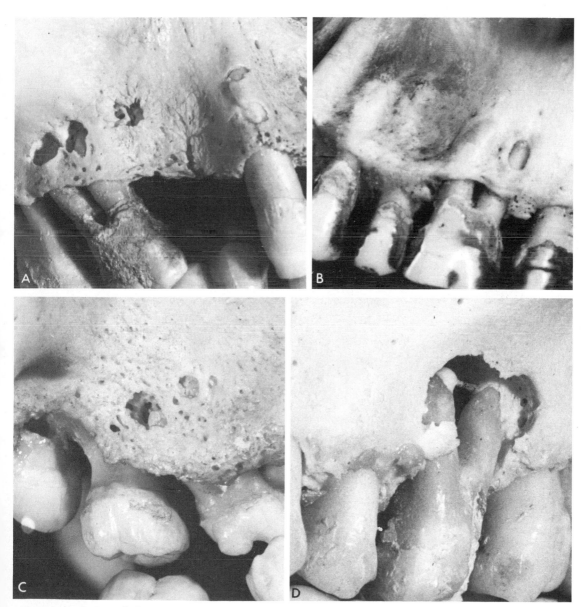

Figure 10–60 Dry skulls showing various fistulas through the maxillary cortical plate over the apices of infected molar buccal roots.

ACUTE TONGUE ABSCESS

In Figure 10–59*A* is illustrated cellulitis of the tongue of unknown origin. There were no sharp teeth or appliances that might have abraded the tongue and permitted the entrance of oral bacteria, nor did the patient remember having bitten his tongue.

The patient first noticed that his tongue was swollen one morning. The tongue gradually increased in size, becoming swollen and very painful. The right side was more swollen and indurated than the left side. The lingual septum did not prevent the spread of infection to the opposite side.

Hourly hot saline mouthwash and 400,000 units of penicillin every 8 hours were prescribed. In 48 hours the abscess ruptured and drained spontaneously along the edge at the junction of the ventral smooth mucosa and the filiform and fungiform papillae midway between the apex and the base. The abscess was located in the posterior third of the tongue.

In Figure 10–59*B* is shown a cellulitis of the tongue in which the swelling and induration were located primarily in the posterior third of the tongue and were confined by the septum linguae mostly to the left side. Again

the cause of this abscess could not be determined.

As can be seen, this patient was edentulous and gave no history of trauma to the tongue either by biting or abrasion from his dentures. Duration when first seen was 3 days. There did not seem to be any point of localization at this time, and the same treatment described above was ordered. Resolution followed.

CHRONIC SKIN FISTULA

In Figures 10–63, 10–66 and 10–68 are shown the end results of three cases of acute mandibular cellulitis and abscesses which were treated improperly with cold applications "to drive the infection in." The patients' parents were told that if cold were used, it would not be necessary to "cut the skin," thus avoiding a scar. Fortunately, however, in spite of continuous cold applications these infections localized and the abscesses ruptured and drained spontaneously extraorally.

The swelling gradually disappeared, and only the draining fistula remained. The fact that there was a source of infection, in these cases a diseased tooth, was forgotten or missed.

(*Text continued on page 497*)

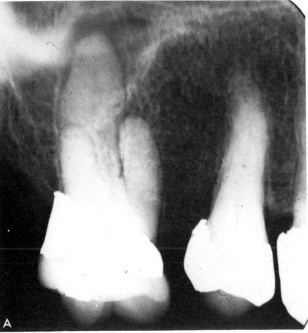
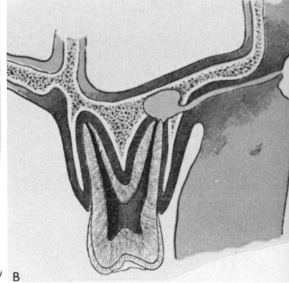

Figure 10–61   Chronically infected teeth have produced extraoral fistulas without an acute cellulitis of the overlying soft tissues, such as is illustrated in this figure and in Figure 10–63. These are exceptional cases.

(*B*, From Black, G. V.: A Work on Special Dental Pathology. Chicago, Medico-Dental Publishing Co., 1920.)

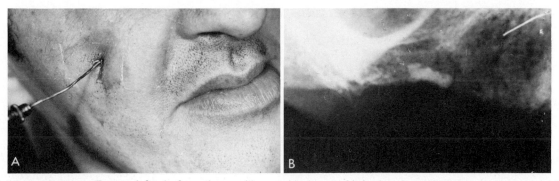

Figure 10–62 *A,* Extraoral fistula from the maxillary residual area of infection shown in the roentgenogram in *B.* Note end of probe in *B* and small fragment of tooth structure. The patient reported that he did not have any pain or swelling. A "pimple" had developed which began to discharge watery pus. Various salves did not cure the "pimple." It was thought that this was a fistula from the maxillary sinus. This was ruled out by failure of a radiopaque oil inserted into the maxillary sinus to exit through the fistula in the soft tissues of the face. Oral radiographs were pronounced normal. *B,* Our probe, through the fistula, contacted bone at an area of radiolucency in the maxilla near a retained piece of root material. Removal of this dentin and curettement of the demineralized bone in this area produced a cure.

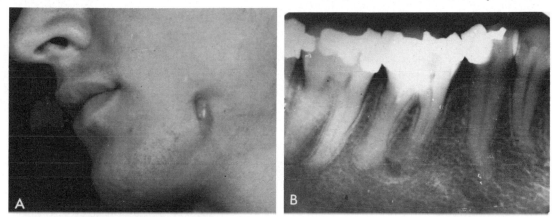

Figure 10–63 *A,* This 25-year-old man had had this draining fistula for over a year, during which time he had been under medical treatment. When a chronically infected mandibular molar (*B*) was extracted, the sinus stopped draining. Study the text on chronic skin fistula.

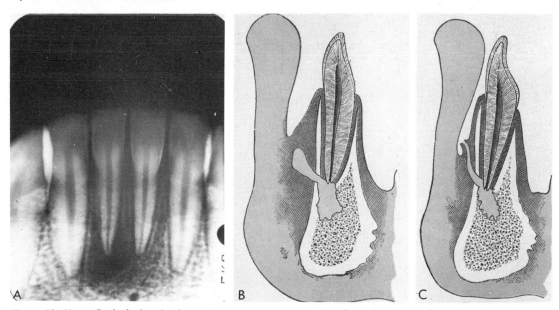

Figure 10–64 *A,* Periapical pathosis. As has been shown, pus, when it reaches the surface of the bone, either raises the periosteum or, as shown in *B*, penetrates it and spills out into the loose soft tissue, with the development of cellulitis, and eventually a large abscess is formed (see Figure 10–51), unless the infection is aborted by the early and adequate administration of antibiotics. If this does not occur, the abscess in the soft tissue either discharges through a fistula intraorally, as shown in *C*, or extraorally, as shown in Figure 10–65.

(*B* and *C,* From Black, G. V.: A Work on Special Dental Pathology. Chicago, Medico-Dental Publishing Co., 1920.)

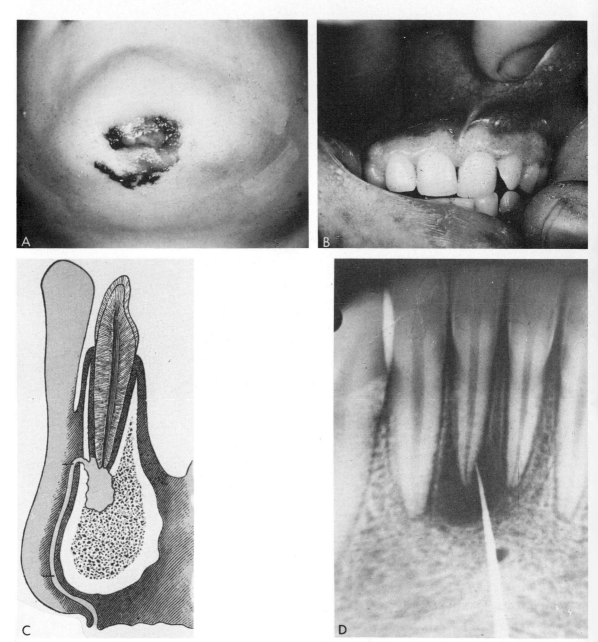

Figure 10–65 *A,* Profusely discharging fistula beneath the mentalis muscle following spontaneous rupture and discharge of an acute cellulitis of the soft tissues over the chin. Patient was told by his dentist that his teeth were negative for periapical infection. He had been under treatment for 6 months by his physician, who had been prescribing massive doses of antibiotics without effect. *B,* Trauma during incisive biting had destroyed the vitality of the lower central and lateral incisors. These teeth were treated, the root canals filled and an apicoectomy performed. Drainage ceased, and subsequently the scar was excised. *C,* Drawing showing pathway of the fistula. *D,* Gutta percha diagnostic point passed into fistulous tract and radiographed.

(*C,* From Black, G. V.: A Work on Special Dental Pathology. Chicago, Medico-Dental Publishing Co., 1920.)

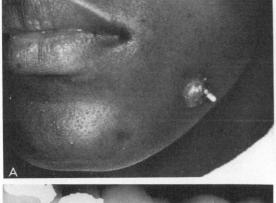

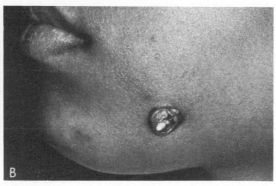

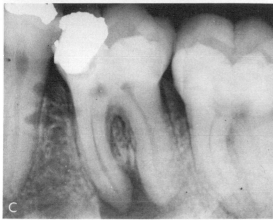

Figure 10–66 This patient gave a typical history of acute pain, followed by extensive swelling of the soft tissues overlying the mandible, spontaneous rupture of the skin and profuse flow of pus, decrease in swelling and continuous minimum drainage from the present extraoral fistula (A and B) for the past year, which has not responded to treatment with antibiotics by the physician. A gutta percha point inserted in the fistula, as shown in A and B, contacted bone. C, The unsuspected and undiagnosed cause. Endodontic treatment was started.

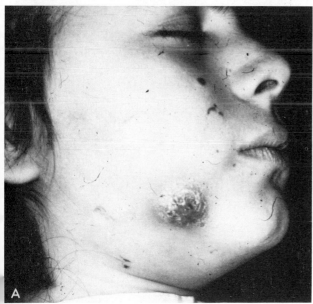

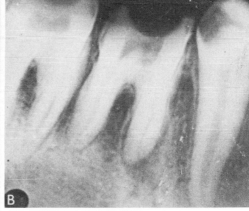

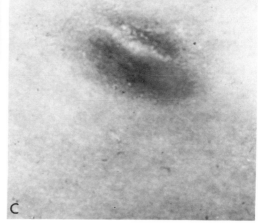

Figure 10–67 A, This patient gave the same history as was detailed in the caption for Figure 10–72. This large, round elevated seminecrotic mass of tissue surrounds the orifice of the fistula, repeatedly closing it until pressure built up, when it would rupture and drain again. The source was an infected first molar, the origin (B) of the initial cellulitis. C, Following the extraction of this tooth, drainage ceased, the fistula closed and this reddish brown, ugly, puckered scar tied down to the inferior border of the mandible resulted. This will remain until it is excised by a plastic surgery procedure.

495

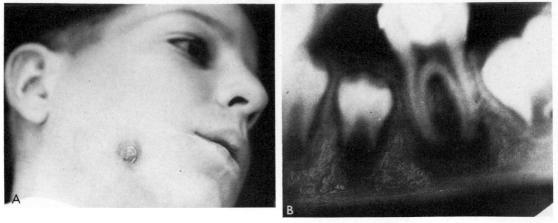

Figure 10–68   *A*, Fistula, present for 5 months, treated with "salves." Small quantities of pus would accumulate beneath the scab. The drainage ceased when a chronically infected deciduous first molar was extracted. *B*, Radiograph reveals periapical pathosis.

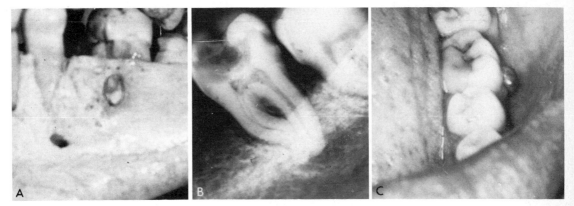

Figure 10–69   *A*, Fistula through the cortical plate of the mandible. *B*, Periapical pathosis. *C*, Fistula through the mucoperiosteal membrane.

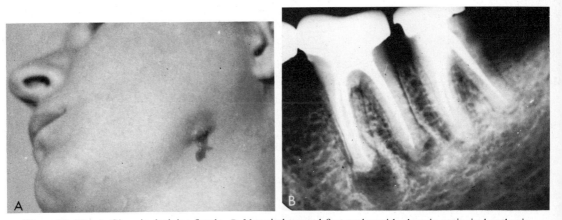

Figure 10–70   *A*, Chronic draining fistula. *B*, Nonvital treated first molar with chronic periapical pathosis.

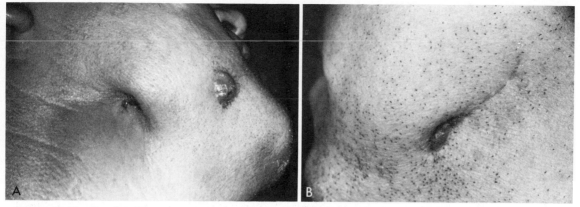

Figure 10–71 *A* and *B*, Two examples of chronically discharging fistulas from residual infection in the mandible. *B*, Scar from an unnecessarily long incision (see Figure 10–50). Note continuing drainage; the original source of infection was not eliminated.

The findings in the dental radiographs of many of these cases at first glance appear to be negative. A careful examination of the film must be made to see if there is a thickened lamina dura about the apex of a tooth. The vitality test should also be used. In other cases visual examination alone reveals an obviously infected mandibular tooth.

After extraction of the offending tooth, drainage promptly ceases. Closure of the fistula follows, and the sinus tract contracts to the cortical plate of the mandible, resulting in an ugly depression in the skin.

Treatment of Fistula. The source of infection is located and removed. The fistula stops draining, closes and contracts to bone, making an unsightly dimple or scar. These are removed by an elliptical incision through the skin around the scar, excising the scar, undermining the skin, and closing.

SPECIAL PROBLEMS RELATIVE TO FACE AND NECK INFECTIONS OF DENTOALVEOLAR ORIGIN

PATIENTS WITH LOW-GRADE INFECTIONS

One at times sees patients with obvious soft-tissue infections that refuse to heal and con-

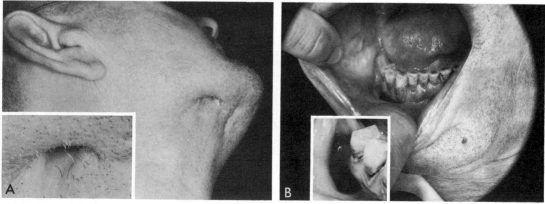

Figure 10–72 This patient gave a history of having been treated for osteomyelitis of the jaw 3 years before, at which time through and through drainage was established, and maintained for many months, with rubber tissue. Drainage of pus finally stopped, but a permanent fistula had been established.

A, Fistula is tied down to the inferior border of the mandible, but does not communicate with the bone. *B*, Intraoral view of the fistula. It was lined with normal-appearing oral mucosa. The patient prevented the escape of fluids from his mouth by constricting the lip and cheek against the mandible when eating or drinking, and refused treatment.

tinue to drain despite wide surgical exposure, massive doses of antibiotics, x-ray therapy and every other conceivable type of treatment. Usually there is some locus of infection present in this type of case, but at times, in spite of the most careful search, nothing can be found. Very often no organisms can be cultured. This type of case may very well be due to one of the uncommon lower organisms, and treatment is often strictly empirical, with local irrigations and through and through drains giving the best results. (See Case Re-

(*Text continued on page 502*)

Case Report No. 6

MIGRATORY ABSCESS

Chief Complaint. A patient was admitted complaining of swelling of the right side of his face, and drainage from an old fistula tied down to the right mandible (Fig. 10–73*A*).

Past History. Seven years before admission the patient had had the lower right third molar removed. The area was swollen at that time, and the extraction was performed under local anesthesia. The swelling subsided but recurred 1 month later. The patient was again hospitalized, and the area was incised and intraoral curettage performed. Three weeks later the right side of the face swelled and ruptured, and drained spontaneously extraorally. A fistula developed when the swelling was gone. Then incision and drainage were performed extraorally, apparently to secure more adequate drainage. Healing was uneventful with the exception of a depressed scar (Fig. 10–73*A*).

Seven years later the maxillary right third molar was removed, followed by extensive diffuse swelling of the right side of the face. Spontaneous drainage occurred intraorally. Intermittent swelling of the face persisted for several months, and drainage finally occurred at the site of the original mandibular fistula.

Present Admission. It was thought at first that this might be a parotid space infection. Injections of radiopaque medium into the sinus tract did not show in this space or in any other definite space.

The swelling and tenderness were most marked in the temporal region.

Antibiotic treatment was instituted, remission of the swelling and drainage followed, and the patient was discharged.

Subsequent Course. In the next 6 months the swelling and tenderness recurred at intervals and promptly disappeared under antibiotic treatment. Radiographic study of the skull failed to show osteomyelitis. There was never any definite localization that would indicate the advisability of incision and drainage until the last admission, when the patient had a well-localized temporal abscess (Fig. 10–73*B*). This was incised and drained, and antibiotic treatment was instituted. However, drainage continued; so through and through drainage between the temporal region and the postzygomatic fossa into the oral cavity was established.

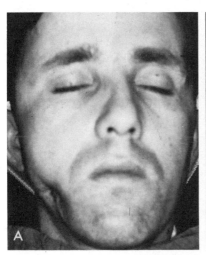
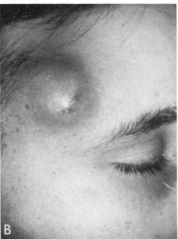
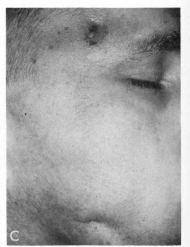

Figure 10–73   Migratory abscess. Study Case Report No. 6 for explanation.

Case Report No. 7

CHRONIC OSTEOMYELITIS OF TRAUMATIC ORIGIN WITH FIBROSIS OF THE LEFT MASSETER MUSCLE DUE TO LOW-GRADE CHRONIC INFECTION*

On October 19, a 34-year-old man was referred to the oral surgery service for diagnosis and treatment of limited motion of the mandible, pain in the left preauricular area and localized subcutaneous abscess of the left mandibular angle region, with associated edema of the left face.

His chief complaint was "locked jaw" and pain in the left face (see Figure 10–74).

The history of the present illness began 8 years previously while the patient was in the armed services in Europe. The patient arose one morning to find that he could not open his mouth and suffered considerable pain and edema of the left face. He reported to his medical officer, who treated him with antibiotics. After 3 days of the treatment a localized subcutaneous abscess formed just below

*Case report prepared by Charles J. Novak, B.S., D.D.S., Resident in Oral Surgery, Veterans Administration Hospital, Pittsburgh, Pa.

and anterior to the ear. The area was incised and drained. Limitation of motion became less severe but persistent. Four months later, the patient again suffered pain and edema in the same region, with limitation of movement, the maximum opening being restricted to 2 cm. He was seen at this time by another medical officer and again treated with antibiotics. The old incision ruptured and drained spontaneously, with resultant cessation of pain and edema. However, limitation of motion persisted, the maximum opening remaining 2 cm. Six months following the second attack the same symptoms recurred. The patient was at this time treated by a dentist. Oral findings were negative for oral foci, and the patient was again treated with antibiotics. A new area of localization of infection occurred inferior to the angle of the mandible, and immediately below the previous incision. Drainage was instituted at this point, and a portion of bone was removed for study. The patient was hospitalized for 8 days, at the end of which time the patient

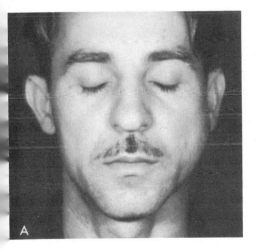

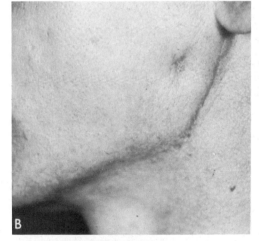

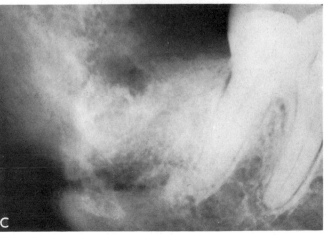

Figure 10–74 *A,* Chronic diffusing osteomyelitis of the mandible, with recurrent cellulitis. *B,* Final residual scars at drainage sites. *C,* Periapical radiograph taken at the time of the patient's hospital admission. (See Case Report No. 7 for details.)

499

stated that he had the greatest motion (the maximum opening at this time was 3 cm.) since the onset of the trouble. The edema subsided and the drainage area healed.

One year later, after the patient had had 3 to 4 days of edema of the left face, a spontaneous rupture and drainage occurred at the old scar sites. Although limitation of motion became more severe, the oral opening being 1 to 2 cm., the patient did not seek aid. The edema subsided, as did the pain, but the trismus persisted. Following this, once each year, usually in the fall, the above sequence of events was repeated. It was always the same: edema with pain, rupture of the old incision, and then remission of symptoms with residual trismus. This continued until the September preceding the present admission, when a new area of localized subcutaneous abscess occurred. Midway between, and just anterior to, the previous wounds the associated trismus occurred in its most severe form, permitting only 0.5 cm. of opening. Edema extended from the temporal region superiorly to the submandibular triangle inferiorly, and from the mastoid area posteriorly to the nose anteriorly. There was ecchymosis of the left infraorbital area. This was the appearance of the patient when first seen in our department.

Oral examination was not thorough at this time because of inaccessibility of the lingual tissues. However, digital and visual examination of the mouth and teeth were attempted. It was found that dentition was partially depleted, the remaining teeth appeared to be in a state of good repair, and the gingival tissues and oral mucosa were normal. The left mucobuccal fold of the maxilla was partially obliterated by edematous buccal tissues in the molar region. This area was tender to palpation.

The patient experienced great pain on attempted mandibular excursion, which was limited to hinge-type movements only. Lymphadenopathy of the left cervical chain and supraclavicular nodes was detected. The patient's temperature at this time was 101° F.

Significant laboratory findings were as follows: white blood count, 14,500; red blood count, 4,600,000; urinalysis, negative; serology and chest film, also negative. Physical examination was essentially negative for systemic disorders. Ear infection was ruled out.

Extraoral radiographs were taken of the jaws. These films disclosed an area of suspicious bone pattern at the angle of the left mandible and a circumscribed radiolucent region, the size of a quarter, in the left ramus. Temporomandibular joints appeared normal, with no evidence of a fracture past or present. In an effort to determine the cause of this condition, the patient was questioned with the idea of trauma's being the initiating factor. When questioned about the possibility of a blow or an accident prior to the initial occurrence of symptoms, the patient remembered having been in-

volved in an automobile accident 6 months prior to the initial attack. He stated that he did not sustain any fractures but was unconscious for 2 hours. On the basis of this evidence, a tentative diagnosis of chronic osteomyelitis of traumatic origin with fibrosis of the masseter muscle due to low-grade chronic infection was made.

Treatment. The following treatment was instituted: crystalline penicillin, 400,000 units three times a day; streptomycin, 0.5 gm. three times a day; hot, wet magnesium sulfate compresses continuously applied to the left face; supportive treatment consisting of multivitamins and a high-calorie liquid diet.

On the second hospital day, the area of localization was incised, a hemostat was inserted and opened to facilitate adequate drainage, and about 10 cc. of purulent exudate was expressed. Culture of the organisms present was positive for *Staphylococcus albus,* and these were susceptible to the antibiotic therapy instituted.

On the sixth hospital day, the patient was afebrile and was taken to the operating room for sequestrectomy of the affected area.

Operation. Under endotracheal anesthesia with Pentothal sodium, 2½ per cent, nitrous oxide and oxygen, and Anectine, the patient was prepared and draped in the usual manner.

A linear incision was made 2 cm. below the inferior border of the left mandible, beginning at the notch and carried posteriorly to the angle, and superiorly to the insertion of the tragus of the ear. The subcutaneous tissues were divided by sharp and blunt dissection. Hemostasis was secured with 000 catgut. The mandibular branch of the facial nerve was identified and elevated out of the operative site. The facial artery and vein were exposed, ligated and severed. By additional blunt and sharp dissection, which was very difficult because of fibrosis of the tissues, the inferior border of the mandible was exposed. The insertion of the masseter muscle was stripped from the angle and elevated superiorly. Immediately below the insertion of the masseter muscle a soft, spongy area the size of a half dollar was found. With sharp curettes the contents of this cavity, which was about 0.5 cm. in depth, were removed. Fibrous tissue and a small amount of serous fluid was expressed.

The masseter muscle fibers adjacent to the ramus were found to be necrotic, and a debridement was done. The tissue removed was sent for histopathologic examination. The masseter muscle was sutured into position, the tissues were approximated in layer and sutured with 000 catgut. A tissue drain was placed and the skin closed by 5-0 interrupted sutures.

A pressure dressing was applied, and the patient left the operating room reacting from the anesthetic and in good postoperative condition.

The patient's postoperative course was uneventful. The second postoperative day the dressing was removed, as were the drain and alternate sutures. The patient was encouraged to exercise his mandible, and to facilitate this exercise he was placed on a semihard diet. On the third postoperative day the remaining sutures were removed. Mandibular branch weakness became evident on this day and was attributed to reaction trauma of this branch.

Biopsy reports returned revealed chronic osteomyelitis, fibrosed skeletal muscle and granulation tissue.

On the sixth postoperative day the patient had 2.5 cm. of intermaxillary space and was discharged to be followed as an outpatient.

After 7 days of physiotherapy, the patient had 3 cm. of intermaxillary space.

Summary. 1. Presented is a case of questionable origin and a problem in differential diagnosis. Possible diagnoses were: (*a*) parotid abscess; (*b*) infected cyst; (*c*) odontogenic infection; (*d*) pathologic condition of the temporomandibular joint; (*e*) fracture; (*f*) osteomyelitis; (*g*) otic infection; (*h*) sinus infection.

2. Final diagnosis, chronic osteomyelitis of traumatic origin with a fibrosis of the left masseter muscle due to low-grade chronic infection, was determined by the radiographic findings and elimination of the above possibilities.

3. Treatment in this case was the elimination of the focus of infection by extraoral sequestrectomy and debridement and antibiotics. Physiotherapy was given to reduce postoperative trismus.

4. This case is an excellent example of inadequate examinations and mismanagement. It serves as a warning to those who would treat symptoms and ignore etiologic factors.

(The reader is also referred to Chapter 25 for additional information on osteomyelitis).

Case Report No. 8

CHRONIC DIFFUSE SCLEROSING OSTEOMYELITIS

James Guggenheimer, D.D.S., Joseph Andrews, D.D.S., and Sidney Spatz, D.D.S.

Chief Complaint. A 50-year old woman was first seen at the dental clinic in February for construction of new complete dentures and evaluation of chronic, intermittent pain in the right mandible and right face.

Past Dental and Medical History. The patient had had her remaining maxillary teeth extracted 4 years previously and the mandibular teeth in October of the year prior to the present admission. A complete upper denture had been constructed but was uncomfortable and appeared to be contributing to the pain. Other than an allergy to penicillin, the remaining history was noncontributory.

Oral Examination. Examination revealed an area of buccal and lingual swelling on the right mandibular alveolar ridge in the area of the first to third molars. The area was tender to palpation, and some erythema was present. Suppurative material could be expressed from a tract on the crest of the ridge. (See Figure 10–76*A*.)

Laboratory Findings. The urine had a specific gravity of 1.012. The white blood count was 9000 per cubic millimeter; microhematocrit, 38.5; and hemoglobin, 13 gm. Lee-White clotting time was 8 min., and rapid plasma reagin (RPR) test was nonreactive. Culture and sensitivity tests were performed. These revealed a mixed aerobic and anaerobic flora with a heavy growth of beta hemolytic streptococci. All organisms were susceptible to erythromycin.

Radiographic Examination and Clinical Course. Radiographs showed numerous irregularly shaped bony densities in the posterior body of the right mandible, as well as in both maxillary tuberosities. (See Figure 10–76*B* and *C*.) Erythromycin was given in daily doses of 1 gm. for the next 2 months, during which time the new dentures were constructed. Antibiotic therapy was then discontinued, and the patient did well for 5 months.

She returned that October with a recurrence of pain, swelling and drainage. At this time there was a small ulceration in the involved area. Erythromycin was begun, and 2 weeks later a segment of the involved bone was removed from the right mandible and submitted for histopathologic examination. (See Figure 10–76*C* and *D*.) The microscopic description mentioned several fragments of dense, irregular, compact bone, some of which showed no osteocytes in the lacunae. The tissue between the bony fragments consisted of a thin fibrous stroma containing a dense infiltrate of plasma cells, lymphocytes and a few polymorphonuclear leukocytes. In some areas, the fibrous element was more pronounced.

The patient did well as long as antibiotics were given, but symptoms recurred each time the drugs were discontinued.

Finally, on December 6, the patient was admitted to the hospital, where, under general anesthesia, the remaining area of sclerotic bone was removed. (See Figure 10–76*E*.) Healing was uneventful, and the erythromycin was discontinued on January 5. She has done well since.

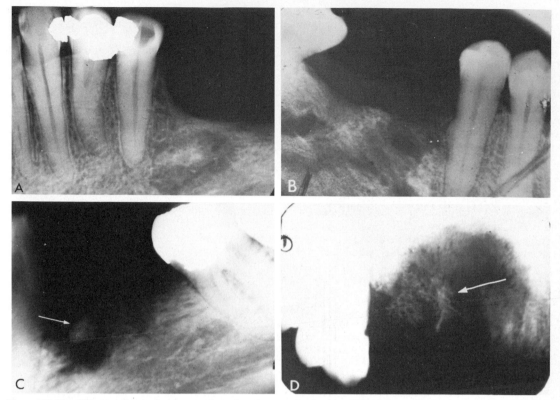

Figure 10–75 These radiographs show osteosclerotic areas in the mandible and maxilla in the process of sequestration. This is known as chronic isolated or diffuse sclerosing osteomyelitis. See Case Report No. 8.

port No. 9 and accompanying figures.) For the more common fungi, such as *Actinomyces,* specific treatment can be used. Histoplasmosis, which is more common than realized, produces oral ulceration that rarely goes on to cellulitis formation.

OSTEOMYELITIS OF THE MANDIBLE

Maxillary osteomyelitis in adults is relatively rare, but mandibular osteomyelitis is far more common. Systemic disease, especially lues, is a common companion of osteomyelitis. This subject is discussed and illustrated in detail in Chapter 25, pages 1630 to 1644.

MANAGEMENT OF THE VERY SICK PATIENT

When a patient presents with a facial abscess and clinically looks and is very sick, management becomes more complex, since we must treat not only the infection but also the deranged physiology. The well-trained oral surgeon is able to do this; the average general practitioner may need help, and he should know where to get it. The *most important* consideration is whether or not it is the infection that is primarily the problem, which means that the patient must be evaluated properly. The very basic minimum requirements are a complete blood count and urinalysis, and most important, an adequate medical history. Hospitalization is indicated. The use of intravenous fluids to overcome dehydration, adequate antibiotic therapy, vitamins, dietary supplements, and so forth, all may be indicated, depending on the individual case. Diabetics require prompt management because of their well-known propensity for getting out of control in the presence of infection. Blood dyscrasias are another major consideration. Generally speaking, infections respond very poorly to treatment in patients with systemic diseases until their primary underlying problem is corrected or relieved.

(*Text continued on page 510*)

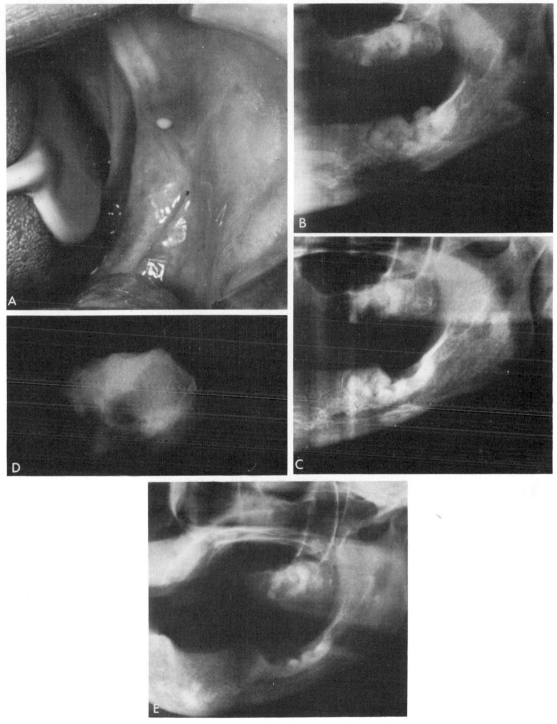

Figure 10–76   Chronic diffuse sclerosing osteomyelitis of the mandible. *A,* Suppurative material expressed from area of bone involvement. *B,* Diffused area of mandibular osteosclerosis in the process of sequestration. *C,* Following excision of a portion of the involved bone. *D,* Roentgenogram of one removed bone segment. *E,* Following second surgical procedure.

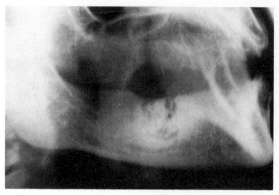

Figure 10–77 A most unusual situation—sequestration of an osteosclerotic area surrounded by condensing osteitis.

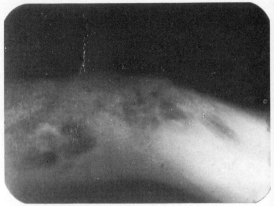

Figure 10–78 A typical radiograph of osteomyelitis of the mandible before sequestration.

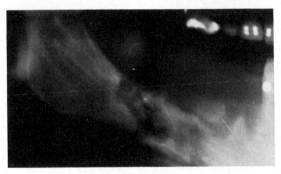

Figure 10–79 Typical radiograph of sequestration in an area of osteomyelitis of the mandible.

Case Report No. 9

PROLONGED UNUSUAL CELLULITIS OF THE FACE AND NECK FOLLOWING EXTRACTION OF A' FIRST MAXILLARY MOLAR

Note: This patient was treated in the preantibiotic and prechemotherapy days.

Patient. J. S., a man age 62, complained of extreme swelling and pain in the left cheek and neck. About 5 weeks previously he had had an upper left first molar extracted. Four days after the extraction he noticed a slight soreness of the left side of the face; this persisted for 2 weeks. Then one morning he awoke with extreme pain in the left cheek, inability to open the mouth, and swelling of the entire left side of the face. All these symptoms gradually and progressively increased. He had chills, fever, and sweats at night for 2 weeks.

He was referred to the Falk Clinic by his dentist, and from there to the Magee-Women's Hospital. His temperature on admission was 101.4° F. at 8 P.M., but later rose to 102° F.

Oral Examination. There was considerable trismus present; the patient could open his mouth only about 2 cm. The tongue had a yellow-white coating, and the oral hygiene was poor. The socket from which the upper left first molar had been extracted was healing normally.

There was no swelling in the pharynx, nor did the patient have difficulty in swallowing or breathing, in spite of the massive swelling and induration involving the side of his face and neck. Infection had not spread into the submaxillary or parapharyngeal spaces.

Extraorally there was an extensive, hard, board-like swelling of the soft tissues of the left side of the face, extending from the zygomatic arch down over the side of the face, over the angle and body of the mandible, and involving the soft-tissue planes of the neck almost to the left clavicle. There were no soft areas that might indicate a localization of pus. (See Figure 10–80.)

Discussion. It was hard to arrive at a conclu-

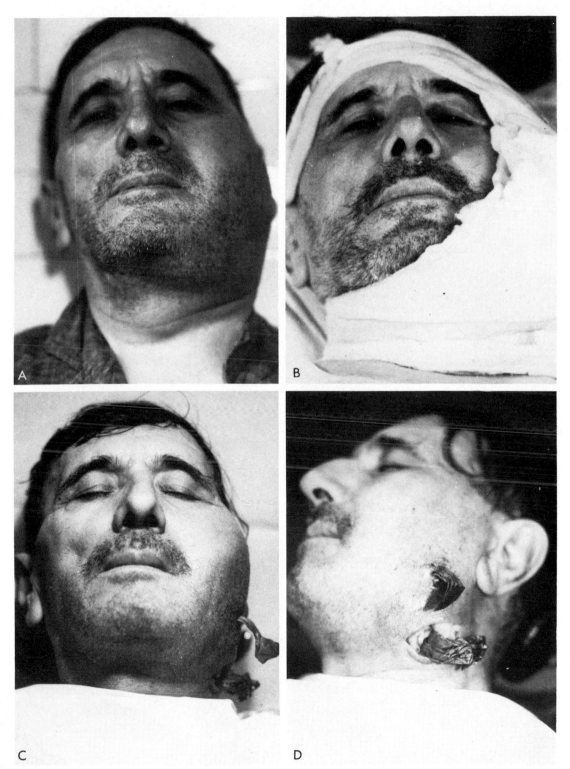

Figure 10–80 Prolonged unusual cellulitis of the face and neck. *A*, Massive brawny induration of the face and neck on the time of admission. *B*, Hot wet dressings applied continuously. (See Case Report No. 9.) *C* and *D*, First incisions for drainage—rubber tissue drains.

(Figure 10–80 continued on following page)

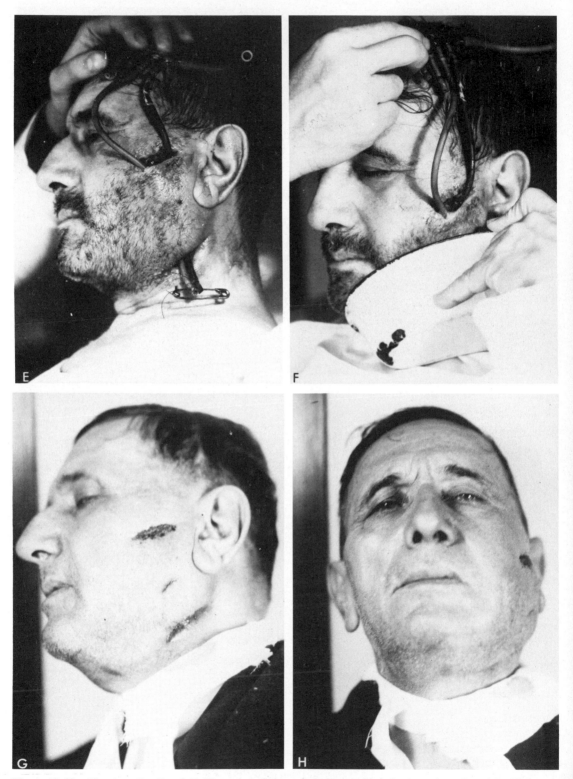

Figure 10–80 (*Continued.*) *E* and *F*, Through and through drainage with irrigating tubes. *G* and *H*, Eight weeks after discharge from hospital: abscess still draining.

(*Figure 10–80 continued on opposite page*)

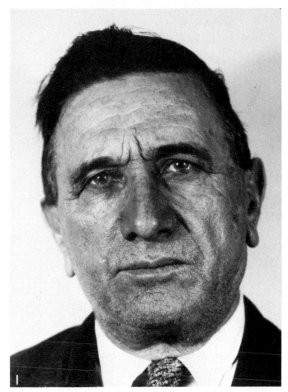
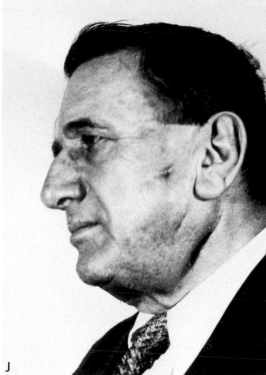

Figure 10–80 (*Continued.*) *I* and *J*, Six months after dismissal from hospital.

sion about this case, even as to diagnostic impressions. Here was an acute cellulitis of the face, of at least 4 weeks' duration, without apparently any suppuration and localization or drainage. Was this (1) a needle-borne infection, (2) an extension of infection from the upper molar that had been extracted or (3) actinomycosis, or was there (4) another source of infection?

Actinomyces hominis is believed to be normally present in the mouth. According to Paget, about 60 per cent of persons affected with actinomycosis show lesions about the head and neck, and of these, in 15 to 20 per cent, the condition follows the extraction of teeth.[25] This anaerobic fungus, lodged in the bottom of a socket after extraction of a tooth, would have been in an ideal incubator, once the blood clot had formed over it.

The slow spreading of the firm, hard, board-like swelling, over a period of weeks, a swelling that did not soften or localize, strengthened our impression that here was, perhaps, a case of actinomycosis.

Orders written on admission were those always written for patients with acute cellulitis of the face, calling for the following: blood count and differential count; urinalysis; sedimentation rate; Wassermann test; lateral jaw radiograph; forced fluids and soft diet; application of hot, wet magnesium sulfate dressings to the face continuously; infrared light (Thermolite) directed on the wet dressings, 1 hour three times a day; sodium hypochlorite, 10 drops with 4 ounces of water, as a mouthwash four times a day; codeine, 1 grain, and aspirin, 10 grains, every 3 hours as needed for the relief of pain. (Today we would add to these orders: penicillin, 600,000 units every 12 hours.)

The day after admission the temperature dropped to normal. The erythrocyte count was 4,250,000; white blood cells, 13,300 per cubic millimeter; hemoglobin, 85 per cent; polymorphonuclear leukocytes, 84 per cent; lymphocytes, 14 per cent; mononuclear leukocytes, 2 per cent. The blood sugar was 101 mg. per 100 cc; nonprotein nitrogen, 33.3; creatinine, 171; chlorides, 379. Findings in the Wassermann and Kahn tests were negative, as were those in the urine.

X-ray Examination. This was negative for evidence of osseous infection in either the maxilla or the mandible.

Course. For the next 4 days the temperature fluctuated between normal and 100° F. The edema and induration increased. There still was no indication of localization either intraorally or extraorally. On the fifth day the temperature rose to 101° F., then dropped to normal the next day, fluctuating again between normal and 100° F., until the ninth day, when it rose to 101.4° F. Now for the next 7 days it fluctuated between normal and approximately 101° F. The patient was very toxic, but there still was no indication for incision and drainage. The edema and induration during this time remained constant. There was no difficulty in swallowing or breathing at any time during his treatment.

On the seventeenth and eighteenth days the temperature touched 102° F., but dropped 2 degrees each morning.

On the twentieth day of admission, a soft area about the size of a quarter was located in the region of the angle of the ramus and body of the mandible, and another similar area halfway between the maxilla and mandible.

Under nitrous oxide and ether anesthesia, these areas were opened and connected subcutaneously. A small quantity of yellow pus with semisolid yellowish bodies was obtained. These looked like the "sulfur granules" seen in actinomycosis. Some of the yellowish bodies were placed between microscope slides, but no grating was heard. However, on staining and examining the smear under high power large numbers of *Leptothrix* were found. A rubber tissue drain was passed into the lower incision and out of the upper (see Figure 10–80C and D).

On culturing, *Staphylococcus albus* was obtained.

Guinea Pig Inoculations. A small amount of material obtained from the jaw of the patient was injected directly into a pocket in the right side of the abdomen of a guniea pig. Forty-eight hours after injection, a small abscess appeared, with a mild amount of induration.

This was removed under anesthesia, but the guinea pig died. Autopsy revealed nothing unusual about the organs of the pig, except for extensive pneumonia. The abscessed area was made up of acute and chronic inflammatory cells surrounding a small amount of necrotic material just beneath the skin. There was nothing about the lesion to suggest anything unusual. The diagnosis was abdominal abscess.

Operative Notes. The patient's temperature dropped to normal and stayed within a degree of normal for the next 4 days. On the twenty-fifth day it rose to 101° F. and again fluctuated up and down

until the twenty-eighth day, when a soft localized area about the size of a quarter was found in the region of the sigmoid notch of the mandible.

Through and through drainage was decided upon, and was established as follows: Under general anesthesia a horizontal incision was made through the skin just beneath the zygomatic process and over the center of the soft area, which was located above the sigmoid notch. A small quantity of thick, yellow pus was obtained. By means of blunt dissection beneath the cutaneous layer, this incision was connected with the incision below the body of the mandible. By means of a curved Kelly forceps, a rubber tube was pulled through the two incisions; then the fibers of the masseter muscle were split, and the sigmoid notch was exposed. A curved Kelly forceps was now passed through the incision below the body of the mandible, along the inner surface of the ramus until the tip was visible in the sigmoid notch. A rubber tube with small openings along the sides was passed into the wound, grasped by the beaks of the Kelly forceps and drawn down along the inner surface of the ramus and out through the lower incision. Dakin's solution was forced through both tubes with a syringe, thoroughly irrigating the wounds. A dressing was applied, and the patient was returned to his room (see Figure 10–80E and F).

Postoperative Course. Postoperatively the wound was irrigated every hour by forcing 75 cc. of Dakin's solution through each tube while pinching off the openings in the lower end of the tube. The solution was then forced through the lateral openings along the length of both tubes, irrigating the tissues. After 2 days there was a marked improvement, and the irrigation was reduced to once every 2 hours from 8 A.M. until 12 midnight.

Improvement was slow but steady, although drainage continued. The patient was discharged 54 days after admission, with moderate swelling but still considerable drainage. The drains were removed at the time the patient was discharged. He was seen in the outpatient department for the next 4 months, until drainage gradually ended. During this period the patient regained his normal weight and strength (see Figure 10–80G to J).

Case Report No. 10

MANAGEMENT OF ACUTE DENTOALVEOLAR ABSCESS IN A PATIENT WITH A HISTORY OF CHRONIC MYELOCYTIC LEUKEMIA*

A 64-year-old white male was admitted to the hospital with a chief complaint of a painful mass

*Case report prepared by Charles J. Tucker, B.S., D.D.S., Resident in Oral Surgery, Veterans Administration Hospital, Pittsburgh, Pa. Patient treated by Medical and Oral Surgery Departments.

of 5 days' duration on the left side of his mandible and submaxillary region.

Past Medical History. The patient had been admitted to this hospital 14 months earlier for malaise, weight loss, weakness and abdominal discomfort. At this time, there was some question about whether the patient had chronic myelocytic

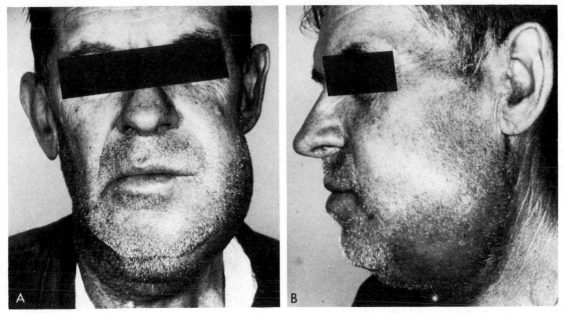

Figure 10–81 Acute cellulitis from a dentoalveolar abscess in a patient with myelocytic leukemia. (See Case Report No. 10.)

leukemia or another myeloproliferative disorder, but on the basis of repeated bone marrow studies, peripheral blood smears, mild anemia, extramedullary hematopoiesis and splenomegaly, a diagnosis of atypical chronic myelocytic leukemia was established. Therapy consisted of radiation (500 R.) to the spleen and the WBC count dropped from the 60,000 to 100,000 per cubic millimeter range prior to treatment to 2000 per cubic millimeter at completion of therapy. He was followed at regular intervals, and the latest hematologic studies, those from 1 month earlier, revealed a hemoglobin of 12 gm., a hematocrit of 41 per cent, a platelet count of 278,000 and a WBC count of 9000, with 77 per cent neutrophils, including 1 juvenile, 13 band, and 63 segmented forms.

Present Findings. The patient was alert, well developed, in no acute distress, but quite uncomfortable from the swelling along the left body of the mandible. His temperature was 99° F., pulse 88 and regular, and blood pressure 118/80. There was a 10- by 8-cm. firm mass over the left mandible, as seen in Figure 10–81, tender, but without local heat or erythema. The patient also had considerable trismus, but a grossly carious first molar could be seen on the left side as well as a bulging of the left mucobuccal fold in the left mandibular molar region. The remaining two mandibular molars on the left side were mobile and tender to percussion, and an oblique roentgenogram of the mandible disclosed radiolucent areas about the apices of these molars. The trachea was slightly deviated to the right, the anteroposterior diameter of the chest slightly enlarged, the liver palpable 3 cm. below the right costal margin and

the spleen 5 cm. below the left costal margin. The remainder of the physical findings were within normal limits.

Hospital Course. From the clinical dental examination and oblique views of the mandible, it was obvious that an acute dentoalveolar abscess was present. However, the absence of any appreciable local heat or redness and the past history of chronic myelocytic leukemia suggested that the cellulitis present might be in part due to an acute leukemic infiltration. If such were the case, surgical intervention had to be reserved for the utmost emergency because of the possibility of intractable bleeding.

Bone marrow studies were ordered to evaluate the hematopoietic status of the patient. The findings were those of a hypoplastic marrow, the majority of the nucleated cells being granulocytes with normal maturation, many platelet masses and few if any definite myeloblasts. The hematologist's impression was that there was no evidence to indicate that the patient was undergoing an acute leukemic flare-up and that the cellulitis was most likely from the dentoalveolar abscess alone and not associated with any leukemic infiltration. The peripheral blood picture also was suggestive of an inflammatory response rather than leukemic infiltration, with the WBC count elevated to 15,600 per cubic millimeter, with 85 per cent neutrophils, including 79 segmented forms and 6 band forms, 2 per cent monocytes, 1 per cent basophils, platelets 322,000, hemoglobin 10 gm. and hematocrit 32 per cent.

The hematologist recommended broad-spectrum antibiotic coverage, investigation of the clotting mechanism and, if that were satisfactory, cautious surgical intervention when fluctuation and pointing ensued.

The clotting mechanism was investigated. A tube of blood showed good clotting and retraction within 1½ hours; bleeding time was 2 minutes, 50 seconds; Lee-White clotting time, 13 minutes, 30 seconds; prothrombin time of patient, 16 seconds, of control, 13 seconds—all within fairly normal limits.

In the interim, the patient had been given tetracyclines, 500 mg. four times a day, and applications of hot, moist soaks. There was a marked increase in trismus, more local heat and redness, a temperature elevation to 102° F. and beginning fluctuation of the mass.

On the third day, the area had become more fluctuant, and in view of acceptable coagulation and bone marrow studies, an extraoral incision and drainage of the most fluctuant and dependent area of the mass were performed. Approximately 50 cc. of foul-smelling, thick, purulent material exuded freely from the site. Cultures were taken, and a rubber dam drain was inserted. The temperature

dropped rapidly from 103° F. prior to incision and drainage to normal on the following day. The swelling resolved rapidly, and the pain subsided the same day. The dressings were changed daily, and the drain was removed on the sixth day; on this same day, the two remaining molars were removed, the sockets were debrided gently and an iodoform dressing was placed for 2 days.

The culture reports indicated gram-positive cocci, with secondary invasion by *Actinomyces;* consequently, the patient was continued on tetracyclines, 250 mg. four times a day, for 6 weeks, the therapy suggested by the medical service. The patient was discharged and followed routinely for his primary problem, *i.e.,* chronic leukemia, and no sequelae of this secondary invasion by *Actinomyces* have occurred.

In summary, this case presented a somewhat cloudy picture of whether this was a cellulitis secondary to dentoalveolar abscess alone or whether leukemic infiltration was present with the dentoalveolar abscess. However, correlation of the various diagnostic studies enabled proper definitive therapy to be carried out.

CAVERNOUS SINUS THROMBOPHLEBITIS

Sicher states, "Of all the communications between the extracranial and intracranial veins, those established by the ophthalmic veins are two types of propagation of a facial thrombophlebitis to the cavernous sinus. One path leads from the anterior facial vein into the superior ophthalmic vein, sometimes, though rarely, into the inferior ophthalmic vein. The infection leads, therefore, into and through the orbit, and finally the thrombophlebitis is transmitted to the cavernous sinus through the superior orbital fissures.

"The second path leads from the posterior facial vein into the pterygoid venous plexus and from here through the inferior orbital fissures into the terminal part of the inferior ophthalmic vein and then immediately through the superior orbital fissure into the cavernous sinus.

"In the first type of ascending facial thrombophlebitis the involvement of the orbit, under the clinical picture of an orbital or retrobulbar cellulitis, precedes the symptoms indicating the involvement of the cavernous sinus. In the second type, intracranial or meningeal symptoms may occur without a previous orbital involvement. In the first type of ascending thrombophlebitis a danger signal

occurs before the ultimate complications arise, while such a warning symptom is lacking in the second type."[30]

DEATH FROM DENTOALVEOLAR INFECTIONS

While the hazards of oral surgery are not as common as in the past, the dentist should be cognizant of them. The venous drainage of the head in part passes into the cavernous sinuses of the skull, and injudicious surgery may produce thrombosis of the cavernous sinuses. The failure to use antibiotics or, worse yet, the use of inadequate dosages may provoke situations in which infectious emboli may lodge in the brain. However, with the current progress in medicine the hazards in this area are definitely on the wane.

Haymaker summarized his findings in 27 cases of fatal intracranial complication of tooth extraction and in one case of transverse myelitis. In nearly all the cases the extractions, undertaken because of periapical abscess, caries, impaction, malposition, painful eruption, and for other reasons, were believed to have initiated or precipitated the infective process.

In only 8 of the 28 cases was there evi-

(*Text continued on page 513*)

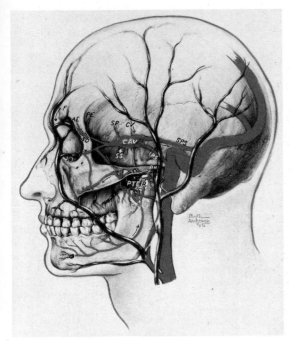

Figure 10-82 The venous tributaries of the cavernous sinus, including those from the teeth. The arrows indicate the direction of the blood flow. Veins of the lower jaw drain via the inferior dental vein into the pterygoid plexus of veins (*PTER*), while those from the upper jaw drain in two directions: the more anterior ones into the anterior facial vein, and the more posterior ones into the pterygoid plexus.

The pterygoid plexus lies in the subtemporal and pterygoid fossae: it surrounds the lateral pterygoid muscle and covers the lateral surface of the medial pterygoid. In addition to the teeth mentioned, the pterygoid plexus drains the fauces, the soft palate, and the pharynx. In ascending infections, complicating tooth extraction, the pterygoid plexus, together with the adjacent pharyngeal plexus (*PH*), is subject to thrombophlebitis. The infection usually reaches the cavernous sinus (*CAV*) by way of the vein of Vesalius (present but not labeled) and often traverses the foramen of the same name, which is situated anteromedial to the foramen ovale; other routes followed from the pterygoid plexus are by way of the foramina ovale and lacerum. On the other hand, a thrombophlebitis of the pterygoid plexus may extend through veins which communicate with the inferior ophthalmic vein.

In cavernous sinus thrombosis following infections of anterior teeth, the thrombophlebitis tends to take the anterior route: i.e., via the anterior facial and its continuation, the angular vein (formed by the union of the supraorbital and frontal veins), and then through the orbit by way of the ophthalmic veins, especially the superior.

Tributaries draining into the cavernous sinus by way of the superior ophthalmic vein (*SO*) are from anterior facial structures (external nose, lips, forehead, eyelids, and cheeks) and from the mucosa of the frontal sinus (*F*), the anterior ethmoidal cells (*AE*), the posterior ethmoidal cells (*PE*), and the upper part of the lateral nasal wall. The cavernous sinus also receives venous blood from the mucosa of the sphenoidal sinus (*SS*), from the superficial inferior cerebral veins (*CV*), and from the sphenoparietal venous sinus (*SP*). The sphenoparietal venous sinus drains the diploe of the lesser wing of the sphenoid and veins of the dura mater. Blood leaves the cavernous sinus chiefly through the superior and inferior petrosal sinuses (*SPS* and *IPS*, respectively). (From Haymaker, W.: Fatal infections after tooth extraction. Am. J. Orthod., *31*;117-118, 1945; modified from Turner and Reynolds.)

Figure 10-83 Pathways followed by infections which ascend from the jaw to reach the intracranial cavity. The most frequent site of penetration of the base of the skull by infections complicating tooth extraction is the greater wing of the sphenoid in the vicinity of the foramen ovale (indicated by the thicker arrow). The extracranial collection of pus is sometimes so deeply situated that its presence is not recognized clinically. The next most frequent cranial structures involved are the sphenoidal sinus and the overlying sella turcica. The infective organism may reach the sphenoidal sinus directly (as indicated by the arrow within the exposed sphenoidal sinus) or by contiguity from the greater wing of the sphenoid bone. (In some cases a sphenoid sinusitis may be the result of retrograde thrombosis from a thrombosed cavernous sinus.) Another route of spread is through the petrous part of the temporal bone. In some cases the infective organism reaches the retrobulbar tissues in the manner indicated, and subsequently may enter the intracranial cavity via the ophthalmic veins or by direct spread through the orbital fissure or canal. (From Haymaker, W.: Fatal infections after tooth extraction. Am. J. Orthod., *31*:117-188, 1945.)

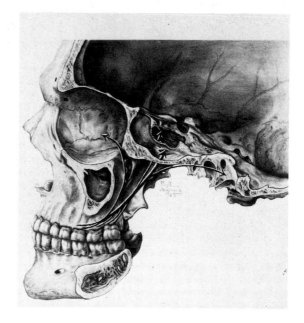

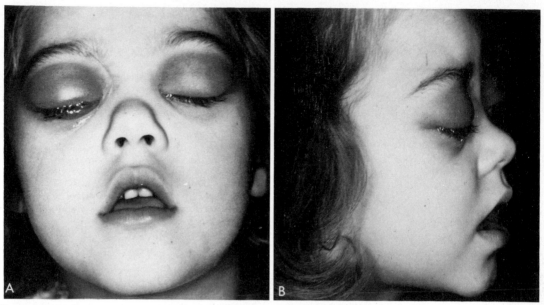

Figure 10–84 Cavernous sinus thrombosis following acute hyperplastic ethmoiditis. The patient was hospitalized 52 days. Penicillin and sulfadiazine were given and the patient recovered after a stormy course.

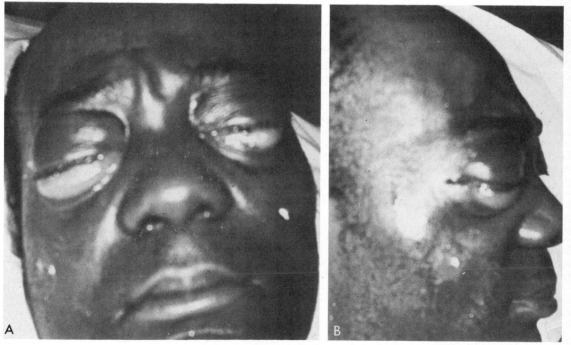

Figure 10–85 Cavernous sinus thrombophlebitis with typical retrobulbar cellulitis producing bilateral proptosis and immobility of eyeballs. The patient responded to penicillin therapy.

Case Report No. 11

CAVERNOUS SINUS THROMBOSIS

Patient. A 20-year-old white female was admitted on February 20 to the Magee-Women's Hospital disoriented and drowsy, and complaining of pain in the head. There was bilateral orbital edema and ecchymosis with proptosis of both eyes, eversion of conjunctivae with bleb formation. On admission there was a definite leukocytosis with increase of polymorphonuclear cells. Red blood count, blood chemistry and sedimentation time were within normal limits.

Course in Hospital. On the day of admission temperature rose to 105.6° F., pulse to 160, and respiration was 36. Temperature continued to remain at a pleateau between 104° and 105° F. for 4 days after admission. During this time, the leukocyte count averaged 20,000 white cells per cubic millimeter. Pulse varied between 90 and 150, ranging usually between 120 and 150. Five days after admission the temperature began to fall by lysis so that gradual downward trend of the temperature was continued, pulse following temperature; by 17 days after admission temperature was varied, with daily rises to less than 100° F. This continued until temperature became normal 26 days after admission, thereafter the course continuing afebrile except for one rise to 99° F. The pulse followed temperature in all phases, averaging between 80 and 90 after the course had become afebrile. Respiration subsided gradually with the temperature and came to average 22 per minute.

The patient was treated with intravenous heparin, doses varying according to coagulation time determination so that an effort was made to keep the coagulation time always above 15 minutes; to effect this, doses between 100 mg. and 250 mg. were administered intravenously at intervals, often as short as 10 hours apart. To supplement the heparin therapy bishydroxycoumarin (Dicoumarin) was used in doses of 300 mg. per day. Confusion in interpretation of laboratory blood studies resulted because it was found that with a bleeding time of 1 minute and a coagulation time of 9 minutes, the prothrombin time was 10 per cent of normal; the prothrombin time was found to be far below normal, while the coagulation time continued within normal limits.

The patient suffered from epistaxis when the prothrombin time was 10 per cent of normal, so Dicoumarin was stopped and a whole blood transfusion of 500 cc. was given. Within 9 days the prothrombin time rose to 70 per cent of normal. Sulfadiazine was also used to supplement this treatment to the level of 5.2 mg. per 100 cc.

There was bilateral postcervical edema with the orbital edema and proptosis. Improvement was concomitant with the following: reduction in proptosis, falling temperature, and reduction of leukocytosis, which were effected after anticoagulant therapy had been maintained over a period of 12 days. Eye grounds at first showed slight papilledema and slight enlargement of the veins, both of which readily subsided before other evidence of improvement appeared.

Laboratory Findings. X-ray of sinuses showed no sinusitis; the nasal accessory sinuses were all clear. Electrocardiogram revealed (1) sinus mechanism with normal conduction time; (2) slurred QRS complexes in all leads. Blood chemistry findings were: sugar, 95 mg. per 100 cc.; nonprotein nitrogen, 31.5 mg. per 100 cc. Serology results were: blood Kahn, negative; Kolmer, negative. Spinal fluid cell count was 4; spinal fluid globulin, negative; spinal fluid culture, negative. Urinalysis findings were negative. Sedimentation time was over 90.

Blood culture demonstrated *Staphylococcus albus,* probably a contaminant. Blood counts were as follows: On February 22, the red cell count was 4,560,000; white cell count, 20,000; hemoglobin, 90 per cent; polymorphonuclears, 66 per cent; lymphocytes, 7 per cent; eosinophils, 27 per cent. On March 1: red cells, 3,260,000, white cell count, 10,100; hemoglobin, 63 per cent; polymorphonuclears, 74 per cent; lymphocytes, 12 per cent; myelocytes, 14 per cent. On March 30: red cells, 3,850,000; white cell count, 10,400; hemoglobin, 74 per cent; polymorphonuclears, 23 per cent; lymphocytes, 24 per cent; eosinophils, 49 per cent; myelocytes, 3 per cent; basophils, 1 per cent. Prothrombin time from February 22 to March 25 averaged 57 seconds, with an average control time of 31 seconds. Coagulation time for the same period averaged 14.7 minutes. Bleeding time averaged 6 minutes. Sulfadiazine level on February 23 was 5.2 mg. per 100 cc.

Consultation Reports. Reports by consultants from the eye, ear, nose and throat, neurological and dental departments were essentially negative. The source of this infection was unknown.

Diagnosis. Cavernous sinus thrombosis.

---

dence of poor oral hygiene. In 19 cases only one tooth was extracted, while in cases with the greatest number of extractions bacteremia did not follow, suggesting, at least in this series, that multiple extraction is not necessarily a cause of fatal intracranial complication.

As many upper teeth were extracted as were lower teeth, yet direct spread of an infective process to the intracranial cavity occurred more often after extractions from the upper jaw than from the lower jaw (10, as compared with 6), while in hematogenous infections the reverse occurred (9, as compared with 5). According to the literature, fatal complications of dental infection in the lower jaw occur approximately twice as often as those in the upper jaw, while those on the left side exceed those on the right side by 3 to 2.

Molars were most frequently extracted. Except for one instance in which a bicuspid was also removed, only molars were extracted in cases in which cavernous sinus thrombosis followed. Infection near molar teeth leading to intracranial complications may be ascribed to anatomic relations: since pus in the posterior part of the jaw has no free access to the oral cavity or to the exterior as it does in the anterior part, it tends to collect between the muscles of mastication and to spread rapidly upward in the fascial planes.

In some of Haymaker's cases pus at the base of the skull was so deeply located that it was not recognized, or could not be reached by surgical means.

In hematogenous infections the most frequently encountered organism was *Streptococcus;* in infections reaching the intracranial cavity by direct spread, *Staphylococcus.* Bacteremia was considered to be the immediate result of extraction in 7 cases and to have occurred shortly after extraction in conjunction with fulminating cellulitis of the jaw in 2 cases, about a month after extraction as the result of surgical intervention in 2 other cases, and at undetermined times in 3 cases.

The infective organism gained access to the cranial cavity by way of the general circulation in 10 cases, and to the spinal cord in 1. Brain abscess occurred in 7 of these 11 cases, and leptomeningitis, choroiditis, lateral sinus thrombosis and transverse myelitis, respectively, in the other 4 cases.

The infective process spread directly to the intracranial cavity in 18 cases. In 8 of these instances there was a suppurative cellulitis that spread to the base of the skull and produced osteomyelitis of the greater wing of the sphenoid bone. Brain abscess occurred in 7 cases, owing to direct spread of the inflammation through the bony cranial wall. There were 9 instances of cavernous sinus thrombosis; in 7 of these cases the venous blood stream enabled the infection to reach the sinus from the extracranial focus, while in the other 2 extension of the inflammation directly through the cranial wall occurred, with secondary invasion of the venous blood stream.

There were 6 instances of intraorbital abscess. Of the paranasal sinuses, the sphenoidal and the maxillary sinuses, in that order, were involved.[16]

DIFFERENTIAL DIAGNOSIS OF FACIAL SWELLINGS

Patients are frequently referred to the dentist because of a swollen face. However, not all swellings of the face are of dental origin. Sudden swelling of the face may be due to angioneurotic edema, as illustrated in the case report in Chapter 25, or to emphysema. Gradually increasing swelling of the face may, of course, be due to tumors or cysts of the hard or soft tissue or to parotid gland involvement, lymphangioma or angioneurotic edema.

Etiology. Three possibilities have been accepted: (1) heredity, (2) food allergy, (3) psychological difficulties.

Sherman states that angioneurotic edema occurs in two forms, "A rare hereditary form, in which involvement of the larynx and viscera is frequent, and a more common sporadic or nonhereditary type, in which visceral lesions are less prominent."

Diagnosis. "The nature of the lesion is generally apparent from the absence of pain and heat and usually of redness. The underlying structures—for example the teeth and sinuses in lesions of the face—should be carefully examined for evidence of infection. Edema persisting for a week or more is rarely angioneurotic edema."

Treatment. "The response of large swellings to symptomatic medication is slow. Epinephrine is indicated, especially if the tongue or larynx is involved. One or two doses of 0.5 ml. of the 1:1000 aqueous solution may be followed by 1.0 ml. of the 1:500 suspension in oil intramuscularly for a prolonged effect. Large doses of the antihistamine drugs are required. Tripelennamine [Pyribenzamine] or diphenhydramine [Benadryl], 50 to 100 mg., may be given every 4 hours.

"When the pharynx or larynx is affected, vigorous treatment and close observation are essential. Preparations should be made for a prompt tracheotomy, if necessary."[29]

In recurrent or persistent cases an effort should be made to determine the cause, which then is eliminated if possible. All infection should be eliminated. Suspected food allergens should be avoided. The factor of emotional stress should be investigated.

OTHER TYPES OF INFECTION OF THE MOUTH AND JAWS

THRUSH (CANDIDOSIS; MONILIASIS)

Several varieties of *Candida (Monilia)*, a higher form of microorganism, are present on about 15 per cent of normal mucous membranes, and active infections are produced because of an increase of virulence of the organism or to debility of the patient. An infection of the oral mucous membranes, thrush, is common. The organism is present in abundance in white patches on inflammatory areas, and is best demonstrated by direct smears. The organism is characterized by the presence of both yeast-like budding forms and long, broad filaments. *Candida* infections may become increasingly important because their growth is apparently enhanced by penicillin and other antibiotics, and none of the currently useful antibiotics or sulfonamide drugs are effective against this organism. Several mild antiseptics are helpful when used locally.

Treatment of Monilia Complications Occurring with Antibiotic Therapy. Oral infection (thrush) is treated with oral nystatin suspension (each cc. contains 100,000 units) by holding 1 cc. in the mouth four times daily before swallowing. Or the lesions may be painted with sodium caprylate solution (N.N.D.), 30.0 cc. Paint on lesions two or three times a day.[12]

VINCENT'S ANGINA

The importance of Vincent's organisms (*Fusiformis dentium* and *Borrelia vincentii*) in oral ulcerations has been greatly overstressed. This fusiform bacillus and the associated spirochete are evidently saprophytes commonly present on mucous membranes. They are naturally present in profusion in any necrotic ulcer, whatever the underlying cause. The tragedy involved in attaching diagnostic importance to the demonstration of such bacteria is the delay involved in more precise determination of the underlying cause of the ulcer. Epidemic stomatitis during World War I was ascribed to these organisms, and since the infections were troublesome among troops, the term "trench mouth" was coined.

ACTINOMYCOSIS*

Actinomycosis is a granulomatous lesion of man and animals. The actinomycetes exist as both saprophytes and pathogens. The organism responsible for human and animal actinomycosis is *Actinomyces bovis*, better known as *A. israelii* when isolated in humans. It is a gram-positive, microaerophilic fungus whose natural habitat is the oral cavity. It grows best under partially anaerobic conditions. This strain is not saprophytic, nor has it been isolated in soil or natural substrates, as was formerly believed.[11, 19, 28] It can be isolated in mucinous plaques, calculus, periodontal pockets, and tonsillar crypts. No direct transmission between man and man or man and animals has been determined, and therefore it is considered to be an endogenous disease.

Actinomyces bovis can gain access and multiply through fracture sites, extraction wounds and periodontal pockets. Organisms have also been found in root canals.[33] Although it is essentially of low pathogenicity, it can multiply and invade tissue under favorable conditions provided by injury or bacterial infections that produce tissue necrosis. It grows well in a suppurative process and in this environment may take over and crowd out its bacterial partner.

The disease manifests itself as three distinct entities: the cervicofacial, thoracic and abdominal types, the cervicofacial variant being the more benign one.

Clinically, cervicofacial actinomycosis may be of the central type, involving bone, or peripheral, involving soft tissue only. The lesion more frequently involves the mandible; however, involvements of the maxilla have been reported. It is a slow-forming lesion that often goes undetected until soft tissue is involved. If radiographs are taken, a radiolucent granulomatous area may be demonstrated.

When it involves soft tissue, very often a hard, painless swelling appears in the third molar areas. Invasion of the soft tissue continues, and the skin surface becomes discolored, taking on a purple hue. The swelling begins to fluctuate and drain, forming mul-

*Prepared by Arthur Mashberg, B.A., D.D.S., Resident in Oral Surgery, Veterans Administration Hospital, Oakland Division, Pittsburgh, Pa.

Case Report No. 12

ACTINOMYCOSIS ("LUMPY JAW") FOLLOWING EXTRACTION OF A MANDIBULAR THIRD MOLAR

A 30-year-old Negro male was treated for cellulitis of the left mandible secondary to pericoronitis involving the lower left third molar. The offending tooth was extracted, and adequate drainage was established. The patient's postoperative course was uneventful except for unrelated medical complaints. The edema had subsided and the patient was asymptomatic. He was then discharged.

Two months later he again appeared on the dental service because of a slowly developing mass in the lower left third molar area. This mass was firm, fixed and hard, measuring 6 cm. in diameter. It was relatively painless (see Figure 10–86).

Findings in radiographs of the mandible were negative. The WBC count was 11,000, with 75 per cent neutrophils. Five days after admission an incision was made to establish drainage, but this was unsuccessful. Twelve days later the mass was fluctuant extraorally and began to show a lumpy or lobulated appearance. Using a Luer-Lok syringe, 1 cc. of pus was aspirated. This was sent to the laboratory for identification of organisms present. The findings were *A. bovis*.

The patient was given tetracycline, 500 mg. four times a day. Soon after, a small amount of pus drained spontaneously, and gradually over a period of 3 weeks there was complete remission of the lesion. Six weeks after admission, the patient was discharged and tetracycline therapy was continued for a total of 8 weeks. He was seen periodically for the next 4 months and showed no evidence of recurrence.

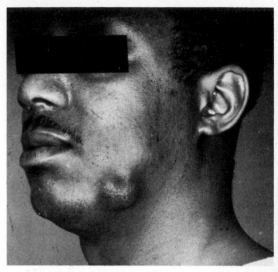

Figure 10–86 "Lumpy jaw" from *Actinomycosis bovis* infection. (See Case Report No. 12.)

Summary. This case of actinomycosis presents the typical history and clinical picture of actinomycosis. Because of early diagnosis and treatment we believe that surgical intervention was avoided. The patient had not yet developed multiple fistulae and extension of the lesion, and responded well to tetracycline therapy. He was finally discharged as cured.

---

tiple fistulae and giving a lobulated or lumpy appearance — hence the term "lumpy jaw." Involvement of the subcutaneous fascial planes may increase the extent of the lesion.

If the process is acute, fever, malaise and purulence make an early appearance. There may be periodic remissions and exacerbations with decreasing severity.

Chronic cases are frequently complicated with pyogenic organisms and therefore may run a long course. Remission of symptoms is no guarantee of complete eradication of disease, since a low-grade infection may continue and go unnoticed. During the active state the sedimentation rate may be elevated, and there is a leukocytosis, with an increase in neutrophils.

The tissue response is typical of a granulomatous lesion, with epithelioid cells, lymphocytes, plasma cells and neutrophils predominating. The characteristic "sulfur granule"

appears in the abscess centers. These are composed of many organisms with interlacing filamentous mycelia and club-shaped peripheries.

Diagnosis can be made by biopsy or bacteriologic studies of cultures and colony growth.

Cervicofacial actinomycosis may require extensive and repeated surgery to remove granulomata and multiple fistulous tracts. Penicillin, 500,000 to 1,000,000 units per day, has been effective therapy in some cases.[39] Tetracycline therapy four times a day, 500 mg., has been employed with success. Whatever the antibiotic used, it should be continued for many weeks or months until it is fairly definite that the entire disease process has been obliterated. In the past potassium iodide had been employed as a therapeutic measure. However, it is now believed to be completely ineffective in treating actinomycotic lesions.[13] In addition to surgical and antibiotic therapy, there have been reports of successful treatment with radiation.

SYPHILIS

Unfortunately this is a reappearing disease, and chancres of the lip, secondary lesions of the mucous membranes, and tertiary lesions or gummas of structures about the oral cavity are beginning to be seen with increasing frequency.

REFERENCES

1. Abramson, D. I.: Vascular Responses in the Extremities of Man in Health and Disease. Chicago, University of Chicago Press, 1944.
2. Anderson, W.: Boyd's Pathology for the Surgeon. 8th ed. Philadelphia, W. B. Saunders Co., 1967.
3. Bancroft, H., and Edholm, O. G.: Effects of temperature on blood flow and deep temperature in the human forearm. J. Physiol., 102:5–20, 1943.
4. Baruch, S.: An Epitome of Hydrotherapy. Philadelphia, W. B. Saunders Co., 1920.
5. Bernier, J. L.: The Management of Oral Disease, pp. 325–327. St. Louis, C. V. Mosby Co., 1955.
6. Black, G. V.: A Work on Special Dental Pathology, Chicago, Medico-Dental Publishing Co., 1920.
7. Burke, J.: Angina ludovici: a translation together with a biography of Wilhelm von Ludwig. Bull. Hist. Med., 7:1115, 1939.
8. Cahn, L. R.: Pathology of the Oral Cavity. Baltimore, The Williams & Wilkins Co., 1941.
9. Carr, M. W.: Acute infections of the face and neck. N.Y. J. Dent., 18:376–385, 1948.
10. Clendenning, L.: In Hashinger, E. H., (Ed.): Methods of Treatment. 8th ed. St. Louis, The C. V. Mosby Co., 1945.
11. Conant, N. F., et al.: Manual of Clinical Mycology. 3rd ed. Philadelphia, W. B. Saunders Co., 1971.
12. Conn, H. J. (Ed.): Current Therapy 1975. Philadelphia, W. B. Saunders Co., 1975.
13. Drill, V. A.: Pharmacology in Medicine. 2nd ed., p. 1188. New York, McGraw-Hill Book Co., Inc., 1958.
14. Gold, R. S., and Sager, E.: Pansinusitis, orbital cellulitis, and blindness as sequelae of delayed treatment of dental abscess. J. Oral Surg., 32:40 (Jan.), 1974.
15. Hall, C., and Morris, F.: Infections of the masticator space. Ann. Otol. Rhinol. Laryngol., 50:1123, 1941.
16. Haymaker, W.: Fatal infections of the central nervous system and meningitis after tooth extraction. Am. J. Orthod., 31:117–188, 1945.
17. Hollinshead, W. H.: Anatomy for Surgeons. Vol. I, Head and Neck. New York, Hoeber, 1954.
18. Johnson, W. S., Devine, K. D., Wellman, W. E., and
19. Fischback, J. E.: Ludwig's angina, concepts of therapy, with report of a case. Oral Surg., 16:1023 (Sept.), 1963.
20. Joklik, W. K., and Smith, D. T.: Zinsser, Microbiology. 15th ed. New York, Appleton-Century-Crofts, 1972.
21. Kovács, R.: Electrotherapy and Light Therapy. 6th ed. Philadelphia, Lea & Febiger, 1949.
22. Laskin, D. M.: Anatomic considerations in diagnosis and treatment of odontogenic infections. J.A.D.A., 69:308 (Sept.), 1964.
23. Lewis, T.: Observations on some normal and injurious effects of cold upon the skin and underlying tissues. Br. Med. J., 2:795, 1941.
24. Meade, S. H.: Diseases of the Mouth. St. Louis, The C. V. Mosby Co., 1941.
25. Nathan, M. H., Radman, W. P., and Barton, H. L.: Osseous actinomycosis of the head and neck. Am. J. Roentgenol. Radium Ther. Nucl. Med., 87:1048 (June), 1962.
26. Paget, J.: On a form of chronic inflammation of bone. (Osteitis deformans.) Med. Chir. Tr. (Lond.), 60:37–63, 1877.
27. Ping, R. S., and Morris, E. E.: Illosone, the propionyl ester of erythromycin. Oral Surg., 13:539–542 (May), 1960.
28. Pollack, H., and Halpern, S. L.: Therapeutic Nutrition. Prepared in collaboration with the Committee on Therapeutic Nutrition, Food and Nutrition Board, National Research Council. Washington, D.C., National Research Council, 1952.
29. Rippon, J. W.: Medical Mycology: The Pathogenic Fungi and the Pathogenic Actinomycetes. Philadelphia, W. B. Saunders Co., 1974.
30. Sherman, W. B.: Angioneurotic edema. In Beeson, P. B., and McDermott, W. (Eds.): Cecil-Loeb Textbook of Medicine, p. 462. 11th ed. Philadelphia, W. B. Saunders Co., 1963.
31. Sicher, H., and DuBrul, E. L.: Oral Anatomy. 5th ed. St. Louis, The C. V. Mosby Co., 1970.
32. Spilsbury, B. W., and Johnstone, F. R. C.: The clinical course of actinomycotic infections. Can. J. Surg., 5:33 (Jan.), 1962.
33. Taffel, M., and Harvey, S. C.: Ludwig's angina: an analysis of forty-five cases. Surgery, 11:841, 1942.
34. Thoma, K. H., and Goldman, H. M.: Oral Pathology. 5th ed. St. Louis, The C. V. Mosby Co., 1960.
35. Thoma, K. H.: Oral Surgery. 5th ed. St. Louis, The C. V. Mosby Co., 1969.
36. Thomas, T. T.: Ludwig's angina: an anatomical, clinical and statistical study. Ann. Surg., 47:161–183, 335–373, 1908.
37. Tiecke, R. W. (Ed.): Oral Pathology. New York, McGraw-Hill Book Co., Inc., 1965.
38. Waite, D. E.: Infections of dental etiology in the mandibular and maxillofacial region. J. Oral Surg., 18:412 (July), 1960.
39. Watkins, A. L.: Research in physical medicine. N. Engl. J. Med., 234:548, 628, 1946.
40. Zitka, E.: Klinische und therapeutische Einfahrungen bei cervicofacialer Actinomykose. Z. Stomatol., 48:67, 1951.

CHAPTER 11

CYSTS OF THE ORAL CAVITY

HAMILTON B. G. ROBINSON, D.D.S., M.S.

The dentist frequently encounters cystic lesions within the jawbones and occasionally within the soft tissues of the oral cavity.

A cyst is a "pouch or sac without an opening, provided with a distinct membrane, and containing fluid or semifluid material, abnormally developed in one of the natural cavities or in the substance of an organ."[35] In a true cyst of the oral cavity, the distinct membrane consists of an epithelial lining within a connective tissue capsule.

Developmental, neoplastic and retention types of cysts occur within the oral cavity, and any of these may be aseptic or infected. The possibility of a cyst should be considered by the dentist in any patient with either a swelling about the mouth or a radiolucent area in the bone. However, this does not mean that all radiolucent areas within the bone, or swellings in the mouth, should be classified as cysts.

Many classifications have been suggested for dental cysts, but most of these groupings have been incomplete or unwieldy. A classification of cysts of the jaw was developed through the cooperative efforts of 20 oral surgeons, oral pathologists, and other interested dentists and physicians.[22] Expanding this to include cysts of the soft tissues and some lesions that have been described more recently, the following classification has been made.

I. Developmental.
  A. Dental origin.
    1. Periodontal (dentoperiosteal, dentoalveolar radicular, dental root, root end).
      a. Periapical.
      b. Lateral.
      c. Residual.
    2. Dentigerous (follicular).*
      a. Cystic odontoma.
      b. Eruption.
    3. Odontogenic keratocyst.
    4. Calcifying odontogenic cyst.
  B. Nondental.
    1. Fissural types.
      a. Nasoalveolar (extra-alveolar).
      b. Median (median palatine, median alveolar, median mandibular).
      c. Incisive canal (nasopalatine).
      d. Globulomaxillary.
    2. Branchial cleft types.
      a. Dermoid and epidermoid.
      b. Branchial cleft (cervical).
      c. Thyroglossal duct.
II. Retention.
  A. Mucous.
  B. Ranula.

In addition to these true cysts, there are a number of lesions that may appear cystic in a radiograph or on clinical examination. These include (a) extravasation cysts (traumatic cysts or traumatogenic cysts); (b) neoplasms resembling cysts radiographically as a result of bone destruction; (c) metabolic dysfunctions resembling cysts as a result of bone destruction; and (d) inflammatory diseases re-

---

*Thoma[33] has suggested the subclassification of circumferential dentigerous cyst, central dentigerous cyst and lateral dentigerous cyst.

ODONTOGENESIS

CYSTS AND NEOPLASM

ORIGIN OF LESIONS

PROLIFERATION

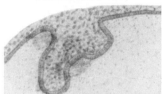

SOLID AMELOBLASTOMA

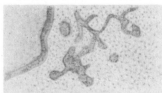

THE AMELOBLASTOMA IS AN EPITHELIAL NEOPLASM WHICH RESEMBLES DENTAL LAMINAE AND ENAMEL ORGANS UNTIL THE PERIOD OF AMELOGENESIS. IT MAY BE DERIVED FROM CELLS OF THE ORAL EPITHELIUM WITH A TENDENCY TO ODONTOGENESIS, FROM REMNANTS OF THE SHEATH OF HERTWIG OR THE DENTAL LAMINA (EPITHELIAL RESTS) OR FROM ABERRANT TOOTH BUDS. IT BEGINS AS A SOLID TUMOR APING THE DENTAL ANLAGE AND ENAMEL ORGAN BUT NEVER FORMS ENAMEL. IT DEGENERATES AT THE EXPENSE OF THE STELLATE RETICULUM TO BECOME A MULTICYSTIC TUMOR.

DIFFERENTIATION

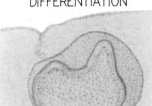

CYSTIC AMELOBLASTOMA

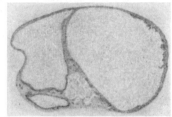

TISSUE FORMATION

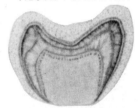

PRIMORDIAL CYST

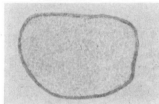

THE PRIMORDIAL CYST IS A CYST OF THE JAW DERIVED FROM THE ENAMEL ORGAN IN ITS EARLY STAGES. BEFORE TISSUE FORMATION BEGINS, THE STELLATE RETICULUM BREAKS DOWN AND FLUID COLLECTS BETWEEN THE INNER AND OUTER ENAMEL EPITHELIUM. THE CYST IS FORMED BY INTERNAL PRESSURE.

TISSUE FORMATION

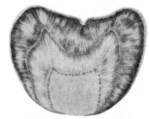

DENTIGEROUS CYST

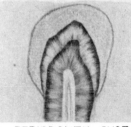

THE DENTIGEROUS CYST IS A CYST OF THE JAW CONTAINING THE CROWN OF A TOOTH. IT IS USUALLY DESCRIBED AS FORMED BY A BREAKDOWN OF THE STELLATE RETICULUM DURING AMELOGENESIS. THIS WOULD PRODUCE HYPOPLASTIC ENAMEL. IT APPEARS TO BE FORMED WITHIN THE REDUCED ENAMEL EPITHELIUM.

ERUPTED TOOTH

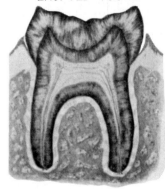

PERIODONTAL CYST

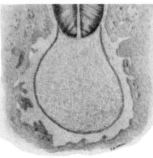

THE PERIODONTAL CYST IS A CYST FORMED IN THE PERIODONTAL MEMBRANE USUALLY AT THE ROOT END OF A PULPLESS INFECTED TOOTH. THE EPITHELIAL LINING IS DERIVED FROM THE EPITHELIAL RESTS (USUALLY REMNANTS OF THE SHEATH OF HERTWIG). THEY ARE COMMONLY THE SEQUELS OF DENTAL GRANULOMATA, IN WHICH EITHER RESTING OR PROLIFERATING EPITHELIUM IS A CONSTANT FINDING.

Figure 11–1 Origin of odontogenic cysts and tumors. (Hamilton B. G. Robinson, School of Dentistry, University of Missouri at Kansas City.)

sembling cysts as a result of bone destruction.

The developmental cysts of the oral cavity are derived from ectodermal remnants. The sheath of Hertwig that outlined the developing roots, the reduced enamel epithelium that connected the tooth bud and oral epithelium, or enamel organs may be the sources of these remnants, as well as inclusions at points of fusion of the primordia of the face and jaw.

DEVELOPMENTAL CYSTS

DEVELOPMENTAL DENTAL CYSTS

Periodontal Cysts.   Periodontal cysts[9, 22, 23] are closed epithelium-lined sacs formed in the periodontal membrane and adjacent structures, usually at the apex of a tooth but sometimes along the lateral surface of its root. The epithelium of these cysts probably is derived from remnants of the sheath of Hertwig or the dental lamina and is stimulated by an inflammatory process or by the same factors that initiated inflammation.

The *radicular* or *periapical* periodontal cyst is usually preceded by a dental granuloma on the apex of a pulpless tooth. The *lateral* periodontal cyst occurs along the side of the root surface, usually as a sequel to a lateral abscess originating in the gingival sulcus, although it may be the result of inflammation progressing from the pulp through a laterally situated pulpal orifice.[32] The *residual* cyst may be left after the extraction of a tooth followed by incomplete enucleation of either of the aforementioned types. Usually cysts that occur lateral to the permanent tooth roots anterior to the first molar, and that contain cementum and dentine, are variants of periodontal cysts at the retained roots of deciduous teeth.

Periodontal cysts may vary in size from a millimeter or less to several millimeters in diameter. Stafne and Millhon[31] found them more common in the maxilla (63 per cent) than in the mandible (37 per cent), and more prevalent in the anterior than in the posterior regions. Of their 500 cases, 151 were the residual type, and 120 of the 349 about roots were on maxillary second incisors. They found the cysts two and one-half times as often on pulpless teeth with untreated pulps as on teeth with filled root canals.

Periodontal cysts are commonly lined by stratified squamous epithelium with a connective tissue capsule. They usually contain a sterile fluid, but, on occasion, may become infected, in which instance they may include pus, seropurulent fluid, sanguinopurulent fluid, semisolid debris, or even solid material. The presence of acute inflammatory cells in the epithelial lining and chronic inflammatory cells in the connective tissue capsule is common.[28] In rare cases, the epithelium is columnar in type, derived from the invasion of the sinuses or the nasal cavity or possibly from metamorphosis of squamous epithelium.

The *odontogenic keratocyst* may appear as a solitary lesion of the jawbones, or there may be multiple cysts.[5] It may also occur as part of the basal cell nevoid syndrome.[9, 16] This cyst is more common in the mandible than in the maxilla, the lower third molar region and ascending ramus being the most usual sites. Almost half of the lesions appear radiographically similar to dentigerous cysts; but histologically the epithelial lining shows marked keratinization. The keratocyst has a high rate of recurrence, and Schofield[25] reported the recurrence of one in a bone graft that had replaced a resected portion of the mandible.

The *calcifying odontogenic cyst* is usually intraosseous, although extraosseous forms have been reported.[14, 18] When bone is involved, the cyst appears as a radiolucent area with varying degrees of radiopaque flecking, depending on the amount of intracystic calcification.[8] The cysts are lined with squamous epithelium, and the elongated epithelial cells of the basal layer show odontogenic characteristics. Scattered between these cells are masses of sheets of epithelial cells and keratin. Large "ghost" epithelial cells are entrapped in the keratin and become calcified. Some authorities distinguish between this cyst and a calcifying epithelial odontogenic tumor (Pindborg tumor).[27] There is a tendency toward recurrence after surgical removal.

In treating periodontal cysts and other oral cysts, the surgeon enculeates the connective tissue capsules and with them removes the closely united epithelial linings. Care must be taken to eliminate the entire epithelium, for any left behind may proliferate to produce a residual cyst. After each successive incomplete operation, the cysts appear to become more invasive.

Oral marsupialization of the cyst (the so-called Partsch operation) is indicated in some cases. See Chapter 12.

Dentigerous Cysts. These are closed epithelium-lined sacs formed about the crowns of unerupted teeth or dental anomalies (odontomas). They usually contain tooth crowns or odontomas, except in unusual cases in which the tooth is removed and the cyst is left behind (causing a residual cyst). These cysts may arise between the reduced enamel epithelium and the tooth or within the reduced enamel or from remnants of odontogenic epithelium. This places their time of development after rather than before the deposition of enamel. The so-called *eruption cysts,* which occur mostly on the third molar teeth, are dentigerous cysts, arising at a late stage of tooth development. The term *follicular cysts* has sometimes been applied to these lesions, but this is confusing.

The term "dentigerous cysts" should be reserved for stratified squamous epithelium-lined connective tissue sacs containing a crown of a tooth or dental anomaly and fluid.[22] The fluid lies between the cyst lining and the tooth. In some instances, an enamel cuticle can be found around the enamel, and it may be present in all dentigerous cysts. Dentigerous cysts may be only slightly larger than the tooth crown, or may become so large as to include a large portion of the maxilla or mandible. In such instances, differentiation from large periodontal cysts may become impossible, and probably is only of academic interest.

The epithelium lining dentigerous cysts has multiple potentials and varies much more than that of other odontogenic cysts. Gorlin observed odontogenic epithelium in 6 of 200 dentigerous cysts and a sebaceous gland in the wall of 1.[11] In 11, the lining was mucoepidermoid. The potentiality of dentigerous cysts to become ameloblastomas has been pointed out frequently.

Primordial Cysts. These cysts are closed epithelium-lined sacs formed through retrogression of the stellate reticulum in enamel organs beginning at a time before any calcified tooth structure has been deposited. Unlike periodontal and dentigerous cysts, they contain no calcified structures.

The term "primordial" has been applied to these cysts because the older term, "follicular," has been indeterminate.[22] Some writers erroneously have called these non-tooth-bearing cysts "dentigerous." The word "primordial" was chosen because it means simplest and most undeveloped in character. Like the other dental cysts, they are lined by stratified squamous epithelium and may be unilocular, multilocular or multiple. A careful clinical and historical study is essential for an accurate diagnosis of this cyst.[23]

DEVELOPMENTAL NONDENTAL CYSTS

Nasoalveolar Cysts. These cysts are formed at the junction of the median nasal, lateral nasal and maxillary processes, *i.e.,* at the base of the nasal alae. They are usually in depressions on the surface of the bone, rather than within the bone substance, and produce asymmetry of the nose and face by their swelling. The cysts are lined with respiratory-type epithelium and contain mucoid fluid. Clinically, they may be mistaken for cysts of dental origin, for dentoalveolar abscesses on the maxillary anterior teeth or for abscesses resulting from an infected hair follicle within the nares.

Palatine Cysts. These are formed in the median fissure of the palate from embryonal remnants.[9] They are lined by stratified squamous epithelium if their anlagen were contributed from the oral side of the fissure; and by ciliated columnar epithelium if their primordia came from the nasal side. These embryonic remnants are simply trapped between the two lateral palatine processes of the maxilla at the time of fusion, and they lie dormant until stimulated by some extrinsic or intrinsic factor. The cysts that occasionally occur between the two maxillary or two mandibular first incisors are not true median cysts, since the bones uniting in these regions have their origin deep within the mesenchyme, with no opportunity for inclusion of epithelial rests. They are probably primordial cysts of supernumerary tooth buds.

Nasopalatine Duct Cysts. Nasopalatine duct cysts, or *incisive canal cysts,* may be located in the incisive canals deep within the bone, or in the soft tissue of the palatine papillae. The latter type have been called *cysts of the palatine papilla (papilla palatina).* The incisive canal is at the place of union of the two lateral palatine processes and the anterior palatine processes. Burket[6] found rudimentary nasopalatine ducts of cystic origin in 21 of 35 human heads examined post-mortem. The stimulus to these developmental remnants may be extrinsic or intrinsic. The connective tissue membranes of these developmental cysts usually contain groups of mucous glands and, commonly, groups of lymphocytes. The epithelium of the lining may be stratified, ciliated columnar, or some transitional type. The cysts are diagnosed by the combined clinical, radiographic and histologic study.[9] Caution should be taken against diagnosing as a cyst a large incisive foramen seen in a periapical radiograph.

Globulomaxillary Cysts. These cysts are found as epithelium-lined sacs between the maxillary second incisor and cuspid. They are formed from epithelial inclusions between the globular (median nasal) and maxillary processes. Clinically, they appear as more or less pear-shaped radiolucent areas between the maxillary second incisor and cuspid, and usually cause a divergence of the roots of those teeth. The adjacent teeth usually have vital pulps, unless they are damaged by an unrelated pulpitis. These cysts may be misdiagnosed as periodontal cysts. It is conceivable that the globulomaxillary cyst may occur between the first and second incisors or between the canine and the first premolars, because the globulomaxillary fissure sometimes passes through these interdental spaces, as evidenced in congenitally formed clefts of the maxilla.

Dermoid and Epidermoid Cysts. Dermoid cysts arise from residual epithelium left in the tissue during union of embryologic processes or implanted by trauma. In the oral cavity they usually are found anteriorly in the floor of the mouth. Clinically they may be confused with ranula. In the wall are one or more skin appendages such as hair follicles, sebaceous or sweat glands. This cyst is not to be confused with the classic teratomas that occur primarily in the ovaries or testes.[2]

Epidermoid cysts are similar, but they contain no definite dermal appendages. Among 54,000 general surgical specimens, Shore[29] observed two dermoid and two epidermoid cysts arising in the floor of the mouth.

Meyer[18] suggested classifying these cysts as (a) epidermoid with an epithelium-lined cavity without skin appendages; (b) dermoid with skin appendages such as hair, hair follicles and sebaceous or sweat glands; and (c) teratoid with skin appendages and, as just noted, mesodermal derivatives such as bone, muscle, respiratory or gastrointestinal tissues.

Branchial Cleft Cysts. These arise from epithelium trapped between the closing branchial arches in the embryo. They are closed epithelial sacs and are usually found anterior to and beneath the sternomastoid muscle[8] or below the ear.

Thyroglossal Duct Cysts. The base of the primitive tongue and thyroid gland directly communicate with one another during development by the thyroglossal duct.[9] This duct normally atrophies during the fifth intrauterine week, but its site persists as the foramen cecum. In rare instances residual tissue may become cystic. These cysts lie beneath the foramen cecum in the floor of the mouth, along the thyroid gland, in the thyroid cartilage at the cricoid cartilage, or in the suprasternal notch.

These cysts occur in the midline of the neck.

RETENTION CYSTS

Mucous Cysts (Mucoceles). Mucoceles are cavities filled with a homogenous, mucin-containing substance that is a product of salivary glands.[4] They occur as soft, somewhat spherical enlargements in the minor salivary glands of the lower lip, buccal mucosa, tongue or floor of the mouth. Apparently, they usually result from obstruction of the ducts, dilatation and rupture of the ducts and pooling of the escaped fluid in the connective tissue. The cyst-like cavity is lined with compressed connective tissue rather than with epithelial cells.

Ranulas. These are cavities of cyst-like nature formed in the floor of the mouth[4, 9] by the rentention of fluid in the sublingual gland or its ducts (more rarely, the submaxillary gland) or in a manner similar to that of mucoceles. The ranula begins its formation on one or the other side of the jaw, and by slow, expansive growth fills the floor of the mouth. As it expands, the overlying tissues achieve a paper thinness, and the lesion becomes blue. It contains a mucoid fluid derived from the secretory cells of the glands.

CYST-LIKE LESIONS

If a radiolucent area in the bone or a swelling of soft tissue is considered indicative of a cyst, almost any lesion may at one time or another simulate a cyst. When a young person receives a blow on the mandible, especially near the angle, a few bone trabeculae may be crushed and hemorrhage then ensues. The reaction will result in a radiolucent area, a cavity without a definite lining and containing blood debris and connective tissue, or even represented as empty bone cavities. These noncystic lesions have been called *"traumatic cysts."* They may occur at the apices of lower anterior teeth under excessive occlusal trauma.

Tumors of any type, malignant or benign, may resemble cysts radiographically and clinically. *Central giant cell tumors of bone* are especially cyst-like in their appearance. *Cementomas* in their early (soft tissue) stages may resemble periodontal cysts.[6]

Xanthomatosis, osteitis fibrosa cystica and other metabolic disturbances may present cyst-like appearances, as may osteomyelitis, actinomycosis, syphilis and other diseases caused by living agents.

REFERENCES

1. Anderson, H. C., Kim, B., and Minkowitz, S.: Calcifying epithelial odontogenic tumor of Pindborg. Cancer, 24:585, 1968.
2. Babbush, C. A., and August, R. V.: Ectopic teeth. A case of bilateral benign cystic ovarian teratomas containing dental and periodontal structures. Oral Surg., 16:586 (May), 1963.
3. Bhaskar, S. N.: Adenoameloblastoma. J. Oral Surg., 22:211–226 (May), 1964.
4. Bhaskar, S. N., Bolden, T. E., and Weinmann, J. P.: Pathogenesis of mucoceles. J. Dent. Res., 35:863–874 (Dec.), 1956.
5. Browne, R. M.: Odontogenic keratocyst: Clinical aspects. Brit. Dent. J., 128:225, 1970.
6. Burket, L. W.: Nasopalatine duct structures and peculiar bony pattern observed in anterior maxillary area. Arch. Pathol., 23:793, 1937.
7. Calman, H. I.: Sublingual branchiogenic cyst. Report of a case. Oral Surg., 16:333 (Mar.), 1963.
8. Camp, L., and Stout, A. P.: Branchial anomalies and neoplasms. Am. J. Surg., 87:186, 1928.
9. Colby, R. A., Kerr, D. A., and Robinson, H. B. G.: Color Atlas of Oral Pathology. 3rd ed. Philadelphia, J. B. Lippincott Co., 1971.
10. Giansanti, J. S., Somerson, A., and Waldron, C. A.: Odontogenic adenomatoid tumor (adenoameloblastoma). Oral Surg., 30:69, 1970.
11. Gorlin, R. J.: The potentialities of oral epithelium manifest by mandibular dentigerous cysts. Oral Surg., 10:271–284 (Mar.), 1957.
12. Gorlin, R. J., Meskin, L. H., and Brodey, R.: Odontogenic tumors in man and animals. Ann. N.Y. Acad. Sci., 108:722–771, 1963.
13. Gorlin, R. J., Pindborg, J. J., Clausen, F. P., and Vickers, R. A.: The calcifying odontogenic cyst—a possible analogue of the cutaneous epithelioma of Malherbe. Oral Surg., 15:1235, 1962.
14. Gorlin, R. J., Pindborg, J. J., Redman, R. S., Williamson, J. J., and Hansen, L. S.: The calcifying odontogenic cyst. Cancer, 17:723–729 (June), 1964.
15. Gorlin, R. J., and Goltz, R. W.: Multiple nevoid basal cell epithelioma, jaw cysts, and bifid rib. New Eng. J. Med., 262:908, 1960.
16. James, P. L., and Fisher, P. L.: Melanotic ectodermal tumor of infancy. Brit. Dent. J., 108:335, 1970.
17. Kronfeld, R.: Adamantinoma. J.A.D.A., 17:681, 1930.
18. Meyer, I.: Dermoid cysts (dermoids) of the floor of the mouth. Oral Surg., 8:1149–1164 (Nov.), 1955.
19. Pindborg, J. J.: Calcifying odontogenic epithelial tumor: Review of the literature and report of an extraosseous case. Acta Odontol. Scand., 4:419, 1966.
20. Robinson, H. B. G.: Histologic study of the ameloblastoma. Arch. Pathol., 23:664, 1937.
21. Robinson, H. B. G.: Ameloblastoma. Arch. Pathol., 23:831, 1937.
22. Robinson, H. B. G.: Classification of cysts of the jaws. Am. J. Orthodont., 31:370, 1945.
23. Robinson, H. B. G., Koch, W. E., and Kolas, S.: Radiographic interpretation of oral cysts. Dent. Radiogr. Photogr., 29:61, 1956.
24. Robinson, H. B. G., and Wallace, W. R. J.: Solid to cystic degeneration in ameloblastoma. Arch. Pathol., 28:207, 1939.
25. Schofield, J. J.: Unusual recurrence of an odontogenic keratocyst. Brit. Dent. J., 130:487, 1971.
26. Schweitzer, F. C., and Barnfield, W. F.: Ameloblastoma of the mandible with metastasis to the lungs. J. Oral Surg., 1:287, 1943.
27. Shafer, W. G., Hine, M. K., and Levy, B. M.: A Textbook of Oral Pathology. 3rd ed. Philadelphia, W. B. Saunders Co., 1974.
28. Shear, M.: Inflammation in dental cysts. Oral Surg., 17:756–767 (June), 1964.
29. Shore, B. R.: Sublingual epidermoid cysts. Ann. Surg., 108:305, 1938.
30. Small, I. A., and Waldron, C. A.: Ameloblastomas of jaws. J. Oral Surg., 8:281–297, 1955.
31. Stafne, E. C., and Millhon, J. A.: Periodontal cysts. J. Oral Surg., 3:102, 1945.
32. Standish, S. M., and Shafer, W. G.: Lateral periodontal cyst. J. Periodont., 29:27–33 (Jan.), 1958.
33. Thoma, K. H.: The circumferential dentigerous cyst. Oral Surg., 18:368–371, 1964.
34. Thoma, K. H., and Robinson, H. B. G.: Oral and Dental Diagnosis. 5th ed. Philadelphia, W. B. Saunders Co., 1960.
35. Webster's New International Dictionary. Springfield, Mass., G. & C. Merriam Co., 1928.

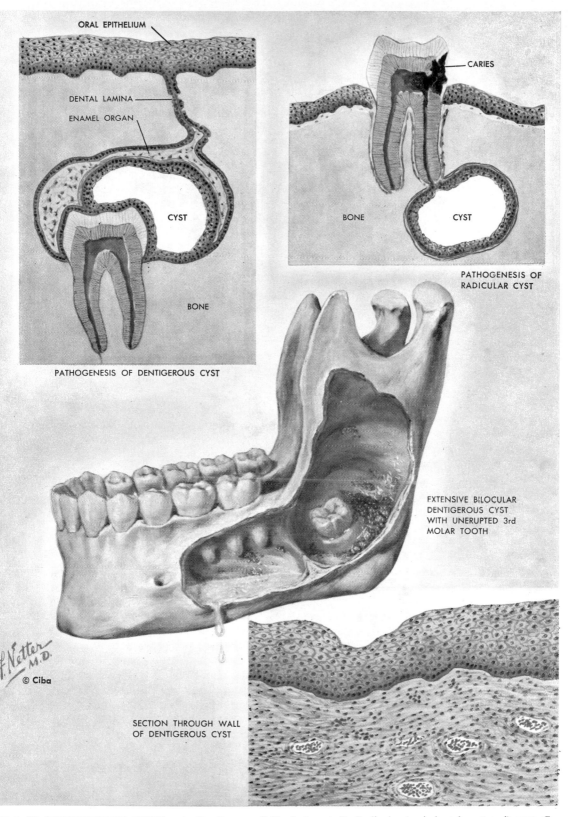

ORAL EPITHELIUM

DENTAL LAMINA

ENAMEL ORGAN

CYST

BONE

PATHOGENESIS OF DENTIGEROUS CYST

CARIES

BONE

CYST

PATHOGENESIS OF RADICULAR CYST

EXTENSIVE BILOCULAR DENTIGEROUS CYST WITH UNERUPTED 3rd MOLAR TOOTH

SECTION THROUGH WALL OF DENTIGEROUS CYST

F. Netter M.D.

© Ciba

Plate III ODONTOGENIC CYSTS. A, Dentigerous (follicular) cyst. B, Radicular (periodontal root end) cyst. C, Pseudo-bilocular dentigerous cyst. The lumen of these cysts is usually filled with a thin watery yellow fluid or a thick creamy whitish fluid which simulates that seen in a soft boiled egg. Older cysts are filled with a light yellowish thick caseous material. Osseous septa arising from the surrounding osseous tissue, when seen on the radiograph, give the viewer the impression that there are loculations in the cyst. This may or may not be true as there may be loculi in the soft tissue, not surrounded by thin osseous walls. D, It is not possible to histologically distinguish this section of the wall of a dentigerous cyst from any other odontogenic cyst. (Drawing from Stern, L.: Cysts. CIBA CLINICAL SYMPOSIA, Vol. 5, No. 3, 1953.)

CHAPTER 12

TREATMENT OF CYSTS OF THE ORAL CAVITY

Regardless of the cause of a cyst, there are three accepted methods of treatment: (1) enucleation of the cyst in its entirety; (2) marsupialization by which the cystic cavity is made a part of the oral cavity; and (3) marsupialization, followed weeks later by enucleation. The "simple bone cyst" (SBC) is "treated" by making a window into the bone cavity. For the specific details of these treatments, see the text that follows.

RADICULAR CYST
(Periodontal, Periapical, Dental Root End, Dentoalveolar Cyst)

The most frequently found small cyst in the oral cavity is the radicular cyst.

It is impossible to tell from a radiograph whether or not the small radiolucent area at the apex of a tooth is a dental granuloma or a cyst. Only histologic examination will reveal whether there is an epithelium-lined cavity in the small (0.5 cm. or smaller) tissue mass, which makes it a true cyst. All periapical granulomas should be carefully removed to insure that those which do contain epithelial cells are thus prevented from continued growth and eventual residual cyst development. All tissue found at the apex or at the root of a tooth should be as carefully removed as though it were known to be a cyst and saved for microscopic examination.

Development of Radicular Cysts. The series of drawings shown in Figure 12–2 illustrates the development of a radicular cyst from a periapical dental granuloma.

In Figure 12–2A, a maxillary cuspid with advanced caries resulting in pulpal infection and necrosis is shown. The noxious substances that have escaped from the root canal into the periapical tissues have stimulated defensive activity by the formation of a mass of acute inflammatory tissue, which is known as a dental granuloma.

Shown in Figure 12–2B are epithelial cells in the strands or clumps commonly found in dental granulomas. These are thought to originate from the ordinarily nonmitosing epithelial remnants of root sheath known as rests of Malassez. Irritating material stimulates these cells into activity.

The cells in the center of the large mass of epithelial cells die because they lack the essentials for life at their distance from the periphery (Fig. 12–2C), and fluid accumulates in the void thus created (Fig. 12–2D). The increase in hydrostatic pressure caused by the fluid accumulation flattens and compresses the epithelial cells lining the fibrous capsule of the cyst. The cyst expands in all directions because this continuous peripheral pressure on the surrounding osseous tissue stimulates osteoclastic activity, and the bone resorbs, just as it does under the pressure of dentures or orthodontic appliances. The cyst will continuously increase in size, because as the fluid

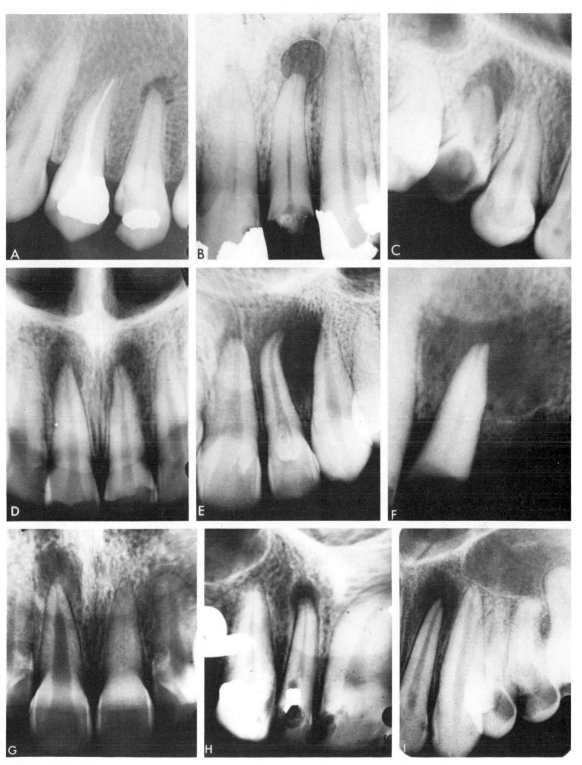

Figure 12–1 These are examples of periapical radiolucencies. These areas usually contain inflammatory hyperplastic tissue and are known as periapical dental granulomas. They are either well circumscribed or have a diffuse border. If these periapical granulomas are not removed at the time of tooth extraction, there is a good possibility that they will develop into radicular cysts, since most of them contain epithelial cells. For that reason the operator must make certain that dental granulomas are removed with curettes at the time of extraction. Some are firmly attached to the apex of one or more roots, and these are removed with the associated teeth at the time of extraction.

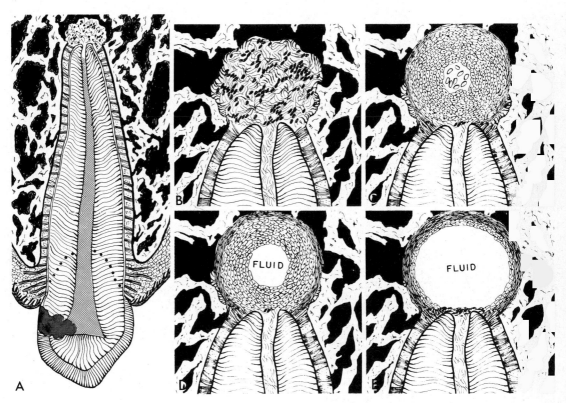

Figure 12–2 Formation of a radicular cyst. (See text for explanation.)

increases, there will be a continuous imbalance of hydrostatic pressure between its contents and the surrounding osseous or soft tissues, resulting from the increased osmolality of the cyst fluid (Fig. 12–2E).

Toller has demonstrated that the "mean osmotic differences between serum and cyst fluid was found to be of the order of 11 mOsm, and this is a sufficient difference in osmotic pressure to account for the observed hydrostatic pressures (70 cm. H_2O) and clinical rates of growth."[81] It is surprising to note that there are those who still think that odontogenic cysts are the direct result of periapical infection or are all infected. Cysts may become infected but this is a secondary episode, not primary. One must remember that radicular cysts develop in periapical dental granulomas and Grossman has shown that in cultures he took of 109 cases of periapical dental granulomas and controls, 93 were negative (85.3 per cent).[37]

Contents of Radicular Cysts. These cysts usually contain a sterile straw-colored fluid with an iridescent sheen imparted by cholesterol crystals. However, they may be infected and contain pus, seropurulent fluid or sanguinopurulent fluid. Occasionally the content is thick and caseous with epithelial and hemorrhagic debris.

SMALL RADICULAR CYSTS

The infected tooth is extracted, if that is the best treatment in the particular case. The *very* small radicular cysts can be enucleated through the root socket by careful insertion of the thin edge of the curette between the connective tissue capsule and the enveloping osseous tissue. Use the largest-sized curette that can be inserted into the cyst cavity. At the start of this "peeling" process, the bowl of the curette is always turned so that the concavity of the bowl is toward the bone. The thin edge of the curette is pushed between the epithelium-lined connective tissue capsule and the bone, starting at the junction of the alveolus and the cystic wall and continuing all around the periphery of the alveolus, stripping the wall away from its attachment to bone and pushing it toward the center of the cystic cavity. When the "equator" of the cystic cavity is reached by this process, the curette is removed and turned so

that the concavity of the bowl of the curette is turned toward the center of the cystic cavity, and by a scooping motion the bowl of the curette is made to slide under the cyst, freeing its capsule from the remainder of its attachment to bone and lifting it out of the bony crypt in the jaw. (See Figure 12–6G, illustrating this technique of enucleation.) If difficulty is encountered when the operator is attempting to remove the cyst from the cavity through the alveolus, he should withdraw the curette and use a mosquito forceps to grasp the cystic wall.

The cavity should now be carefully examined to make certain *that all of the cystic membrane has been removed.* A suction tip and a good light are essential. The parts of the cavity that are not visible should be carefully explored wih the curette. If remnants of the capsule lined with epithelial cells, or a portion of a dental granuloma containing epithelial cells, are left behind, there will be a recurrence of the cyst from the former, or a development of a cyst from the latter. Remaining segments of a dental granuloma without epithelial cells are replaced by bone.

LARGE RADICULAR CYSTS

Very large radicular cysts should be marsupialized if enucleation might (a) produce fistulas into the maxillary sinus or nasal cavity, (b) result in the loss or devitalization of teeth other than those already involved, (c) traumatize neurovascular bundles, or (d) cause a fracture.

Large radicular cysts revealed by radiographic examination almost always appear to involve several teeth. It is extremely important, however, *that only the nonvital teeth be removed or treated.* Tooth vitality can be ascertained only by carefully checking all the teeth with an electric pulp tester. Entirely too many sound, healthy teeth have been extracted because, in the radiograph, the roots *appeared* to be involved in the cystic cavity. *Extract only the nonvital teeth.* Even in some cases of nonvital teeth it is desirable and good practice to fill the root canals and retain these teeth. In some cases the cyst is enucleated and an apicoectomy is performed (see the case shown in Figure 12–22). Bone will eventually fill in around the roots of the teeth.

(*Text continued on page 539*)

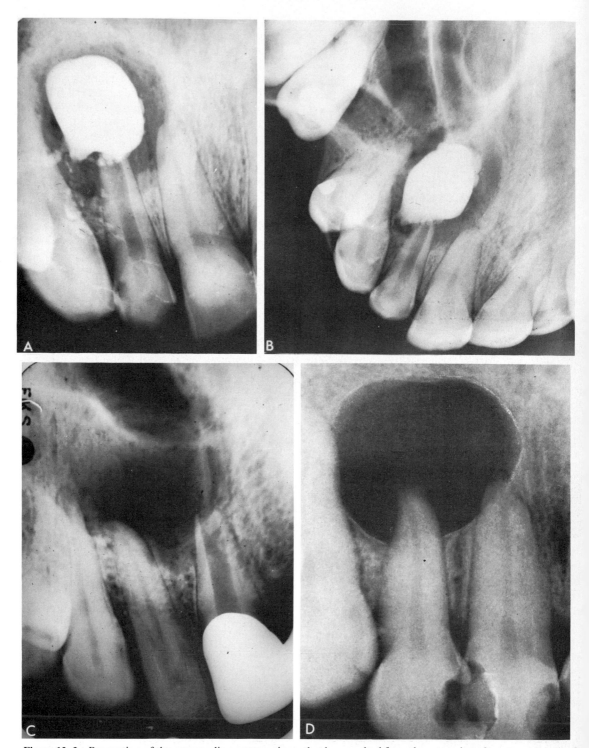

Figure 12–3   Resorption of the surrounding osseous tissue that has resulted from the expansion of a cyst, as described in Figure 12–2.

A and *B*, The pulpal vitality of these lateral incisors was destroyed, probably by trauma, before the roots were completely formed. This is demonstrated by the wide root canal with the incomplete apex. Radiopaque fluid was injected into these cysts. Note the thick cyst walls.

C and *D*, A typical radicular cyst, globular in shape, with well-defined borders surrounded by a thin sclerotic line of osseous tissue.

(Figure 12–3 continued on opposite page)

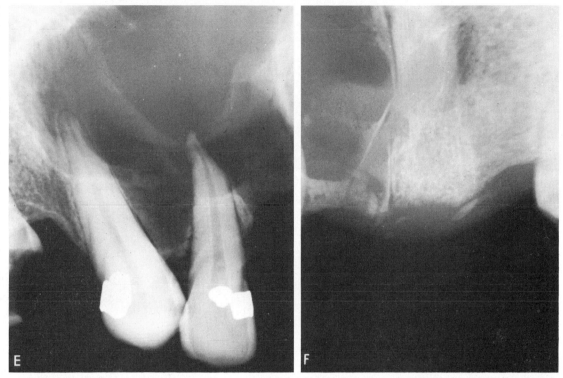

Figure 12–3 *(Continued.) E* and *F,* A very large radicular cyst that developed about the apex of the lateral incisor, whose vitality has been lost for some unknown reason. The expansion of this cyst is extensive in all directions, including the apical area of the cuspid, although the apex of the cuspid still is covered with bone, up to the floor of the nasal cavity, and, as is shown in *F,* anteriorly to the midline of the maxilla.

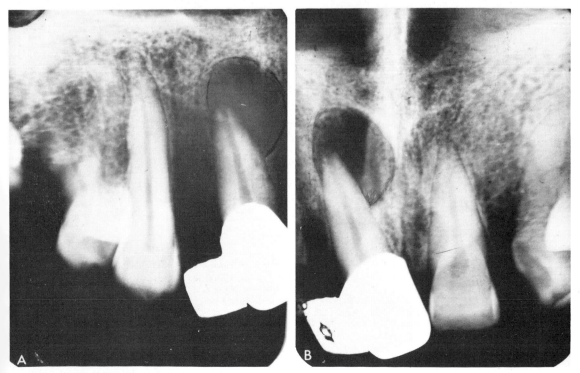

Figure 12–4 A well-circumscribed radicular cyst about the apex of the left central incisor.

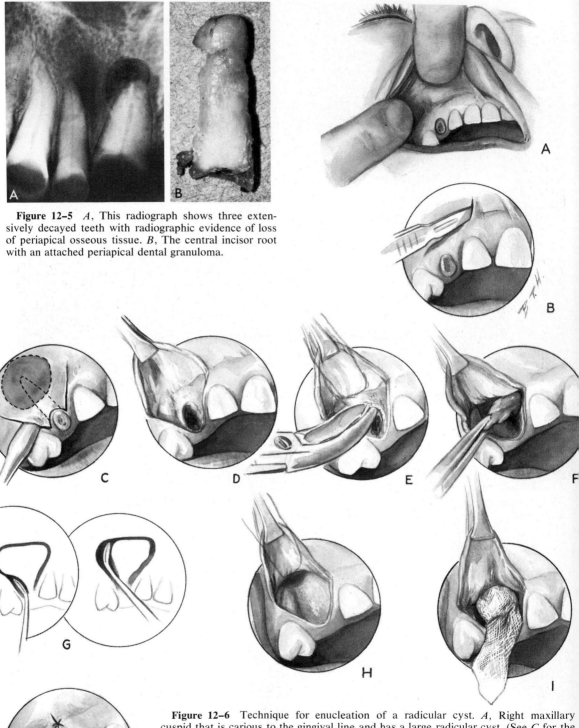

Figure 12-5 *A,* This radiograph shows three extensively decayed teeth with radiographic evidence of loss of periapical osseous tissue. *B,* The central incisor root with an attached periapical dental granuloma.

Figure 12-6 Technique for enucleation of a radicular cyst. *A,* Right maxillary cuspid that is carious to the gingival line and has a large radicular cyst. (See *C* for the outline of this cyst.) *B,* Start of incision for the mucoperiosteal flap. *C,* Incision completed and periosteal elevator inserted to elevate and reflect the mucoperiosteal flap. *D,* Flap reflected and held back by the Allis forceps, exposing the thin cortical bone. *E,* Thin cortical bone removed with end-cutting rongeurs.

F, Cystic membrane grasped with a hemostat. *G,* With the curette the cystic membrane is stripped from the bony crypt. *H,* Cyst has been completely enucleated, and the bony margins have been rounded. *I,* Cystic cavity is filled with iodoform gauze. If the cystic cavity is small and is filled with a blood clot, this dressing is not necessary. *J,* Mucoperiosteal flap is replaced and sutured into position. Note the iodoform gauze drain.

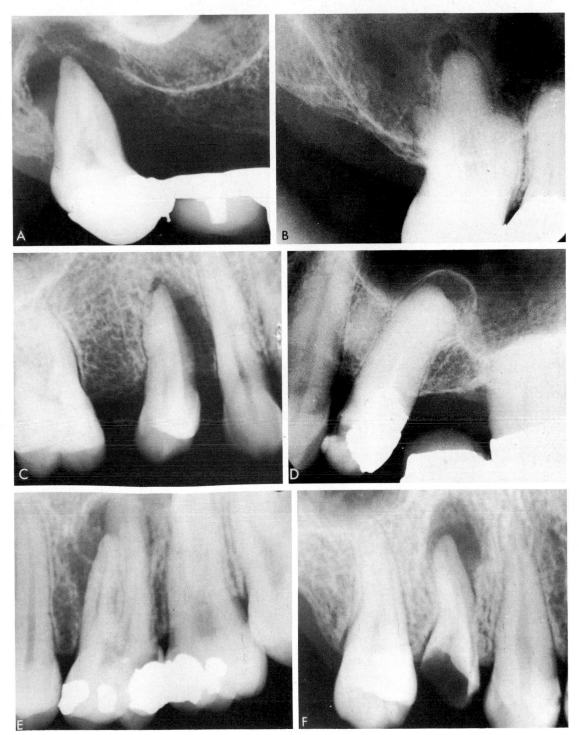

Figure 12–7 Examples of periapical radiolucent areas on the apices of maxillary molars and bicuspids. Some of these areas are well circumscribed with sclerotic borders, while others have irregular diffused borders, representing different densities in the bone that influence the resorption rate of bone. *A* through *D* also illustrate the proximity of some radiolucent areas to the maxillary sinus.

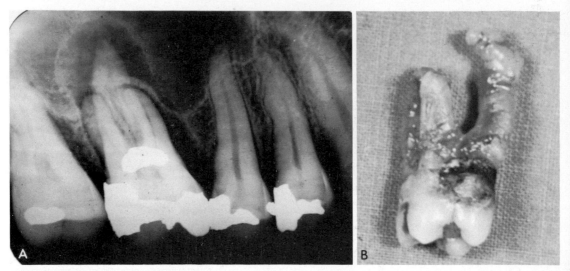

Figure 12-8 *A*, A maxillary molar with a large area of periapical radiolucency surrounded with a clear-cut sclerotic border. *B*, The molar shown in *A* with the attached periapical dental granuloma.

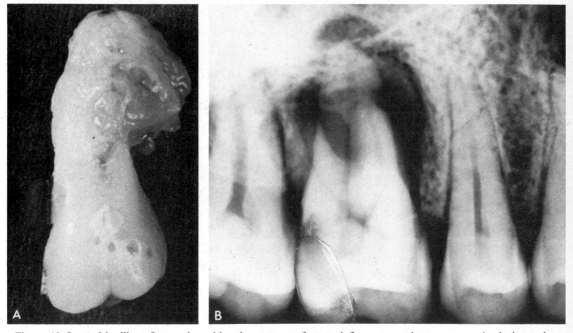

Figure 12-9 *A*, Maxillary first molar with a large mass of acute inflammatory tissue, commonly designated as a periapical dental granuloma. *B*, Radiograph of a maxillary first molar with a large area of periapical radiolucency, indicating the probability of a periapical granuloma such as that shown in *A*.

Figure 12-10 Periapical dental radiographs with examples of periapical lesions of the mandibular anterior teeth and mandibular bicuspids. It will be noted that the radiolucent areas involving the roots of these teeth may involve the lateral surface and therefore could possibly be periodontal cysts (*A* and *I*). They are either well circumscribed (*E*, *F* and *H*) or have diffused borders (*B*, *C* and *D*). Some are small (3 to 4 mm. in diameter); others are quite extensive and involve up to three or four anterior teeth. These radiolucent areas probably represent destructive processes and at operation will be found to contain kinds of acute inflammatory tissue that are commonly known as periapical granulomas or periodontal granulomas. Most dental granulomas contain individual epithelial cells, or clumps or strands of them, from

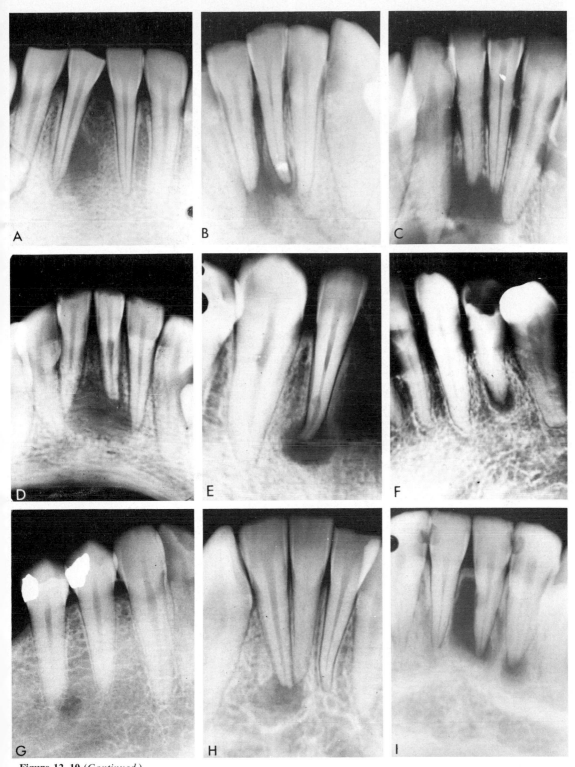

Figure 12–10 (*Continued.*)
which the radicular cysts shown in subsequent illustrations can develop. As has already been pointed out, these collections of acute or chronic inflammatory tissue (dental granulomas) should be removed at the time of surgery, whether that surgery involves extraction of the teeth or periapical treatments, such as apicoectomies. The reason for removing this tissue, of course, is to avoid the possible development of residual cysts. The radiolucent area in *G* is the mental foramen, which is projected over a portion of the apex of the second mandibular bicuspid by the angle of the x-ray tube when this radiograph was made.

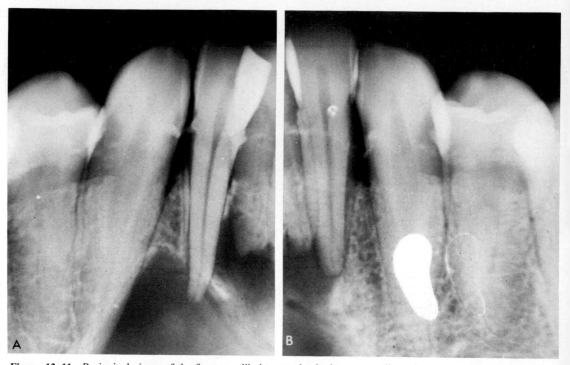

Figure 12–11 Periapical views of the four mandibular anterior incisors, revealing a large central radiolucent area in bone that involves all mandibular incisor apices, but only the central incisor apices show irregular resorption of their roots. The resorption of the roots of teeth from the pressure of cysts or periapical granulomas is not common. It is of interest to note that while the apices of both the mandibular right and left lateral incisors appear to be involved in this radiolucent area, there is no evidence of resorption of their apices. The most logical explanation is that the apices of these two teeth are either anterior or posterior to the extensive radiolucent area in the bone. (This theory was supported by the fact that both of these teeth were vital.)

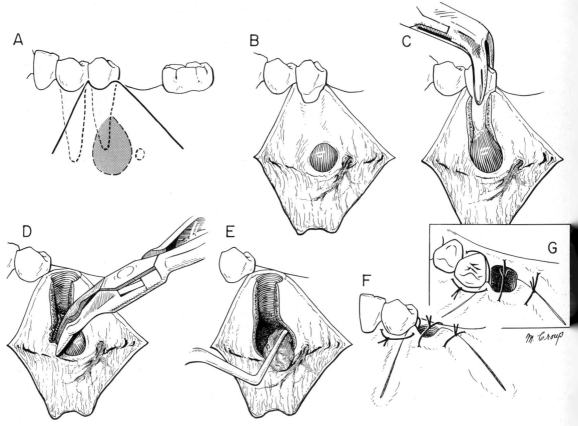

Figure 12–12 *See opposite page for legend.*

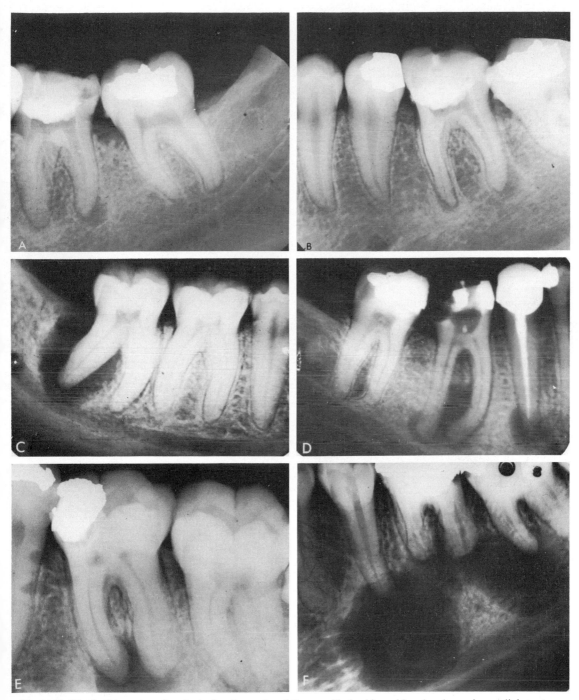

Figure 12–17 In this series of periapical radiographs of the mandibular bicuspid and molar region, radiolucent areas can be seen about the apices of the molar teeth and also about one bicuspid root. These radiolucent areas are either diffused or have clear-cut sclerotic borders. These proved to be periapical granulomas, which were removed at the time surgery was carried out.

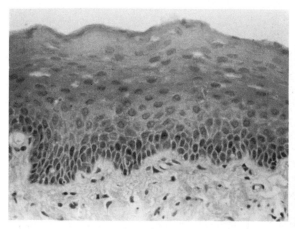

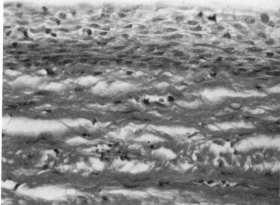

Figure 12–18 A section of normal stratified squamous epithelium from the buccal mucosa.

Figure 12–19 A fibrous cyst wall, in which the lining of stratified squamous epithelial cells has been compressed by the osmotic pressure of the fluid within the lumen of the cyst. Below the compressed epithelium is the fibrous capsular wall of the cyst.

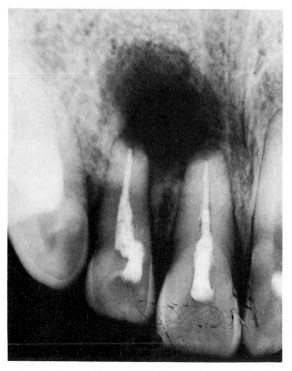

Figure 12–20 The left central incisor and lateral incisor with excised root apices and inadequate root canal fillings. In spite of the treatment of the root canals and the apicoectomies, there is a large radiolucent area with diffused borders present. It probably represents a periapical granuloma or perhaps a cyst.

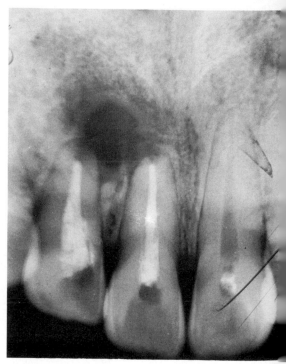

Figure 12–21 Following re-treatment and filling of the central and lateral incisor roots, and the surgical removal of a large periapical granuloma, the original area of radiolucency has materially reduced in size but shows a well-circumscribed area of osseous sclerosis about the periphery. When a periapical lesion penetrates both the lingual and the labial or buccal cortices, the bone will never completely fill in. All too frequently a dentist unfamiliar with the history of a case like this will subsequently diagnose it incorrectly as a residual area of infection. This is not true. Such areas can be positively identified by passing a needle in a syringe through the soft tissue filling one of these voids from the labial to the lingual side (see Figure 12–23).

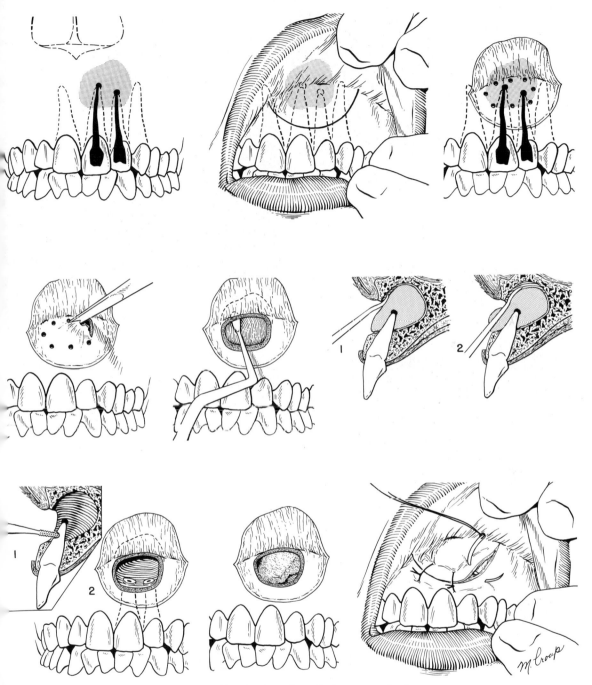

Figure 12–22   Enucleation of a radicular cyst, and apicoectomy.

The larger radicular cysts (over 0.5 cm. in diameter) that are to be enucleated should not be removed through the alveolus. It is impossible to reach with a curette every portion of the cavity through the alveolus; hence there is a great possibility of not removing all the epithelium-lined sac, with the result being

subsequent recurrence. (See Figure 12–12 for correct technique.)

In the removal of large radicular cysts a large mucoperiosteal flap should be reflected, exposing the alveolar bone overlying the cystic area. The operator makes a window through the bony plate by cutting out the thin

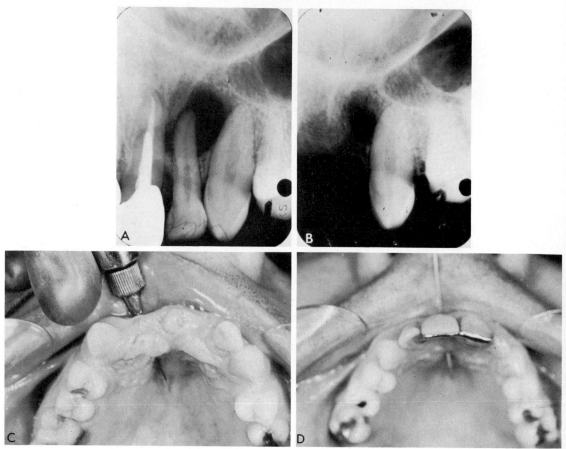

Figure 12–23 *A*, Both the right central and lateral incisors shown here were extracted. When the radicular cyst was removed, it was discovered that both labial and palatal cortical bones had been resorbed. *B*, Three years later, during a routine oral radiographic examination, he was told by his dentist that he had a residual cyst. *C*, When both cortices are destroyed, bone does not fill the cavity. This fact is shown in the radiograph in *B* and proved by passing a needle through the fault from the labial to the lingual side, as shown in *C*. *D*, A similar case.

bone, first using a bur or a chisel and then enlarging the opening by cutting the thinned-out bone with bone shears or a crosscut fissure bur. This process is continued until solid bone is reached and an adequate-sized window for that particular cyst has been made. The cyst is then "shelled out" by means of the largest-bowled curette that will fit into the bony crypt. The reason for using a large-bowled curette is to prevent puncturing the cystic wall.

After the epithelium-lined sac has been removed, the cavity is examined, the alveolar process is smoothed, and the cavity is irrigated with normal saline solution. A drain is inserted, and the soft tissue flap is replaced and sutured with black silk. There is no need to pack the cavity with iodoform gauze. As granulation takes place, the cavity can be irrigated with diluted Dakin's solution to keep it clean.

MARSUPIALIZATION (PARTSCH OPERATION) FOR LARGE CYSTS

The operation of marsupialization has been known as the Partsch operation, after the German surgeon who was supposed to have originated the technique. However, at the University of Istanbul a few years ago Chevket Ö. Tagay first called my attention to the fact that it was an American dentist by the name of John S. Smith, from Lancaster, Pennsylvania, who in 1885 was the first to publish this basic technique that has been modified and improved by others since.[71]

Marsupialization of an oral cyst is the

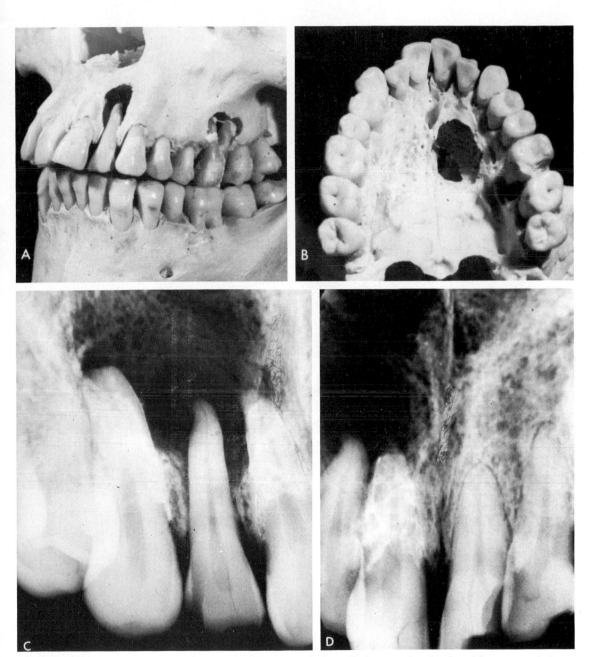

Figure 12-24 *A*, This anatomic specimen demonstrates a large radicular cyst that developed from a nonvital maxillary lateral incisor. By gradual expansion over the years and resultant pressure erosion, it has destroyed not only a small area of the labial cortical plate but, as shown in *B*, a large area of the palatine bone of the maxilla. Furthermore, the osseous floor of the nasal cavity has also been eroded. An attempt to enucleate this cyst would have created a naso-oral fistula. It would have been technically impossible to free the cyst lining from the mucoperiosteum of the palate, even with sharp dissection, and be absolutely certain that not a shred of stratified squamous epithelium remained. If it did, a recurrent cyst would develop. This case was one in which marsupialization was clearly indicated. *C* and *D*, Radiographs of *A*.

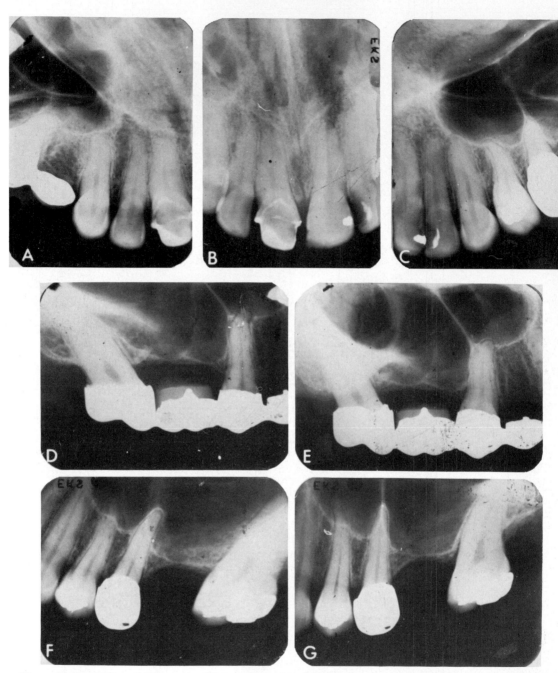

Figure 12–25 Differential diagnosis of the maxillary sinus from a cyst is best accomplished by radiographing the entire maxillary arch and comparing the side on which a cyst is suspected, from the radiographic findings, with the radiographs of the opposite side. Supplement these radiographs with vitality tests on *all* maxillary teeth. *A* to *C,* In this case a supposed large radicular cyst was diagnosed by routine radiographs of the crowned upper right bicuspid. *F* and *G,* However, the mistaken diagnosis was readily corrected when the rest of the maxillary arch was radiographed, as shown in *D* and *E.* It should also be noted that the lamina dura is very distinct above the apex of the suspected right bicuspid, a situation which would be nonexistent if this tooth had been the source of the suspected cyst.

The maxillary sinuses (*D, E, F, G*) in this case are exceptionally large. Note that on both sides they approximate the apices of the cuspids. The characteristic W formation due to the long septum in both sinuses is visible in this case. Another valuable diagnostic method that should always be used in case of doubt is to attempt to aspirate fluid from the suspected cyst with a syringe on which has been mounted a 20 gauge needle.

If the oral surgeon draws in air and readily reinjects air, he has penetrated the maxillary sinus, not a cystic cavity or a tumor.

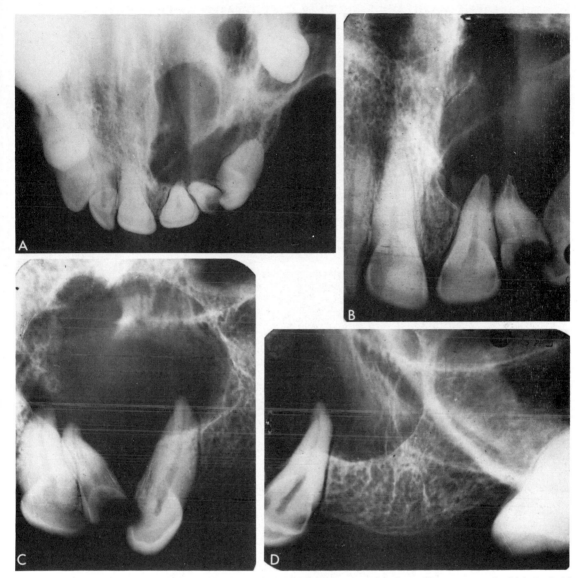

Figure 12–26 This large maxillary radicular cyst, which simulated a globulomaxillary cyst and which probably originated from the filled nonvital lateral incisor, expanded and destroyed the vitality of the central incisor. The cuspid was vital, and the apex was covered with a thin layer of bone, as shown in the occlusal view. No bone was over the central incisor. This case was treated by marsupialization and an apicoectomy of the lateral incisor.

surgical procedure whereby the cyst is made an accessory compartment of the oral cavity. In odontogenic, fissural and hemorrhagic "simple bone cysts" (SBC's), this permits the escape of the fluid contained in the cyst, whose hydrostatic pressure of 70 cm. H_2O in the odontogenic and fissural cysts and 5 cm. H_2O in hemorrhagic cysts,[81] had been continuously exerted on the cyst capsule. This pressure was in turn transmitted to the enveloping bone, which stimulated osteoclastic activity, resulting in resorption of bone, progressive enlargement of the bony cavity, and thus ex-

pansion of the cyst in all directions. When the cyst is marsupialized and drainage is maintained by keeping the opening into the cyst cavity patent with an obturator (see Figure 12–36 for details of this technique), these osteoclasts become osteoblasts and new bone is steadily laid down all around the remaining capsule, until the bone cavity is *completely filled with osseous tissue,* which is much more radiopaque than the surrounding bone. The capsule steadily diminishes in size, until it disappears altogether as the bone fills in around it.

(Text continued on page 550)

LARGE MAXILLARY RADICULAR CYST TREATED BY ENUCLEATION

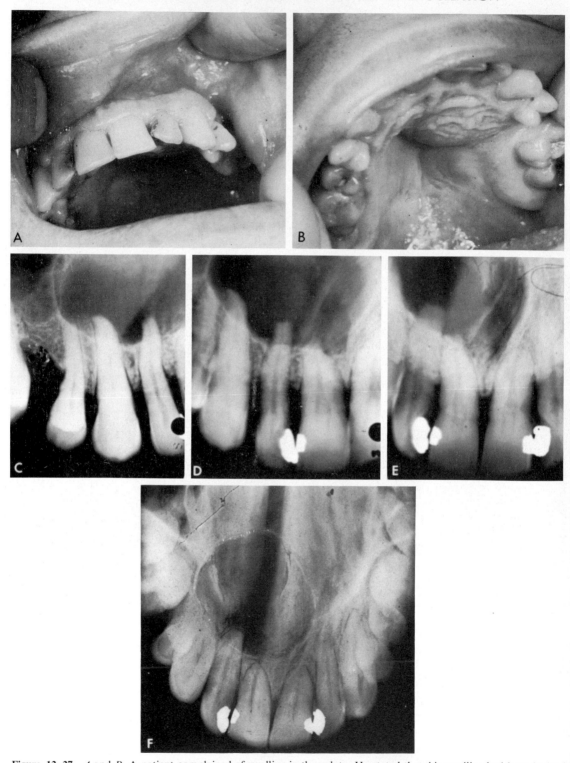

Figure 12–27 *A* and *B*, A patient complained of swelling in the palate. He stated that this swelling had been incised and drained three times. There was, as shown here, a soft, fluctuant swelling in the palate. There was no labial swelling. All teeth were vital except the left lateral incisor.

C to *F*, Periapical and occlusal radiographs revealed a large radiolucent area. A diagnosis of a radicular cyst was made.

(Figure 12–27 continued on opposite page)

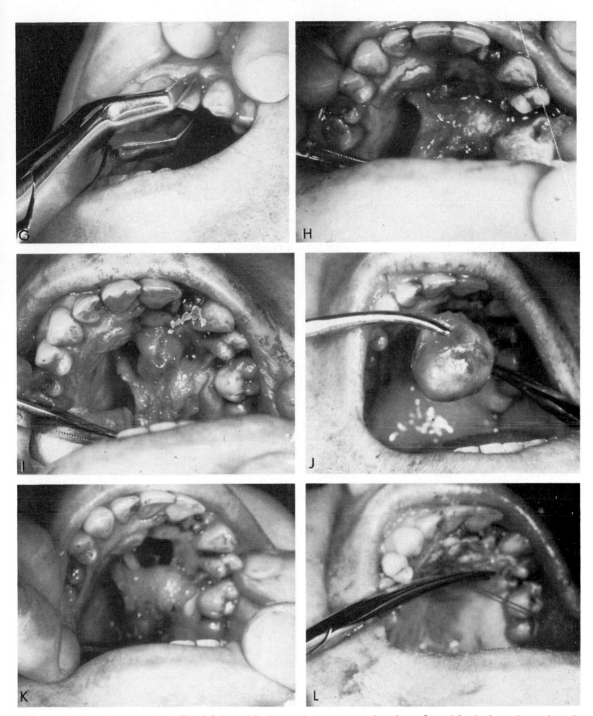

Figure 12–27   (*Continued.*) *G*, The left lateral incisor *only* was removed, and pus flowed freely from the socket; *do not remove teeth which are vital even though radiographically they appear to be involved in the cystic cavity. H*, A palatal flap was turned back—the same type of flap that is used to expose the palatal bone prior to the removal of a palatally impacted cuspid (see Chapter 5). *I*, As the mucoperiosteal flap was reflected, it drew with it the cyst membrane; there were only two points of firm attachment of this cyst: (1) around the apex of the left lateral incisor socket, and (2) the palatal mucoperiosteal membrane where the previous incisions had been made for drainage. *J*, The radicular cyst completely enucleated and carefully freed from its attachment to the mucoperiosteal flap. *K*, Crypt of radicular cyst. *L*, Bony crypt filled with iodoform gauze, and mucoperiosteal flap replaced and sutured in position.

(*Figure 12–27 continued on following page*)

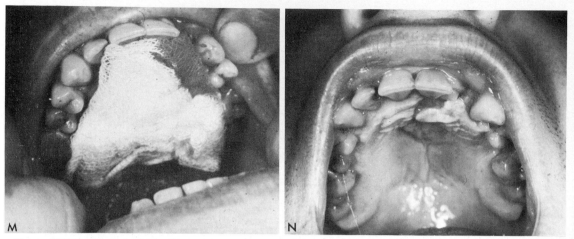

Figure 12–27 *(Continued.) M,* The palate packed with gauze; this should be kept in position for 10 hours. *N,* Appearance of the wound 3 days postoperatively.

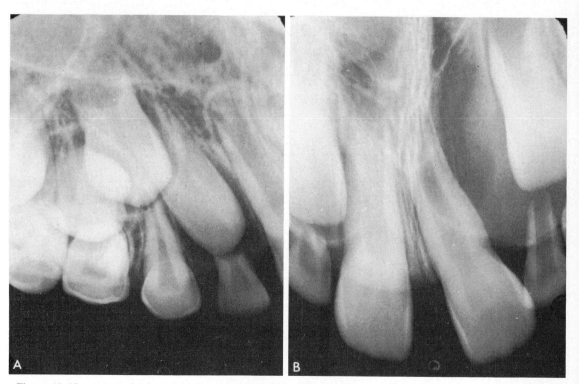

Figure 12–28 *A* to *D,* Periapical radiographs of an 8-year-old child with a large radicular cyst originating from the nonvital deciduous maxillary right lateral incisor, whose dental pulp was devitalized by trauma when he was 2 years of age. The cyst has moved the erupting permanent lateral incisor distally and the partially formed root of the permanent right central incisor mesially.

E, Posteroanterior (Waters' position) view of the maxilla, showing the size and shape of the radicular cyst and lateral incisor. One must remember in viewing this radiograph that the lateral incisor and cyst are *not in* the maxillary sinus, but in *front* of it. Thus the maxillary sinus is projected over the radicular cyst and unerupted permanent lateral incisor when the radiograph is taken.

Treatment: Extraction of the right deciduous central and lateral incisors and enucleation of the cyst are required. The permanent maxillary lateral incisor crown was clearly visible at the lateral surface of the bony crypt after the cyst had been removed. A drain was placed in the bony cavity, and the labial flap was replaced and sutured. In 3 months the lateral incisor erupted, and the patient was referred for orthodontic work.

(Figure 12–28 continued on opposite page.)

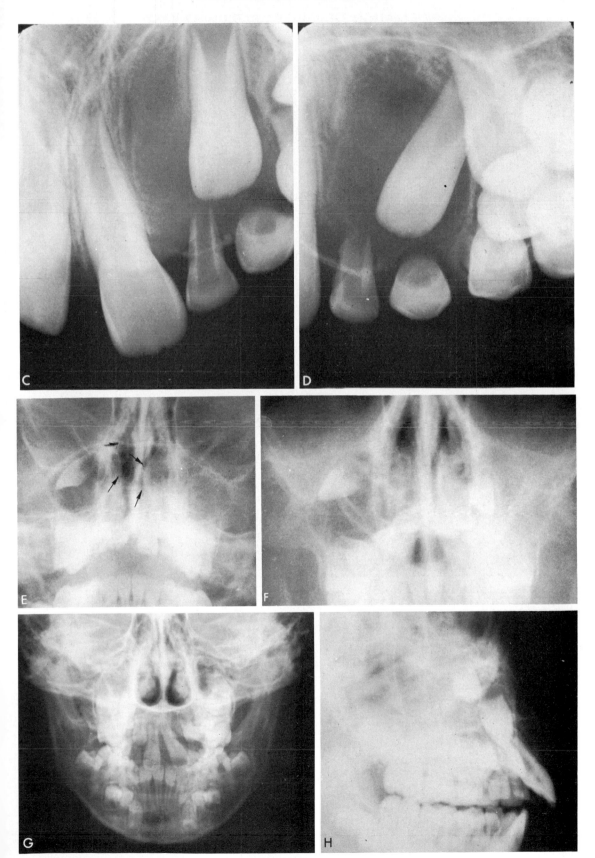

Figure 12–28 *(Continued.)*

ENUCLEATION OF A LARGE RADICULAR CYST

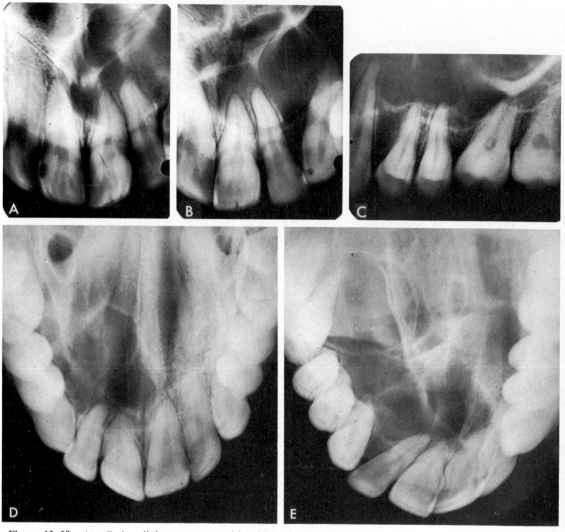

Figure 12-29 *A* to *C,* A radiolucent area resulting from a large radicular cyst, which apparently originated from the nonvital lateral incisor, the only tooth in the area of the cyst which includes the central incisor, lateral incisor, cuspid, first and second bicuspid, and the first molar, which is nonvital.

D and *E,* The occlusal films indicate the extensive area of this cyst. It is in close proximity to the floor of the nasal cavity and has extended into the maxillary sinus.

F, The orifice of the fistula is illustrated here between the right lateral incisor and the maxillary cuspid.

G, A large semicircular incision is made through the mucoperiosteal membrane starting over the apex of the left maxillary central incisor carrying the incision down towards the gingival line and posteriorly just above the necks of the teeth to the most distal point above the right maxillary first molar and angled up toward the mucobuccal fold.

H, The mucoperiosteal flap is reflected exposing the fistulous tract and the area of destruction of the labial cortical bone around the fistula.

I, A portion of the alveolar bone has been removed and the cyst capsule has been pushed back from the labial and buccal cortical plate of bone with a curette.

J, The area through the buccal cortical plate is shown with the wall of the cyst as it is being enucleated just beneath the retractor and the index finger.

K, Considerable difficulty was encountered around the apices of the lateral incisor, cuspid, bicuspid and first molar. As the cyst was enucleated, it brought with it an attached eggshell thickness of bone, which proved to be the floor of the maxillary sinus. Visual examination of the sinus showed a perforation into what little of the maxillary sinus was present.

(Figure 12-29 continued on opposite page.)

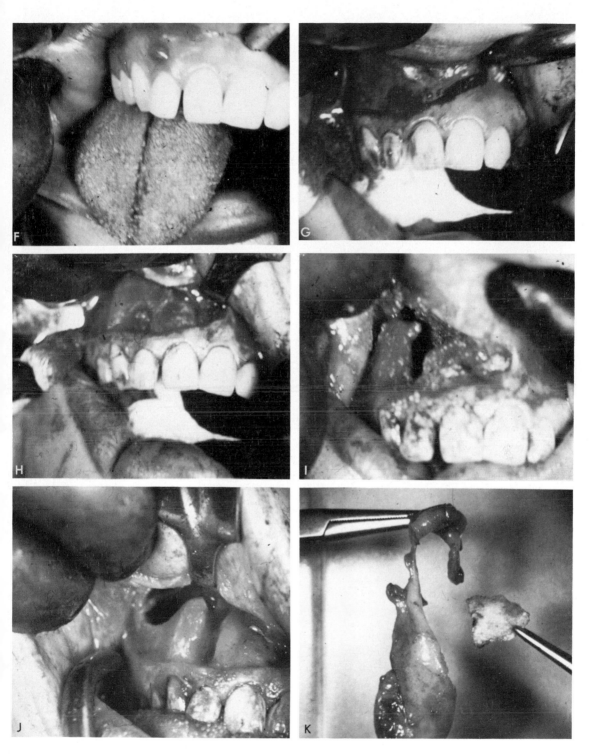

(Figure 12–29 continued on following page)

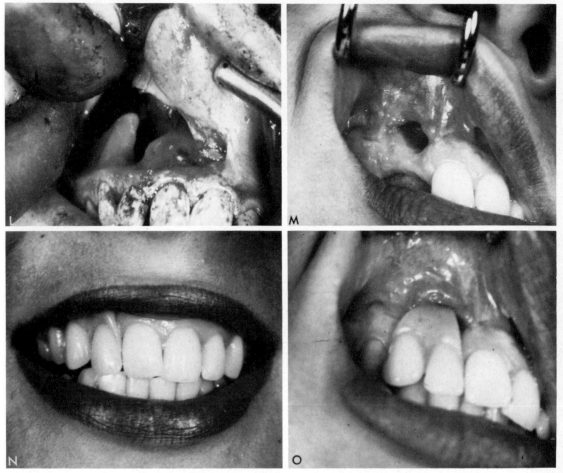

Figure 12–29 *(Continued.)* *L,* The area occupied by the cyst was very extensive. The nasal cavity was approximated with only a thin layer of bone separating the nasal cavity from the cyst wall. Only a small portion of the maxillary sinus was left, and this, as has been described, was unfortunately inadvertently opened. The apices of the teeth enumerated in the previous caption were exposed. It was obvious that the technique decided upon for the treatment of this cyst, namely, enucleation, was an error. This cyst should have been marsupialized.

M, Postoperatively there was one episode after another of acute infection, in spite of all accepted methods of treatment (no antibiotics were available at this time). It was necessary to extract all the teeth on the right side of the maxilla before the infection ceased, and even when this area of the maxilla was edentulous there continued to be areas in which subperiosteal infection periodically developed, requiring incision and drainage.

N and *O,* A partial denture that was inserted during the early treatment of this cyst. As additional teeth were extracted, they were added to this partial denture.

Technique of Marsupialization. As Howe says, "There can be no doubt that the poor opinion of this technique held by many authorities is due at least in part to the fact that in the past it has often been performed badly and that only an inadequate opening has been obtained. If the dentist makes only a small window in the lesion, rapid shrinkage of the annular scar surrounding the ostium occurs and is soon followed by recurrence of the cyst. For this reason any technique of marsupialization must be designed to ensure the patency of the ostium by producing an adequate opening surrounded by the minimum amount of scar tissue.

"Before making an incision the dental surgeon must utilize all the clinical and radiographic evidence available to him to estimate the extent of the cyst. This assessment enables him to design a mucoperiosteal flap, the shape and size of which are related to the size of the ostium which will be left at the end of the operation."[41]

STANDARD TECHNIQUE. When the corti-

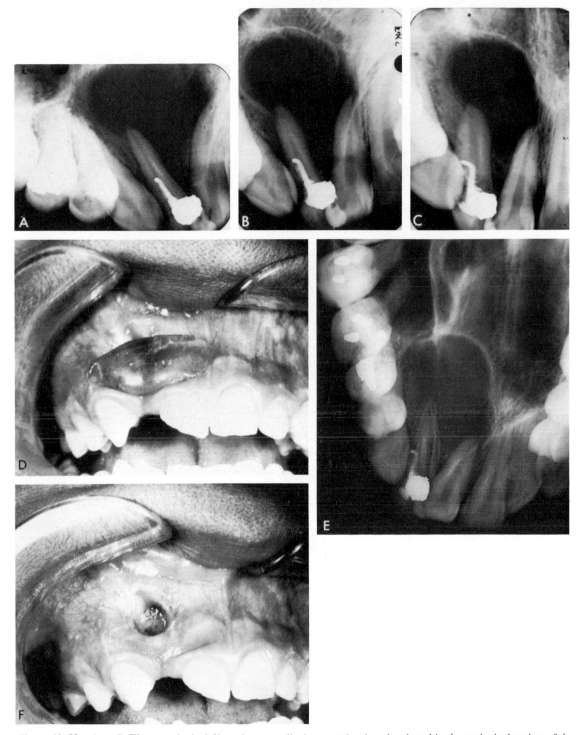

Figure 12–30 *A* to *C*, These periapical films show a radicular cyst that has developed in the periapical region of the nonvital infected lateral incisor. The radiolucent area is surrounded by a thin, sclerotic border. The occlusal film (*E*) and the palpation of the floor of the nasal cavity with a large ball burnisher revealed the absence of bone between the floor of the nasal cavity and the cyst. Therefore, marsupialization of the cyst was elected to prevent the near certainty of creating a nasal fistula if this cyst were enucleated.

D, A plastic obturator was inserted into the cyst during the day to prevent the entrance of food at mealtime and was removed at night. This obturator assured patency of the opening into the cyst while bone was filling in behind the cystic wall.

F, The cystic cavity is almost completely filled with bone. It is not necessary to continue to use the obturator when such a degree of filling has taken place.

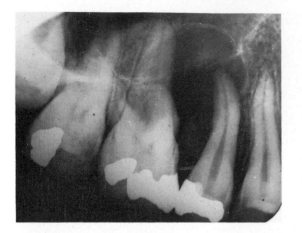

Figure 12–31   This large radicular cyst arising on the maxillary left second bicuspid has also invaded the interseptal space between the bicuspid and the maxillary first molar. In such a situation, in view of the proximity of the cyst to the mesial buccal root, as well as to the lingual root, it is judicious to marsupialize even a comparatively small cyst such as this to avoid exposing the apices of the molar and bicuspid. Exposure would destroy the blood supply to the buccal roots of the molar.

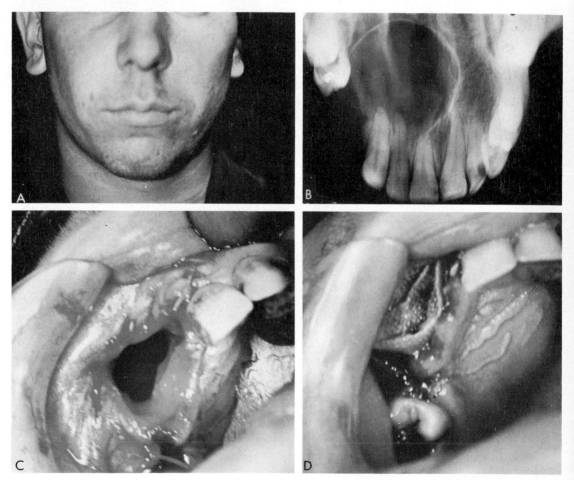

Figure 12–32   *A*, Note the swelling of the right side of the upper portion of the face. *B*, The radiograph reveals a large radicular cyst approximating the floor of the nasal cavity. There was also resorption of the osseous tissue palatally, and expansion of the palatal tissue, as is shown in *D*. *C* and *D*, Marsupialization was indicated in this case because of the adherence of the cystic capsule to the palatal mucoperiosteal tissue and the buccal tissue and in addition the proximity of the cyst to the floor of the nasal cavity. The loss of bone between these two cavities clearly indicated marsupialization as the treatment of choice rather than an attempt to enucleate the cyst. With the latter technique there would be the great possibility of not being able to remove it in its entirety because of its adherence to the tissues just enumerated, as well as the possibility of creating a naso-oral fistula during removal of the cyst wall.

(Figure 12–32 continued on opposite page)

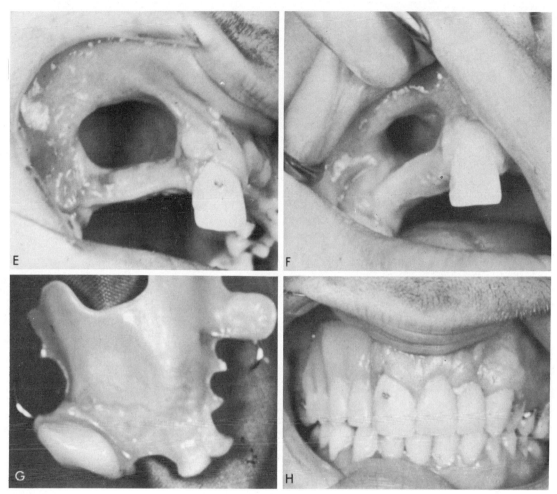

Figure 12–32 *(Continued.) E,* A view of the cystic cavity, which is smaller than originally because of the filling in of bone all around the cystic capsule. *F,* Marked (95 per cent) reduction of the original void in the maxilla. In view of the fact that the buccal bone as well as the palatal bone had been resorbed by the pressure of the cyst, complete filling in of bone will not progress much beyond what is seen here 8 months postoperatively. *G* and *H,* Partial denture, which also acted as an obturator in preventing the entrance of food during the filling of this cyst.

cal bone over the cyst is *thick,* the following technique is used. (Study Figures 12–51 to 12–53 and 12–60.)

Make a flap so that the edges of the mucoperiosteal flap extend along the edges of the proposed opening (ostium) into the cystic cavity; reflect the flap so that the bony plate overlying the cystic cavity is exposed. With burs or chisels and rongeurs carefully remove overlying bone, taking care not to penetrate the cystic cavity. When the predetermined size of the "window" into the cystic cavity is reached, take a pair of sharp scissors, pierce the cystic sac near the bony margin, and cut out the exposed cystic wall. Aspirate the cystic contents. Fold the mucoperiosteal flap into the cavity, and suture this flap to the cys-

tic membrane (see Figure 12–33). Fill the cavity with iodoform gauze. This is to aid in the union of the membranes. Do not change this packing for 72 hours. To reduce the absorption of oral fluids into the iodoform gauze, cover the gauze with a thick mixture of zinc oxide and eugenol. Cover this with Burlew "dry foil."

After initial healing has taken place (usually 1 week), take an impression of the cavity and make an acrylic obturator. The purpose of the obturator is to keep food out of the cavity during meals. It is removed at night to prevent aspiration or swallowing. This must be reduced in size as the cavity fills in with bone (see Figure 12–36).

MODIFIED TECHNIQUES.   The author has

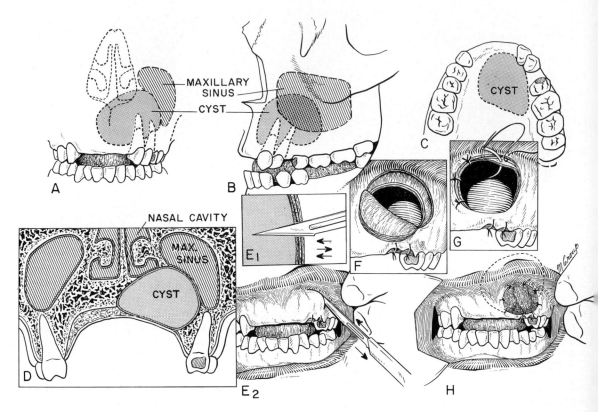

Figure 12–33 Marsupialization of a maxillary cyst. *A* to *D,* Note, in various views, the position of the cyst with respect to nasal mucosa and antral membrane. To enucleate this cyst invites disaster because it is virtually impossible to separate a cyst from either the membrane of the nose or antrum without perforating the membrane or leaving cystic epithelium behind. The consequences of enucleation are naso-oral or antro-oral fistulas or recurrence of the cyst.

Technique: The nonvital teeth are extracted and a window is made higher up in the mucobuccal fold rather than through the socket, in order to minimize food impaction. The window technique is done as follows: E_1, A No. 15 scalpel is inserted through the thin eggshell-like buccal plate directly into the cyst. It passes through mucosa, periosteum, bone and cyst wall. E_2, Using a back and forth motion to cut bone, mucoperiosteum and cyst wall in one clean line, a circular hole about the size of a dime is cut in the labial plate. *F,* Incision is half completed; the flap is retracted, and the interior of the cyst is visualized. At this stage small curved scissors are sometimes handier than a scalpel for removing the rest of the flap. *G,* The circle of tissue is now removed, and with interrupted sutures, the oral mucosa is sutured to the cystic membrane in an edge-to-edge relationship. The cystic membrane is usually, though not always, thick enough to hold sutures. (If it is very thin, the suturing is omitted.) The oral and cystic epithelia are thus apposed and become continuous during healing. *H,* The cystic cavity is packed loosely with iodoform gauze, which acts as an obturator. When healing of the incision takes place an acrylic obturator can be constructed, and this is gradually reduced in size as the cystic cavity shrinks. Some surgeons wait until the cystic cavity has shrunk enough to allow its enucleation without danger to the sinus or nasal membranes, while others do no secondary procedure of enucleation but merely allow the cavity to shrink slowly until it disappears.

modified this technique in those cases in which the cysts have very thin overlying cortical bone. The reader is referred to Figures 12–33 and 12–112 for a description of this modified technique, as it has been used in large hemorrhagic solitary bone cysts (SBC's).

When I presented this technique ("excision of a labial or buccal disc") at the Dental School at the University of Turkey, what I had considered an original modification of the then current marsupialization technique (see Figures 12–109 and 12–110 of Smith, Partsch, Blum and others, I was surprised to find that Professor Tagay was using the same "new technique," with a modification for those cases in which *no bone* exists between the cyst capsule and overlying mucoperiosteal tissue, which is an improvement over my technique, particularly in these cases. An excerpt from his article follows:

"We want only to present and discuss a

modification of this method [Partsch] whose indication is limited to cases in which bone apposition does not go parallel with loss of bone structure, *i.e.,* where the bony layer which separates the cystic mucosa from the buccal mucosa has completely disappeared and the cyst is largely expansive toward the buccal floor, the cheek, and the lip, and adherent to the environing tissues. This modification makes the original Partsch operation [a modification of Dr. Smith's] still easier and safer and presents fewer drawbacks for the doctor as well as for the patient. This modification consists of the following:

"After having carefully determined the limit of the cyst and the place of the incision to be made, I put in four to six sutures, according to the dimensions of the cyst, exactly at the level of this limit, and prior to making the incision. These sutures are applied with a curved needle, in a direction perpendicular to that of the incision to be made later on (I find it important to mention this, because when operating in a very vascular region, such as the lips, the cheeks or the buccal floor, these sutures may also serve as a sort of prophylactic ligature). By doing this the cyst mucosa is already sutured to the buccal mucosa. The hanging up (suspension) of the cystic membrane is assured before the incision is made, and I thus avoid the retraction of the cyst, which usually happens during the operation. I then make the incision at the level of the sutures and thus I easily cut a large window in the cyst. As usual, I fill the cavity with iodoform gauze. We wait for the epithelialization of the cystic borders with the buccal mucosa, and a week later we remove the gauze and the sutures, as we do in the original Partsch operation."*

Discussion. Many reasons have been advanced to discourage the conservative treatment (marsupialization) of these large dental cysts, none of which is of sufficient merit to cause this method to be discontinued. For instance, some practitioners state that the cyst will recur because the membrane has not been enucleated. I have never clinically observed this over a period of 48 years *if the opening into the cyst cavity was maintained* until bone had completely filled in around the capsule, thus gradually *obliterating the cavity and its capsule.* I have seen any number of cysts recur when enucleated and the wound sutured tight at the time of operation. The inconvenience to the patient of a large opening in the buccal or labial alveolus has likewise been set forth as a reason for not advocating the conservative method. I have yet to hear a patient complain for that reason, since actually the wound requires very little attention once the patency of the opening has been established, except for irrigation at the same time daily oral hygiene is performed.

In the case of dentigerous and other cysts, the remote possibility that an ameloblastoma or the very rare epidermoid carcinoma could develop in the cyst membrane has been advanced as an argument against marsupialization. The author made a survey of the Diplomates of the American Board of Oral Pathology, and all but two oral surgeons stated that marsupialization of dentigerous and other cysts was not contraindicated because of this remote possibility.

Another argument advanced for enucleation by some is that serial histologic examination of the cyst membrane can be made to rule out ameloblastoma or carcinoma. Chaudhry* advises that it would require thousands of serial sections in a large cyst to rule out this possibility and that such a procedure is not practical. Furthermore, of what immediate value is this information after the cyst membrane is enucleated? Further surgery is not indicated, as proliferations in the cyst wall do not prove invasion into the surrounding osseous tissue. I am referring to those cysts that "shell out" readily and do not have to be "dug out" with the curette, thus proving that there is invasion of this cystic tumor into the investing bone.

All cystic or other osseous cavities should be followed periodically by roentgenographic examination to learn whether they have recurred. If so, additional surgery is indicated. For a further discussion of ameloblastomas, see Chapter 13.

---

*From Tagay, C. Ö.: About the surgical treatment of paradental cysts. A modification of the method of marsupialization. Inf. Dent., *31*(13):381–386 (Mar. 27), 1949.

*Anand P. Chaudhry. Personal communication.

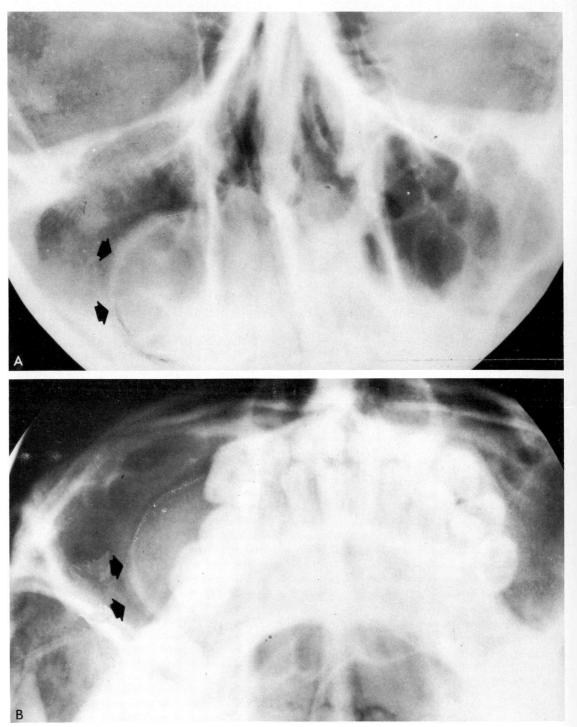

Figure 12–34　*A* and *B*, These posteroanterior radiographs of the skull reveal a large residual cyst which extends into the maxillary sinus with a wide sclerotic border.

(Figure 12–34 continued on opposite page)

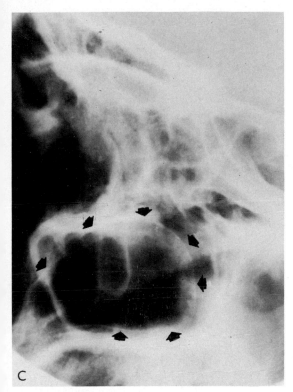

Figure 12–34 *(Continued.)* *C*, A lateral head radiograph shows the extent of the cyst's growth into the maxillary sinus. This cyst was marsupialized.

Summarizing the benefits of marsupialization of large dental cysts:

1. The contour of the oral tissues is preserved practically intact.

2. Teeth that may radiographically appear to be involved in the cystic process are usually vital, and these are never removed. If clinical tests as well as actual operative examination indicate involvement, root treatment alone or with resection may be resorted to at the time of marsupialization.

3. Anesthesia resulting from surgical trauma to or actual severance of a large nerve is eliminated.

4. Hemorrhage is rare, since the large blood vessels are not likely to be disturbed by manipulative methods.

5. By preservation of the contour of hard and soft tissues, as well as the teeth, there is no problem of prosthetic devices.

6. The potential danger of surgical fracture in the mandible is avoided in the especially large cysts by the absence of

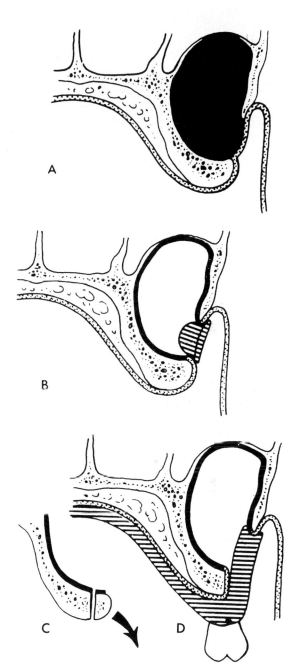

Figure 12–35 Methods of maintaining the patency of the opening of a marsupialized cyst.

A, A large cyst in an edentulous maxilla in which a portion of the buccal cortical bone has been completely resorbed and is covered only with the mucoperiosteal membrane.

B, The marsupialized opening into the cyst, into which an acrylic plug has been inserted.

C and *D*, Method for use of a denture to cover this opening during the replacement of the lost bone around the wall of the cyst. It is quite possible to also use a maxillary denture, even the patient's own denture, without removing the segment of bone which is illustrated in *C*. (From Howe, G. L.: Minor Oral Surgery. Bristol, England, John Wright & Sons, Ltd., 1971.)

LARGE ACRYLIC OBTURATOR FOR MARSUPIALIZED RESIDUAL CYST OF THE MAXILLA

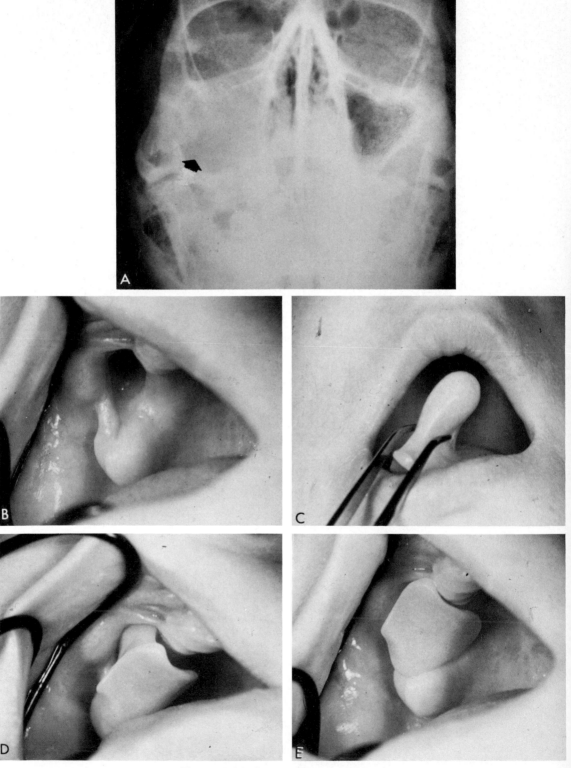

Figure 12–36 *See opposite page for legend.*

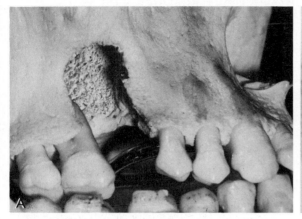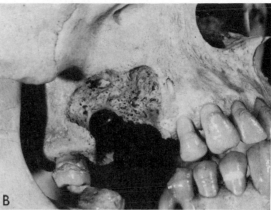

Figure 12–37 Two anatomic specimens in which there had been large residual cysts. In *A* it is interesting to note that while there was extensive pressure erosion of osseous tissue, the floor of the maxillary sinus retreated as the cyst enlarged. *B,* Shows an unusual area of destruction of bone, the dense lingual cortical plate, in addition to the buccal cortical plate and cancellous bone.

manipulation, which tends to insult further a previously weakened jaw.

7. Since the cystic membrane becomes a part of the oral mucous membrane, there hardly can be a recurrence unless this cyst is only one loculation of a multilocular cyst.

8. The time element in the healing of this wound cannot be advanced as a serious problem because the patient is entirely oblivious to and has no control over Nature's measures in the regeneration of bone.

9. The possibility of creating oral fistulas into the maxillary sinus or nasal cavity by the enucleation of the cystic capsule is removed.

RESIDUAL OR RECURRENT CYSTS

As already stated, if any portion of an epithelium-lined connective tissue capsule or a dental granuloma containing epithelial cells is left in the bone, a residual cyst will most likely develop in that area. Also, after the extraction of a tooth, any irritant left behind that could stimulate epithelial cells in the periapical region might result in the formation of a residual cyst. Careful postextraction periapical curettage is essential to remove any of these potential factors.

Roentgenographically, residual cysts in edentulous jaws usually appear as round radiolucent areas with clear-cut sclerotic borders. (See Figure 12–47.) If teeth are ad-

Figure 12–36 *A,* This posteroanterior view of the maxillary sinuses reveals the right maxillary sinus to be completely filled with a residual cyst. This patient had an edentulous maxilla with buccal thinning and resorption of the cortical plate.

B, Four-week postoperative view of a Partsch operation for a large residual maxillary cyst that had practically obliterated the maxillary sinus cavity. A Partsch operation was selected in this case because of the great possibility of creating an antro-oral fistula if the cyst membrane had been enucleated.

C, An acrylic plug with a saddle was constructed to prevent the entrance of food into the cyst cavity during the time the cavity was filling in. This plug, of course, does not begin to fill the entire cyst cavity. It is gradually reduced in size as the cavity fills in. It is left out at night.

D, The plug partially inserted into the cyst cavity. *E,* The plug and saddle seated in place. Once a day the patient removes the plug and irrigates the cavity. When the periphery of the opening heals, a full maxillary denture is constructed with a short extension into the cystic cavity. The denture is removed at night. As the cyst fills in with bone, the extension is reduced until it is completely removed.

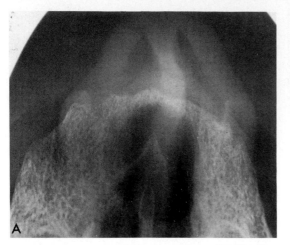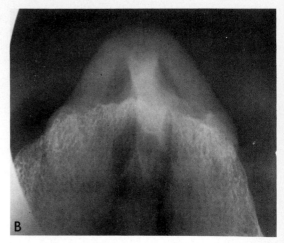

Figure 12–38 *See opposite page for legend.*

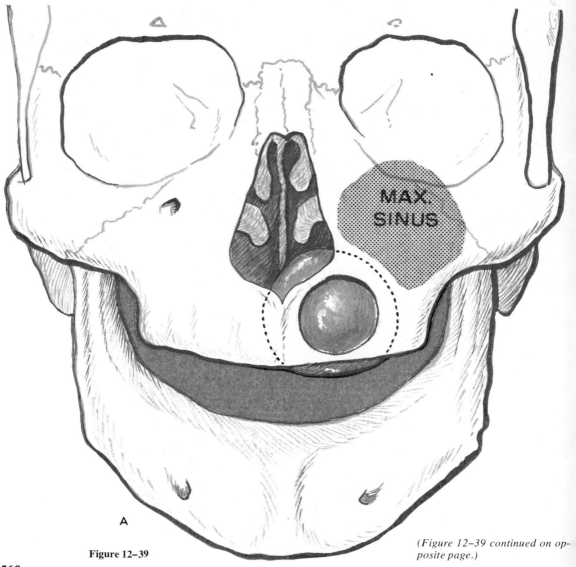

A

Figure 12–39

(Figure 12–39 continued on opposite page.)

Figure 12-38 *A,* This radiograph shows a large radiolucent area in the anterior maxilla. Labial exploratory palpation revealed a loss of labial cortical plate in this area. Palpation of the palatal mucoperiosteal membrane over this area also revealed an absence of osseous tissue. Palpation of the floor of the nasal cavity showed that bone was missing and only soft tissue separated the nasal cavity from the cyst wall. (See Figure 12-39 for location.) *B,* Radiograph 1 year after performance of the procedure illustrated in Figure 12-30.

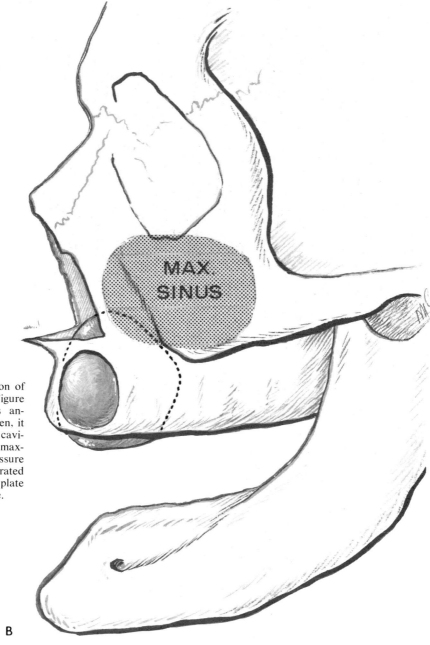

Figure 12-39 The location of the residual cyst shown in Figure 12-38*A* in the edentulous anterior maxilla. As can be seen, it has extended into the nasal cavity, deflected the floor of the maxillary sinus, and caused pressure resorption that has penetrated through the labial cortical plate and through the palatal bone.

B

Figure 12-39 *(Continued.)*

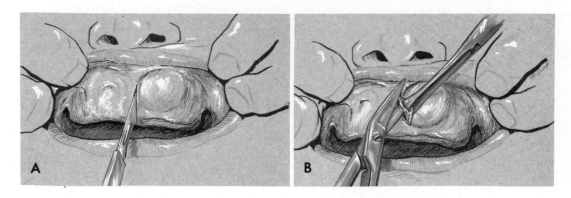

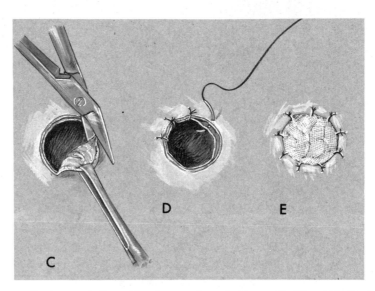

Figure 12–40   Marsupialization was indicated for the cyst shown in Figures 12–38 and 12–39. *A,* With a No. 11 Bard-Parker blade, an incision was made through the mucoperiosteum and cyst capsule at the edge of the osseous tissue where the cyst capsule protruded through the cortical plate, elevating the mucosa. In some cases there is a very thin "eggshell" thickness of expanded cortical bone over the cyst capsule. For these a disc of mucoperiosteum, thin bone and cyst capsule can easily be removed together as just described. *B,* Into this incision one cutting edge of a No. 9 Dean's scissors is inserted, and a disc of mucoperiosteal membrane, thin bone, if present, and cyst capsule is excised as shown in *C. D,* Suturing of the mucoperiosteal membrane with the cyst wall. *E,* The suturing has been completed about the periphery with interrupted sutures, and a loose dressing of iodoform gauze has been inserted. This gauze is removed within 48 hours, and the cavity is irrigated daily. Shrinkage of the soft tissue will occur. Bone will only partially fill in this cavity, because in cases such as this in which the labial cortical plate, the bony floor of the nasal cavity and the palatal bone are all perforated by the cyst, there will never be a complete filling in of osseous tissue. These spaces are filled with dense fibrous tissue. (See Figure 12–38*B*).

jacent to the origin of the residual cyst, they will affect the shape of the radiolucent area as the cyst expands, because roots of teeth do not usually resorb as does bone. Small residual cysts should be enucleated, and if large residual cysts encroach on or invade the max-illary sinus, nasal cavity or orbital cavity, or involve neurovascular bundles, they should be marsupialized.

Postoperative Treatment of Cystic Cavities. An extensive literature over the years advocates the use of bone and bone substitutes in

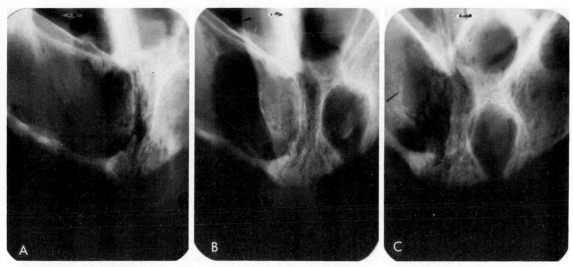

Figure 12–41 In these three periapical radiographs of an edentulous anterior maxilla are two well-circumscribed radiolucent areas, one large and one small, the left one of which appears to involve the floor of the nasal cavity. Both of these proved to be residual cysts; the large one was marsupialized, and the small one, which was completely encased in osseous tissue, was enucleated.

the filling of osseous defects caused by neoplasms, cysts, trauma, congenital diseases and surgical intervention. The aims of this replacement include restoration of morphologic contour, mechanical strength and function; elimination of dead space to reduce postoperative infection; prevention of ingrowth of soft tissue; and the enhanced retention of prosthetic devices where applicable.

Some of the materials used for these purposes are autogenous, homologous and heterogenous organic bone, their anorganic derivatives and cartilage (see Chapter 23). Alloplasts (bone substitutes) investigated include calcium salts, polyvinyl sponge, glass, polyurethane, cellulose, metals, plastics, hemihydrate of calcium sulfate (plaster of paris) and urinary tract mucosa. None of these materials has been universally acceptable.

Bone Chips in Cystic Cavities. Packing large cystic cavities in the maxilla and mandible with bone chips obtained from a bone bank appears, according to some authorities, to aid in the healing of these cavities and reduce somewhat postoperative depressions in the jaws.

TECHNIQUE. Following enucleation of the cystic membrane, a piece of frozen cancellous or cortical bone cut into small fragments with a pair of bone shears is firmly packed into the bony crypt. The soft tissue flap is then replaced and sutured.

While we have used this technique in a small series of cases, we are not overly impressed with the claimed advantages over the standard technique of cyst treatment.

The author's clinical results with so-called osteogenic substance to stimulate bone growth have been very disappointing. Mitchell and Shankwalker found that "despeciated calf bone paste, calcium hydroxide and gelatin mixtures appeared to delay the healing of small surgical wounds in monkey tibias. Anorganic bone is rather inert ... and in the surgical wounds of the tibia, it alone remained unresorbed in the healed wounds. . . . It is concluded that the untreated control wounds, as studied, healed better in all respects than did the treated bone wounds."[53]

"Sponges" in Cystic Cavities. My experience with starch or fibrin foam sponges in large cystic cavities, even when the sponges were soaked in thrombin and penicillin, has not been good. These agents furnish an ideal matrix for the growth of bacteria, with subsequent chronic or acute infection. They have not aided in healing but materially retarded it. Ultimately, this foul-smelling foreign material must be washed away from the cystic cavity to permit normal healing.

(Text continued on page 581)

ENUCLEATION OF BILATERAL PALATAL RESIDUAL CYSTS AND A MESIODENS

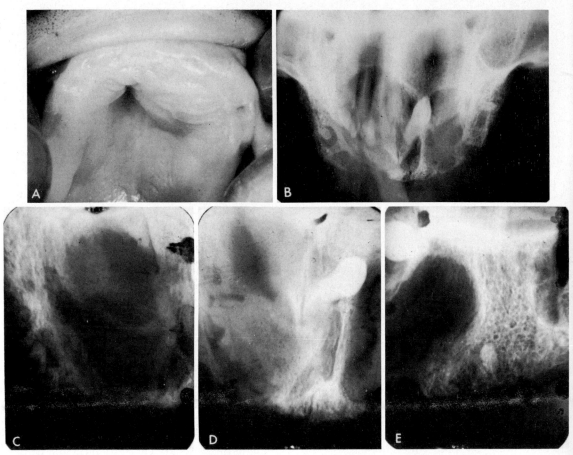

Figure 12–42 *A,* Residual cysts of the maxilla. The patient complained of a progressively increasing unilateral palatal swelling. *B,* Occlusal intraoral radiographs revealed two radiolucent areas in the palatal bone which had the appearance of residual cysts. In the midline of the palate there appeared to be a rudimentary central incisor (mesiodens). At first glance it appeared that the radiolucent areas, one or both, might be a dentigerous cyst. At operation there was no connection between the cysts and the mesiodens. *C* to *E,* Regular intraoral periapical radiographs of this case. Note the mesiodens in *D* and *E. F,* An incision was made on the crest of the ridge through the mucoperiosteal membrane from the left first molar region to the right first molar region, and the full thickness of the flap was reflected from the palate, exposing an eggshell thickness of bone overlying the cysts. This was expanded over the left cyst but not the right one. *G,* The thin palatal bone was removed with bone shears, exposing the thick capsule of each cyst. The small (right) cyst was enucleated from its crypt with large-bowled curettes. The left (larger) cyst was exposed and enucleated. Beneath this cyst was a rudimentary cuspid that was removed (see arrow). Iodoform gauze drain was placed in the crypts for 72 hours. The palatal flap was replaced and sutured with a continuous 00 black silk suture. *H,* The appearance of the line of incision 1 week later. The blood clot in the left palatal crypt broke down because of infection, and a large abscess developed. This was drained through the original line of incision, and the cavity remained open as it filled with bone. The right (smaller) crypt healed without trouble. *I,* The two cysts and the rudimentary cuspid.

(Figure 12–42 continued on opposite page)

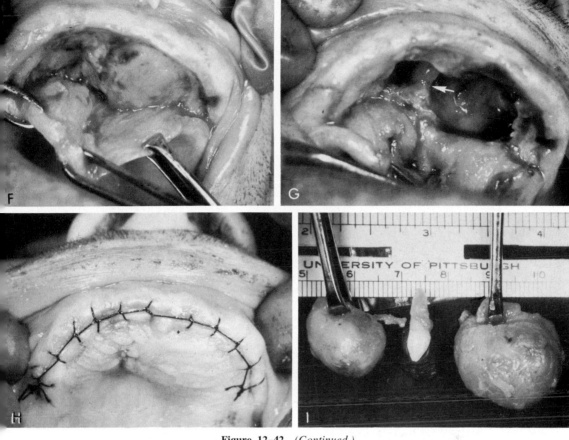

Figure 12-42   *(Continued.)*

Figure 12-43 The well-circumscribed radiolucent area near the lingual root of the left maxillary first molar is a well-defined nasolacrimal canal. It is not a residual cyst nor is it the greater palatine foramen, for which it is often mistaken. Occasionally these radiolucent areas are superimposed over the lingual root of a maxillary molar, usually the first or second, and are misinterpreted as being indicative of a loss of periapical osseous bone due to a pathologic condition.

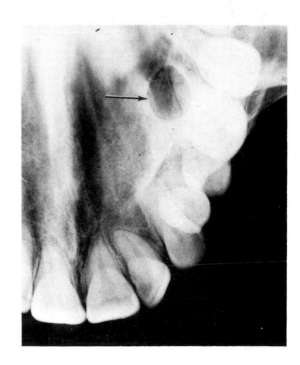

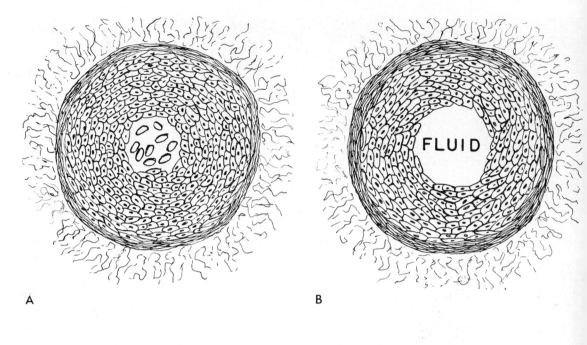

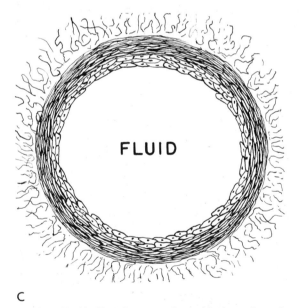

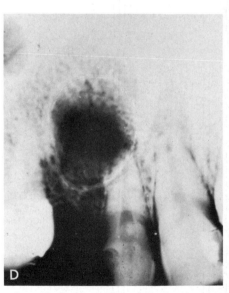

Figure 12–44 Development of a residual cyst from the retention of a periapical granuloma, following the extraction of a tooth. *A*, The periapical granuloma contains a large clump of residual epithelial cells. The cells in the center have died because of lack of oxygen, food and water. As time goes on, as seen in *B*, an accumulation of fluid occurs as a result of the greater osmotic pressure within the capsule. In *C* can be seen the gradual flattening of the epithelial cells lining the capsule. This continuous pressure from within the epithelium-lined fibrous capsule onto the surrounding bone stimulates osteoclastic activity. This process results in a gradual expansion of the cyst to the very large sizes already illustrated. *D*, The radiographs of such a residual cyst with a clear-cut sclerotic border.

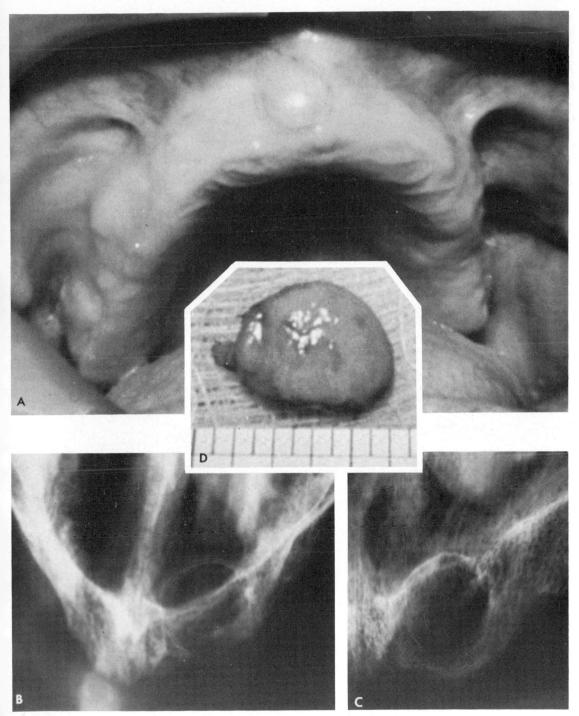

Figure 12–45 *A*, Expansion of a residual cyst through the labial cortical plate of an edentulous maxilla. *B* and *C*, Occlusal and periapical radiographs indicating the extent of the cyst as it has expanded. Palpation of the floor of the nasal cavity does not reveal any loss of bone in that area. There was not any encroachment on the nasal cavity by this cyst, although the radiographs, particularly the occlusal, suggest it. Note that the periapical radiograph (*C*) shows osseous tissue between the cyst and nasal cavity. Therefore, the cyst, which is shown in *D*, was enucleated, following the raising of the labial flap and excision of the cortical bone.

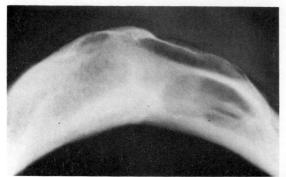

Figure 12–46 An unusually shaped radiolucent area is revealed in this occlusal film of an edentulous mandible in the region of the symphysis. The labial cortical plate appears to be depressed and thinned out. The multilocular radiolucent area probably represents a residual cyst caused when the thin labial cortical plate was depressed by a blow that this patient received on his chin in a fist fight. At operation it was found that there were actually two cysts in this area; both were enucleated.

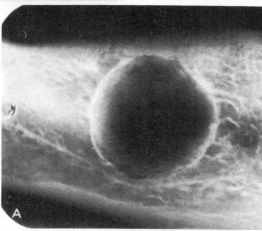

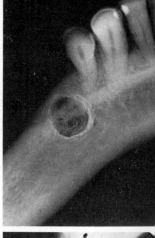

Figure 12–47 *1*, Examples of residual cysts of the mandible. *A*, Periapical and occlusal views of a circular residual cyst of the body of the mandible. *B*, Periapical and occlusal views of a smaller residual cyst with a clear-cut sclerotic border in the bicuspid area. *C*, Circular residual cyst in the molar area of the mandible. The occlusal view shows a very dense, expanded cortical plate. The treatment for all of these residual cysts was enucleation and primary closure of the wound.

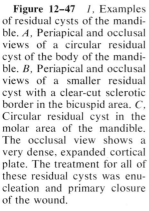

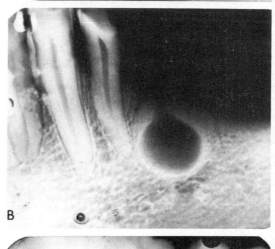

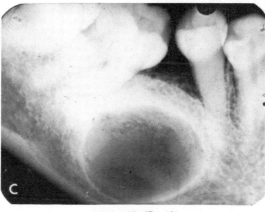

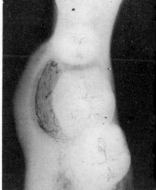

Figure 12–47 *(1)*

(Figure 12–47 continued on opposite page)

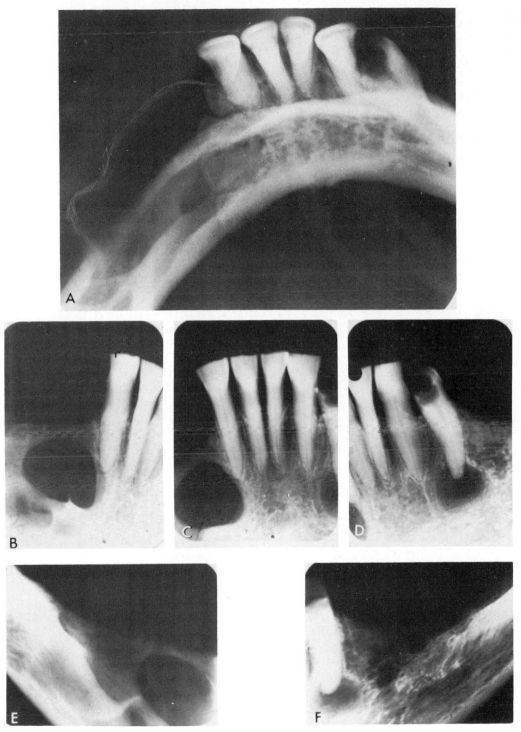

Figure 12–47 *(Continued.)* *(2)*

Figure 12–47 *(Continued.)* 2, Another example of a residual cyst and a small radicular cyst. *A*, Occlusal view indicates the expansion of the buccal cortical plate. *B* to *F*, Periapical dental radiographs of the mandibular teeth show the extent of the cyst anteriorly and posteriorly, superiorly and inferiorly and the relationship with the teeth and inferior alveolar canal. Of interest also is the round jet-black radiolucent area just distal to the left lateral incisor. This is usually indicative of complete loss of the lingual cortical bone in that particular area. The well-circumscribed radiolucent area at the apex of the carious right cuspid may be a large periapical granuloma or a small radicular cyst.

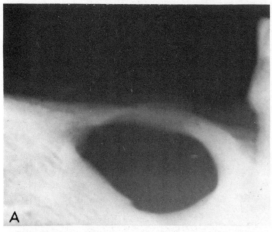

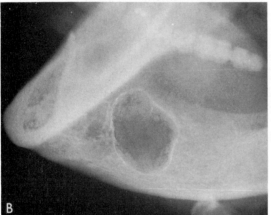

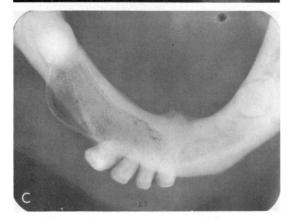

Figure 12–48 In this figure we have three areas of radiolucency in edentulous areas of the mandible. In *A*, please note the jet-black radiolucent area with sharp, well-defined margins. This indicates that there is not any buccal or lingual cortical plates of bone over this area. A needle can be passed freely from buccal to lingual and this really does not represent a residual cyst at all. It is a healed bone defect following surgery for a cyst in which both the buccal and lingual cortical plates of bone had been eroded by cystic pressure. In these cases the author has never seen a complete filling in of bone. *B*, A well-circumscribed sclerotic area of bone surrounding a radiolucent area which probably represents a residual cyst. *C*, An occlusal view of another case in which a large residual cyst has been present for many years gradually expanding anteriorly, posteriorly and buccally as well. This case was marsupialized.

Figure 12–49 *A*, Posteroanterior radiographic view of the mandible, revealing a radiolucent area in the left body of the mandible. *B*, The left lateral oblique radiograph of the body of the mandible shows the anterior–posterior extent of this radiolucent area, which extends in both directions from beneath the roots of the second molar. The sclerotic border of this particular radiolucent area appears to pass over the apical third of the roots, which indicates that the radiolucent area could be either buccal or lingual to the roots. It is very likely on the buccal side. This radiolucent area also extends to the very narrow inferior border of the mandible. Note that the neurovascular canal has been deflected downward and thinned by the pressure of the contents of this radiolucent area, which proved to be a residual cyst. Because of the approximation to the inferior alveolar canal and the possibility of disturbing its contents even to the point of severing the neurovascular bundle contained therein, the cyst was marsupialized.

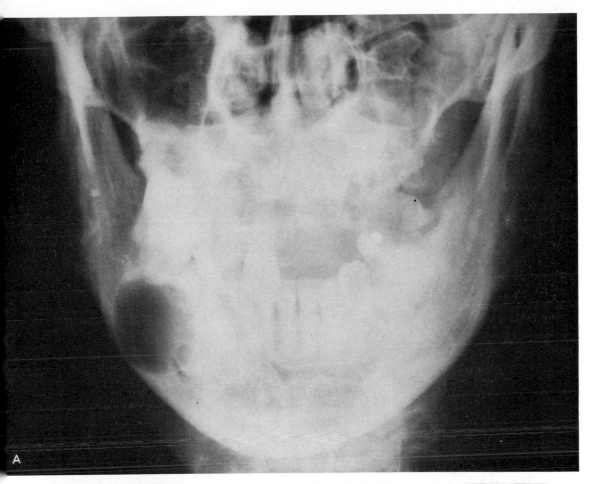

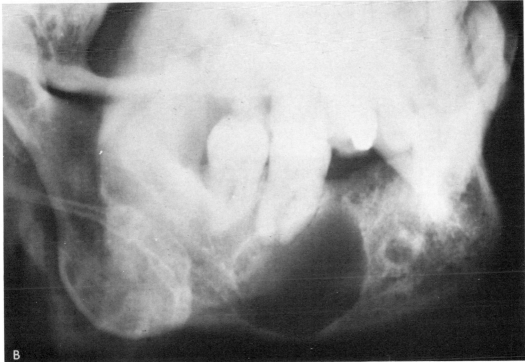

Figure 12–49 *See opposite page for legend.*

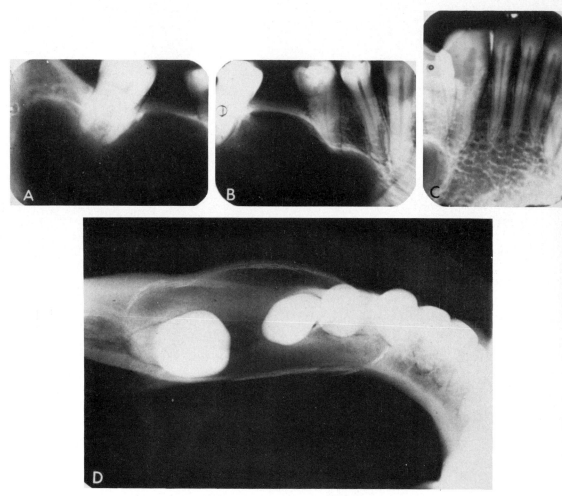

Figure 12–50 *A* to *C,* These periapical radiographs show a large radiolucent area extending from beneath the apex of the mandibular left first bicuspid inferiorly to the lower border of the mandible, posteriorly beneath the second bicuspid, then sweeping up almost to the crest of the edentulous ridge between the second bicuspid and the second molar, down beneath the apices of the second molar and distally into the third molar area, which is also edentulous, and then down again to the inferior border of the mandible. *D,* The occlusal film of this particular area shows that the buccal expansion has produced a thin cortical plate as the result of the hydrostatic pressure of the contents of what proved to be a multilocular residual cyst. A marked thinning of the lingual cortical plate was also evident. This residual cyst, in all probability, was the result of failure to remove a periapical granuloma present at the apices of the lower left first molar when that tooth was extracted, so long ago that the patient could not remember the year. This case is similar to the one shown in Figure 12–99. See Figure 12–51 for the operative technique used in these cases.

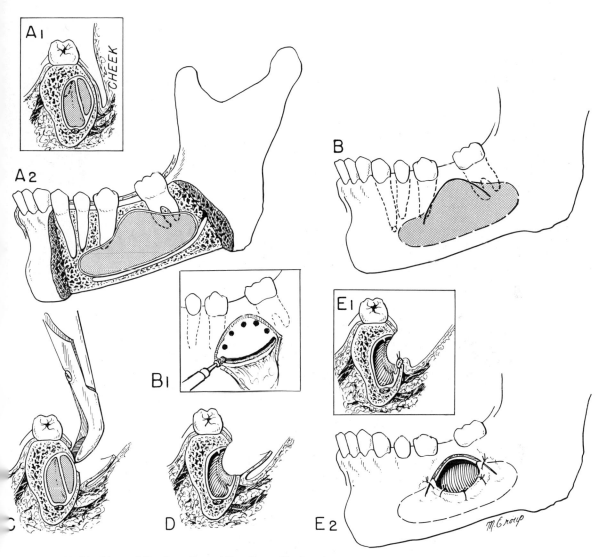

Figure 12–51 Marsupialization of a multilocular residual cyst.

A_1, Cross section showing a soft-tissue partition and the bulging cortical plate, as well as the relationship of the cyst to the inferior alveolar canal, which has been pushed downward.

A_2, Extent of the cyst—the teeth on either side were all vital. Note again the relationship of the inferior alveolar neurovascular bundle to the cyst. This is adherent to the cystic wall, and the possibility of severing the bundle and its contents, if the cystic membrane is enucleated, is very real. Also, the nerve and blood supply to the adjacent teeth would be disrupted. For these reasons marsupialization is indicated.

B, The mucoperiosteal tissue is reflected after a semicircular incision is made along the superior border of the bulged cortical plate.

B_1, If the cortical plate is thick, with a spear-pointed drill a series of holes is drilled through the cortical bone. They are then connected with a crosscut fissure bur.

C, If the bone is thin, the mucoperiosteal flap is reflected, and the thin cortical bone is cut away with a bone rongeur.

D, A window is cut through both cyst walls, and the contents of the cyst are removed—in this patient a waxy caseous material was found.

E_1, Buccal flap is cut off just about at the inferior bony border of the cystic cavity.

E_2, Buccal flap is sutured to cyst lining.

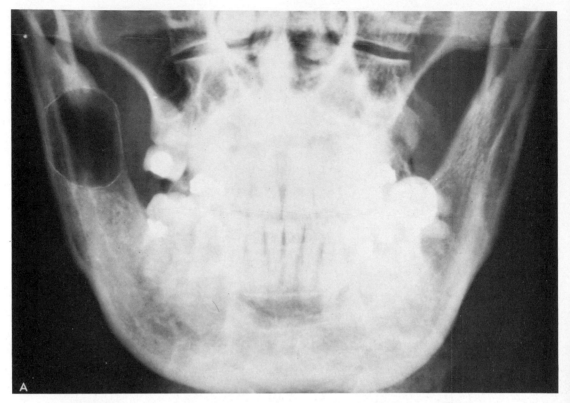

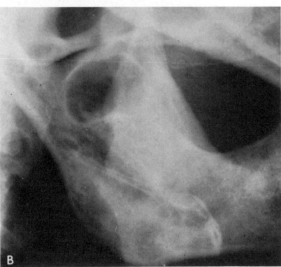
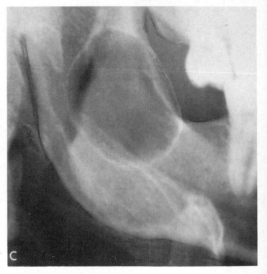

Figure 12–52 Radiographs of three separate cases, illustrating the positions of residual (or recurrent) cysts in the vertical ramus of the mandible.

A, Posteroanterior view of the maxilla and mandible. In the left vertical ramus halfway between the inferior border and the sigmoid notch is a well-circumscribed area of radiolucency surrounded by a sclerotic osseous line. This, in all probability, is a recurrent cyst; the patient reported that she had had surgery for a cyst in this area some 8 years previously. Many of these cases are actually the result of an unsuccessful attempt to enucleate the cyst in its entirety. Failure to remove all the cyst by the enucleation process, leaving behind some of the epithelium-lined cystic wall, even though the osseous tissue fills the cystic cavity, permits the epithelial remnants to continue to increase in size, and a recurrent residual cyst develops.

B, Left lateral oblique radiograph of the vertical ramus of the mandible. In its superior third, in contact with and just below the sigmoid notch, there is a well-circumscribed radiolucent area with a dense sclerotic border. This proved to be a cyst. The comments made concerning cystic development in *A* apply equally well in this particular area and in *C*.

C, A fairly long oblong radiolucent area in the middle and lower third of the vertical ramus, with anterior expansion that is bordered by a sclerotic white line encircling the entire radiolucent area. Here again, the patient had had an operation for a cyst in this area some years before. He was told that the cyst was "completely removed" at that time.

Treatment: In these particular cases in which there has been a history of recurrence, I select marsupialization as the treatment of choice, even though admittedly it is difficult to maintain the patency of the openings. This is necessary so that the cyst does not heal over before osseous tissue has been deposited around the circumference of the cyst and the cavity has been almost completely obliterated by this growth. Recurrences, when marsupialization is the operation of choice, in the majority of cases occur simply because of failure to maintain this patency.

574

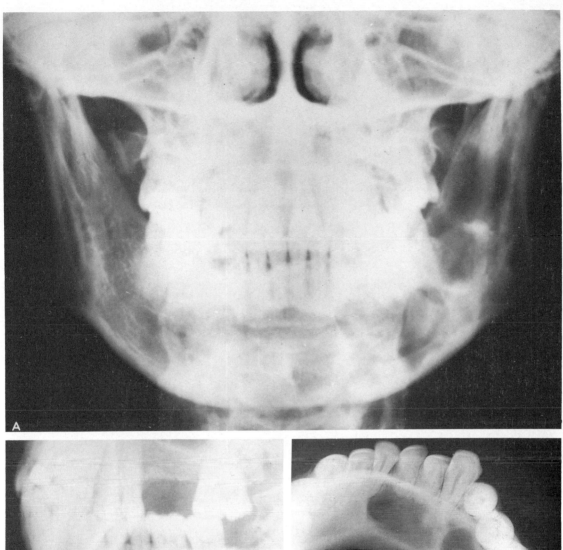

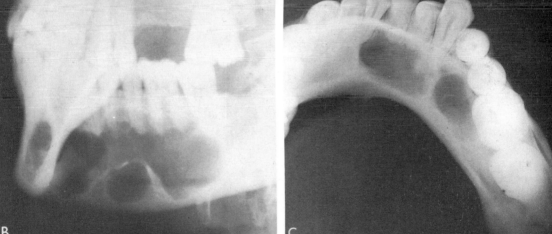

Figure 12–53 Radiographic series for one patient. *A*, Posteroanterior view of the maxilla and the mandible. Three radiolucent areas that seem to be separated by osseous partitions can be seen in the right vertical ramus. There is also a radiolucent area in the symphysis.

B, Oblique radiograph of the right body of the mandible. In this view the radiolucent areas can be seen more distinctly, almost in their complete circumference. The teeth in this area are all vital, and the areas seem to be separated.

C, Occlusal radiograph of the anterior right two-thirds of the mandible that gives an almost completely undistorted view of the symphysis. Both the radiolucent areas indicating loss of osseous structure and the very thin labial cortical plate remaining can be seen.

In this case all four of these areas were labially marsupialized. We were not able to determine the cause of these "cysts" because there was no evidence in the mandible of any reason for them to develop. The lining of these lesions was a very thin, almost fibrous, membrane. The patient, who was in her late forties, did not return as she was instructed to do after the first 4 months. Attempts to get in touch with her and have her return were unsuccessful. About 15 years later we learned from a colleague of ours that the patient had come to his office for a checkup on her mandible, and she once more had "cysts" in these same areas (which he treated). This is one of the cases in which the patient failed to return for care; as a result the openings healed over, and the "cysts" recurred.

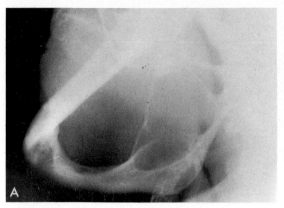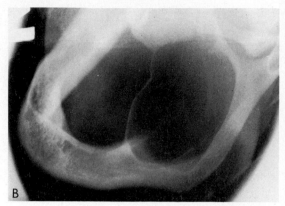

Figure 12–54 *A,* A very large residual cyst in the vertical ramus of a 72-year-old edentulous male. This cyst was marsupialized.

B, A very widely expanded residual cyst of the vertical ramus in a 66-year-old female. This case was treated by marsupialization.

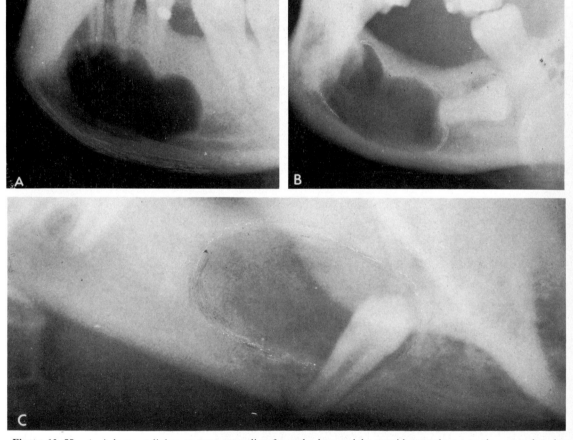

Figure 12–55 *A,* A large radiolucent area extending from the lower right cuspid area almost to the second molar. This radiolucent area is well circumscribed, and we thought it represented a radicular cyst because the mandibular cuspid had a large filling and was nonvital. Because of the approximation of the bicuspids to this radiolucent area, as well as its relationship to the neurovascular bundle in the inferior alveolar canal, marsupialization was the treatment of choice and was carried out.

B, Another large radiolucent area in the corpus of the mandible, in which no teeth are involved. The horizontally impacted and unerupted second bicuspid was never completely formed because the thick capsule of this residual cyst, as it proved to be, had blunted the tooth-forming organ. There is also a small radiolucent area about the crown of this bicuspid, and so there are actually two cysts in this area, a large, almost multilocular, residual cyst, and a much smaller dentigerous cyst. Treatment included the marsupialization of the large cyst for reasons of preventing any injury to the neurovascular bundle, and the horizontally impacted bicuspid, along with the small cyst about its crown, was surgically excised.

C, Another dentigerous cyst involving the crown of an unerupted bicuspid at the lower border of the mandible. This was also treated by marsupialization, and the crown of the tooth was exposed. Because the patient was in her teens, the bicuspid was moved into position by orthodontic treatment.

576

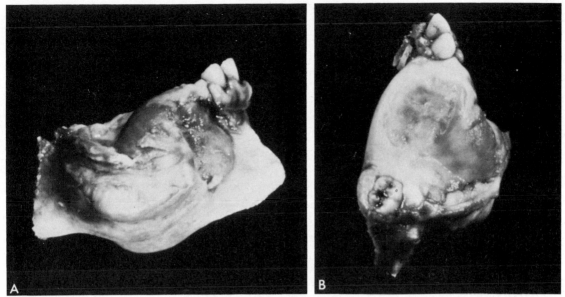

Figure 12-56 In these photographs we see the unfortunate sequelae of a partial resection of the mandible without a prior diagnosis of the lesion that existed in this particular patient's jaw. *A,* Without even the benefit of a radiograph—merely on the presence of this large swelling—the general surgeon resected this portion of the patient's right mandible from the right lateral incisor posteriorly to the third molar. *B,* The interior of the mass, which proved it to be a residual cyst. A biopsy taken from the cyst wall revealed stratified squamous epithelium. The treatment indicated in this case was marsupialization, or even possibly enucleation of the cyst. Certainly surgical excision of this portion of the mandible was not indicated. (Courtesy of Dr. Leo March.)

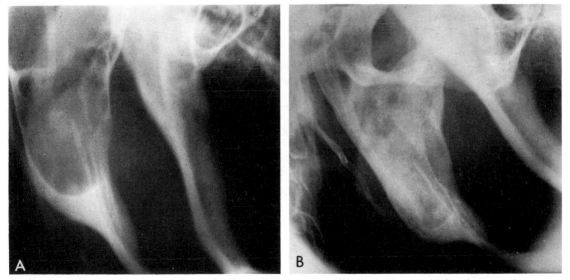

Figure 12-57 *A,* Left oblique radiograph of an edentulous mandible in a 70-year-old female (note the extreme resorption of the body of the mandible). This cyst was marsupialized. *B,* Ramus 18 months later completely filled in with osseous tissue. (Courtesy of Dr. Lester R. Cahn, New York City.)

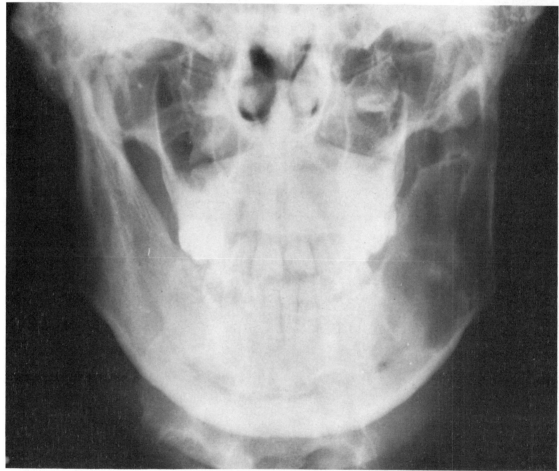

Figure 12–58   Large residual cyst of the left body and vertical ramus of the mandible. This cyst was marsupialized to avoid possible injury to the inferior alveolar neurovascular bundle.

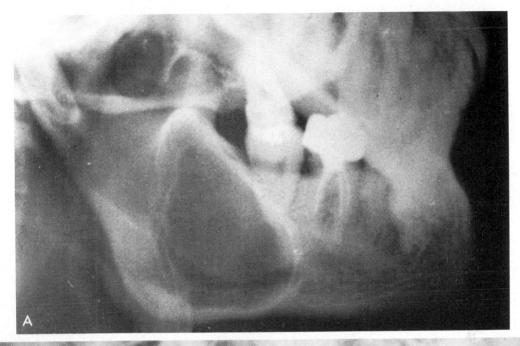

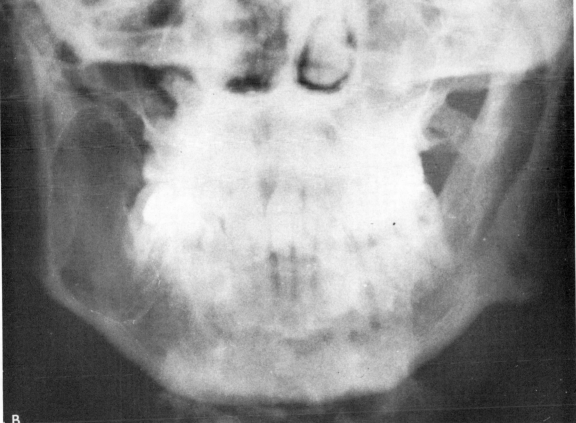

Figure 12–59 Still another case of a large cyst that developed in the third molar area of the mandible. This patient had had a nonimpacted third molar removed from this area many years before. This is probably a residual cyst.

MARSUPIALIZATION OF A VERY EXTENSIVE RESIDUAL CYST OF THE MANDIBLE

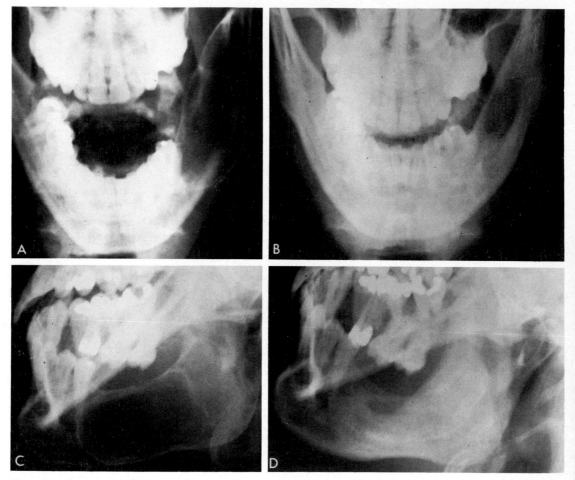

Figure 12–60 *A* and *C*, Posteroanterior roentgenogram (*A*) of the mandible of a 29-year-old man reveals the extent of destruction of bone caused by what appears to be a very large residual cyst involving both the body and vertical ramus of the mandible. Note the thin, bulging buccal cortical plate. Striations give the impression that this is a multilocular cyst. However, when the cystic cavity was marsupialized, these striations proved to be septa extending into the cavity. Oblique roentgenogram (*C*) of the right mandible shows the extent of destruction of osseous tissue in the vertical ramus up to the sigmoid notch and in the horizontal ramus (body) to the inferior border. The neurovascular bundle containing the inferior alveolar artery, vein and nerve has been displaced and is undoubtedly adherent, at least in some areas, to the fibrous cystic wall.

B and *D*, Twenty months following marsupialization, the cystic cavity is 90 per cent filled in with osseous tissue. Note how the inferior alveolar canal has been displaced inferiorly and posteriorly from its normal position. *Note:* This patient had had an unerupted impacted lower right third molar and the erupted first and second molars removed 5 years before the time of this marsupialization, by another dentist. It is apparent that the presence of the cyst was not recognized at that time. (Courtesy of Richard J. King, D.D.S., Butler, Pa.)

ENUCLEATION OF A LARGE MANDIBULAR RESIDUAL CYST

Patient. A 38-year-old white man presented himself at the dental school with a decided prominence of the right side of the lower jaw. Intraoral examination revealed a large swelling of the right mandible, extending from approximately the cuspid to the molar regions. The mouth was edentulous. Digital manipulation of the enlarged portion of the mandible resulted in a crepitant sound similar to that of crackling parchment. Periapical and occlusal radiographs revealed a large cyst that, slowly enlarging, had caused buccal expansion and thinning of the buccal cortical plate (Fig. 12–61A to E). The pressure atrophy extended inferiorly also until only ⅛ inch of the lower border of the mandible remained. It was surprising that spontaneous fracture of the mandible had not occurred. The patient was sent to the Eye and Ear Hospital for removal of the cyst under general anesthesia. (Study Figure 12–61).

Laboratory Reports. Findings were essentially negative.

Operative Notes. Under general anesthesia, the inferior alveolar, lingual and long buccal nerves were blocked with 2 per cent procaine, 1:100,000 epinephrine solution. An oropharyngeal partition was then placed. With a No. 15 blade an incision was started in the right lower third molar area along the crest of the ridge to approximately the right lateral region and then at a 45-degree angle to the mucobuccal fold. The buccal mucoperiosteal tissue was reflected with periosteal elevators until the entire thin, bulging bony covering of the cyst was exposed. At one point on the buccal surface of the mandible, over the cyst, the bone had completely resorbed, and the cystic membrane was visible. Starting at this point, the point of the bone shear was gently worked between the thin buccal plate and the cystic sac, in order to cut away the buccal bone, care being taken not to penetrate the cystic sac. Because of the eggshell-like quality of the bone, it was possible to remove a large portion also simply by placing a periosteal elevator between the bone and the cystic membrane and, with upward pressure, fracturing segments of the thin, bony plate. Other pieces of the bony wall that were denser had to be trimmed with the bone shears and removed by means of a hemostat.

After the entire plate had been removed, exposing the buccal surface of the cyst, which had not yet been penetrated, the periosteal elevator with the spoon edge against the bone was gradually worked between the bony wall and the cystic membrane on the lingual, mesial, distal and inferior surfaces of the cyst. Alternating with a large-bowled curette, the entire cyst, still intact, was freed, except for an attachment to the sheath containing the inferior alveolar nerve, artery and vein. (See the specimen, Figure 12–61H and I.) In dissecting the cyst from the neurovascular bundle,

the latter was inadvertently torn at its exit through the mental foramen. This resulted in massive hemorrhage, which was controlled by gauze pressure on the inferior neurovascular bundle held for approximately 5 minutes. When this was done, the entire cyst was removed. The cut ends of the mandibular neurovascular bundle were approximated with sutures. The flap was sutured back into place after an iodoform gauze drain had been placed into the cavity.

Because of the large amount of destruction of bone, great care had to be used to prevent a fracture of the mandible during the operation, especially when placing the mouth prop. For the same reason good relaxation of the muscles of the mandible was maintained by the anesthetist. The patient was taken from the operating room in good condition.

Note: A better technique for this case would have been oral marsupialization.

When the cyst was cut into after its removal, the contents were found to be yellow caseous material. The cyst was sent to the laboratory for biopsy.

Pathologist's Report. The cyst was 4 cm. at its greatest diameter, sausage-shaped, smooth and thin-walled, but dense. The contents were caseous and nonpurulent, with no hair or teeth. Some old blood was present in the cyst contents. The wall was fibrous with some inflammatory reaction, and lined with cuboidal cells; there were many layers, but they were regular. No budding or papillary elongations into the cystic cavity were found. The structure was that of a follicular cyst.

Postoperative Course. An ice bag was applied to the face for the first 24 hours only; then Biolite (infrared) was applied for heat, 20 minutes three times a day. Sodium hypochlorite, 10 drops in 6 ounces of water, was used as a mouthwash four times a day.

There was bleeding from the operative wound that could not be controlled by application of thrombin packs. Under local anesthesia, one catgut suture was applied and two others were tightened; thereafter, the bleeding was controlled.

On the day after operation there was marked edema of the right cheek and buccal mucosa because of the extensive bleeding into the muscle planes from the wound. There was also considerable ecchymosis. There was intense numbness of the right half of the lower lip, about which the patient complained bitterly.

On the second postoperative day the edema was somewhat less; there was still slight bleeding from the tissues. By the third postoperative day the edema was still less, all bleeding had stopped, and the ecchymosis was more marked. The patient continued to make progress, and was discharged on the fourth postoperative day, to be seen at the Dental School thereafter.

(Text continued on page 584)

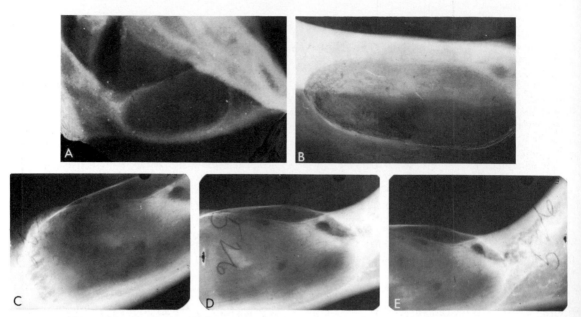

Figure 12–61   *A,* A large radiolucent area completely occupies the left body of this edentulous mandible. The area extends from the crest of the edentulous ridge to the inferior border of the mandible, and from the cuspid region to that of the third molar. *B,* In this occlusal film a marked expansion of the buccal cortical plate can be seen. A considerable thickness of the lingual cortical plate is still present. The circumscribed radiolucent area in the upper right side is the mental foramen. The inferior alveolar canal cannot be seen in this view. *C* to *E,* Periapical views, from anterior to posterior, of this radiolucent area, presenting more detail than that seen in the previous films. The circular radiolucent area in the upper right side in each of the three views represents the mental foramen of the inferior alveolar canal as it exits almost on the crest of the ridge. On close examination of the radiograph, one can see what might represent the compressed inferior alveolar canal beneath this large residual cyst. However, this is by no means certain, and I have never personally seen an inferior alveolar canal that was compressed to the small diameter indicated by the black line beneath the cyst and just above the sclerotic inferior border of the mandible.

F, The flap has been reflected and the overlying thin bone removed, exposing the thick capsule of this cyst. With a periosteal elevator the cyst was freed from its crypt and elevated, as seen in *G.* At this point we could see that the inferior alveolar neurovascular bundle was adherent to the inferior portion of the cystic capsule. As we lifted the cyst from the bottom of the bony crypt, the attached neurovascular bundle was clearly visible. By blunt dissection with the rounded tip of the periosteal elevator, we were able to free the neurovascular bundle from its anterior attachments posteriorly to a point at which we could see the attachment on the cystic capsule only with difficulty. However, we proceeded by sense of touch, gently we thought, severing the attachment of this bundle from the capsule of the cyst. However, we failed to remember that all the pressure we were applying at this posterior point to free the neurovascular bundle was being transmitted along the bundle until it passed through the mental foramen, where its lumen was considerably smaller. Suddenly, and almost instantaneously, the oral cavity filled with blood. It was obvious what had happened. We had torn completely through the bundle at the mental foramen, severing the bundle and the inferior alveolar artery. The cyst was removed because it was now fortunately free from the bunde. The massive hemorrhage was controlled by packing this large mandibular crypt with 1-inch iodoform gauze and applying considerable finger pressure on it for 5 minutes before the bleeding ceased. When the packing was gently removed, we saw that the neurovascular bundle was resting in the bottom of the bony crypt, and it had indeed been torn apart at the point where it normally would exit through the mental foramen.

H, The inferior border of this intact cyst and the fibrous connection of the cystic wall to the neurovascular bundle can clearly be seen as two ridges of tissue extending from the anterior to the posterior end of the cystic capsule. *I,* The cyst was opened, and this very thick, creamy material exuded from it. *J,* The neurovascular bundle was picked up with a suction tip and lifted from the bottom of the osseous cavity, as can be seen here. The neurovascular bundle was sutured, end to end, as is shown in *K.* However, union did not take place, and the patient had permanent anesthesia of the lower lip and was quite irate. This particular case clearly illustrates the necessity of marsupializing cysts in which this danger is present. Nothing is lost either by marsupializing in these cases until bone has filled in completely, as it will do and as has been illustrated, or, if the oral surgeon is concerned about the remote potentiality of a pathologic lesion's developing in the cystic wall, enucleating what remains of the wall after it has shrunk while the bone filled in beneath and around it. This avoids the danger of severing the neurovascular bundle, as we did here, or creating antrooral fistulas or naso-oral fistulas, as we have also unfortunately done in the past. In my opinion these complications can be prevented in practically 100 per cent of these cases by the marsupialization of these cysts.

(Figure 12–61 continued on opposite page)

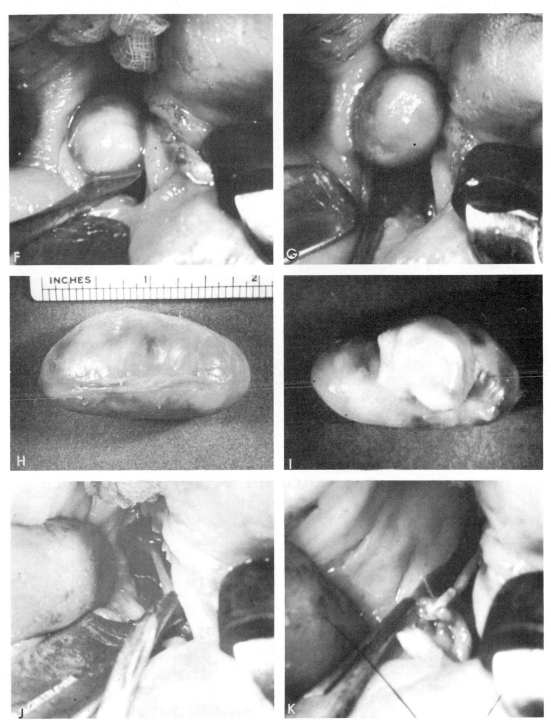

Figure 12–61   *(Continued.)*

CONCLUSIONS

This patient was very unhappy with the accidental severing of his right neurovascular bundle and the resulting postoperative complications, and in particular the intense numbness in the right half of his lower lip and cheek. The outlook for eventual return to normalcy, we frankly told him, was poor, and this proved to be the case. He left our area 2 years later with no return of sensation, although it did not "bother" him as much as formerly.

Treatment in this case should have been marsupialization. Cysts this large are not rare in this region, and we had successfully enucleated others, but the point is that as long as it is impossible to determine preoperatively whether or not a neurovascular bundle or nerve trunk is involved in any large cyst in the jaws, the ever-present possibility of injury to the nerve or blood supply should be avoided by marsupializing these cysts. (See Figure 12–60 as a case in which injury was avoided.)

This is in the patient's best interests and additionally will not give rise to the possibility of a malpractice suit.

DENTIGEROUS (FOLLICULAR) CYSTS

Dentigerous cysts that can be enucleated without postoperative morbidity should be enucleated. The same rule applies to any cyst. Large dentigerous cysts should be marsupialized if enucleation and tooth removal might result in the destruction of the nerve and blood supply to adjacent teeth, involve adjacent anatomic structures, such as the maxillary sinus, the nasal cavity, or the orbital cavity, involve major neurovascular bundles, such as the inferior alveolar one, or possibly result in the fracture of the mandible.

Dentigerous cysts, large or small, that contain the crowns of teeth which can serve a useful purpose should be marsupialized, and with orthodontic aid the teeth should be moved into the dental arch.

(Text continued on page 588)

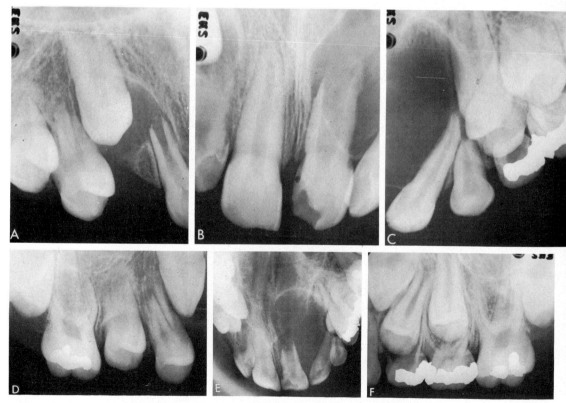

Figure 12–62 *A* to *C,* Periapical radiographs of the maxillary anterior teeth reveal an unerupted left maxillary permanent cuspid with a small dentigerous cyst about its crown. The right maxillary central incisor, whose crown was fractured by a fall, is nonvital and is incompletely formed, as indicated by the large pulp chamber and canal. The large radiolucent area between this central incisor and the left maxillary cuspid is a radicular cyst, which has developed about the apex of the central incisor. In *C* note the distal displacement of the left maxillary lateral incisor and cuspid by the radicular cyst.

D to *F,* Periapical radiographs of the maxillary bicuspid and molar area, and an occlusal view of the anterior maxilla.

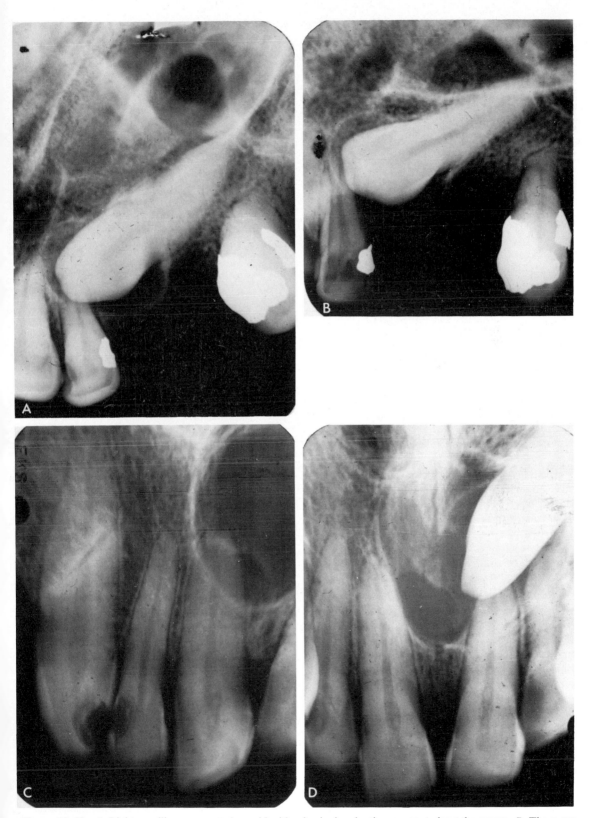

Figure 12–63 *A*, Right maxillary unerupted cuspid with a beginning dentigerous cyst about the crown. *B*, The x-ray tube has been moved distally, and the cuspid has moved in the same direction, which indicates that the unerupted cuspid is located on the palatal side of the arch. *C*, This is a portion of a dentigerous cyst that, as can be seen in *D*, has developed about the crown of an unerupted maxillary cuspid.

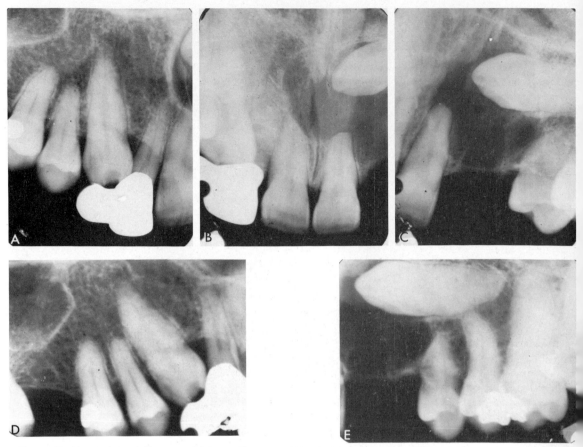

Figure 12–64   *A,* A partially erupted left maxillary cuspid is situated beneath the pontic of a bridge that is attached to the left maxillary lateral incisor, as seen also in *D.* *B,* A dentigerous cyst above the maxillary central incisors, which is causing some resorption of the root of the right central incisor. *C,* The maxillary cuspid associated with the dentigerous cyst lies in a horizontal position above the roots of the bicuspids, as shown also in *E.*

Figure 12–65   *A* to *E,* These periapical radiographs reveal the presence of a large maxillary dentigerous cyst above the roots of the maxillary anterior teeth and superior to the nasal floor, which is producing resorption of the apical third of the left central incisor root. The cyst, including the crown and most of the root of the right maxillary cuspid, then extends posteriorly over the bicuspids and molar.

F, The occlusal film reveals the extent of the cyst's growth into the palate, where it approximates the floor of the maxillary sinus and nasal cavity. Digital and instrumental exploration of the floor of the nasal cavity with a large ball burnisher proved that there were areas in which the bone was resorbed between the epithelial membrane of the nasal cavity and the capsule of this large dentigerous cyst. It is evident, from the radiographic examination, that the maxillary sinus has also been invaded by the cyst. This diagnosis is confirmed in *G,* the Waters' position posteroanterior radiograph of the maxillary sinus.

H, The maxillary cuspid (after its removal), with a 90-degree curvature of the apical third of the root. *I,* The obturator in place through the marsupialization opening. *J,* The obturator removed, revealing the large opening into the cyst that was marsupialized. An attempt to enucleate this cyst would have exposed the apices of all the teeth that were in this area. Enucleation would very likely have involved the nasal cavity and the maxillary sinus, creating fistulas. In my opinion there was no question whatsoever as to the absolute necessity for marsupialization of this particular dentigerous cyst. *K,* The cystic cavity has almost completely been filled in by bone. *L,* Periapical views of the maxillary anterior teeth showing the osseous tissue filling in the space formerly occupied by the large dentigerous cyst.

M, These radiographs again show the obliteration of the cystic cavity by normal osseous tissue. The radiolucent area that is above the second bicuspid is the depression in the buccal cortical plate shown in *K.* This radiolucent area is not due to any alteration in the osseous structure; it is simply a decreased amount of osseous tissue in this area because the cavity has not yet been completely filled in.

N, Occlusal film, if compared with the occlusal film in *F,* reveals the complete healing of the defect caused by the pressure of this dentigerous cyst.

MARSUPIALIZATION OF A LARGE MAXILLARY DENTIGEROUS CYST

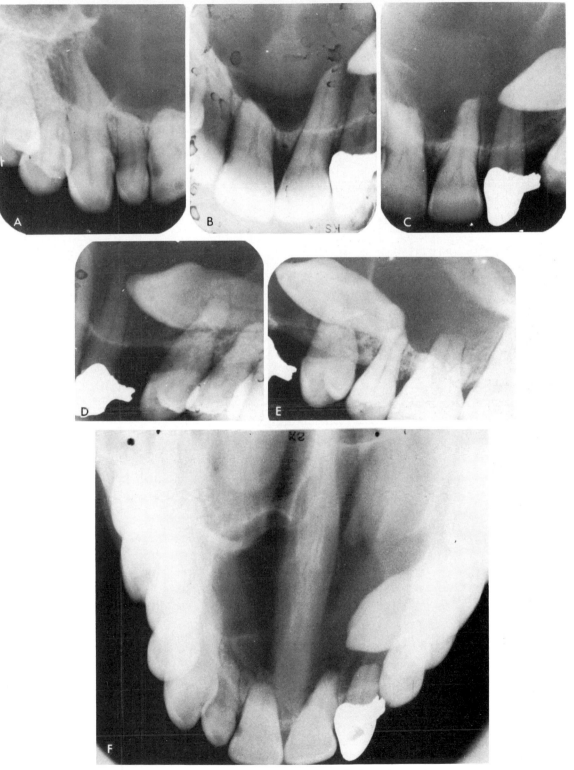

Figure 12–65 *See opposite page for legend.*

(Figure 12–65 continued on following page)

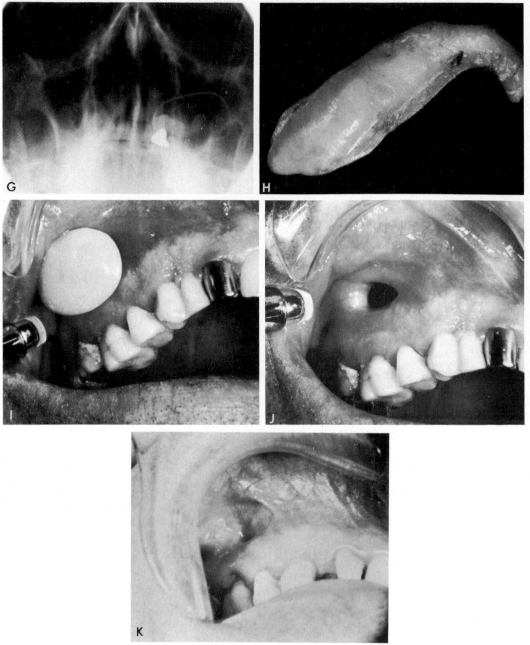

Figure 12–65   *(Continued.)*

(Figure 12–65 continued on opposite page)

To gain access to these cysts, it is necessary to make an adequate-sized mucoperiosteal flap. The edges of this flap should extend widely enough to obtain good access to the cystic cavity. The accompanying photographic case reports give a detailed description of the operative technique.

For a discussion of the remote possibility that dentigerous cysts may develop into ameloblastomas, see Chapter 13.

(Text continued on page 604)

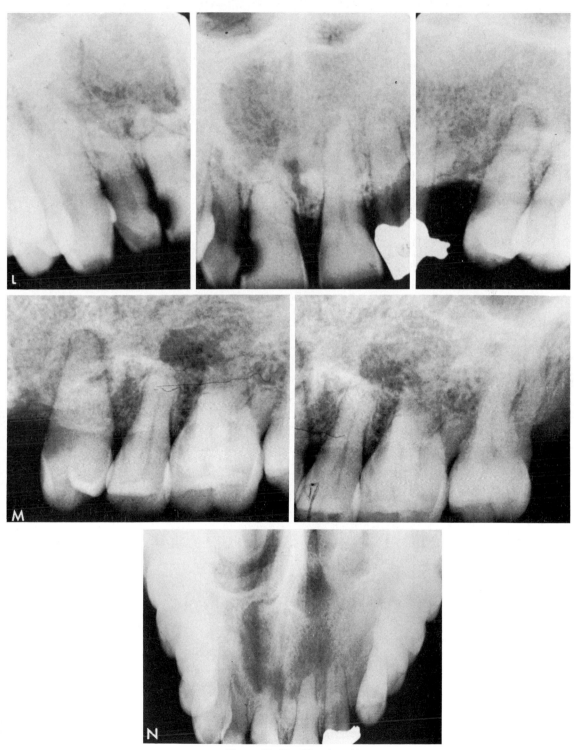

Figure 12–65 *(Continued.)*

MARSUPIALIZATION OF A LARGE DENTIGEROUS CYST ARISING FROM A RUDIMENTARY SUPERNUMERARY MAXILLARY LATERAL INCISOR IN A TWELVE-YEAR-OLD FEMALE

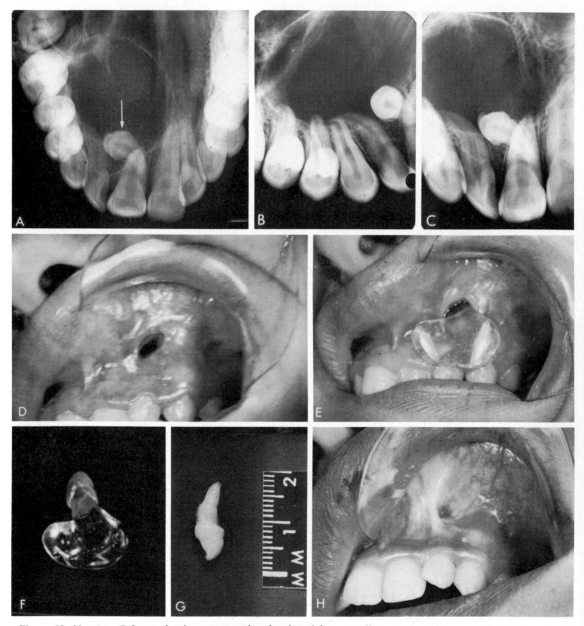

Figure 12–66 *A* to *C*, Large dentigerous cyst that developed from a rudimentary supernumerary lateral incisor. All teeth were vital, and it was very evident that enucleation of this cyst would devitalize the partially formed right lateral incisor, cuspid and both bicuspids. In addition, there was a very good possibility that either an antro-oral or naso-oral fistula or both would be created by enucleation. The technique of choice here was labial marsupialization and removal of the supernumerary lateral incisor. *D*, The small marsupialization opening into the cystic cavity was maintained by the obturator shown in *E* and *F*. *G*, Supernumerary tooth after removal. *H*, The original 1.5-cm. opening slowly closed and finally was maintained at this size until the cavity completely filled in with bone.

Frequently, particularly on the maxilla, and in young patients especially, it is not easy to maintain the patency of the opening. Patients will leave the obturator out and the opening closes so that the obturator cannot be replaced. This requires excision of soft tissue, which is best accomplished by the radiosurgical loop. When the opening maintains itself and closes slowly as the cavity fills in, no obturator is required. See Figure 12–67 as an example of this situation.

(*Figure 12–66 continued on opposite page*)

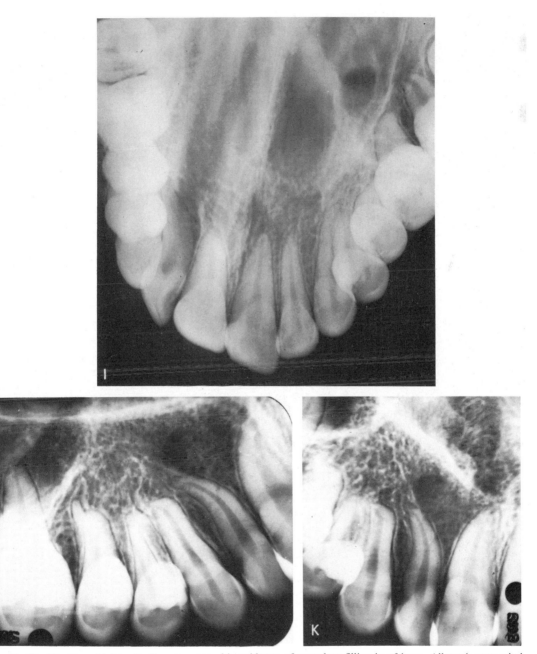

Figure 12–66   *(Continued.) I* to *K,* Roentgenographic evidence of complete filling in of bone. All teeth were vital. The radiolucent area mesial to the apex of the lateral incisor is the healed depression in the labial cortical plate shown in *H.*

MARSUPIALIZATION OF A LARGE DENTIGEROUS CYST WHICH INVOLVED THE PERMANENT LEFT MAXILLARY CENTRAL AND LATERAL INCISORS AND CUSPID IN A TEN-YEAR-OLD MALE

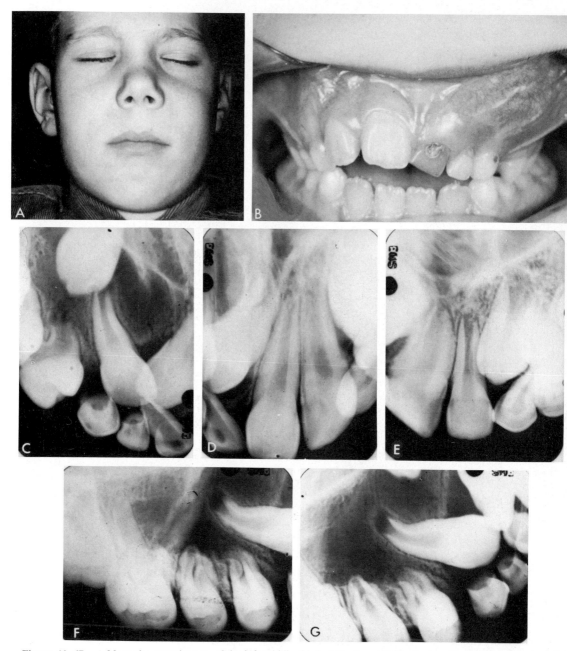

Figure 12–67 *A,* Note the prominence of the left middle third of the face. *B,* Marked expansion and thinning of the labial and buccal cortical bone. The carious discolored primary left central incisor was nonvital. The primary left lateral incisor and cuspid were loose. *C* to *G,* Roentgenograms reveal a large radiolucent area containing the left maxillary permanent central and lateral incisors and cuspid. The nonresorbed root of the nonvital primary incisor, whose root canal was not completely formed when the vitality of the pulp was destroyed, suggests that vitality was lost at approximately the age of 7. Possibly a radicular cyst had originally developed about the apex of this tooth and gradually over the years involved the three permanent teeth, preventing their eruption. (Possibly three dentigerous cysts had joined, but this would be most unusual.) In any event to prevent the loss of the three permanent teeth and the destruction of the nerve and blood supply to the partially formed premolars (bicuspids), whose partially formed roots were already being deflected by the cystic wall, marsupialization was the operative technique clearly indicated.

(Figure 12–67 continued on opposite page)

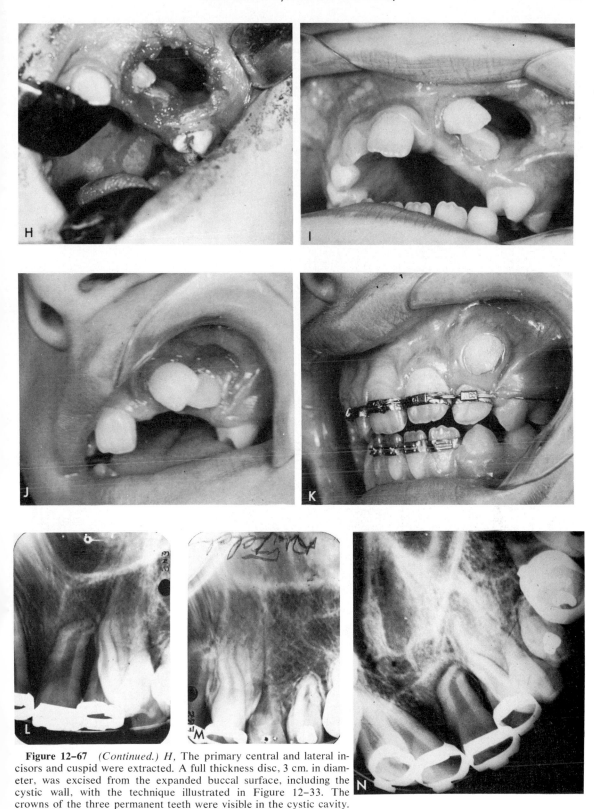

Figure 12–67 *(Continued.)* *H*, The primary central and lateral incisors and cuspid were extracted. A full thickness disc, 3 cm. in diameter, was excised from the expanded buccal surface, including the cystic wall, with the technique illustrated in Figure 12–33. The crowns of the three permanent teeth were visible in the cystic cavity. *I*, Eight weeks later the central and lateral incisors were partially erupted. No obturator was necessary. *J*, Nine months after marsupialization these teeth were fully erupted, in malposition, and the cystic cavity was filled in with bone. Orthodontic treatment was started. *K*, Two years after operation and orthodontic treatment, the cuspid was beginning to erupt. *L* to *N*, Roentgenograms demonstrate a complete filling in of normal bone.

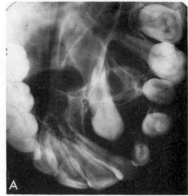

Figure 12–68 *A*, Dentigerous cyst surrounding a right maxillary cuspid. *B* to *D*, Periapical radiographs showing the extent of this dentigerous cyst and its relationship to the roots of the teeth of the right side of the maxilla. Note the deciduous cuspid still in place, with a partially resorbed root. The treatment here is to extract the deciduous root and marsupialize the cyst, not disturbing the unerupted cuspid. It is then allowed to erupt. This patient was only 8½ years of age.

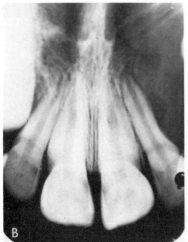
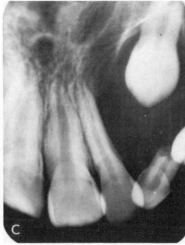
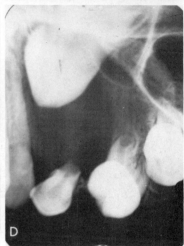

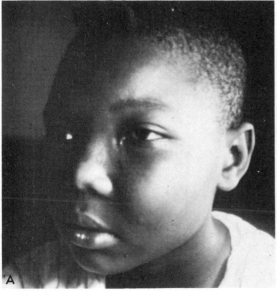
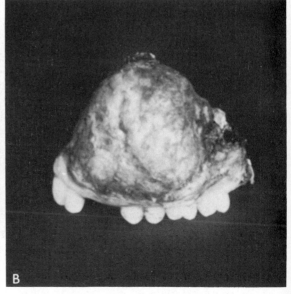

Figure 12–69 *A*, Twelve-year-old boy with marked enlargement of the left maxilla. *B*, Without a biopsy a diagnosis of a "tumor" of the left maxilla was made, and it was resected by the general surgeon. Note the absence of two maxillary teeth in the specimen. The enlargement was caused by a dentigerous cyst. Marsupialization of this cyst should have been the treatment of choice. (Courtesy of Dr. Leo March.)

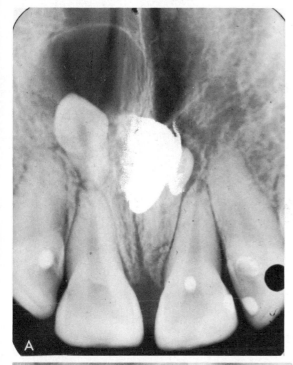

Figure 12-70   The periapical radiograph shown in *A* reveals bilateral mesiodentes in the midline of the maxilla. The mesiodens on the left has developed a large dentigerous cyst about the crown. *B*, A mesiodens in the edentulous maxilla is shown in this radiograph. *C*, Another edentulous maxilla in which the retained mesiodens has a small dentigerous cyst developing about the crown.

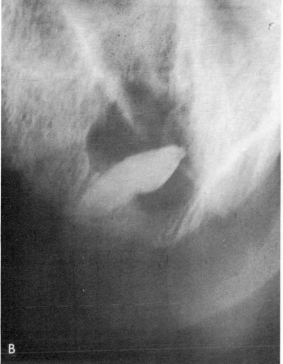

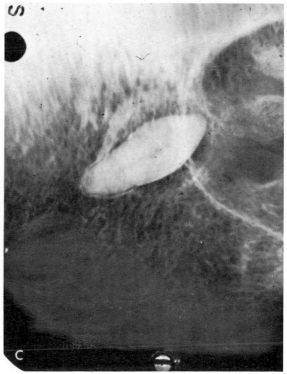

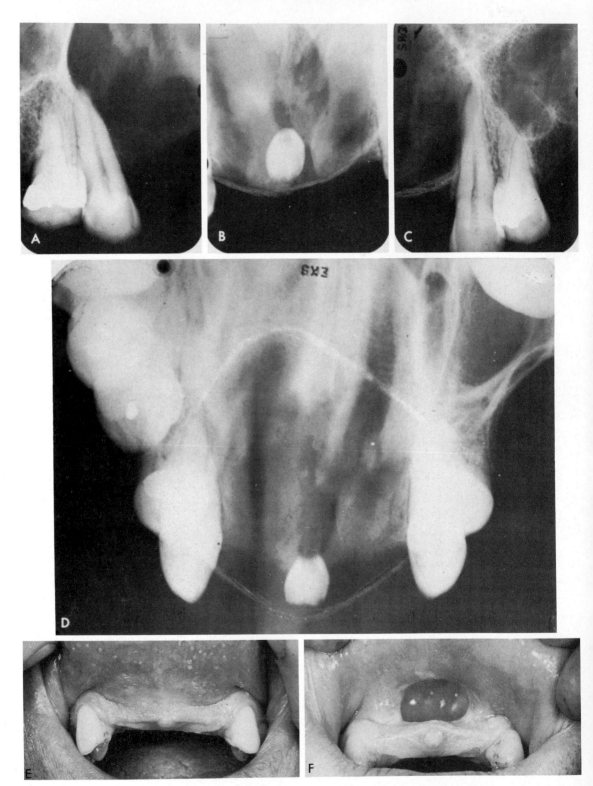

Figure 12–71 *A* to *C*, These periapical radiographs of the anterior maxilla reveal a large dentigerous cyst that has developed about the crown of a mesiodens. *D*, The palatal extension of this dentigerous cyst. Nasal exploration revealed an absence of osseous structure in the floor of the nose, which lay directly over this cyst. *E*, The obliteration of the labial sulcus by the protrusion of this cyst. *F*, This cyst was marsupialized, as an attempt to enucleate it would have resulted in a naso-oral fistula; in addition, because the cystic wall was adherent to the overlying soft tissues, it would have been most difficult to be sure that all of it was removed. The cavity shown in *F* is the result of the failure of this patient to return for the final removal of the obturator, which projected slightly into this cystic cavity. Following the removal of this projection the sulcus returned to normal.

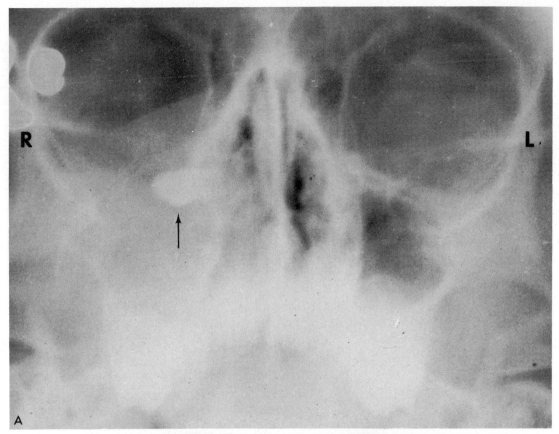

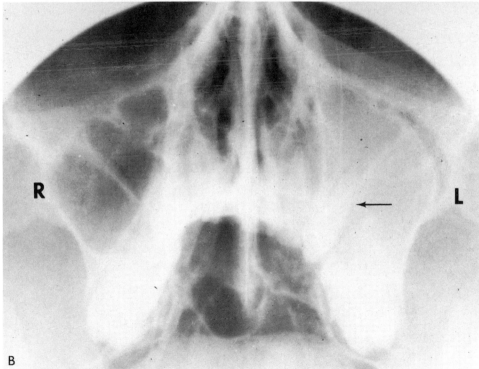

Figure 12–72 Posteroanterior radiographs of the maxilla taken in Waters' position. *A*, A dentigerous cyst about the crown of an unerupted right maxillary cuspid, now located just below the floor of the orbit. The cyst has completely filled the maxillary sinus. *B*, Another dentigerous cyst that has developed about an unerupted left maxillary cuspid and almost completely filled the maxillary sinus.

In each of these cases a large window was opened into the cyst, the unerupted cuspid was removed, and the patency of the opening of the cyst was maintained with an obturator until the cystic cavity had completely filled with bone.

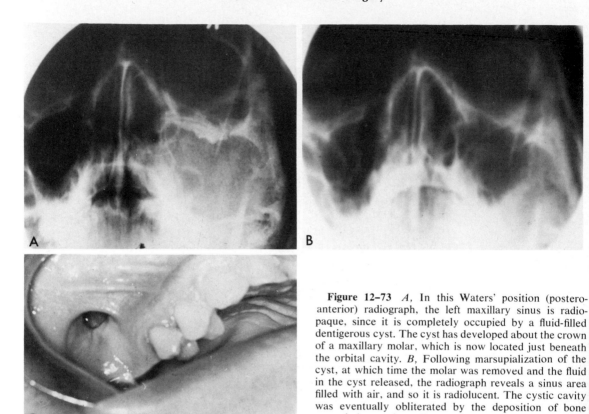

Figure 12–73 *A,* In this Waters' position (postero-anterior) radiograph, the left maxillary sinus is radio-paque, since it is completely occupied by a fluid-filled dentigerous cyst. The cyst has developed about the crown of a maxillary molar, which is now located just beneath the orbital cavity. *B,* Following marsupialization of the cyst, at which time the molar was removed and the fluid in the cyst released, the radiograph reveals a sinus area filled with air, and so it is radiolucent. The cystic cavity was eventually obliterated by the deposition of bone around the cystic wall. *C,* This photograph shows the location of the opening into the maxillary sinus created at the time of marsupialization. This opening was maintained by means of an acrylic obturator until the cystic wall was completely obliterated by the filling of bone around the periphery of the cystic wall.

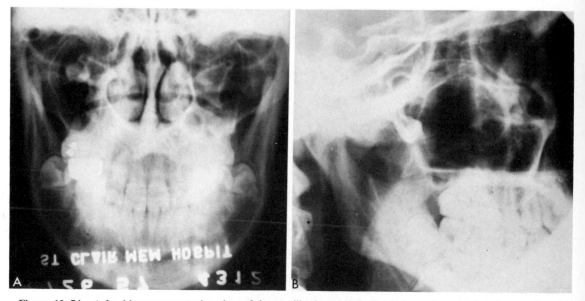

Figure 12–74 *A,* In this posteroanterior view of the maxilla the partially formed maxillary third molar was found in a dentigerous cyst high up on the distal surface of the right maxilla, as is shown in this radiograph. *B,* Lateral head radiograph of this 16-year-old female shows the location of the third molar distal to and high up on the posterior surface of the right maxilla. This cyst was marsupialized, permitting the tooth to move slowly down to where it could be removed easily as the cyst filled in.

JAW CYST–BASAL CELL NEVUS–BIFID RIB SYNDROME
(GORLIN-GOLTZ SYNDROME)

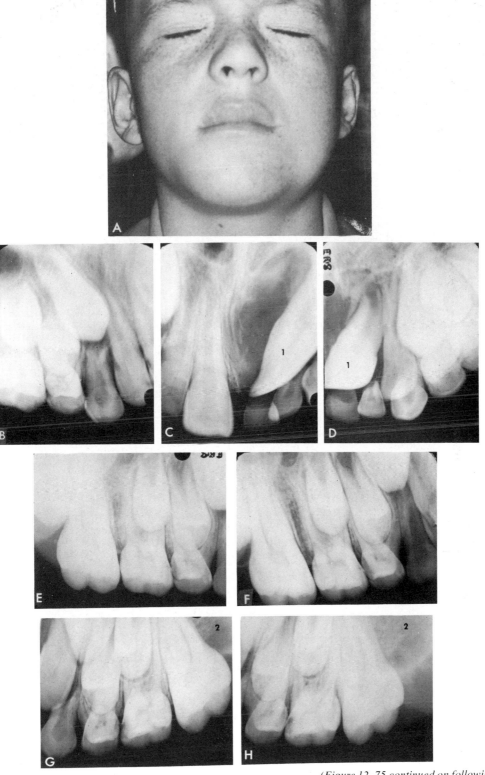

(Figure 12–75 continued on following page)

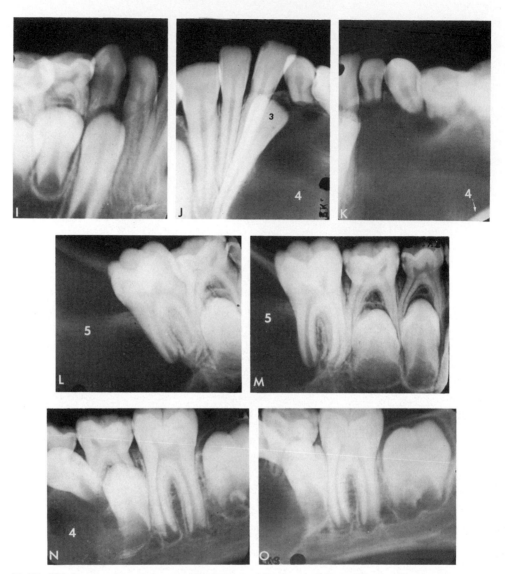

Figure 12–75　This is a complex syndrome with many possible abnormalities besides the dental and osseous anomalies. *A,* Note the minor mandibular prognathism, mild hydrocephalus, wide nasal bridge and hypertelorism. *B* to *R,* Multiple dentigerous keratocysts of the maxilla and mandible. Note that the cysts and their associated unerupted teeth are numbered consistently throughout the various radiographs so that the same number refers to the same tooth and cyst in all.

These keratocysts are no different from those not associated with the syndrome and the potential for recurrence is the same. Because they usually occur early in life, there is extensive displacement of developing teeth. As a conservative oral surgeon, I am not in accord with those who urge surgical removal of all these cysts. Judgment is used to decide which to remove and which to marsupialize. It has been shown that the recurrence rate of these cysts is less following marsupialization than following removal. The results of both techniques are demonstrated in the photographs and radiographs that follow.

Please note the remarkable eruption into almost normal position of the maxillary and mandibular teeth in those areas in which these cysts were marsupialized.

(Figure 12–75 continued on opposite page)

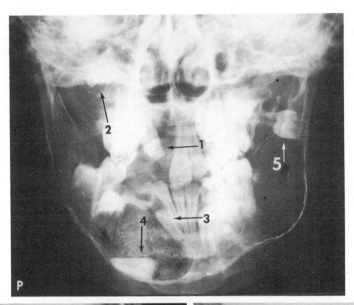

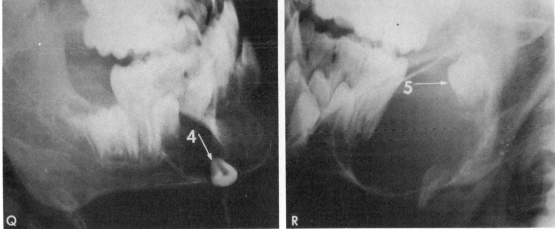

Figure 12–75 *(Continued.)*

Figure 12–75 *(Continued.)* *S,* Eruption of the right permanent central and lateral incisors prevented by the large dentigerous cyst shown in *C* and *D*. *T,* Deciduous maxillary lateral and central incisor extracted and cyst marsupialized. *U,* Mandibular right deciduous lateral incisor, cuspid and first molar were extracted (see radiographs *J, K, P* and *Q*) to permit the possible eruption of the grossly displaced permanent right lateral incisor, cuspid (at the inferior border of the mandible) and the first and second bicuspids. The remarkable *untreated* spontaneous movement of these permanent teeth is shown in *X*. *V* and *W,* Two views of a large dentigerous cyst enucleated from the right body of the mandible was followed by the poor result also shown in *X*. The patient was lost to the follow-up of our service for several years before returning at the time the panoramic radiograph *X* was made. His parents reported that he had had "several teeth extracted" from the right jaws (for reasons unknown) in the interval since we had seen him last.

(Figure 12–75 continued on following page)

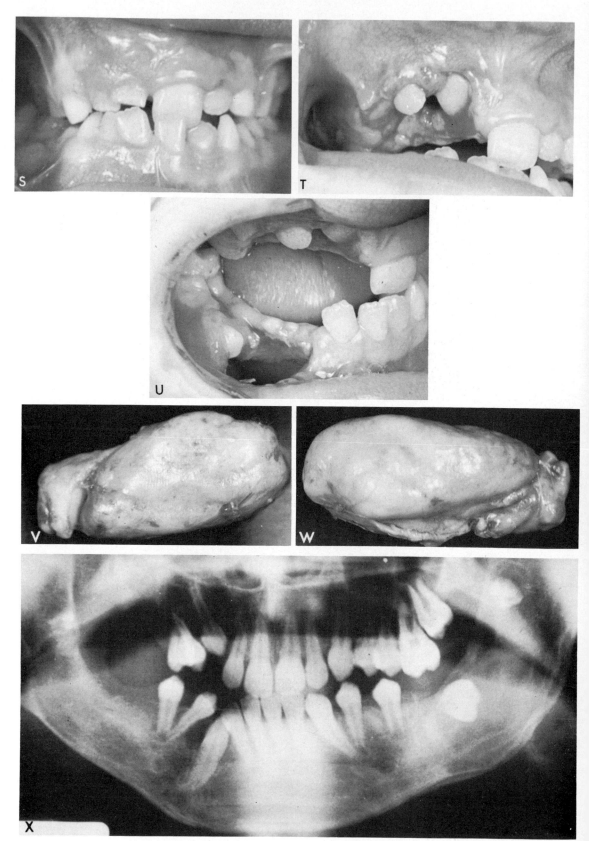

Figure 12–75 *(Continued.)*

JAW CYST–BASAL CELL NEVUS–BIFID RIB SYNDROME IN A 7-YEAR-OLD MALE

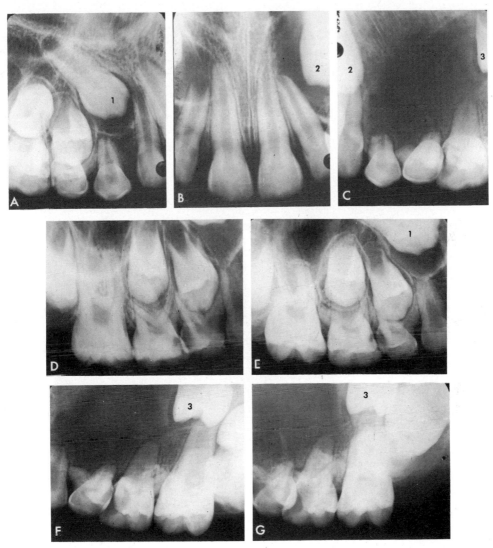

Figure 12-76 Multiple dentigerous keratocysts in both the maxilla and mandible in a 7-year-old male. These were part of the complex of symptoms for which this patient is at present under treatment. These cysts were treated by marsupialization to permit the eruption of the teeth, with orthodontic guidance. Again, impacted and unerupted teeth are numbered consistently throughout this series so that any one number refers to the same tooth in all the radiographs.

(Figure 12-76 continued on following page)

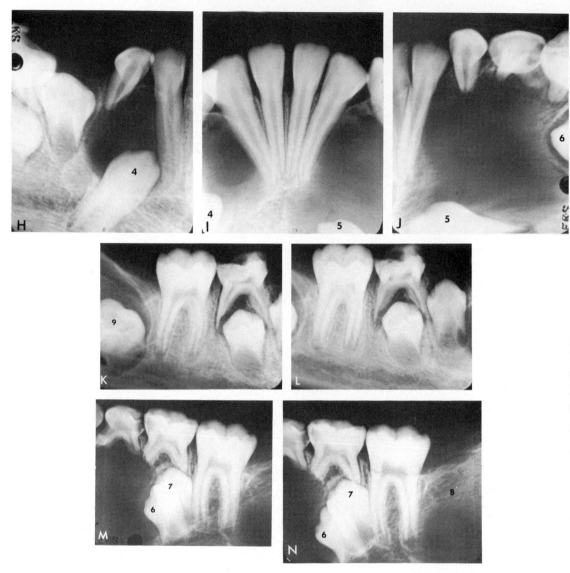

Figure 12–76 *(Continued.)*

(Figure 12–76 continued on opposite page)

Central Dentigerous (Follicular) Cyst. This is the most common form of the dentigerous cyst; it covers the crown, which is centrally located.

Lateral Dentigerous (Follicular) Cyst. This cyst differs from the central dentigerous form only in location. It does not cover the crown but is displaced to one side.

Multilocular Dentigerous (Follicular) Cyst. This cyst develops from a number of small cysts that coalesce; it is usually found in the mandibular third molar area.

Etiology. In discussing the sources of dentigerous (follicular) cysts, Tiecke says, "The cause of all follicular cysts is unknown, although two theories include perifollicular inflammation from any cause and retrograde changes in the stellate reticulum of the enamel organ. These proposals have merit, but the high incidence of dentigerous (follicular) cysts in the mandibular third molar and maxillary cuspid regions suggest an inherent or congenital weakness in the enamel organ of these teeth."[80]

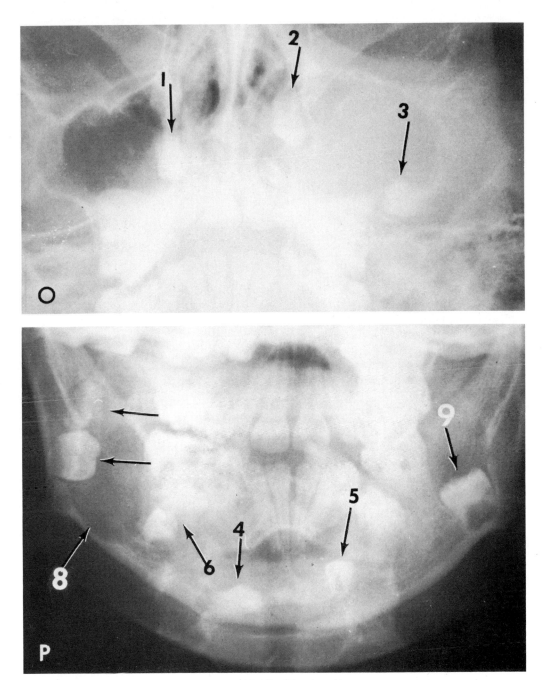

Figure 12–76 *(Continued.)*

(Figure 12–76 continued on following page)

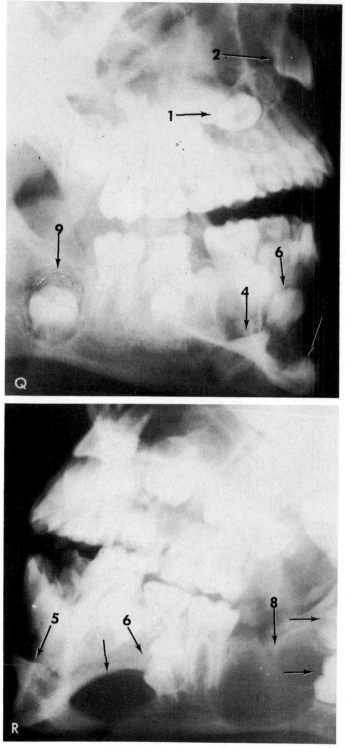

Figure 12–76 *(Continued.)*

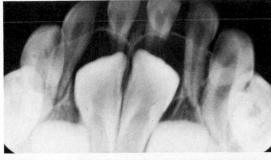

Figure 12–77 Central dentigerous cysts around the crowns of the mandibular permanent central incisors.

Figure 12–78 *A,* Lateral dentigerous cyst involving the crown of the permanent mandibular second bicuspid. *B,* Multilocular dentigerous cyst involving the crowns of the permanent mandibular cuspid and first and second bicuspids.

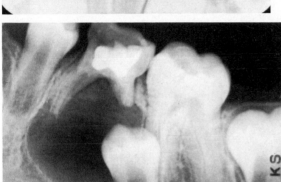

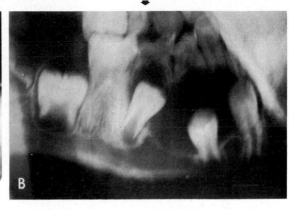

Case Report No. 2

LARGE MANDIBULAR DENTIGEROUS CYST

In this 18-year-old girl the operation planned was the marsupialization of a dentigerous cyst in the mandible involving the unerupted left second bicuspid (Fig. 12–79).

The operation was performed under general anesthesia, which was supplemented with local anesthesia.

With a Bard-Parker scalpel and No. 15 blade, a 45-degree angle incision was made between the cuspid and the lower first bicuspid for a distance of 1 cm. toward the mucobuccal fold, and continued posteriorly around the cervix of the first bicuspid, across the vacant space between the first bicuspid and first molar, around the neck of the first molar and then diagonally toward the mucobuccal fold for about 2.5 cm. With a periosteal elevator, the mucosa was gently separated from the bony cystic capsule, which had a glistening white appearance. As more of the buccal mucosa was dissected away from the bulging cystic wall, the layer of cortical plate, of eggshell thickness, covering the buccal surface of the cyst was exposed. This thin bone was carefully removed by bone shears and hemostats, exposing the cystic membrane. The distal third of the cystic capsule was constricted, thus giving the appearance of two separate cystic cavities. However, it was discovered later that it was composed of only one.

A piece of this thin cystic wall, about 2 cm. long and 1 cm. wide, was cut out with tissue scissors, as a Partsch operation was planned. When the cystic capsule was punctured, a watery fluid and white material oozed forth. This material looked like partially boiled egg albumin and curdled milk. A sample of this material was sent to the laboratory for culture, and the remaining contents were removed with suction. The entrance to the cavity was enlarged, and the buccal portion of the cystic capsule was cut out with scissors. The cavity was about the size of a walnut and extended beneath the root of the first bicuspid and distally under the roots of the first molar. The crown of the second bicuspid was visible through the cystic wall on the bottom of the cavity.

While photographs were taken of the operation, excessive retraction with hemostats of a portion of the cystic capsule unfortunately enucleated the entire capsule and unerupted bicuspid. For this reason, marsupialization, which had been contemplated, could not be performed. The cystic sac was sent to the laboratory for examination. There was a perforation through the lingual cortical plate about the size of a penny, and the lingual mucoperiosteum was visible. The cavity was loosely filled with iodoform gauze and sutured with 000 silk sutures. The patient was removed from the operating room in good condition.

(Text continued on page 623)

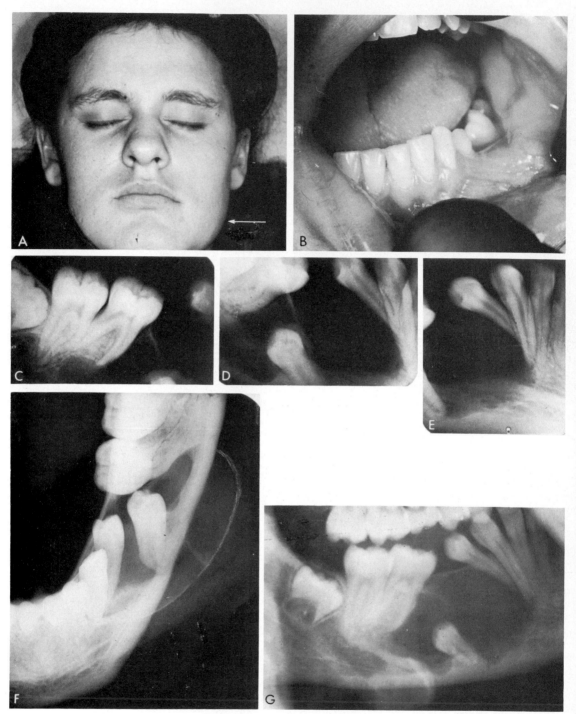

Figure 12–79   Dentigerous cyst. (See Case Report No. 2 for details.)

A, The patient presented the complaint that the left side of her jaw was becoming larger than the right side. *B,* Oral examination revealed a marked bulging of the left cortical plate. The intraoral radiograph revealed a large dentigerous cyst. *C* to *E,* Periapical radiographs of the dentigerous cyst associated with the mandibular second bicuspid. Note the loss of bone distal to the first bicuspid and mesial to the second molar, and the inferior displacement of the second bicuspid by the expansion of this cyst. *F,* The intraoral occlusal film shows the thin expanded buccal cortical plate. *G,* Left lateral jaw radiograph reveals the extent of resorption of bone due to the expansion of the dentigerous cyst. Note the relationship to the inferior border of the mandible.

(Figure 12–79 continued on opposite page)

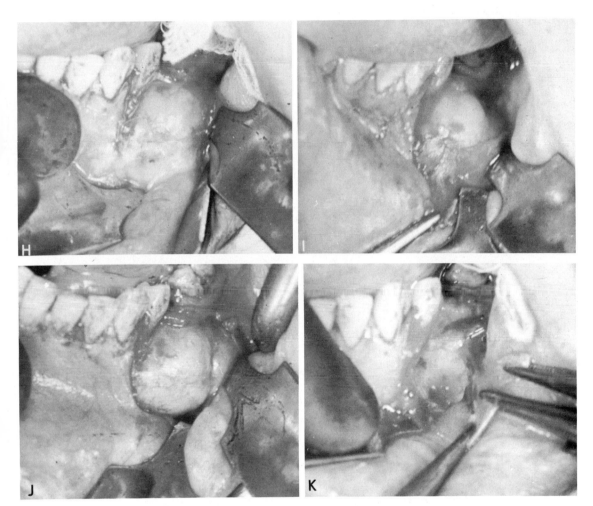

Figure 12–79 *(Continued.) H,* Incision between the left cuspid and the first bicuspid to the mucobuccal fold. *I,* The mucoperiosteal membrane reflected, exposing the thin buccal cortical bone. *J,* The thin cortical bone removed, exposing the cystic wall. *K,* The cystic wall is incised, grasped with hemostats, and reflected. The cyst was filled with a whitish material the consistency of the white of a soft-boiled egg.

(Figure 12–79 continued on following page)

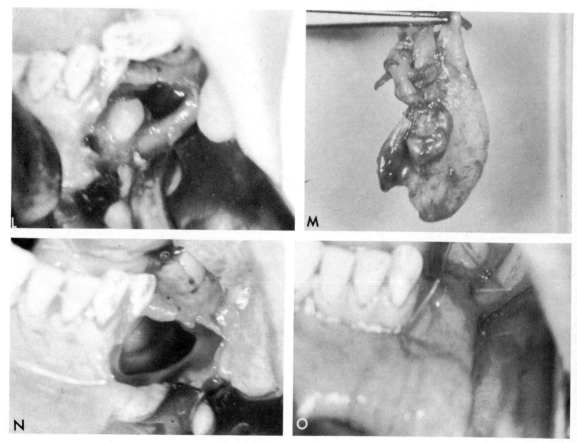

Figure 12–79 *(Continued.) L,* Marsupialization had been planned for this dentigerous cyst, but inadvertently too forceful traction by the assistant on a portion of the cystic capsule wall, which was being cut out as a window into the cyst, dislodged the capsule and its attached bicuspid *(M)* from the crypt in the mandible. An attempt was made to save the bicuspid by cutting it free from the capsule and replacing it in its small alveolus. Unfortunately, this failed. *N,* With the cystic capsule and second bicuspid removed, it could be seen that a round section of the lingual cortical bone was resorbed as a result of cystic pressure, exposing the sublingual space. *O,* The cavity was loosely filled with ½-inch iodoform tape, the buccal flap was replaced and sutured to the lingual mucoperiosteal membrane, with a strip of the iodoform tape protruding from the cavity at the line of closure to act as a drain.

DENTIGEROUS CYST WHICH PROVED TO BE AN AMELOBLASTOMA

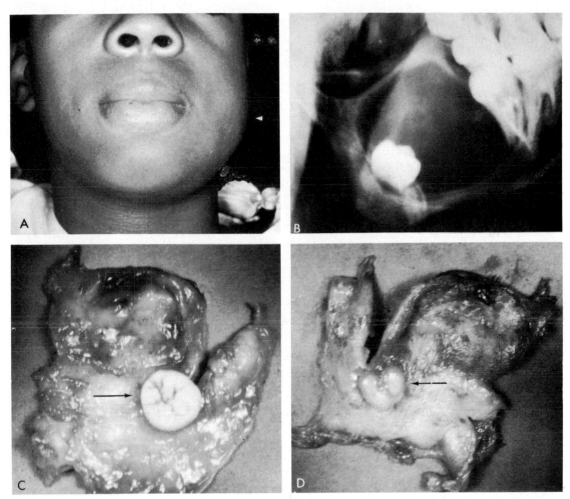

Figure 12–80 *A*, This patient, aged 15, was brought in because her mother had noticed that the left side of her jaw was larger than the right side. *B*, Lateral jaw radiograph revealing a dentigerous cyst. The first and second permanent molar roots were covered with bone and were vital. The cyst was buccal to these teeth. Enucleation was elected; because of the buccal expansion, there was little or no danger of destroying the vitality of the molars or the continuity of the inferior alveolar neurovascular bundle. In addition, the partially formed third molar was not essential and was a potential impacted tooth. *C*, The cyst "shelled out" easily after exposure without exposing the molar roots or the neurovascular bundle. Histopathologic examination of the large mural proliferations shown in this figure proved that this was an ameloblastoma. No further surgery was indicated. The patient was examined for several years with no sign of recurrence. Subsequent attempts to get the patient to return were fruitless. *D*, Reverse side of cyst capsule showing the ends of the partially formed roots.

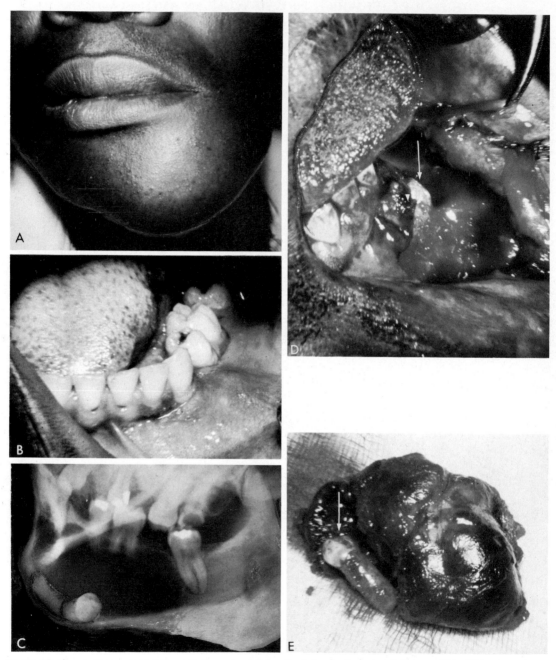

Figure 12–81 *A*, Expansion of the soft tissues overlying the left anterior area of the mandible. This expansion was due to the pressure of the expanded bone beneath the soft tissue. *B*, Intraoral view showing the complete obliteration of the anterior labial and buccal sulci by the expansion of the labial and buccal cortical bone beneath the soft tissue. *C*, An oblique radiograph of the left body of the mandible, including a portion of the symphysis, reveals this large radiolucent area containing an unerupted bicuspid at the lower border of the mandible, thereby raising the possibility that this was a dentigerous cyst. The diagnosis was confirmed by aspiration of straw-colored fluid through the thin buccal cortical plate. *D*, Opening into the area of the cyst showing the crown of the bicuspid projecting into the cyst. *E*, The enucleated cyst with the bicuspid whose follicle developed into the dentigerous cyst. (This surgery was performed by Dr. Leo March, of Kingston, Jamaica, who also contributed these photographs.)

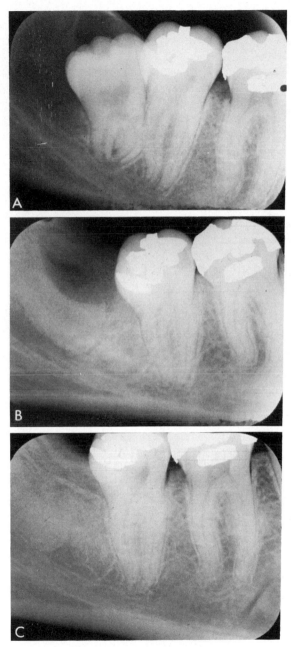

Figure 12–82 *A,* Periapical radiograph of the mandibular molar area showing an unerupted vertically impacted third molar. The large radiolucent area about the third molar proved to be a dentigerous cyst at operation. The tooth was removed intact with the cyst about its crown. Although, as can be seen in *A,* the wall of the dentigerous cyst did approximate the inferior alveolar neurovascular bundle, osseous tissue separated the two, and no damage was done to the neurovascular bundle. *B,* Periapical radiograph 6 months later revealing that the osseous crypt produced by the dentigerous cyst has been filled in by 50 per cent. *C,* One year later the osseous crypt was completely filled in with normal bone.

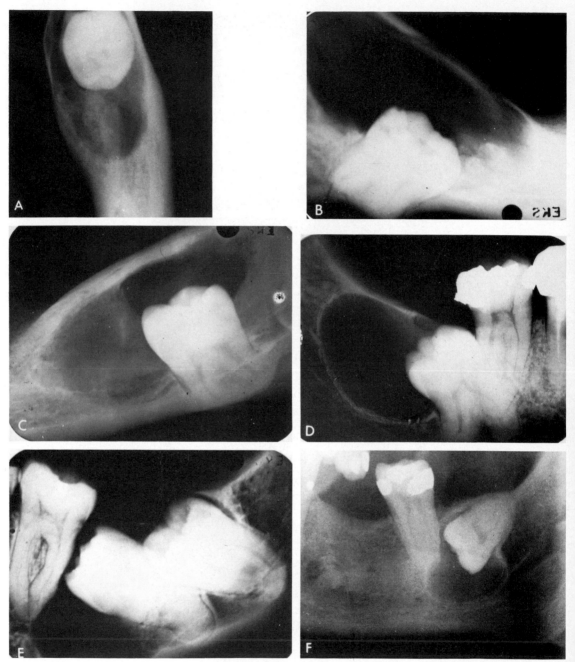

Figure 12–83 *A,* Occlusal view of this dentigerous cyst shows the expansion and thinning of the lingual cortical bone. Also it reveals that the third molar is closest to the buccal side. *B,* From this periapical view we see that the molar roots project through the inferior border of the mandible and *incorrectly* appear to be inclined lingually.

C, Central dentigerous cyst of the mandibular third molar. *D* to *F,* Examples of lateral dentigerous cysts of mandibular second and third molars.

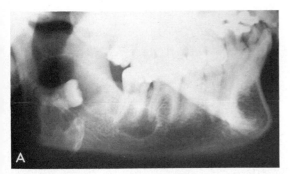

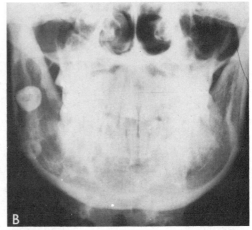

Figure 12–84 *A,* An unusual dentigerous cyst about the crown of an unerupted mandibular third molar well back in the vertical ramus. Also of interest in this left lateral oblique radiograph is the well-circumscribed area of radiolucency that involves the distal root of the first molar and the mesial and distal roots of the second molar, clearly outlined with sclerotic border. This area simulates very closely the idiopathic area seen in Figure 12–119, and we suspected that possibly it was of the same origin, namely, a follicular cyst that had developed from a tooth follicle, or that it could be a simple bone cyst (SBC).

B, The posteroanterior view of the mandible revealed the buccal-lingual relationship of the horizontally positioned mandibular third molar. It was shown to be closer to the buccal than to the lingual side. A radiolucent area in the molar region with a clear-cut sclerotic border may also be seen. The opaque object lateral to this radiolucent area is not an irregular tooth form but a button from this patient's dress (note the four radiolucent areas representing four holes in the button).

The treatment was to expose the dentigerous cyst involving the third molar and to enucleate it with the tooth. It was not adherent to the neurovascular bundle and was removed simply by tugging on the capsule. The radiolucent area beneath the molars was marsupialized with a small opening. The cavity was empty. This established the diagnosis of a simple bone cyst (SBC). (See page 641.) Patency of the small opening was maintained for a week.

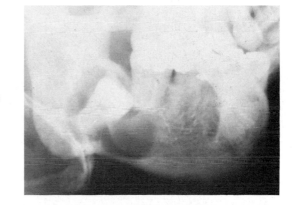

Figure 12–85 A mesioangularly impacted third molar and dentigerous cyst that appeared to be multilocular. The cyst was opened and the impacted molar removed. Gentle tugging on the cystic wall did not result in its enucleation. Apparently there was fusion between the cystic wall and the neurovascular bundle, so the cyst was marsupialized until bone had filled in around the periphery and over the neurovascular bundle, at which time what was left of the cystic wall was removed. Actually, we cannot see any legitimate reason for removing the cystic wall at this time, but because of concern expressed by the patient, that there was "diseased tissue in this area," we enucleated what was left.

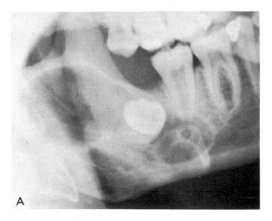

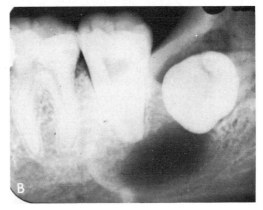

Figure 12–86 Multilocular dentigerous cyst. *A,* This case illustrates the absolute necessity for lateral (oblique) jaw radiographs in order to determine the extent of the cysts. *B,* The small intraoral film is woefully inadequate in this case.

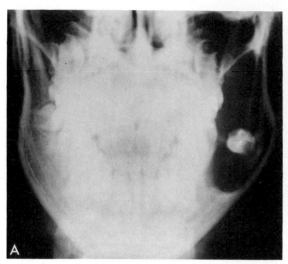

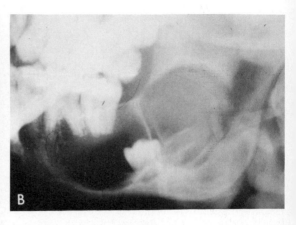

Figure 12–87 *A,* Posteroanterior view of a very large dentigerous cyst involving the body and vertical ramus of the mandible. The third molar has been displaced downward and laterally, approaching closely the inferior border of the mandible. *B,* The lateral oblique radiograph of this area reveals that the cyst approximates the inferior border of the mandible and is two-thirds the height of the vertical ramus and extends from the anterior external oblique ridge posteriorly to two-thirds the width of the ramus. Because of the impossibility of determining whether or not the first and second molars, which were vital, were involved in this cyst, it was marsupialized until sufficient bone had filled in to cover these roots. At that time the cyst was enucleated, and the third molar was removed. It must be noted also that this period of waiting had permitted bone to fill in around the circumference of the cyst, preventing the possibility that the neurovascular bundle might be torn because of possible fusion between the neurovascular bundle and the cystic capsule. (Courtesy of Dr. Nicholas Berman.)

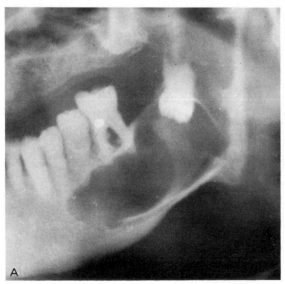

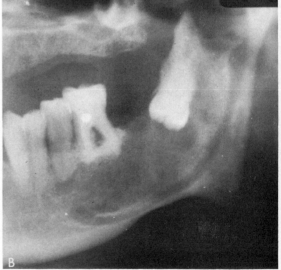

Figure 12–88 *A,* The lateral oblique radiograph of the right body of the mandible and the vertical ramus shows a large dentigerous cyst about the mandibular third molar. The molar is inverted in the vertical ramus of this 69-year-old patient. This cyst was marsupialized for reasons that should be apparent. *B,* Eighteen months later the cystic cavity had completely filled in with bone, and the third molar was not visible. We decided to do nothing further in this case. The patient has been observed for the last 3 years, once a year, and there is no indication of a recurrence of the cyst, and the patient is symptomless.

Figure 12–89 *A,* A lateral oblique radiograph of the mandible reveals a mesioangularly impacted third molar, with a large cyst extending beneath the molar and superiorly into the ramus and inferiorly to the lower border of the mandible.

B, The posteroanterior view reveals the very thin expanded buccal cortical plate and inferior border of the mandible. By palpation it was determined that there was no bone in a large area of the lingual cortical plate.

ENUCLEATION OF A LARGE DENTIGEROUS CYST OF THE MANDIBLE

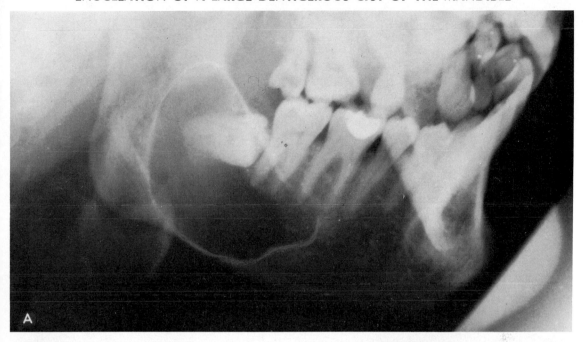

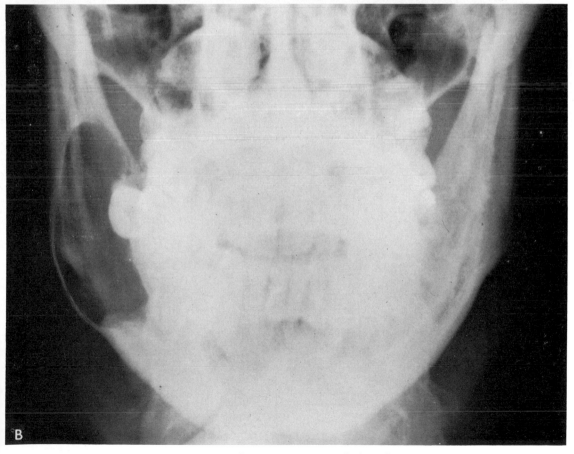

Figure 12–89   *See opposite page for legend.*

(Figure 12–89 continued on following page)

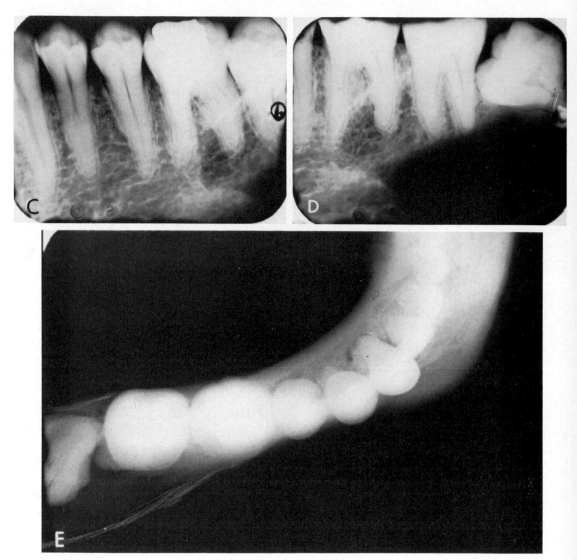

Figure 12–89 *(Continued.)* C and D, Periapical views of this area.

E, Occlusal film in which both the thin buccal cortical plate and lingual cortical plate are visualized. Because of the potentiality for a fracture during surgery, splints were applied preoperatively, as can be seen in F and G. The second molar was nonvital. It was decided to remove it as well as the impacted tooth. A buccal flap was reflected, buccal bone was removed around the second molar and the impacted third molar. More bone was removed than usual because we wanted to reduce as much as possible the resistance of these teeth to their removal by forceps. It was our intention to marsupialize this cyst, but during the surgical procedure the cystic wall was easily dislodged, and with gentle tugging the cyst in its entirety, as shown in H, was enucleated. No damage was done to the neurovascular bundle, which was visible in the lateral wall of the bone cavity.

(Figure 12–89 continued on opposite page)

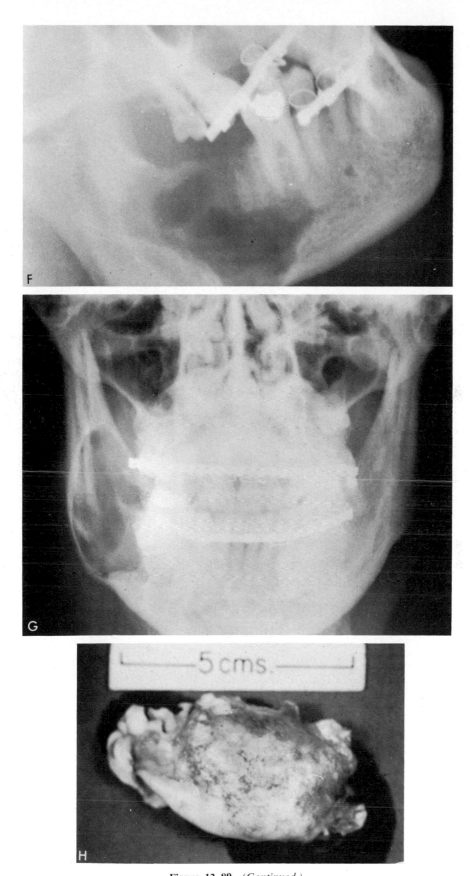

Figure 12–89 *(Continued.)*

(Figure 12–89 continued on following page)

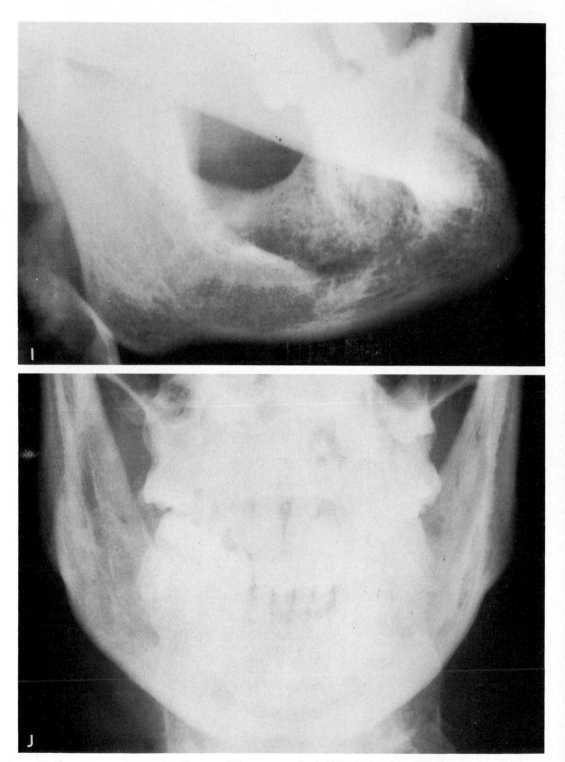

Figure 12–89 *(Continued.)* *I* to *M*, The mandible a year and a half later, showing complete filling in of the bone.

(Figure 12–89 continued on opposite page)

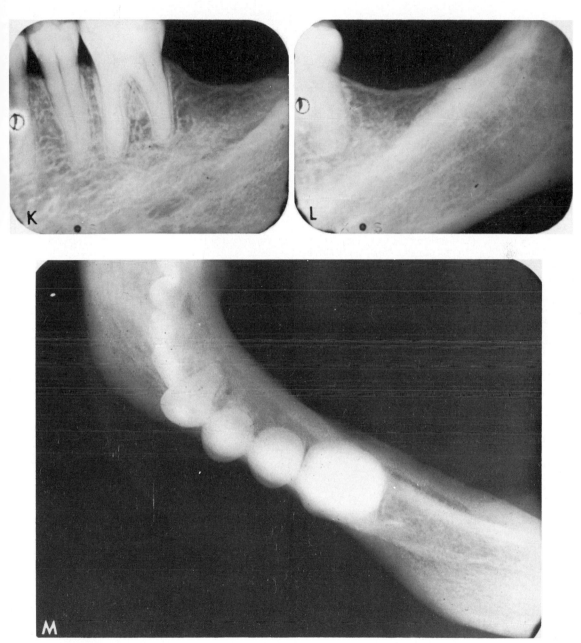

Figure 12–89 *(Continued.)*

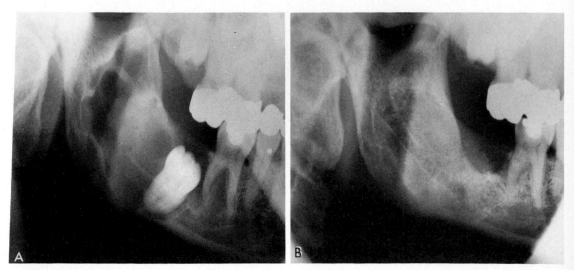

Figure 12–90   *A,* This follicular (dentigerous) cyst in a 35-year-old woman was marsupialized. When the lesion was reduced to a small size it was easily enucleated, together with the impacted tooth. I say impacted because, during the reduction period, this tooth erupted to such an extent that the crown could be seen impacted against the second molar. I am quite convinced that this tooth would have been completely erupted if the second molar had not been present. *B,* Appearance when almost completely filled in with bone. (Photographs and legend courtesy of Dr. Lester R. Cahn, New York City.)

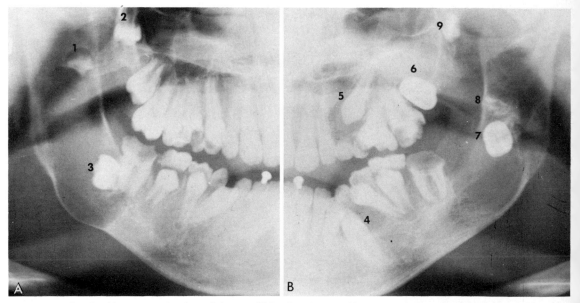

Figure 12–91   In this panoramic view of the mandible of a 10-year-old, we see nine areas of the maxilla and mandible in which there are various-sized dentigerous cysts about the crowns of second and third mandibular molars (*1, 3, 7* and *8*), a mandibular cuspid *(4)*, maxillary third molars (*2* and *9*), a maxillary bicuspid *(6)* and a maxillary cuspid *(5)*. The treatment in this particular case was multiple marsupialization operations in an attempt to facilitate the eruption of as many of these unerupted teeth as possible.

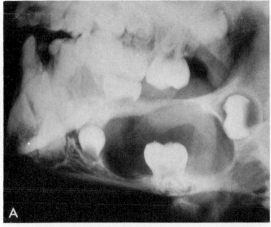

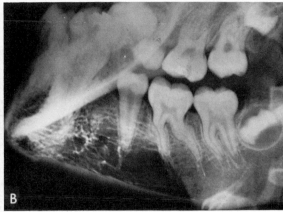

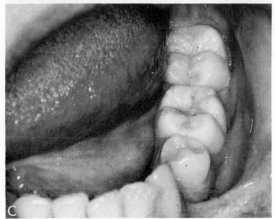

Figure 12–92 *A*, Large dentigerous cyst of 7-year-old child treated conservatively (marsupialized) and fitted with a cyst plug. *B*, Development of /678̄ 6 years later. *C*, The teeth are in correct occlusion without orthodontic treatment. (From B. W. Fickling, C.B.E., F.R.C.S., F.D.S.: Cysts of the jaws: A long-term survey of types and treatment. Proc. Roy. Soc. Med., *58*[11]:847–854 [Nov.], 1965.)

PRIMORDIAL CYST
(Simple Follicular Cyst)

This rare cyst when found is usually in the mandibular third molar area. It develops through cystic degeneration and liquefaction of the stellate reticulum before any calcified enamel or dentin has formed.[67] This cyst can develop in the tooth follicle of any of the deciduous (temporary), permanent, or supernumerary teeth (See Figures 12–93 to 12–95.)

ODONTOGENIC KERATOCYST

While any cyst of the oral cavity may have keratinization of the epithelial lining of its capsule, the odontogenic cysts—dentigerous, primordial and lateral periodontal—are those most frequently found with the characteristically very thin lining of squamous epithelium, usually with parakeratosis, no more

than six or eight cells thick, and only occasionally showing rete pegs and having a rippled surface. The connective tissue capsule often shows small islands of epithelium that may be seen as small cysts.[67]

Keratocysts are not commonly seen. Studies have shown that only 3 to 6 per cent of all jaw cysts have keratinization, while 20 per cent of primordial cysts are keratinized.[67]

They may occur at any age! In his series of 104 patients with keratocysts, Browne found that the average age was 35 years; 79 per cent of these cysts were in the mandible, 50 per cent were in the third molar and ascending ramus area, and 40 per cent were in third molar dentigerous cysts. Only 21 per cent were in the maxilla.[12, 13]

The major cause for concern in these cysts is their high rate of recurrence. Regretfully, some authors have felt that keratocysts had a greater potential to undergo neoplastic transformation than did other odontogenic cysts. This has not been demonstrated.

The early reports on the recurrence rate of

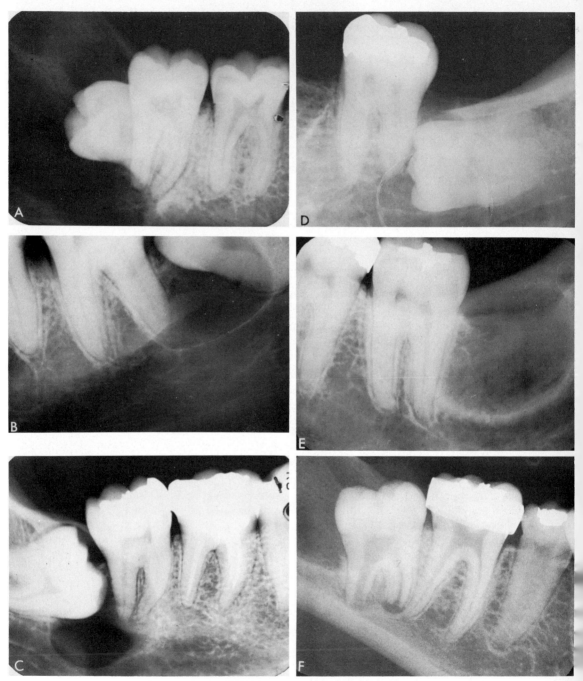

Figure 12–93 *A* to *F,* A series of periapical radiographs of the mandibular molar area in which dentigerous cysts developing about the crowns of impacted mandibular third molars can be seen.

In *E,* there appears to be a primordial (simple follicular) cyst developing. The other third molars in this patient's maxilla and mandible were present, and she had never had a tooth extracted from this area; therefore, our conclusion was that this radiolucent area must be a simple follicular cyst developing from a tooth-forming organ in which no calcification had occurred.

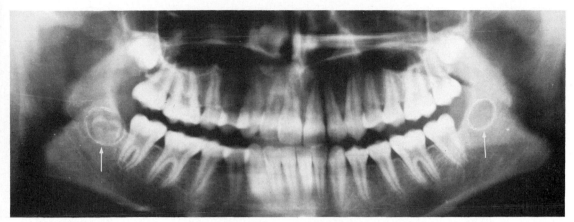

Figure 12–94 This panoramic film of a 10-year-old male shows the formation of the enamel occlusal surface in the left mandibular third molar crypt. In the right body of the mandible in the third molar crypt, which in all probability contains a tooth-forming organ, no evidence of any calcification is seen. This is the early state of the development of a simple follicular cyst, a cyst which develops in the dental follicle and can, as will be illustrated, fully occupy the vertical ramus and extend even into the body of the mandible. It is obvious that when such a situation is encountered, the early removal of the dental follicle is indicated. Note that the formation of the maxillary third molar crowns is well-advanced.

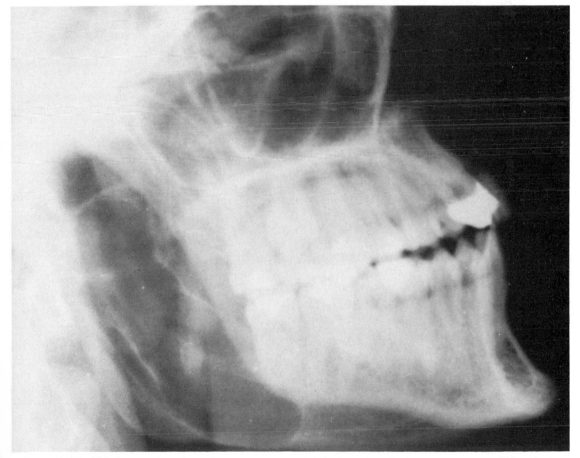

Figure 12–95 This is a semitrue lateral radiograph of the left body and vertical ramus of the mandible. The large radiolucent area, which extends beneath the apices of the left mandibular second molar and posteriorly across the third molar area and which completely occupies the ramus anteriorly, posteriorly and superiorly to the sigmoid notch, and inferiorly to the inferior border of the mandible, was diagnosed as a simple follicular cyst. The patient had not had a tooth extracted from this area, and all other third molars were present and fully formed. The cyst was marsupialized.

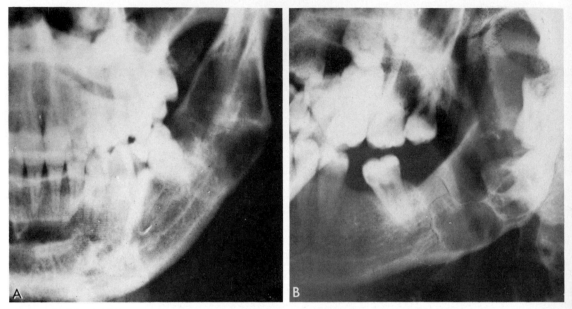

Figure 12–96 *A,* This posteroanterior radiograph of the right side of the maxilla and mandible shows radiolucent areas of the right body of the mandible extending up into the vertical ramus, with septa extending out into the radiolucent area. *B,* Although some of the cervical spine is superimposed over the vertical ramus in the right oblique view, the septa can be seen extending into the radiolucent area for a considerable distance, giving it a multilocular appearance. The radiolucent area is seen to extend well up into the vertical ramus, reaching the coronoid process and sigmoid notch. This was originally diagnosed by the roentgenologist as a possible ameloblastoma. Our biopsy proved that it was not an ameloblastoma but an epithelium-lined cyst. The patient had had a lower right third molar extracted 2 years previously, but she stated that as far as she knew, there was not a cyst in this area. There was a good possibility that the cyst was present at the time of extraction, because no extraoral radiographs of this jaw had been made. The only films taken were the small, intraoral dental films that she held with her fingers. This case points up once more the necessity of having periapical radiographs that include as much of the surrounding osseous tissue as possible, particularly in the third molar area. Admittedly, this is a rather difficult area in which to get intraoral periapical radiographs far enough posteriorly to show much of the bone distal to the third molar. In these cases, of course, it is mandatory to have an extraoral oblique film of the mandible or a panoramic film made.

keratocysts were as high as 58 per cent. Eversole and associates in their study of 70 keratocysts reported a 25 per cent recurrence, Browne reported 21 patients out of 81, also a 25 per cent recurrence rate.[13] None of Eversole and coworkers' cases of keratocysts underwent transformation to ameloblastoma or carcinoma. They concluded that there was no greater potential for keratocysts to undergo neoplastic transformation than there was for other odontogenic cysts.[27]

Treatment. The high rate of recurrence may very well be because these cysts are difficult, if not impossible, to enucleate in their entirety, because the cyst wall is very thin and friable and tears easily. This means that fragments of this thin capsule are left behind on the osseous walls of the bony cavity, where they develop into a "recurrent" cyst. Another factor to be considered in the treatment of these cysts is that in the larger cysts,

particularly those in the mandibular third molar and ascending ramus area, there frequently is complete resorption of the cortical bone between the cyst capsule and contiguous soft tissue, which further complicates enucleation and increases the possibility of postoperative infection in one of the adjacent anatomic spaces, as, for example, the pterygomandibular. While Browne in his report did not find any "significant difference in the recurrence rate"[13] following any of the three main methods of treatment—(1) marsupialization, (2) enucleation and primary closure or (3) enucleation and packing open—I personally am of the opinion that the best interests of the patient are served by marsupializing these large cysts. All cysts, large or small, particularly those in bone, should be radiographed annually for at least 5 years to ascertain whether or not there is a recurrence.

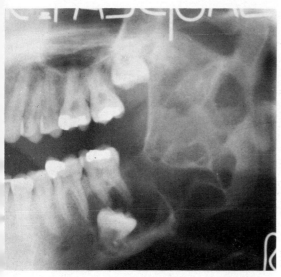

Figure 12–97 Panoramic radiograph of a dentigerous keratocyst that simulated the appearance of an ameloblastoma. The capsule with its epithelial lining was diagnosed as a keratocyst. (Courtesy of Dr. Harry N. Pasqual.)

CALCIFYING ODONTOGENIC CYST
(Gorlin Cyst, Keratinizing Cyst, Calcifying Epithelial Odontogenic Cyst)

This lesion has an unusual combination of the features of a cyst and a solid tumor. It has been, and still is, misdiagnosed as one of the forms of ameloblastoma. Like this tumor, the great majority of the calcifying cysts are found in the mandible. (See Case Report No. 3, which concerns an exception to the rule because the cyst is in the maxilla.)

Radiographs reveal a well-circumscribed radiolucent area, in which there are variable amounts and sizes of a radiopaque material scattered throughout (see Figures 12–98 and 12–99). Cases have been reported in which the cyst is associated with a complex composite odontoma or an ameloblastic odontoma, or "there is a rare variant in which melanin is present within the odontogenic epithelium. Finally, it is recognized that carcinomatous transformation in this lesion can occur."[67] *Treatment:* Enucleation.

Case Report No. 3

TREATMENT OF A PIGMENTED CALCIFYING ODONTOGENIC CYST OF THE MAXILLA*

Patient. A 14-year-old female patient was admitted to Eye and Ear Hospital. The patient's chief complaint was a swelling on the left side of the face for the past 2 years. It was for the most part painless but continued to increase in size (see Figure 12–98A and B). Three months earlier the patient had been admitted to a hospital, where the area was "incised and drained," but the area remained approximately the same size. It was painless except when pressure was applied externally. Findings in her past medical history were essentially negative, except for a tonsillectomy and adenoidectomy, the removal of some cysts from her leg, and the usual childhood diseases.

Physical Examination. This revealed a well-developed, well-nourished female in no acute distress. Blood pressure, 90/60, pulse 68, full and regular. Head, nontender swelling over left maxillary sinus. Neck, no node palpable. Ear, nose, and throat, findings negative. Lungs, clear to palpation and auscultation. Heart, good quality, no murmur heard. Abdomen, no masses, tenderness, or scars. Extremities, no deformities or edema.

Laboratory Examination. Findings in the routine blood and urine examinations were well within normal limits. The patient was suspected of having a tuberculous lesion of the left lung, but further examination results were negative, and the patient was cleared for surgery.

Dental Examination. Previous dental history was unremarkable. Tongue, cheeks and floor of the mouth were normal. Gingival tone and color were good. The missing teeth were maxillary left 3, 4 and 8. Dental radiographs revealed that the mandibular left and right 8 were impacted. Also there was a large radiolucent area in the left maxilla containing the cuspid and first bicuspid, which were displaced superiorly to the periphery of the radiolucent area. This area did not have a clear-cut border, and it had a "snowflake" appearance (see Figure 12–98C to E). The patient had an antro-oral fistula in the area of the impaction.

Operative Report. With general and local anesthesia, the following procedure was performed: With a No. 15 Bard-Parker blade, an incision was made along the crest of the ridge to the midline, extending from the molar area. It was then carried

---

*Case report prepared by Charles E. Stoner, Oral Surgery Resident, Presbyterian-University Hospital, Pittsburgh, Pa.

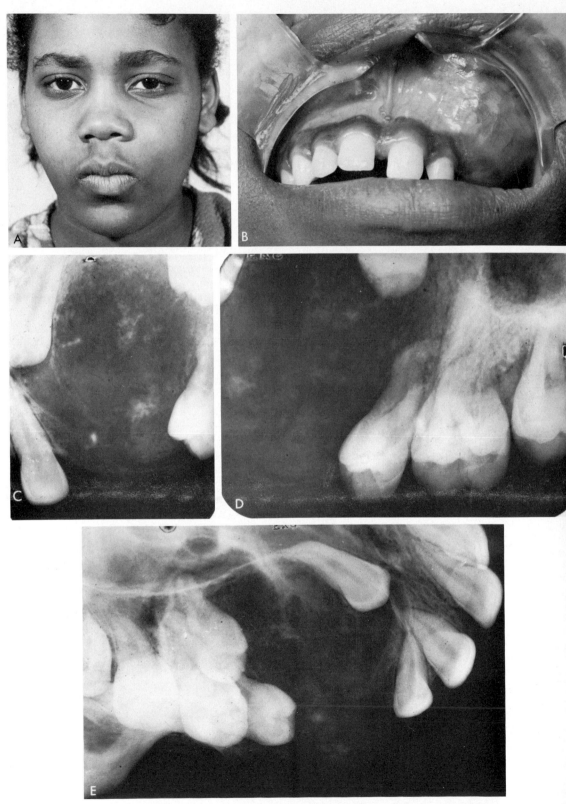

Figure 12–98 *A* and *B*, Swelling from a pigmented calcifying odontogenic cyst. See Case Report No. 3. *C* to *E*, Note the islands of calcified radiopaque material that are scattered throughout the radiolucent area of this cyst.

to the labial mucosa. The tissue was reflected a distance of approximately 15 mm. In the area of the fistulous tract a great deal of difficulty was encountered in reflecting the tissue because of an extensive fibrous process. This was in approximately the left bicuspid region. When the mucosa was finally reflected, it was found that the tumor mass was protruding through an eroded portion of the cortical bone, measuring approximately 8 mm. in diameter. The following teeth were then extracted: maxillary left 1, 2, 5 and 6, to allow for greater access in removal of further cortical bone. The bone was found to be extremely soft and granular. A window measuring 3 cm. in length and 1 cm. in width was finally obtained. With periosteal elevators and a large-bowled curette, the mass was enucleated from its bony crypt. There was some fibrous attachment, but no extreme difficulty in its enucleation was encountered. When finally removed, the mass was found to be roughly circular. The tumor measured approximately 3 cm. in diameter. The specimen was sent to the laboratory for examination. The impacted cuspid revealed by radiographic study was found to be in the medial wall of the bony crypt. At the removal of the tumor there was found to be some attachment to the tooth. With Apexo elevators the impacted tooth was luxated and removed with a No. 286 forceps. There was found to be a slight perforation into the left antrum at the deepest portion of the tumor crypt. It was also found that the greatest growth of the tumor mass was laterally, thereby encroaching on the left antrum, but very little. All bone was found to be soft. The anterior wall of the antrum was depressed into the sinus. This was opened and completely removed with biting forceps. The bone was very soft. The lining membrane of the antrum was thickened. It was removed completely with a curette. The antrum itself was large. A nasoantral window was made and the antrum packed with tincture of benzoin gauze carried through the nose. The mucosal flap was trimmed and the remnant of the left alveolus was shaped and smoothed with bone rongeurs and bone files. The flap was approximated and sutured into position with 000 black silk. The fistulous tract was also sutured slightly with two interrupted black silk 000 sutures. The patient was taken from the operating room in good condition.

Final Laboratory Diagnosis. Pigmented calcifying odontogenic cyst (A. P. Chaudhry, Oral Pathologist).

Postoperative Course. On the day of surgery the patient was given aqueous penicillin daily with 1 gm. of streptomycin. Postoperative condition the same day was good. The temperature of the patient never exceeded 37.5° C. at any time. The second postoperative day the antral packing was removed. On the fourth postoperative day the nose was clear, and the edema was subsiding. On the fifth postoperative day the sutures were removed, and the area was healing well. The patient was discharged on the seventh day. She was to be seen in 2 weeks.

Final Diagnosis. 1. Pigmented calcifying odontogenic cyst of the left maxilla. 2. Impacted left maxillary cuspid. 3. Chronic hyperplastic maxillary sinusitis (left).

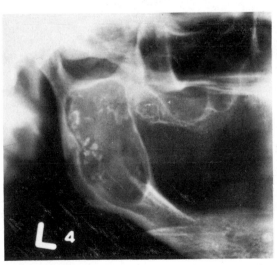
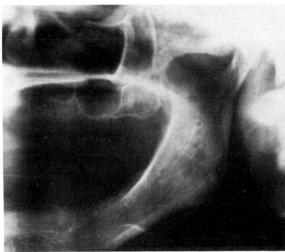

Figure 12–99 In this panoramic film of an edentulous mandible in an adult, a large radiolucent area is seen completely filling and expanding the osseous tissue of the left vertical ramus. Calcified bodies are distributed along the posterior and superior walls of this radiolucent area.

The cystic capsule was exposed by the removal of overlying bone and enucleated with curettes around the periphery. A portion of the loose capsule was grasped with a hemostat, followed by gentle traction. Strangely enough, the neurovascular bundle was not adherent to the cyst, although it was readily visible lying in a shallow groove in the medial wall of the bony crypt. *Histologic report*: Calcifying odontogenic cyst. Healing was uneventful.

CYSTS OF THE ORAL MUCOSA IN THE NEWBORN
(Epstein's Pearls, Bohn's Nodules)

Small, white, raised, multiple nodules from the size of a pinhead to 2 to 4 mm. are frequently seen in the alveolar and palatal mucosa of newborns. According to Cataldo, "The most common site is along the palatal raphe and the least common site is the mandibular mucosa. However, 80 per cent of the infants examined have cystic nodules on the maxillary, mandibular or palatal mucosa."[17]

The majority are inconspicuous and we usually notice only the larger ones. No treatment is indicated, as they do not interfere with the eruption of teeth; they become superficial and rupture and drain spontaneously within a few months.

ERUPTION CYSTS IN THE NEWBORN

In Figure 12–100 are shown several cases of eruption cysts in newborns. These cysts are present at the time of birth; they usually rupture spontaneously and exfoliate the partially formed crown. Marsupialization, accomplished by cutting off the tops of these cysts, has not prevented exfoliation of the partially formed tooth (about three-fifths of the crown of the incisors and proportionately less of the posterior teeth), as was hoped.

Treatment. Marsupialization of those

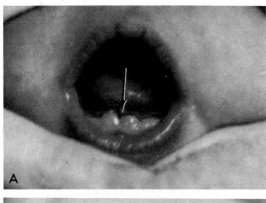
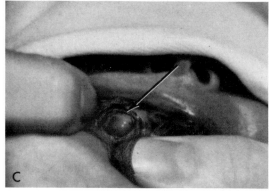
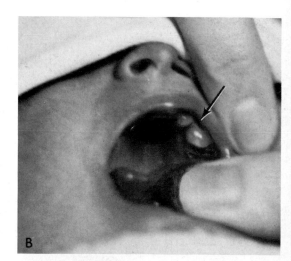
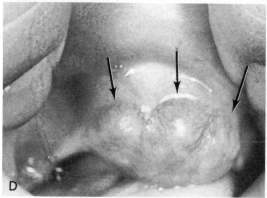

Figure 12–100 Eruption cysts in newborn babies. *A,* Four-day-old baby with eruption cysts of the deciduous central incisors. *B,* Large eruption cyst in the deciduous cuspid and first bicuspid area. Baby 1 week old. *C,* In this newborn the eruption cysts over the maxillary deciduous central incisors have ruptured. Cuspid cyst is still intact. *D,* Multiple large eruption cysts on the anterior maxillary ridge of a 4-week-old baby. A cyst can be observed at the tip of each of the three arrows. See the text for treatment of these cysts.

cysts that do not rupture spontaneously should be performed. If the partially formed crown is mobile, remove it.

PREMATURE ERUPTION OF PRIMARY TEETH

Occasionally prematurely erupted loose primary teeth at birth are associated with not only a cyst but a tumor of the mandible. If there is a swelling of the mandible, a roentgenogram should be made of this area. The tooth or teeth are extracted, a small flap reflected and an incisional biopsy taken if tumor tissue is present. Definitive treatment is based on the pathology report.

INFECTED CYSTS

The contents of oral cysts are originally sterile. They may become chronically or acutely infected secondarily. The chronically infected ones are usually symptomless, but some develop fistulas that attract the patients' curiosities and they seek consultation. These cysts with low-grade infection usually have capsules (sacs) that may be slightly thickened but are not necrotic.

Treatment. The cause of the cyst should

be removed, and enucleation or marsupialization, whichever is indicated in that particular case, carried out. Treatment of an acutely infected cyst accompanied by pain, swelling (if the pus has escaped from the bony cavity) and temperature includes incising and draining it and administering appropriate and adequate antibiotic treatment based on a culture of the pus. No other surgery is indicated until the acute infection has subsided and remained subdued for at least 3 weeks, drainage and irrigations of the cavity having been maintained during this period.

In many of these cases the patient has a history of recurrent acute infections or recurrent cysts in this area. The reason for the latter is the retention in this area of the epithelial elements mentioned above.

In those cysts that have had acute infectious episodes and that have been incised and drained, or have drained spontaneously, the cyst capsule is, for the most part, already destroyed, and only a few scattered remnants of the epithelium-lined sac remain. The repeated acute infections result from bacteria retained in this warm, dark cavity containing an excellent "broth"; in short, it is an ideal incubator. This is particularly true when drainage and irrigation have not been maintained for several weeks. However, even in this last situation, to prevent recurrences of a cyst, it is necessary to marsupialize these areas.

Cauterization — either chemical or thermal — of cyst cavities, in an attempt to destroy any remaining epithelial elements, or to render the cavity "sterile," is, in my opinion, contraindicated. As a rule, marsupialization prevents both recurrence of the cyst and infection.

CARCINOMA IN ODONTOGENIC CYSTS (ODONTOGENIC SQUAMOUS CELL CARCINOMA)

Gorlin states: "Over 80 case reports of squamous cell carcinoma arising in pre-existing dental cysts may be found in the literature. However, one must be extremely stringent in evaluating these reports. Carcinoma of the jawbones is usually due to spread from carcinoma of the overlying epithelium. Any case report in which there is overlying ulceration must therefore be eliminated from consideration. Moreover, carcinoma may be metastatic to the jawbones and, therefore, careful search for a primary lesion must be

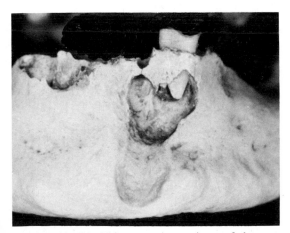

Figure 12–101 This anatomic specimen of the symphysis of the mandible shows a rather large area of loss of cortical bone. Because the carious lateral incisor root projects into this area, one can assume that the pressure of a radicular cyst on this dense bone stimulated osteoclastic activity, producing the resorption of bone to the inferior border of the mandible. One can also speculate that this was a fistulous tract, such as is illustrated in Figure 12–102, although this is certainly a very large area of resorption for a sinus tract beneath the periosteum.

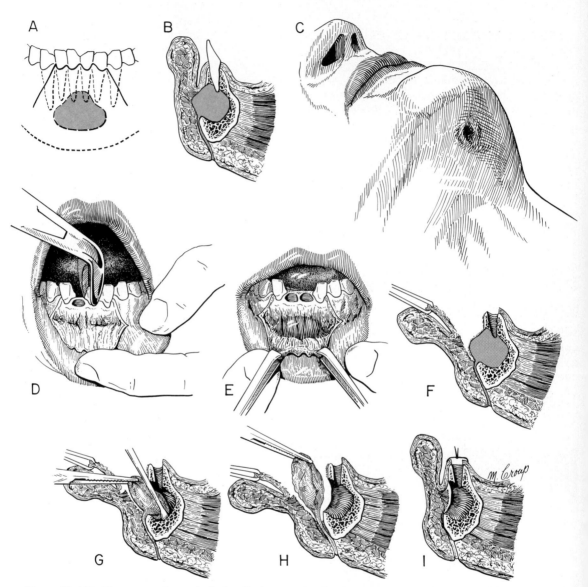

Figure 12–102　Treatment of a periapical radicular cyst that has become chronically infected and has developed a fistulous tract. *A,* Large radicular cyst (copied from a radiograph) that had originated from mandibular central incisors whose vitality had been destroyed by a blow. *B,* The cyst eroded through the labial cortical plate and expanded into the soft tissues overlying the symphysis. Then it became acutely infected, with additional swelling, and finally spontaneously ruptured and drained, leaving a chronic fistulous tract draining through the soft tissues beneath the symphysis, as shown in *C. D,* Making a flap and extracting the two nonvital central incisors. *E,* Dissecting the mentalis muscle fibers away from the cystic wall. *F,* The cyst exposed. *G* and *H,* The cyst is then enucleated from its bony crypt. The sinus tract is freed toward the inferior border of the mandible and two thirds of its length cut off. *I,* The flap is replaced and sutured into position. The fistulous tract will close spontaneously. There will be, however, a depressed scar tied down to the inferior border of the mandible. This can be eliminated, after healing, by an elliptical incision around the scar down to bone and including the periosteum. This elliptical bit of tissue is removed. The cutaneous tissue is then undermined in all directions and approximated with sutures.

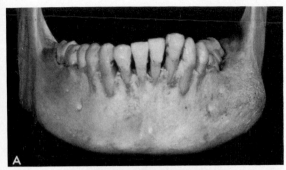

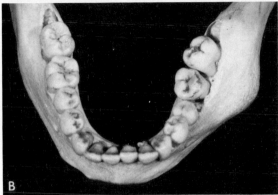

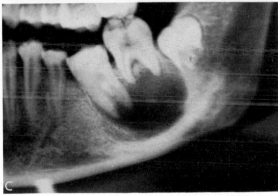

Figure 12-103 Anatomic specimen. *A* and *B,* Marked expansion of the buccal cortical plate of the left corpus (body) of the mandible in the region of the lower left first, second and third molars. *C,* A lateral jaw radiograph of the specimen reveals a large circular radiolucent area involving the first and second molars. The evidence in this dry specimen is inconclusive as far as a diagnosis of the cause for the expanding lesion. It is of interest to note condensing osteitis about the central area of radiolucency. This bodily defensive activity, which is shown by the deposition of calcium salts throughout the cancellous bone surrounding the radiolucent area, is not usually seen in areas in which there are cysts or tumors. Perhaps the lesion was an infected primordial cyst.

as 'a malignant change in a dentigerous cyst' by Bradfield and Broadway.[10]

"Moreover, the photomicrographic evidence in many reported cases has been so poor as to defy diagnosis.

"One must rule out the possibility that the jaw 'cyst' does not represent cystic degeneration of an epithelial neoplasm or that the cyst and tumor are *independent* but in close [proximity] to each other.

"When all these requirements are considered, there are fewer than 30 cases which meet the criteria.[4, 10, 28, 34, 39, 45, 47, 50, 52, 55, 69, 76, 88]

"The median age is 57 years, and there is a 2:1 male predilection. The mandible has been the site over twice as often as the maxilla (Gardner,[34] Shear[69]).

"Perforation of the cortical plate and a rapid increase in jaw size are important clinical features. The bony expansion is firm, smooth, hard, and usually nontender. Pain is variable and lip paresthesia is not a feature.

"Roentgenographically, the radiolucent lesions are oval or round with jagged, indistinct borders. Roots of adjacent teeth exhibit resorption, and the teeth may become loose."*

Others concur with Gorlin's skepticism of the literature. Tiecke states, "Of 48 cases reported in the literature, only 8 were acceptable to this author.[80] Bernier states, "In over 41 years as a practicing oral pathologist, over half of which was spent at the Armed Forces Institute of Pathology, I have not personally seen a squamous cell carcinoma arising in an odontogenic cyst. It is not unusual, however, to see epithelial changes occurring in such cysts, but these must be related to the behavior of the lesion. Squamous cell carcinoma is established as an entity when it behaves as a malignant tumor. I do not say that such a lesion cannot occur, but I have not seen one and the literature is not convincing to me."[7]

OSSEOUS REPLACEMENT FOLLOWING TREATMENT OF ODONTOGENIC CYSTS

Marsupialization vs. Enucleation. It has long been stated, and repeated from author to author, particularly by those who have been

---

made. In addition, all epithelial tumors arising from the odontogenic apparatus and the antral mucosa must be eliminated. For example, a calcifying odontogenic tumor was reported opposed to, or lukewarm toward, marsupialization of cysts, and therefore have had little if any experience with this technique, that "cysts fill in with bone more quickly following enucleation than following marsupialization."

During my first 20 years of practicing oral surgery, I am sorry to say, I believed all the unjustified criticisms leveled against marsupialization of cysts by most of the "authorities" in this country and so enucleated all cysts, large and small, regardless of the morbidity that such a technique does create in a percentage of the cases of large cysts. As chance will operate, I had a series of patients in a short period of time with distressing postoperative complications that could have been avoided *if* I had marsupialized these cysts rather than enucleated them. Being aware that my colleagues overseas *did not* criticize this technique, and, as a matter of fact, *unhesitatingly used* marsupialization as the treatment of choice in large cysts, I tried and used marsupialization in large cysts for the next 28 years while practicing and teaching oral surgery. Would that I could make amends to those patients from the first 20 years who suffered because of my unquestioned belief in the statements of many of the "authorities" of that day, belief in whom, to my great sorrow, continues today in some areas.

Time Required for Filling in of Bone. Having had extensive experience with both enucleation and marsupialization, I have formed the opinion that there is little, if any, difference in the healing time of large cystic cavities, regardless of the technique used. Actually, one must consider that with marsupialization much time may be gained and the patient may avoid the suffering, complications and inconvenience that might have ensued if enucleation had been carried out. The surgeon may save the time he would have lost, to say nothing of his mental distress, in the treatment of those complications. In the first two decades of life large cystic cavities in bone, as a rule, should be completely filled with new bone within 6 to 12 months following marsupialization, depending on the size of the cyst. (See Figures 12–66 and 12–67.)

As the patient's age increases, there is a surprisingly small increase in the time necessary for the obliteration of cystic cavities with new bone. Taking into consideration the size of the cystic cavity, the average time for

complete healing runs from a year to a year and a half as an average, even in the largest cysts in patients in the third, fourth and fifth decades of life, and even in those of 60 years or more. (See Figures 12–64, 12–88 and 12–90.) This rapid healing is remarkable, considering that some large cysts (shown in cases illustrated in this chapter) have taken 10 to 20 years to develop. These required only a year and a half or two to fill in completely with new bone.

The exceptions to the rule are those cysts in which portions of the cortical plates on both the labial or buccal and lingual sides of the alveolar ridge have been completely resorbed because of cyst pressure. These cysts do not completely fill in with bone. On post-treatment radiographic examination a radiolucent area will be seen in the center; this is filled with a comparatively thin but dense fibrous tissue. (See Figures 12–23 and 12–38.)

Conclusion. If a large or small cystic cavity in the bone has not been completely obliterated, according to radiographic examination, by the times just indicated for the different age groups, regardless of the technique originally employed, the radiolucent area should be explored. There may be a recurrent cyst developing.

POSTOPERATIVE RADIOGRAPHS

In all cyst cases, postoperative radiographs should be taken annually until the cystic cavity has been completely filled with bone.

The following statement by the American Dental Association should allay the fears of those dentists or patients and their families who are concerned about the effects of patient exposure to radiation in dentistry and medicine:

"Dental x-rays are an essential part of the best possible dental care. Dental x-ray examinations made with modern methods and safeguards pose no known or documented danger to the patient. The amount of radiation from such x-rays which reaches the gonadal area, for example, is less than that received from natural sources, such as cosmic rays from outer space and background radiation from the earth. Dental x-ray equipment manufacture and use are both monitored by Federal and state laws which the dental profession has supported and helped formulate. Just as each person's general and oral health situation is different, the frequency of x-ray use cannot be governed by norms universal to all patients. Only the dentist well-trained in radiation practice can examine the patient and determine the minimum number and frequency of x-rays for the diagnosis and prevention of oral diseases."[3]

RADIOLUCENT AREAS IN THE MANDIBLE AND MAXILLA THAT MAY RADIOGRAPHICALLY SIMULATE ODONTOGENIC CYSTS

In the differential diagnosis of odontogenic cysts the following must be considered:
1. Normal anatomic structures, such as the nasopalatine, greater palatine and mental foramina; lacrimal duct; maxillary sinus; and nasal cavity.
2. Such lesions as osteoporotic bone marrow defect, idiopathic (static) bone cavity,[74] solitary bone cyst (SBC), and aneurysmal bone cyst (see later in this chapter).
3. Odontogenic tumors (see Chapter 13):
   A. Periapical dental granuloma

B. Periapical cemental (fibrous) dysplasia, stage one.
C. Ameloblastoma. (This tumor *should not be called a multilocular cyst!* Too many jaws have needlessly been resected because roentgenologists have stated in their reports, "multilocular cyst [ameloblastoma]," and without confirming this report with a biopsy, the surgeon has resected the jaw.)
D. Fibroma.
E. Myxoma.
4. Benign nonodontogenic tumors (see Chapter 13):
   A. Central giant cell granuloma.
   B. Fibro-osseous (cementous) dysplasia.
   C. Cherubism.
   D. Neurofibroma and neurilemmoma (intraosseous).
   E. Benign osteoblastoma.
   F. Central hemangioma.
5. Malignant tumors:
   A. Metastatic tumors.
   B. Fibrosarcoma.
   C. Osteolytic osteosarcoma.
   D. Multiple myeloma (Figs. 12–105 to 12–107).
   E. Plasmacytoma (a plasma cell type

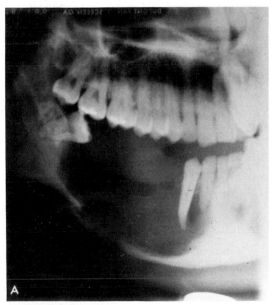
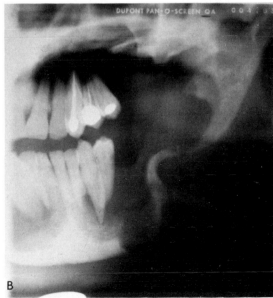

Figure 12–104 Right and left panoramic views of the mandible of a young adult male in which massive bilateral osteolysis of the mandible took place, resulting in a pathologic fracture on one side. The cause remains unknown. (From Malter, I. J.: Massive osteolysis of the mandible: Report of a case. J.A.D.A., *85*:148–149 [July], 1972).

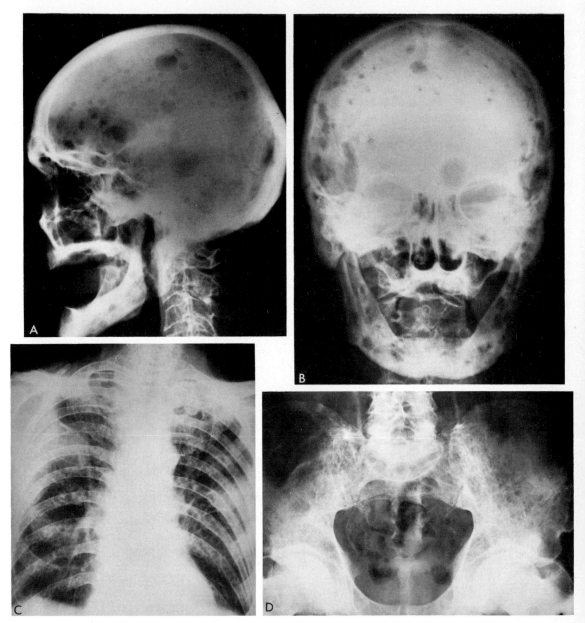

Figure 12–105   A patient whose series of radiographs of the skull, chest and pelvis show the multiple small and large well-circumscribed radiolucent areas found in the osseous structures of the three skeletal divisions that are associated with multiple myeloma (plasma cell myeloma). (See also Figure 13–186.)

A, Lateral radiograph of the skull. Note lesions in the cervical vertebrae also. *B,* Posteroanterior view, showing clearly the punched-out areas in the skull and mandible seen in multiple myeloma. *C,* Multiple small radiolucent areas in the ribs and clavicles due to plasma cell myeloma. *D,* Multiple osteolytic areas in the ribs, lumbar vertebrae and bones of the pelvis typical of multiple myeloma.

of multiple myeloma); see Case Report No. 4.

    F.   Reticulum cell sarcoma of bone.

6. Metabolic disturbances, such as hyperparathyroidism (osteitis fibrosa cystica); see Case Report No. 5 and Figure 12–107.

7. Destruction of bone caused by microor-

ganisms, as in osteomyelitis, actinomycosis and syphilis (see Chapters 10 and 25).

8. Disturbances of the reticuloendothelial system, such as in eosinophilic granuloma of bone, Hand-Schüller-Christian disease, Letterer-Siwe disease and Gaucher's disease.

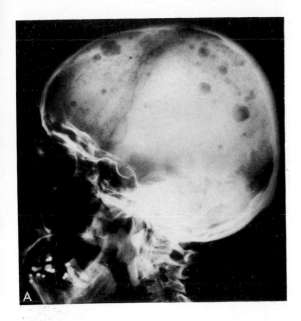

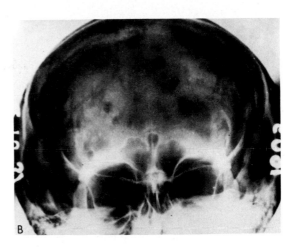

Figure 12–106 *A*, Lateral view, and *B*, a posteroanterior view of the skull of another patient with multiple myeloma. Note the various-sized osteolytic lesions of this disease.

Case Report No. 4

MULTIPLE MYELOMA (PLASMACYTOMA) INVOLVING THE WHOLE SKELETON

A woman, aged 44, had a chief complaint of a painful swelling in the lower right jaw.

History. The patient had been referred by her dentist because of continued swelling of the lower right jaw, in spite of the fact that he had extracted two teeth from this area, several months before, and also had lanced it several times since.

Oral Examination. There was a large rounded swelling in the lower right molar area, with marked expansion of the buccal cortical plate. This plate was as thin as an eggshell. The overlying mucosa was darker in appearance than the rest of the oral mucosa.

The clinical impression was that of a large radicular cyst.

Radiographic Findings. The small intraoral dental films were not informative. They suggested a tumor, or a multilocular cyst or an ameloblastoma, or metabolic disease of the mandible. The posteroanterior and lateral jaw films of the mandible revealed several cyst-like areas in the body of the right mandible with irregular outlines. Surrounding these large radiolucent areas, in fact all through the rest of the body of the mandible, and up into the ramus, were radiolucent areas about the size of a pea. In some areas there was fusion and overlapping of these areas. From the radiographs it was impossible to differentiate between metastatic carcinoma and multiple myeloma. Study Figure 12–107.

A biopsy was taken from the crest of the tumor, which bled freely.

Pathologic Laboratory Report. Macroscopically, the specimen consisted of unidentified tissue. There were three firm nodular pieces of tissue ranging from 0.5 to 1.5 cm. in length and stained a deep brown.

Microscopically, there were two portions of tissue. One of them was covered by stratified squamous epithelium overlying a dense connective tissue, in which were a few skeletal muscle fibers and a small spicule of bone. In the depths of the section was an infiltration of cells identical with the structure seen in the second piece of tissue. Here the architecture revealed a compact mass of cells, with no particular arrangement, moderately vascular, and with little stroma. The cells were almost all of the same type, showing a pink cytoplasm, with an eccentrically placed nucleus typical of a plasma cell. An occasional mitotic figure was seen; at times, the cells contained two nuclei.

Depending on the presence of similar lesions in the other bones of the body, the diagnosis of multiple myeloma was withheld until such finding was established, and a pathologic diagnosis of plasmacytoma was made.

In view of this report, the patient was referred to her physician, who advised her to go to the hospital for additional study. However, she was fearful of hospitals and did not go for 3 months.

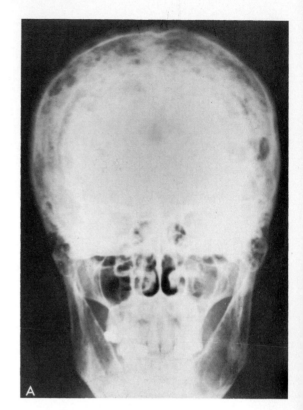

Figure 12–107 *A*, A posteroanterior radiograph of the skull, the maxilla and the mandible, showing medium- to large-sized areas of radiolucency in the osseous structures. This is a case of multiple myeloma (plasmacytoma, plasma cell myeloma) that also involves the whole skeleton. (See Case Report No. 4.) *B* and *C*, Right lateral oblique views of the mandible that again show these diffuse radiolucent areas throughout the cancellous bone.

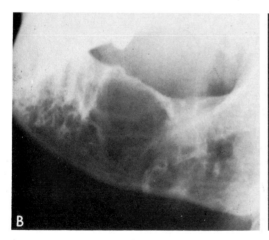

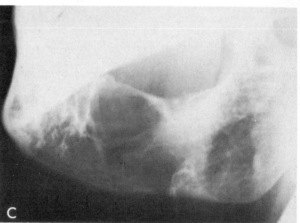

Admission Notes. When the patient finally entered the hospital, the swelling on the right jaw had been present for 5 months. For the past 6 weeks she had been confined to bed with a bad backache. She was unable to walk, since walking aggravated the backache. The backache was not present when the patient did not move.

Physical Examination. Blood pressure was 150/80. The lower right jaw showed an absence of molars, with a round, smooth tumor continuous with the tumor that was felt and seen externally. It was the size of a walnut and felt as if it were cystic. The teeth were in fair repair. Deep palpation over the sacroiliac region revealed tenderness.

Laboratory Report. The urine had a specific gravity of 1.010; examination revealed albumin, 3 plus; three white blood cells per high-power field, with occasional epithelial cells.

Blood studies were as follows: erythrocytes, 3,170,000 cells per cubic millimeter; leukocytes, 7750; polymorphonuclear leukocytes, 61 per cent; lymphocytes, 38 per cent. Blood chemistry showed a blood sugar level of 101 gm. per 100 cc.; nonprotein nitrogen, 46.5 gm.; creatinine, 1.88 gm.; chlorides, 330 gm.; serum albumin, 3.79 gm. per 100 cc.; serum albumin, 2 gm. The sedimentation rate was over 90. Results of Wassermann and Kahn tests were negative. The icteric index was 5.

No plasma cells were seen in a smear for such cells. The Bence Jones protein was positive.

Diagnosis. This was determined as plasma cell cytoma involving the whole skeleton.

Course. The patient died 5 months later.

X-ray Report. There were multiple radiolucent areas, varying in size from that of a pinhead to 1.5 cm. in diameter, scattered throughout the skull. No evidence of bone production was detected. Large cystic areas were noted throughout the body and ramus of the right mandible.

Multiple small radiolucent areas were present in the ribs and clavicles; the sternal end of the right clavicle was largely destroyed. An old fracture with the fracture line still evident, accompanied by considerable bone proliferation, was noted on the left eighth rib posteriorly 2 inches lateral to the spine. There were also multiple radiolucent areas in both humeri and both femora, and in both innominate bones. There was marked destruction of the left ilium along the ileopectineal line, including the entire lower three-fifths of the ilium along the medial line, adjacent to the sacrum. There was also marked destruction of the left side of the sacrum.

The conclusion was as follows: multiple radiolucent areas involving the entire bony skeleton, the appearance indicating a destructive process, without any new bone proliferation. The appearance was that which is seen in multiple myeloma.

Additional roentgen studies of the legs and right foot showed no positive evidence of involvement of the bones in these parts by the neoplastic lesions. Several small areas of destruction were seen in the bones of forearms. Views of the left mandible revealed destructive changes similar to but less marked than those of the right mandible. Films of the lateral thoracic and lateral lumbar spine showed only slight evidence of involvement of the upper thoracic vertebral bodies. and no positive evidence of lesions in the lumbar spine, which showed demineralization.

This examination of additional parts of the bony framework showed evidence of lesions of multiple myeloma in the radii and ulnae, thoracic and lumbar spines and left mandible.

Case Report No. 5

HYPERPARATHYROIDISM (OSTEITIS FIBROSA CYSTICA)

A 17-year-old girl was admitted to the Magee-Women's Hospital in June.

Chief Complaint. Vomiting.

1. Patient began vomiting 23 months ago.
2. Patient always feels tired.
3. Patient broke her leg on February 11; fell on ice while walking.
4. She broke her knee three weeks ago.
5. She feels pain in her left shoulder when she moves.
6. Previously her knees would hurt when moved.
7. Patient's gums have bled on brushing for 2 years.
8. Amenorrhea—she had one or two periods at 13 years of age, none before or since.

The patient had visited the Pittsburgh Diagnostic Clinic 20 months prior to the present admission. This was their diagnosis at that time:

1. Cyclic vomiting, etiology undetermined, probably functional.
2. Amenorrhea, probably functional.
3. Renal abnormalities, etiology undetermined.

Oral Examination. There is a 2-cm. bulging of the left half of the symphysis of the mandible extending from the gingival line of the central and lateral incisors, cuspid and first bicuspid almost to the inferior border of the mandible, which is firm but not osseous. The labial cortical plate has been eroded. The teeth are firm. (See x-ray report on oral films.)

Laboratory Reports. Blood nonprotein nitrogen, sugar, phosphorus, acid phosphatasc and plasma CO_2 were all normal. Blood calcium was 15.6 gm. per 100 cc., and alkaline phosphatase was 42.1 Bodansky units. Urinalysis was negative. Leukocyte count was 14,700. Basal metabolic rate was normal. Sedimentation rate was slightly elevated. Renal function was poor.

X-ray Conclusions

1. Generalized decalcification involving all of the osseous structures examined. This finding was most marked in the skull and pelvis. However, the long bones are involved as well as the vertebral bodies.
2. Cystic lesion of the mandible producing destruction at the roots of the left cuspid and first bicuspid. Absence of lamina dura about the roots of the teeth. Generalized demineralization of the cancellations in the mandible (see Figure 12–108).
3. Old fracture through the neck of the left femur and fracture of the distal end of the left femur.
4. These findings, generalized decalcification

and cystic changes with evidence of pathologic fractures, suggest the probability of hyperparathyroidism.

Diagnostic Biopsy of Tumor of Mandible. A semicircular soft tissue flap was reflected over the bulging area, exposing a rubbery brownish-red mass. A 1-cm. plug block was excised from the tumor.

Histopathologic Report. The tumor is composed of osteoblasts, and osteoclastic giant cells are present in great numbers. No bony spicules are found in the biopsy specimen. *Diagnosis:* Giant cell tumor of the mandible (hyperparathyroidism).

Final Diagnosis. Hyperparathyroidism.

Treatment. Parathyroidectomy. No oral surgery is indicated. The osteolytic lesions will be gradually filled in with bone following the parathyroidectomy.

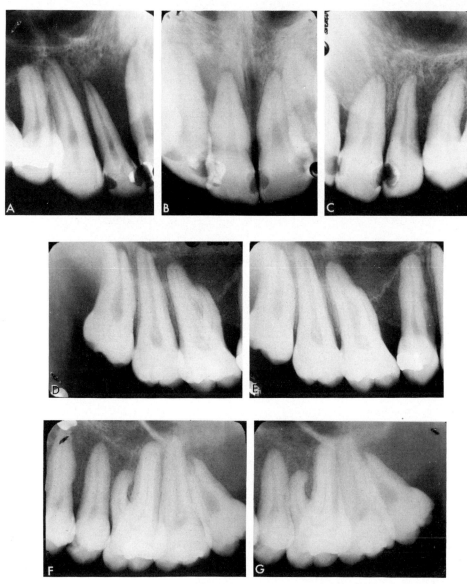

Figure 12–108 In making a differential diagnosis of cysts of the jaws, one should consider the oral findings in hyperparathyroidism (osteitis fibrosa cystica, or von Recklinghausen's disease of bone), such as shown in these periapical dental radiographs of a 23-year-old female who had primary hyperparathyroidism. (See also Figure 13–185.) The disease is characterized by a generalized reduction in the radiographic density in the bone, which gives it a "ground glass" appearance. Cyst-like areas are seen where the trabeculae are mostly destroyed. In disease of long standing there is often the formation of giant cell tumors. The absence of the lamina dura is evident in many of these teeth. This is not pathognomonic of the disease.

(*Figure 12–108 continued on opposite page*)

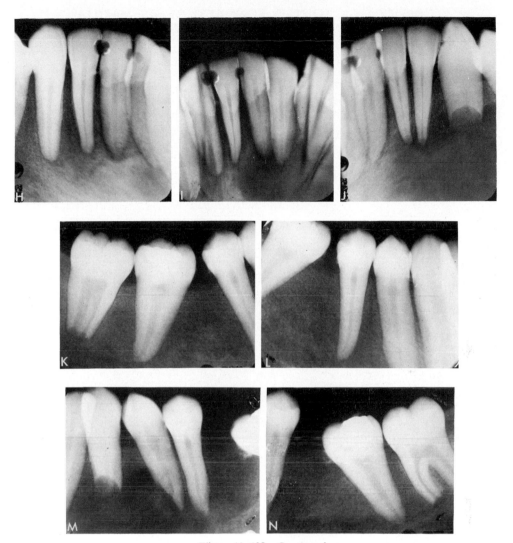

Figure 12–108 *Continued.*

SOLITARY BONE CYST (SBC)
(Simple Bone Cyst, Hemorrhagic Cyst, Extravasation Cyst, Traumatic Cyst, Progressive Bone Cavity, Unicameral Bone Cyst)

Hopefully, we can all agree to drop these confusing names for what is essentially one specific entity, a cavity in bone, with or without fluid, of unknown etiologic cause; it is not life-threatening, and it is easy to treat.

A cyst has been defined as "an abnormal space or sac containing gas, fluid, or a semi-solid material."[75] It appears that the solitary bone cyst (SBC) meets these requirements.

However, at least in Europe, the following criteria proposed by Rushton in 1946 "must be met":

"1. The cyst should be single, have no epithelial lining and show no evidence of acute or prolonged infection.
2. The cyst should contain principally fluid and not soft tissue.
3. The walls of the cyst should be of bone, which is hard, though possibly thin in parts.
4. The pathologic and chemical findings should be consistent with a diagnosis of SBC.

These criteria were adopted to rule out cases in which an epithelial lining, once present, might have been destroyed by infection

HEMORRHAGIC SOLITARY BONE CYST OF THE MAXILLA
TREATED BY ORAL MARSUPIALIZATION

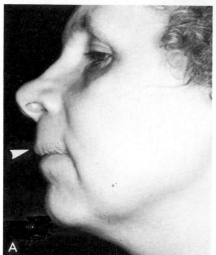

Figure 12-109 *A,* Hemorrhagic solitary bone cyst of the maxilla. The patient complained that her upper jaw was getting bigger, thus forcing her lip out. *B,* An occlusal radiograph revealed an extensive radiolucent area in the palate. *C,* A brownish fluid was aspirated from this area. The presence of hemosiderin indicated that this was a hemorrhagic cyst. *D,* To outline the cystic area radiographically a radiopaque oil was injected into the cavity. *E,* To prevent the iodized oil from escaping, the mucosa at the point of the needle puncture was closed with a hemostat. The occlusal film, as shown here, only partially outlined the cystic area, because not all the cystic fluid had been aspirated. It can be seen occupying the space above the heavier radiopaque oil and the sclerotic border surrounding the cyst.

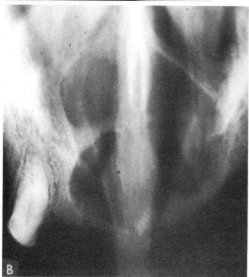

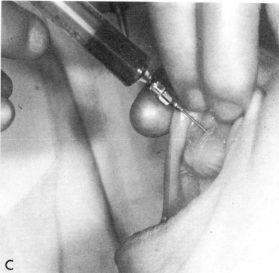

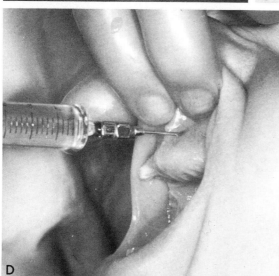

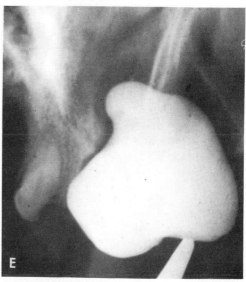

(Figure 12-109 continued on opposite page)

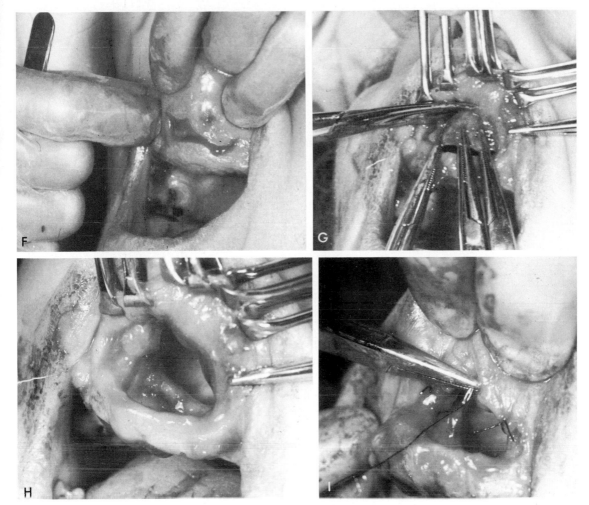

Figure 12–109 *(Continued.)* *F*, A large semicircular incision was made from the left bicuspid area to the right bicuspid area close to the crest of the anterior maxillary ridge. The mucoperiosteum was reflected, the thin cortical plate removed and the cystic capsule exposed.

G, An incision was made along the exposed margin of the cystic wall, which was then grasped with hemostats. With a No. 9 Dean's scissors a window was cut in the cystic wall. Marsupialization of this cyst was elected because of the great possibility of creating nasal and maxillary sinus fistulas if an attempt had been made to enucleate the entire thin cystic wall. Exploration of the cystic cavity revealed the absence of a bony wall separating the cyst cavity from either the nasal or antral cavities.

H, A view into the cystic cavity after a labial portion of the capsule had been excised. Note the depth and size of the cavity and the bony septa projecting into the cavity from the palate.

I. The mucoperiosteum is turned into the cystic cavity and sutured to the capsule of the cyst. We do not use this technique anymore because the new technique, described in Figure 12–112, is not only better but takes less time.

(Figure 12–109 continued on following page)

and to rule out variations of osteitis fibrosa, local or general, characterized by giant-cell tumors, large polycystic formations or diffuse porosis and hyperostosis."[70]

Etiology. The cause of these cysts is unknown, but there are many theories: (1) degeneration of bone tumors, (2) faulty calcium metabolism, (3) low-grade infection, (4) local disturbance in bone growth, (5) venous obstruction, (6) excessive osteolysis, (7) multiple causes, and (8) intramedullary hemorrhage. This last theory is the most widely accepted. It is thought that as a result of trauma an intramedullary hematoma develops, and "normally an organization of the blood clot takes place, but in this case there is a failure, the clot undergoes liquefaction and a cavity is formed."[70] This theory leaves a lot of unanswered questions, which of course makes it unacceptable to many.

Clinical Findings. The great majority of solitary bone cysts reported have been found in the mandible in the first two decades of life. Very few have been found in the maxilla.

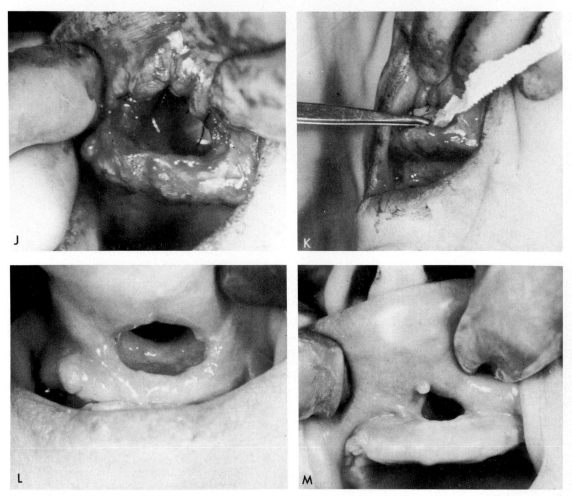

Figure 12–109 *(Continued.)* *J*, The mucoperiosteum has been sutured to the cyst capsule. *K*, The cavity filled with iodoform gauze. A quick-curing acrylic plug is a very good way to keep fluid and food out of the cavity during healing as well as to maintain the patency of the opening while bone is filling in. *L*, Appearance of the cystic cavity 6 weeks after operation. *M*, Appearance of the cystic cavity 10 months after operation. Note how fast the cavity has filled in.

Sieverink, as the result of his worldwide review of the literature, states, "SBCs in the maxilla are extremely rare."[70] Four are reported in this chapter, two in patients in the fifth decade, one in a patient in the seventh, and one in a patient in the eighth. (See Figures 12–109, 12–110, 12–112 and 12–113.) Radiographic findings are not pathognomonic.

(See same figures and their legends.) However, classic examples of the radiolucency of solitary bone cyst in the mandible are shown in Figures 12–84, 12–117 and 12–118. The teeth involved are vital, and there is no erosion of the roots. Most of the solitary bone cysts are discovered by routine radiographic examination, as they are usually symp-

Figure 12–110 Hemorrhagic solitary bone cyst of the anterior edentulous maxilla.

A and *B*, Expansion of the maxillary labial cortical bone.

C, A large semicircular incision was made from the sulcus in the region of the left maxillary cuspid down approximately to the crest of the ridge, across the anterior ridge to the opposite cuspid area and then up to the labial sulcus. With a periosteal elevator the mucoperiosteal flap was reflected and held back with two Allis forceps, as shown. It is of interest to note that the mucoperiosteal flap could be dissected away from this thin cystic wall without rupturing it, which was surprising.

D, Removal of additional cortical bone. Actually, this was not necessary because the cyst was to be marsupialized, but it did reveal the width of the cyst and the manner in which the cyst bulged forth from its crypt.

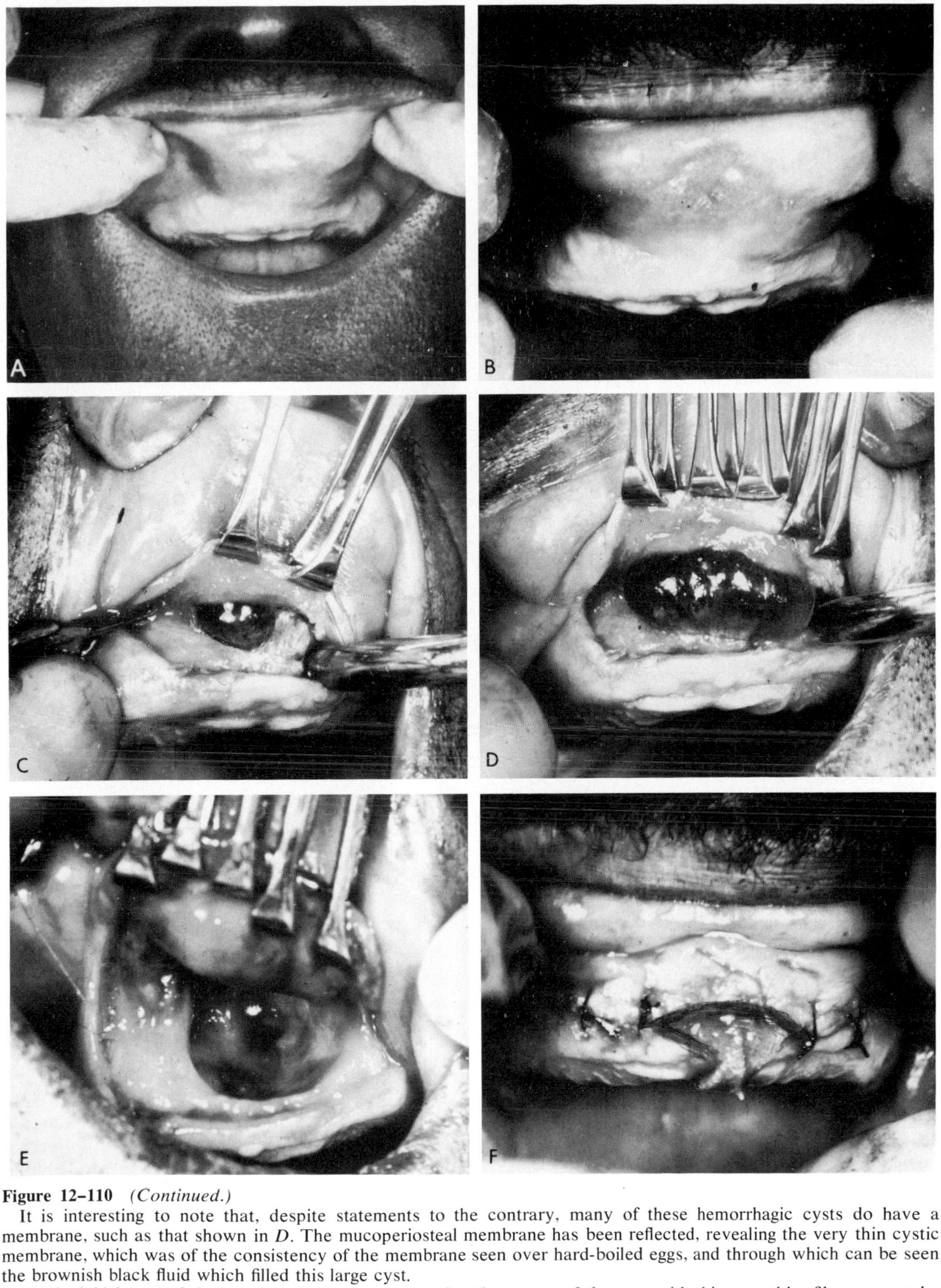

Figure 12–110 *(Continued.)*

It is interesting to note that, despite statements to the contrary, many of these hemorrhagic cysts do have a membrane, such as that shown in *D*. The mucoperiosteal membrane has been reflected, revealing the very thin cystic membrane, which was of the consistency of the membrane seen over hard-boiled eggs, and through which can be seen the brownish black fluid which filled this large cyst.

E, The labial area of the cystic wall cut away, exposing the extent of the cyst with this very thin, fibrous capsule. This cyst was filled with brownish black fluid similar to but darker than that which was shown in the previous hemorrhagic cyst. Visual examination of the inner surface of the capsule revealed many fine capillaries, with very slight oozing of blood. The flap was replaced and, as shown in *F*, sutured on the right and left, but a large opening was kept in the middle. The cavity was filled temporarily with iodoform gauze until a denture with a labial extension into the mar-supialized cyst could be constructed. The extension would maintain the opening while bone was laid down around the periphery of the cystic capsule, and the capsule shrinks as the cavity is gradually obliterated.

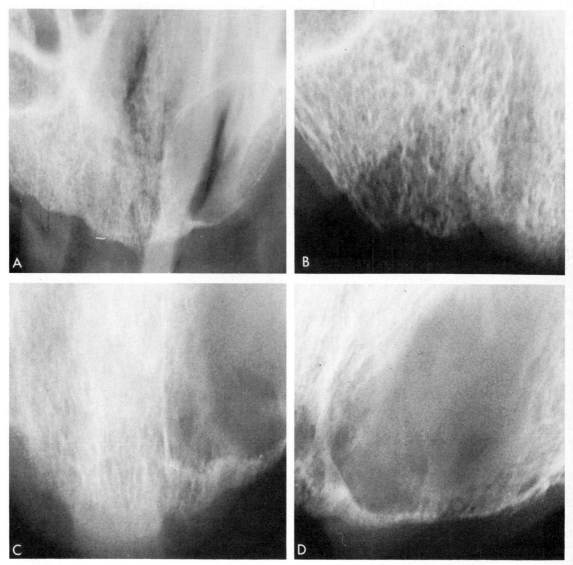

Figure 12–111   This series of periapical radiographs of the edentulous anterior maxilla show a well-circumscribed radiolucent area with an osteosclerotic border in the region of the maxillary left lateral incisor, cuspid and bicuspid. The close relationship of this radiolucent area to the maxillary sinus is obvious in *A*. Aspiration from this cavity did not reveal a reddish brown fluid but rather a straw-colored fluid with cholesterin granules. This residual cyst was readily enucleated without the involvement of the maxillary sinus because it was completely surrounded with a thin layer of bone.

tomless, except when a patient notices an abnormal swelling in his jaw, as happened in the four maxillary cases in this chapter. In addition to swelling, others have reported pain, paresthesia at the mental foramen, a fistula, and a fracture of the mandible.

Differential Diagnosis.   All those lesions of bone that produce radiolucent areas on the radiograph must be considered. This includes all the odontogenic cysts and the tumors and diseases found in bone and listed on pages 635 and 636 for differential diagnosis of cysts.

While it is necessary to consider all these factors and arrive at a tentative diagnosis, the fact remains that the only method by which a positive diagnosis can be made is by opening the radiolucent area surgically.

Treatment.   A mucoperiosteal flap is reflected over that area of the radiolucency in the jaw that will permit creating an opening through the bone and that will not result in injury to the roots of teeth or other anatomic structures. If the cavity is empty, the flap is replaced and sutured. Some surgeons advocate curettage to induce bleeding. To do so is to invite damage to the nerve and blood supply to the teeth or even the neurovascular bundle if the lesion is in the mandible. At one time we advocated the insertion of a ¼-inch iodoform gauze dressing into the cavity. This was not damaging but simply delayed healing and has been discontinued.

The four hemorrhagic solitary bone cysts described in this chapter were marsupialized. These cysts were all filled with a brownish red sanguineous fluid (the color was caused by hemosiderin pigment). These all had smooth, bony walls covered with a glistening thin connective tissue lining in which the eroded capillaries were clearly visible and from which there was a very slow seepage of blood. Within an hour after these cysts were open, the oozing of blood from the capillaries ceased. To have sutured the flaps back into place instead of marsupializing would have perpetuated the cyst, in my opinion.

Toller's work describes the process of development of hemorrhagic solitary bone cysts. He has found the intracystic pressure of 5 cm. H_2O to be about the same as capillary pressure.[83, 84] (This is low compared to the fluid pressure in odontogenic cysts, which is 70 cm. H_2O.[81]) The osmotic tension of the hemorrhagic solitary bone cyst fluid is higher than that of the blood of the patient; therefore, small expansile pressure is present. As a result of this low pressure, capillaries can exist in the connective tissue cyst wall, and erosion of these capillaries due to pressure atrophy, could account for periodic hemorrhage into the cyst. He concludes that in all probability the hemorrhagic solitary bone cyst increases in size by this continuing small expansile pressure.[83, 84] This is my reason for marsupializing these cysts.

Sieverink's conclusions from the review of the literature, supported by his eight presented case reports, were the following:

"1. The SBC in the jaws must be conceived as the same entity as the SBC elsewhere in the skeleton. With regard to the clinical findings and response to treatment, the SBC in the jaws belongs to the group of SBC's found in unusual and infrequent location.

2. A reason for the infrequent finding of a SBC after the second decade of life could be the increasing incidence of extraction of teeth as the patient grows older. After the . . . extraction of a tooth in the area of the SBC a bleeding possibly takes place in the lesion and healing occurs.

3. The SBC has no influence on vitality of teeth. In all [eight] patients presented teeth reacted [proved] on vitality tests.

4. A SBC is seldom diagnosed in an edentulous area. An explanation is given, for a part, in conclusion 2. There can be no explanation given, however, that [tells why] the SBC always has some extensions from the ascending ramus to the teeth-bearing area or the reverse.

5. The minimal size of a SBC in the jaws is 1 cm. SBC's smaller than 1 cm. possibly remain undiagnosed.

6. The SBC has a low intracystic pressure [5 cm. H_2O] in comparison with [that of] an odontogenic cyst [70 cm. H_2O]. Divergence of roots is exceptional; root resorption is never seen. Eruption of teeth is not disturbed, and germs are never pushed aside.

7. The only method to establish the diagnosis SBC is exploration of the lesion.

8. The best and most simple method of treatment is exploration of the lesion. The contact of the bloodclot with the healthy connective tissue of the flap is sufficient for healing of the cyst.*

9. The constituents of the fluid in a SBC resemble serum; not all SBC's contain a fluid; the lesion may be empty. Of the eight cases presented, only two SBC's contained a fluid. The presence or absence of a fluid possibly depends on the time of existence of the lesion.†

10. There seems to be no relationship between the existence of a connective tissue lining of the SBC and the recurrence rate; in most cases a lining is absent. In none of the eight patients with a SBC was a lining present.‡

11. The traumatic origin of the SBC must

---

*AUTHOR'S NOTE: While I am in accord with this statement for empty SBC's, I prefer, for reasons already stated, to marsupialize the hemorrhagic SBC's.

†AUTHOR'S NOTE: The eight patients were teen-agers.

‡AUTHOR'S NOTE: The cysts in five out of our seven patients had a lining. See Figures 12–109, 12–110, 12–112, 12–113 and 12–118.

HEMORRHAGIC SOLITARY BONE CYST OF THE MAXILLA TREATED BY ORAL MARSUPIALIZATION

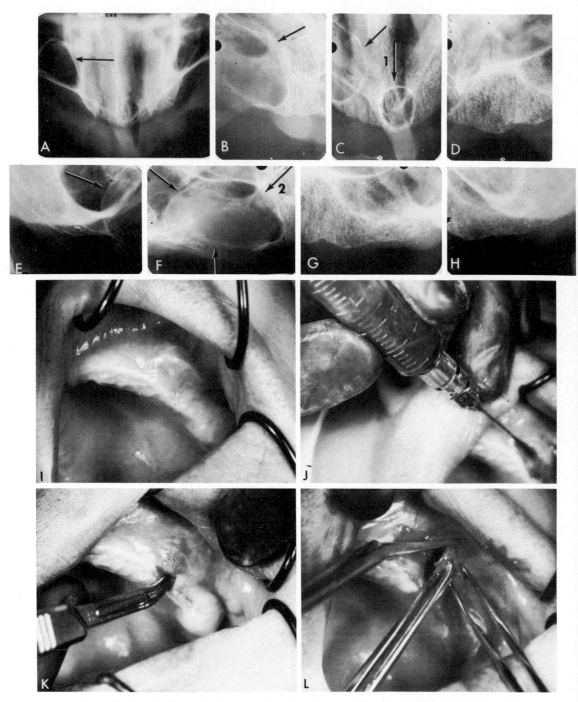

Figure 12–112 *A*, Occlusal radiograph of an anterior edentulous maxilla with a well-circumscribed sclerotic border that extends into the maxillary sinus. (See arrow.) *B*, Periapical radiograph also revealing the sclerotic border that surrounded this cyst. *C*, Arrow *1* points to a well-circumscribed area of radiolucency in the nasopalatine region with a clearly defined osteosclerotic border. This was a nasopalatine cyst whose enucleation is illustrated in Figure 12–125. *D*, The right cuspid region of this same patient.

(Figure 12–112 continued on opposite page)

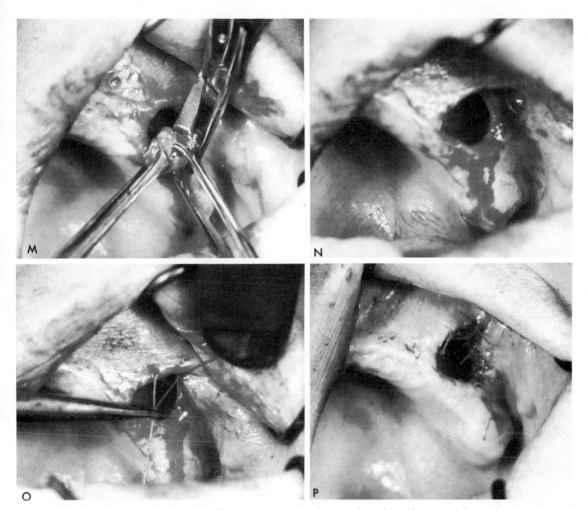

Figure 12-112 *(Continued.)* *E* and *F,* The arrows point to the complete circumference of the osteosclerotic border outlining the cyst (*2*) shown in *A* and *B.* It must be recognized, of course, that even though this osteosclerotic border is so well defined in the lateral radiograph, this is not proof that the labial, buccal or lingual surfaces of this cyst are also covered by bone. One must not take it for granted that when he sees such an osteosclerotic border, he can, with impunity, proceed to enucleate the cyst without the possibility of creating a nasoalveolar or an antro-oral fistula. *G* and *H,* Periapical radiographs of the right cuspid, bicuspid and molar areas of the edentulous maxilla to compare with those of the left side. In the diagnosis of cysts of the maxilla, both in edentulous areas and in areas containing teeth, it is imperative to radiograph both sides of the maxilla as well as the anterior maxilla so that a careful comparison of the anatomic structures on both sides can be made. It is only by doing so that one is able to discover differences that help in diagnosing the presence of a cyst in either maxilla.

I, Hemorrhagic solitary bone cyst of the maxilla. The patient had noticed a light brown soft swelling in the left molar region of his edentulous maxilla.

J, A reddish brown fluid (due to the hemosiderin) was aspirated. A diagnosis of hemorrhagic cyst was made.

K, A new technique for the Partsch operation for cysts was decided upon. In this case the window into the cystic cavity was to be made by cutting through the thin cortical bone and cystic membrane, and all removed in one piece. The above-mentioned structures were incised with a No. 12 Bard-Parker blade at the inferior border of the cyst. The No. 11 Bard-Parker blade is also very satisfactory for this incision.

L and *M,* With Allis forceps placed in the incision, the combined cystic membrane, thin cortical bone and mucoperiosteal tissue were grasped and held while the window was cut out of the buccal surface of the cyst with a No. 9 Dean's scissors.

N, In this view can be seen the mucosa, the cystic capsule and the cystic cavity.

O, The oral mucosa and cystic capsule are sutured together around the periphery.

P, Suturing of cystic capsule and oral mucosa completed.

(Figure 12-112 continued on following page)

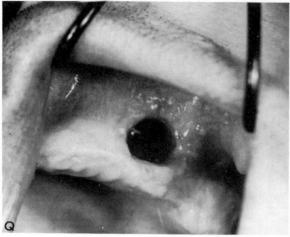
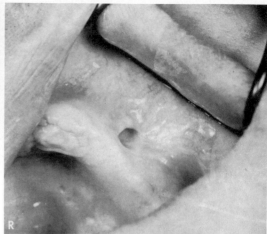

Figure 12–112   *(Continued.) Q*, Appearance 2 weeks later. *R*, Appearance 6 months later.

be conceived as very doubtful. This origin was refuted by, among others, Moore and associates,[54] and in only one case definite maxillofacial trauma (boxing) was present.

12. The initial lesion is still an enigma. The SBC is always just discovered in its full evolution. In the literature,[29] only one case was found in which an enlarging of the lesion was seen when no treatment was instituted.*

13. Most SBC's in the jaws are discovered accidentally. Seven of the eight proved SBC's reported were discovered after examination of the jaws for another reason.

14. With the rise of routinely taken panoramic roentgenograms of the jaws, more data can be expected with regard to the age of the patients and SBC's in evolution.''*

---

*AUTHOR'S NOTE: In four of our hemorrhagic cysts, there was a history of years of a small but steady enlarging of our cysts, resulting in disfigurement ranging from upper lip protrusion to distortion of one half of the middle third of the face. (See Figures 12–109, 12–110 and 12–113.)

---

*Reproduced with permission from Sieverink, N. P. J. B.: The Simple Bone Cyst. Leiden, The Netherlands, Stafleu-Tholen, 1974.

Figure 12–113   *A*, Very large hemorrhagic solitary bone cyst of the left maxilla that has distorted the facial contour of this 73-year-old woman. (See Case Report No. 6.)

B, Posteroanterior roentgenogram of the head reveals complete obliteration of the left maxillary sinus, invasion of the nasal cavity, resorption of the left cortical bone and alveolar ridge, and erosion of the palatal process of the left maxilla. (See also Figure 12–114.)

C, Intraoral view of the hemorrhagic cyst that has by expansion stimulated resorption of the labial and buccal cortical bone, the maxillary anterior alveolar process, and the palatine bone of the anterior maxilla. Ten cc. of brownish red fluid was aspirated and sent to the laboratory.

D, The cyst was marsupialized by cutting out a disc from the labial and buccal surface of the extensively expanded mucoperiosteum and cystic wall (seen in *C*). When the cyst was opened, a large quantity of brownish red fluid with cholesterin granules escaped. After the fluid had been evacuated, the mucoperiosteal membrane, together with the cystic capsule, was approximated with interrupted black silk sutures.

E and *F*, The patient's facial appearance *(E)* and intraoral appearance *(F)* 2 weeks postoperatively. It is obvious from both of these photographs that changes have already taken place in the contour of the patient's face, resulting in a marked improvement in her appearance. This patient was 73 years old at the time of operation and lived until the age of 80. Normal facial contour returned, but the cavity never did completely fill in with bone. The patient irrigated the small cavity in the maxilla and was able to wear a full upper denture very satisfactorily. (See Figure 12–114 for the size and location of this cyst in relation to other anatomic structures and the specific surgical technique for its marsupialization.)

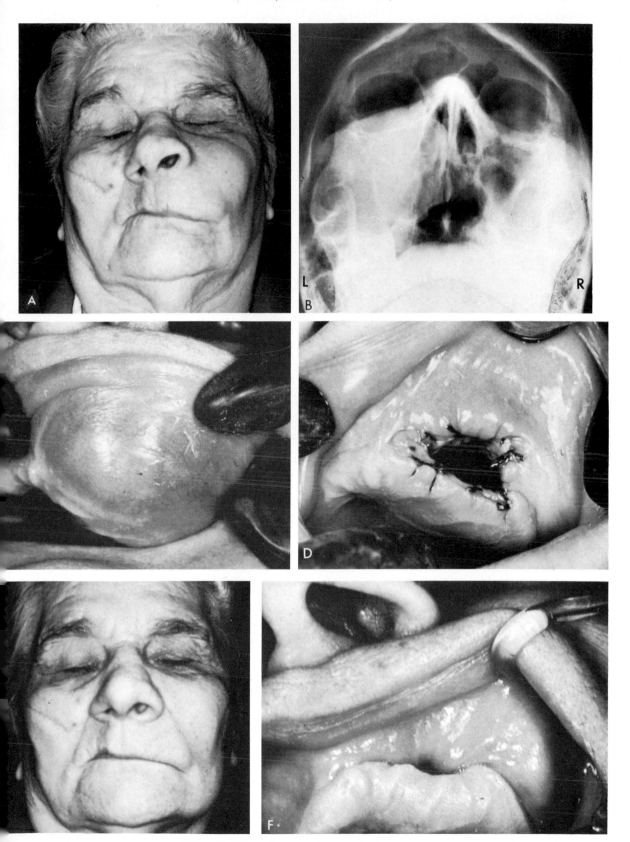

Figure 12–113 *See opposite page for legend.*

HEMORRHAGIC SOLITARY BONE CYST OF THE MAXILLA*

Patient. A 73-year-old white female came to the dental clinic of the South Side Hospital with a chief complaint of "swelling on the left side of the face."

History of Chief Complaint. For a period of 15 years the patient had noticed a small swelling in the left side of the maxilla over the cuspid region. The patient recalled that at that time a young boy in her neighborhood had struck her in the face with a stone while she was hanging the family wash in the yard. The patient's maxillary denture had been broken by the impact of the blow, and within a period of 2 days a small nodule had appeared on the gingival tissues, which the patient referred to as a "blood blister." The involved area was always tender to palpation, and it had slowly increased in size over the years. Because of the patient's fear of hospitals and surgeons she refused to have the lesion treated.

Hospital Admission Notes. The patient was admitted to the South Side Hospital. Physical examination revealed a well-developed female in no acute distress. Her blood pressure was 165/90 and physical findings were essentially negative. The oral surgical resident who recorded the admission history had some difficulty in communicating with the patient because the expansile lesion, which was now protruding from the maxilla out of the mouth, greatly impaired the patient's speech and her ability to pronounce words clearly.

Consultations with the ear, nose, and throat as well as the plastic surgery services were requested.

Excerpts from the plastic surgeon's consultation stated, "I believe this is a mixed tumor with recurrent hemorrhage into it. I do not know whether it would be reasonable to remove the lesion or not, because of its size. . . . This patient refused surgery (on the very day of surgery) 10 years ago. Now the lesion is very large in size."

Oral Examination. Examination revealed an edentulous female with asymmetry of the left half of the middle face because of a bulging mass in the left maxilla that had distorted the face and left nostril (see Figure 12–113A). There was a large globular mass, measuring 13 cm. in its greatest diameter, protruding from the left body of the maxilla. The lesion appeared to be quite vascular, and it extended from the central incisor region posteriorly to the area of the first molar. The alveolar ridge could not be identified (see Figure 12–113C). The lesion was compressible and painful to palpation. There was no impairment of vision on the affected side, but the lateral margins of the nose were distorted, and there was invasion of the nasal cavity by the protruding mass.

Roentgenograms. The posteroanterior view

(Fig. 12–113B), as well as a true lateral jaw x-ray, showed obliteration clouding of the left maxillary sinus, with gross downward displacement and erosion of the palatine process of the maxilla. Invasion into the nasal cavity was noted. The lesion extended to the base of the skull.

Laboratory Findings. An aspiration biopsy of the lesion was attempted. At this time 10 cc. of clear brownish red fluid was withdrawn from the lesion. The fluid appeared to contain hemosiderin, and this finding was confirmed by the hospital pathologist. All of the other indicated laboratory studies were within normal limits.

In view of the clinical and radiographic findings, as well as the patient's own history, a final diagnosis of a hemorrhagic cyst of the maxilla was established.

Operation. The patient was operated on under local anesthesia. The cyst was marsupialized by means of a modified Partsch operation (Fig. 12–114). The interior of the cystic cavity was exposed by excision of a circular disc of tissue, measuring approximately 4 cm. in diameter, from the labial aspect of the lesion. This disc contained both oral mucosa and the adherent cystic wall. No bone was present in the area. A total of 63 cc. of hemorrhagic fluid was aspirated from the interior of the lesion. Visual examination of the cavity confirmed that it extended posteriorly to the cranial base. Digital exploration disclosed no osseous wall medially or laterally, and only about one third of the palatal process of the maxilla was present. The epithelial lining of the cyst was sutured to the oral mucous membrane, and an iodoform gauze drain (measuring a total of 10 yards in length!) was inserted into the open cystic space.

Postoperative Course. The patient's postoperative course was relatively uneventful. One yard of the gauze drain was removed each day for 10 days. After 10 days an acrylic obturator was constructed to maintain the patency of the cystic cavity, which appeared to be closing rapidly. The patient's facial deformity regressed markedly.

The patient was instructed to irrigate the cystic cavity with warm water each day. She was discharged on the fourth postoperative day and was seen at periodic intervals over a period of 2 years, during which time the cystic cavity diminished in size.

Pathology Report. The specimen of tissue presented for evaluation consists of a piece of

---

*Case report prepared by Ross P. Cafaro, Jr., D.D.S., Senior Staff, South Side Hospital, Pittsburgh, Pa., and Associate Professor, Department of Anesthesiology, University of Pittsburgh School of Dental Medicine.

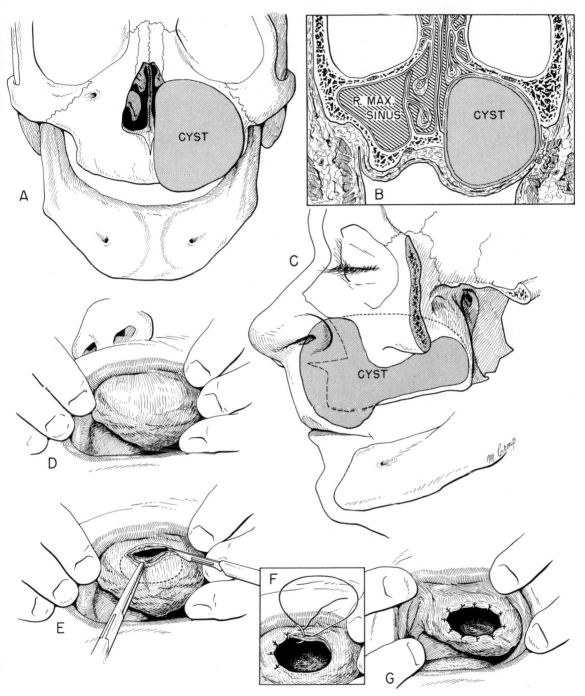

Figure 12–114 *A*, Extent of the cyst medially and laterally in the left maxilla. *B*, Sagittal section showing the pressure erosion of the floor of the nasal cavity, the palatal process of the maxilla and the lateral maxillary wall. *C*, Lateral view reveals the anteroposterior extension of the cyst and complete obliteration of the maxillary sinus. *D*, Anterior bulge of the cyst. All osseous structure in this area was resorbed because of the stimulation of the osteoclasts by the steady pressure exerted on the surrounding bone by the gradually increasing size of this cyst. *E*, With a No. 11 Bard-Parker blade a disc of soft tissue composed of the oral and cystic membranes is excised. *F* and *G*, Oral mucosa and cystic membrane are sutured together. See Case Report No. 6 and Figure 12–113.

smooth, glistening membrane tissue varying in thickness from 2 mm to 3 mm. The entire specimen is taken for sectioning.

In sections of the tissue there are recent evidences of hemorrhage, some inflammatory cells and cholesterol crystals. One surface is covered by adult intact stratified squamous epithelium (this was the labial surface of the excised disc), and within the underlying fibrous connective tissue stroma there is a suggestion of a cyst wall lined by dense granulation tissue. No evidence of malignancy is seen here.

Dr. Leonard B. Meyers, the hospital pathologist, confirmed the diagnosis: hemorrhagic cyst of the maxilla with chronic inflammation.

Summary and Discussion. This case of a hemorrhagic cyst of the maxilla was interesting from both a diagnostic and surgical aspect.

From a surgical standpoint, the value of the modified Partsch operation for the marsupialization of large cysts has once more been demonstrated. To attempt enucleation of the cystic membrane in this case, without causing further injury to the vital structures and normal tissue in the proximal areas and the adjacent nasal and orbital cavities, would have been surgically impossible.

ANEURYSMAL BONE CYST
(Aneurysmal Giant Cell Tumor, Ossifying Hematoma, Hemorrhagic Osteomyelitis)

This lesion, which is most commonly found in long bones and vertebrae, has rarely been located in the jaws, and then only in patients under 20 years of age. Its importance is in its differential diagnosis from other cysts of the jaws that it simulates very closely on roentgenograms. Unfortunately, it does not have the characteristic soap-bubble appearance seen in long bones. While pain is associated with long-bone lesions, regrettably this is not a symptom with the jaw lesions.

The solid portion of the lesion is similar to the central giant cell granuloma or the "brown tumor" of hyperparathyroidism.

As Tiecke explains, "This lesion should not be confused with rare vascular lesions that occur within bones, such as arteriovenous fistula or angiomatous tumors, which connect with the vital circulation in the area. Surgical intervention in such cases may produce uncontrollable hemorrhage and death of the patient, whereas the bleeding associated with the aneurysmal bone cyst, though excessive, can be controlled."[80]

Treatment. Surgical enucleation is required.

Case Report No. 7

ANEURYSMAL BONE CYST IN THE MAXILLA FOLLOWING THE EXTRACTION OF THE LEFT MAXILLARY FIRST MOLAR

H. Serrano Roa, D.D.S.

A 12-year-old boy was referred to the Department of Estomatology in the Roosevelt Hospital, Guatemala City, with the following history: 15 days before, the first permanent molar had been extracted, and it had bled until 24 hours later, when hemorrhage was controlled. Three days after that a growth started in the maxilla, rapidly reaching the size of a nut, with no pain.

The patient (Fig. 12–115C), who was in good general health and cooperative, had facial asymmetry caused by the intraoral growth, which was 3 by 4 cm. in the molar area of the maxilla (Fig. 12–115D). The round surface was covered by a slightly pale mucosa with small papillae in the area of the socket from which the molar had been ex-

tracted. The growth was well limited in the palate. The roentgenogram from the maxilla showed a lesion with radiolucent areas and the bone expanded. A biopsy was taken, and the microscopic examination caused much controversy among several pathologists at our hospital and the medical staff from a cancer institute at which the case was also presented. New biopsies were taken, but the discussion was not resolved. Because the evolution, history, x-rays and clinical characteristics were compatible with the diagnosis of aneurysmal bone cyst given by one of the pathologists, a decision was made to treat the lesion as benign.

Under general anesthesia, after the patient's external carotid had been tied through a Weber-

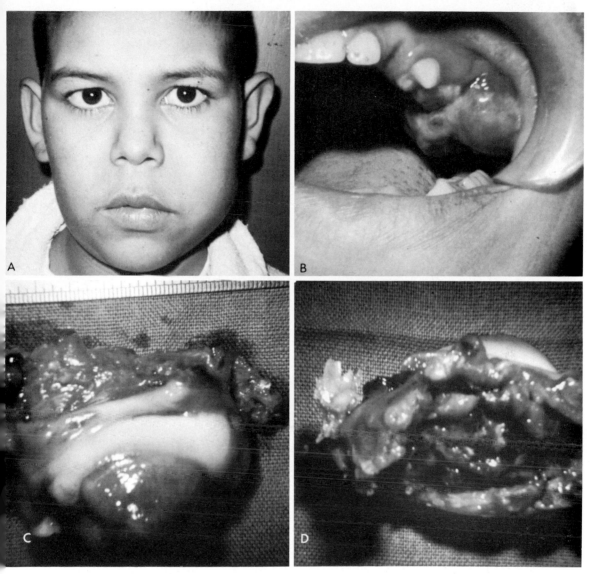

Figure 12–115 Aneurysmal bone cyst of the maxilla. *A* and *B*, Extraoral and intraoral clinical appearance preoperatively. *C* and *D*, Resected specimen. (See Case Report No. 7 for details.)

Fergusson type incision, the cyst was exposed and enucleated. Hemorrhage was controlled after the enucleation (Figs. 12–115*E* and *F*).

Grossly, the lesion was soft and contained numerous blood-filled spaces. After curettage of the normal osseous wall, the wound and skin were closed. The histopathologic report from a study of the specimen indicated an aneurysmal bone cyst of the maxilla. The patient satisfactorily uses a prosthesis, which fills the portion taken from the maxilla.

IDIOPATHIC BONE CAVITIES

These are symptomless, unilateral, ovoid, well-demarcated radiolucent areas surrounded by a dense margin below or slightly overlapping the inferior alveolar canal (see Figures 12–116 and 12–119). They have been called mandibular embryonic bone defects, latent bone cysts, static bone defects, static bone cavities, aberrant salivary gland defects, con-

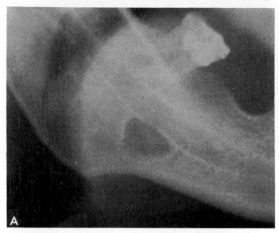

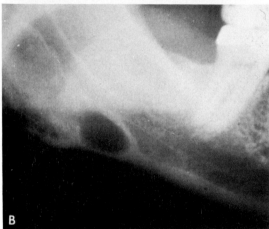

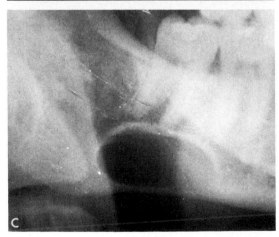

Figure 12-116 Three idiopathic bone cavities of the inferior border of the mandible in the region of the ascending vertical ramus. Please note in each example that the cavity is beneath the inferior alveolar canal. These have been called latent bone cysts, static bone defects, congenital defects and similar names. Certainly they are not cysts, and surgical interference is not indicated. See the text for additional information.

genital defects, and now idiopathic bone cavities. Etiologic factors suggested are developmental anomalies, trauma, chronic trauma (particularly chronic pressure from adjacent anatomic structures), lymphadenitis, and aberrant salivary gland tissue.

At operations have been found lymph node tissue, a lobe of the submandibular gland, empty bone cavity, lymphatic and fatty tissue, and fibrous and fibromatous connective tissue.

Operative interference is not recommended by some authors inasmuch as these bone cavities are apathogenic. Instead they periodically examine these areas radiographically. Others justify surgical intervention to establish a diagnosis, and particularly in those cases in which there is not a clear-cut osseous border.

This author surgically investigates only those radiolucent areas below the mandibular canal *without* a definite white border. (Compare Figures 12-117 and 12-118.)

FISSURAL (SUTURAL) CYSTS

Median Cysts. The origin of these cysts—that is, the palatal median, anterior maxillary median, mandibular median, nasoalveolar median and globulomaxillary median—is thought to be the entrapment of a portion of the epithelial covering of the embryonic processes at the time of closure. Here they persist as epithelial rests and develop into cysts in the same manner as do the odontogenic cysts.

Crist has challenged this concept as an explanation of the globulomaxillary and nasoalveolar cysts as fissural cysts. His conclusion and summary are:

"An etiologic and histologic study of the globulomaxillary cyst was made. Documentation from the literature concerning embryology revealed that facial processes do not exist per se and that ectoderm does not become entrapped in the facial fissures of the nasomaxillary complex.

"The results of this study indicate that the globulomaxillary cyst should be removed from the category of orofacial fissural cysts, since modern embryologic concepts do not support such an origin. On the basis of mate-

(Text continued on page 660)

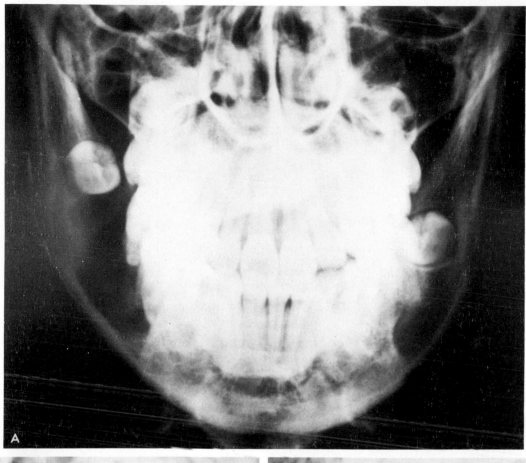

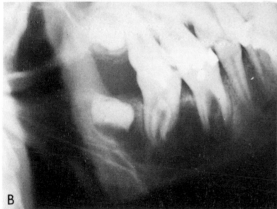

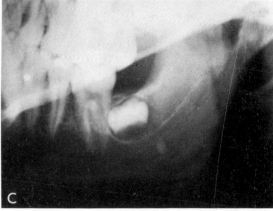

Figure 12–117 The radiographs of this 14-year-old girl show radiolucent areas in the left body of the mandible and a smaller but similar area in the right body of the mandible beneath the molar teeth. These diffuse areas of radiolucency very clearly envelop the roots of the left first and second molars. Both of these teeth are vital, as was the first molar on the right side. The tentative diagnosis in this particular case was "extravasation cysts" (hemorrhagic solitary bone cysts).

The treatment was to turn back a small flap, drill through the buccal cortical plate, creating an opening (3 to 5 mm. in diameter) into what proved to be an open space in the cancellations of bone. A strip of 1/4-inch iodoform gauze was placed into these cavities and removed a week later. The cavities were irrigated with normal saline when the patient came in for postoperative examinations. The patient was instructed to irrigate these areas with an ear syringe, which she did until the openings closed 3 weeks later. The patient was requested to return for follow-up observations and radiographs, which she did for a few months, at which time she was given an appointment for 6 months later. Unfortunately, she failed to return, and attempts to locate her were unsuccessful. *Final diagnosis:* Empty solitary bone cyst.

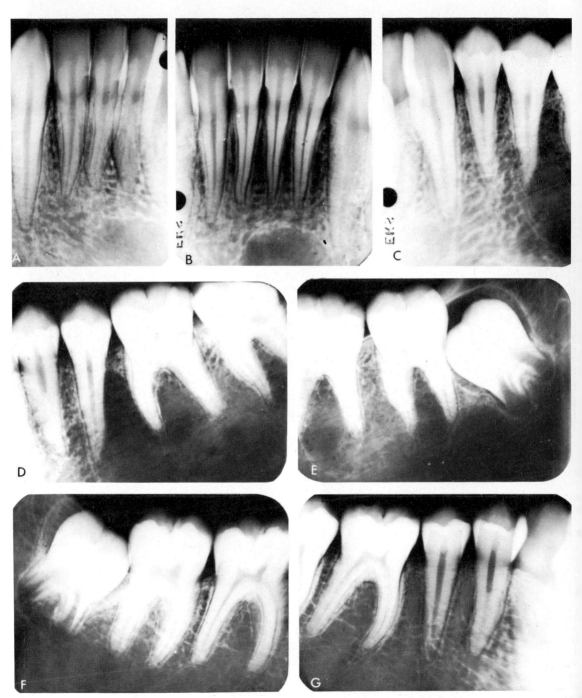

Figure 12–118   In this 16-year-old male the periapical radiographs of the anterior mandibular area (*A* to *C*), the right molar and bicuspid area (*D* and *E*), and the left molar and bicuspid area (*F* and *G*), all reveal distinct radiolucent areas. The bicuspid and molar areas are diffuse as compared with the fairly well circumscribed radiolucent area beneath the lower anterior teeth that has a sclerotic border.

(*Figure 12–118 continued on opposite page*

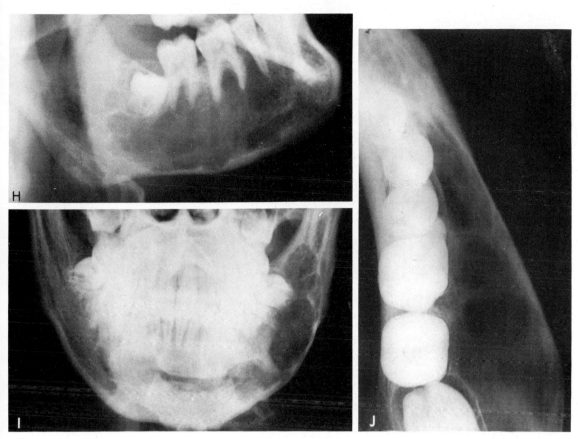

Figure 12–118   *(Continued.)*

H, This left oblique radiograph shows the large, diffuse radiolucent area more distinctly, including its entire periphery, with a scalloped edge along the inferior border of the mandible. Distally it has a rather distinct border, and there are also several smaller radiolucent areas extending distally to the crown of the lower left impacted third molar.

I, The posteroanterior radiograph of the mandible indicates the buccal extent of this radiolucent area, as well as the extension of the radiolucency distally in the impacted lower third molar. The scalloped buccal margin of this radiolucent area is clearly outlined.

J, An occlusal radiograph of the right body of the mandible shows the buccal extent as well as the lingual extent of the radiolucent area, which appears to be compartmentalized.

Treatment: This particular area was opened into by the reflection of a mucoperiosteal flap and drilling through the thin cortical bone well beneath the apices of the first and second molar. Lining this empty cavity was a very thin membrane the thickness and consistency of the membrane found over a hard-boiled egg. It was avascular and very difficult to remove without tearing. The attempt was made only to remove enough membrane for a biopsy. *Diagnosis:* Fibrous tissue.

Note: These cavities have been called traumatic, or extravasation, or hemorrhagic solitary bone cysts, which I personally feel is incorrect. This particular cavity was devoid of any fluid or caseous material. It was just an open space in the mandible. In my opinion, a hemorrhagic solitary bone cyst is one that is filled with blood or blood-tinged fluid, and the capillaries in the fibrous wall of the epithelium-lined cyst are so close to the surface that they exude small quantities of blood into the cavity to mix with the usual fluid of cysts of odontogenic origin. I cannot accept the theory that these idiopathic cavities are the results of trauma to the bone that resulted in bleeding into the osseous cancellations, and then the blood also was resorbed, leaving behind these cavities. Originally, most surgeons made large openings into these areas and packed them with iodoform gauze. That, too, was our technique in the early encounters with these "cysts." However, we, as well as others, have found that it is really only necessary to make a small opening into the cavity and do nothing more than what was described in this case, namely, put a small wick of iodoform gauze in for a few days and then take it out. Following this, for some unknown reason, these cavities gradually fill in with bone. It has been speculated by some individuals that if these were really left they would eventually fill in with bone. We have not so far carried out this "watchful waiting" (nonoperative) treatment.

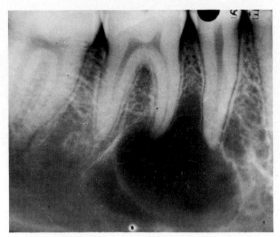

Figure 12–119 A mandibular idiopathic radiolucent area surrounded by a clear-cut sclerotic border. This almost has the appearance of being multilocular. Because the cause of this radiolucent area was unknown, conservative treatment was carried out. In all probability it was a follicular cyst, arising in a supernumerary tooth follicle in the region of the apex of the second bicuspid and first molar. The follicle did not lay down any calcified material to form what might have been a rudimentary supernumerary bicuspid but instead a follicular cyst developed. We rationalize this conclusion on the basis of the clear-cut sclerotic border just described. (We had entertained the thought that this might be a so-called "hemorrhagic cyst," but it is not very often that one sees a well-circumscribed sclerotic border in a radiolucent area when the lesion is a hemorrhagic solitary bone cyst in the mandible.)

The treatment employed here was to open a small window into this cavity (marsupialization). Fluid was found to be present, which substantiated the tentative diagnosis of a follicular cyst. Only pseudo "hemorrhagic cysts" are empty cavities in bone. As explained in the legend for Figure 12–118, a hemorrhagic cyst, in my opinion, is one that really contains blood or blood elements in fluid, and I do not believe that explanations about blood resorption are plausible (see Figure 12–118). I have no explanation myself for these idiopathic voids in the mandible, but certainly there is no need for extensive surgery in treating them. Note similarity to Figure 12–84, which was a "true" solitary bone cyst (SBC).

rial reviewed in this study, an odontogenic origin appears far more likely.

"The nasoalveolar cyst has traditionally been considered the soft-tissue counterpart of the globulomaxillary cyst. In consideration of the embryology of this region and the histologic pattern noted in this lesion, an origin from the nasolacrimal duct appears probable."[20]

Until this opinion is more widely adopted, we will continue to classify these as fissural cysts.

Cysts of the Nasopalatine Region. In the nasopalatine duct, cysts of the incisive canal and nasopalatine papilla develop that are considered to be fissural cysts.

These arise from epithelial remnants in the incisive canal and are relatively common. They are usually lined with stratified squamous epithelium. However, if they arise in the upper portions of the canal, ciliated epithelium may be present, and if in the lower portion, perhaps cuboidal epithelium.

Nasopalatine (incisive canal) cysts are classically described as being "heart-shaped" in their roentgenographic appearance (see Figure 12–121). The shadows responsible for this image are cast by the frequently divergent roots of the central incisors, and the superimposition of the nasal spine over the superior portion of the radiolucent area of the cyst. This is not always pathognomonic of nasopalatine cysts, as was proved in the case described in Figure 12–121 and shown in Figure 12–123.

Cysts of the nasopalatine canal frequently rupture and drain spontaneously. In these cases the following history is presented: the patient complains that periodically he experiences several days of marked soreness in the roof of his mouth "just back of the front teeth." This soreness disappears abruptly, accompanied with "a salty taste" in his mouth. Several weeks, or months, later he experiences the same train of events. The explanation for this repeated sequence is that the

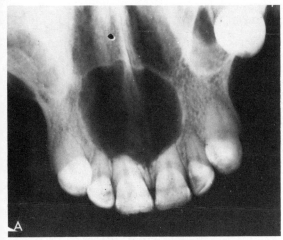

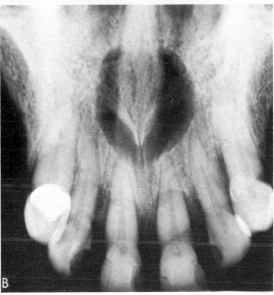

Figure 12–120 *A*, A large palatal median cyst with a distinct sclerotic border. Note the blunting of the maxillary central incisors due to cystic wall pressure stimulating resorption of the apical thirds of these teeth. *B*, Another example of a palatal median cyst of the maxilla.

fluid tension in the cyst builds up, stretching the overlying palatine papilla and surrounding mucoperiosteal tissue, which produces the tenderness and soreness (see Figure 12–122). Then the stretched tissue ruptures, the cyst fluid mixed with a small quantity of blood escapes into the mouth, giving rise to the salty taste. The overlying mucoperiosteal tissue and palatine papilla heal, the cyst fills up

again, and the reported series of events recurs. Or, as illustrated in Figure 12–122*B*, occasionally at the time the cyst ruptures it becomes chronically infected and the patient becomes aware that pus continuously oozes from the spot in which formerly there were swelling and pain.

Treatment. Marsupialization is the preferred treatment for large fissural cysts and enucleation is preferred for small ones.

INCLUSION CYST

While the fissural cysts can in one sense be called inclusion cysts, this term is used primarily to indicate cysts that do not originate in the epithelium covering the embryonic processes at suture lines. Instead, they may develop from trauma or the entrapment of surface, odontogenic or glandular epithelium.[80]

Surface Epithelial Origins. Those cysts originating in the surface epithelium generally involve the soft tissue and are round, fluctuant, freely movable swellings. However, they may be found in bone, where they simulate residual cysts or simple follicular cysts. Treatment is enucleation or marsupialization, depending on size and location.

Odontogenic Epithelial Origins. Epidermal inclusion cysts of odontogenic origin are extremely rare. They are hard, tumor-like swellings found in the soft tissue with a white roughened surface. Treatment is excision.

Glandular Epithelial Origins. Epidermal inclusion cysts of glandular origin arise in either salivary or sebaceous glandular tissue.

SEBACEOUS GLANDS. The sebaceous inclusion cysts are extremely rare and probably arise from Fordyce's granules in the buccal mucosa and lips. Treatment is excision.

SALIVARY GLANDS. Inclusion cysts of salivary glandular origin involve either (1) lymph nodes or (2) bone. Those in lymph nodes are swollen and found mostly in the parotid region, where they are misdiagnosed frequently as neoplasms. Those in bone are from inclusion of salivary gland tissue within the body of the mandible. They are seen as discrete, well-circumscribed radiolucent areas in the mandibular molar area.[80] Treatment is surgical removal. (See Figures 12–146 to 12–151.)

MARSUPIALIZATION OF A MEDIAN ALVEOLAR CYST

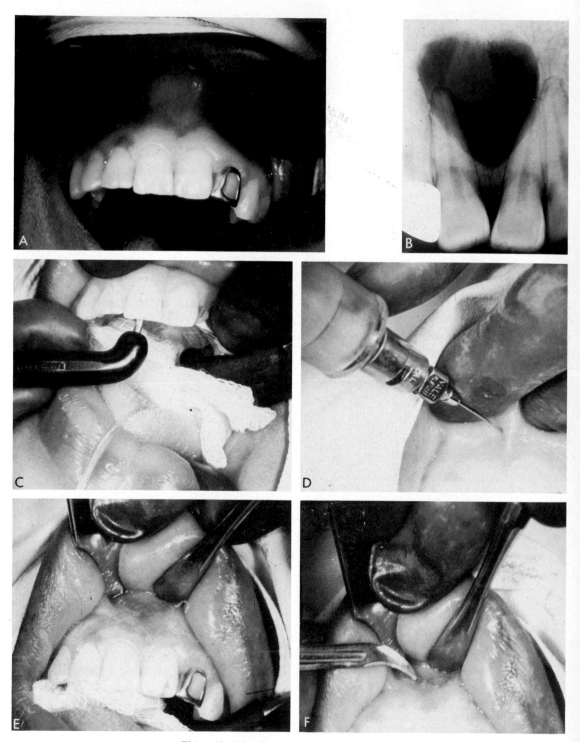

Figure 12–121   *See opposite page for legend.*

(Figure 12–121 continued on opposite page)

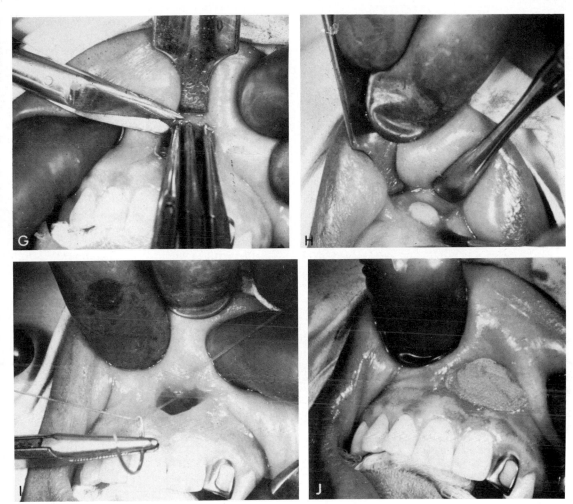

Figure 12-121   *(Continued.)*

Figure 12-121   *A,* In the mucolabial fold there was a distinct swelling that was readily compressible. The typical eggshell thickness of bone could be felt over this area.

B, Median alveolar cyst. The radiolucent area was discovered in a routine radiographic examination. It was thought at first to be a nasopalatine duct cyst. There was no sign on the palate, however, that would have indicated a loss of osseous tissue or soft-tissue swelling, indicative of a large nasopalatine cyst. At operation no neurovascular bundle was seen within the cyst, and there was not any palatal numbness following the labial marsupialization of this cyst. *Diagnosis:* Anterior median palatal cyst.

C, All the teeth were vital.

D, A sterile, light yellow creamy fluid was aspirated from the cyst.

E, Because of the danger of creating a naso-oral fistula, marsupialization was elected. A semicircular mucoperiosteal flap over the cyst was reflected.

F, With a No. 12 Bard-Parker blade an incision was made through the thin cortical plate of bone and cystic wall. Note that in this case the thin layer of cortical bone was not removed first before penetrating the cystic membrane.

G, Three hemostats were inserted into the incision, and the thin cortical plate with its attached cystic wall was grasped. Then with No. 9 Dean's scissors an oral window was cut out of the labial cortical plate and attached cystic wall.

H, When the window was removed, the remaining yellow creamy cystic fluid could be seen.

I, The fluid was aspirated, and the mucoperiosteal flap was sutured to the cystic membrane.

J, The cystic cavity was filled with iodoform gauze.

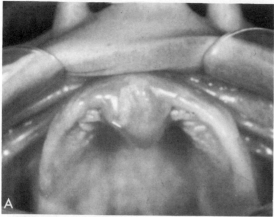

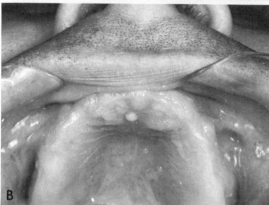

Figure 12–122 *A*, Large cyst of the nasopalatine papilla. Such cysts are radiographically negative. This cyst produced an unusually large swelling into the oral cavity without spontaneous rupture. Marsupialization was the indicated operative procedure because technically it would be practically impossible to enucleate all the epithelium-lined capsule. *B*, Drainage from an infected nasopalatine cyst or a cyst of the nasopalatine papilla. Radiographic examination is necessary for differentiation.

CYSTS OF THE FLOOR OF THE MOUTH

Though they are rather infrequent, both congenital and acquired cysts may develop in the floor of the mouth or may involve it secondarily. These include the ranula (by far the most frequent) and mucocele (both of which are retention cysts), dermoid cyst, thyroglossal duct cyst (which extends from the foramen cecum of the tongue into the deep fascia toward the thyroid isthmus) and cystic ectasis of the salivary ducts. These cysts are all slow-growing and are mostly round or ovoid in shape. (See text and figures beginning page 685.)

Symptoms. These include (1) difficulty in speech, mastication, or swallowing; (2) interference with normal dentition; (3) swelling in the floor of the mouth or in the submental region.

Differential Diagnosis. One should exclude the presence of acute infection, particularly when there is submaxillary swelling. Cellulitis of the floor of the mouth is distinguishable by its acute rapid development, rise in temperature, pain, leukocytosis, and the like. The possibility of lipoma, fibroma, hemangioma, carcinoma or sarcoma must be excluded. Congenital cysts are not actually cysts of the floor of the mouth, but occasionally they grow so large as to become visible in this region. The thyroglossal cysts of the Bochdalek duct are among the congenital cysts found most frequently encroaching on the floor of the mouth. Branchial tumors may also appear as cysts in the floor of the mouth.

(Text continued on page 685)

Figure 12–123 *A* and *B*, Clear-cut sclerotic borders are a frequent radiographic finding of nasopalatine cysts. The cysts shown in *A* and *B* appear to have developed in the two major lateral canals of the anterior palatine system of canals. Those in *C*, *D*, *E*, *F* and *G* probably developed in the two minor canals located in the median line.

Stafne has observed that a "cyst of the incisive canal that has an appreciable size by extension upward and posteriorly into the palate (see Figure 12–120), . . . because of its location, might be referred to as a median cyst; however, in the removal of such a cyst, the incisive canal has been obliterated and the contents of the canal are situated within the capsule of the cyst; therefore, it is most plausible to infer that they arise in the incisive canal."[72] This is an acceptable theory; however, the neurovascular bundle is demonstrated within the lumen of the large cyst shown in Figure 12–120. There are "median cysts" in which there are no neurovascular bundles, and it is reasonable to assume that these have arisen from trapped epithelial elements in the incisive or median palatine osseous fusion lines. Figures 12–120 and 12–121 illustrate such cases.

Treatment: Marsupialization of the large cysts and enucleation of the small cysts. With a few exceptions, such as the one shown in Figure 12–121 (study this case), the surgical approach should be palatal. Delayed healing and possible devitalization of the anterior teeth, if present, usually result from the labial operative approach.

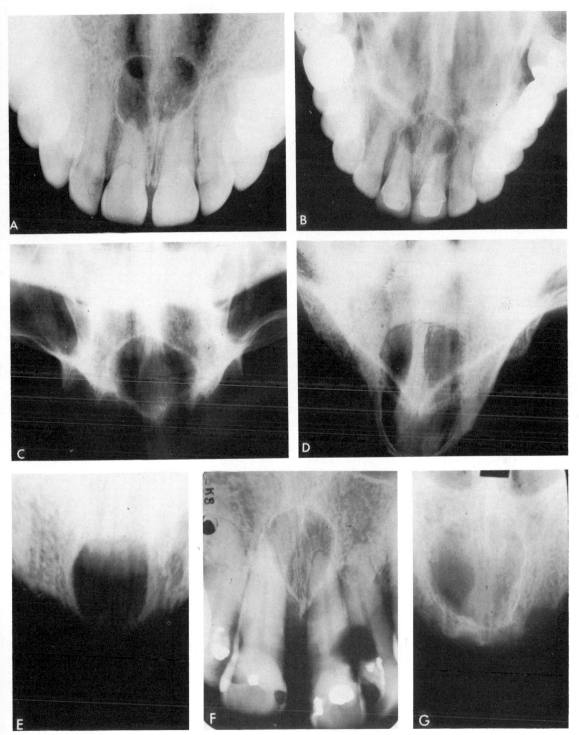

Figure 12–123 *(See opposite page for legend.)*

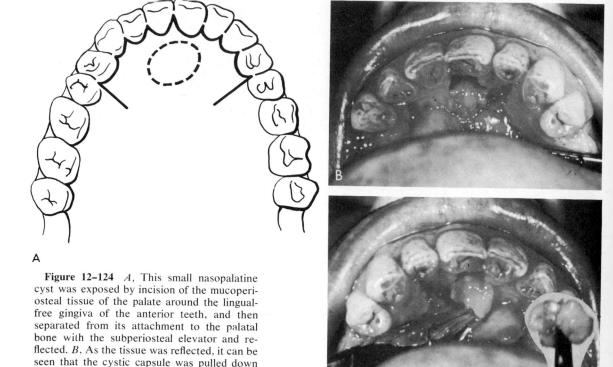

A

Figure 12–124 *A,* This small nasopalatine cyst was exposed by incision of the mucoperiosteal tissue of the palate around the lingual-free gingiva of the anterior teeth, and then separated from its attachment to the palatal bone with the subperiosteal elevator and reflected. *B,* As the tissue was reflected, it can be seen that the cystic capsule was pulled down from its cavity in the palatal bone because of its fibrous attachment to the mucoperiosteal membrane of the palate.

C, The cyst was completely enucleated from its crypt, and the connection with the soft tissue was severed with scissors and removed as shown. The flap was replaced and sutured between the necks of the teeth from the lingual to the labial surface. The insertion of a previously constructed palatal surgical template to hold the flap firmly in place, by clasps or wires through the interproximal spaces, is recommended. Because of the incidence of recurrence of these cysts, it was thought that we must be leaving behind, on the inner surface of the mucoperiosteal membrane, some segments of epithelial tissue. If there is any doubt of this at the time of operation, we now excise a small portion of the mucoperiosteal tissue, as illustrated in Figure 12–129 *H* and *I.*

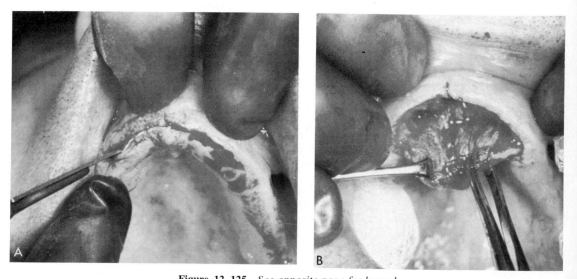

Figure 12–125 *See opposite page for legend.*

(Figure 12–125 continued on opposite page)

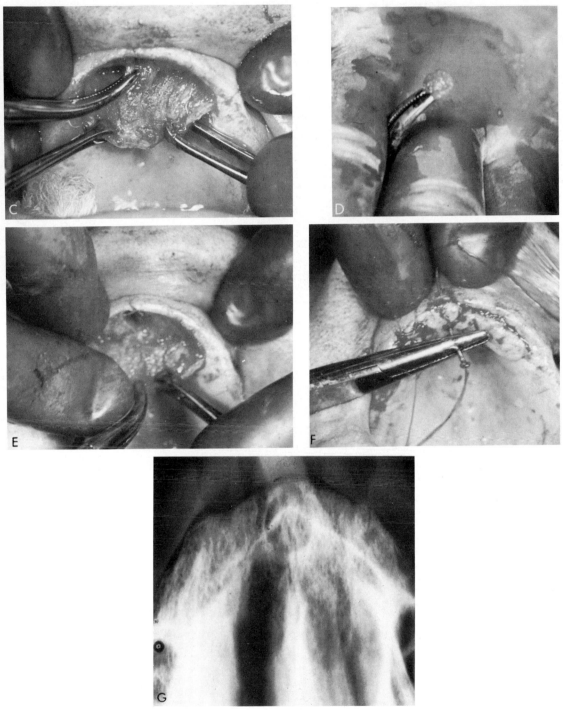

Figure 12–125 *A*, Mucoperiosteal tissue is incised along the crest of the anterior maxillary alveolar ridge from cuspid to cuspid area for removal of a small nasopalatine cyst. *B*, Care is taken to make certain that the full thickness of the palatal mucoperiosteal tissue is freed from its attachment to bone and reflected. Note that the cystic capsule is attached to the mucoperiosteum. *C*, The capsule of the cyst and the neurovascular bundle that it contains are grasped with curved mosquito forceps. *D*, By blunt and sharp dissection the small cyst is freed from its attachment.

E, The small crypt in the palatal bone. *F*, Mucoperiosteal flap is sutured into place with black silk. The denture is inserted to hold the flap in contact with the palatine bone. If the flap is large, as is necessary for removal of larger nasopalatine or median cysts, the denture should be fixed to the alveolar ridge with screws or wires through the labial flange and alveolar ridge.

G, Preoperative occlusal radiograph of the palate with a well-circumscribed small nasopalatine cyst.

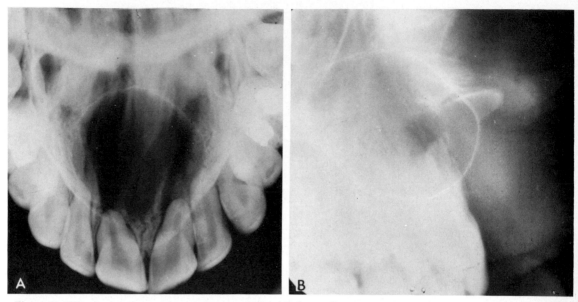

Figure 12–126 A very large nasopalatine cyst (*A*) with forward extension of the nasal spine (*B*). It was treated with marsupialization and a cyst plug (obturator) from a palatal approach. Vitality of all teeth was preserved. (From B. W. Fickling, C.B.E., F.R.C.S., F.D.S.: Cysts of the jaws: A long-term survey of types and treatment. Proc. Roy. Soc. Med., *58*[11]:847–854 [Nov.], 1965.)

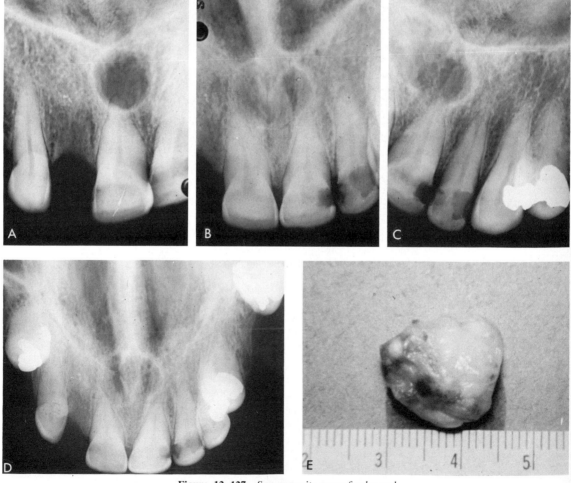

Figure 12–127 *See opposite page for legend.*

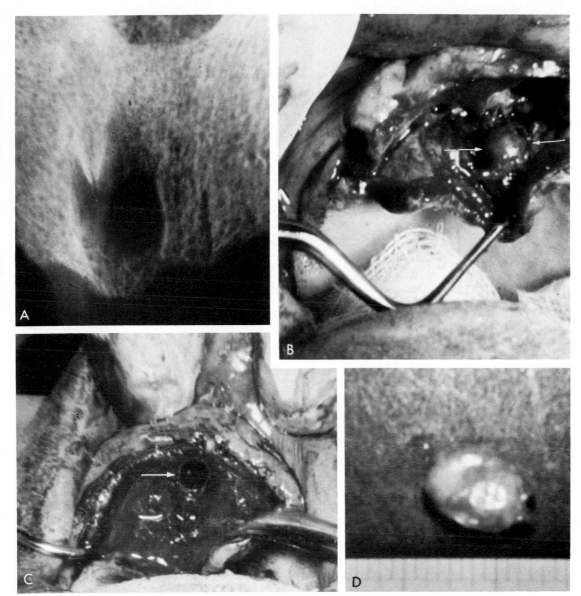

Figure 12–128 *A*, Radiographs of the edentulous anterior maxilla that reveal a rather irregularly shaped radiolucent area in the region of the nasopalatine foramen. This was diagnosed as a nasopalatine cyst. *B*, A palatal flap was reflected by incising along the crest of the edentulous ridge from cuspid to cuspid and then freeing the mucoperiosteal membrane from the palatal osseous tissue. As the flap was reflected, it can be seen that the globular nasopalatine cyst was completely withdrawn from the nasopalatine canal because it was adherent to the overlying mucoperiosteal tissue.

C, The nasopalatine crypt that contained the cyst is shown here; the cyst was dissected free from the palatal surface of the mucoperiosteal tissue. *D*, Intact cyst that was severed from its attachment to the palatal tissue. On physical examination it was felt that no epithelial tissue was left on the inner surface of the palatal flap.

Figure 12–127 *A, B* and *C*, Periapical dental radiographs of the maxillary anterior teeth reveal a well-circumscribed radiolucent area that proved to be a nasopalatine cyst. Note how the radiolucent area was superimposed over the apices of the right and left central incisors in the radiographs of the lateral incisors and cuspids. *D*, Occlusal radiograph of the maxilla showing a large nasopalatine cyst. *E*, Cyst after enucleation by the palatal approach. Note the irregular and nodular surface, which is unusual.

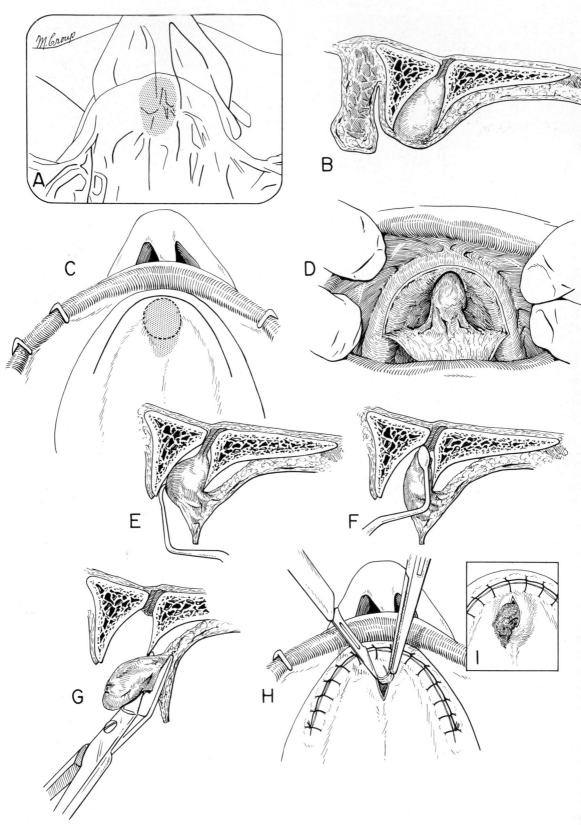

Figure 12–129 *See opposite page for legend.*

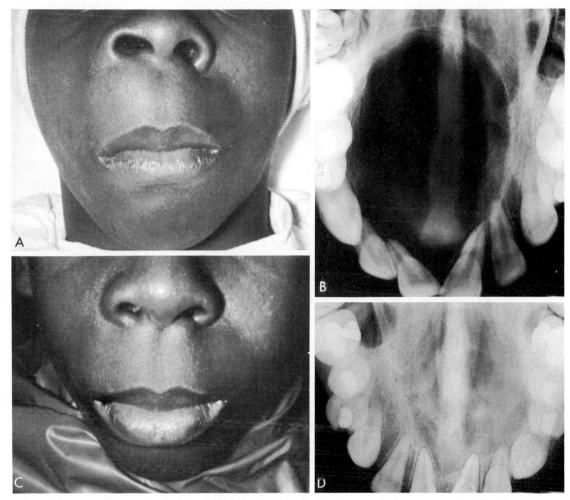

Figure 12–130 *A,* Pronounced protrusion of the upper lip in this 13-year-old boy was produced by the very extensive median anterior maxillary cyst (incisive canal cyst), shown in the radiograph *(B).*

"Operation: The Partsch or marsupialization technique was the procedure of choice. Enucleation of such a cyst invites disaster, since it is virtually impossible to separate the cyst from either the membrane of the nose or the antrum without perforation or without leaving cystic tissue behind. In other words, the consequences of enucleation are likely to be naso-oral or antro-oral fistulas or recurrence of the cyst."

Normal contour of the lip *(C)* and complete obliteration of the cystic cavity with normal bone having filled in the area *(D)* 1 year after operation.

The technique of marsupialization employed by Drs. Saunders, Wisniewski and Soumera is illustrated in Figure 12–40. (From Saunders, L. A., and Wisniewski, H.: Extensive incisive canal cyst. Report of a case. Oral Surg., *26*[3]:284–290 [Sept.], 1968.)

Figure 12–129 Nasopalatine cyst. *A,* Drawing made from an occlusal radiograph shows a large nasopalatine cyst, also known as incisive canal cyst. *B,* Cross section showing extent of the cyst in the canal. *C,* An incision is made along the crest of the ridge extending from the bicuspid area on one side along the midpoint of the crest of the ridge to the bicuspid area on the opposite side of the maxilla. *D,* The mucoperiosteal flap has been reflected, and as it is reflected, the cyst is partially pulled from its bony crypt. *E* and *F,* Use of the curette to free the cyst from its crypt down to the neurovascular bundle in the nasal palatine canal, where the vessels are severed from the cystic wall. *G,* The cyst has been enucleated from the bony crypt but is still closely adherent to the mucoperiosteal membrane. It is severed from the mucoperiosteal membrane, with scissors, at its base. However, it is impossible to be certain that all the epithelial tissue has been removed by this process, and so in *H,* we make an elliptical incision after the mucoperiosteal membrane has been replaced and sutured as shown. This elliptical incision is made over the nasopalatine area. In this opening a small dressing of ¼-inch iodoform gauze is placed.

In this technique, it will be seen that we not only enucleate the nasopalatine cyst but actually marsupialize the cavity as well. The reason here for the enucleation plus a semimarsupialization is to help prevent recurrences. It is true that a small amount of food will get into the cavity in the initial healing stages with this technique, but only for a short period of time. Transitory numbness of the anterior mucoperiosteal palatal membrane follows this operation and lasts approximately 4 to 6 months.

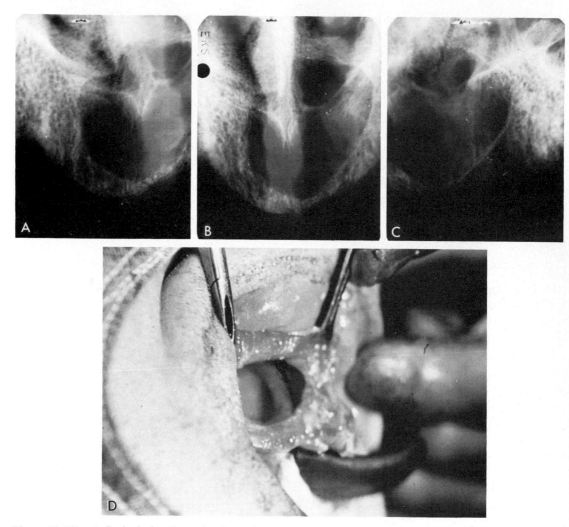

Figure 12-131 *A,* Periapical radiograph of an edentulous anterior maxilla with a large radiolucent area having a clear-cut, partially circumscribed sclerotic border that had invaded the nasal cavity. *B* and *C,* In view of the lack of bone in the floor of the nasal cavity, marsupialization of this median cyst was elected because of the very great risk of creating a naso-oral fistula if enucleation were attempted. This proved to be an especially fortunate choice because when the flap was reflected, *D,* and an opening was made through the capsule into this large cyst, the neurovascular bundle *was seen passing through the center of the cyst!* If an attempt had been made to enucleate this cyst, a very severe massive hemorrhage would have occurred when this bundle was severed as it entered into and passed out of this median cyst. Some authors have stated that they have never seen a neurovascular bundle involved in a cyst. Here is such an example, rare though it may be. This author has seen cyst capsules with fibrous adherence to neurovascular bundles on several occasions. (See Figure 12-54.)

The potential for severe hemorrhage when large cysts are enucleated from this area is ever-present.

Figure 12-133 *A* and *B,* Radiographs of a typical "globulomaxillary cyst," first described by Thoma as a fissure cyst that had "developed from entrapped nonodontogenic ectodermal rests found in the globulomaxillary suture." (See text.) Crist calls this classification "an embryologic misconception."[20]

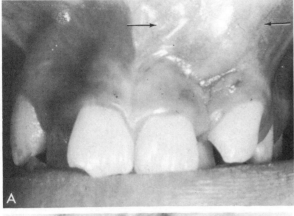

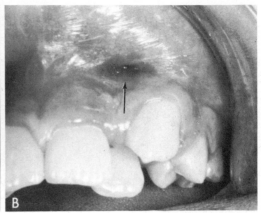

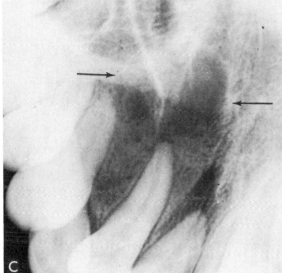

Figure 12–132 *A*, Between the arrows is the swelling of the labial vestibule as a result of the expansion of a nasoalveolar cyst from the suture line into the soft tissue not covered with bone. *B*, Several months after the marsupialization procedure, the opening into the cyst has been almost completely obliterated. *C*, Osseous sclerotic border outlining the depression in the maxilla caused by the pressure of the fluid contents of this cyst. While the cyst developed as a result of trapped epithelial cells in the suture line, the cyst was not completely covered with bone. This is the usual situation with nasoalveolar cysts. Therefore, the cyst expands immediately into the soft tissue from the suture line. The treatment of the cyst should obviously be marsupialization because of the difficulty of completely dissecting out the thin cystic wall from the soft tissue of the cheek.

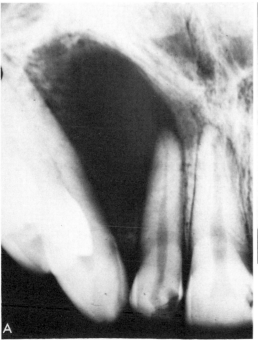

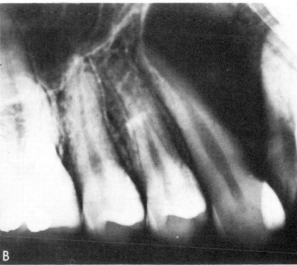

Figure 12–133 *See opposite page for legend.*

GLOBULOMAXILLARY CYST TREATED BY ORAL MARSUPIALIZATION

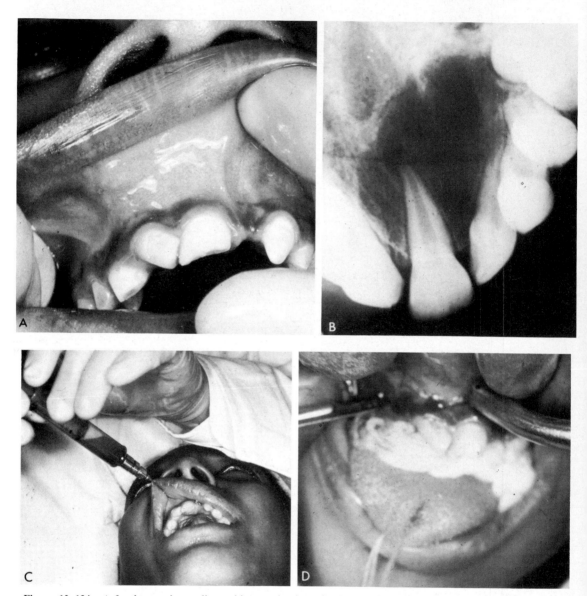

Figure 12–134 *A*, In the routine radiographic examination of a 9-year-old patient, a "globulomaxillary cyst" was suspected. *B*, Both these teeth were vital, and a diagnosis of "globulomaxillary cyst" was made. The usual location of these cysts is between the lateral incisor and the canine. Note how the cyst extends down between the roots of these teeth.

C, Sterile straw-colored fluid was aspirated from the cavity.

D, Under general anesthesia a large semicircular incision was made through the mucoperiosteum.

E, When the bony covering was removed, the cystic capsule was visible.

F, With No. 9 Dean's scissors the thin bony plate covering the cyst was cut out.

G, The thin bone was cut and lifted with a hemostat.

H, To prevent exposure of the roots of the central and lateral incisors, marsupialization of the cyst was elected. We can see into the cystic cavity because of a large window cut out of the labial wall of the cystic capsule.

I, The mucoperiosteum is sutured to the cystic membrane.

J, Appearance of the cystic cavity 4 weeks later.

(Figure 12–134 continued on opposite page)

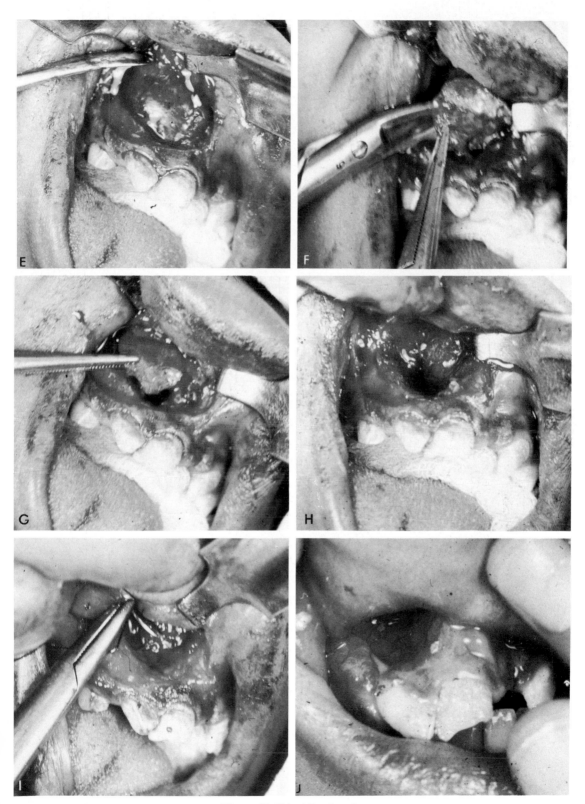

Figure 12–134 *(Continued.)*

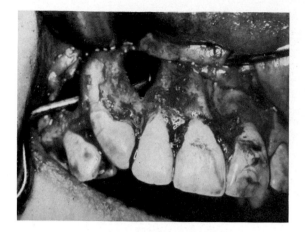

Figure 12–135 This illustration demonstrates the extent of a "globulomaxillary cyst" that extended lingually and distally to the maxillary cuspid. The apex of the cuspid was covered with bone; therefore, the nerve and blood supply to this tooth was intact. The treatment here was a simple marsupialization with an opening left to the distal and to the mesial sides of the cuspid. The area filled in uneventfully with osseous tissue.

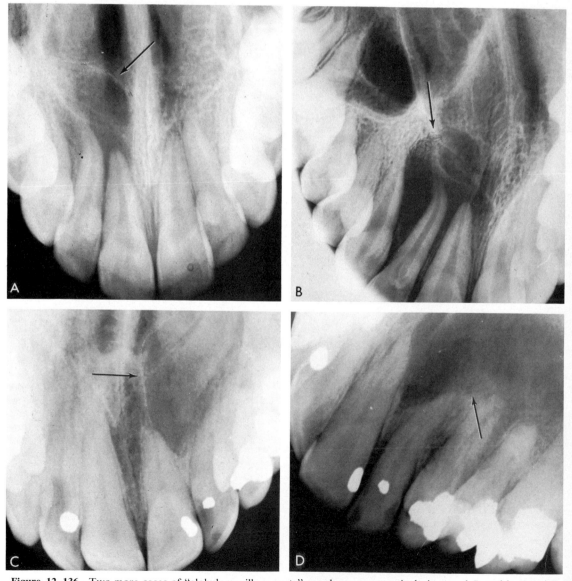

Figure 12–136 Two more cases of "globulomaxillary cysts" are shown consecutively in *A* and *B*, and in *C* and *D*.

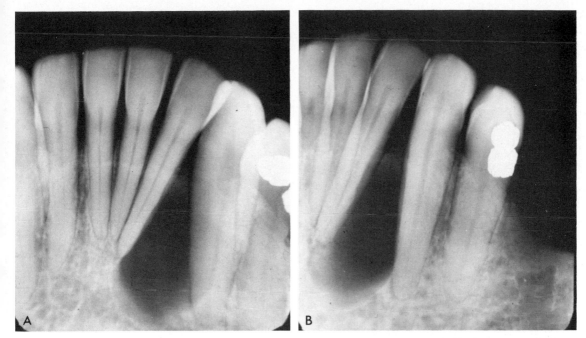

Figure 12–137 *A*, Radiolucent area between the right mandibular lateral incisor and cuspid. The pressure of this expanding lesion resulted in a deflection of the root of the lateral incisor. *B*, This V-shaped radiolucent area between the lateral incisor and cuspid simulates that which is seen in the maxilla and which we recognize as a so-called globulomaxillary cyst. The etiologic factor in the development of this radiolucent area was not known. Both teeth were vital. It is possible, of course, that this could have been a follicular cyst that developed from a supernumerary tooth germ. There was no physical evidence that the patient had any of the systemic diseases that affect bone. Furthermore, the diseases that include resorption of bone as one of their symptoms do not usually produce a separation of the roots of teeth.

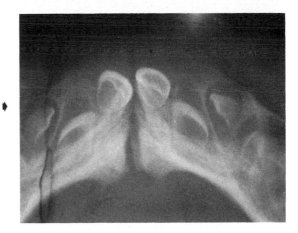

Figure 12–138 Mandibular occlusal radiograph of a 4-day-old infant. Only the enamel caps of the anterior deciduous incisors have been formed. Note that the fusion lines in the midline (symphysis area) are still open in the newborn. The trapping of epithelial remnants when these two osseous bodies close and fuse together as a solid unit can and does give rise to the fissural cysts that are occasionally seen in the symphysis of the adult mandible.

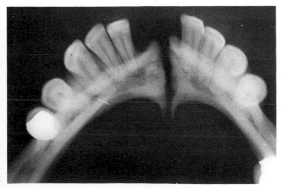

Figure 12–139 An occlusal film of the symphysis of the mandible in an adult in which there is no bony fusion labially, lingually, superiorly or inferiorly. (See also Figures 12–140 and 12–141.) Further details of this most unusual case and the surgical treatment eventually used are described in the article by the contributors of this illustration. (From Weinberg, S., Moncarz, V., and Van de Mark, T. B.: Midline cleft of the mandible. J. Oral Surg., *30*[2]:143 [Feb.], 1972. Copyright by the American Dental Association. Reprinted by permission.)

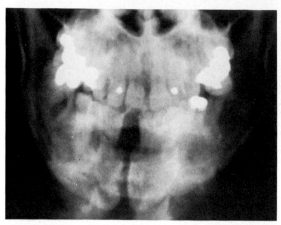

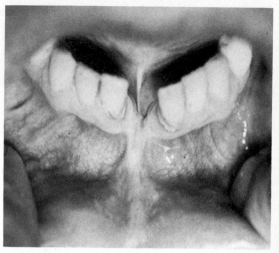

Figure 12–140 Anteroposterior radiograph of the same mandible shown in Figure 12–139. Note the midline absence of bone from the superior border of the mandible through the inferior border. This void was filled with dense fibrous tissue. (From Weinberg, S., Moncarz, V., and Van de Mark, T. B.: Midline cleft of the mandible. J. Oral Surg., *30*[2]:143 [Feb.], 1972. Copyright by the American Dental Association. Reprinted by permission.)

Figure 12–141 In this patient the lingual frenum and the mentalis muscle are both inserted into the cleft of the symphysis of the mandible. See radiographs in Figures 12–139 and 12–140. (From Weinberg, S., Moncarz, V., and Van de Mark, T. B.: Midline cleft of the mandible. J. Oral Surg., *30*[2]:143 [Feb.], 1972. Copyright by the American Dental Association. Reprinted by permission.)

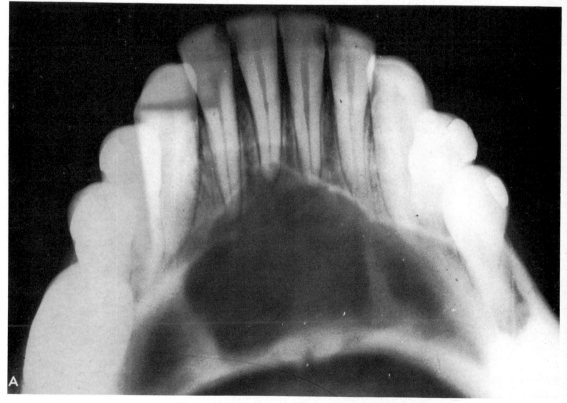

Figure 12–142 *See opposite page for legend.*

(*Figure 12–142 continued on opposite page*)

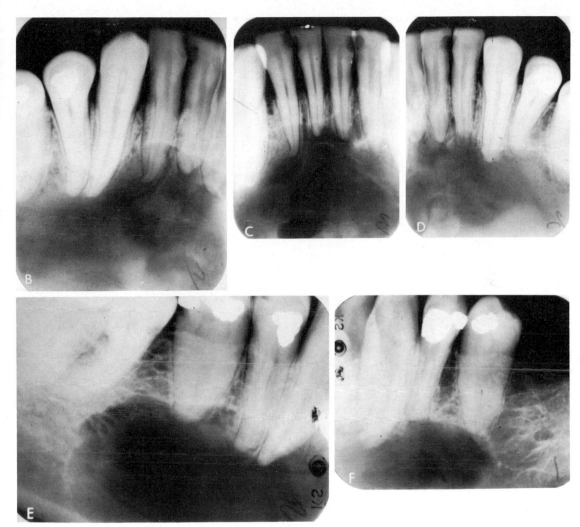

Figure 12–142 *(Continued.)*

Figure 12–142 *A*, In this semiocclusal radiograph of the symphysis of the mandible, there is a very large radiolucent area surrounded by a clear-cut sclerotic border. This radiolucent area extends from the mesial side of the right first molar roots forward to the symphysis, across to the opposite side, ending at a point just over the apex of the left second bicuspid on the opposite side (see periapical films, *B* to *F*). All these teeth being vital, the conclusion is inescapable that this is a fissural, or inclusion, cyst. Fissural cysts, as have already been described, develop in areas of fusion in the facial bones in which the membrane covering the bone was not completely lost or resorbed when the bones fused, thereby trapping a portion of this epithelial membrane within the lines of fusion.

This collection of epithelial cells multiplies, forming a large group of cells in which a fissural cyst develops in the same manner that radicular, periodontal or dentigerous cysts develop. In brief, the collection of fluid in the center of the cells, which now line a fibrous capsule, increases the hydrostatic pressure against the surrounding bone, which consequently is resorbed. The cyst continues to expand until the pressure within the cyst is removed either by marsupialization or by enucleation of the capsule of the cyst itself. In this case, marsupialization, to prevent the possible devitalization of all these teeth, is clearly the treatment of choice.

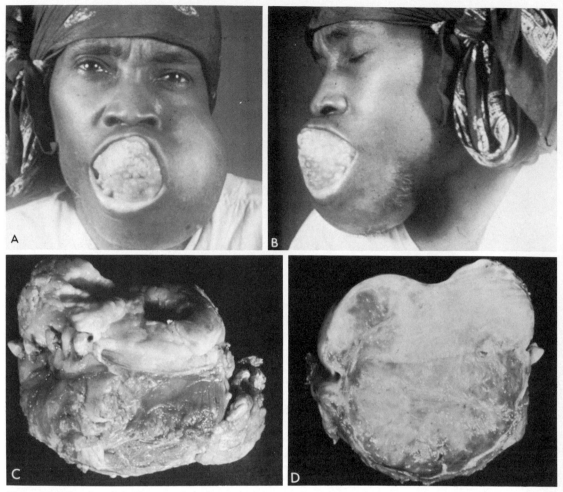

Figure 12–143 *A* and *B*, Front and profile views of a Jamaican with a very large mass, arising from the anterior region of the mandible, that obviously prevented normal mastication. No biopsy was taken of this growth either before or after surgery. *C,* The symphysis of the mandible between the right and left molars was resected by a general surgeon. *Preoperative diagnosis:* "Tumor of the mandible." *D,* This surgical specimen was sectioned sometime later and found to be an epithelium-lined cyst of the mandible. It appeared to have been a fissural cyst that had expanded the mandible labially and lingually. As it expanded lingually and superiorly, the patient traumatized the mucoperiosteal tissue overlying this cyst during mastication for many, many years, producing the thick, fibrous superior capsule of the cyst shown in *C.* It is obvious that the radical surgery used to "treat this case" was not necessary. This patient could have been treated by simple marsupialization, thus sparing her this crippling operation. (Courtesy of Dr. Leo March.)

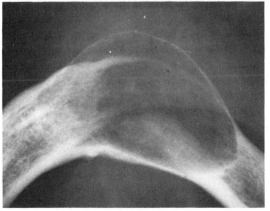

Figure 12–144 The radiolucent area in this occlusal film of an edentulous mandible could be either a residual cyst or a fissural (inclusion) cyst of the symphysis of the mandible. Note the thin, expanded cortical plate and the thin lingual plate that, as yet, had not been expanded. It is recognized that the labial plate expands much more rapidly than the lingual cortical plate because of the difference in the density of the labial and lingual osseous tissues.

Figure 12-145 In this oblique radiograph of the mandible in the region of the symphysis, we have a cross-sectional view of the symphysis in which the expanded labial and lingual cortical plates are both demonstrated. It is of interest to note that the cyst is surrounded by a rather dense and thick sclerotic border of bone. These anterior teeth are all vital. *Diagnosis:* Fissural (inclusion) cyst of the mandible. *Treatment:* Marsupialization, in order to protect the vitality of the mandibular anterior teeth.

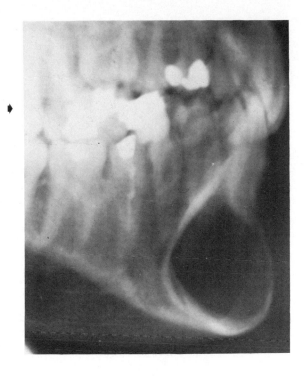

Figure 12-146 Anatomic positions of an epidermal inclusion cyst in the floor of the oral cavity. *A* and *C*, Sublingual position: Occlusal and lateral views, respectively, of a cyst located above the mylohyoid muscle. *B* and *D*, Submental position: Occlusal and lateral views, respectively, of a cyst located below the mylohyoid muscle. (See text on page 661.)

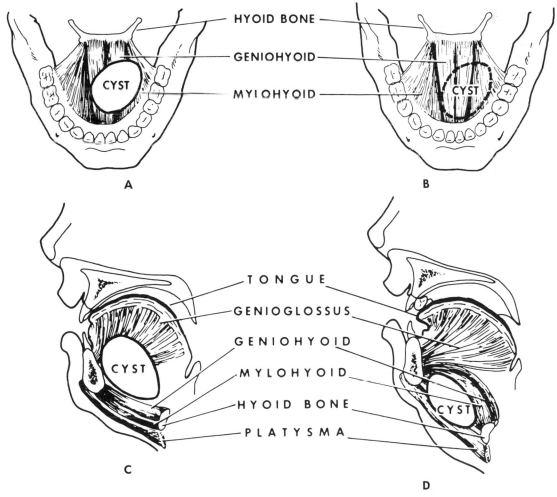

HYOID BONE

GENIOHYOID

MYLOHYOID

CYST

A

B

TONGUE

GENIOGLOSSUS

GENIOHYOID

MYLOHYOID

HYOID BONE

PLATYSMA

CYST

C

D

Figure 12-146

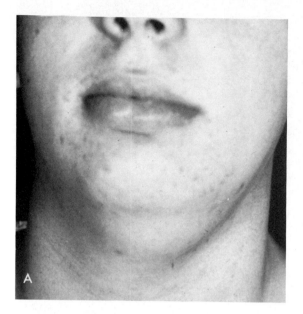

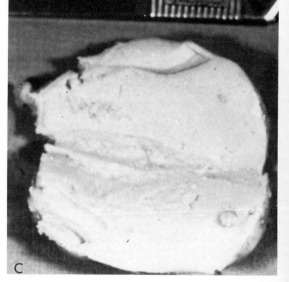

Figure 12–147 An unusual epidermal inclusion cyst that extended from the submental space, as shown in *A*, through the mylohyoid muscle and into the sublingual space, elevating the mucosa of the floor of the oral cavity, as shown in *B*. *C*, The cyst is cut open, exposing its caseous contents. This cyst had the superficial appearance of a mixed tumor (pleomorphic adenoma): however, it was not hard like a mixed tumor but rather was soft and mushy to finger pressure and felt like dough.

Photographic Case Report

INCLUSION CYST INVOLVING THE SUBLINGUAL AND SUBMENTAL SPACES

Marvin E. Pizer, D.D.S., M.S.

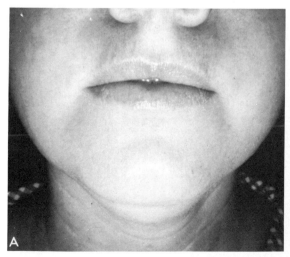

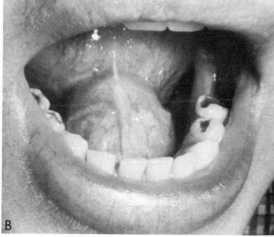

Figure 12–148 *See opposite page for legend.*

(Figure 12–148 continued on opposite page)

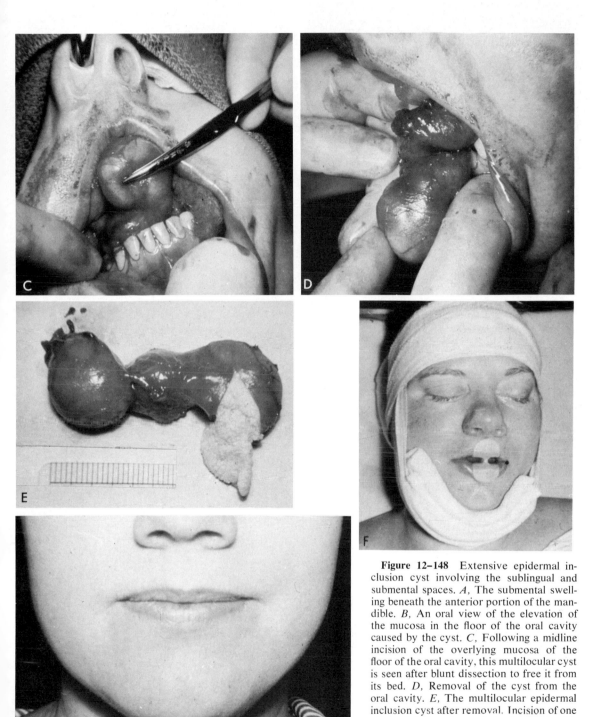

Figure 12–148 Extensive epidermal inclusion cyst involving the sublingual and submental spaces. *A*, The submental swelling beneath the anterior portion of the mandible. *B*, An oral view of the elevation of the mucosa in the floor of the oral cavity caused by the cyst. *C*, Following a midline incision of the overlying mucosa of the floor of the oral cavity, this multilocular cyst is seen after blunt dissection to free it from its bed. *D*, Removal of the cyst from the oral cavity. *E*, The multilocular epidermal inclusion cyst after removal. Incision of one of the lobules shows it to be filled with thick, caseous debris. *F*, Immediate postoperative appearance. *G*, Final appearance after surgery.

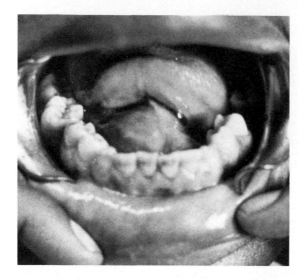

Figure 12–149 Another example of a midline epidermal inclusion cyst in the sublingual anatomic position.

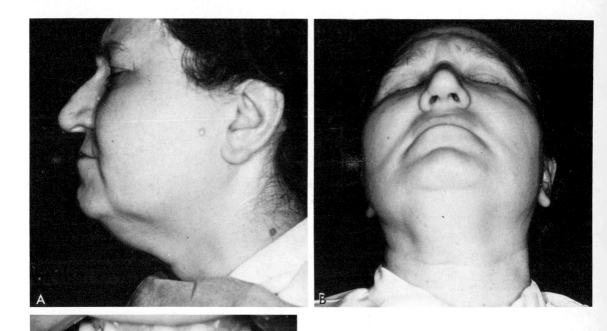

Figure 12–150 *A,* Lateral photograph of a patient with an epidermal inclusion cyst that did not produce submental swelling. *B,* Anterior view of the same patient; neck contour is normal. *C,* Elevation of the floor of the oral cavity caused by the pressure of a sublingual epidermal inclusion cyst.

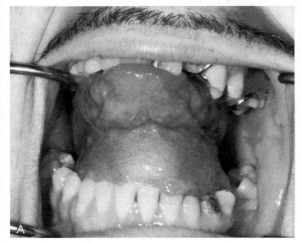

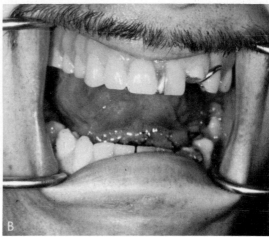

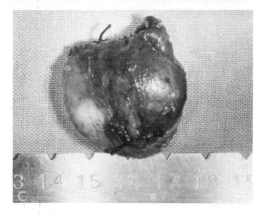

Figure 12–151 *A*, Comparatively large sublingual epidermal inclusion cyst. *B*, Intraoral appearance following the extirpation by blunt dissection of this globular epidermal inclusion cyst. *C*, The cyst following removal.

(Text continued from page 664)

MUCOUS RETENTION CYSTS

RANULA

A ranula is a thin-walled, bluish, transparent retention cyst located beneath the tongue in the anterior floor of the oral cavity. It is due to obstruction of the duct of the submandibular gland, the incisive gland of Suzanne or one of the ducts of the sublingual salivary glands (Rivini's glands).

Etiology. The cause of these retention cysts is under discussion. The theory of obstruction in the duct is disputed by Standish and Shafer because retention cysts failed to develop when they ligated ducts of submandibular and sublingual glands in rats.[67] However, I would answer that in the human there is a slow, gradual closure of these ducts as the lumen is narrowed by flocculent material, so that there is a small but continuous pressure on the walls of the duct as the discharge of saliva is inhibited. This gradually produces an expansion of the duct walls as the lumen is

narrowed and finally closed. I personally cannot believe that ranulas are the result of "traumatic severances of a salivary duct," a theory of theirs that is physically logical in the production of mucoceles.

These cysts are filled with a thick, crystalclear mucoid fluid. They are not painful and are soft and fluctuant. They form slowly and are generally found on one side of the midline. Occasionally they rupture spontaneously, but they slowly recur.

Treatment. Simple incision and drainage results in recurrence. The introduction of a seton to establish a permanent opening frequently fails. Marsupialization is the treatment of choice. This consists in excision of the anterior-superior wall of the cyst, and suturing of the cystic wall to the mucous membrane in the floor of the oral cavity, as in the Partsch operation.

Attempts to enucleate these cysts completely without rupturing the cystic wall are nearly impossible because of the wall's thinness. Such attempts should be limited to

(Text continued on page 689)

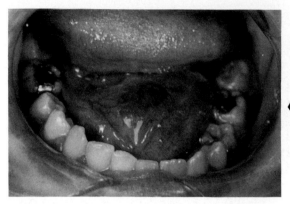

Figure 12–152 Note the difference in clinical appearance between the mucosa of the floor of the oral cavity overlying this midline ranula as compared with that overlying the previously illustrated sublingual epidermal inclusion cyst. By palpation one can also be helped to make the differential diagnosis between a retention cyst of salivary secretions and a sublingual epidermal inclusion cyst. Whereas a ranula feels soft and is readily compressed, a sublingual epidermal inclusion cyst has the previously described doughy or mushy feeling and is not readily compressed by the palpating fingers.

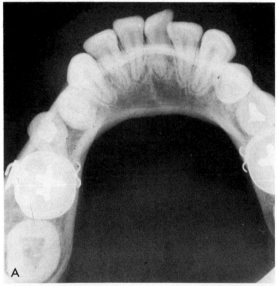

Figure 12–153 Extensive multilocular ranulas. *A*, Occlusal view before radiopaque material was introduced into this large multilocular ranula. *B* and *C*, The occlusal radiograph *(B)* and the lateral oblique radiograph *(C)* show the multilocular ranula filled with radiopaque oil. (Courtesy of Marvin E. Pizer, D.D.S., M.S.)

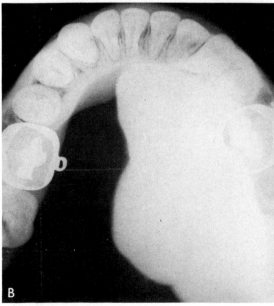

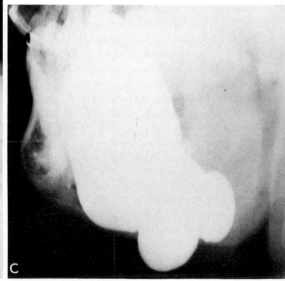

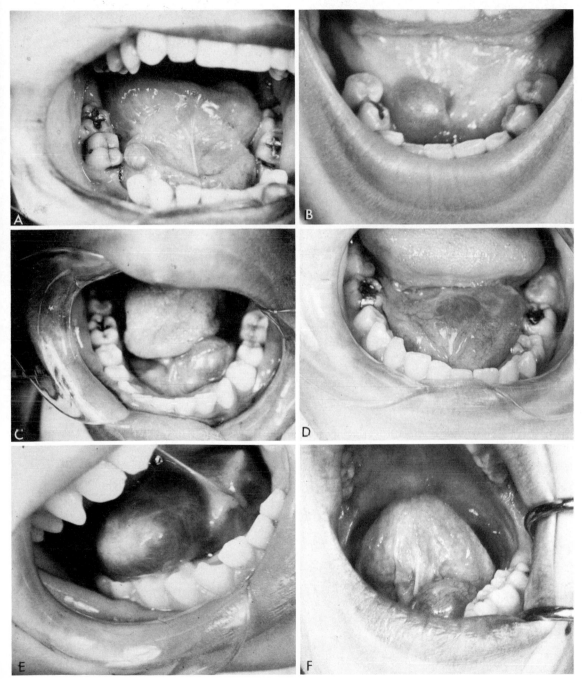

Figure 12–154 Examples of salivary retention cysts (ranulas) in the floor of the oral cavity. *A* and *B*, Cysts of the sublingual gland. *C* to *F*, Cysts from the submandibular gland, the sizes indicating how long the ducts have been blocked. As a rule these cysts are unilateral. An exception is seen in *D*, which shows a cyst that has expanded to include both sides of the floor of the mouth.

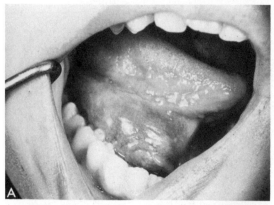

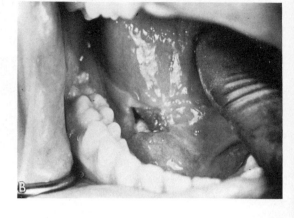

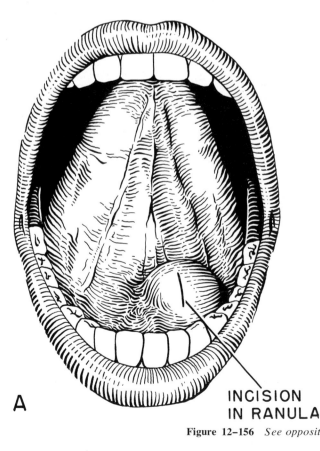

Figure 12–155 *A*, A ranula in the right floor of the oral cavity. *B*, A small piece of iodoform gauze is placed in the lumen of the cyst for the first 24 hours after marsupialization (see Figure 12–156 for technique). This area usually is not sutured, except perhaps for one suture distally and one suture anteriorly to reduce the size of the opening. *C*, The appearance of the floor of the oral cavity 4 weeks following surgery. The submandibular duct is patent.

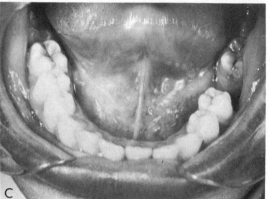

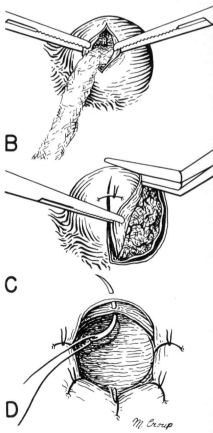

INCISION
IN RANULA

Figure 12–156 *See opposite page for legend.*

MARSUPIALIZATION OF A RANULA

A modified Partsch operation for a salivary ranula of the floor of the mouth was performed on a woman patient. (Study Figures 12–154 to 12–156.)

Technique. Under general anesthesia, the oral cavity having been prepared, the mouth opened, the tongue secured in routine manner, and the oropharyngeal partition inserted, the mucous membranes overlying the ranula, which was located to the left of the midline, were prepared with tincture of Merthiolate. The ranula was moved up into clear view by extraoral pressure beneath the left body of the mandible. A portion of the mucous membrane overlying the crest of the ranula, which appeared to be 1.5 cm. wide and 5 cm. long, was incised with a No. 15 Bard-Parker blade, and an attempt was made to incise the overlying mucous membrane without penetrating the cystic wall. This was thought to be impossible because of the thinness revealed by the translucency of the tissues in this area, the ranula having the typical bluish gray cystic appearance. After the incision was carried posteriorly for a distance of about 1 cm. without penetrating the cyst, the cystic wall suddenly ruptured, and immediately the contents of the cyst flowed out into the oral cavity and were aspirated by the suction. The contents were of the thick, clear, mucilaginous, ropy saliva type. The thick material stretched from the cystic cavity to the suction tip for a distance of 4 cm. without the ropy saliva's breaking.

After the cystic contents of the cavity were evacuated, the cavity was packed with plain selvage gauze to outline the extent of the cystic cavity. Next, the overlying mucous membranes and adherent cystic wall were removed around the periphery of the cystic cavity, as it was revealed by the gauze packing, with a pair of scissors. It was then found that the cystic cavity was approximately 3 cm. deep. After this the cystic wall was picked up where it was adherent to the mucous membrane lying in the oral cavity, and, with hemostat and needle passed through the cystic lining and then through the membranous lining of the floor of the mouth, it was tied. Sutures were placed through the cystic wall and the floor of the oral cavity entirely around the periphery of the cystic cavity, except in the lingual surface of the mandible, where the cystic wall and mucous membrane were adherent. The cavity was filled with iodoform gauze, and the patient left the operating room in good condition.

---

small mucoceles in which the mucous gland is also extirpated.

TECHNIQUE FOR MARSUPIALIZATION OF A RANULA. (See Figure 12–156.) If local anesthesia is selected, the lingual nerve should be anesthetized, with the same technique as that used when the inferior alveolar nerve and the lingual nerve are anesthetized, except that the needle is not carried back to the mandibular sulcus. The needle penetrates the mucous membrane only $1/8$ inch, and then 0.5 cc. of anesthetic solution is slowly deposited.

The patient places the tip of the tongue against the palate as far posteriorly as possible. If general anesthesia is used, the tongue is held up and back.

A $1/2$-inch incision is made through the mucosa and cystic wall.

The clear, thick mucoid fluid is removed with suction.

The cystic cavity is now filled with sterile $1/4$-inch selvage-edge gauze until the cystic cavity is completely outlined. A single suture is passed through the middle of the incision.

The gauze-filled cystic cavity is pushed up by finger pressure from beneath the mandible.

With a pair of No. 9 Dean's scissors, the operator begins at one end of the original in-

---

Figure 12–156 Marsupialization of a ranula. *A*, Ranula located beneath the tongue in the anterior floor of the oral cavity. *B*, After fluid is removed with suction, the cystic cavity is filled with $1/4$-inch selvage-edge gauze until the cavity is completely outlined. *C*, A single suture is placed through the middle of the incision. The mucosa and cystic membrane are cut from the top of the gauze-filled cavity. *D*, Several sutures are placed around the periphery to join the cystic wall to the mucosa of the floor of the oral cavity.

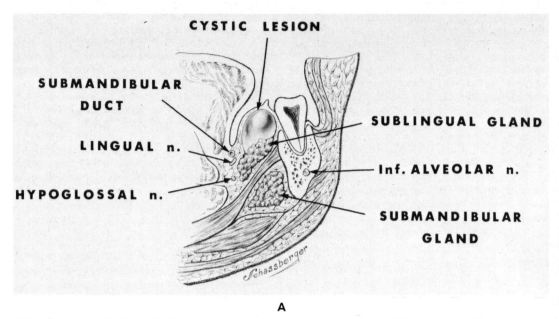

A

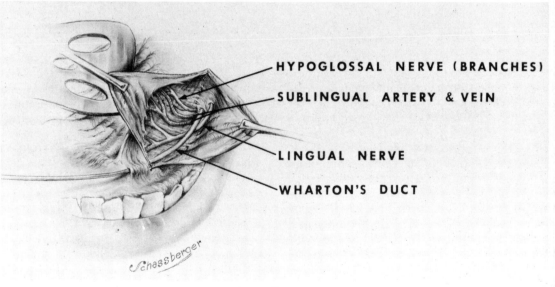

B

Figure 12–157 Anatomic structures involved in a ranula and its treatment. (From Catone, G. A., Merrill, R. G., and Henny, F. A.: Sublingual gland mucus-escape phenomenon—treatment by excision of sublingual gland. J. Oral Surg., 27(10):774–786 Oct., 1969. Copyright by the American Dental Association. Reprinted by permission.)

(Figure 12–157 continued on opposite page)

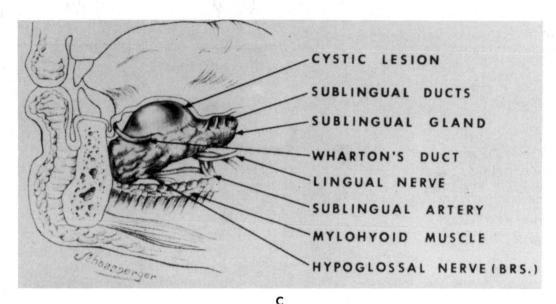

CYSTIC LESION

SUBLINGUAL DUCTS

SUBLINGUAL GLAND

WHARTON'S DUCT

LINGUAL NERVE

SUBLINGUAL ARTERY

MYLOHYOID MUSCLE

HYPOGLOSSAL NERVE (BRS.)

C

Figure 12–157 *(Continued.)*

cision and cuts the mucosa and cystic membrane from the top of the gauze-filled cystic cavity around the greatest perimeter of the cyst.

In most cases only a few sutures are needed around the periphery to join the cystic wall to the mucosa of the floor of the oral cavity.

MUCOCELE

These are small retention cysts that occur in the oral mucosa, most frequently on the lower lip, occasionally on the palate and rarely on the upper lip. These have been thought to be caused by a blockage of the mucous glands or their ducts. (See Figures 12–159 and 12–160.)

Recent investigations of Shafer, Standish and Bhaskar "appear to indicate that traumatic severance of a salivary duct, such as that produced by biting the lips or cheek or pinching the lip with extraction forceps, permits a continuous pooling of saliva in the tissues and the development of a well-demarcated cavity which is histologically identical with the natural retention cyst."[67]

Treatment. In the average case, marsupialization suffices. Occasionally it is necessary to excise the gland if there is recurrence.

In very small mucoceles, the mucous gland is extirpated. When this is done, it is immaterial if the small cyst is ruptured during surgery.

TECHNIQUE. (See Figures 12–161 to 12–163 and their legends.)

DERMOID CYSTS (DERMOIDS) OF THE FLOOR OF THE MOUTH*

IRVING MEYER, D.M.D., M.Sc., D.Sc.

The majority of dermoids are developmental cysts derived from epithelial debris or rests enclaved during the midline closure of the bilateral mandibular (first) and hyoid (second) branchial arches. Some of these cysts

*Reproduced in part with permission from Meyer, I.: Dermoid cysts (dermoids) of the floor of the mouth. Oral Surg., 8:1149–1164 (Nov.), 1955; copyrighted by The C. V. Mosby Co., St. Louis.

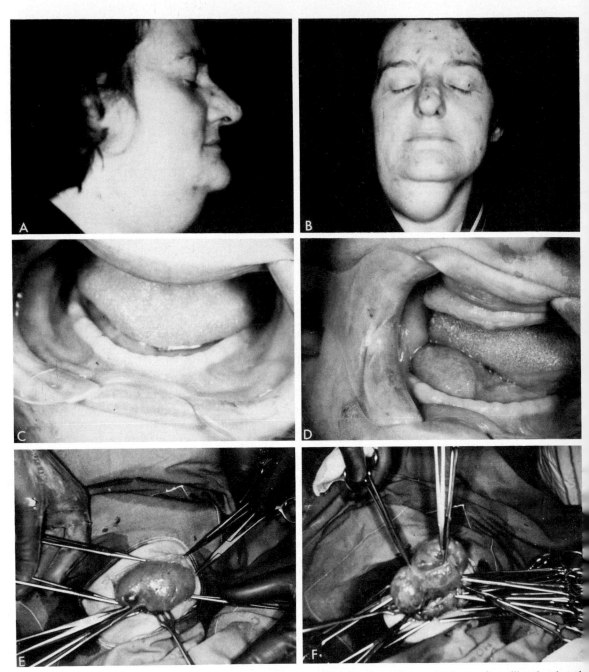

Figure 12–158 *A* and *B*, Profile and full face views of the extensive submaxillary and submental swelling developed slowly over a period of 3 to 4 years. *C*, Note the absence of any intraoral swelling. The retention cyst is below the mylohyoid muscle. *D*, However, when extraoral pressure was applied to the submaxillary swelling, a portion of the cyst was forced around the posterior border of the mylohyoid muscle into the sublingual space. *E*, Partial enucleation of the submaxillary retention cyst. *F*, Enucleation of the submaxillary retention cyst and extirpation of the submaxillary gland.*

*Another example of cooperation between specialists for the patient's benefit is demonstrated in this case. The skills and knowledge for the diagnosis and treatment of this patient were supplied by T. B. McCullough, M.D., and B. L. Silverblatt, M.D., of the Otolaryngology service, and W. H. Archer. D.D.S., and S. S. Spatz, D.D.S., of the Oral Surgery service of the Eye and Ear Hospital, Pittsburgh, Pa.

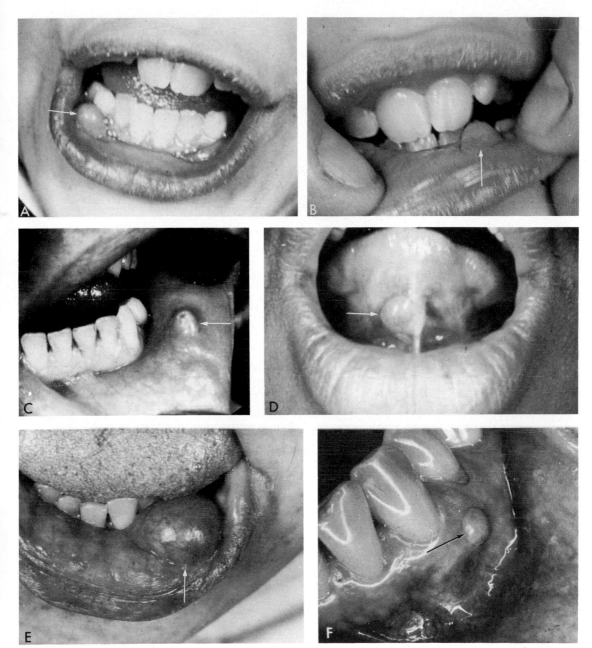

Figure 12–159 Various examples of retention cysts of the oral mucosa and in particular of the lip, where these retention cysts are probably most frequently seen. These retention cysts of small mucous glands, wherever they occur in the mucosa of the oral cavity, are known as mucoceles.

A and *B*, Small mucoceles of the lip in two youngsters, one 6 and the other 8 years of age.

C, A mucocele with a hyperkeratotic surface. Note the dense white tissue, in the center of which is a dark spot. This represents an area in which this patient's dentist had incised and drained this small cyst on half a dozen different occasions.

D, A mucocele in an unusual location along the lingual frenum just at the point at which it is attached to the ventral surface of the tongue.

E, A large mucocele on the lip of a 26-year-old woman.

F, A mucocele in a most unusual position, that is, arising from the dense mucoperiosteal membrane of the labial surface of the mandible just beneath the gingival line of the lateral incisor and cuspid. (*F*, Courtesy of Dr. Ernesto Muller M., Caracas, Venezuela.)

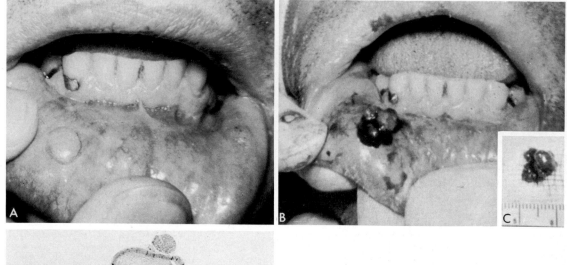

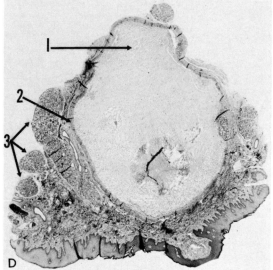

Figure 12–160 *A*, A well-circumscribed mucocele of the lip that is flattened out somewhat by the tensing of the lip with the two fingers. *B*, An incision is made around the cyst, and by blunt dissection the overlying mucosa and the cyst, as shown in *C*, were removed. The mucosa is then closed with sutures. *D*, The photomicrograph shows mucoid material *(1)* in a circumscribed cavity bordered by a fibrous wall *(2)* with no epithelial lining. Several mucus gland lobules *(3)* are present at the periphery of the specimen. (*D*, Courtesy of Billy N. Appel, D.D.S., Oral Pathologist.)

may be formed by remnants of the tuberculum impar of His which, together with the lateral processes from the inner surface of each mandibular arch, form the body of the tongue and floor of the mouth. These developments take place during the third and fourth weeks of embryonic life. (See Figures 12–164 to 12–166.)

CLASSIFICATION

Using the terms *dysontogenetic, epidermoid, dermoid, teratoid,* or *teratoma,* and the germ layer hypothesis of development of these cysts as suggested by various authors, including Ewing, Boyd, Colp, and so forth, I propose the following classification on histopathologic considerations of these cysts of the floor of the mouth:

Dysontogenetic Cysts of the Floor of the Mouth
(a) Epidermoid
(b) Dermoid
(c) Teratoid
(a) *Epidermoid cyst of floor of mouth:* An epithelium-lined cavity surrounded by a capsule with no skin appendages present.
(b) *Dermoid cyst of floor of mouth:* An epithelium-lined cavity with skin appendages of hair, hair follicles, sebaceous glands, sweat glands, and so on, present in the underlying connective tissue. This is a compound cyst.
(c) *Teratoid cyst of floor of mouth:* An epithelium-lined cavity with the following elements present in the capsule: (1) skin appendages including hair follicles, sebaceous glands, sweat glands, keratin,

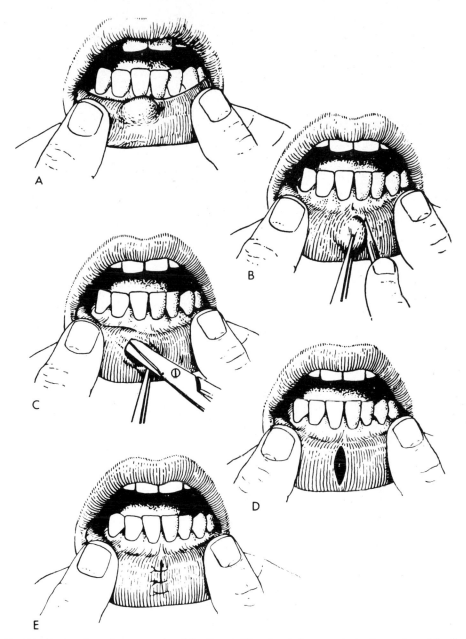

Figure 12–161 Extirpation of a mucocele of the lip. *A*, The elevated mucocele in the center of the lip held by the thumb and finger of the assistant. *B*, The cyst is grasped in dissecting tweezers and the overlying mucosa is incised completely around the periphery. *C*, The attached mucous glands are separated from their attachments by blunt dissection. *D*, Resulting defect. *E*, Sutures inserted. (From Howe, G. L.: Minor Oral Surgery. Bristol, England, John Wright & Sons, Ltd., 1971.)

and so forth; (2) connective tissue derivatives such as fibers, bone, muscle, blood vessels, and so on; and (3) respiratory and gastrointestinal tissues. This is a complex cyst.

Because of its long usage and presence in the literature, *dermoid* should be retained as a clinical term for all types of dysontogenetic or developmental cysts of the floor of the mouth. The acquired traumatic implantation cyst of the floor of the mouth is excluded from this proposed classification.

(Text continued on page 700)

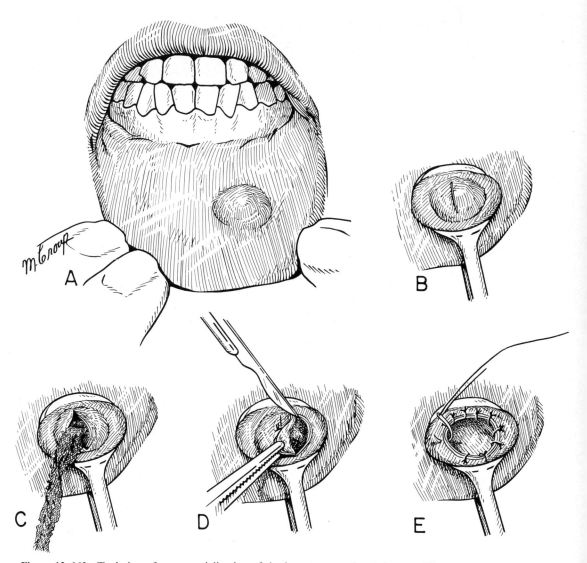

Figure 12–162   Technique for marsupialization of the larger mucoceles. It is very difficult to be certain that the entire cystic wall and involved glands are removed by the surgical excision of these cysts. For that reason marsupialization is indicated.

A, The lip is extended and pulled down with the fingers. Because of the four hands in this very small operating area, this is an awkward position and for that reason the technique which follows was developed. *B*, The placing of the Chalazion forceps. This is also known as a Desmarres clamp. An incision is then made into this cyst as shown, and the contents are evacuated. *C*, The cavity is next filled with ¼-inch iodoform gauze. *D*, The incision is closed with a single suture, or more if needed, and then a circle of overlying mucosa is removed with the scalpel. *E*, The mucosa of the lip is sutured to the cystic wall, and the clamp is removed.

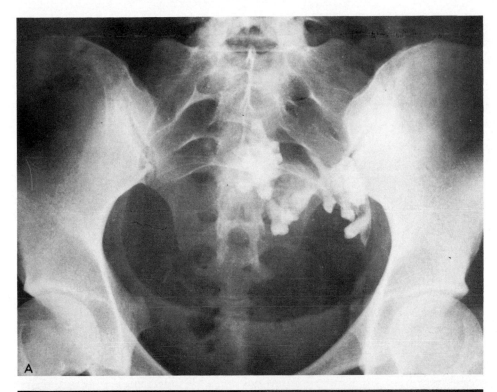

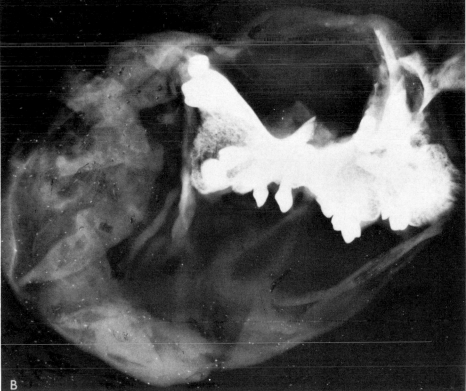

Figure 12-165 *A*, Radiograph of a female pelvis with a large dermoid cyst (benign cystic teratoma) of the left ovary with a large segment of bone (mandibular) containing many malformed teeth. *B*, Radiograph made after the cyst had been removed and the soft caseous material that filled it had been evacuated. Fifteen teeth of various forms had erupted and were firmly held in alveoli in the bone segment; dermal appendages, hair and sweat and sebaceous glands were also present in the cystic wall.

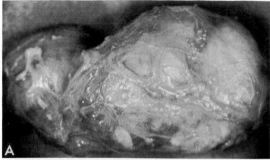

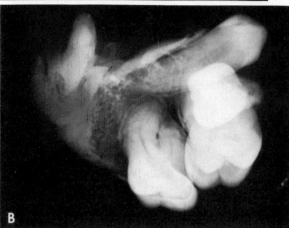

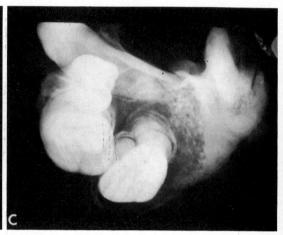

Figure 12–166 *A,* Large dermoid cyst of the ovary. *B* and *C,* These two radiographic views of the specimen clearly show well-formed teeth in their alveoli in the "mandibular" bone, which is covered with a mucoperiosteal membrane.

CLINICAL ASPECTS AND DIFFERENTIAL DIAGNOSIS

Clinically, dermoids of the floor of the mouth are frequently quite striking in their appearance. Those presenting themselves intraorally, or sublingually, may actually displace the tongue upward toward the palate until difficulty in eating, speaking, and even

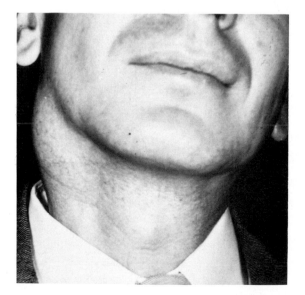

breathing may occur; those presenting extraorally, or submentally, usually appear as pendulous masses beneath the mandible. The cysts generally have a "dough-like" feel, but may feel cystic, depending on the consistency of the contents, which may vary from a cheesy, sebaceous-like substance to a more liquefied material. Hair, nails, keratin, and so forth, may be present, depending on the type

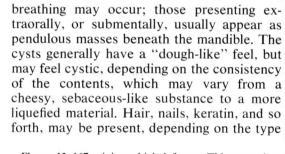

Figure 12–167 A branchial cleft cyst. This cyst arises from epithelial remnants of a branchial cleft, usually located between the second and third branchial arches. These cysts "usually occur at the angle of the jaw"[86] but may be seen at any point from the front of the external auditory canal to the clavicle. And they occur at any age; the youngest patient seen by Ward and Hendrick[86] was 5 months; the oldest was 79 years. "They develop as painless, at first inconspicuous, swellings along the anterior border of the sternomastoid muscle. They may grow to a very large size from a globular mass in the upper anterior triangle of the neck just below the angle of the jaw, and they may enlarge and become elongated as they follow the course of the sternomastoid muscle growing just under the anterior edge.

They may bulge into the floor of the mouth at the base of the tongue but seldom, if ever, bulge into the pharynx. Drainage of these cysts only creates a persistent sinus." Fistulous openings, which may result from these cysts, are illustrated in Figure 12–169.

Treatment consists of the complete extirpation of the cyst, with special care that all epithelium-bearing tissue is removed. If any is left behind, there will be a recurrence. "Contraindicated is incision and drainage, radiation or the injection of sclerosing solutions."[86]

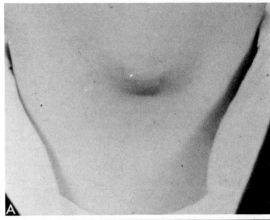

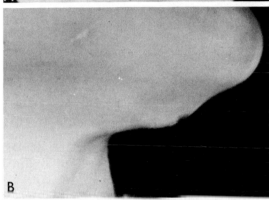

Figure 12–168 *A* and *B*, Thyroglossal tract cyst. This cyst in the neck develops from remnants of the stratified squamous epithelium–lined thyroglossal duct. Frequently they are located in the midline between the geniohyoid muscles. It is pointed out that "the thyroglossal duct cyst or fistula occurs in or near the midline any place from the foramen cecum at the base of the tongue to the suprasternal notch and that these abnormalities are the most frequent pathologic lesions situated in this region." The treatment of the cyst is the surgical excision of the entire sinus or fistula. Ward and Hendrick stress that they should not be incised and drained, nor treated by radiation or by the injection of sclerosing solutions.[86] There is a high rate of recurrence of the cyst because of the failure to remove all of the tract, which is lined by stratified squamous, columnar or transitional epithelium up to the foramen cecum at the base of the tongue. To leave any of this tissue behind guarantees recurrence of the cyst.

of cyst being dealt with. Some have frank pus present because of acute infection. These lesions vary in weight from 1 gm. to several hundred grams, and may vary in size from a small pea-sized growth to one the size of a large grapefruit. Sinus tracts may develop from these cysts to open either intraorally into the floor of the mouth or extraorally into the skin beneath the chin. Dermoids may undergo malignant degeneration and may metastasize to lymph nodes.

The differential diagnosis of dermoids of the floor of the mouth include: (1) ranula, (2) unilateral or bilateral blockage of Wharton's duct, (3) thyroglossal duct cyst, (4) cystic hygroma, (5) branchial cleft cysts, (6) acute infection or cellulitis of the floor of the mouth, (7) infections of submaxillary and sublingual glands, (8) benign and malignant tumors of the floor of the mouth and adjacent salivary glands, and (9) normal fat mass in the submental area. The clinical diagnosis is inconclusive.

TREATMENT

The treatment of dermoid cysts of the floor of the mouth is surgical. Aspiration may be used for temporary relief. Aspiration and sclerosing agents, as definitive therapy, are not good; these may lead to even more difficulties, including acute infection and cellulitis of the surrounding area. There have been no reports of the use of radiation, but it can readily be assumed that this would not be effective.

The surgical approach can be made either intra- or extraorally, depending on the position of the cyst in relation to the mylohyoid and platysma muscles. Those lying between mylohyoid and oral mucous membrane (sublingual position) are best removed by an intraoral approach; those lying between my-

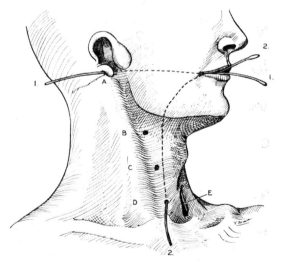

Figure 12–169 Sites at which branchial and thyroglossal fistulous openings may appear. *A*, Opening of a fistula auris of the first (hyomandibular) cleft. Sound *1* indicates its communication with the oral cavity. *B* and *C*, Possible locations of an opening of a cervical fistula originating from the position of the second pharyngeal pouch. *D*, Opening of a fistula of third pouch origin; sound *2* has been passed through it from the mouth. *E*, Opening of a thyroglossal duct fistula.

(From Ward, G. E., and Hendrick, J. W.: Tumors of the Head and Neck. Baltimore, The Williams & Wilkins Co., 1950; based on Corning, 1921.)

lohyoid and platysma (submental position) are approached through a transverse incision through skin, fascia and platysma. Usually the cysts are readily shelled out by blunt dissection, with difficulty being encountered only if there has been matting down of tissue from previous treatment by aspiration or sclerosing solutions or episodes of infection.

SUPPLEMENTARY READING

Calcifying Odontogenic Cysts

Abrams, A. M., and Howell, F. V.: The calcifying odontogenic cyst. Report of four cases. Oral Surg., 25:594 (Apr.), 1968.

Chaves, E.: The calcifying odontogenic cyst. Oral Surg., 25:849, 1968.

Johnson, R. H., and Topazian, R. G.: Calcifying odontogenic cyst: Report of case. J. Oral Surg., 26:394 (June), 1968.

Komiya, Y., Susa, A., and Kawachi, H.: Calcifying odontogenic cyst. Report of a case. Oral Surg., 27:90 (Jan.), 1969.

Overgaard, R. H., and Holland, P. S.: The calcifying odontogenic cyst. A case report. Br. J. Oral Surg., 5:169 (Nov.), 1967.

Ulmansky, M., Azaz, B., and Sela, J.: Calcifying odontogenic cyst: Report of cases. J. Oral Surg., 27:415 (June), 1969.

Dentigerous Cysts

Alvares, O., Olech, E., and Silverglade, L. B.: Lingual mandibular bone cavity concomitant with a dentigerous cyst. A clinical and histologic report. Oral Surg., 27:252 (Feb.), 1969.

Bloom, J. Y.: Infected dentigerous cyst simulating tuberculous osteomyelitis of mandible. Case report. J. N.J. Dent. Soc., 39:809 (Apr.), 1968.

Dresser, W. J., and Segal, E.: Ameloblastoma associated with a dentigerous cyst in a 6 year old child. Report of a case. Oral Surg., 24:388 (Sept.), 1967.

Duquette, P., and Goebel, W. M.: Radiographic superimposition and suspected dentigerous cyst. Oral Surg., 37:306 (Feb.), 1974.

Gebrig, J. D., and Freedman, D. L.: Impacted third molar and dentigerous cyst of the condylar neck of the mandible: Report of case. Oral Surg., 26:609 (Sept.), 1968.

Gilbert, A. G.: Dentigerous cyst of the maxillary antrum: Case report. J. Can. Dent. Assoc., 34:132 (Mar.), 1968.

Hutton, C. E.: Occurrence of ameloblastoma within a dentigerous cyst. Report of a case. Oral Surg., 24:147 (Aug.), 1967.

Lee, K. W., and Loke, S. J.: Squamous cell carcinoma arising in a dentigerous cyst. Cancer, 20:2241 (Dec.), 1967.

Paul, J. K., Fay, J. T., and Stamps, P.: Recurrent dentigerous cyst evidencing ameloblastic proliferation: Report of case. Oral Surg., 27:211 (Mar.), 1969.

Quinn, J. H., and Fournet, L. F.: Dentigerous cyst with

mural ameloblastoma: Report of a case. J. Med. Genet., 27:662 (Aug.), 1969.

Santangelo, M. V.: Concrescence associated with a dentigerous cyst. Oral Surg., 26:769 (Dec.), 1968.

Small, E. W.: Ciliated epithelium lining a mandibular dentigerous cyst: Report of case. J. Oral Surg., 25:260 (May), 1967.

Small, E. W.: Mandibular dentigerous cyst in a 6 year old child. Report of a case. Oral Surg., 23:320 (June), 1967.

Smith, N. H.: Multiple dentigerous cysts associated with arachnodactyly and other skeletal defects. Report of a case. Oral Surg., 25:99 (Jan.), 1968.

Stoneman, D. W.: Dentigerous cyst. Oral Health, 57:191 (Mar.), 1967.

Stroh, E., Friedman, J., and Levy, K.: A large dentigerous cyst in a nine year old child. A case report. N.Y. Dent. J., 35:223 (Apr.), 1969.

Via, W. F., Jr.: Dentigerous cyst involving the maxillary sinus. Oral Surg., 24:629 (Nov.), 1967.

Follicular Cysts

McCann, C. F., Mallett, S. P., and Houghton, J. D.: Recurrent follicular cyst of mandible. Report of a case. Oral Surg., 23:391 (Mar.), 1967.

Newman, G. W., and Rafel, S. S.: Treatment of a pseudo–class 3 malocclusion and associated follicular cyst: Report of case. J.A.D.A., 80:340 (Feb.), 1970.

Rakower, W.: Successful conservative management of a large follicular cyst of the mandible. N.Y. J. Dent., 40:13 (Jan.), 1970.

Globulomaxillary Cysts

Brown, P. R.: An unusual case of globulomaxillary cyst. Oral Surg., 24:719 (Dec.), 1967.

Di Conza, P. J., Rasi, H., and Fischer, L. A.: Bilateral globulomaxillary cysts. Report of a case. N.Y. Dent. J., 35:228 (Apr.), 1969.

Johnston, W. C., and Stoopack, J. C.: Globulomaxillary cyst invading the maxillary antrum. Report of a case. Oral Surg., 22:675 (Nov.), 1966.

Mehrotra, M. C.: Globulomaxillary cyst. J. Indian Med. Assoc., 51:397 (Oct.), 1968.

Saracino, S. F., and Kleinman, M.: An unusually large globulomaxillary cyst treated by marsupialization and enucleation. Oral Surg., 25:298 (Mar.), 1968.

Keratocysts

Bang, G.: Keratocysts, skeletal anomalies, ichthyosis, and defective response to parathyroid hormone in a patient without basal-cell carcinoma. Report of a case. Oral Surg., 29:242 (Feb.), 1970.

Hjorting-Hansen, E., Andreasen, J. O., and Robinson, L. H.: A study of odontogenic cysts with special reference to location of keratocysts. Br. J. Oral Surg., 7:15 (July), 1969.

Panders, A. K., and Haddlers, H.: Solitary keratocysts of the jaws. Oral Surg., 27:931 (Dec.), 1969.

Rud, J., and Pindborg, J. J.: Odontogenic keratocysts: A follow-up study of 21 cases. J. Oral Surg., 27:323 (May), 1969.

Torres, I.: Keratocyst of the mandible: Report of case. Oral Surg., 27:965 (Dec.), 1969.

Mandibular Cysts

Amar, H.: Gingival cyst. Report of a case. Oral Surg., 22:578 (Nov.), 1966.
Chesnay, G.: Mandibular cyst and supernumerary premolars. Oral Surg., 37:654 (Apr.), 1974.
Conklin, W. W.: Hidden cyst. Oral Surg., 37:138 (Jan.), 1974.
Lemmer, J., and Shear, M.: Unusual presentation of a dental cyst. Oral Surg., 26:333 (Sept.), 1968.
Loscalzo, L. J., and Marcotullio, R. G.: The multilocular cyst: A surgical approach. Oral Surg., 24:559 (Oct.), 1967.
Martinelli, C., and Rulli, M. A.: Periapical cyst associated with actinomycosis. Oral Surg., 24:817 (Dec.), 1967.
Tucker, W. M., Pleasants, J. E., and MacComb, W. S.: Decompression and secondary enucleation of a mandibular cyst: Report of a case. J. Oral Surg., 30:669 (Sept.), 1972.

Median Cysts

Courage, G. R., North, A. F., and Hansen, L. S.: Median palatine cysts. Review of the literature and report of a case. Oral Surg., 38:745 (May), 1974.
Buchner, A., and Ramon, Y.: Median mandibular cyst—a rare lesion of debatable origin. Oral Surg., 37:431 (Mar.), 1974.
Durdi, A. R.: Distribution of midpalatine cysts: A reevaluation of human palatal closure mechanisms. Oral Surg., 26:41 (Jan.), 1968.
Morgan, G. A., and Morgan, P. R.: Maxillary mid-line radiolucencies. Differential radiological interpretation. J. Ont. Dent. Assoc., 46:245 (June), 1969.
Stout, F. W., and Collett, W. K.: Etiology and incidence of the median maxillary anterior alveolar cleft. Oral Surg., 28:66 (July), 1969.
Swindle, P. F., and Maher, W. P.: Blood vessels of median palatal fissural cysts. Oral Surg., 27:368, (Mar.), 1969.
Thornton, W. E., Allen, J. W., and Byrd, D. L.: Median palatal cyst: Report of a case. J. Oral Surg., 30:661 (Sept.), 1972.

Maxillary Cysts

Cramer, J. R., White, R. P., Jr., and Berkowitz, R. P.: A surgical approach to the large maxillary cyst. J. Med. Genet., 27:665 (Aug.), 1969.
Howell, R. A.: Two cases of lateral periodontal cyst. Oral Surg., 23:183 (Feb.), 1967.
Kendrick, V. B.: An unusual cyst of the maxilla. J. N.C. Dent. Soc., 52:31 (Jan.), 1969.
Seward, M. H., and Seward, G. R.: Observations on Snawdon's technique for the treatment of cysts in the maxilla. Br. J. Oral Surg., 6:149 (Mar.), 1969.
Smith, H. W.: Cystic lesions of the maxilla. 1. Classification and clinical features. Arch Otolaryngol., 88:315 (Sept.), 1968.
van der Kwast, W. A., and van der Waal, I.: The mucosal cyst of the maxillary sinus. J. Oral Surg., 32:396, 1974. (Abstr.)
Wigglesworth, J.: Fissural cysts in the lateral incisor

region of the maxilla. Trans. Congr. Int. Assoc. Oral Surg., 153, 1967.

Nasoalveolar Cysts

Bull, T. R., McNeill, K. A., and Milner, G.: Naso-alveolar cysts. J. Laryngol. Otol., 81:37 (Jan.), 1967.
Santora, E., Jr., Ballantyne, A. J., and Hinds, E. C.: Naso-alveolar cyst: Report of case. Oral Surg., 28:117 (Feb.), 1970.
Walsh-Waring, G. P.: Naso-alveolar cysts: aetiology. Presentation and treatment. Six cases are reported. J. Laryngol. Otol., 81:263 (Mar.), 1967.

Nasolabial Cysts

Brandao, G. S., Ebling, H., and Faria e Souza, I.: Bilateral nasolabial cyst. Oral Surg., 37:480 (Mar.), 1974.
Crawford, W. H., Jr., Korchin, L., and Greskovich, F. J., Jr.: Nasolabial cysts: Report of two cases. Oral Surg., 26:582 (Sept.), 1968.
Roed-Petersen, B.: Nasolabial cysts. A presentation of five patients with a review of the literature. Br. J. Oral Surg., 7:84 (Nov.), 1969.

Nasopalatine Cysts

Cerine, F. C., Sine, G. W., and Benton, E. C.: Bone regeneration following enucleation of nasopalatine duct cyst. J. Periodont., 38:398 (Sept.–Oct.), 1967.
Danziger, A., Arthur, A., and Salman, S.: Nasopalatine cyst: Report of a case. Ann. Dent., 25:82 (Sept.), 1966.
Francis, T. C., and Archard, H. O., Jr.: Nasopalatine duct cyst with epidermoid features: Report of case. Oral Surg., 25:263 (May), 1967.
Freedman, G. L., Hooley, J. R., and Funk, E. C.: Unusual radiographic appearance of a probable incisive canal cyst. J. Can. Dent. Assoc., 34:317 (June), 1968.
Saunders, L. A., Wisniewski, H., and Soumerai, S.: Extensive incisive canal cyst. Report of a case. Oral Surg., 26:284 (Sept.), 1968.

Primordial Cysts

Fay, J. T.: Extensive development of a primordial mandibular cyst. Oral Surg., 28:510 (Oct.), 1969.
Parnell, A. G.: Primordial cyst of the jaw: Case report. J. Can. Dent. Assoc., 34:61 (Feb.), 1968.
Soskolne, W. A., and Shear, M.: Observations on the pathogenesis of primordial cysts. Br. Dent. J., 123:321 (Oct.), 1967.

Radicular and Residual Cysts

Ahlstrom, U., Johansen, C. C., and Lantz, B.: Radicular and residual cysts of the jaws. A long term roentgenographic study following cystectomies. Odontol. Rev., 20:111, 1969.
Balfour, R.: Radicular cyst (infected). J. Clin. Stomatol. Conf., 7:106 (Mar.), 1966.

Stoneman, D. W.: Suppurating residual cyst. Oral Health, *59*:41 (Jan.), 1969.

Solitary Bone Cysts (SBC)
(Hemorrhagic, Traumatic, Extravasation, Unicameral Cysts)

Fein, S., and Mohnac, A. M.: Submandibular gland extravasation cyst: Report of an unusual case. J. Oral Surg., *31*:551 (July), 1973.

Fordyce, G. L.: Haemorrhagic cysts of the mandible. Br. J. Oral Surg., *2*:80, 1964.

Moore, C. R., Steed, D. L., and Jacoby, J. J.: Traumatic bone cyst. J. Oral Surg., *28*:188 (Mar.), 1970.

Sapone, J., and Hansen, L. S.: Traumatic bone cysts of jaws: Diagnosis, treatment, and prognosis. Oral Surg., *38*:127 (July), 1974.

Schofield, I. D. F.: An unusual traumatic bone cyst. Oral Surg., *38*:198 (Aug.), 1974.

Sieverink, N. P. J. B.: The Simple Bone Cyst. Leiden, The Netherlands, Stafleu-Tholen, 1974.

REFERENCES

1. Abrams, A. M., et al.: Nasopalatine cysts. Oral Surg., *16*:306 (Mar.), 1963.
2. Amaral, W. J., and Jacobs, D. S.: Aberrant salivary gland defect in the mandible: Report of a case. Oral Surg., *14*:748, 1961.
3. American Dental Association: A.D.A. Lead. Bull., *IV*(25):4 (Dec. 23), 1974.
4. Angelopoulos, A. P., et al.: Malignant transformation of the epithelial lining of the odontogenic cysts. Oral Surg., *22*:415–428, 1966.
5. Becker, M. H., Kopf, A. W., and Lande, A.: Basal cell nevus syndrome: Its roentgenologic significance. Review of the literature and report of four cases. Am. J. Roentgenol. Radium Ther. Nucl. Med., *99*:817 (Apr.), 1967.
6. Bergenholtz, A., and Persson, G.: Idiopathic bone cavities: A report of four cases. Oral Surg., *16*:703 (June), 1963.
7. Bernier, J. L.: Personal communication, January 1975.
8. Bernstein, H. F., Lam, R. C., and Pomije, F. W.: Static bone cavities of the mandible: Review of the literature and report of a case. Oral Surg., *16*:46, 1958.
9. Bhaskar, S. N.: Bone lesions of endodontic origin. Dent. Clin. North Am., 521–533 (Nov.), 1967.
10. Bradfield, W. J., and Broadway, E. S.: Malignant change in a dentigerous cyst. Br. J. Surg., *45*:657–659, 1958.
11. Bramley, P. A., and Browne, R. M.: Recurring odontogenic cysts. Br. J. Oral Surg., *5*:106 (Nov.), 1967.
12. Browne, R. M.: The odontogenic keratocyst: histological features and their correlation with clinical behavior. Br. Dent. J., *131*:249, 1971.
13. Browne, R. M.: The odontogenic keratocyst: Clinical aspects. Br. Dent. J., *128*:225, 1970.
14. Browne, R. M., and Miller, W. A.: Rupture strength of capsules of odontogenic cysts in man. Arch. Oral Biol., *14*:1351 (Nov.), 1969.
15. Burtschi, T. A., and Stout, R. A.: Bilateral nasoalveolar cysts. Oral Surg., *16*:271 (Mar.), 1963.
16. Carr, B. M., and Mohnac, A. M.: Simple ameloblastoma within a follicular cyst of the maxilla. Oral Surg., *15*:1136 (Sept.), 1962.
17. Cataldo, E.: Cysts of the oral mucosa in newborns. Am. J. Dis. Child., *116*:44–48 (July), 1968.
18. Choukas, N. C., and Toto, P. D.: Etiology of static bone defects of the mandible. J. Oral Surg., *18*:16, 1960.
19. Cook, T. J., and Zbar, M. J.: Arteriovenous aneurysm of the mandible. Oral Surg., *15*:442 (Apr.), 1962.
20. Crist, T. F.: The globulomaxillary cyst: An embryologic misconception. Oral Surg., *30*(4):515–526 (Oct.), 1970.
21. Cunningham, C. J., and Penick, E. C.: Use of a roentgenographic contrast medium in the differential diagnosis of periapical lesions. Oral Surg., *26*:96 (July), 1968.
22. Dent, R. J., and Wertheimer, F. W.: Hyaline bodies in odontogenic cysts: A histochemical study for hemoglobin. J. Dent. Res., *46*:629 (May–June), 1967.
23. Dewberry, J. A., Jr.: The use of the pulpal space of a tooth in the conservative treatment of a large area of rarefaction. Oral Surg., *25*:869 (June), 1968.
24. Dorland's Illustrated Medical Dictionary. 25th ed. Philadelphia, W. B. Saunders Co., 1974.
25. Ebling, H., and Wagner, J. E.: Calcifying odontogenic cyst. Oral Surg., *24*:537 (Oct.), 1967.
26. Ebling, H., and Wagner, J. E.: Aneurysmal bone cysts of the mandible: report of a case. Oral Surg., *18*:646 (Nov.), 1964.
27. Eversole, L. B., Sabes, W. B., and Rovin, S.: Oncogenic potential of odontogenic cysts. University of Kentucky Paper presented at the Annual Meeting of the American Academy of Oral Pathology, Montreal, 1973.
28. Falkmer, S., et al.: Carcinoma arising in odontogenic cyst of the jaw. Odontol. Tidskr., *65*:220–231, 1957.
29. Fordyce, G. L.: Haemorrhagic cysts of the mandible. Br. J. Oral Surg., *2*:80–85, 1964.
30. Fordyce, G. L.: The probable nature of so-called latent haemorrhagic cysts of the mandible. Br. Dent. J., *101*:40, 1956.
31. Frankl, Z.: Clinical aspects and pathology of cysts of the jaws. Histopathology of the cysts of the jaws. Leucoplakic changes of the epithelial lining of the cysts. Dent. Delin., *20*:12 (Spring), 1969.
32. Frankl, Z.: Clinical aspects and pathology of cysts of the jaws. Surgical therapy. Dent. Delin., *19*:7 (Autumn), 1968.
33. Frankl, Z.: Clinical aspects and pathology of cysts of the jaws. Dent. Delin., *19*:11 (Summer), 1968.
34. Gardner, A. F.: The odontogenic cyst as a potential carcinoma; a clinico-pathologic appraisal. J.A.D.A., *78*:746–755, 1969.
35. Giunta, J. L., and Wisner, B. W.: Conservative management of mandibular incisors with a large area of bone involvement: Report of a case. 68-8. U.S. Naval Submar. Med. Cent. 1–6, 16 April, 1968.
36. Gorlin, R. J., and Goldman, H. M.: Thoma's Oral Pathology. 6th ed. St. Louis, The C. V. Mosby Co., 1970.
37. Grossman, L. I.: Bacteriologic status of periapical tissue in 150 cases of infected pulpless teeth. J. Dent. Res., *38*(1):101–104 (Feb.), 1959.

38. Grupe, H., Jr.: Epithelial rests in periodontal membrane explants. J. Periodontol., *39*:42 (Jan.), 1968.

39. Hankey, G. T., and Pedlar, J. A.: Primary squamous cell carcinoma of mandible arising from epithelial lining of dental cyst. Proc. R. Soc. Med., *50*:680–687, 1957.

40. Hjorting-Hansen, E.: Heterogeneous bone implants in the treatment of odontogenic cysts. Trans. Congr. Int. Assoc. Oral Surg., 357–365, 1967.

41. Howe, G. L.: Minor Oral Surgery. Bristol, England, John Wright & Sons, Ltd., 1971.

42. Howell, F. V., and De La Rosa, V. M.: Cytologic evaluation of cystic lesions of the jaw: A new diagnostic technique. J. South Calif. Dent. Assoc., *36*:161 (Apr.), 1968.

43. Jacobs, M. H.: The traumatic bone cyst. Oral Surg., *8*:940, 1955.

44. James, P.: Malignancies arising in odontogenic cysts. Trans. Congr. Int. Assoc. Oral Surg., 135–140, 1967.

45. Kay, L. W., and Kramer, I. R. H.: Squamous cell carcinoma arising in a dental cyst. Oral Surg., *15*:970–979, 1962.

46. Killey, H. C., and Kay, L. W.: An analysis of 471 benign cystic lesions of the jaws. Int. Surg., *46*:540 (Dec.), 1966.

47. Ködel, G.: Karzinomatöse Umwandlung einer odontogenen Kieferzyste. Dtsch. Zhan Mund Kieferheilkd., *43*:97–105, 1964.

48. Korchin, L.: Dermoid cyst with lingual sinus tract. Report of a case. Oral Surg., *37*:175 (Feb.), 1974.

49. Lalonde, E. R., and Leubke, R. G.: The frequency and distribution of periapical cysts and granulomas. An evaluation of 800 specimens. Oral Surg., *25*:861 (June), 1968.

50. Lee, K. W., and Loke, S. J.: Squamous cell carcinoma arising in a dentigerous cyst. Cancer, *20*:2241–2244, 1967.

51. Lefebvre, J., and Chaumont, P.: Eosinophilic granuloma of the oral cavity in infants. J. Radiol. Electrol., *39*:705–712 (Mar.), 1959.

52. Mårtensson, G.: Cysts and carcinoma of the jaws. Oral Surg., *8*:673–681, 1955.

53. Mitchell, D. F., and Shankwalker, G. B.: Osteogenic potential of calcium hydroxide and other materials in soft tissue and bone wounds. J. Dent. Res., *37*:6 (Nov.-Dec.), 1958.

54. Moore, C. R., Steed, L. L., and Jacoby, J. J.: Traumatic bone cyst. J. Oral Surg., *28*(3):188–195 (Mar.), 1970.

55. Morrison, R., and Deeley, T. J.: Intra-alveolar carcinoma of the jaw. Br. J. Radiol., *35*:321–336, 1963.

56. Olech, E.: Ranula. Oral Surg., *16*:1169 (Oct.), 1963.

57. Patterson, S. S.: Endodontic therapy: Use of a polyethylene tube and stint for drainage. J.A.D.A., *69*:711 (Dec.), 1964.

58. Penhale, K. W.: Cysts of the maxilla and mandible; diagnosis and treatment. J. Oral Surg., *1*:138, 1943.

59. Peterson, L. W.: Cystic cavity in the mandible: Report of a case. J. Oral Surg., *2*:182, 1944.

60. Pindborg, J. J.: Variations in odontogenic cyst epithelium. Trans. Congr. Int. Assoc. Oral Surg., 120–127, 1957.

61. Richard, E. L., and Ziskind, J.: Aberrant salivary gland tissue in mandible. Oral Surg., *10*:1086, 1957.

62. Rushton, M. A.: Solitary bone cysts in the mandible. Br. Dent. J., *81*:37, 1946.

63. Salman, L., and Salman, S. J.: Decompression of odontogenic cysts. N.Y. Dent. J., *34*:409 (Aug.-Sept.), 1968.

64. Schultz, W. F.: Multiple pathologic entities on a single film. Oral Surg., *29*:223 (Feb.), 1970.

65. Seidner, S.: Conservative treatment of inoperable cysts of the oral cavity: Report of five cases. Schweiz. Mschr. Zahnheilk., *68*:116–119 (Feb.), 1958.

66. Seltzer, S., Soltanoff, W., and Bender, I. B.: Epithelial proliferation in periapical lesions. Oral Surg., *27*:111 (Jan.), 1969.

67. Shafer, W. G., Hine, M. K., and Levy, B. M.: A Textbook of Oral Pathology. 3rd ed. Philadelphia, W. B. Saunders Co., 1974.

68. Sharp, G. S., and Helsper, J. T.: Radiolucent spaces in the jaws. A new guide in diagnosis. Am. J. Surg., *118*:712 (Nov.), 1969.

69. Shear, M.: Primary intra-alveolar epidermoid carcinoma of the jaw. J. Pathol., *97*:645–651, 1969.

70. Sieverink, N. P. J. B.: The Simple Bone Cyst. Leiden, The Netherlands, Stafleu-Tholen, 1974.

71. Smith, J. S.: Am. J. Dent. Sci., Scr. 3, *XIX*(6): (Oct.), 1885.

72. Stafne, E. C.: Oral Roentgenographic Diagnosis. 4th ed. Philadelphia, W. B. Saunders Co., 1975.

73. Stafne, E. C.: Value of roentgenograms in diagnosis of the jaws. Oral Surg., *6*:82, 1953.

74. Stafne, E. C.: Bone cavities situated near the angle of the mandible. J.A.D.A., *29*:1969, 1942.

75. Stedman's Medical Dictionary. 22nd ed. Baltimore, The Williams & Wilkins Co., 1972.

76. Stokke, T., and Koppang, H. S.: Squamous cell carcinoma arising in mandibular cyst. Acta Odontol. Scand., *26*:667–670, 1968.

77. Stoneman, D. W.: Swelling of the jaws, a radiologic consideration. Oral Health, *57*:553 (Aug.), 1967.

78. Stoneman, D. W.: Healing cyst. Oral Health, *57*:261 (Apr.), 1967.

79. Thoma, K. H.: Case report of a so-called latent bone cyst. Oral Surg., *8*:963, 1955.

80. Tiecke, R. W.: Oral Pathology. New York, McGraw-Hill Book Co., Inc., 1965.

81. Toller, P. A.: Newer concepts of odontogenic cysts. Int. J. Oral Surg., *1*:3–16, 1972.

82. Toller, P. A.: Origin and growth of cysts of the jaws. Ann. R. Coll. Surg. Engl., *40*:306 (May), 1967.

83. Toller, P. A.: The growth of radioactive isotope and other investigations in a case of hemorrhagic cyst of the mandible. Br. J. Oral Surg., *4*:86–93, 1964.

84. Toller, P. A.: Experimental investigations into factors concerning the growth of cysts of the jaws. Proc. R. Soc. Med., *41*:681–688, 1948.

85. Toller, P. A., and Holborow, E. J.: Immunoglobulins and immunoglobulin-containing cells in cysts of the jaws. Lancet, *2*:178 (26 July), 1969.

86. Ward, G. E., and Hendrick, J. W.: Tumors of the Head and Neck. Baltimore, The Williams & Wilkins Co., 1950.

87. Whinery, J. G.: Progressive bone cavities of the mandible; a review of the so-called bone cyst and a report of three cases. Oral Surg., *8*:903, 1955.

88. Whitlock, R. I. H., and Jones, J. H.: Squamous cell carcinoma of the jaw arising in a simple cyst. Report of a case. Oral Surg., *24*:530–536 (Oct.), 1967.

89. Whitlock, R. I. H., and Summersgill, G. B.: Ranula with cervical extension. Oral Surg., *15*:1163 (Oct.), 1962.

CHAPTER 13

TREATMENT OF ORAL
NONMALIGNANT TUMORS AND
LESIONS

Nonmalignant tumors or abnormal growths in the oral cavity are found in the following order of frequency:

First are lesions arising from the gingival tissues or mucoperiosteal membrane of the alveolar process of the maxilla or mandible. These include hyperplasias, fibromas, pyogenic granulomas, fibromatoses, pregnancy tumors, papillomas, peripheral giant cell reparative granulomas, hemangiomas, diphenylhydantoin sodium (Dilantin sodium) gingival hyperplasia, peripheral giant cell tumors, and neuromas.

Secondly, on the cortical bone of the maxilla or mandible, growths such as various exostoses, torus palatinus, torus mandibularis, chondroma, osteochondroma, osteoma, or diffuse hyperostosis may be found.

Third are the hyperplasias of the labial and/or buccal vestibular mucosa and lingual mucosa that may develop as the result of long-continued trauma from a loosely fitting denture; also in this group are hypertrophy of the fibrous mucoperiosteal tissue (alveolar gingiva) of edentulous maxillary and mandibular ridges from denture trauma, peripheral giant cell reparative granulomas, and peripheral giant cell tumors may develop.

Fourth, within the cancellous portion of the maxilla or mandible the following tumors may be found: diffuse hyperostosis, known as fibro-osteoma, ossifying fibroma, osteoid osteoma, osteoclastomas (central giant cell tumor), central giant cell reparative granuloma, ameloblastomas, myxomas, odontomas, localized enostosis, such as sclerotic bone (osteosclerosis, bone whorls).

Fifth, tumors may be found on or beneath the mucosa of the cheek: fibromas, neurofibromas, lipomas, fibropapillomas, hemangiomas, focal epithelial hyperplasias (epulis fissuratum), mixed tumors (pleomorphic adenomas) and amputation or traumatic neuromas.

Sixth, on the palate: fibromas, fibromatosis, fibropapillomas, myxofibromas, rhabdomyomas, acute inflammatory papillary hyperplasia, mixed tumors (pleomorphic adenomas) and soft tissue plasmacytomas are found.

Seventh, on or in the tongue: papillomas, hemangiomas, rhabdomyomas, myoblastomas, leiomyomas and lymphangiomas may develop.

Eighth, nonmalignant tumors found in the floor of the oral cavity are: mixed tumors (pleomorphic adenomas), myxofibromas, dermoid cysts.

BIOPSY

Most benign tumors or abnormal growths are readily diagnosed, visually, digitally and radiographically, by the trained oral surgeon or diagnostician.

When there is a doubt in the mind of the clinician or diagnostician as to the identity of the tumor, then a preoperative biopsy is indicated. However, it is imperative that a competent pathologist examine microscopically all tissue that is removed from the oral cavity, even though clinically it appears to be nonmalignant. As a general rule, the more nearly the tumor tissue resembles the surrounding normal tissue in color and texture, the more likely it is to be benign. However, Grade I malignancies and metastatic tumors are often an exception to this rule.

Indications for Biopsy. Rovin has made the following observations on biopsy decisions: "Whether a lesion should undergo biopsy or be treated or observed is decided by the presence or absence of an obvious cause of the lesion. For example, if a jagged tooth or ill-fitting dentures appear to have caused an ulceration, then the cause of the ulcer should be removed and the lesion observed for a short period of time. Similarly, swellings and keratinized or erythematous areas for which there is an apparent cause should be observed after elimination of the source of irritation or infection.

"If there is an ulcer, swelling, red or white discoloration or other change for which there is no clinical explanation, a period of observation will be of little or no value: a biopsy is indicated. At this time the patient should be informed of the necessity to have the lesion examined microscopically in order to ascertain the nature of the disease. Patients with lesions that are to be observed should be informed that a biopsy may be necessary at a subsequent visit. If the dentist who first observes the lesion does not do the biopsy, it is his responsibility to see that the patient is referred to a dentist who will.

"Once it has been decided to treat or to observe a lesion, under no circumstances should the waiting period to the next appointment exceed 7 to 10 days. At the end of that time, if the lesion is worse, has not responded to treatment or shows no evidence of healing, a biopsy should be performed. *It should be kept in mind that cancerous lesions do not heal.*"*

Biopsy Technique. Rovin has also made the following outline of biopsy technique:

"1. The area or areas that are the most representative of the disease process when the lesion is too large to be entirely removed are to be selected. Incomplete removal of a lesion is called an *incisional biopsy.*

2. It is better to make deep, narrow biopsies rather than broad, shallow ones, because superficial changes may be different from those deeper in the tissue (Fig. 13–1). An invading carcinoma may be missed by a shallow biopsy, which shows only superficial necrosis. Several

specimens from the same lesion may be necessary (Fig. 13–2).

3. The specimen should include surrounding normal tissue.

4. Elliptical sections with cuts converging to a **V** in the underlying normal tissue are desirable (Figs. 13–2 and 13–3).

5. If the lesion is small, its complete removal, or an *excisional biopsy,* is indicated (Fig. 13–3). A lesion 1 cm. or less usually can be readily removed. However, this is variable and will depend on the skill and confidence of the dentist.

6. The specimen is placed into a container with 10 per cent formalin (4 per cent formaldehyde). Specimen jars with fixative are provided by most oral pathology departments of dental schools or by other pathology laboratories.

7. Each specimen is to be labeled and the history form which accompanies the specimen container carefully completed. It is essential that the history and description of the lesion be as complete and accurate as possible. *Help the pathologist to help you!* Diagnostic errors are made less likely by good histories.

8. The specimen jars are carefully wrapped and mailed in cylindrical mailing containers often provided by the pathology laboratory."*

---

* Reprinted with permission from Rovin, S.: The role of biopsy and cytology in oral diagnosis. Dent. Clin. North Am., 429 (July), 1965.

Figure 13–1 The desirable *incisional* biopsy is one that is deep and narrow (*left*) rather than broad and shallow (*right*). The former biopsy reveals the deeper changes that may be more significant than those revealed by the shallower biopsy. (From Rovin, S.: The role of biopsy and cytology in oral diagnosis. Dent. Clin. North Am., 429–434 [July], 1965.)

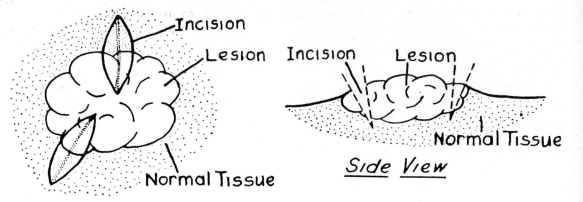

Figure 13–2   Incisional biopsy. More than one biopsy may be necessary to demonstrate the nature of the disease in larger lesions. In the left illustration the dotted lines represent the inferior borders of the incisions that converge to form a V in the deep part of the tissue as they are viewed from the surface. The side view in the right illustration shows the convergence of the incisions in the underlying tissues. (From Rovin, S.: The role of biopsy and cytology in oral diagnosis. Dent. Clin. North Am., 429–434 [July], 1965.)

ORAL EXFOLIATIVE CYTOLOGY

Introduction and Indications for Use.   Oral exfoliative cytologic specimens (the oral "Pap" smear) are diagnostic aids in detecting early cancer. The technique is designed to demonstrate malignant changes in cells taken from surfaces of carcinomatous lesions and achieves its greatest importance in those cancers which do not appear clinically suspicious. *Thus far, it should be considered only as an adjunct to the biopsy: it is a preliminary examination procedure, and the resulting diagnosis does not constitute a final diagnosis.*[68] When in doubt, take a biopsy. Rovin[69] reports that in smears taken from 65 proven oral carcinomas, 17 of the smears were *negative,* giving a *false negative rate of 26 per cent!* He further reports *false positive* specimens, particularly in reparative or severely inflamed epithelium. Shapiro and Gor-

lin also report a high rate of false positives and negatives. They concluded that "intraoral exfoliative cytology must be reserved for (1) use with biopsy or (2) lesions that are so very innocent clinically that biopsy is contraindicated."[76] With this conclusion the author most heartily concurs.

Cytologic Technique.   To obtain specimens for accurate cytologic diagnosis, the following steps should be taken:

1. The sample of cells is more readily obtained if first the lesion is moistened either by the patient's saliva or with saline or water applied by the dentist.
2. The lesion is firmly scraped with a tongue blade, spatula or similar instrument. Several passages of the scraping instrument may be necessary to obtain an adequate specimen.
3. The scrapings are spread over the surface of a glass slide. Usually two slides

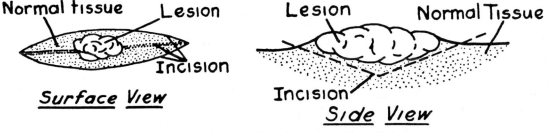

Figure 13–3   Excisional biopsy. The complete removal of a lesion by making elliptical surface incisions that converge to a V in the underlying tissues is illustrated. The elliptical surface incisions are demonstrated in the left illustration by the solid lines drawn around the normal tissue. The convergence of the incisions in the underlying tissue is shown by the dotted lines in the left drawing and by the dashed lines in the right drawing. (From Rovin, S.: The role of biopsy and cytology in oral diagnosis. Dent. Clin. North Am., 429–434 [July], 1965.)

are prepared for each area to be smeared.

4. The slides are immediately immersed in fixative or are flooded with fixative and allowed to air dry. If the slides are immersed, they are removed after 30 minutes and allowed to air dry. Ninety-five per cent ethyl alcohol is one of many suitable fixatives that can be used.

5. After drying, the slides are sent to the cytology laboratory for diagnosis. The methods used to handle mailed specimens will differ, and it is best to follow the directions given by the laboratory that will handle your smears.

EXOSTOSES

Localized circumscribed bony outgrowths on the cortical plate of bone are called exostoses. These are relatively common, and they include the torus palatinus, torus mandibularis, and bony overgrowths or outgrowths of the alveolar ridges of the maxilla and mandible.

A few examples are shown in Figures 13–4 and 13–5.

TORUS PALATINUS (PALATAL OSTEOMA)

Torus palatinus is a benign osseous outgrowth of the hard palate that is usually bilateral, is situated along the median palatine suture and extends laterally from it, involving the maxillary palatal process and rarely the palatine bone. Such bony growths are generally symmetrical, of various sizes and shapes and made up of two major bony parts, right and left, which may again be divided into two or more segments. The segments are covered with thick cortical bone with cancellous dullary centers. Most of these tori extend back to the junction of the palatine bone with the palatal process of the maxilla (Fig. 13–4A).

These osseous growths are lodged only on the oral side of the palate; they have no counterpart on the nasal side. The downward enlargement of the diploë produces the palatal tori, and the palatine processes of the maxilla are not bent. The enlargement is gradual, with the most rapid growth period being the second and third decades of life.

Torus palatinus has been noted in both

(*Text continued on page 715*)

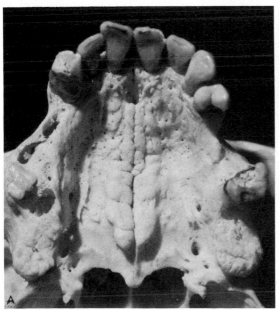 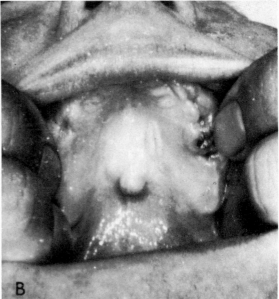

Figure 13–4 *A*, Torus palatinus of the nodular type. Note the osseous segmented bilateral outgrowths that meet at the midline. In the greater percentage of these cases the growth extends back to the palatine bone.

B, This is a most rare type of lobular torus palatinus. The author has never seen another one either personally or illustrated.

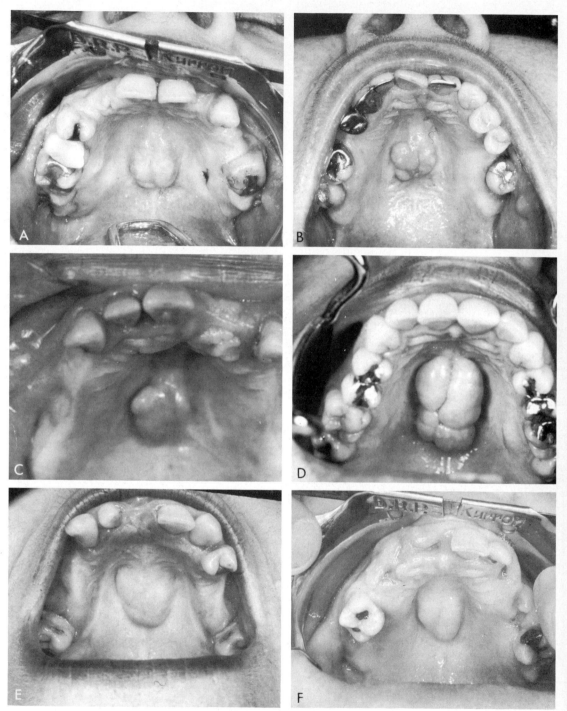

Figure 13–5 Examples of torus palatinus. These benign bony protuberances in the midline of the palate range in size from small, smooth, convex outgrowths to large nodular ones.

A, B and C are medium-small nodular tori palatini. D is a large nodular one, while E and F are medium-sized, smooth and convex bony outgrowths. These are not as common as the nodular type.

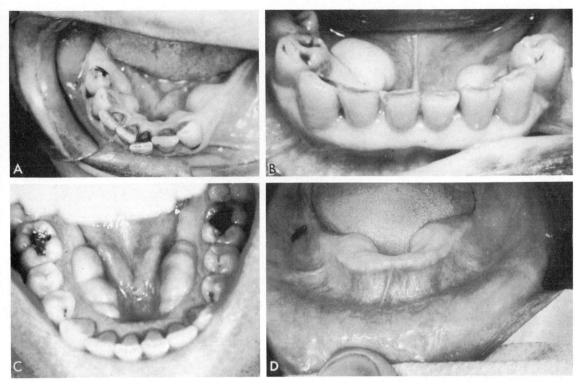

Figure 13–6 Torus mandibularis. This condition is usually bilateral and is found on the lingual surface of the mandible in the region of the bicuspids and molars. Excision permits full coverage of the denture-bearing area, aiding retention and increasing efficiency of a mandibular full denture. Removal is necessary if a lingual bar for a partial denture is to be adapted. *A* and *C* show multinodular bilateral mandibular tori; *B* and *D*, bilateral lobular torus mandibularis.

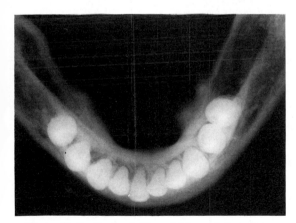

Figure 13–7 Occlusal film of bilateral lingual torus mandibularis.

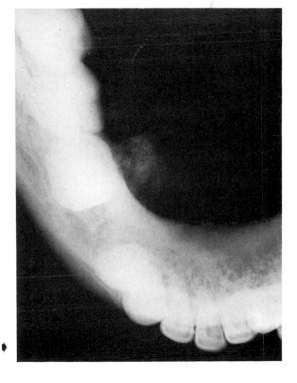

Figure 13–8 Osteoma, recurrent, on lingual surface of mandible.

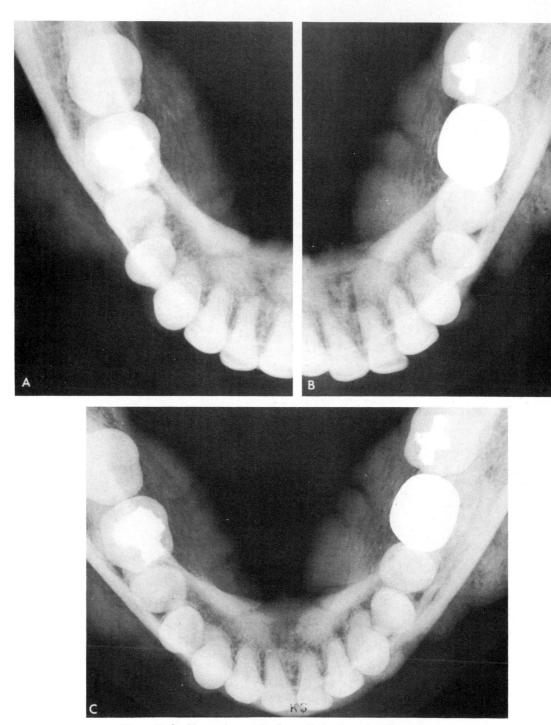

Figure 13–9   Unusual example of mandibular lingual and buccal exostoses.

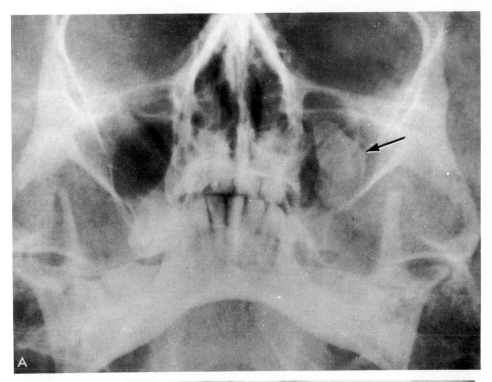

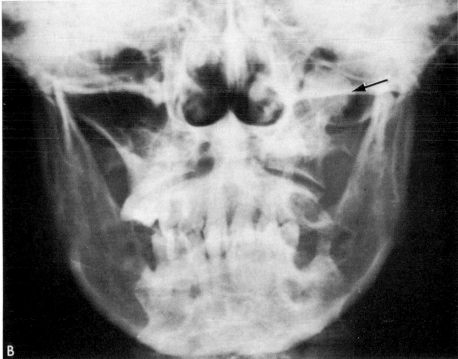

Figure 13–10 *A,* Posteroanterior radiograph, with the nose and chin in contact with the cassette (Waters' position). Note the large osteoma in the maxillary sinus.

B, Posteroanterior radiograph of the same skull with the nose and forehead in contact with the cassette. Note the different projection of the same osteoma on this film. This is the standard view taken to show the mandible, maxilla, nose and maxillary sinuses. The patient was symptomless and obviously no treatment was indicated.

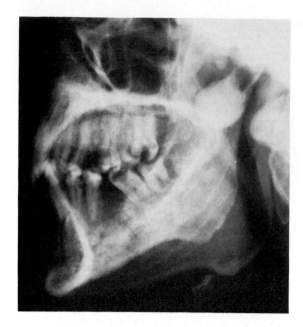

Figure 13-11 Osteoma of the vertical ramus.

Photographic Case Report

OSTEOCHONDROMA OF THE MAXILLA

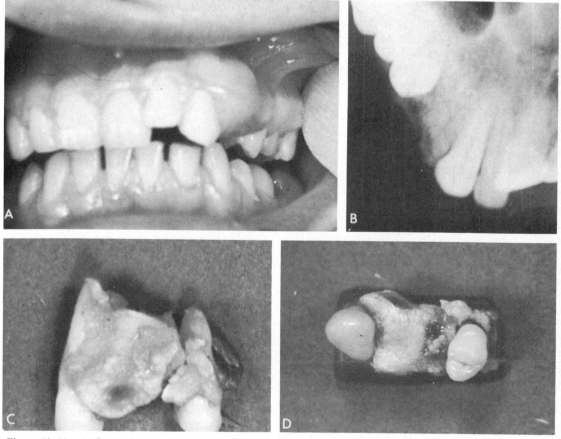

Figure 13-12 *A,* Cortical type of a rare maxillary osteochondroma, a slow-growing benign, painless tumor which can enlarge and separate the teeth, as illustrated here.

B, Periapical radiographs reveal mottled calcification evenly distributed throughout the tumor.

C and *D,* Because they have a tendency to recur, wide excision is indicated, and in this case a block section of the maxilla including the cuspid and first bicuspid was excised.

(*Figure 13-12 continued on opposite page.*)

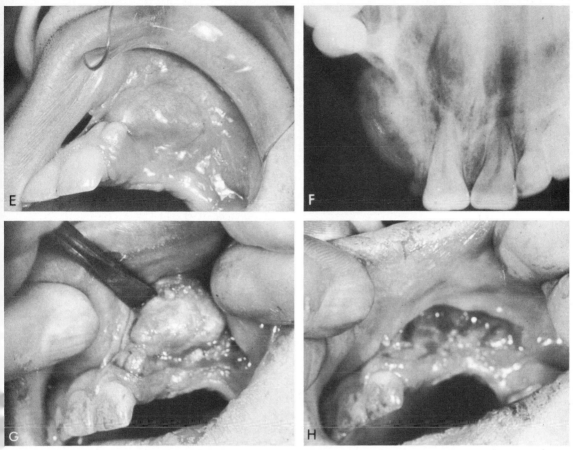

Figure 13–12 *(Continued.)* *E*, In spite of this wide excision nodular growths recurred higher on the buccal cortical plate within 9 months.

F, The occlusal radiograph reveals the well-circumscribed cortical osteochondroma and the mottled appearance (like ground glass) of the growth.

G, The mucoperiosteal membrane was reflected and with chisels and burs these growths were removed with hopefully adequate surrounding bone (*H*) to prevent a recurrence. Patient returned periodically for the next 6 months and then was lost to follow-up, although he was told to have his jaw examined periodically wherever he was and to send us a report.

sexes at all ages, among all races and cultures but not in the same frequency. Palatal tori have been observed in 5.59 per cent of newborns by Moore in his study[55] and from 20.9 per cent by Kolas et al.[48] to 24.2 per cent by Miller and Roth[54] in their respective studies of adults. In studies of certain racial groups by Hooton[40] and Woo,[94] the percentage of occurrence was found to be even higher. The cause is unknown but thought to be familial in many instances. The average ratio of male to female has been found by most investigators to be approximately 1:2 for both infants and adults.

The fact remains that for an unknown reason the osteoblasts along this line of fusion in the palate continue to lay down bone instead of ceasing their activity, and, as a result,

various forms of osseous outgrowths slowly but continuously grow from the palate.

Classification. The following are the four main kinds of torus seen:

1. The convex, sessile, smooth bilateral outgrowth, usually symmetrical in outline (see Figure 13–5*E* and *F*).

2. The nodular torus, a semifused mass of various sizes and numbers of semipedunculated osseous protuberances, as shown in Figure 13–5*A* to *D*.

3. The lobular torus, most likely a nodular torus which by a more rapid growth is quite large and has very marked undercuts (see Figure 3–66). The base is pedunculated but this is difficult to visualize in the larger lobular tori until some of the segments have been exposed by

the reflection of the mucoperiosteal membrane (see Figure 13–4).

4. The spindle torus, which is much less common than the first three. It is a long, thin, rounded ridge in the midline, or it may have a tapered form such as that shown in Figure 3–67D. This is an unusually large spindle torus palatinus.

TORUS MANDIBULARIS
(MANDIBULAR EXOSTOSES)

Mandibular tori are usually bilateral osseous outgrowths found on the lingual surfaces of the mandible in the region of the bicuspids. They may consist of several nodules ranging in size from that of a BB shot to that of a hazelnut and are composed of solid cortical bone. They should be removed to facilitate the construction of full or partial mandibular dentures when necessary. Figures 13–6 and 13–7 show examples of mandibular tori.

Surgical Treatment of Torus Palatinus and Torus Mandibularis. The reader is referred to Chapter 3 (pages 199 to 201) for a description of the surgical technique for the removal of these bony growths and the reasons therefor.

BONY OUTGROWTHS IN THE
MANDIBULAR MOLAR REGION

In many mandibles a shelf-like projection of bone, called the "linguomandibular balcony," projects sharply at the lingual gingival margin of the mandibular molars, particularly in the second and third molar region. This bony outgrowth may be narrow and sharp, or broad and slightly rounded. In either case there is a marked undercut. This is an exaggerated continuation of the internal oblique ridge, and as such there is little, if any, reduction in size owing to normal resorption following the extraction of the mandibular molars. For this reason, when extracting mandibular molars, it is necessary to reflect the lingual mucoperiosteal tissue and reduce this shelf with sharp bone chisels and a mallet or with a bur (see Chapter 3).

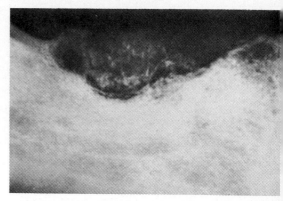

Figure 13–13 Chondroma involving the mandible. (From Stafne, E. C.: Oral Roentgenographic Diagnosis. 4th ed. Philadelphia, W. B. Saunders Co., 1975.)

CHONDROMA AND OSTEOCHONDROMA

Tumors of cartilage in the maxilla are considered to be extremely rare and only slightly less so in the mandible, where they are found in the region of the mental foramen, the coronoid or the condyle. The case shown in Figure 13–12 is one of the very rare ones seen in the maxilla. Chaudhry, Robinovitch and Mitchell[21] reviewed the English literature between 1912 and 1959 and only found 18 cases in the mandible or maxilla.

Stafne discusses this subject as follows: "A chondroma consists primarily of cartilage. In some instances it may become an osteochondroma, and eventually an osteoma by replacement of the cartilage with bone. There may be roentgenographic evidence, therefore, of linear and mottled calcification within the lesion."[87] These lesions are uncommon in the jaws. When seen they are usually on the cortex (see Figures 13–12 and 13–13), and less frequently in the medulla.

Treatment. While benign, they have a tendency to recur unless radically excised to make sure the entire tumor has been removed.

In spite of the innocent microscopic appearance of many chondromas, they behave as low-grade chondrosarcomas, as Case Report No. 1 demonstrates. In this particular instance the services of five pathologists were sought. It was only after their evaluation that a seemingly benign tumor (chondroma) was labeled as malignant (chondrosarcoma) by three of the five.

CHONDROSARCOMA OF THE ANTERIOR MAXILLA

Patient. A well-developed, well-nourished 45-year-old white male (occupation, fireman) was admitted to Eye and Ear Hospital on January 1.

Chief Complaint. "Persistent swelling in the roof of the mouth."

Past History. Thirteen years earlier the patient had noticed a mass on the labial cortical bone above his maxillary central incisors. He was examined by an oral surgeon, who extracted the maxillary central and lateral incisors and excised the osseous tumor. No pathology report.

The patient described the tissue as being "shrimp-like." It had caused no discomfort and, except for being visible, was asymptomatic. It was first noticed while he was brushing his teeth and it had increased in size until the lip was slightly elevated. At the time of its excision, the mass was the size of a cherry.

The next year a partial denture was constructed while the patient was in the Army. Three years later the lesion had recurred and extended over the periphery of the denture. At no time was pain a factor.

Three years after that the mass was ¾ inch by ½ inch. It extended from the labial edge to the palate in the midline of the alveolar ridge. He said it felt as though it was "under my nose."

The tumor was excised by a general surgeon at another hospital in that year. Pathology report—*Macroscopic:* This specimen consisted of three firm, white nodular pieces of tissue, the largest measuring 1.5 cm. in its greatest dimension, and the smallest 0.75 cm. The pieces had a nodular, smooth, glistening surface, were almost spherical in shape, and showed what appeared to be small pedicles or bases, at which point they had been excised. They were very firm to palpation.

Sectioning revealed only a firm, white, apparently encapsulated central core.

Microscopic: Sections showed a squamous epithelial covered nodule with marked calcification of the central area. The tumor was composed largely of calcified fibrous tissue, with a few areas of true bone formation.

Diagnosis: Osteochondroma—gingiva (E. L. Heller, M.D., Pathologist).

Following this operation the patient had his remaining teeth extracted and a full denture constructed. Since then there has been a gradual recurrence until now, 6 years later, he can't insert his denture.

Intraoral Examination. On the anterior maxillary alveolar ridge to the left of the maxillary midline is a slightly elevated oval mass 1.5 cm. in diameter. To the right side of midline is a similar area, less regular in dimensions. Epithelium remains intact, tissue is normal in color. Both areas are firm but not hard. Remainder of oral soft tissues are unremarkable.

Extraoral Examination. Normal facial contours. No cervical or submaxillary nodes palpable.

Medical Evaluation. Essentially negative. Acceptable for surgery.

Anesthesia. Pentothal Sodium with endotracheal nitrous oxide and oxygen.

Preoperative Impression. Osteochondroma.

Operative Technique. With use of a No. 15 Bard-Parker blade, an incision was made over the crest of the maxillary edentulous alveolar ridge extending from the left to the right premolar regions. Labial and palatal mucoperiosteal flaps were reflected permitting complete visualization of the anterior palate and maxilla. Clinically noted were several shiny lobulated areas connected by a

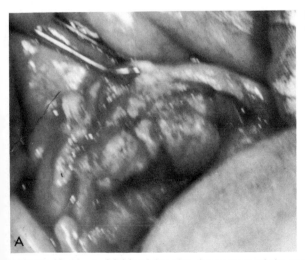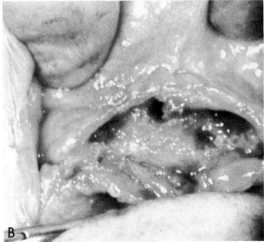

Figure 13–14 *A,* Multinodular chondrosarcoma of the anterior maxilla. The first histopathologic report indicated chondroma, as did the report following the wider excision of the first recurrence. *B,* Postoperative site after wide excision, including what little was left of the maxillary alveolar process, a portion of the palatine bone, up to and including the anterior portion of the osseous floor of the nasal cavity.

stroma of fibrous connective tissue interspersed between. The primary areas of involvement lay adjacent to the nasopalatine foramen and on the crest of the anterior alveolar ridge. See Figure 13–14A. With use of rongeurs, chisels, and curettes, wide excision of the involved bone up to the floor of the nasal cavity was completed in an attempt to insure against recurrence. See Figure 13–14B. The cavity was then filled with iodoform gauze saturated with a sclerosing solution. The gauze was maintained in position by sutures passed over the packing and through the labial and lingual soft tissue flaps.

Pathology Report. *Macroscopic:* Specimen consists of a biopsy from the palate labeled (1) Superficial, (2) Deep. The first portion of the specimen consists of eight ragged, irregular pieces of tissue amounting to 2 by 1 by 1 cm. The cut surface of these is smooth, glistening, and grayish white with firm areas. The second portion consists of six ragged fragments of similar tissue amounting to approximately 1 cm. Half of these are bony fragments.

Microscopic: The sections show irregular fragments of tissue composed of hyaline stroma and spaces containing oval cells with finely granular pink cytoplasm and round dark nuclei. No mitoses are present. There are a few fragments of bone.

Note: We believe that this is a low-grade malignant neoplasm that is prone to local recurrence but rarely metastasizes.

Diagnosis: Chondrosarcoma of palate.

Note: The specimen was submitted to four other outstanding pathologists for their opinion. Pathologist No. 1 reported, "Chondroma." Pathologist No. 2 reported, "On histologic criteria alone one might consider a diagnosis of low-grade chondrosarcoma. However, in view of the history and location, this becomes a bit speculative." Pathologist No. 3, "Chondrosarcoma." Pathologist No. 4, "Chondrosarcoma."

Hospital Course. Uneventful. The patient was discharged January 28.

Subsequent Course. The patient was admitted on ear, nose and throat service November 2 for more definitive surgical excision of the tumor from the nasal vault. On completion of this procedure, the patient was returned to the dental service for outpatient care.

PLEOMORPHIC ADENOMAS (MIXED TUMORS) OF THE ORAL CAVITY

The various theories concerning the formation of pleomorphic adenomas (mixed tumors) are described in the excellent article on mixed tumors by Cheyne, Tiecke and Horne.[24] In the oral cavity they are found in palate, cheek, lips, oropharynx and tongue. They have even been found in the nares and mandible. Tumors in the submaxillary or sublingual glands grow slowly and possess a thickened capsule. Mixed tumors which arise outside of the glands undoubtedly start in accessory salivary tissue in the oral tissues. Those in the palate, lips, cheek and fornix of the vestibule are quite benign, easily removed and seldom recur.

Chaudhry and associates conclude in part as a result of their analysis of 1414 intraoral minor salivary gland tumors that "pleomorphic adenoma appears to be the most common tumor arising from the intraoral minor salivary glands. Next in order of frequency are cylindromatous adenocarcinoma, mucoepidermoid tumor and adenocarcinoma."[23]

Treatment. Chaudhry and associates make the following observations on treatment of pleomorphic adenoma: "Pleomorphic adenoma is a slow-growing tumor with no unusual tendency to recur. There is no evidence that long-standing benign tumors may undergo malignant transformation.* In general enucleation seems to be an adequate method of treatment. In case of clinical or microscopic evidence of invasion, local excision of the tumor and the overlying mucosa is satisfactory. The prognosis is excellent. Radical surgical excision or radiation therapy is not indicated."[23]

PLEOMORPHIC ADENOMAS OF THE LIP AND PALATE

These tumors are sometimes mistaken for torus palatinus. One point of differentiation is that they do not arise in the midline of the palate. They are smooth, semispherical, well circumscribed, and covered with normal mucosa. A frequent site is to the lingual side of the molars or in the soft palate. They normally grow slowly and should be completely removed.

Recurrence after removal is unusual. While

*AUTHOR'S NOTE: There is always an exception. See Case Report No. 5, in which a mixed tumor of the palate of 37 years' growth in a 59-year-old male exhibited malignant changes. However, the technique of treatment of these tumors as indicated above is satisfactory.

Photographic Case Report

PLEOMORPHIC ADENOMA OF THE LIP ("MIXED" TUMOR)
Abdel K. Attar, D.M.D.

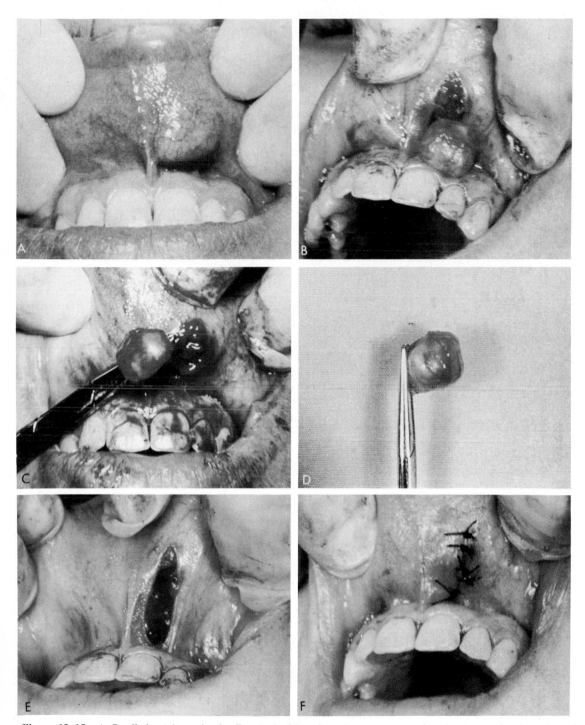

Figure 13–15 *A*, Small, hard lump in the lip. *B*, Incision through mucosa exposing the encapsulated semiround tumor. *C* and *D*, Removal of tumor by blunt dissection. *E* and *F*, Incision closed with silk sutures.

SMALL PALATAL PLEOMORPHIC ADENOMA ("MIXED" TUMOR)
THEODORE R. PALADINO, D.M.D.

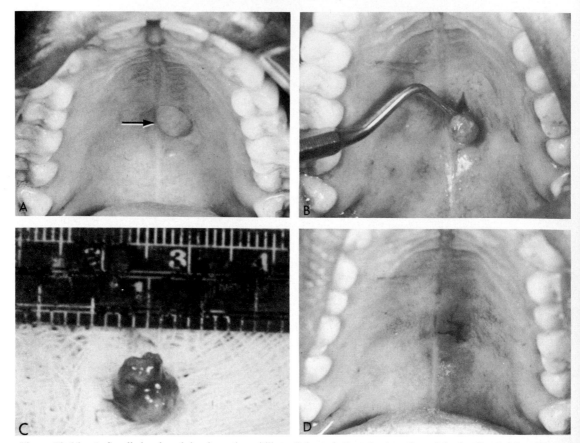

Figure 13–16 *A*, Small, hard nodule along the midline of the palate at the junction of the hard and soft palates. *B*, Incision through the palatal mucosa; with blunt dissection the tumor is freed from its loose attachment to the submucosal tissues and elevated with a curette. *C*, Small, nodular encapsulated tumor after removal. *D*, Palatal mucosa closed with two silk sutures.

Diagnosis: Pleomorphic adenoma.

many of these tumors are well encapsulated, as in the case shown in Figures 13–19 and 13–23, and are readily shelled out, others are more difficult to remove. In these cases the tumor bed should be thoroughly coagulated.

If the tumor is above the anterior palatine artery, coagulation is superficial. The patient should be informed of the possibility of recurrence, and should return if there is any sign of a new growth.

Case Report No. 2

MIXED TUMOR OF ACCESSORY SALIVARY GLAND IN THE LIP

Patient. A normally developed, well-nourished 57-year-old white male (employed by U.S. Steel) presented as an outpatient at Magee-Women's Hospital on August 9.

Chief Complaint. "Persistent soft-tissue swelling in the upper lip."

Intraoral Examination. Examination revealed an 0.5-cm. solitary, circumscribed mass in the vermilion border of the maxillary lip slightly to the right of midline. There were no observable areas of focal irritation. Palpation of the enlargement did not produce discomfort. The remainder of the oral soft tissues are unremarkable.

Extraoral Examination. Examination revealed a normal facial symmetry with no palpable cervical or submaxillary nodes.

ADENOID CYSTIC CARCINOMA (CYLINDROMA; ADENOCYSTIC CARCINOMA, BASALOID MIXED TUMOR)

ABDEL K. ATTAR, D.M.D.

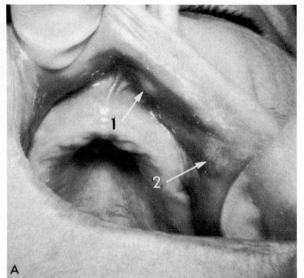

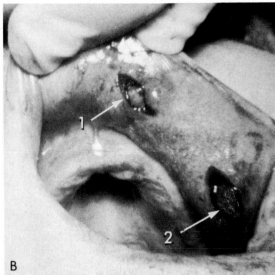

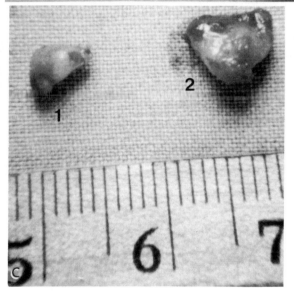

Figure 13–17 *A,* This patient reported that she had two painless, small, hard nodules in her cheek (*1* and *2*). Preoperative impression was pleomorphic adenomas. *B,* Tumors exposed. There was not excessive fixation to the surrounding soft tissues, nor was there any evidence of invasion of the deeper tissues. They were easily removed by blunt dissection. *C,* Tumors *1* and *2*. Note the smooth capsule and the seminodular shapes.

Histopathology report: Adenoid cystic carcinoma (acinic cell adenocarcinoma). No nodes were palpable. This situation occurs in about 30 per cent of these cases.

Preoperative Impression. Fibroma of the upper lip.

Anesthetic. Local (infiltration).

Operative Technique. With a No. 15 Bard-Parker blade, a 1.5-cm. vertical incision was made in the vermilion border of the maxillary lip overlying the mucosal enlargement. The flap was retracted with plastic hooks, and with blunt and sharp dissection, the mass was freed from its submucosal attachments and excised in toto. Closure was completed with 000 black silk sutures of interrupted tie.

Postoperative Impression. Fibroma.

Pathology Report. *Macroscopic:* The specimen included a mucocele and consisted of a single piece of material measuring 0.5 cm. in diameter. It was round in contour and presented a glistening, grayish white surface. It had a moderately firm consistency.

Microscopic: The tumor was composed of cells that had scant pink cytoplasm and small uniform nuclei, and these cells formed conglomerate masses with intermingled areas of myxomatous tissue, some of which had lacunae and resembled cartilage. A margin of tissue was about the tumor, but the margin on one side was quite thin. Included in the section were several mucous glands.

Diagnosis: Mixed tumor of lip of salivary gland origin (R. H. Fennell, Jr., M.D.).

Postoperative Course. The patient was discharged August 9th.

Case Report No. 3

MIXED TUMOR OF THE PALATE

Patient. This patient was admitted to Magee-Women's Hospital and was found to be a normally developed, well-nourished, 30-year-old white female. Occupation—housewife.

Chief Complaint. "Localized palatal enlargement."

History of Present Illness. The existence of a small palatal mass had first been noticed 6 to 12 months prior to the present admission. During the interim, it had gradually increased in diameter, asymptomatically.

Past Medical History. Negative history of systemic diseases. The patient had no allergies, and this was her first hospital admission.

Intraoral Examination. A freely movable, soft-tissue mass, approximately 1.5 cm. in diameter, was found at the posterior junction of the hard palate, immediately adjacent to the greater palatine foramen (see Figure 13–18A). The epithelium remained intact, and the dentition was well maintained. The remainder of the oral mucous membranes were unremarkable.

Extraoral Examination. Normal facial symmetry. No adenopathy.

Laboratory Report. All hematology and urinalysis findings fell within normal limits.

Preoperative Impression. Mixed tumor of the hard palate.

Anesthesia. Pentothal sodium with endotracheal nitrous oxide and oxygen.

Operative Technique. With a No. 15 Bard-Parker blade, a 2-cm. anteroposterior incision was made through the palatal mucosa overlying the mucosal enlargement. Blunt dissection was used in carrying the incision into the submucosal layer, whereby the tumorous mass was freed from its tissue attachments and shelled from its base in toto. Care was taken not to traumatize the anterior palatine artery, which lay just beneath the tumor. A small segment of ½-inch iodoform gauze was inserted to facilitate drainage, and the wound was closed with 00 catgut sutures of interrupted tie.

Postoperative Impression. Mixed tumor.

Pathology Report. *Macroscopic:* The tumor mass from the hard palate was an ovoid structure that measured 1.5 cm. by 1.2 cm. in diameter. It appeared to be covered with a capsule that was smooth for the most part and pale grayish pink. At places it presented some fibrous tags. The mass was moderately firm in consistency and the cut surfaces presented a gray, granular, rather friable tissue.

Microscopic: Study of microscopic sections prepared from this tissue justified the diagnosis recorded.

Diagnosis: Mixed tumor of heterotopic parotid gland tissue of soft palate.

Hospital Course. The drain was removed 1 day after surgery. The remainder of the course was uneventful, and the patient was discharged 2 days postoperatively.

Case Report No. 4

MIXED TUMOR OF THE HARD PALATE*

Patient. This patient was admitted to Eye and Ear Hospital and was found to be a normally developed, well-nourished, 38-year-old white female. Occupation—housewife.

Chief Complaint. "Palatal swelling."

History of Present Illness. A palatal enlargement had first been noted on a routine dental examination 1 month prior to the present admission.

Past Medical History. The patient had had the usual childhood diseases and no allergies. She had previously been hospitalized for breast biopsy, with resultant negative findings.

Intraoral Examination. Examination revealed a 1-cm. raised, smooth, firm but fleshy, well-demarcated mass located slightly to the left of midline on the hard palate (see Figure 13–18B). No areas of focal irritation were visible that could be attributed to the localized palatal mass. The patient's dentition was well restored. The remainder of the oral soft tissues were unremarkable.

Extraoral Examination. Normal facial symmetry. No adenopathy.

Medical Evaluation. Blood pressure was 110/80. No breast masses were found, and the lungs were clear. A normal sinus rhythm was heard, and no murmurs. The patient was deemed acceptable for surgery.

Preoperative Impression. Mixed tumor of the hard palate.

Anesthesia. Pentothal sodium with endotracheal nitrous oxide and oxygen.

Operative Technique. With a No. 15 Bard-Parker blade, a 2-cm. anteroposterior incision was

---

*Case report prepared by Paul H. Iverson, Oral Surgery Resident, Magee-Women's Hospital.

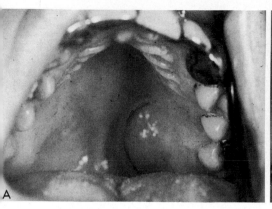
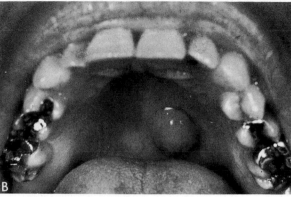

Figure 13–18 *A,* Pleomorphic adenoma ("mixed" tumor) of the palate (see Case Report No. 3). *B,* Pleomorphic adenoma ("mixed" tumor) of the palate (see Case Report No. 4).

made through the palatal mucosa overlying the mucosal enlargement. Blunt and sharp dissection were used in carrying the incision into the submucosal layer, whereby the tumorous mass was freed from its tissue attachments and shelled from its base in toto. Closure was completed with 000 black silk sutures of interrupted tie.

Postoperative Impression. Mixed tumor.

Pathology Report. *Macroscopic:* The specimen submitted in formalin consisted of an ovoid piece of tissue measuring 0.8 by 0.7 by 0.6 cm. It was a grayish white, papillary piece of tissue which on one surface was covered by a dark brown, roughened tissue. The cut surface was dull and grayish white.

Microscopic: The sections showed a partly encapsulated nodule consisting of densely packed round or oval epithelial cells with dark nuclei and scant cytoplasm. A few areas showed a somewhat whorled arrangement. Several small areas of hyalinization were seen.

Diagnosis: Mixed tumor of the palate.

Hospital Course. The patient was discharged the second day after operation.

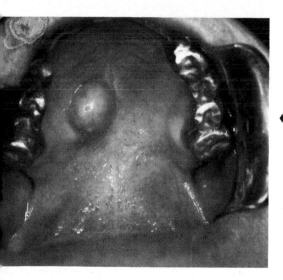

Figure 13–20 Pleomorphic adenoma produced this diffuse swelling of the right soft palate. (Courtesy of L. R. Marmins, M.D., Eye and Ear Hospital, Pittsburgh, Pa.)

Figure 13–19 Small, encapsulated pleomorphic adenoma of the palate.

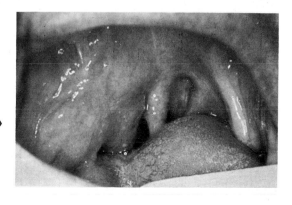

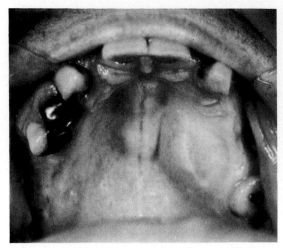

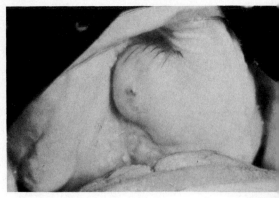

Figure 13–22   Sessile pleomorphic adenoma ("mixed" tumor) with a biopsy wound.

Figure 13–21   Wide-spreading palatal pleomorphic adenoma. Note the clear line of demarcation of the spread of the tumor beneath the mucosa. This generally indicates an encapsulated tumor. (The indentation of the covering mucosa is the biopsy site.)

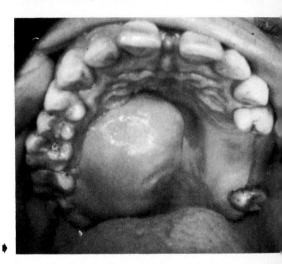

Figure 13–23   Large pleomorphic adenoma ("mixed" tumor) of the palate.

Case Report No. 5

MIXED TUMOR OF THE PALATE*

Patient. This patient was admitted to Eye and Ear Hospital and was found to be a normally developed, well-nourished, 59-year-old white male. Occupation — electrician.

Chief Complaint. "Difficulty in breathing and swallowing. Inability to focus left eye."

History of Present Illness. The patient had first sought medical advice at the age of 21 following a 9-year observation of a persistent, slowly developing palatal enlargement. Its existence was, at that time, attributed to a cystic lesion, and he was advised not to have it removed. Since its onset, the median mass had gradually increased in diameter by asymptomatic nodular expansion on its lateral borders, and by now was approximately 7 by 5 by 5 cm. in size. Normal masticatory movements had become impossible to execute, and patient was

maintained on a soft to liquid diet. Breathing an swallowing had in the same manner become in creasingly difficult, and the simple performance c these functions had recently kept him in a nightl state of partial insomnia. He was now having di ficulty with the lateral rotation of his left eye, an he complains of a 1-week history of diplopia.

Past Medical History. The patient had had th usual childhood diseases. He had also had trauma tic cataract of the right eye for 30 years, but n allergies. This was his first hospital admission.

Intraoral Examination. Examination revealed

*Case report prepared by Paul H. Iverson, Ora Surgery Resident, Magee-Women's Hospital, Pittsburgh Pa.

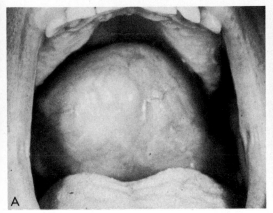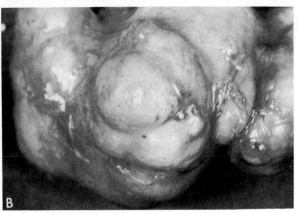

Figure 13–24 *A,* A large pleomorphic adenoma that originated from salivary gland tissue of the soft palate. *B,* Note the encapsulated nodular surface. There were malignant changes in the center of the tumor and metastases to the lung. It had been growing for 37 years.

massive, firm, nodular, palatal enlargement extending anteriorly from the midline of the hard palate, posteriorly to the oropharyngeal region and laterally to the lingual borders of the maxillary alveolar ridges. Its vertical height extended inferiorly to the posterior border of the anterior two-thirds of the tongue (see Figure 13–24). The mucosal epithelium remained intact, and apart from a mild generalized gingivitis, the remainder of the oral soft tissues were unremarkable. Hygiene was poor, and examination of the throat was impossible.

Extraoral Examination. Examination revealed a normal facial symmetry with no palpable nodes. The patient has a cataract of the right eye and impaired lateral movement of the left.

Medical Evaluation. Blood pressure was 130/70, pulse 80/min. A normal sinus rhythm with no murmurs was heard. The chest is clear, and reflexes are physiologic. The patient was acceptable for surgery.

Ophthalmology Consultation. The sudden onset of diplopia is due to a paralysis of the left abducens nerve, affecting the left lateral rectus muscle.

He has a grade I–II arteriosclerosis of the retinal vessels, and this is possibly on a vascular basis but a toxic cause or a tumor must be ruled out (J. M. Evans, M.D.).

Reports. *Roentgenology:* Mouth: Examination of the remaining teeth failed to reveal any periapical infection or retained root tips. Sinuses: There was an opaque shadow rather circumscribed, oval in shape and measuring about 1.5 by 2.5 cm. It was seen in the posterior ethmoid region. It was quite dense. If this condition is pathologic, we are not sure just what its nature is. There was no other pathologic condition noted about the bones of the face or the accessory nasal sinuses. Bones of the skull: Further examination with a base view did not reveal any destruction of bone at the base of the skull.

Laboratory: All findings of hematology, chemistry, serology and urinalysis fell within normal limits.

Preoperative Impression. Mixed tumor of palate.

Anesthetic. Local.

Operative Technique. With a No. 15 Bard-Parker blade, an 8 cm. anteroposterior incision was carried through the mucosal tissue overlying the mesial aspect of the palatal mass. While I was exercising extreme care in an attempt to preserve the continuity of the capsular lining, the overlying mucosal tissue was relieved of its submucosal attachments, reflected laterally and held with Allis forceps, thus exposing the entire diameter of the massive lesion. With blunt and sharp dissection, the entire tumor mass was then freed from its submucosal and periosteal attachments and enucleated in toto (see Figure 13–24). Following excision, the tumor was seen to have eroded the palatine bone and extended into the nasal cavity and nasopharyngeal region. The wound edges were then repositioned, excess tissue was excised, closure was completed with interrupted sutures of 000 black silk and a pressure pack was placed over the surgical site.

Postoperative Impression. Mixed tumor.

Pathology Report. *Macroscopic:* This specimen submitted in Formalin is a previously cut 7.5 by 5 by 4.5 cm. very firm, nodular mass. The surface is grayish white and smooth except for a few attached fibers. The cut surface is pale white without any special gross structure. *Microscopic:* Multiple sections show the bulk of this well-circumscribed mass to be made up of dense hyaline collagenous tissue containing varying sized groups of squamous cells. These are either lining spaces or in solid groups. The squamous cells are polygonal and have large rounded nuclei with prominent nucleoli. Mitoses vary considerably in different areas, but in some places up to two per high-powered field are seen. Keratinoid material is seen, but not intercellular bridges. In other areas there are small glands lined by cuboidal cells and surrounded by loose myxomatous stroma. A few areas of pseudocartilage are seen. *Note:* There are a few remnants of ordinary mixed tumor which establish the origin of this growth. The areas of solid cellular proliferation and marked hyalinization suggest malignancy. *Diagnosis:* Mixed tumor (salivary gland type) of palate — malignant (R. S. Totten, M.D.).

Hospital Course. A moderate amount of vascular seepage continued postoperatively for the first 24 hours. By 48 hours the patient could swallow with relative ease and was free of respiratory difficulty. By the sixth postoperative day, the oral tissues were healing satisfactorily, edema had nearly subsided and discomfort was minimal. Patient was discharged 8 days after the operation.

Subsequent Course. Four days following previous discharge, the patient was readmitted to Eye and Ear Hospital for evaluation of persistent left orbital pain. Neurologic examination at that time was negative except for the finding of sixth nerve paralysis. The possibility of existing malignancy was reaffirmed, the patient was treated palliatively and was discharged 6 days later.

PLEOMORPHIC ADENOMAS OF THE OROPHARYNX AND PAROTID GLAND

See Chapter 14 for discussion of the treatment of mixed tumors in the parotid gland, as well as Case Report No. 6 here.

Case Report No. 6

MIXED TUMOR OF THE SOFT PALATE, OROPHARYNX AND PAROTID GLAND*

Patient. This patient was admitted to Eye and Ear Hospital on September 3 and was found to be a normally developed, well-nourished, 31-year-old white female in no acute distress. Occupation — housewife.

Chief Complaint. "A swollen cheek and a growth in my mouth and throat." (See Figure 13–25*A* and *B*).

History of Present Illness. The patient first noticed the existence of a slowly growing localized enlargement nearly 8 years prior to present admission. During this interim, she was under frequent medical attention and was receiving weekly "injections" in an attempt to "reduce the lump." Because of its persistent enlargement, however, she was twice referred to another surgeon and on an outpatient basis underwent incisional biopsies of the tumor mass. Pathology reports in both instances were returned with the following: "Essentially normal mucous membrane showing mild exudative inflammation involving connective tissue. Fragments of stratified squamous epithelium. The lesion shows no evidence of neoplasia." Thereupon the patient was given further appointments for additional "medical treatments." On the absence of her attending physician, she eventually sought additional medical help and from there was referred to the office of W. H. A. During the entire course of growth, the enlargement continued to remain asymptomatic, although by now it interfered with chewing and speech. Swallowing was not difficult but did necessitate thorough mastication of food, which in turn necessitated a prolonged time in eating.

Past Medical History. Usual childhood diseases. No allergies or previous surgery.

Oral Examination. Examination revealed a hard, regular, nontender mass protruding from the right cheek and posterior border of the soft palate. The enlarged mass extended into the oral-nasal-pharyngeal region, pushing forward the entire soft palate and occluding a considerable portion of the posterior half of the oral cavity (see Figure 13–25*B*). The airway remained unobstructed, although examination of the throat was impossible. All maxillary teeth were missing.

Extraoral Examination. Examination revealed unilateral facial asymmetry, with pronounced enlargement and hardness of the soft tissues adjacent to the right intermaxillary arches. The inability of

---

*This interesting case illustrates the value of bringing together special skills from three specialties — oral surgery, plastic surgery and otolaryngology — for the ultimate benefit of the patient (J. C. Gaisford, M.D., B. L. Silverblatt, M.D., and W. H. Archer, D.D.S.). Case report prepared by Paul H. Iverson, Oral Surgery Resident, Magee-Women's Hospital, Pittsburgh, Pa.

the patient to maintain a normal vertical intermaxillary relationship resulted in the facial features appearing somewhat elongated. The neck was generally supple, with no cervical or submaxillary nodes palpable. The skin was clear, with no areas of focal inflammation.

Medical Evaluation. Blood pressure was 130/80; pulse was 88/min. and regular; respirations were 20/min. Lungs were clear. The patient had a normal sinus rhythm with no murmurs. Findings in the additional systemic review were essentially negative. The patient was considered acceptable for surgery.

Laboratory Findings. All findings of CBC and differential bleeding time, coagulation time, urinalysis, serology, fasting blood sugar, and nonprotein nitrogen fell within normal limits.

Preoperative Impression. Mixed tumor of palate.

Operation. Incisional biopsy.

Anesthetic. Pentothal sodium with endotracheal nitrous oxide and oxygen.

Operative Technique. With a No. 15 Bard-Parker blade, a vertical incision was carried over the midline of the palatal mass extending from the posterior to the anterior borders. With blunt dissection and use of periosteal elevators, the overlying mucosa was reflected laterally exposing a well encapsulated, hard, lobular, massive tumor. With sharp dissection, a broad incisional biopsy was undertaken in order to assure a representative sample for histologic evaluation and to enlarge the oropharyngeal space pending subsequent definitive surgery. The mucosal flaps were then repositioned and closed with interrupted sutures of 00 plain catgut.

Pathology Report. *Macroscopic:* This specimen consisted of two irregularly shaped pieces of tissue submitted as tumor of palate. The specimens measured 3 by 2.3 by 2.5 cm. and 3 by 3 by 1 cm., respectively. On one aspect of the larger piece was an area with a cratered contour. The base of this contained tiny villous-like processes. On section both pieces were similar, pearl gray in color, rubbery in consistency and cut with an increased resistance. *Microscopic:* The section consisted entirely of a neoplasm composed of irregular cords of epithelium in areas showing attempted gland formation alternating with broad basophilic deposits of cartilage-like material. *Diagnosis:* Mixed tumor of the palate. *Note:* The lesion showed no histologic evidence of malignancy (E. L. Heller, M.D.).

Hospital Course. Uneventful. The patient was discharged on September 7.

Subsequent Course. On November 25 the patient was readmitted to Eye and Ear Hospital for definitive surgical treatment of the tumor mass. Following is a narrative summary of her second admission.

November 27 — A transverse tracheostomy was performed under pentothal anesthesia and a No. 5 tracheal tube was inserted between the third and fourth tracheal rings.

November 28 — The entire parotid oropharyngeal tumor was excised. Operative technique was as follows.

An incision was made in the superior portion of the right ear, at the approximate height of the helix, then curving in a wide fashion behind the ear and extending down under the right mandible, approximately to the midline of the symphysis. Skin flaps were then retracted. This was done with sharp dissection, all bleeding points being ligated as the dissection proceeded. The skin over the tumor was then completely freed so that the subcutaneous tissue and all muscle were dissected from the tumor mass. The right facial nerve was found to run entirely over the mass and with meticulous care was dissected free and saved intact. The upper end of the tumor was then dissected free with blunt and sharp dissection, all bleeding points being clamped and ligated. The dissection was then carried below where the tumor was found to extend over and under the mandible (see Figure 13–25). The tumor was dissected free from the mandible, but it was impossible to get the portion that was under the mandible and under the palate extending down to the posterior pharynx without resection and separation of the mandible. Therefore, a subperiosteal resection was made, in the second molar area. The tumor was then, with blunt dissection, dissected free from the mandible, hard palate and posterior pharynx, and removed in one piece (see Figure 13–25D). Two holes were then drilled in each end of the mandible, and with a criss-cross wire the mandibular body was reunited. The mucous membrane was then closed with 000 chromic catgut interrupted sutures. The subcutaneous tissues were then brought together on the outside skin incision with 000 chromic catgut, buried, and then closed with 5–0 black silk sutures (see Figure 13–25E and F). The area high in the nasopharynx, where the tumor was excised, was packed with gelfoam and a pressure dressing was applied to the face. During the procedure, the patient received 1000 cc. of blood and 2000 cc. of saline.

On December 5, following a satisfactory postoperative period of recovery, the intermaxillary arches were stabilized to assure immobility of the mandibular fracture and provide palatal support and comfort to the patient by re-establishing a normal vertical intermaxillary relationship. This was accomplished by insertion of a previously prepared maxillary splinting denture which was retained in position by bilateral pin fixation in the region of the canine eminence, and an application of an Erich arch bar on the mandible followed by intermaxillary closure with use of elastics.

December 5 — Roentgenologist's Report: There was considerable soft tissue swelling noted in the region of the right mandible and extending posteriorly and downward from this site. A column of

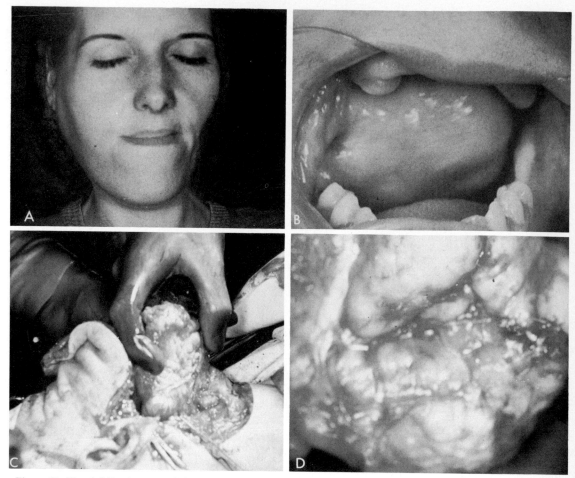

Figure 13–25 *A,* Mixed tumor of the parotid gland that apparently started in the retromolar lobe because the patient had first noticed a lump in her throat about 10 years ago. *B,* The tumor completely filled the oropharynx and part of the oral cavity.

(*Figure 13–25 continued on opposite page.*)

air was noted within the soft tissue and within this column of air was a mottled density which apparently represented a partial opacified packing. The right mandible was fixed in good alignment at its point of separation by two wire loops.

On the lateral film, there appeared to be some soft tissue swelling within the oropharynx projecting from the posterior wall, which could have been superimposed shadows (D. A. Hout, M.D.).

Pathology Report. *Macroscopic:* This specimen consisted of a mass of tissue measuring 9.5 by 8 by 4 cm., submitted from the right neck. It was submitted in a fixed state. It was gray in color with areas of reddish discoloration. The surface was grossly irregular with papules of various sizes projecting from the surface. In most areas the mass seemed to be within these irregularities and fairly well encapsulated. When the mass was cut

the tissue was found to be white in color, rather firm in consistency and homogeneous in appearance, with the exception of the middle of this large mass, where there was a cystic area which exuded yellowish fluid. This area was lined with shaggy, irregular soft lining. Section was submitted for microscopic study. An elongated, roughly ovoid, grayish white piece of tissue was submitted as a right submaxillary gland. This tissue measured 2 cm. in length, 0.5 cm. in width. The tissue was cut along its long axis and the interior was found to be made up of small strands of whitish tissue surrounding and demarcating several round, reddish brown areas. These transections were submitted as a whole for microscopic study.

Microscopic: Both sections showed a partially encapsulated tumor, the center of which was an admixture of cartilaginous material along with fi-

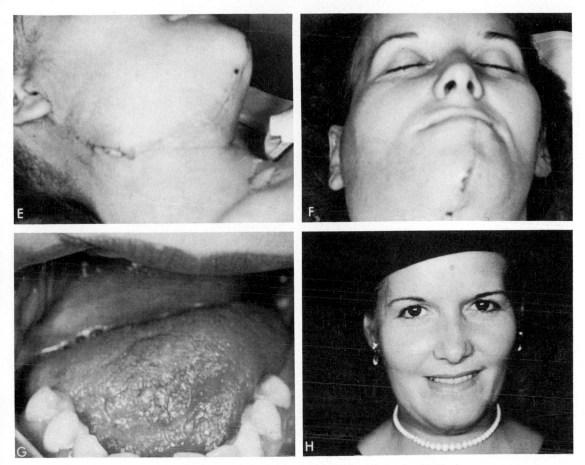

Figure 13–25 *(Continued.)* *C* to *G,* See case report No. 6 for full details. *H,* Final appearance.

brous and collagenous connective tissue. In some areas, this was quite vascular and throughout there were distributed small aggregates and clumps of epithelial cells, most of which were polyhedral with round hyperchromatic nuclei. In some areas of the tumor, the epithelial cells were arranged in an alveolar-like or duct-like fashion. Sections of lymph nodes showed intact capsules and a fairly well maintained architecture. Sinusoidal spaces were distended and filled with a proliferation of reticuloendothelial cells as well as an infiltration of chronic inflammatory cells. No tumor cells were noted throughout.

Diagnosis: Mixed tumor of the parotid gland. Chronic hyperplastic lymphadenitis—cervical (E. L. Heller, M.D.).

Follow-up. (See Figures 13–25*G* and *H.*) No recurrence followed.

PLEOMORPHIC ADENOMAS IN THE MUCOBUCCAL FOLD

These tumors are most frequently seen in the palate, but many cases have been reported in the lips. The mixed tumor illustrated in Figure 13–26 was located in the mucobuccal fold.

ENUCLEATION OF A PLEOMORPHIC ADENOMA (MIXED TUMOR) FROM THE FORNIX OF THE RIGHT MANDIBULAR VESTIBULE (MUCOBUCCAL FOLD)

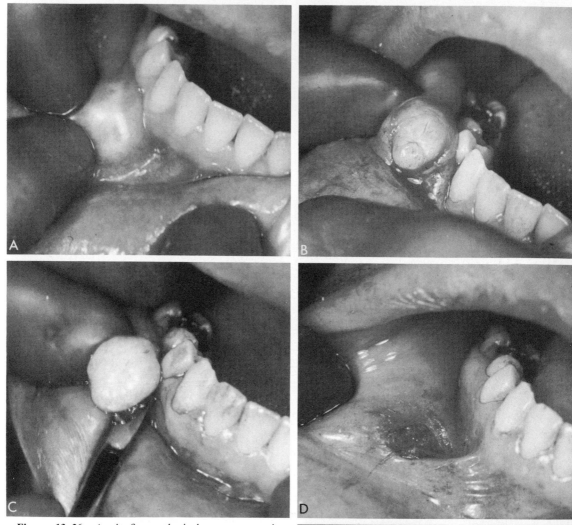

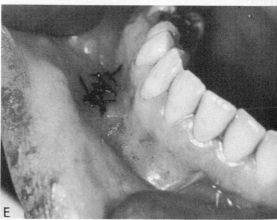

Figure 13–26 *A,* A firm spherical mass approximately 2 cm. in diameter freely movable in the mucobuccal fold opposite the mandibular right cuspid and bicuspid area. *Provisional diagnosis:* Mixed tumor.

B, An incision over the tumor through the mucosa exposed the encapsulated tumor.

C, With the periosteal elevator the tumor was easily shelled out. Pathology report, macroscopically, revealed that the specimen consisted of a white globular firm tumor 1.5 cm. in diameter. On section, the tumor consisted of solid-appearing stroma. Microscopically, there was an epithelial growth with small glandular structures in places. Elsewhere pseudocartilage was developing. The tissue was surrounded by a fibrous capsule. *Diagnosis:* Mixed tumor.

D, The tumor bed after the tumor was removed; no tumor tissue visible.

E, The mucosa closed with interrupted black silk sutures.

MIXED TUMOR OF ACCESSORY SALIVARY GLAND IN THE
PTERYGOMANDIBULAR SPACE*

Patient. This patient was admitted to Magee-Women's Hospital September 12 and found to be a normally developed, somewhat obese, 51-year-old female. Occupation—housewife.

Chief Complaint. The patient complained of soft tissue swelling in the posterior region of the mouth, difficulty in swallowing and annoyance in mastication.

History of Present Illness. Ten years ago the patient had observed a painless, freely movable nodular growth located slightly posterior and lingual to the anterior border of the right mandibular ascending ramus. After that time it persisted and gradually increased its diameter. Discomfort was minimal, paresthesia absent.

Past Medical History. The patient had had the usual childhood diseases, and no allergies. She had been hospitalized previously for full-mouth extraction and is a gravida VI, para VI, with full-term deliveries.

Twenty-six years ago a physician informed her that she had a "leaky heart." Six weeks following her first full-term delivery she developed rheumatism and migratory polyarthritis and with a succeeding pregnancy 5 years later had bronchial pneumonia. Two years ago she developed "asthmatic" attacks with persistence of exertional and paroxysmal nocturnal dyspnea. Six months ago she was told that her blood pressure was high and was placed on a low-salt diet. At present, she has two-pillow orthopnea, dyspnea after six to eight stairs and pitting pretibial edema.

Intraoral Examination. Examination revealed a 2.5-cm. oval, well circumscribed, hard solitary mass located anterior to the right tonsillar fauces. The epithelium was intact. The patient was now wearing a full maxillary denture that imparted continual traumatic irritation to the area in question, producing an indentation in the mass (see Figure 13–27).

Extraoral Examination. Normal facial symmetry was observed. There were no cervical or submaxillary nodes palpable.

Medical Evaluation. *Physical findings:* Blood pressure 174/96, pulse 84/min., respirations 20/min.

Heart: Point of maximum impulse is 1 cm. left of the midclavicular line in the sixth intercostal space; normal sinus rhythm with occasional premature systole; grade III-IV harsh presystolic murmur at apex, transmitted widely but not to the neck. No thrills.

Lungs: Clear to percussion, palpation and auscultation.

Pitting pretibial edema. No costovertebral angle tenderness. Pallor of the skin and mucous membranes.

Impression: Hypertensive cardiovascular disease and rheumatic fever with cardiac enlargement, congestive failure and mitral stenosis. Benign hypertension.

Recommendations: More complete evaluation prior to surgery, including ECG, chest films, and possible investigation of apparent anemia.

Reports: Posteroanterior and left lateral views of the chest indicate there is moderate enlargement of the left ventricle and left auricle. The lungs are clear, except for slight bronchovascular accentuation in the mesial segments of both lower lobes. ECG interpretation is as follows: 1, Sinus mechanism with normal conduction time. 2. Abnormal P waves. 3. Occasional ventricular premature beats and supraventricular premature beats. 4. Possible left ventricular hypertrophy. Additional investigation of possible anemia was not pursued.

Final Evaluation: No evidence of failure now. Acceptable for surgery. Institute antibiotic coverage.

Laboratory Findings:

Hematology:	12th	15th	17th	20th
Hgb.	8 g.	9 g.		10.5 g.
Hct.		35		
RBC	4.2 m.	3.95 m.	3.75 m.	3.5 m.
WBC	7,800	9,200		8,200
Platelets			282,400	
Bld. Time	2'30″		2'30″	
Coag. Time	4′		3′	

Differential: Poly-63, Eos-6, Lymph-29, Mono-2.
RBC Morphology: Marked hypochromia, slight polychromia, Rouleaux tendency.

Urinalysis: S.G. 1.016, albumin and sugar negative.

Preoperative Diagnosis. Mixed tumor of minor salivary gland.

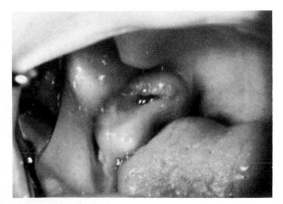

Figure 13–27 Pleomorphic adenoma ("mixed" tumor) in the pterygomandibular space (see Case Report No. 7 for further details).

*Case report prepared by Paul H. Iverson, Oral Surgery Resident, Magee-Women's Hospital, Pittsburgh, Pa.

Operation: The patient was premedicated one-half hour before the operative procedure with Nembutal, 1½ grains, and atropine sulfate, 1/150 grain. Antibiotic coverage with procaine penicillin was instituted 5 days prior to surgical intervention. The patient was draped in the customary manner and the oral mucous membranes prepared with tincture of zephirin. Anesthesia was accomplished by inferior alveolar nerve block and local infiltration with xylocaine, 2 per cent.

An incision was made from the retromolar region over the crest of the ridge, over the mixed tumor. A periosteal elevator was used to retract the tissue and to free the mucosa from the encapsulated mixed tumor. The tumor was shelled out completely. The edges of the wound were apposed by 000 Dermol.

Pathology Report: *Macroscopic:* The specimen consisted of a piece of tissue measuring 3 by 2 by 1.5 cm. The specimen was semifirm in consistency and had a slightly friable appearance. It was pinkish gray and contained a couple of blue-dome cysts that measured 7 mm. in diameter. There was a small amount of soft, fibrous tissue attached to the specimen. On cutting into the specimen, it had a slightly granular feel and appeared to be soft and friable.

Microscopic: The tumor was made up of sheets of cells that were rather uniform and little acinar formation was evident. Though mitoses were present, they were inconspicuous, and the cells were rather uniform. It was impossible to establish that the tumor was completely circumscribed, though it was in part.

Diagnosis: Mixed tumor of salivary origin (R. H. Fennell, M.D.).

Hospital Course. Uneventful. The patient was discharged on September 20.

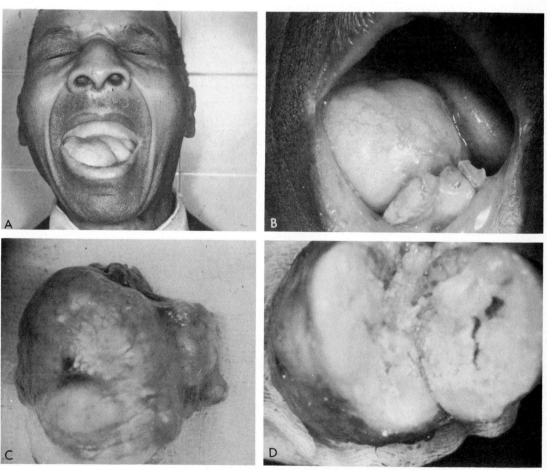

Figure 13–28   *A,* A large pleomorphic adenoma ("mixed" tumor) of the floor of the oral cavity, present for at least 30 years that the patient can remember. *B,* Close-up of the tumor shown at left. *C,* Mixed tumor removed by blunt dissection. *D,* Tumor sectioned. There were no malignant changes.

PLEOMORPHIC ADENOMAS OF THE FLOOR OF THE ORAL CAVITY

Figure 13–28 illustrates a mixed tumor of the floor of the oral cavity. These are very rare, and this is the only case the author has ever seen. This tumor was enucleated without much difficulty other than in access. It was encapsulated and above the mylohyoid muscle.

Case Report No. 8

EXCISION OF A PLEOMORPHIC ADENOMA IN THE SUBMANDIBULAR GLAND

MARVIN E. PIZER, D.D.S., M.S.

Patient. A healthy 48-year-old white female was admitted to Alexandria Hospital.

Chief Complaint. A mass in the left side of the neck.

History of Present Illness. The patient feels a hard mass about the size of a walnut in the left submandibular space. The mass is freely movable, of 3 years' known duration, with some growth suspected during that time. The mass is painless to palpation and does not change in size or produce pain when the patient is eating. (See Figure 13–29A).

Past Medical History. The patient presents a surgical history of hemorrhoidectomy, appendectomy, removal of tonsils and adenoids and a benign breast tumor. Medically, the patient is taking a diuretic for ankle edema and has had a tendency to bleed excessively when cut.

Intraoral Examination. Soft and hard structures of the oral cavity are normal, with the exception of a firm mass that is felt during palpation of the posterior left floor of the mouth while the fingers of the other hand support the mass from the neck side. Occlusal and lateral jaw films are unrevealing.

Extraoral Examination. There is a protruding firm mass in the left submandibular region that is evident on visual examination. There is no cervical lymphadenopathy.

Physical Examination. Complete physical and laboratory workup were performed with emphasis on bleeding studies. These were all normal with the exception of a slight increase of capillary fragility. A mass on the patient's back was found and thought to be a cyst, and she was advised to have this removed.

Operative Technique. The patient was prepared and draped in the usual fashion, and under endotracheal anesthesia the procedure that follows was performed. The mass in the left submandibular triangle was identified, and a submandibular incision following the anatomic position of the anterior and posterior belly of the digastric muscle was made. The incision was carried through skin, subcutaneous tissue, platysma muscle and superficial and deep fascia until the mass was identified. With sharp and blunt dissection the entire mass, which was found to be incorporated in the submandibular gland, was removed. This tumor was found to be most indurated on the medial aspect. During retraction of the mylohyoid muscle anteriorly to aid in removal of the deep portion of the submandibular gland, an atropic submandibular duct was noted entering into the floor of the mouth. This duct was doubly ligated and then cut between the ties. All bleeding having been controlled, the wound was closed in layers. (See Figure 13–29B to D.) A thyroid drain was inserted and the skin closed with 5–0 interrupted silk sutures; a gauze pressure pack was placed. Dr. Robert Adeson then proceeded to remove the tumor from the patient's back.

Pathology Report. *Macroscopic:* (1) The specimen consists of a reddish brown submandibular mass that measures 4.5 by 3.0 by 3.0 cm. The capsule appears intact, and on section there is a well circumscribed tumor mass that is grayish tan and firm. It cuts with slight resistance and measures 3.2 by 2.5 by 2.2 cm. (2) The specimen consists of a tan cyst that contains cheesy material. It measures 1.5 cm. in diameter.

Microscopic: Sections of the submandibular gland show an encapsulated tumor mass. It is composed of connective tissue elements and epithelial cells. The neoplastic epithelial cells are present in regular ductal or acinar arrangements in which the cells tend to be cuboidal or columnar. A few of the acini contain amorphous mucinous material. In other areas the epithelium appears in some solid sheets or as isolated strands and cords. The cells are fairly well differentiated. The connective tissue stroma is present in some portions of septa, and in other areas there is fibrous connective tissue that is loose and shows foci of mucinous tissue interspersed with stellate cells. There are scattered islands of hyaline material and masses of cartilage-like tissue present. The tumor appears benign, and the adjacent submandibular gland shows slight compression but no invasion. A section of the second specimen shows a cyst that contains keratin material and is lined by stratified squamous epithelium.

Diagnosis: (1) Benign mixed tumor, left submandibular gland. (2) Epidermal inclusion cyst, back (Dee R. Parkinson, M.D.).

Postoperative Course. The patient was followed in the hospital, and on the second postoperative day the drain was removed; on the fourth postoperative day alternate sutures were removed, and the patient was discharged from the hospital. On the seventh postoperative day, in the office, the remaining skin sutures were removed. The patient has been followed on a 6-month basis, free of disease, and it is now 4 years since surgery.

Final Diagnosis. Benign mixed tumor, left submandibular gland. Epidermal inclusion cyst, back.

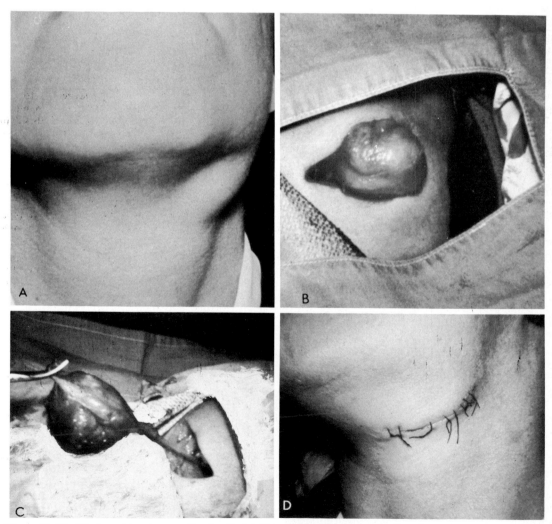

Figure 13–29 Pleomorphic adenoma (benign "mixed" tumor) in the submandibular gland. See Case Report No. 8 for details.

ODONTOGENIC TUMORS*

Cahn writes, "The classification of tumors of the jaws has become extremely complicated and bewildering, and the adopted nomenclature frequently has led to unnecessarily drastic surgical procedures.

"For example, most of the oral pathology textbooks contain in their classification malignant odontogenic tumors which have not been shown conclusively to exist.

"The hyphenated names implying that the reaction within the stroma of an ameloblastoma represents a different neoplasm, for example, hemangio-ameloblastoma, and that the entire growth is made up of two different tumors, is a misconception.

"Perez-Tamayo well describes such thinking when he writes: 'To create complicated names for tumors of varied morphology but single histogenesis is a pernicious pastime of ivory tower histopathologists who in this way pretend to escape reality.'[61]

"The term odontogenic tumor is used . . . to signify a tumor composed of cells whose primary purpose is to form tooth structures. In other words an odontogenic tumor is one which in its evolution produces a tooth or teeth, or tooth structures in disorganization, or which contains progenitors of these calcified structures."[16]

Histologically, there are three basic groups of odontogenic tumors: (1) those in which the tumor element is epithelial, (2) those in which the tumor element is mesenchymal, and (3) those which are a combination of the two.

The following is a simplified classification by Cahn and Tiecke:[17]

1. Epithelial odontogenic tumors:
   a. Simple ameloblastoma.
   b. Adenoameloblastoma.
   c. Melanoameloblastoma.
2. Mesenchymal odontogenic tumors:
   a. Odontogenic myxoma and fibroma.
   b. Dentinoma.

c. Cementoma—cementifying fibroma.
3. Mixed odontogenic tumors:
   a. Ameloblastic fibroma.
   b. Ameloblastic hemangioma.
   c. Ameloblastic neurinoma.
   d. Ameloblastic odontoma.
   e. Complex composite odontoma.
   f. Compound composite odontoma.

Gorlin, Chaudhry and Pindborg[35] classify odontogenic tumors as follows:

Epithelial odontogenic tumors
  No inductive (causing to occur) change
    in the connective tissue
    Ameloblastoma
    Ameloblastic adenomatoid tumor
      (adenoameloblastoma)
    Calcifying epithelial odontogenic
      tumor
  Inductive change in connective tissue
    Ameloblastic fibroma and ameloblastic
      sarcoma
    Dentinoma
      Immature (fibroameloblastic type)
      Mature
    Ameloblastic odontoma and ameloblastic odontosarcoma
    Complex odontoma
    Compound odontoma
Mesodermal odontogenic tumors
  Odontogenic myxoma and fibroma
    (fibromyxoma)
  Cementifying fibroma (cementoma)
    Periapical fibrous dysplasia type (periapical osteofibrosis)
    Gigantiform type (multiple or large cementifying fibromas)

AMELOBLASTOMA (ADAMANTINOMA, ADAMANTOBLASTOMA)

This tumor may arise from the remnants of the dental lamina and of the enamel organ, from the basal layer of the oral mucous membrane, or from the epithelial lining of dentigerous cysts.

Frequent mention is made of the dentigerous cyst as a potential ameloblastoma. The same is equally true of the dental follicle, which invests the crowns of unerupted impacted mandibular third molars. The complete removal of these follicles is a practical technical impossibility when they are adherent to the overlying mucosa. Therefore, portions of this "potentially dangerous tissue are left in the wounds of hundreds of thousands of pa-

---

*The author made a survey of the Diplomates and Fellows of the American Academy of Oral Pathology, asking whose classification of odontogenic tumors they would recommend for inclusion in this book. The great majority suggested Gorlin, Chaudhry and Pindborg's,[35] with Cahn and Tiecke's[17] second. It was interesting to note that many of those who selected that of Gorlin et al. noted that this classification was more meaningful for the graduate student and suggested Cahn and Tiecke's as better suited to the undergraduate student. For this reason both classifications are included.

tients who have impactions removed each year, and yet how many ameloblastomas per year develop in these areas postoperatively? Only one or two have been reported.

Many authors quote Cahn's article of 1933,[14] "Dentigerous cyst as a potential adamantinoma." In 1965 he advised me[16] that he had just seen a second one in a dentigerous cyst after reporting this one 32 years before.

I have seen only one (see Figure 12–80) in 48 years.

Based on this statement of possible ameloblastoma formation, reiterated over the ensuing years, thousands of large dentigerous cysts which encroached on teeth and other anatomic structures were enucleated, creating countless dental cripples because of needless loss of adjacent teeth, antro-oral or naso-oral

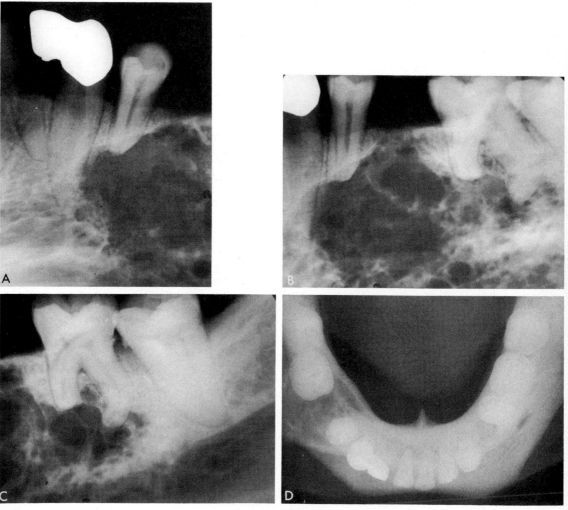

Figure 13–30   *A* to *C,* Intraoral views show the small multilocular or multicystic appearance of this tumor. Note in the bicuspid area the absence of a clear-cut bony wall. Instead, there is a diffuse radiolucent area indicating an infiltration in this area rather than a pressure atrophy such as is seen near the crest of the ridge. Note also the destruction of the apices of the first bicuspid and the mesial root of the second molar. This tumor was excised by removing a block section of bone down to the inferior border of the mandible and what was thought to be an adequate amount of bone anteriorly and posteriorly beyond the margins of the tumor. Seven years later, this patient had two additional operations in another city to excise recurrent tumor. Eleven years after the first operation, extensive recurrence of ameloblastoma was observed, and the patient returned to this city, where, by combined plastic and oral surgery, a partial resection of the mandible and insertion of an iliac crest bone graft were carried out. A portion of the graft was lost owing to infection. Another attempt to insert a bone graft is planned.

D, Occlusal view showing the expansion of the buccal and lingual cortical plates.

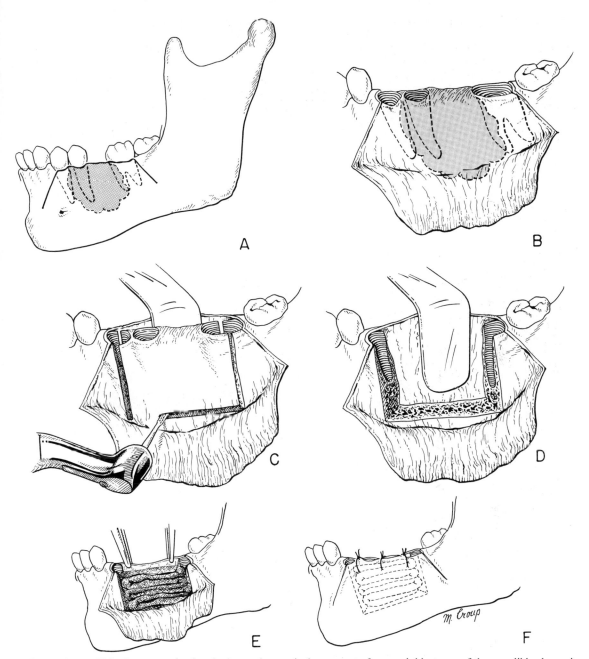

Figure 13–31 This diagrammatic sketch shows the surgical treatment of an ameloblastoma of the mandible shown in Figure 13–30.

A, The broken line is the outline of the tumor. The heavy black line is the outline of the buccal flap.

B, The buccal mucoperiosteal flap is reflected. The lingual mucoperiosteal membrane is loosened and reflected without making any vertical incisions.

C, The teeth involved in the tumor are extracted. Vertical cuts are made anteriorly and posteriorly at least 1 cm. beyond the border of the tumor.

D, The vertical cuts extend, in this case, through the inferior alveolar canal. Bleeding is controlled by compressing bone into the canal with a blunt, rounded instrument. The patient should be informed, prior to surgery, that the lip on the side involved will be permanently numb after the operation. The vertical cuts are connected by a horizontal cut made with the saw, access permitting. If not, then burs are used in the contra-angle handpiece.

E, A superficial coagulation of the exposed bone is done, and then the cavity is packed with iodoform gauze saturated with Carnoy's solution.

F, The soft tissues are sutured over the gauze. The dressing and sutures are removed in 3 days. Cavity is irrigated daily by the patient until it is epithelialized.

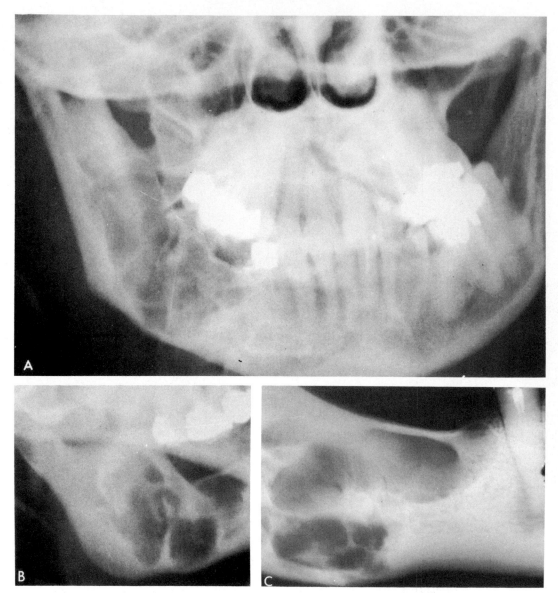

Figure 13–32 *A*, Posteroanterior view of the mandible and ramus showing an extensive multicystic ameloblastoma. Many circular compartments are clearly visible. Monocystic ameloblastomas are found occasionally, and they simulate in appearance the radicular or follicular cyst except that the margin is irregular and lobulated.

B, Left lateral jaw radiograph. Note the lobulated notches about the periphery. These are due to variations in the rate of growth of the different areas of the tumor, causing an irregular resorption of bone due to the pressure of that area of the tumor against the bony crypt.

C, Intraoral films show more clearly the multicystic appearance of this typical ameloblastoma. From these views the likelihood of a pathologic feature of the mandible is realized. Extraoral radiographs are shown in *A* and *B*.

fistulas, and anesthesia of the mandibular nerve. The author regrettably produced his share of these cripples in his early career.

In summary, the potential risk of postoperative morbidity in the enucleation of large dentigerous cysts is not justified in view of the *remote possibility* of the development of an ameloblastoma. These cysts should be marsupialized, with enucleation delayed until sufficient bone has filled in to prevent postsurgical complications when the membrane is enucleated.

At the time of marsupialization, the interior of the cyst should be examined visually and with large ball burnishers to determine whether there are mural proliferations. If these are present, enucleate the cyst regardless of potential morbidity.

Ameloblastomas are central benign embryonal type neoplasms derived from cells with a potentiality for enamel formation. These tumors are usually slow-growing, occur more frequently in the body or ramus of the mandible than in the maxilla, and may or may not be encapsulated. They can occur at any age, but are seen more frequently between ages 20 and 30. This is probably due to the fact that although they have been slowly growing for many years, they are not discovered until either a routine oral radiographic examination is made or the patient observes that one side of his jaw or face is larger than the other. As it enlarges, the tumor may expand the cortical plate of bone to the extent that it ruptures its bony confines and invades the investing soft tissues or neighboring structures, such as the maxillary sinus, the orbit, and even the base of the brain. These neoplasms at first are solid but later become cystic at the expense of their stellate cells. Early diagnosis with radical operation without destroying the continuity of the mandible will avoid recurrences to a large degree. These are benign tumors, but because of their invasive tendency and frequent recurrence they are considered to be, and are, more serious tumors that are fraught with potential complications if not completely eradicated.

Treatment. The preferred treatment for ameloblastoma is radical excision, conserving (when possible) the inferior border of the mandible. The excision is carried beyond the neoplasm into healthy tissue. This should be followed by electrodesiccation, or by treatment of the wound with phenol followed by 95 per cent alcohol. The possibility of recurrence is ever present, and the patient should be carefully instructed in the necessity of periodic examination for many years postoperatively. However, Young and Robinson stress the fact that most authorities agree on conservative treatment of the early small lesion occurring from birth to 9 to 10 years of age.[95]

Figure 13–30 illustrates a case of ameloblastoma of the right body of the mandible, and other examples follow.

Case Report No. 9

AMELOBLASTOMA (ADAMANTINOMA) OF THE MANDIBLE

History. A woman, age 28, was admitted to hospital for pregnancy at term. While in the hospital, she complained of pain and swelling in the lower right jaw.

Oral Examination. There was marked swelling in the lower right body of the mandible, which was edentulous distal to the lower right cuspid. The swelling was firm; the color of the mucosa was normal. Lateral jaw x-ray films were ordered.

Report on Radiographs. There was a large multilocular cyst involving the right lower jaw. The lesion extended from the bicuspid region back to the third molar region. The unerupted mandibular third molar was contained in this cyst. See Figure 13–33A and B.

Diagnosis. The right lateral jaw radiograph revealed what appeared to be a typical polycystic ameloblastoma of the body and ramus of the mandible containing an unerupted third molar in the ramus. The margins were clear-cut and well defined. The extent of the destruction of the osseous structure made a pathologic fracture of the mandible a good possibility. A soft diet was recommended.

Operation. Under general anesthesia, the mucoperiosteal tissue overlying the tumor was incised, beginning along the external oblique line about halfway up the ramus and carrying the incision along the crest of the tumor mass, until the first bicuspid area was reached. At this point the incision was carried down to the mucobuccal fold at a 45 degree angle.

The mucoperiosteal tissue was reflected buccally from the tumor. In some places the bone was destroyed and the dissection was difficult. After reflecting the flap, the bone, thin in some areas, thicker in others, was removed with bone rongeurs. Then by means of a large-bowled curette, the tumor, which was quite solid, was removed with difficulty from its crypt. (Technique today is to remove the tumor and surrounding bone in block section.) In the lower second molar

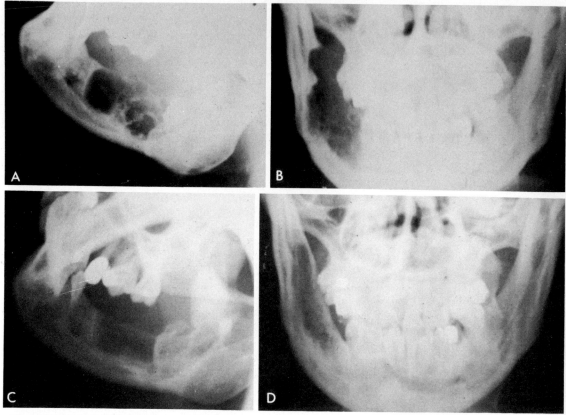

Figure 13–33 Neoplastic cysts, ameloblastoma (adamantinoma), of the mandible. *A,* Lateral jaw radiograph of a polycystic ameloblastoma. *B,* Posteroanterior radiograph. *C,* Lateral jaw radiograph taken 1 year after removal of ameloblastoma. Note that bone is filling in. *D,* Posteroanterior radiograph taken 1 year after removal of ameloblastoma. Note how the lingual cortical plate has filled in.

region, the lingual cortical plate was destroyed by pressure for an area about the size of a dime in the region of the inferior border of the mandible.

About 0.5 cm. of good bone was removed from the circumference of this lesion and the remaining bone was coagulated. At this point the only bone remaining in this area was the inferior border of the mandible.

The third molar had to be removed separately. It was lying horizontally in the buccal plate of the ramus about one third up the length of the ramus. The soft tissues were replaced and sutured in position with 000 catgut.

The mass removed was firm. The anterior-posterior surface was smooth, but the distal surface was rough and looked like small grapes. On cutting through the mass, bonelike masses were encountered in the substance of the tumor.

Pathology Report. *Macroscopic:* The specimen consisted of a mass of white firm tissue 4 cm. in diameter. One surface was smooth and regular; the opposite surface was rough and granular, with the appearance of bunches of grapes. On section, the

external portion was softer than the midportion. Frozen section was performed and the specimen pronounced nonmalignant.

Microscopic: Two sections were examined microscopically. A collagenous connective tissue separated smaller and larger cysts, some containing cellular structures, others almost devoid of their structures. The lining of the cells was a columnar epithelium with the nuclei distal to the base line. A few of the cysts were true cysts with cavities. Most of them, however, were filled with a cellular structure which varied from an embryonal connective tissue cell up to an epithelial cell, which grew rapidly and at times gave a suggestion of epithelial pearl formation. At other times the cells resembled a poor attempt at the formation of osteoid tissue. Islands of cells were growing through the stroma, apparently not enclosed in an epithelial envelope. Islands of bone were present in the stroma of the periphery.

Diagnosis: Ameloblastoma of the mandible.

Postoperative Course. When the pathology report confirmed the preoperative diagnosis, consideration was given to the possibility that perhaps there had been some proliferation of epithelium in the spongiosis or haversian system of the cortex or through the lingual opening in the lingual cortex as already mentioned. For this reason, it was decided to place 100 mg. of radium in the cavity for 6½ hours. A curved lead shield was made to cover the mandible over the bony crypt during treament, to protect the rest of the mouth. There was a normal amount of slough following this treatment.

The patient returned periodically for checkups,

and her radiographs over a period of 3 years showed the bone cavity practically filled in with new bone and no sign of a recurrence.

Subsequent Course. The patient left the city and eleven years after operation I was advised by an oral surgeon from another city that this patient had a recurrence. Ten years after her second operation (21 years from the first operation) she had a second recurrence. The first recurrence was 3 cm. from the first operative site. The second was in the ramus.

Case Report No. 10

RECURRENT AMELOBLASTOMA OF THE RIGHT MANDIBULAR BODY

Patient. The patient was admitted to Magee-Women's Hospital on March 11 and was found to be a normally developed, husky, 36-year-old white male in no acute distress. Occupation—carpenter.

Chief Complaint. "Cyst of right lower jaw."

History of Present Illness. Prior to present admission, the patient had twice undergone surgical procedures in the area of involvement. The first was to remove a tooth within the center of the cystic area, but the operation was not concluded. In a short period of time, the area became filled with granulation tissue which protruded from the alveolar socket. A second surgical undertaking was attempted while the patient was hospitalized in his home town. The jaw was surgically opened, but because "the mandibular nerve and artery were visualized within the fibrous mass," the surgeon elected not to continue the procedure. Referral followed shortly.

Past Medical History. Usual childhood diseases and chronic tonsillitis. No allergies. Previous surgery confined to dental procedures.

Oral Examination. Reveals a small proliferative mass in the retromolar region of the right mandibular body. The adjacent mucosa is mildly inflamed and edematous and the dorsal surface of the tongue appears to have a migratory glossitis. Several teeth are missing and multiple operative restorations are required. There exists mild bilateral inflammation in the tonsillar fauces with marked tonsillar hypertrophy. The remainder of the oral mucous membranes are unremarkable.

X-Ray Examination. Dentigerous cyst of mandible (see Figure 13–35*A*).

Extraoral Examination. Reveals a normal facial symmetry with no cervical or submaxillary nodes palpable.

Medical Evaluation. Blood pressure 110/80, Pulse 84/min. and full and regular. Heart sounds are of good quality with no murmurs. Lungs are

clear. Remainder of the systemic review is unremarkable. Patient is acceptable for surgery.

Family History. Father died of cardiovascular disease at an early age. All additional family members are alive and well.

Social History. The patient denies use of cigarettes or intake of alcohol. He remains physically quite active.

Laboratory Findings. All tests of hematology and urinalysis fall within normal limits.

Preoperative Impression. Dentigerous cyst of right body of mandible.

Anesthetic. Pentothal sodium with endotracheal nitrous oxide and oxygen.

Operative Technique. Following incision and reflection of a mucoperiosteal flap, the cystic wall was freed from its attachment to the mandible mesially, buccally and distally by means of large curettes. On the lingual, the cortical plate was destroyed and the cyst was found attached to the lingual mucoperiosteum. With blunt and sharp dissection, the attachment was freed and the cyst and third molar were removed intact. Sulfanilamide crystals were inserted into the cavity followed by a loose packing with ½-inch iodoform gauze.

Operative Note: The mandibular canal and its contents were forced inferior to the cyst wall and were not observed in the tumor mass.

Postoperative Impression. Dentigerous cyst.

Pathology Report. *Macroscopic:* The specimen consisted of an irregular piece of tissue measuring 2.5 cm. in length. Its one surface was coarsely granular. The rest was firm and rubbery. *Microscopic:* The surface was covered by a papillomatous arrangement of stratified epithelium growing in a loose vascular stroma infiltrated with chronic inflammatory cells. The growth was very active. Deeper was an epithelial tumor composed of spindle-shaped cells arranged at right angles around the periphery of each island. The islands

MARSUPIALIZATION OF A CYST OF THE MANDIBLE WITH AN INTRALOCULAR AMELOBLASTOMA: AN ATTEMPTED CONSERVATIVE TREATMENT

LAKANA SRIVIROJANA, D.D.S.

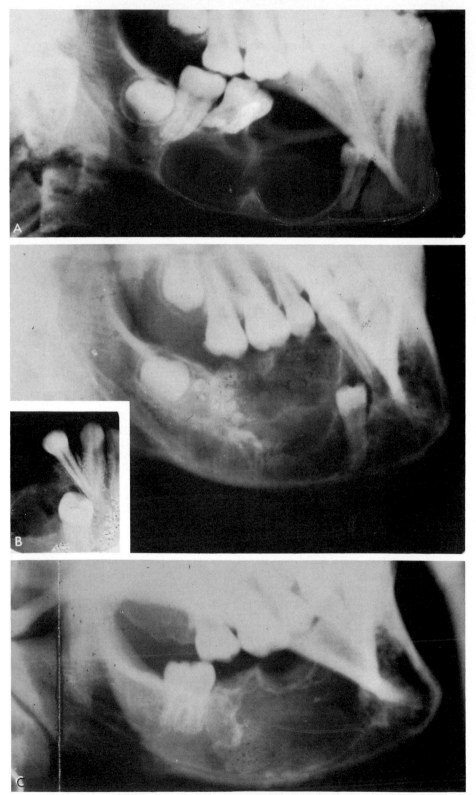

Figure 13–34 *See opposite page for legend.*

(Figure 13–34 continued on opposite page)

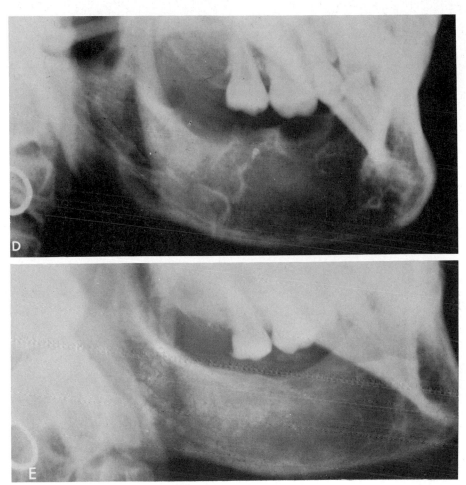

Figure 13–34 *(Continued.)*

Figure 13–34 A 14-year-old girl from southern Thailand was seen in the dental school clinic with a swollen jaw, which she stated had slowly been getting larger for the past 4 years. She now had pain when eating, and there was a distasteful fluid draining from the swelling intraorally.

A, This oblique radiograph revealed a large radiolucent area which contained an unerupted second bicuspid. A biopsy through the crest of the swelling between the first bicuspid and first molar was diagnosed as ameloblastoma. Two weeks later the first and second molars were extracted, and a large ovoid opening extending from the second molar alveolus to the distal surface of the first bicuspid was made into the cavity in the mandible, excising a portion of the cyst wall and "granulation-like" tissue and surrounding thin bone. The second bicuspid was not extracted for fear of fracturing the mandible. The bone cavity was examined periodically by her provincial dentist, and the patient irrigated the cavity daily.

B, A year later, on the patient's return to the dental clinic, the opening into the bone cavity was almost closed and it was necessary to enlarge it. A year later this opening again was enlarged and at this time the unerupted bicuspid, which did not show any signs of erupting, was removed. The patient did not return for 4 years.

C, On her next visit (this was 6 years after the first operation) the radiograph revealed a scalloping of the crest of the ridge and a well-circumscribed radiolucent area in a mottled area of bone that had a fairly well-defined border. At operation a recurrent ameloblastoma in a residual cyst was found.

D, The third molar was extracted, and the soft and bony tissue found in this area and anterior to the first bicuspid was excised and removed with rongeurs and curettes.

The department of oral pathology reported that microscopic examination showed "fibrous connective tissue with reactive bone and sequestra."

Diagnosis: "Subacute osteomyelitis and reactive bone." *E*, This radiograph taken a year later shows normal bone and no sign of recurrence.

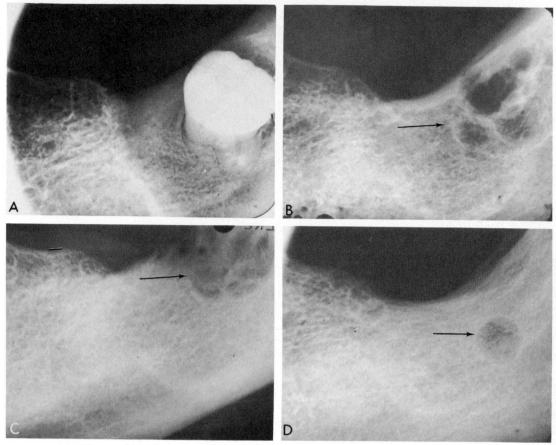

Figure 13–35   See Case Report No. 10 for details on this recurrent ameloblastoma of the mandible.

were surrounded by heavy hyaline masses which separated the tumor cells and the surrounding stroma. Still deeper were mucous secreting glands, some of them showing compression atrophy. Minute spicules of bone were present in the deepest portions of the growth. *Diagnosis:* Adamantinoma (ameloblastoma) (M. Cohen, M.D.).

Hospital Course. Uneventful. Patient was discharged on March 14.

Subsequent Course. Eight years later, following a periodic radiographic examination in the area of previous involvement, a suspicious lesion (see Figure 13–35B) was observed in the right posterior mandibular region and the patient was referred to the office of W. H. A. On December 11, he was admitted to Eye and Ear Hospital with a preoperative diagnosis of ameloblastoma. Following is a narrative summary of his second admission.

December 12 – A block section of the cystic lesion was performed. Operative technique consisted of the reflection of a large mucoperiosteal flap and the excision of the lesion and bone, anterior, posterior and inferior to the lesion. Note that the pathologist did not find any tumor in the bone.

Pathology Report. *Macroscopic:* This speci-

men consisted of three separate specimens which consisted of several pieces of irregular pinkish gray and red tissue and bone. The smallest specimen measured approximately 8 mm. and the largest measured 2.5 cm. in greatest diameter. The specimens were labeled 1, 2, and 3 and were submitted in their entirety. Since a portion of specimen No. 1 consisted of bone fragments, the bony fragments were submitted for decalcification. *Microscopic:* Sections revealed a dense collagenous stroma containing irregular clusters of epithelial cells distributed as alveolar masses and elongated cords. The cells were basophilic and the peripheral layer disposed in palisade stellate. Mitoses were not noted. No involvement of bone fragments by the tumor was evident and a separately submitted mass (specimen No. 3) consisted of dense scar tissue free of tumor *Diagnosis:* Adamantinoma (Ameloblastoma) – mandible (E. L. Heller, M.D.).

Hospital Course. Uneventful. Patient was discharged the day following surgery.

Subsequent Course. Following a three-year period of apparent inactivity, the cystic lesion again presented itself during routine radiographic examination (Fig. 13–35C). The patient was readmitted to Eye and Ear Hospital, and under local anesthesia a block alveolar resection encompassing the ameloblastic lesion was accomplished. It is of interest to note the apparent difficulty encountered in categorizing the present lesion microscopically.

Pathology Report. *Macroscopic:* This specimen consists of a fragment of moderately firm, tannish white tissue received in formalin. It measures 0.5 cm. in greatest diameter and is somewhat granular on the surface. *Microscopic:* The section shows a dense fibrous stroma containing a few nests and strands of epithelial cells. In the center there is an irregular cyst cavity, lined with squamous epithelium. In the lumen there is cellular and acellular pigmented debris. *Diagnosis:* Paradental cyst of mandible, inflamed.

Amended Report. Review of the material removed three years before showed a small cystic adamantinoma with prolongations of epithelium from its margin similar to those seen in this material. In view of this I believe the lesion must be considered as a recurrence of adamantinoma. *Diagnosis:* Adamantinoma of mandible, recurrent (R. S. Totten, M.D.).

Hospital Course. Uneventful. Patient was discharged after 2 days.

Subsequent Course. Almost 3 years thereafter, patient was again readmitted to Eye and Ear Hospital following radiographic evidence of a small cystic recurrence (Fig. 13–35D). Under local anesthesia, a block surgical resection of bone was again taken from the right posterior mandibular body. Pathology report follows:

Pathology Report. *Macroscopic:* Part 1 is labeled as a separate nodule and consists of a 0.2 by 0.2 by 0.2 cm. reddish tan nodule which is firm. Part 2 is labeled "main tumor mass" and consists of seven fragments of bone, having a pinkish gray cortex and a pinkish tan cancellous portion, in which there are several grayish pink nodules of firm tissue. Together these fragments of bone are 2 by 1.5 by 0.7 cm. *Microscopic:* Within the marrow spaces there are clear areas surrounded by two or more layers of small cells with clear cytoplasm and small round to oval nuclei. The outermost layer has cells whose nuclei are radially arranged. Adjacent to these cells is an eosinophilic homogenous thin layer surrounded by loose and dense fibrous tissue. This tissue occupies the majority of the marrow spaces; however, there are a few foci of marrow cells which are not remarkable. The separately submitted specimen contains similar tumors. *Diagnosis:* Recurrent ameloblastoma of right mandible (R. S. Totten, M.D.).

Hospital Course. The patient made an uneventful recovery and was discharged.

Follow-up. To date, 8 years later, no osteolytic activity in this area of the mandible has been revealed.

COMMENT

Here is a patient who had four recurrences of an ameloblastoma in the same area of the body of the mandible over a 14-year period in spite of what was considered to be adequate surgery, in view of the fact that the pathologist did not find tumor tissue in the bone removed from around the tumor. This case proves the absolute necessity of following these patients with periodic roentgenographic examination for at least 5 years.

Case Report No. 11

EXTENSIVE AMELOBLASTOMA (ADAMANTINOMA) OF THE MANDIBLE

ROGER A. HARVEY, M.D.,
AND EUGENE R. ELSTROM, R.T.

History. This 41-year-old female was admitted to the hospital because of a hard mass on the left mandible. The patient stated that she had noticed this gradually growing larger during the past 5 years.

Physical Examination. Normal, with the exception of the hard mass mentioned above.

Radiographic Examination. A lateral jaw radiograph (Fig. 13–40) revealed multicystic areas throughout the region formerly occupied by the roots of the molar and bicuspid teeth. The superior margin of the bone appeared to be broken through, but there were no radiating bone spicules. The areas of pathosis seemed to be made up of at least three central foci of activity with numerous areas about them.

Radiograpic Diagnosis. Tumor of left mandible, multicystic in character.

(*Text continued on page 749*)

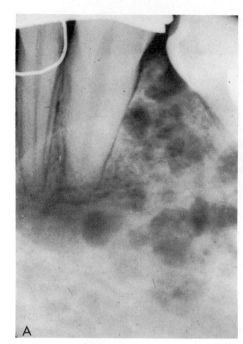

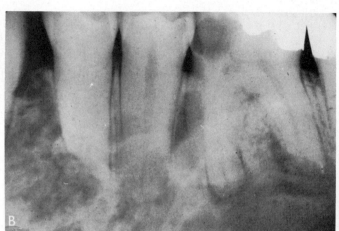

Figure 13-36 Another example of the radiographic appearance of an ameloblastoma of the mandible. Note the resorption of the apex of the second bicuspid.

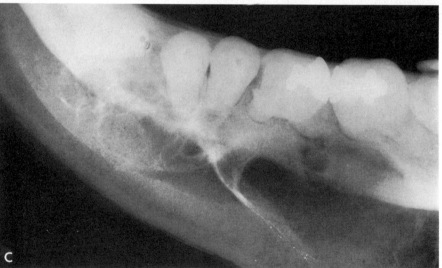

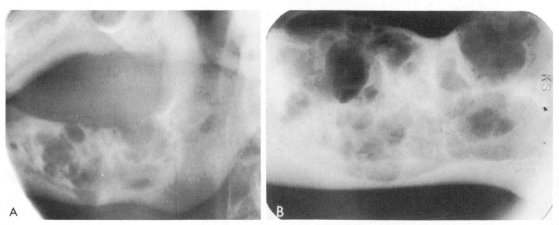

Figure 13-37 *A,* This oblique radiograph of the mandible is not a good diagnostic film. *B,* Note the markedly improved diagnostic quality of this intraoral film. It is recommended that, whenever possible, extraoral radiographs be supplemented by intraoral films.

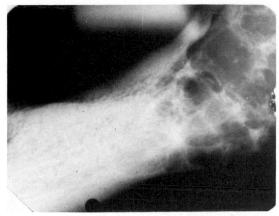

Figure 13–38 In this extensive ameloblastoma of the vertical ramus it is surprising that no fracture took place through the mandible during mastication. Resection of the ramus is necessary.

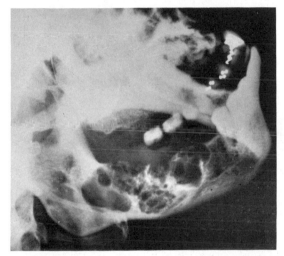

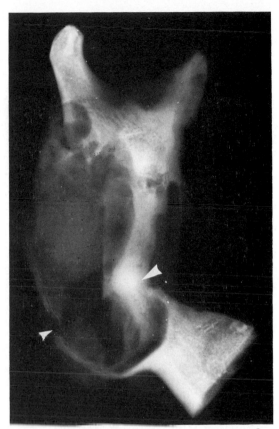

Figure 13–39 Vertical ramus resected because of an extensive ameloblastoma. Note that this ramus did spontaneously fracture during mastication. (Courtesy of Alvin F. Gardner, D.D.S.)

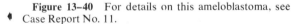

Figure 13–40 For details on this ameloblastoma, see Case Report No. 11.

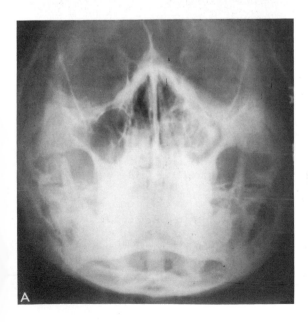

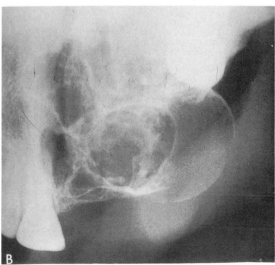

Figure 13–41 Ameloblastoma of the maxilla. The patient refused surgery.

Photographic Case Report

ENUCLEATION OF A RESIDUAL MAXILLARY ANTERIOR CYST WITH AN INTERLOCULAR AMELOBLASTOMA
Francis M. S. Lee, B.D.S.

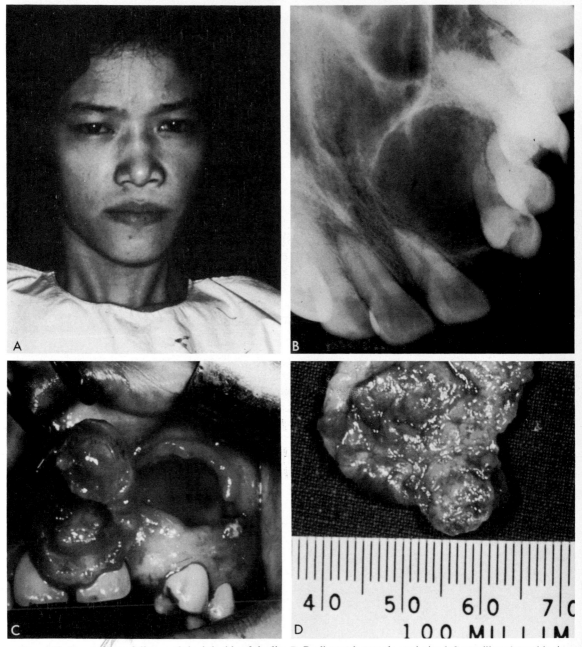

Figure 13–42   *A,* Note fullness of the left side of the lip. *B,* Radiograph reveals a missing left maxillary lateral incisor and a well-circumscribed radiolucent area that could possibly be a residual cyst that developed from a retained periapical granuloma of the left lateral incisor at the time of extraction. *C,* The mucoperiosteal membrane has been reflected, thinned cortical bone around the periphery of the lesion was removed and the lesion opened into by turning back a labial circular section of the capsule. *D,* The inner surface of the capsule had an area of proliferation of hyperplastic tissue that a biopsy revealed as an ameloblastoma. This area was excised.

(Figure 13–42 continued on opposite page)

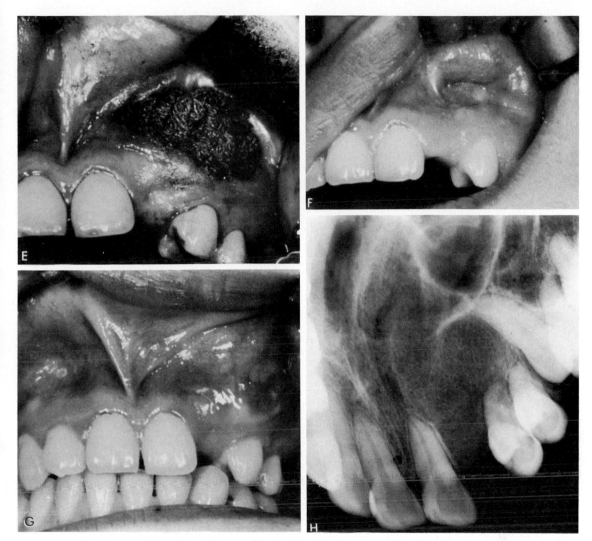

Figure 13–42   (*Continued.*) *E*, The cavity was filled with iodoform gauze. *F*, Postoperative view several weeks later. Cavity almost completely filled in with bone. *G*, Six months later complete healing with normal labial contour. *H*, Radiograph of the area shows normal cancellous bone. There has not been a recurrence 5 years later.

Operation.   The left ramus and the posterior three fourths of the body of the mandible were resected.

Pathology   Report. *Macroscopic:* Specimen consisted of three pieces of bone which, when joined, formed the ramus and body of the left mandible. No teeth were present. There was a fusiform swelling of the fragment representing the body of the bone which was 3 cm. in length, 2.5 cm. in width, and approximately 2 cm. in height. Directly posterior to the mass there was half of a large open cavity about 2 cm. in diameter. The overlying alveolar soft tissue was nodular and firm. There was a loss of mucosa over one area, 1.5 cm. by 0.6 cm. The other two pieces of bone were essentially normal. Representative sections were taken and decalcified.

Microscopic: Extending down from the submucosal tissues and invading the mandibular bone over a wide area were nests of epithelial cells. These nests had a row of radially directed cells which enclosed a loose reticular fibrous tissue. In areas, cystic degeneration of these spaces had occurred and fat-laden macrophages had accumulated. The bone was eroded by this tumor and there was active osteoclastic resorption in areas where tumor cells were proliferating adjacent to the bone.

Final Diagnosis.   Adamantinoma involving the left mandible.

AUTHOR'S COMMENT

While this is an extensive ameloblastoma and it does closely approach the inferior border of the mandible at one point, in my opinion the continuity of the mandible should have been preserved by taking out a block section from the body of the mandible containing the tumor. A hemisection of the mandible is a radical, major, crippling operation for a benign tumor in a 41-year-old woman. In the event of recurrences, additional surgery could have been performed, leaving as a last resort a hemisection of the mandible.

Case Report No. 12

AMELOBLASTOMA OF SYMPHYSIS OF THE MANDIBLE*

History. The patient, a 51-year-old man, had his 6 remaining mandibular anterior teeth extracted in the office of a local oral surgeon. It should be noted that this procedure was done without preoperative radiographs. The postoperative course was uneventful. Approximately 3 years later the patient went to see his family dentist for extraction of his remaining maxillary teeth and the construction of a full upper and lower denture. During the routine preprosthetic examination, the dentist noticed a swelling in the anterior part of the mandible. Upon digital pressure, a milky fluid was expressed from this area. A circular opening into this area to "establish drainage" was made at this time (see Figure 13–44A). Routine intraoral radiographs were taken and the patient was referred to me.

Oral Examination. In the expanded symphysis of the edentulous mandible, there was a circular opening into a cavity which collected food and debris and served as a source of irritation. The area of labial expansion extended from the region of the right cuspid to the left cuspid. The cortical plate was thinned and was easily compressed.

Roentgenographic Examination. Roentgenograms revealed a large multilocular cystic area of the symphysis of the mandible. The labial cortical plate was expanded and thinned. In the left cuspid and premolar area there was a thinning and expansion of the lingual cortical plate. There were many small cystic areas in or around the larger cystlike areas. This lesion had the radiographic appearance of an ameloblastoma (Figs. 13–43 and 13–44).

A biopsy was performed, and the diagnosis was "ameloblastoma of the mandible with chronic inflammation and reactive hyperplasia."

The patient was admitted to the Eye and Ear Hospital.

Physical Examination. The routine medical history and physical examination revealed no systemic disease.

Operative Notes. Under thiopental sodium and endotracheal nitrous oxide and oxygen anesthesia, an incision was made in the mandible, extending from the second premolar on the right to the second premolar on the left. This tissue was reflected on both the lingual and the labial surfaces. In spite of the large size of this tumor, a conservative approach was decided upon in order to preserve the continuity of the mandible. I planned to excise the tumor with a reasonable amount of bone beyond the periphery, including the labial and lingual cortical bone, and leave only the inferior border of the mandible. This was accomplished after the expanded bone overlying the tumor was exposed by the reflection of large mucoperiosteal flaps labially and lingually and by means of burs, chisels, and rongeurs. The bone and tumor were excised. The inferior alveolar canal was cut through bilaterally; bleeding was controlled by coagulation and packing. To destroy any tumor tissue which might have invaded the cancellations beyond the area excised, the surgical site was thoroughly coagulated with a ball coagulating tip. The cavity was then filled with iodoform gauze saturated with Carnoy's solution. The gauze was held in position by sutures passed over the packing and through the labial and lingual soft tissue flaps. The patient was removed from the operating room in satisfactory condition.

Pathology Report. The specimen consisted of 10 pieces of moderately firm, irregularly shaped, grayish tan tissue submitted in Formalin. Portions of each tissue were covered by opaque, tannish white, somewhat granular membrane, and attached to many of the pieces were large fragments of bone. In the aggregate, this specimen measured 7 by 5 by 2.5 cm. The cut surface of most of the fragments was pale tannish white, smooth, and somewhat granular.

Microscopic: The tumor was composed of a dense fibrous connective tissue lined by stratified squamous epithelium with marked acanthosis. Within the connective tissue were large sheets and columns of epithelium of epidermoid type and

---

*From Archer, W. H.: Ameloblastoma of symphysis of the mandible. Oral Surg., *12*:1055–1060 (Sept.), 1959.

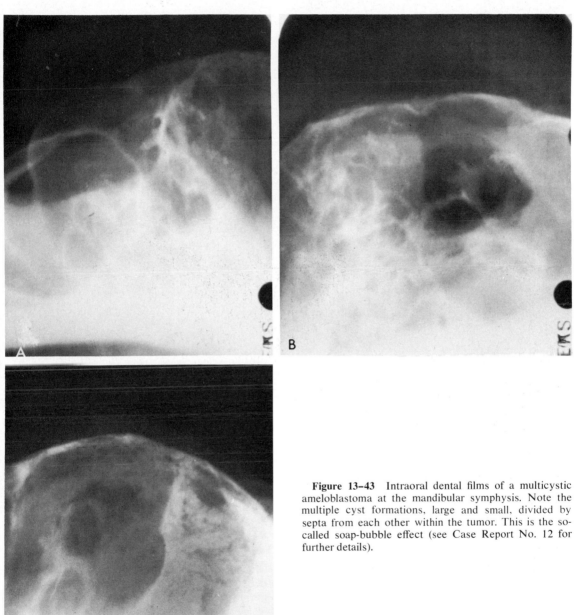

Figure 13–43 Intraoral dental films of a multicystic ameloblastoma at the mandibular symphysis. Note the multiple cyst formations, large and small, divided by septa from each other within the tumor. This is the so-called soap-bubble effect (see Case Report No. 12 for further details).

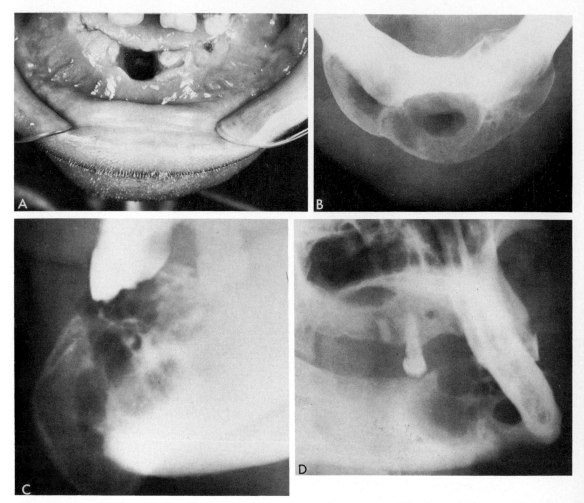

Figure 13–44 *A*, Edentulous mandibular symphysis expanded by a large multicystic ameloblastoma. The opening was made by the patient's dentist to "establish drainage." *B*, An intraoral occlusal film that shows the extent of the expanded thin labial cortical bone. Also on the left lingual incisor to bicuspid area is another expanded and thinned area of lingual cortex. This is an unusual finding in this region of the mandible. *C*, This true lateral radiograph of the mandible discloses the extent of the labial and inferior expansion of the ameloblastoma. *D*, Left extraoral oblique roentgenogram of the left horizontal ramus symphysis. One of the characteristics of multicystic ameloblastoma is the breakdown of the septa between small cysts, thus producing larger and larger cysts. This is illustrated very well in this figure.

areas of basal cells which encircled groups of large vacuolated cells connected by cytoplasmic bridges. There were scattered areas of lymphocytic and polymorphonuclear leukocyte infiltration. Bony trabeculae were seen surrounding the tumor mass.

Diagnosis: Ameloblastoma of the mandible (R. S. Totten, M.D., Pathologist).

Postoperative Course. The postoperative course was satisfactory, and the patient was discharged from the hospital 4 days after admission. He was to receive follow-up treatment in the office. The wound appeared as shown in Figure 13–45*A* when the dressing was removed 10 days after the

operation. Eight weeks after the operation the wound contained large lobules of pyogenic granulation tissue, covering a loose sequestrum (Fig. 13–45*B*). This sequestrum was the anticipated end result of the extensive coagulation carried out at the time of operation. The sequestrum was removed (Fig. 13–45*C*). The wound now epithelized rapidly and healed well.

Follow-up. Two years later, there is no visual or radiographic evidence of a recurrence of the tumor (Fig. 13–45*D*). The mandible will be radiographed annually for the next 5 years in order to discover early any radiographic evidence of recurrence.

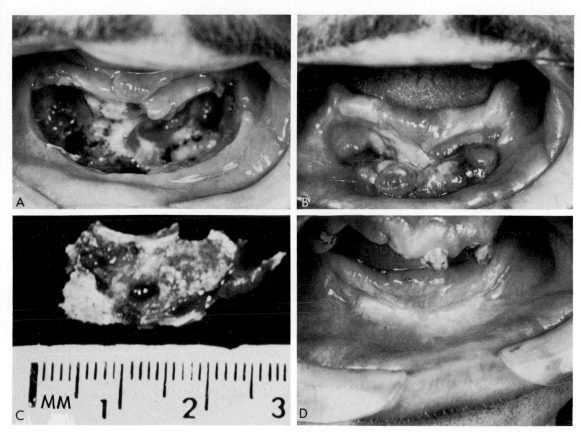

Figure 13–45 *A*, The appearance of the wound when the dressing was removed 10 days postoperatively. *B*, Large multilobules of pyogenic granulation tissue covering the loose sequestrum intentionally produced at the time of operation by the use of the coagulator; this is 8 weeks postoperatively. *C*, Sequestrum. *D*, Clinical appearance 1 year later.

Case Report No. 13

ADENOAMELOBLASTOMA

RICHARD G. TOPAZIAN, D.D.S.

Patient. A 15-year-old South Indian girl was first seen in May, complaining of a swelling over the anterior aspect of the left maxilla. This lesion had first been noted 2 months previously.

Oral Examination. Examination revealed a firm, nontender swelling that measured approximately 4 by 4 cm. The swelling was oval in shape and extended from the lateral margin of the left external naris posteriorly. Intraorally, it extended into the buccal sulcus from the lateral incisor, to the first premolar region, to a point 1 cm. above the gingival margin. There was moderate deflection of the lateral aspect of the left external naris.

Radiographic Examination. Radiographic examination revealed a radiolucent area, approximately 3 by 3 cm., involving the crown and part of the

root of the unerupted left maxillary cuspid (Fig. 13–46*A*). All teeth were vital. The preoperative diagnosis was a follicular cyst.

Operative Notes. Following induction of general anesthesia, the left maxilla was infiltrated with 1 per cent procaine-containing epinephrine. A linear incision was made 0.5 cm. above the gingival margin, from the left second molar to the left central incisor. The mucoperiosteum was reflected, exposing the tumor, which was covered by a thin shell of bone. This overlying bone was removed with rongeurs. The defect was filled with a grayish tissue of liver-like consistency. This tissue was not adherent to the cavity walls and was easily removed with the cuspid tooth, which was in intimate relation to the tumor. The walls of the

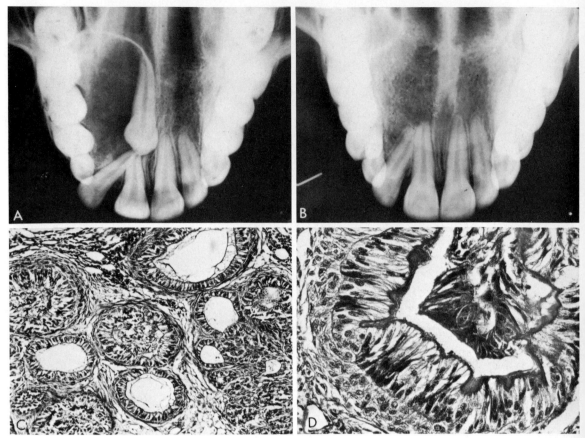

Figure 13–46   Adenoameloblastoma. (See Case Report No. 13 for details.)

defect were curetted and treated with phenol followed by alcohol. The margins were smoothed with bone files, and the incision was closed with interrupted sutures. The maxillary sinus was not continuous with the defect.

Clinical Course. Microscopic examination revealed the typical pattern of adenoameloblastoma (Fig. 13–47*C* and *D*). Sutures were removed on the sixth day following surgery, and the patient made an uneventful recovery. The patient was followed for 3½ years without recurrence (Fig. 13–47*B*).

Case Report No. 14

ADENOAMELOBLASTOMA IN AN ODONTOGENIC CYST

H. Serrano Roa, D.D.S.

Patient. An 18-year-old female in the twenty-eighth week of pregnancy was referred to the Department of Estomatology in the Roosevelt Hospital of Guatemala, Central America, for a swelling in the left maxilla.

Examination. Examination showed a deformity in the face (Fig. 13–47*A*) from an enlargement in the left maxilla that was hard and painless (Fig. 13–47*B*). X-ray examination of the left maxilla showed a unilocular cyst, about 3 by 3 cm. in diameter, in the superointernal angle. The lateral incisor was contained within the cyst (Fig. 13–47*C*). General evaluation of the patient indicated findings within normal limits.

Operative Notes. Under local anesthesia an intraoral curved incision was made from the midline of the maxilla to the region of the first upper left molar; the mucoperiosteum was detached by

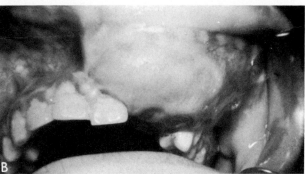

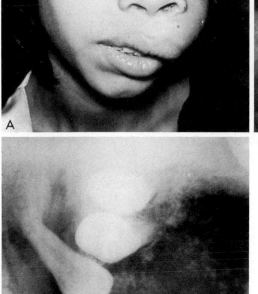

Figure 13–47 Adenoameloblastoma. (See Case Report No. 14 for details.)

means of periosteal elevators, when a thin, cystic wall came into view. Enucleation of the growth was performed, with a little flow of yellow liquid. Gross examination of the resected specimen showed a thin and regular capsule, but in the superointernal angle where the lateral incisors were in contact with a portion of the capsule, there was an increase in thickness. The specimen was sent to the pathology department with the recommendation that they do several sections, and especially where the capsule had adjoined the teeth.

Pathology Report. The pathologist's report indicated that the specimen was an odontogenic cyst with adenoameloblastoma in two areas.

Conclusions. We felt that the complete cnucleation of the capsule in this patient was sufficient treatment. There has not been a recurrence.

AMELOBLASTIC ADENOID TUMOR

Gorlin and associates state: "Ameloblastic adenoid tumor (adenoameloblastoma, cystic compound odontoma, and tumor of the enamel organ epithelium) is a benign tumor and is treated conservatively."

CALCIFYING EPITHELIAL ODONTOGENIC TUMOR

"Calcifying epithelial odontogenic tumor is extremely rare and is apparently invasive and may recur, behaving like an ameloblastoma."[35]

Treatment. Radical excision is the treatment for this tumor.

AMELOBLASTIC FIBROMA AND AMELOBLASTIC SARCOMA

Ameloblastic Fibroma. Gorlin and associates state that: "The ameloblastic fibroma is frequently mistakenly diagnosed as an ameloblastoma. It is not commonly seen in individuals over 21 years of age. The clinical behavior is benign. It does not infiltrate and can be curetted or 'peeled off' from its bony cavity."[35]

Ameloblastic Sarcoma. Gorlin and associates have found that: "Ameloblastic sarcoma (sarcoma ameloblasticum, ameloblastosarcoma, adamantinoma sarcomatoides and malignant ameloblastoma) is most common in young adults, grows rapidly and frequently is painful. This may lead to tooth extraction with subsequent growth of the tumor from the socket. Destruction of the alveolar process may cause loosening of the teeth."[35] The usual treatment is radical excision.

Discussion. Shira and Bhaskar in a case report of an ameloblastic fibroma in a 6-month-old child state: "In recent years a malignant counterpart of this lesion, namely the ameloblastic sarcoma, has been described. The ameloblastic sarcoma, of which about 11 cases so far have been reported, is said to grow far more rapidly than its benign counterparts; it has occurred in patients 13 to 52 years of age and is believed to develop in some instances from an ameloblastic fibroma. The ameloblastic sarcoma is characterized by a mesenchymal stroma which is said to show pleomorphism, but the epithelial islands in this stroma do not show malignant features. Since mesenchymal tissue during early development grows as rapidly as, if not faster than the malignant tissue, it is not inconceivable that some of the so-called ameloblastic sarcomas are really ameloblastic fibromas. In any event, before a diagnosis of ameloblastoma or ameloblastic sarcoma is made in a child and radical treatment contemplated, one must be certain that such radical treatment is justified."[80]

Case Report No. 15

AMELOBLASTIC FIBROMA

Richard G. Topazian, D.D.S.

Patient. An 11-year-old South Indian boy was first seen on June 10, complaining of pain and swelling of the right lower jaw. Two years earlier, he had noticed a small swelling of the gingiva behind the lower right first molar. The swelling had slowly increased in size, causing a noticeable facial deformity. There was occasional oozing of blood from the growth intraorally. The tumor had been curetted twice intraorally at another hospital.

Physical Examination. Extraorally, a firm, nontender, diffuse, central expansion involving the entire right body of the mandible from the premolar region to the angle could be palpated. Intraorally, an oval mass of tissue measuring 3 by 3 cm. was seen in the mucous fold behind the first molar (Fig. 13–48A). The second molar was missing.

Radiographic Examination. Lateral oblique radiographs revealed a partially erupted second molar and a developing third molar on the normal side. On the involved side, a radiolucent lesion with irregular margins could be visualized. It involved the mandible from the first molar to the angle region, and the major part of the ramus, excluding the condyle (Fig. 13–48B). The second and third molars were missing. Occlusal films revealed a cystic lesion with expansion of both the lingual and buccal plates of bone (Fig. 13–48C).

Clinical Course. A biopsy was performed intraorally under local anesthesia. Histologic examination resulted in a diagnosis of ameloblastic fibroma (Fig. 13–48D).

Operative Notes. On June 18, under general anesthesia, an incision was made 2 cm. below the inferior mandibular border, from the angle to the canine region. The thin lateral cortex of the mandible was exposed and removed, revealing a well-encapsulated fibrous tumor, which was readily and completely removed from its bony bed. The body and ramus had been considerably enlarged mediolaterally by the lesion. The oral mass was removed en bloc with the major specimen after incision of the mucosa around it. The defect was packed with gauze, the end of which protruded into the mouth, and the wound was closed in layers. The pack was removed in 10 days and the defect irrigated periodically.

Postoperative Course. The patient was last seen 6 months after surgery. Clinically and radiographically normal healing had occurred (Fig. 13–48E). The patient was lost to subsequent follow-up.

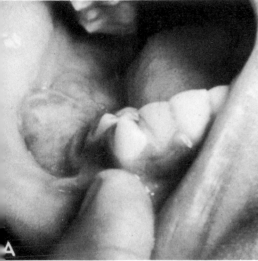

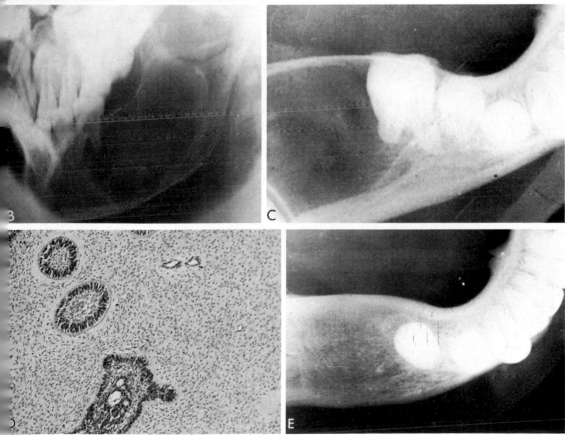

Figure 13–48 Ameloblastic fibroma. (See Case Report No. 15 for details.)

DENTINOMA

Gorlin and associates make the following observations: "Dentinoma may be mature or immature. The former may be called the fibroameloblastic type, essentially an ameloblastic fibroma in which there is dentine or osteodentin. It is frequently encapsulated and 'shells out' easily from the surrounding bone."[35]

Ryba and Kramer report a case of an infant who at birth had two lower incisors erupted which were both shortly lost. Thirteen weeks later there were two tumor-like masses projecting from this area. Radiographs showed calcified material in both masses. An ellipse of mucosa bearing the two swellings was excised and submitted for histological study. This showed that the "masses resulted from the continued growth of the dentine papilla, with the formation of both regular and irregular dentine, and continued activity of Hertwig's sheath."[71] This is a most rare case.

MYXOMA

These tumors are usually located centrally in the maxilla or mandible in tooth-bearing areas and frequently are associated with unerupted teeth. The presence of collagen fibers makes such a tumor a fibromyxoma. They expand the bone and radiographically they show a trabeculation which is similar to that of central giant tumors, ossifying fibromas and even ameloblastomas (see Figures 13–50 and 13–52). In brief, the radiographs are not particularly diagnostic.

Treatment. The treatment consists of enucleation and curettage, at times followed by

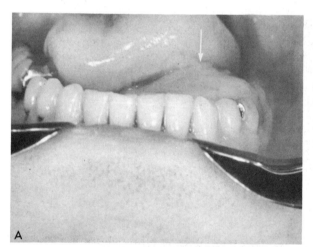

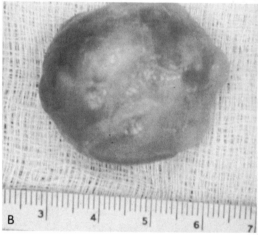

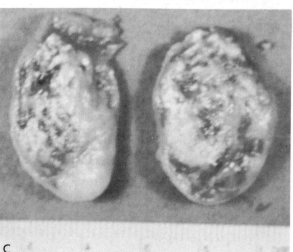

Figure 13–49 According to Shafer, Hine and Levy, "the intraoral soft tissue myxoma is an extremely rare lesion. The majority of oral cases undoubtedly represent only myxomatous degeneration in a fibrous tumor, and cannot be considered true myxomas."[75] Quantitatively, the encapsulated tumor shown here had more myxomatous tissue than fibrous.

A, This fibromyxoma was located in the soft tissue of the floor of the oral cavity above the mylohyoid muscle. *B*, Tumor was removed, after the covering mucosa was incised, by blunt dissection. *C*, Note the shiny, sticky surfaces of the two halves of the tumor.

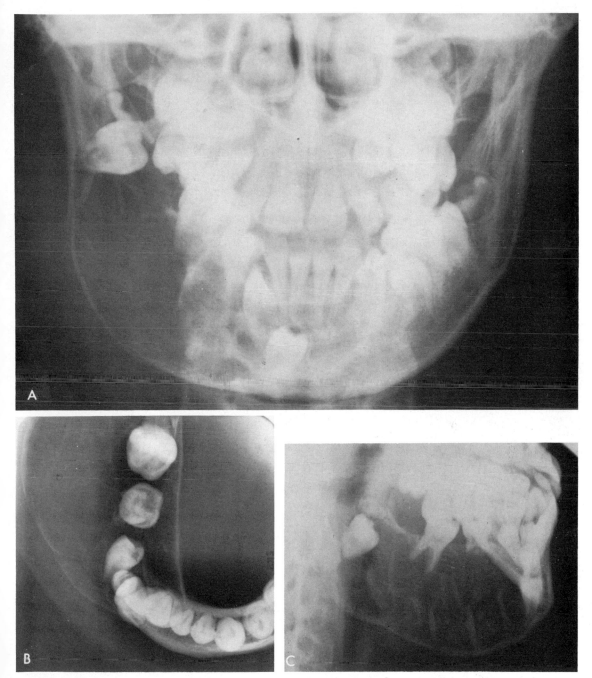

Figure 13–50 *A*, Odontogenic fibromyxoma arising from the second premolar, which has been displaced anteriorly and inferiorly to a position in the symphysis anterior to the cuspid, and the second molar, which also has been displaced distally and buccally. *B*, The expansion and thinning of the buccal and lingual cortical plates are clearly shown. The striations throughout the tumor are similar to those seen in central giant cell tumors. *C*, In this oblique view of the tumor it radiographically resembles osteoid osteoma.

chemical or electric cautery, while en bloc resection has been used for extensive lesions. The tumor is not radiosensitive. Prognosis is excellent, but recurrences are common (25 per cent) if therapy is too conservative. (See Case Report Nos. 16 and 17 (myxomas of the maxilla) and 18 (myxofibrosarcoma of the mandible.)

Case Report No. 16

RECURRENT MYXOMA OF LEFT MAXILLA

Patient. A normally developed 12-year-old white female presented to Eye and Ear Hospital with a complaint of "cyst in the upper jaw."

History of Present Illness. Six months prior to admission, the patient observed mobility of her maxillary left deciduous cuspid and attributed it to the normal eruptive forces of the secondary dentition. Instead of being exfoliated, the tooth was retained and, approximately 4 months later, an asymptomatic mucosal enlargement developed adjacent to it. She was taken to her family dentist who observed, on radiographic examination, a large radiolucent area, and a tentative diagnosis of "cyst" was established.

Past Medical History. The patient had had the usual childhood diseases. She was allergic to penicillin and had been hospitalized previously for pneumonia at the age of 3 and tonsillectomy and adenoidectomy at the age of 5.

Oral Examination. This revealed a 3-cm. long expansile lesion of the left maxillary alveolar ridge extending distally from the lateral incisor to the first molar region. The area was firm and nonfluctuant and on palpation it gave evidence of both buccal and palatal expansion of the cortical bone. The mucous membrane was intact and the remainder of the oral soft tissues were unremarkable.

Physical Examination. Revealed a normal facial symmetry with mild palpable lymphadenopathy of the left submaxillary nodes. The skin was clear and dry and there were no areas of focal inflammation. Blood pressure was 110/70, pulse 84/min., and respirations were full and regular. The heart

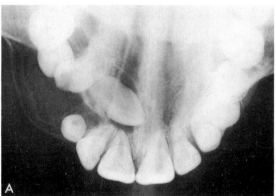

Figure 13–51 *A*, The occlusal view of the maxilla reveals a marked bulging of the left maxillary cortical plate. Beneath this bulge is a radiolucent area that contains a malpositioned cuspid and first bicuspid. Note the retained deciduous cuspid in this 12-year-old female.

B to *D*, The dental radiographs reveal a radiolucent area containing an impacted and displaced maxillary left cuspid and first bicuspid.

(Figure 13–51 continued on opposite page)

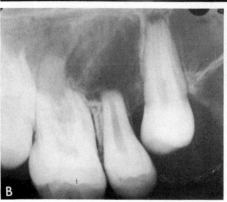

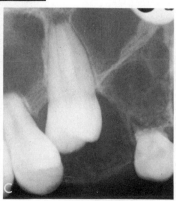

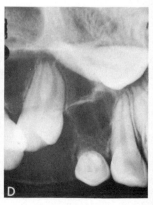

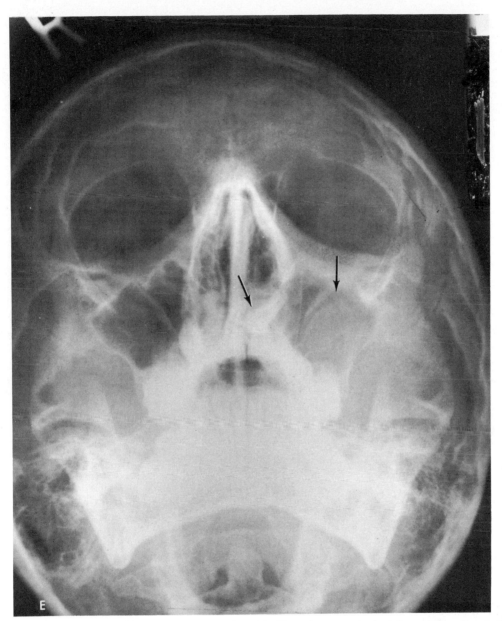

Figure 13–51 *(Continued.)* *E,* The Waters' view of the maxillary sinus reveals the left maxillary sinus to be very cloudy in comparison to the right. Within this area of the left maxillary sinus an unerupted cuspid is contained. This tumor was occupying the maxillary sinus.

(Figure 13–51 continued on following page)

showed a normal sinus rhythm with no murmurs. The lungs were clear and the reflexes were physiologic.

Laboratory Findings. There is a mild elevation of the white cell count to 10,000. All additional findings of hematology and urinalysis were within normal limits.

Radiographic Examination. Maxilla—The right maxilla showed normal dental development. On the left side a radiolucent area is discernible along the alveolar margin in the bicuspid region. This alveolar margin bulges slightly (Fig. 13–51A). The

crown of the left upper first bicuspid is enclosed within the radiolucent area. This tooth is unerupted. The upper left second bicuspid is erupted and lies along the posterior margin of the radiolucent area (Fig. 13–51B to D). There are also some radiolucent changes around the upper left cuspid which is unerupted and impacted with its crown close to the apex of the roots of the maxillary incisors. This tooth is angled toward the midline. The primary upper left cuspid remains in the alveolus. This area may well represent a dentigerous cyst. There is considerable clouding of the left maxillary

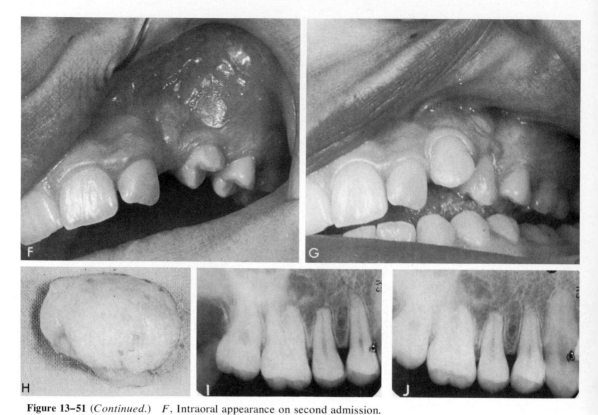

Figure 13–51 (*Continued.*)   *F*, Intraoral appearance on second admission.
G, Left maxillary cuspid and first bicuspid erupting into normal position.
H, Specimen from the left maxillary cuspid and bicuspid area at the second operation.
I and *J*, Radiographs of operative area showing eruption of teeth and normal healing of bone in the former tumor site.

antrum on the lateral projection. A rounded shadow is seen arising from the floor on the anterior wall of the left antrum (D. A. Huot, M.D.).

Preoperative Impression. Giant cell tumor of maxilla.

First Operation. A large semicircular incision was carried anteriorly high in the mucobuccal fold from the region of the left second molar to the crest of the ridge in the region of the cuspid. The incision then turned upward into the mucolabial fold, finally ending in the region of the left central incisor. The mucoperiosteum was reflected upward, revealing the thin, expanded buccal cortical plate. There were no areas of perforation. The thin alveolar bone was removed with rongeurs, exposing a whitish, firm tumor mass with irregular polypoid projections along its external surface. With careful blunt dissection, the mass was freed from its adjacent alveolar attachments and was enucleated from its bony crypt. The tumor measured approximately 4 by 3 cm. (Fig. 13–51*H*). Further examination of the bony defect revealed the permanent maxillary cuspid and first bicuspid to be displaced lingually and superiorly and the lateral wall of the maxillary sinus was exposed, thus revealing a large section of its intact membranous lining. The deciduous cuspid root, which was totally resorbed, was removed. The surgical defect

was then loosely filled with iodoform gauze and the mucoperiosteal flap was repositioned and closed with interrupted sutures of 000 black silk.

Postoperative Impression. Myxofibroma of the left maxilla.

Pathology Report. *Macroscopic:* This is an irregular, firm tumor measuring 3.5 by 2.5 by 2.5 cm., submitted in Formalin. Its external surface is dull, white, and shows irregular polypoid projections along one area. Its cut surface is smooth, glistening, pearly white, and shows fine trabeculations. There are several small areas of bone attached to the external surface, and a small 1- by 0.5-cm. area of cartilage on the external surface.

Microscopic: The sections show a uniform fibrous growth. In addition to spindle-shaped and fusiform fibroblasts there are a few large lymphocytes, macrophages and plasma cells. The matrix is loose reticular substance which is lightly basophilic.

Diagnosis: Myxoma of maxilla (R. S. Totten, M.D.).

Postoperative Course. A moderate amount of postoperative edema developed, although recovery continued uneventfully and the patient was discharged. The patient failed to return for follow-up observation.

Subsequent Course. Five years later, the patient was again admitted to Eye and Ear Hospital with a possible recurrence of the myxomatous lesion in the left maxilla. One month prior to this date she had developed a series of moderate headaches. Radiographic evidence suggested a possible recurrence of the myxoma (Fig. 13–51E). The oral examination revealed that the maxillary left cuspid and second bicuspid were not erupted (Fig. 13–51F). She was admitted to the hospital for observation, exploration and possible excision of the lesion.

Radiographic Findings. January 12—There is a large area of radiolucency beginning posterior to the maxillary left first bicuspid and continuing to the third molar area. The floor of the maxillary sinus on this side is very indistinct (Fig. 13–51E). The apical portion of the root of the maxillary left second bicuspid is incompletely developed. The maxillary right and left third molars are impacted and the mandibular right and left third molars are impacted.

Second Operation. A semicircular incision was made over the labial-cortical plate extending from the cuspid area to the first molar area and carrying the incision down to within 0.5 cm. of the gingival line in the premolar region. This flap was reflected and it was seen that a small portion of the labial cortical plate had been eroded by the tumor, the tumor tissue being visible in this area. The small opening was enlarged until a cavity approximately 1 cm. long by 0.5 cm. at its widest portion was exposed and a small apparent recurrent myxoma was removed with a curette. When this small recurrent myxoma was removed, it was observed in the depths of this bony crypt that there were apparently other myxomatous lesions beyond this particular area. The opening was enlarged and it was observed that a very large tumor mass elevated the floor of the maxillary sinus upward and forward, almost obliterating the antral cavity. As the myxoma was removed with large curettes the third molar was approached and it was apparent that this myxoma had originated from the impacted, unerupted maxillary third molar. An incision was made over the crown of the impacted third molar and the mucoperiosteum was reflected. Myxomatous tissue was found to be adherent to the third molar, filling this particular area as well as the area already described. The third molar was removed with the adjacent myxomatous tissue. The cavity was carefully explored for remnants of tumor tissue and none were found. Iodoform gauze was inserted into the large defect which measured approximately 5 cm. in length by 4 cm. at its greatest width. The mucoperiosteum was then repositioned and closed with a drain being permitted to protrude from beneath the flap.

Pathology Report. *Macroscopic:* The specimen is submitted in 2 parts: (1) Myxoma of left maxilla, (2) Polypoid tissue of maxilla. Part 1 consists of a multinodular mass of pale gray, semitranslucent tissue in about 8 pieces plus 1 molar tooth. The

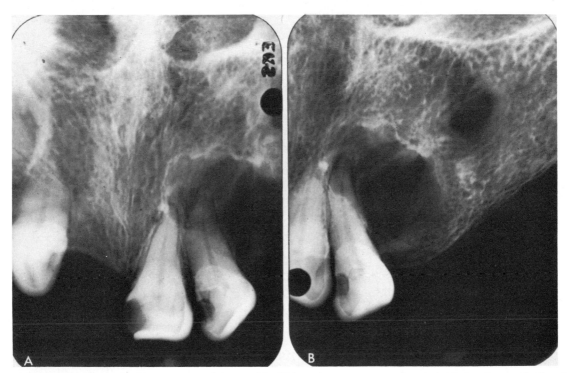

Figure 13–52 Recurrent fibromyxoma of the maxilla. This patient was operated on twice before by enucleation of the tumor and packing with iodoform gauze saturated with Carnoy's solution. This time a block section containing the central and lateral incisor and the tumor was excised.

soft tissue measures in aggregate 2 by 2 by 1.5 cm. and the tooth measures 1.1 cm. long and is 0.8 by 0.7 cm. in cross-section dimensions at the crown. To this is attached a small amount of tissue similar to that described above. The soft tissue has a large amount of tenacious, clear, mucoid material on it. Part 2 consists of a mass of multinodular blood-tinged, pale gray, firm, semitranslucent tissue in about 10 pieces.

Microscopic: Part 1 is composed entirely of a myxoid connective tissue with abundant fine fibrils interwoven so that the intervening substance appears vacuolated. Part 2 is similar to part 1.

Diagnosis: Myxoma of left maxilla (R. S. Totten, M.D.).

Postoperative Course. The patient's hospital course was uneventful and she was discharged to be followed as an outpatient. Subsequent intraoral photographs were taken. Within a year after the second operation the grossly impacted maxillary cuspid and the unerupted displaced first bicuspid had erupted into practically their normal positions in the arch without any orthodontic aid (Fig. 13–51*G*). See Figure 13–51*I* and *J* for the 1-year postoperative periapical radiographs.

Case Report No. 17

MYXOMA OF LEFT MAXILLA*

Patient. A 37-year-old white woman was admitted to the hospital for the removal of an impacted, unerupted maxillary left third molar and adjacent tumor.

History. The patient first noticed swelling and tenderness in the left posterior area of the maxilla 4 years previously. She reported this to her dentist, who neglected to radiograph the area. He stated that the maxillary left second molar was "pyorrhetic" and extracted the tooth. The patient recovered uneventfully, except that she noticed recurrent swelling and soreness of the area. One month prior to the present admission, swelling, larger than heretofore, developed in the left maxillary molar area which persisted for a longer period and was accompanied by pain which was

aggravated by swallowing. Antibiotic treatment effected a recovery. Radiographs taken of the area disclosed an impacted, unerupted maxillary left third molar and irregular radiopaque and radiolucent patterns anterior to the third molar (Fig. 13–53*A*). The patient was referred for surgery.

Examination. There were several swollen left submaxillary lymph nodes. Intraorally, the left maxillary molar area was expanded to the size of a walnut. The mucosal tissue appeared normal and light pink in color. The preoperative diagnosis was "impacted left maxillary third molar and a central

*From Archer, W. H.: Myxoma of left maxilla. Oral Surg., *13*:139–141(Feb.), 1960.

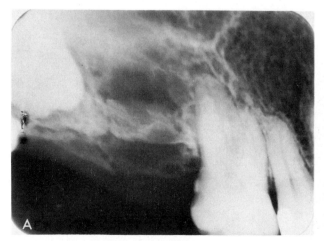
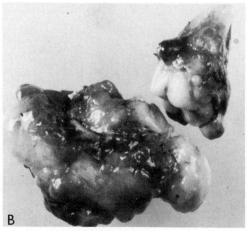

Figure 13–53 *A,* Radiograph reveals an unerupted maxillary third molar and irregular radiopaque and radiolucent areas suggestive of fibromyxoma or giant cell tumor. *B,* Maxillary third molar and myxoma enucleated from the left maxilla. See Case Report No. 17 for details.

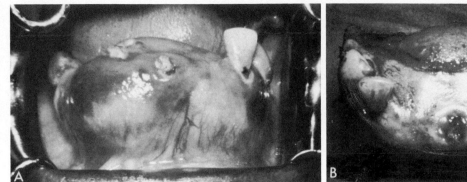

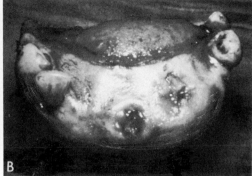

Figure 13–54   *A*, Odontogenic fibromyxoma (myxofibroma, odontogenic myxoma) of the anterior mandible. *B*, Tumor excised; note that it shells out easily. (Courtesy of Dr. Leo March.)

tumor anterior and superior to this tooth." It was believed that the tumor might be a fibromyxoma or a central giant cell tumor, with chronic secondary infection.

Surgical excision of the impacted, unerupted maxillary left third molar and of the tumor was recommended.

Operation.   Under thiopental sodium and nitrous oxide and oxygen anesthesia, a wide mucoperiosteal flap over the area was reflected with a periosteal elevator, exposing thin expanded cortical bone. Enough buccal bone was removed with a chisel and rongeurs to permit good visualization of the maxillary left third molar. The molar was eas-

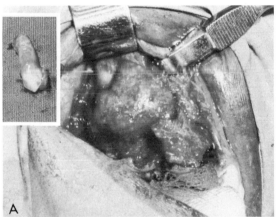

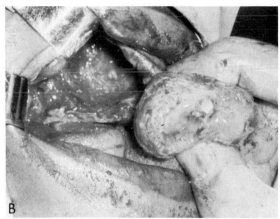

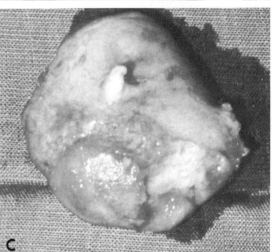

Figure 13–55   *A*, Mucoperiosteal tissue has been reflected, exposing the large anterior maxillary odontogenic myxofibroma. *B*, Tumor is easily shelled out of its bed. *C*, Tumor that contained several maxillary anterior teeth.

(See also Figure 12–91 for a case of an enormous odontogenic myxofibroma of the maxilla that had developed on the surface of a cyst because of the trauma of mastication.) (Courtesy of Dr. Leo March.)

ily removed with elevators. A cartilaginous, whitish, semifirm tumor was noted anterior to the third molar alveolus. The tumor was fully exposed by the removal of the thin cortical bone with which it was covered. Clinically, the tumor was considered to be a fibromyxoma. It was grasped with Allis forceps and enucleated with a periosteal elevator. The tumor extended to the floor of the maxillary sinus but not into it, although the intact lining membrane of the sinus was exposed. The tumor was approximately 3 cm. long and 2 cm. wide (Fig. 13–53B). The alveolus of the third molar was debrided; the flap was repositioned, and the wound was closed with 000 silk sutures. The tumor was sent to the pathology laboratory for histopathologic examination. The patient was removed from the operating room in good condition.

Pathology Report. The mass of tissue measured 3.0 by 1.5 by 1.5 cm. This material was jellylike at the edge with some harder or fibrous areas at the center. Actually, on section, areas that resembled cartilage were encountered.

Microscopic examination of the tumor showed it to be composed of myxomatous tissue in which there was a large amount of connective tissue matrix and intercellular substance. The nuclei were widely separated and were small and uniform.

Diagnosis. Myxoma (John C. Henthorne, M.D.).

Postoperative Course. The patient had an uneventful recovery and was discharged three days after admission. She was seen periodically for two years. The ridge was completely healed, with a wide depression marking the site of the tumor. There was no visual or radiographic evidence of a recurrence.

Case Report No. 18

MYXOFIBROSARCOMA OF THE MANDIBLE

Patient. A 55-year-old Negro male carpenter entered the Magee-Women's Hospital complaining of "burning at the right side of the face and swelling of the mouth."

History. About 2 months previously the patient had first noticed a small knot-like swelling on the right side of his face in the mental foramen region. It was not particularly painful but occasionally caused a burning sensation.

One month later he had visited his dentist, who had lanced the swelling intraorally. By this time it had grown larger. Blood had exuded from the incision, and the patient had been referred to the University of Pittsburgh School of Dentistry,

where a complete examination was performed. From there he was admitted to the hospital for further evaluation.

Physical Examination. Extraoral examination revealed swelling extending from the cuspid to the molar region, which was constantly burning and aching. The lower right side of his lip had a burning sensation also, but there was no paresthesia. This swelling was hard and firm, lying opposite the mandible. There were no palpable submaxillary nodes nor any submaxillary swelling.

On admission the patient's temperature was 99.4°F., pulse 88, respiration 20, and blood pressure 128/80. All laboratory examinations, which

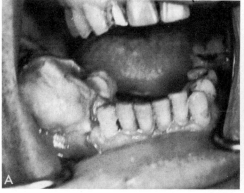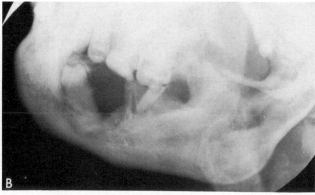

Figure 13–56 *A,* Fibrosarcoma of the mandible. (See Case Report No. 18 for more details.) *B* to *F,* Radiographs of the fibrosarcoma of the mandible. *G,* Note the arch bars attached to the maxilla and mandible. The tumor increased rapidly in size after the biopsy was taken. *H,* Resected body of the mandible, with tumor, from midline to the angle. *I,* Occlusal view of the tumor.

(*Figure 13–56 continued on opposite page*)

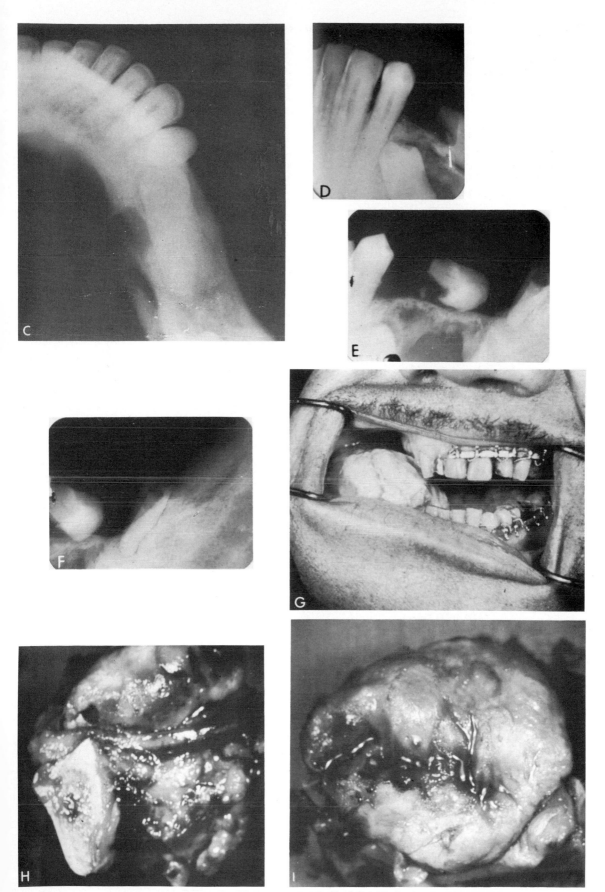

Figure 13–56. *(Continued.)*

included complete blood count, blood chemistry, serology and urinalysis, were within normal limits with the exception of a white blood count of 12,600 and hemoglobin value of 11.5 gm. (76 per cent).

Intraoral examination revealed a large swelling, 45 by 35 mm., extending from the mandibular right cuspid region to the second molar area (see Fig. 13–56A). It completely filled the mucobuccal fold and extruded over the remaining teeth. The mass reached the midregion of the cheek and interfered with occlusion. Imprints of the maxillary teeth could be seen at the superior portion. The growth had also caused an expansion of the lingual cortical plate and covered the first bicuspid. The mass was freely movable at the surface but was firmly attached at its base. It was soft when palpated but was not painful or tender. The edges were of a grayish slough. The patient's tongue was heavily coated with a brown discoloration that was probably due to his excessive smoking, and he complained of excessive salivation.

Radiographic Study. A long-bone survey and chest plate revealed no abnormalities. There was nothing suggestive of metastatic malignancy. Posteroanterior and left lateral views of the mandible were taken. The right half of the mandible showed a large ovoid radiolucent area extending from the ramus to the anterolateral border (Fig. 13–56B). This area was multiloculated and contained one complete bicuspid tooth and what appeared to be retained roots in the first and second molar regions (Fig. 13–56D to F). The mandible was hollowed out to a variable depth at the site of the bicuspid tooth. Almost the entire superoinferior dimension of the bone was eroded, so that only a thin shell remained at the inferior margin.

In addition to the teeth, the radiolucent area contained scattered densities having a granular appearance suggestive of debris. The compartments of the radiolucent area were sharply circumscribed in contour at the periphery, except at the anterolateral angle, where there was a suggestion of a break through the cortex into the medullary canal. The lingual cortex is sharply perforated (Fig. 13–56C). The interior of the cystic area contained islands of bone in the molar region. These changes were most suggestive of a dentigerous cyst, but it was difficult to exclude a malignant lesion.

Pathology Report. A biopsy was taken and on the following day the tumor had increased in size, and at the end of the fifth postoperative day it was at least five times its original dimensions (Fig. 13–56G). Pathology reports revealed the lesion to be a myxofibrosarcoma.

Treatment. Metallic arch bars were wired to the maxilla and the mandible as far as the midline on the left side. These were to be used for stabilization. A right mandibular resection from angle to midline was performed (Figs. 13–56H and I). Examination of the specimen showed an adjacent cervical node to be involved. Subsequently a right radical neck dissection was performed. Pathology studies revealed no evidence of metastasis of the primary sarcoma to the cervical region.

The postoperative course was uncomplicated. The left portion of the mandible was placed into occlusion and held by elastics attached between the arch bars. This method of stabilization was not satisfactory, and an acrylic splint was made which enabled the patient to open his mouth and to eat without having the left section swing to the midline.

ODONTOMA

The term "odontoma" has been applied to any growth originating from tooth structures, or from those embryonal structures from which the tooth develops. Cahn[15] classifies these tumors as hard or soft.

Soft Odontoma. The soft odontoma is a growth made up of cells that form enamel, dentine and cementum in which no actual tooth substance (enamel, cementum or dentine) is produced. When islands and strands of enamel epithelium are found in the mesenchymal matrix, it is difficult to distinguish these structures from those found in the ameloblastoma.

The reader is referred to oral pathology texts[75, 90] for a detailed description of these epithelial odontogenic tumors.

Hard Odontoma. Hard odontomas include radicular odontoma, cementoma, compound odontoma, complex odontoma, cystic odontoma, and geminated odontoma.

The radicular odontomas in the gross have the typical appearance of a tooth with apical excementosis. On sectioning the tooth it will be observed that the bulbous apical third of the root is made up of dentine, cementum and enamel. Figure 13–57 is an unusual radicular odontoma. In this case the entire root is made up of a mass of dentine, enamel and cementum.

COMPOUND ODONTOMA

The compound odontoma is made up of many rudimentary diminutive tooth forms

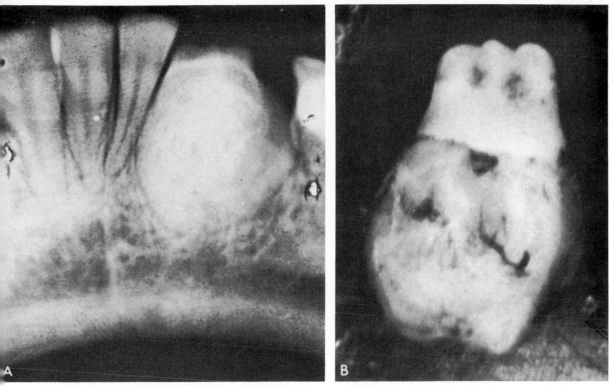

Figure 13–57 An unusual radicular odontoma (see text). *A*, Radiograph of the odontoma in place. *B*, Photograph of the specimen after removal. Note the convolutions of the various tooth elements that make up the abnormal root. (Courtesy of Dr. Harry J. Field, Newark, N.J.)

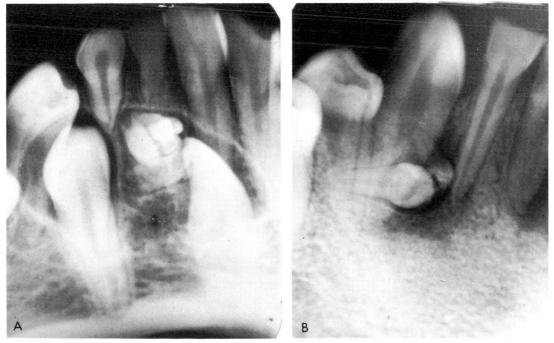

Figure 13–58 *A*, This small cystic odontoma, located in the anterior region of the mandible beneath the deciduous lateral and cuspid teeth, was found in a 6-year-old child. The dentigerous cysts (right and left) were separate and distinct cysts and did not communicate with the cystic odontoma. In this particular patient the cystic odontoma was removed, the unerupted cuspid and lateral incisor, whose eruption had been prevented by the cystic odontoma, were both marsupialized, and eventually the teeth erupted to a point from which they could be moved by the orthodontist into their normal positions in the arch.

B, A small cystic odontoma containing a rudimentary lateral incisor and cuspid located in the anterior region of the mandible in a 12-year-old child. The cyst and supernumerary teeth were removed. One might actually consider this as a dentigerous cyst.

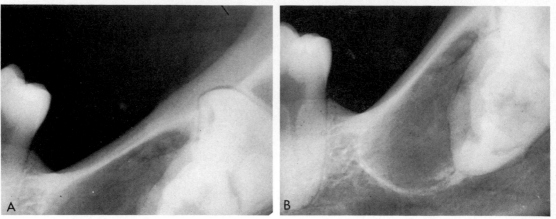

Figure 13–59 *A* and *B*, Periapical radiographs of the molar area in a 26-year-old male that reveal a compound complex cystic odontoma. Treatment was excision of the odontoma together with the cyst wall.

complete with enamel crowns and cementum-covered roots and is frequently associated with unerupted teeth. The normal enamel organ splits into many small enamel organs, which in turn develop into miniature tooth-forming organs, which then produce the rudimentary tooth forms. Frequently they are small masses of tooth structure with no resemblance to a normal tooth. They are generally united by fibrous connective tissue.

These tumors do not increase in size once the various elements have formed calcified masses.

Treatment. Treatment of the compound odontoma includes surgical removal, with care being taken not to disturb the unerupted tooth or teeth.

Figure 13–61 illustrates the technique for the surgical removal of a compound odontoma. In this patient, a labially malposed lateral in-

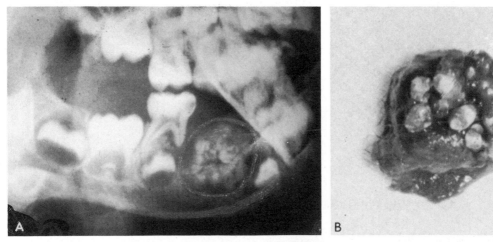

Figure 13–60 *A*, A cystic odontoma in the body of the mandible in a 5-year-old child. *B*, The specimen after excision and after the superior surface of the cyst wall was removed. Inside we see multiple rudimentary supernumerary teeth. (Courtesy of Dr. Leo March.)

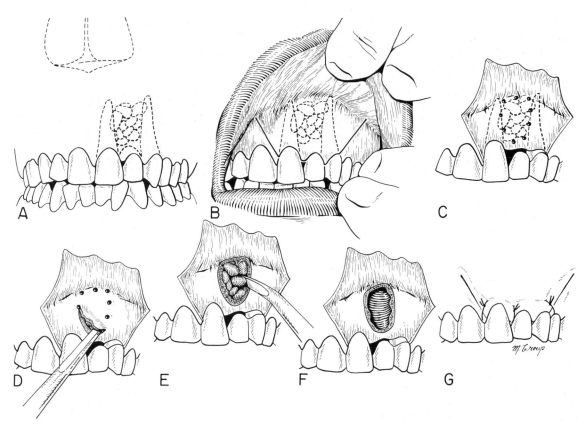

Figure 13-61 Removal of a compound odontoma. A, Position of tumor beneath a bridge pontic. B, Flap outlined. C, Flap reflected and holes drilled in cortex, avoiding the roots of the adjacent teeth. D, Connecting holes with chisel to remove bone. E, Multiple components and fibrous connective tissue enucleated. F, Area thoroughly debrided of all tissue and rudimentary teeth. G, Flap sutured.

cisor, which had been deflected from its normal path of eruption by this tumor, had been extracted several years prior to this operation and a bridge constructed. Radiographs were not taken before the extraction.

Figures 13-62 to 13-67 illustrate examples of compound odontoma.

COMPLEX ODONTOMA

This tumor does not have the appearance of tooth structure, but is a semi-round, hard, calcified mass of enamel, dentine and cementum mixed together without the anatomic arrangement found in normal tooth structure. Generally there is associated with this mass a normal tooth which has been displaced and its eruption prevented. These tumors vary in size from 0.5 cm. to 5 cm. in circumference. They expand and thin out the cortical plates of bone even to the extent of complete destruction of the cortical bone.

Treatment. These tumors are surrounded by a thin membrane and when small shell out easily, once the overlying bone has been removed to the circumference of the tumor. However, when large and irregular in outline, they must be sectioned and removed in small segments, because a fracture of the mandible or maxilla would result if an attempt were made to elevate the entire mass from its crypt. (See Figure 13-73.)

CEMENTIFYING FIBROMA (CEMENTOMA)

A cementoma appears on the radiograph in the early stage of its development as a radiolucent area about the apex of a vital tooth, most frequently a mandibular incisor. It is also called a "periapical osteofibrosis" or "periapical fibrous dysplasia." The vitality test will rule out the possibilities that the radiolucent area is filled with granulation tis-

(Text continued on page 775)

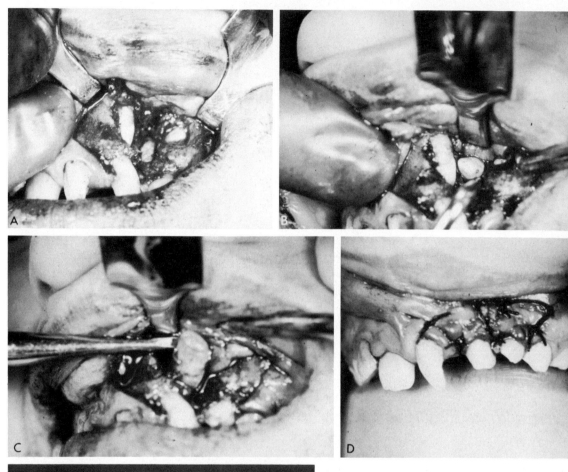

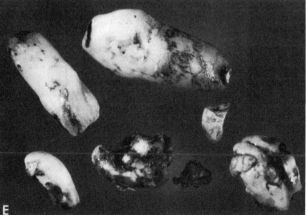

Figure 13–62 Removal of a compound odontoma, according to the technique in Figure 13–61. *A,* Labial flap reflected. Labial cortical bone removed and exposure of some of the rudimentary tooth forms. *B,* Elevation of one of the larger mesiodentes in this compound odontoma of the anterior maxilla. *C,* Removal of a large rudimentary tooth form; care was taken, of course, not to disturb the teeth that had erupted, even though they were also devoid of a normal crown. They can be crowned to restore a normal appearance. *D,* Tooth forms, single and fused, that were removed from this patient.

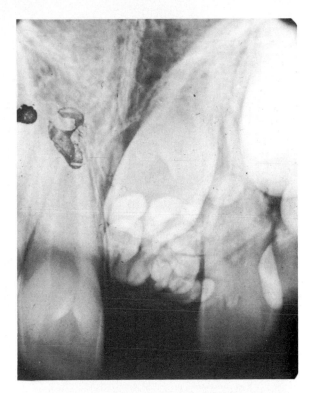

Figure 13-63 Compound odontoma in the right central incisor area. The eruption of the central incisor has been prevented.

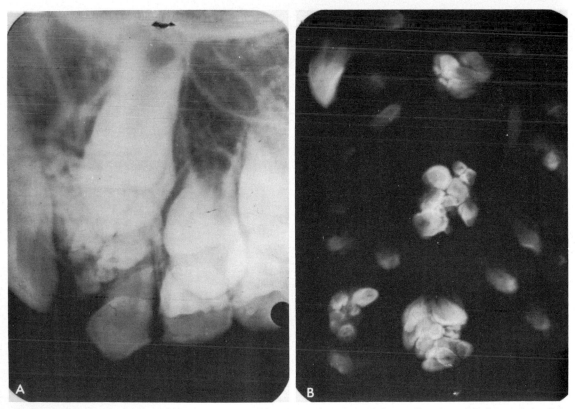

Figure 13-64 Cystic composite odontoma preventing the eruption of the right maxillary lateral incisor and the right cuspid.

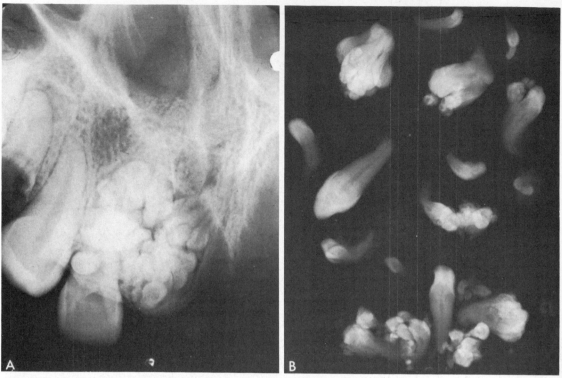

Figure 13–65 *A,* Large compound odontoma of the anterior maxilla. *B,* Specimens, single and fused, of small and large rudimentary tooth forms removed from their bed in the maxilla.

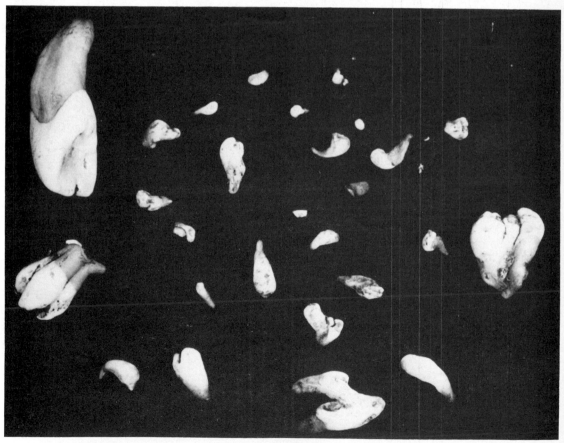

Figure 13–66 *See opposite page for legend.*

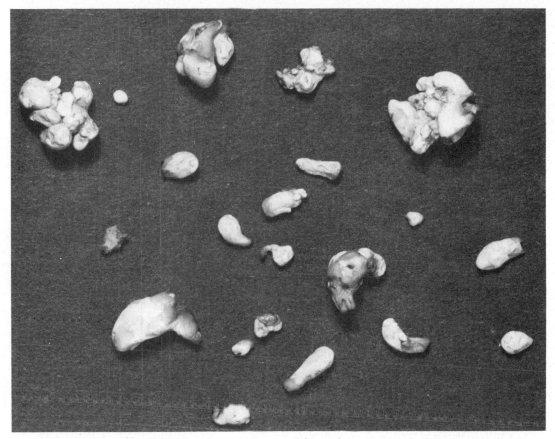

Figure 13–67 More than 60 rudimentary teeth removed from a large compound odontoma in the maxilla.

sue or that it is a small radicular cyst because in these cases the teeth are nonvital. Eventually the fibrous tissue in these areas is replaced by cementum (see Figures 13–75 to 13–80). Occasionally multiple cementomas involve a considerable area of bone.

Treatment. There is no indication for the removal of these tumors unless they are distorting an edentulous area and would produce "high spots" which would interfere with denture comfort.

GEMINATED ODONTOMA

When two buds and subsequently two enamel organs are given off from the same epithelial cord of a primary tooth, the result is the formation of two similar separate teeth or a single oversize tooth from the simultaneous development of the two teeth which fuse from incisal edge to the apex (see Figures 2–99 and 2–125). This development is known as *gemination* (twin teeth), and the end result is known as a geminated odontoma. This condition should be differentiated from concrescence (see following section).

HYPERPLASIA OF THE CEMENTUM

A diffuse thickening of the cementum over the entire root may take place. This is known as *hypercementosis.*

A localized area of thickening of the cementum may take place, usually about the apex of the tooth. This is known as *excementosis.*

Figure 13–66 Small and large, single and fused, rudimentary tooth forms removed from a large compound odontoma.

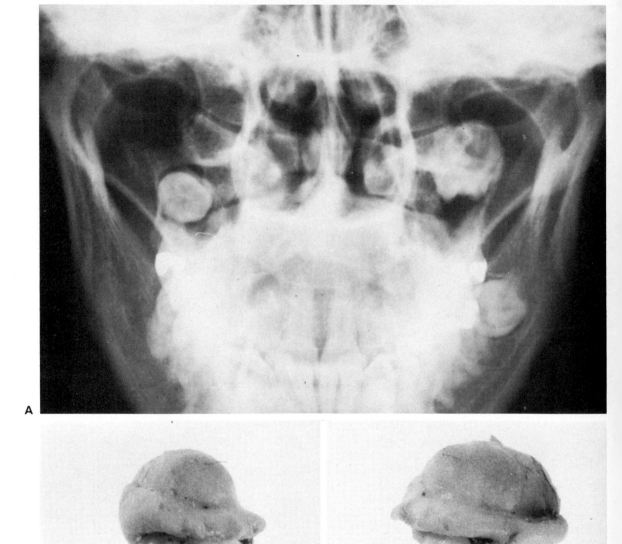

Figure 13–68 *A*, This large cystic odontoma was located in the maxillary sinus. *B*, The complex odontoma after removal.

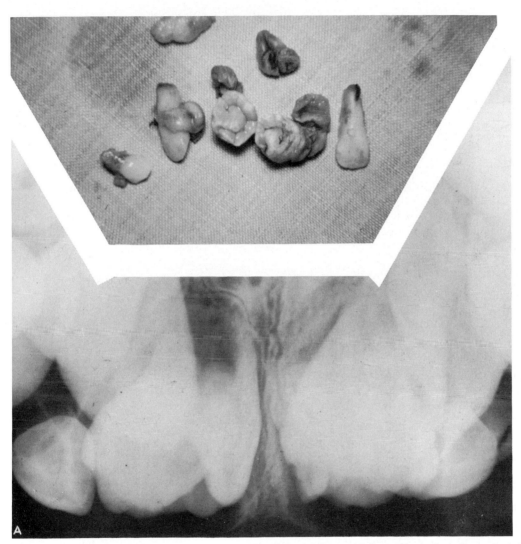

Figure 13–69   *A*, Compound odontoma (*above*) containing bilateral dentes in dente (shown in radiograph, *below*), which were removed from the anterior maxilla of an 8-year-old.

(*Figure 13–69 continued on following page*)

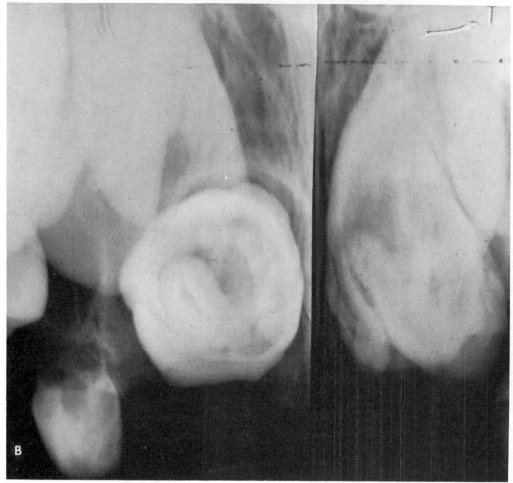

Figure 13–69 (*Continued.*)   B, Anterior maxillary radiographs clearly reveal the structure of the bilateral mesiodentes.

(*Figure 13–69 continued on opposite page*)

The additional layers of cementum are laid down as the result of irritation from either a low-grade infection or the degree of traumatic stress to which the tooth has been subjected.

The presence of hyperplasia of the cementum is revealed by the radiograph. These teeth, when extracted, must first have sufficient bone removed about the root to permit delivery of the tooth without fracturing a large segment of alveolar bone, or perhaps fracturing the maxillary tuberosity and the floor of the maxillary sinus.

CONCRESCENCE

Concrescence is the fusion of the cementum of the roots of normally developing teeth whose tooth-forming organs are in contact at the time this portion of the tooth structure is being laid down. Figure 2–98 shows examples of concrescence.

FIBROMA

The fibroma is a benign, well-defined connective tissue tumor, either pedunculated or sessile, frequently found in the oral cavity. Fibromas are either soft or hard in consistency. The hard fibromas have a white to grayish stroma of connective tissue made up principally of thick interlacing bundles of collagen fibers. In the soft fibroma, there is a greater vascularity and the collagen fibers are loosely arranged.

Fibromas arise from the deep layers of the mucosa or from the periosteum of the jaws. Hard fibromas of the sessile type that are

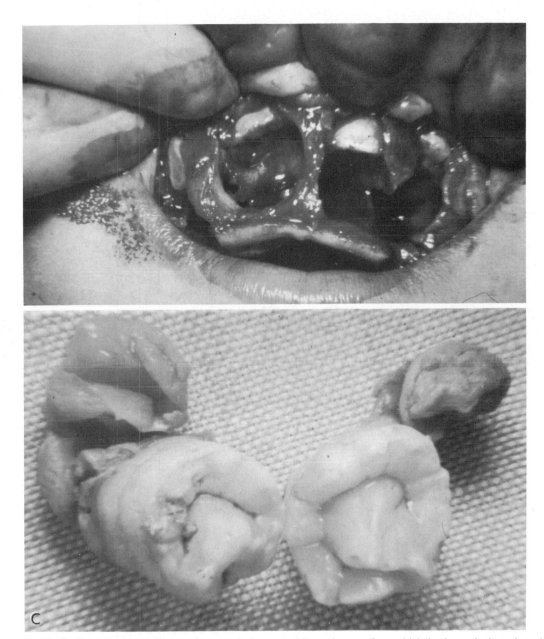

Figure 13-69 *(Continued.)* *C,* Upper photograph shows the bilateral crypts from which the dentes in dente have been removed; these are shown in the lower photograph. In the upper photograph note the incisal thirds of the right and left maxillary incisors, whose normal eruption was prevented by the odontomas. (Courtesy of H. Serrano Roa, D.D.S.)

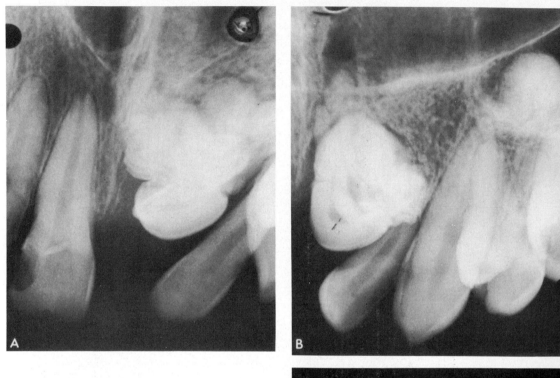

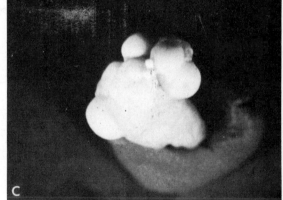

Figure 13–70 *A* and *B*, Radiographs of a compound odontoma of the anterior maxilla. *C*, Odontoma after removal.

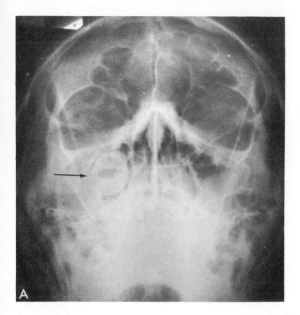

A

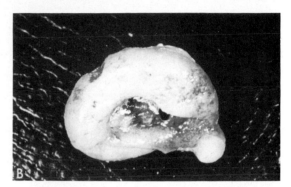

B

Figure 13–71 *A,* Ameloblastic fibro-odontoma in the right maxillary sinus. Note the well-circumscribed radiolucent area (*arrow*) containing a single large, round radiopaque mass. Tissue typical of an ameloblastic fibroma surrounded the odontoma.

B, The unusually shaped odontoma, an admixture of dental tissues. The concavity in the center contains some of the tumor tissue. *Treatment:* Enucleation. These tumors do not invade bone locally, nor do they recur.

located around the necks of the teeth frequently extend through the interproximal space to the lingual, labial or buccal surfaces. These tumors arise not only from the periosteum, but from the periodontal membrane as well. This fact must be kept in mind when removing these tumors, or there will be recurrences. The technique for treatment of these tumors is discussed in the legends to Figures 13–82 and 13–83.

(*Text continued on page 791*)

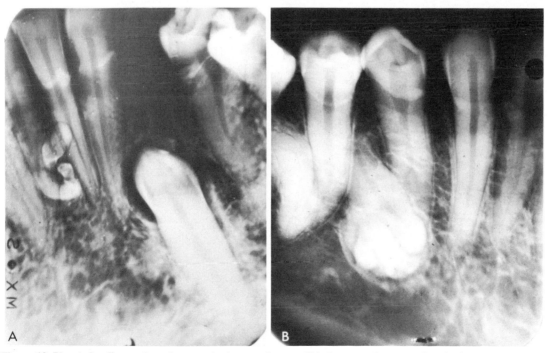

A   B

Figure 13–72 *A,* Small complex odontoma in the anterior mandible between the roots of the incisors. *B,* Compound odontoma between the mandibular bicuspids.

EXCISION OF A LARGE MANDIBULAR COMPLEX ODONTOMA AND IMPACTED SECOND MOLAR

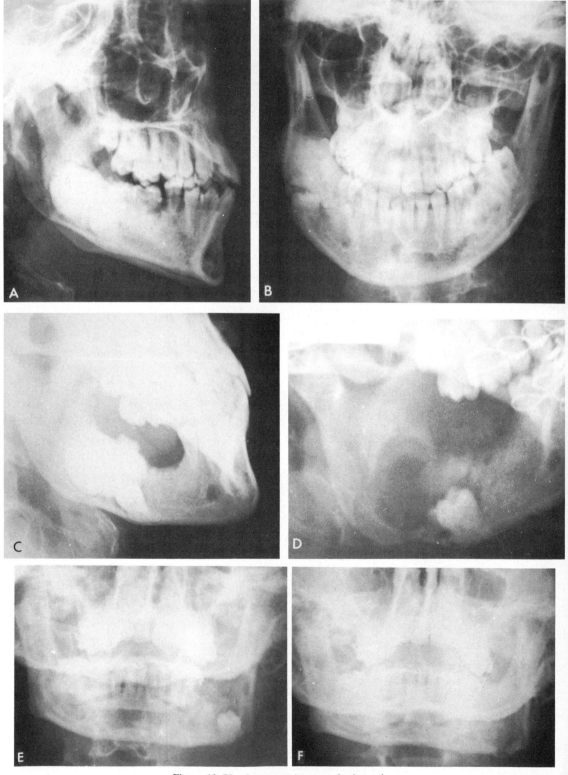

Figure 13–73 *See opposite page for legend.*

(*Figure 13–73 continued on opposite page*)

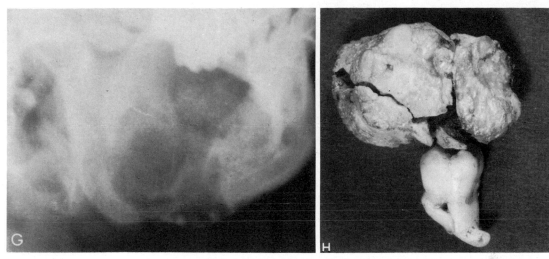

Figure 13–73   (*Continued.*)

Figure 13–73   *A*, A true lateral jaw film in which the opposite horizontal ramus was superimposed over the horizontal ramus containing the complex odontoma and tooth showed that superiorly and inferiorly there was only a thin margin of cortical bone at the inferior border of the mandible. This view made it clear that extreme care had to be taken to prevent a fracture of the mandible when removing this tumor. It is equally apparent that this tumor could not be "shelled out" but had to be carefully sectioned with crosscut fissure burs and removed a section at a time.

B, Posteroanterior view of the mandible, showing the bulging and thinning of the buccal cortical plate. As already stated, a large portion of the lingual cortical plate had been destroyed.

C, Lateral jaw radiograph of a large complex odontoma and unerupted impacted second molar lying at the inferior border of the mandible, in a female patient 18 years of age. In this case the lingual cortical plate of bone was completely destroyed by pressure atrophy. The covering mucosa became irritated and inflamed, bacteria from the oral cavity gained entrance into the sublingual and submaxillary spaces, and abscesses in these areas developed, necessitating intraoral incision and drainage.

D, It was anticipated that a fracture of the mandible would most likely occur during removal of the tumor; hence, prior to the first operation, Stout wiring for fracture reduction was placed around the maxillary and mandibular teeth so that intermaxillary elastics could readily be placed if a fracture should occur, in spite of all precautions taken to prevent such an event. The posterior fragment would have to be reduced and fixed in position with extraoral fixation. This, plus intermaxillary elastics, would have been the combined treatment necessary to secure a good result.

In this figure the cavity in the mandible following the removal of the complex odontoma is shown. To remove this tumor three separate operative periods of 1 hour each of careful cutting with crosscut burs were necessary. Considerable hemorrhage from the inferior alveolar artery was encountered when the distal inferior section of the tumor was removed. This was controlled by careful packing plus finger pressure along the internal surface of the ramus in the vicinity of the mandibular sulcus.

Second molar was removed a week later.

E, Posteroanterior view of the mandible, showing the complex odontoma removed, but the second molar still in position.

F, Posteroanterior view of the mandible immediately after the removal of the complex odontoma and second molar. Note the thin osseous inferior border of the mandible.

G, Lateral jaw radiograph showing the complete removal of the complex odontoma and the second molar without fracture of the mandible. This was a matter of good luck as well as a slow and careful technique. As can be seen in this radiograph, there were several spots along the inferior mandibular border in which the cortical bone had been eroded. The patient was placed on a liquid diet for several weeks and then on a soft diet. She was warned explicitly what would happen if she violated these instructions. She was also urged to be exceedingly careful to avoid any form of trauma to her jaw. Intermaxillary elastics were not placed on her jaws, but the wiring was left in place for 3 months before removal.

H, Photograph of the complex odontoma and second molar after removal. Some pieces are missing, since they were sectioned.

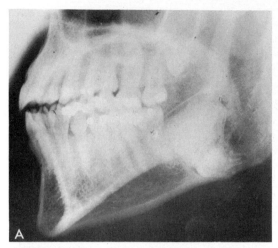

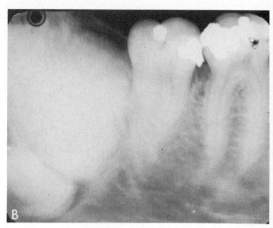

Figure 13–74 *A,* Oblique radiograph showing an ameloblastic odontoma, in agreement with the pathologist's report on the soft tissue surrounding the superior aspect of the compound odontoma. *B,* Periapical radiograph of an ameloblastic odontoma.

Treatment: Controversial. Radical excision of a portion of the mandible is advocated by some. Others, including myself, elect conservative *enucleation.* This is done by cutting the dental tissues into sections, as is done with large odontomas, and removing them in sections, along with the investing soft tissues. Those that I have treated were not invasive of the surrounding bone and "shelled out" easily. They are followed for several years by radiographic examination. I have not seen a recurrence. If there were, then radical surgery could be carried out.

(*A,* Courtesy of Dr. Herbert A. Eckert.)

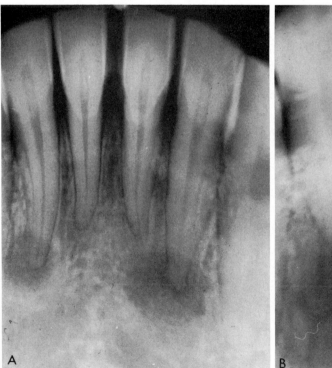

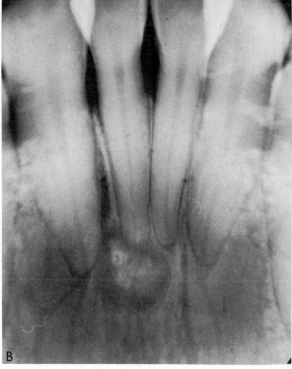

Figure 13–75 *A,* Soft periapical osteofibrosis. *B* and *C,* Cementomas at the apices of the lower incisors. All these teeth were vital. The osteolytic stage is shown at the apex of the right lateral incisor in *C.* The tumor here is composed of cellular tissue that grows at the expense of bone. The tumor about the apices of the left central and lateral incisors has reached the cementoblastic stage in which the tumor has started to form cementum.

(*Figure 13–75 continued on opposite page*)

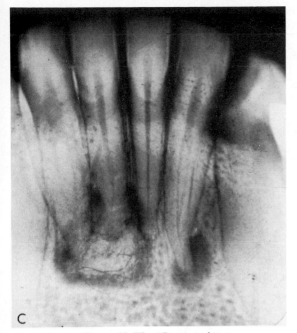

C

Figure 13-75 *(Continued.)*

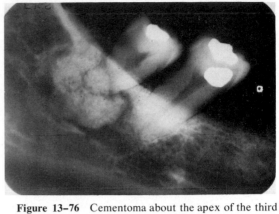

Figure 13-76 Cementoma about the apex of the third molar. This tumor is in the cementoblastic stage.

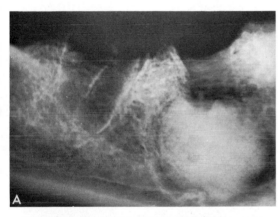

A

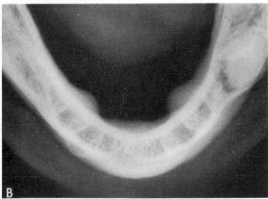

B

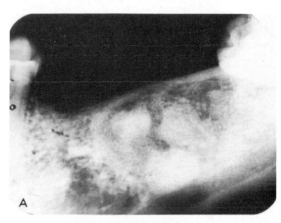

A

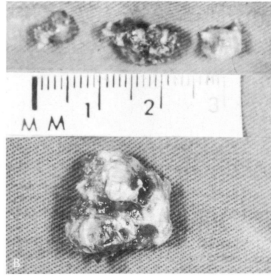

B

Figure 13-77 *A,* Large, well-circumscribed cementoma beneath the alveolus of a recently extracted molar. The ovoid dense radiopaque area is surrounded by a band of varying radiolucent areas. The band is the diagnostic clue that this is a cementoma and not condensing osteitis, osteosclerosis or endostosis, which are continuous with the surrounding osseous tissue. *B,* Occlusal view that discloses buccal expansion due to the growth of the cementoma.

Figure 13-78 *A,* Multiple cementomas in the body of the mandible. These are in the cementoblastic stage in which the tumor has started to form cementum. *B,* Cementomas removed.

785

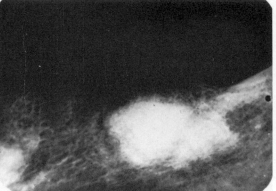

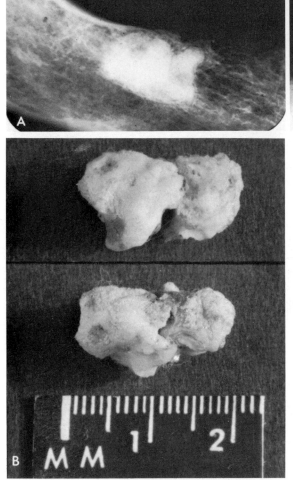

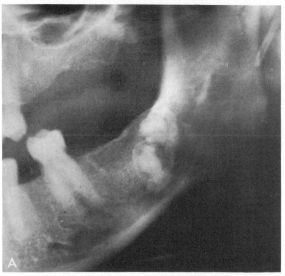

Figure 13–79 *A*, Cementomas in the right and left bodies of an edentulous mandible. *B*, Cementomas after surgical excision.

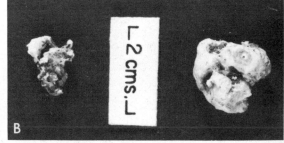

Figure 13–80 *A*, Growing mandibular cementomas. *B*, Cementomas that were removed.

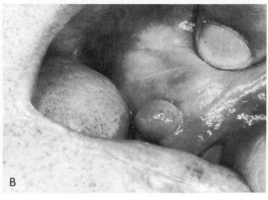

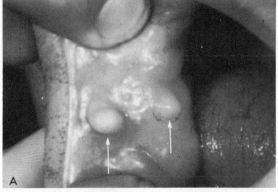

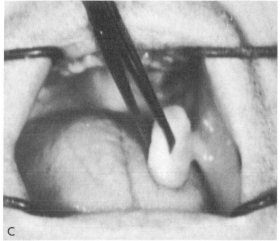

Figure 13-81 *A*, In this unusual case there are two fibromas. The one near the commissure of the lip is firm and well developed. Just posteriorly is another smaller fibroma in the early stages of development. It is softer and does not have a pedunculated base as yet. *B*, A hard pedunculated fibroma, illustrating how spherical these tumors can become. This fibroma arises from the mucosa just above the mucobuccal fold. Note the relationship of the tumor to the crest of the edentulous mandibular ridge, and the smooth, shiny surface. *C*, A large pedunculated fibroma of the cheek.

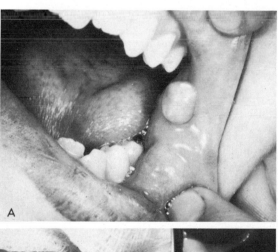

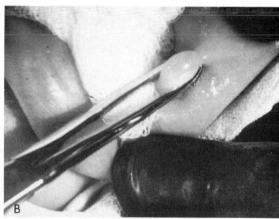

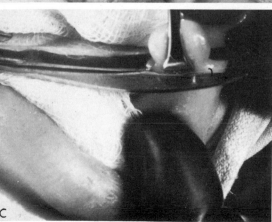

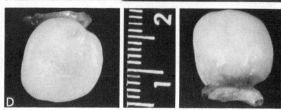

Figure 13-82 *A*, Another example of the typical semihard, sessile spherical fibroma of the cheek. *B*, The fibroma flattens easily when grasped with the Allis forceps. *C*, With the scissors cutting between the jaws of the Allis forceps and the buccal mucosa the tumor is excised, and the buccal mucosa is closed with silk sutures. *D*, Resected specimens.

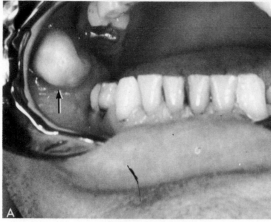

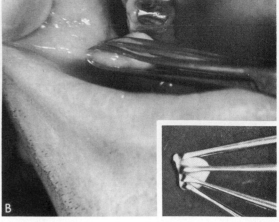

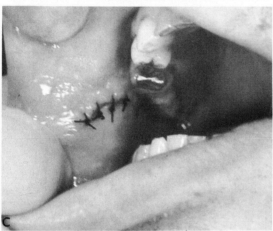

Figure 13–83 *A*, A semispherical soft fibroma of the mucosa of the right cheek. Note the indentation in the upper portion caused by the pressure of the maxillary first molar on the tumor. It is apparent that because of the location of these tumors they may become traumatized and ulcerated. That this condition is not seen more frequently is surprising.

B, After infiltrating the base of the pedicle with local anesthetic solution, the base of the pedicle is grasped with a series of Allis forceps. Make certain that the orifice or any portion of the parotid (Stensen's) duct has not inadvertently been grasped by an Allis forceps. If the tumor is situated where this possibly might occur, then a filiform bougie, or soft metal probe, should first be passed into the duct before grasping the fibroma. Note how readily this soft fibroma flattens out under the Allis forceps. Hard fibromas do not compress this readily. *Inset:* Soft fibroma after removal, showing the manner in which Allis forceps are attached to the base.

C, With the No. 9 Dean's scissors sever the pedicle along the edge of the Allis forceps. Caution the assistant not to create traction on the handles of the Allis forceps during this procedure, but to hold the forceps still; otherwise a large section of mucosa will be cut away. The edges of the mucosa are then undermined and approximated with interrupted silk sutures.

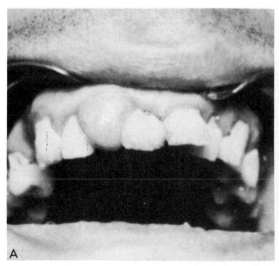

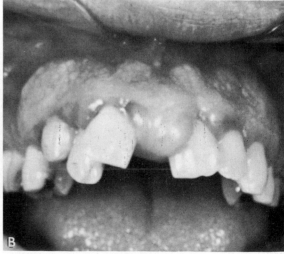

Figure 13–84 *A*, This sessile hard fibroma in this male adult had been present for over 5 years, according to the patient. It had been growing slowly, gradually displacing the left central incisor, and had pushed the left central incisor labially and the left lateral incisor lingually. Note, however, that the pressure of the growing fibroma did not displace the right lateral incisor, which was backed up by the cuspid with its long and firmly embedded root.

(Figure 13–84 continued on opposite page)

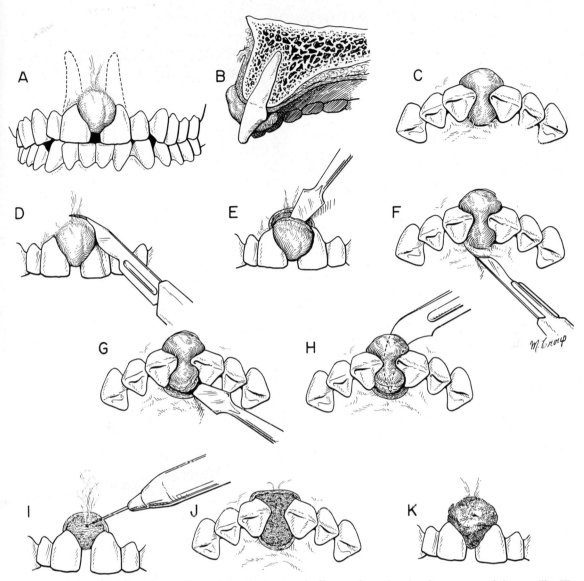

Figure 13–85 Excision of a sessile peripheral odontogenic fibroma from the alveolar process of the maxilla. The fibroma was located between the central incisors, thus producing a diastema. *A,* Anterior view of lesion. *B,* Cross-sectional view of the lesion. *C,* Occlusal view of lesion. *D* to *G,* An incision is made down to the bone on the labial and palatal aspects (with a No. 15 BP scalpel) and the mass elevated away from the bone with a periosteal elevator. *H,* The interproximal attachments are incised with a No. 12 BP scalpel and the lesion removed *in toto.* *I,* The bone is fulgurated to remove any remnants of the lesion. Extreme care must be observed to destroy all tumor tissue around the cervical line of the incisors. *J,* Area following fulguration. *K,* Fulgurated area covered with protective pack of cotton fibers, zinc oxide and eugenol. Dressing left in place 2 weeks.

Figure 13–84 *(Continued.)*

The poor oral hygiene is very apparent. There was destruction of the gingival third of the interseptal bone between the right lateral and central incisors. This was thought, however, to be due to periodontal disease, which was prevalent in this mouth, and not to the fibroma.

While some fibromas have invasive tendencies, this is the exception rather than the rule. The opposite is true with peripheral giant cell tumors.

B, Another example of a sessile hard fibroma (peripheral odontogenic fibroma), in this case between the maxillary central incisors. Note the separation of the incisors.

EXCISION OF A FIBROMA FROM THE ALVEOLAR PROCESS OF THE MAXILLA

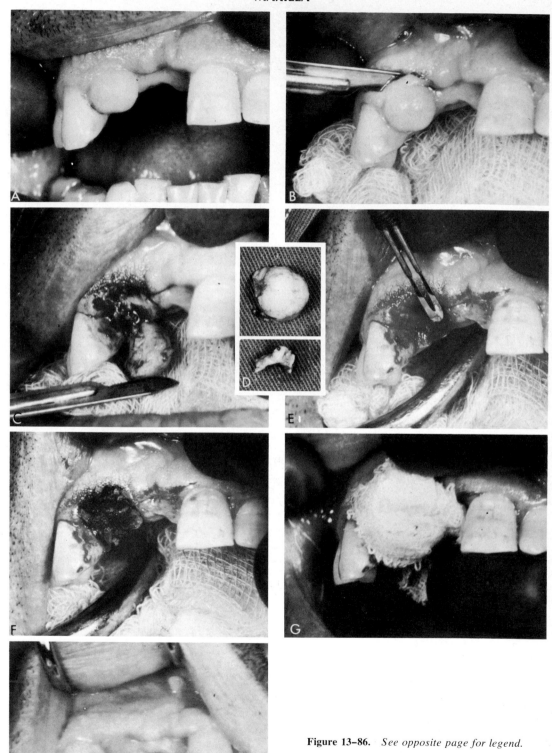

Figure 13–86. *See opposite page for legend.*

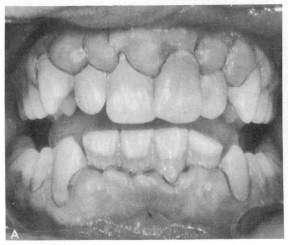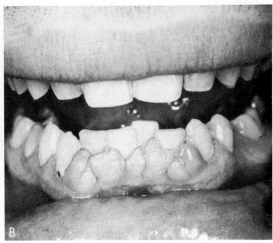

Figure 13-87 Labial fibromatosis gingivae around the necks of the maxillary and mandibular six anterior teeth. The irregularity of these teeth facilitated the retention of food debris and this, with poor patient oral hygiene, caused chronic irritation and inflammation of the gingival tissues, resulting in the very evident chronic gingival fibromatosis. Treatment indicated is prophylactic therapy followed by daily oral hygiene. When the chronic irritation is removed, a gingivectomy is indicated. (See Figure 13-90.)

The most common site is probably the cheek (Figs. 13-81 to 13-83). When fibromas occur here, they are pedunculated spherical tumors covered by smooth, normally pink mucosa. They may be caused by cheek biting, are slow-growing and may attain the size of a walnut.

Fibrosarcoma, the malignant counterpart of the fibroma, is rare in the oral cavity (see Figure 13-200 and the accompanying case report).

BENIGN NEUROGENIC TUMORS

Tumors of nerve tissue may arise from the nerve sheaths—endoneurium, perineurium (*Text continued on page 799*)

Figure 13-86 *A,* This patient had been advised that if the adjacent teeth were removed, this tumor (peripheral odontogenic fibroma) would disappear. When this prophecy failed to materialize, the patient sought relief elsewhere.

This hard, spherical fibroma had its origin in the periosteum and the periodontal membrane. Tumors in this area have the highest rate of recurrence simply because the entire base has not been removed or destroyed. This is due to the difficulty of gaining access to the entire base when the teeth are present.

For this reason some oral surgeons advise, in the treatment of these tumors, removal of adjacent teeth and then removal of the fibroma. This is unnecessary.

The author never extracts the adjacent teeth in these cases *unless* there is a definite indication for their extraction, such as extensive destruction of interseptal bone, which is occasionally seen. It is possible to remove these tumors carefully with the knife and then to destroy every cell that has been missed, by use of appropriate-sized electric cauteries that will fit into the interproximal spaces. When this is done carefully and thoroughly, there will not be a recurrence and valuable functioning teeth are saved.

B, With a small sharp knife—the No. 15 Bard-Parker blade is used here—an incision is made several millimeters beyond the base of the tumor completely through the mucoperiosteal membrane, firmly contacting bone entirely around the fibroma. *C,* The tumor turned back from its base. *D,* Tumor after removal. An additional small piece of tissue was removed on the palatal side to make certain that the entire base was removed. *E,* The osseous base and soft tissue periphery are cauterized. Extreme care must be taken to cauterize the periodontal membrane carefully and thoroughly without overheating the tooth or teeth in those patients in whom two or more teeth are present. *F,* The base has been adequately cauterized. This, of course, means that a thin sequestrum of bone will eventually be cast off, but it also means that the possibility of recurrence of the fibroma is remote. *G,* Iodoform gauze coated with zinc oxide and eugenol is packed over the operative site. This reduces the postoperative pain. *H,* Postoperative view after healing of ridge.

Note: While the actual cautery was used in this case, the fulguration current is equally effective, and there is less danger of destroying too much bone. COAGULATING CURRENTS REQUIRE EXTREME CAUTION IN THEIR USE TO AVOID EXCESSIVE LOSS OF BONE.

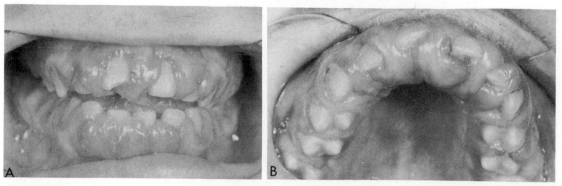

Figure 13–88 *A,* Massive gingival fibrous hyperplasia in an 18-year-old epileptic female who, for the past 14 years, has been receiving diphenylhydantoin sodium therapy. *B,* The disfiguring growths have separated and displaced both maxillary and mandibular teeth, producing malocclusion. These growths should have been periodically reduced during the past, thus preventing the present condition.

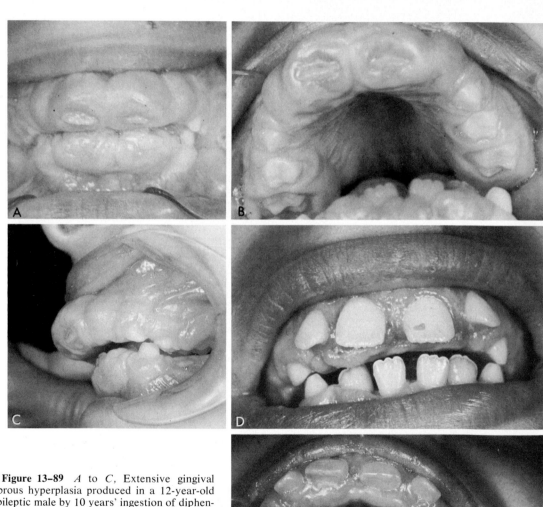

Figure 13–89 *A* to *C,* Extensive gingival fibrous hyperplasia produced in a 12-year-old epileptic male by 10 years' ingestion of diphenylhydantoin sodium. The teeth are practically completely covered with the growth, which has grossly displaced them. Note the marked overjet and overbite. *D* and *E,* The appearance of the teeth and gingival tissue 4 weeks after surgical excision of the hyperplasia by the technique described in Figure 13–90. As the hyperplasia recurs it will be excised as soon as it extends 2 mm. beyond the gingival line.

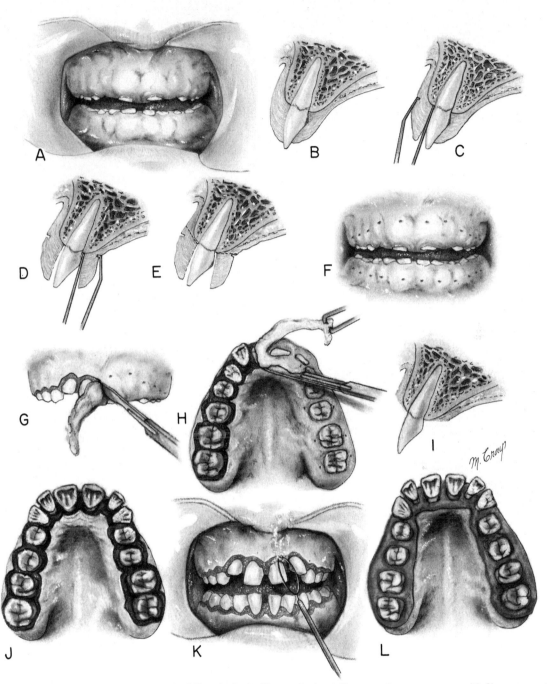

Figure 13-90 Technique for removal of fibrous gingival hyperplasia. *A*, Preoperative appearance, with fibrous growth covering all but incisal edges and occlusal surfaces of teeth. *B*, Cross section, showing massive growth practically covering maxillary central incisor. *C*, The straignt tip of a Crane-Kaplan pocket marker is inserted along the labial, buccal and lingual surfaces of each tooth to the depth of the hyperplastic growth. *D* and *E*, The instrument is now compressed, and the sharp right-angle tip cuts into the fibrous tissue, creating a bleeding point. *F*, The line of nicks corresponds to the gingival line, which is the termination line for the labial, buccal and lingual incisions. *G* and *H*, These incisions are made on both sides of the arches with the No. 15 Bard-Parker scalpel, starting the cut 3 mm. *above* the line of nicks and beveling toward the gingival line, producing a slanted incision. *I* and *J*, The incisions through the interseptal spaces are completed with the No. 12 Bard-Parker hook-shaped scalpel. *K*, Additional beveling is carried out with a radio-surgical knife. Exactly the same procedure is carried out on the mandible.

L, After this procedure, a thick mixture of eugenol and zinc oxide powder into which cotton fibers are incorporated is placed around the necks of the teeth to cover the exposed raw surface. This medicated cement dressing is allowed to remain in place for 96 hours, at which time it is removed.

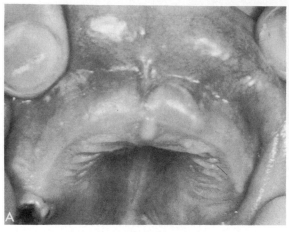
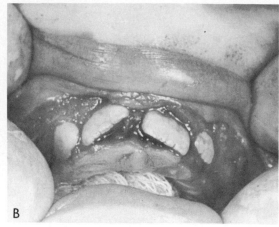

Figure 13-91 *A*, Dense fibrous hyperplasia (fibromatosis) of the mucoperiosteal membrane over the anterior maxillary ridge in a 9-year-old boy who had lost his deciduous anteriors and molars owing to gross caries before he was 6 years of age. His permanent lower anterior teeth erupted on schedule, and he has been traumatizing the mucoperiosteal tissue of the edentulous anterior maxilla at meal times for over 3 years. This has produced the dense, thick, fibrous mucoperiosteal membrane that has blocked the eruption of the permanent maxillary anterior teeth.

B, Treatment is the wide excision of this tough membrane over the crowns of the unerupted teeth and, if necessary, *careful* removal of alveolar bone up to the height of contour of the crowns of the incisors to facilitate normal eruption, as is shown here.

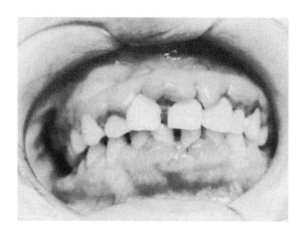

Figure 13-92 Typical gingival hypertrophy in acute monocytic leukemia seen in an 18-year-old female who, 5 months prior to this visit, had noticed slight gingival bleeding. Three months before this visit, she had observed gingival swelling that had slowly increased. She died 3 months after this photograph was taken. (Courtesy of H. Clayton Sato, D.D.S., M.D.)

Figure 13-93 Gingival hypertrophy in acute myelogenic leukemia. This patient was a 23-year-old female who died 5 months after she first complained of feeling weak and tired. Next she noticed changes in the gingival tissues, gradual swelling, bleeding, ulceration and soreness in her entire mouth.

The types of gingival hypertrophy in monocytic and myelogenic leukemia are different. The monocytic is harder; in myelogenic, the gingiva is softer and more flabby in its texture, bleeds easily, and when ulceration starts, there is a breaking down of gingival tissues, leaving raw, bleeding surfaces. Compare Figures 13-92 and 13-93. (Courtesy of H. Clayton Sato, D.D.S., M.D.)

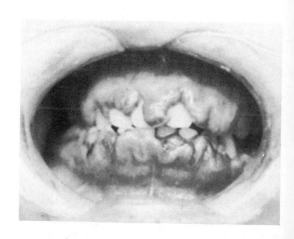

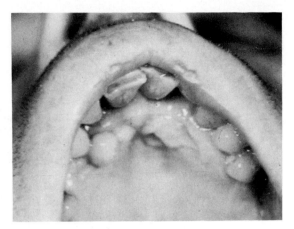

Figure 13–94 An unusual pedunculated odontogenic fibroma arising on the lingual gingival surface near the maxillary cuspid. *Treatment:* Excision of the tumor at the pedicle and cauterization of the base.

Photographic Case Report

FIBROMA OF THE PALATE AND ANTERIOR MAXILLARY PROCESS

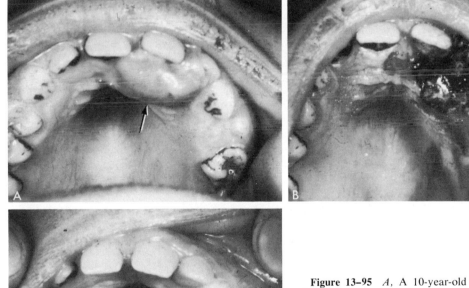

Figure 13–95 *A,* A 10-year-old boy was brought to the clinic for treatment of a large, sessile hard fibroma, which not only was spreading over the palate but was creeping through the interproximal spaces to the labial surface of the anterior maxilla, deflecting the permanent central incisors and permanent left lateral incisor. If the technique advocated by some oral surgeons, namely, the extraction of the involved teeth, were carried out, this patient would become a dental cripple early in his life.

B, The tumor was carefully and completely excised, along with the periosteum, from the palate, from between the involved teeth and from the labial surface of the anterior maxilla. Then the soft-tissue periphery and the entire osseous base and interproximal spaces were cauterized with an electric cautery; a zinc oxide and eugenol dressing was placed over the entire operative area. This dressing materially helps in reducing postoperative pain.

C, Eight weeks after the operation the area is covered with new mucoperiosteal membrane. The displaced teeth are moving back into position.

Photographic Case Report

EXCISION OF A MANDIBULAR FIBROMA OF THE INTERDENTAL SPACE

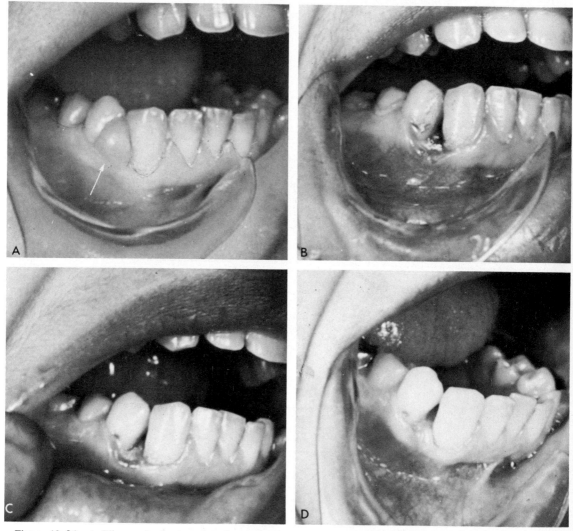

Figure 13–96 *A*, Fibroma in the interdental area that has not separated the teeth as yet. *B*, Fibroma excised, base coagulated. One week later zinc oxide and eugenol dressing is removed. *C*, Small loose, bony sequestrum ready for removal 2 weeks postoperatively. *D*, Final healing.

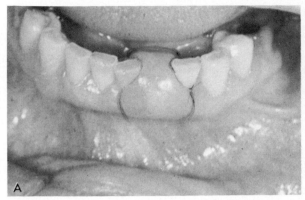
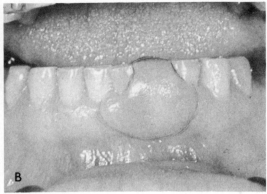

Figure 13–97 *A,* Occlusal view of a long-standing, very dense, hard mandibular odontogenic fibroma in a 66-year-old female. During its slow growth it has separated the lower anterior left central and lateral incisors, shifting all the teeth in the arch as well. Attention is directed to the generalized abrasion of all the mandibular teeth (although not shown here, the maxillary teeth were also abraded) and the absence of any injury to the tough surface of this fibroma, even though it is subjected to the same trauma as the teeth on either side.

B, Labial surface of this tumor, which was observed during an oral examination. The patient did not know exactly how long it had been present, but knew it had been "for years." When assured that the growth was benign, the patient was, as were we, satisfied not to institute any surgery unless future examinations indicated a specific reason for its excision.

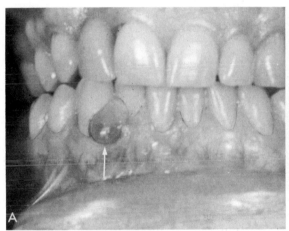
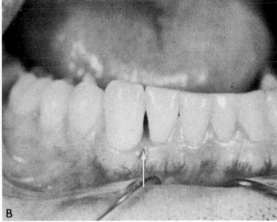

Figure 13–98 *A,* Neurofibroma that in appearance simulated a peripheral giant cell tumor because of its light and dark shades of red and pink. The growth was also not as hard as a fibroma. However, there was not any evidence of resorption of alveolar bone. This might have been because the lesion was only 6 weeks old. *B,* View 4 weeks after simple excision of the lesion, including the mucoperiosteum, and minor superficial coagulation of the osseous surface to control slight bleeding. To our surprise the oral pathologist found that it was a peripheral neurofibroma. There was not a recurrence, which is a frequent sequela in these cases.

Figure 13–99 Peripheral ossifying fibroma. (Courtesy of Alvin F. Gardner, D.D.S.)

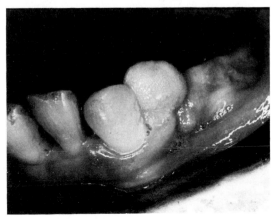

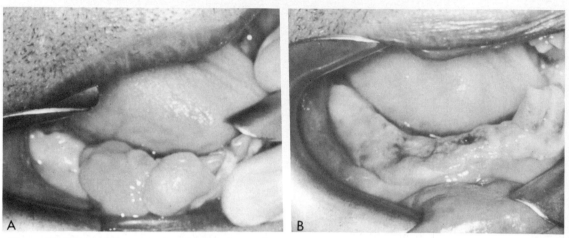

Figure 13–100 *A,* Fibroma and peripheral giant cell tumor on the crest of the mandibular ridge. *B,* Both tumors were excised, and the crest of the ridge was cauterized.

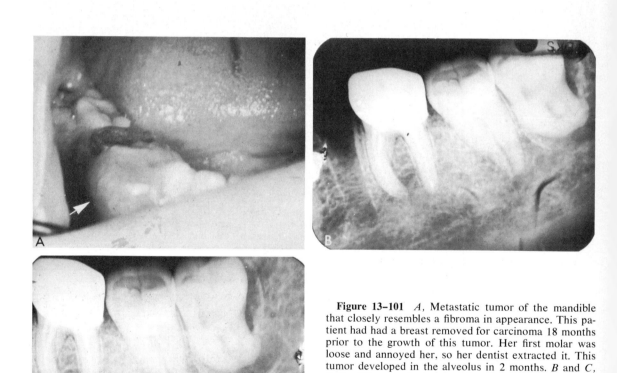

Figure 13–101 *A,* Metastatic tumor of the mandible that closely resembles a fibroma in appearance. This patient had had a breast removed for carcinoma 18 months prior to the growth of this tumor. Her first molar was loose and annoyed her, so her dentist extracted it. This tumor developed in the alveolus in 2 months. *B* and *C,* Both of these periapical dental radiographs show diffuse, small, distinct osteolytic lesions. There were metastases to most of the bones of the skeleton.

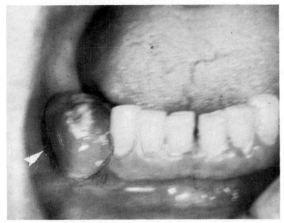

Figure 13–102 Large metastatic tumor of the mandible. This patient had carcinoma of the uterine cervix.

and epineurium. In the oral cavity we find the neurofibroma, neurofibromatosis (Recklinghausen's disease), and schwannoma originating from nerve sheaths. Tumors may also arise from the nerve cell. The amputation and traumatic neuromas develop from the nerve cell.

In outline form these tumors are listed by Shklar and Meyer as follows:
1. Neurofibroma.
   a. Single lesion (neurofibroma).
   b. Multiple lesions (neurofibromatosis; Recklinghausen's disease).
2. Schwannoma (neurinoma; neurilemoma; perineural fibroblastoma).
3. Neuroma (amputation neuroma; traumatic neuroma).[82]

NEUROFIBROMA

While the single neurofibroma may be found in any area of the oral cavity, it is most frequently found on the tongue as a pedunculated firm mass. In other areas it is a firm, round mass, which protrudes somewhat from the soft tissue in which it is located. Neurofibromas involving the mandibular nerve are rare. These may produce pain and paresthesia. Stafne illustrates such a case in Figure 13–106.

Treatment. It is removed by surgical excision. If a large nerve enters the tumor, it should be joined after the tumor is removed. See Figure 13–98 for illustration of a symptomless neurofibroma which grew in the labial dental interseptal space.

NEUROFIBROMATOSIS

This is a difficult problem. Shklar and Meyer[82] recommend:

Treatment. Any lesion subject to obvious and continuous trauma should be removed, because of the possibility of malignant transformation. Any obvious increase in the size or ulceration of a lesion should be investigated immediately with complete excision of the lesion. If malignant change has occurred, the prognosis is poor, for many of these resulting sarcomas appear to metastasize early in the course of development.

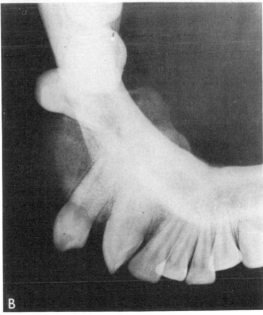
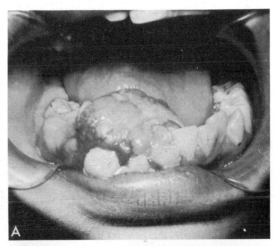

Figure 13–103 Ossifying fibroma. (Courtesy of H. Serrano Roa, D.D.S.)

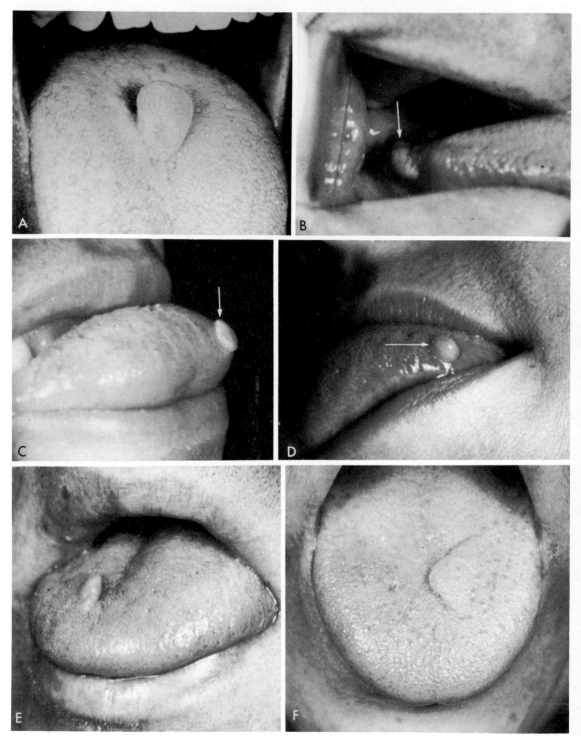

Figure 13–104   *A, C* and *D*, These are three examples of "irritation fibromas" of the tongue. They consist mostly of collagenous connective tissue. Irritations associated with mastication give rise to these tumors. *Treatment:* Surgical excision at the base.

B, Papilloma on the lateral surface of the base of the tongue. *E* and *F*, Healed traumatic injuries of the tongue that were never closed with sutures.

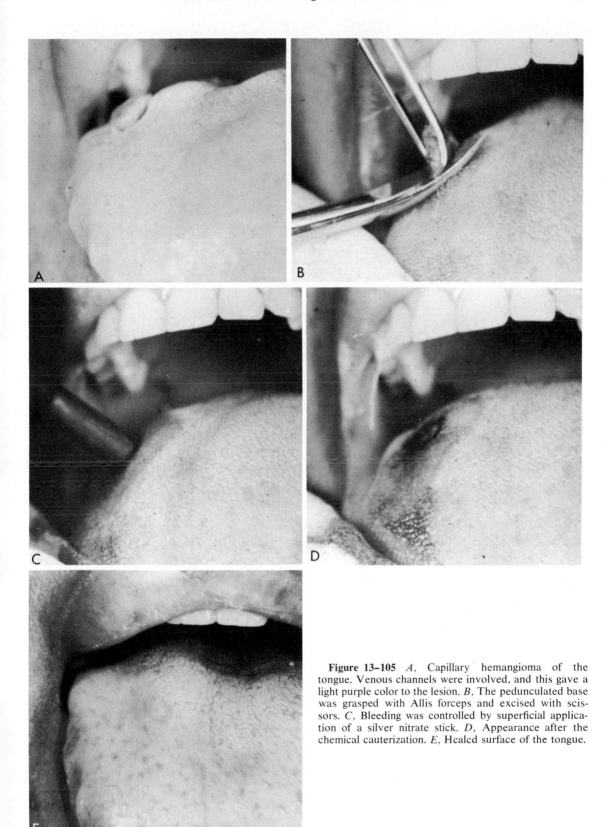

Figure 13–105 *A,* Capillary hemangioma of the tongue. Venous channels were involved, and this gave a light purple color to the lesion. *B,* The pedunculated base was grasped with Allis forceps and excised with scissors. *C,* Bleeding was controlled by superficial application of a silver nitrate stick. *D,* Appearance after the chemical cauterization. *E,* Healed surface of the tongue.

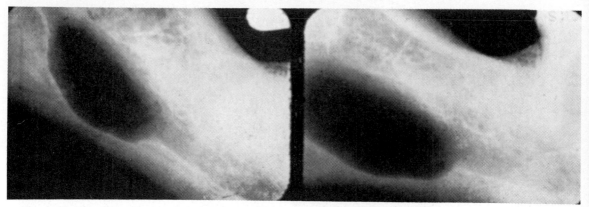

Figure 13–106   Neurofibroma of the inferior dental nerve, showing bulbous enlargement of the mandibular canal and increased growth. The roentgenogram on the left was made 10 years prior to the one on the right. (From Stafne, E. C.: Oral Roentgenographic Diagnosis. 4th ed. Philadelphia, W. B. Saunders Co., 1975.)

Case Report No. 19

NEUROFIBROMATOSIS

A. E. McDonald, D.D.S.

A 63-year-old black female was referred for full stomatoplasty for marked uneven ridge resorption in both the maxilla and mandible. She was in no acute distress, but clinical examination in the office showed diffuse gross nodules growing on the face and neck and all of the body's surfaces, with marked impairment in movement of the left hand because of a large nodular growth on the wrist.

(See Figure 13–107.) The mass was located on the radial aspect and was approximately 5 to 7 cm. in diameter. Oral examination revealed marked resorption of the dental ridges, with diffuse nodular masses dispersed about the mucosa. The oral masses in no way compared with those on the body, being only about 1.5 to 2 mm.^{2} in size. Blood pressure was 120/70; pulse was 90, with

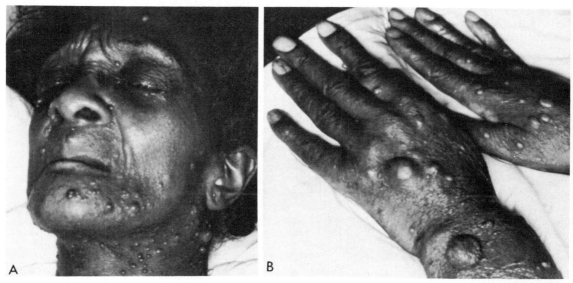

Figure 13–107   Neurofibromatosis, marked by soft tumors (neurofibromas) dispersed over the surface of the entire body, as well as the dental ridges. (See Case Report No. 19 for details.)

some signs of coupling; respirations were 20 per min., and the skin was somewhat dry. A tentative diagnosis of neurofibromatosis was made, and the patient was scheduled for hospitalization and stomatoplasty.

Physical examination in the hospital revealed a moderately nourished 63-year-old black female with a chief complaint of ill-fitting dentures. Her family history was unremarkable. The patient's medical history showed no major incidence until neurofibroma had begun to appear about 7 years before. She had sought no treatment of any kind until her chewing became difficult because her dentures were not fitting anymore. She had now been wearing the same full upper and lower dentures for 10 years. Auscultation revealed mild cardiomegaly but no untoward heart sounds.

Because the patient seemed more disturbed by the inability to use her left hand than the inability to chew, a medical-surgical consultation was obtained. As a result, an excisional biopsy of the mass on the left wrist was decided upon. *Diagnosis:* Neurofibroma of the wrist (von Recklinghausen's disease).

SCHWANNOMA

This tumor develops in the submucosal tissue as a firm painless mass. It is a semiresilient lesion not as hard as the fibroma and simulates a lipoma in appearance and on palpation.

Treatment. The encapsulated schwannoma is "shelled out," care being taken to separate it from the associated nerve without cutting the nerve.

NEUROMA

Amputation Neuroma. Bernier states: "The amputation neuroma is common in the region of the mental foramen of the mandible. The frequent surgery relating to the extraction of teeth is, no doubt, responsible for its development. The lesion is a bulbous enlargement which occurs at the ends of nerves when they are divided, brought about by ac-tive proliferation of Schwann cells and the nerve sheaths. With age, this intermingling of structures becomes scarlike in character and often quite painful. Pressure on the mass, such as from dentures, may initiate pain or, if present previously, accentuate it. The amputation neuroma is not considered a true neoplasm; however, its clinical significance in the oral regions is worthy of special note."[7]

Treatment. Bernier also writes that the treatment of amputation neuroma "depends largely upon the location of the mass and whether or not it is producing symptoms. Since it may bring about marked discomfort, removal may be the only choice. Subsequent formation of another mass is a distinct possibility and should be borne in mind. Alcohol injections are worthwhile in selected cases, particularly when a surgical approach is difficult. Avoidance of pressure and other 'triggering events' is of great importance."[7]

Case Report No. 20

RECURRENT NEUROMA OF THE VESTIBULE OF THE MANDIBLE*

Patient. The patient, who presented himself as an outpatient at Magee-Women's Hospital, was found to be a normally developed, well-nourished 41-year-old white male.

Chief Complaint. "Irritation of the lower lip."

History of Present Illness. Patient first noticed a small localized nodule within the left mucobuccal fold 2 years ago, which he attributed to a "blood blister." Pain was produced when mild pressure was applied to the mucosa overlying the mental foramen. Denture insertion also produced this same pain and consequently the patient was un-able to wear his mandibular denture. At this time, he had a surgical excision of the mass, which proved to be a peripheral proliferation of the neurovascular fibers localized in an area approximately 4 mm. from the mental foramen. Etiology was attributed to local irritation by the mandibular

---

*Case report prepared by Paul H. Iverson, Oral Surgery Resident, Magee-Women's Hospital, Pittsburgh, Pa.

denture. Five months later he developed a spontaneous rupture and drainage in the same area as operated. Remission followed, and he did not return for further definitive care until this admission, when he has again presented with an "aching lump" in the left mucobuccal fold that "persistently drains causing a bitter taste."

Oral Examination. Reveals a small hard nodule located in the mucobuccal fold adjacent to the mandibular left bicuspids. Discomfort is produced on palpation. Patient is edentulous. Remainder of oral soft tissues are unremarkable.

Extraoral Examination. Normal facial symmetry. No adenopathy.

Preoperative Impression. Neuroma.

Anesthetic. Local (inferior alveolar and long buccal nerve blocks—left).

Operative Technique. The mucosa was incised over the elongated nodule and by blunt dissection was freed from the surrounding tissue. The mental foramen was identified, and it was obvious that this was a neuroma of the terminal branch of the mental nerve.

Postoperative Impression. Neuroma.

Pathology Report. *Macroscopic:* The specimen is labeled neuroma. It consists of an irregularly shaped fragment of soft tissue which is red, and represents a fibroid nodule. It measures 1.0 by 0.3 by 0.2 cm.

Microscopic: Peripheral nerve bundles in fibrous tissue.

Diagnosis: Neuroma (F. D. Beyer, Jr., M.D.).

Postoperative Course. The patient's immediate recovery was quite satisfactory, although partial paresthesia did persist for a period of several months.

Subsequent Course. A year later, in April, sensations had returned but the patient was now experiencing intermittent pain which seemed to be increased in frequency on exposure to cold weather. By September of the same year, a discrete hard nodule, approximately 1 cm. in diameter, could be palpated in the mucobuccal fold adjacent to the mandibular molars. Surgical excision was again undertaken with a biopsy report as follows:

Microscopic: Specimen submitted for examination is composed of fibrous connective tissue stroma in which there is a tangled mass of nerve fibers. Numerous. Vascularity moderate.

Diagnosis: Neuroma (mandible) (R. Tiecke, D.D.S., Oral Pathologist).

To date, there is no sign of recurrence. Patient has remained asymptomatic.

MYOMA

(MYOBLASTOMA, LEIOMYOMA, RHABDOMYOMA, FIBROMYOMA, ADENOMYOMA)

This is a relatively rare benign muscle tissue tumor, most frequently found in the tongue or lips. A few have been reported as arising from the mandibular or maxillary mucosa. Such a case is described in the accompanying case report of a myoblastoma in a newborn. The tumors are reported as being 0.5 cm. in diameter with a maximum size of 1.5 cm. The one reported here was multilobular with an average size of 1.5 cm. They may occur at any age, but in 155,862 births at the Magee-Women's Hospital in the last 38 years, only one myoblastoma in a newborn has been brought to my attention. A case of rhabdomyosarcoma, the malignant counterpart of rhabdomyoma, is illustrated in Figure 13–227.

Treatment. The myoblastoma is not encapsulated and so is removed by a wide elliptical incision around the base to insure complete removal.

Case Report No. 21

CONGENITAL MYOBLASTOMA OF THE NEWBORN*

Patient. This patient, a newborn white female, 72 hours old, had been delivered at Magee-Women's Hospital. Delivery was uneventful, and findings in the physical examination of the baby were essentially negative except for the presence of a pedunculated tumor on the labial aspect of the dental ridge of the maxilla in the right lateral incisor region (see Figure 13–108).

*Case report prepared by Charles J. Ganley, D.D.S., M.S. Assoc. Staff., and Abdel Moneim El Attar, B.Ch.D., Oral Surgery Resident, Magee-Women's Hospital, Pittsburgh, Pa.

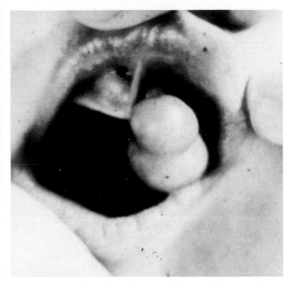

Figure 13–108 Bilobular myoblastoma in a newborn. See Case Report No. 21.

The lesion measured approximately 2.5 by 2.0 cm. in diameter. Upon palpation it was found to be firm in consistency and movable, and it contained 2 lobes. It was pink, identical in color to that of the supporting mucosa. The tumor protruded from the mouth when the lips were in contact.

Surgical Procedure. The patient was taken to the operating room for surgical excision of the lesion. Infiltration anesthesia was induced with lidocaine hydrochloride, 1.5 per cent, without vasoconstrictor. The tumor was grasped with an Allis tissue forceps and an elliptical incision was made about the base of the lesion extending down to the bone. The specimen was removed *in toto* and submitted to the pathologist for histologic evaluation. Interrupted sutures of 000 black silk were inserted so as to reapproximate the edges of the wound. The patient's postoperative course was uneventful.

Pathologic Findings. The tumor measured approximately 2.5 by 2.0 by 1.5 cm. in cross-sectional diameter and was comprised of 2 encapsulated lobes, the largest of the lobes being 1.5 cm. in diameter. The specimen was covered by an intact, smooth, grayish white capsule. The sectioned tissue revealed 2 firm yellowish gray nodules.

The histopathologic appearance of the tumor was characteristic of a granular cell myoblastoma of the newborn (congenital epulis). The tissue was covered with stratified squamous epithelium which demonstrated parakeratosis and atrophy with loss of rete pegs. The tumor was composed of large polyhedral-type cells which contained a pink-staining granular cytoplasm with prominent eccentrically placed nuclei. The tumor was separated from the overlying epithelium by dense collagenous fibers. A delicate thin network of collagenous fibers was noted throughout the stroma of the tumor mass. The periphery of the specimen was marked with numerous dilated hyperplastic blood vessels.

Diagnosis: Myoblastoma of the mucosa of the anterior maxillary ridge.

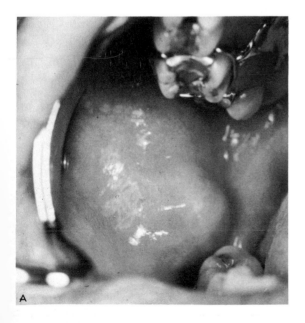

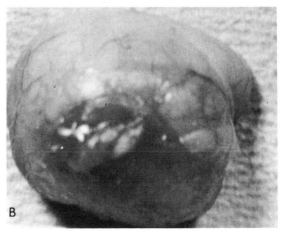

Figure 13–109 *A*, Lipoma of the medial surface of the cheek. *B*, Lipoma after enucleation. (See Case Report No. 22.)

LIPOMA

These rare tumors arise in the adipose tissue of the oral cavity and are made up largely of fat tissue. In a fibrolipoma the adipose tissue is greatly infiltrated with strands of fibrous connective tissue. They are found in the cheeks, tongue and floor of the mouth. They are a soft, slow-growing benign tumor usually located beneath the oral mucosa. The one shown in Figure 13–109 was a spherical tumor although they also are found as a mass of grape-like lobes. The surface is smooth, except where it may be attached by a pedicle to adjacent muscle fibers, yellowish white and streaked with blood vessels.

Treatment. After exposure they are bluntly dissected free from the surrounding structures. Sharp dissection is required if a pedicle is present.

Case Report No. 22

LIPOMA OF THE CHEEK*

Patient. A 62-year-old white man presented complaining of a "swelling" in his right cheek (see Figure 13–109).

History. This swelling started 3 months ago after the extraction of the lower right first molar and since that time has increased in size.

Oral Examination. Examination revealed a missing lower right first molar tooth. Opposite the extraction site a semisolid nonmovable mass about 2.5 cm. in diameter was found.

Physical Examination. This was essentially negative.

Tentative Diagnosis. Lipoma.

Operative Procedure. Under local anesthesia a 3 cm. horizontal incision was made, with a No. 15 Bard-Parker blade, in the mucosa of the right cheek. The incision was held open with Allis forceps and the specimen was "shelled out" and cut from its only attachment to the buccinator muscle by scissors, and removed. The incision was closed with 000 black silk suture.

The specimen was a spherical, well circumscribed, encapsulated, soft yellowish mass of tissue measuring 2.5 cm. in diameter.

Microscopic Diagnosis. Lipoma.

---

*Prepared by Charles A. Clark, D.D.S., Oral Surgery Resident, Magee-Women's Hospital, Pittsburgh, Pa.

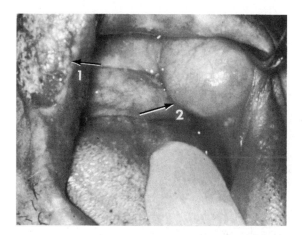

Figure 13–110 *1,* Epidermoid carcinoma of the right upper corner of the lip. *2,* Large lipoma of the left cheek.

LYMPHOMA

GIANT FOLLICULAR LYMPHOMA

Giant follicular lymphomas are malignant tumors of lymphoid tissue. Although they are extremely rare in the oral regions they may simulate normal lymphoid tissue. For this reason they have been included in this chapter on benign lesions of the oral cavity.

The soft palate, the tonsils, the submental and submaxillary lymph nodes, and the parotid gland have been described as initial sites of the disease.

An enlargement of the lymph nodes occurs as a result of a multiplication of the cells of the lymph nodes. This condition is accompanied by enlargement of the spleen and other lymph nodes throughout the body. Locally the lesions can be excised with the knife or electrosurgically. They are radiosensitive. Case Report No. 23 presents a case treated by radiation therapy.

Case Report No. 23

GIANT FOLLICULAR LYMPHOMA OF THE ORAL CAVITY*

History. This patient, a 68-year-old white male, had had maxillary and mandibular full dentures constructed. Six months later he had noticed a small mass in the left maxillary vestibular fornix which was asymptomatic. The patient had returned to his dentist for possible denture adjustment. The dentist found no denture irritation and referred him to an oral surgeon. However, the patient did not report until 2½ years later, at which time the lesion in the left maxillary vestibule (mucobuccal fold) measured 3 by 4 cm. (see Figure 13–111). A biopsy of the lesion resulted in a diagnosis of giant follicular lymphoma. Multiplicity in other areas was not determined.

Treatment. Irradiation therapy through several ports totalled 5000 R. in air.

Subsequent Course. Two years later, the patient was still asymptomatic, with no mouth lesions and no enlargement of liver, spleen or nodes.

---

*Case report prepared by Samuel Byers, D.D.S., Senior Oral Surgery Resident, Veterans' Administration Hospital, University Drive, Pittsburgh, Pa.

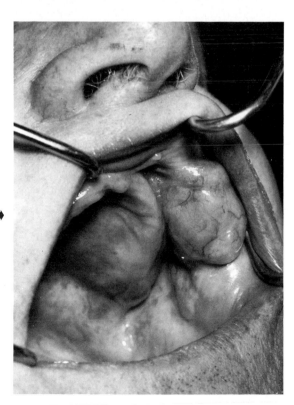

Figure 13–111 Giant follicular lymphoma of the left maxillary vestibular fornix. See Case Report No. 23.

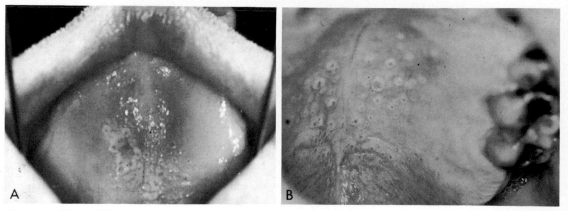

Figure 13–112   *A*, Nicotina stomatitis. The irritants associated with smoking, such as heat, smoke, and the chemicals in the burning tobacco, produce hyperkeratosis (white rings) about the excretory ducts of the palatal mucous glands. *B*, Another case of palatal nicotina stomatitis. In this palate the hyperkeratosis around many of the duct orifices has coalesced with that of other ducts.

INFLAMMATORY PAPILLARY HYPERPLASIA (PALATAL PAPILLOMATOSIS, VERRUCOUS PAPILLOMATOSIS)

Occasionally beneath partial or full dentures there is an extensive area of warty, inflamed mucosa. The palatal mucosa may be covered with small spherical masses of epithelium varying in size from that of a berry seed to that of a BB shot. When located beneath relief areas of dentures, multiple papillomas retain their round form, but under denture pressure these areas are flattened out. (See Figure 13–114 *A*, *B* and *C*). These epithelial

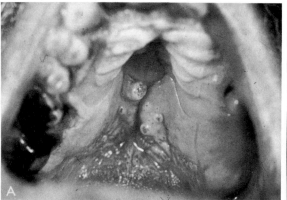

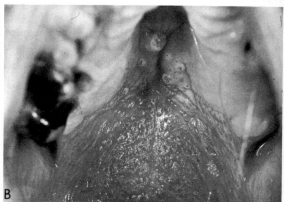

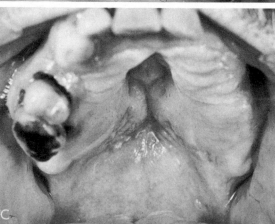

Figure 13–113   Acute palatal nicotina stomatitis in a patient who smoked two to three packs of cigarettes daily.
A, A partial denture has covered part of the palate, thus protecting the underlying mucosa. However, the unprotected areas have been severely damaged by the heat and smoke, as is shown by the swollen, hyperkeratotic orifices of the ducts. These are completely closed, thus forming small intraductal cysts. *B*, The soft palate is acutely inflamed and raw. *C*, Treatment consisted of cutting of the swollen orifices of the ducts, thus opening and draining the small retention cysts, the patient's complete cessation of smoking and his maintenance of normal oral hygiene. It took 5 weeks for the palatal tissues to heal as shown in this photograph.

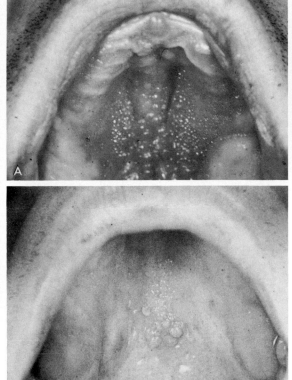

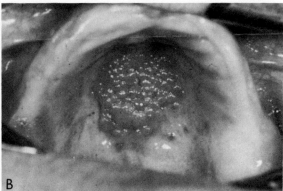

Figure 13-114 *A* and *B*, Examples of acute inflammatory papillary hyperplasia of the palate (palatal papillomatosis). The cause of this lesion is unknown, but it is seen only under maxillary dentures, which may or may not fit well. The lesions do not disappear when the denture is removed for a few days, but the inflammation does disappear, as shown in *C*. New dentures should not be made until this papillary hyperplasia has been surgically excised.

outgrowths are the result of an inflammatory hyperplasia produced by a denture whose palatal surface is rough, or they may develop from palatal inflammation as the result of continuous night and day wearing of the denture. While the traumatically induced inflammation will disappear if the patient stops wearing the denture, the papillomatosis will remain. The fabrication of a new denture will not produce a cure either. Surgical excision of these "numerous small vertical projections each composed of parakeratotic or sometimes orthokeratotic stratified squamous epithelium with a central core of connective tissue"[75] down to the corium is necessary. Unfortunately, these cases have been treated too radically in the past, as they were diagnosed, according to Shafer, "by the inexperienced as epidermoid carcinoma. However, most authorities now agree that true epithelial dysplasia and malignant transformation do not occur in palatal papillomatosis."[75] For example, the end result of a too-radical treatment of this benign condition can be the loss of palatal osseous tissue producing naso-oral fistulas.

Treatment. The technique for removal is shown in Figure 13-115. The papillomatosis, as shown in Figure 13-115*A*, is confined to the relief area of the denture. Figure 13-115*B* is a cross section showing the multiple pedicle bases. A biopsy is taken with a scalpel before excision of this lesion with a radiosurgical loop. The best method for removal is to plane off the papillary projections until the corium, the dense white fibrous tissue beneath the epithelium, is reached as is shown in Figure 13-115*C* to *E*. It is not necessary to remove the full thickness of the mucoperiosteal membrane to prevent recurrence.

After surgery, it is necessary to remove the cause of irritation, which is usually in ill-fitting or rough denture. To protect the raw palatal surface, as seen in Figure 13-115*E*, and to prevent postoperative pain, a thin wash of zinc oxide and eugenol is spread over the palatal portion of the denture which then is immediately inserted as shown in Figure 13-115*F*. The denture is allowed to remain in the mouth for the next 72 hours, at which time it is removed and the hardened zinc oxide dressing is scraped from the palatal portion of the denture. The palatal portion of

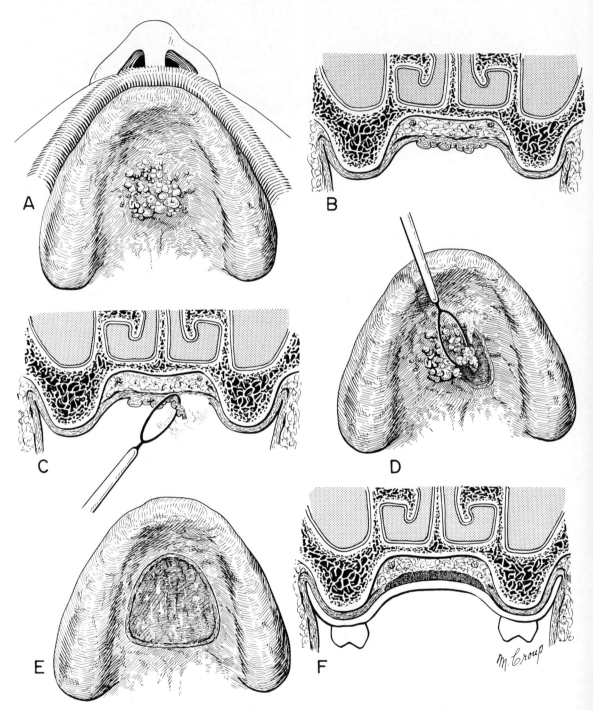

Figure 13–115 Excision of inflammatory papillary hyperplasia (papillomatosis of the palate) with the radiosurgical loop. See text for description of technique.

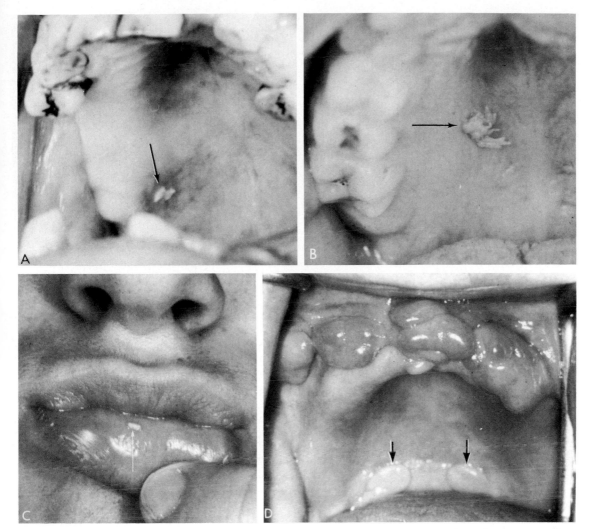

Figure 13–116 *A, B* and *D,* Papillomas (benign epithelial tumors) of the palate with the typical cauliflower-like growth and pedicle base. *C,* Papilloma of the lip. (See Figure 13–118 for treatment.)

the denture is then polished to make certain that all pointed, sharp or irregular surfaces are removed.

When the raw surface of the palate has been epithelialized, a new denture can be constructed for the patient or the old denture can be rebased. It is essential that the palatal portion be extremely smooth, with no irritating surfaces, and that the patient be advised not to wear the denture at night. The patient should be seen postoperatively at 6 months, a year, and 2 years to determine whether there is a recurrence.

PAPILLOMAS

The papilloma is a small, soft or hard, sessile or pedunculated, warty or cauliflower-like epithelial hyperplastic growth which may occur on any surface of the oral mucosa. They emerge from the oral epithelium and are probably most frequently seen on the mucosa of the hard or soft palate or uvula, then the lips, and next the tongue.

The soft papilloma is usually pedunculated. It is flabby, and when it occurs on the palate beneath a prosthetic device, it is flattened out

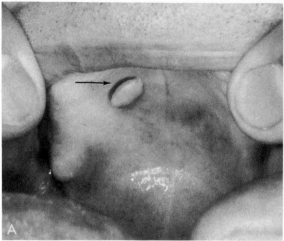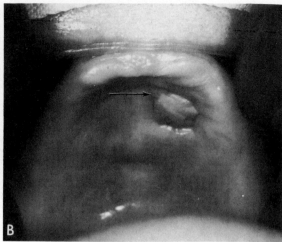

Figure 13-117 *A*, An unusual papilloma because it is round and smooth, with no visible branching or cauliflower-like growth. *B*, Typical palatal papilloma with the narrow pedicle. It is plastered against the palate by the maxillary full denture. See Figure 13-118 for its appearance when hanging by the stalk for excision.

by the pressure of the denture. They are usually very small, measuring only a few millimeters in diameter, but occasionally one is seen that is a centimeter or more wide. Soft papillomas are found in all age groups.

Hard papillomas are usually seen as verrucous outgrowths, or a single point of proliferation in areas of hyperkeratosis.

While the possibility of malignant degeneration is remote, papillomas arising from the tongue or cheeks which have a fixed base and induration of the underlying tissues should especially be regarded with suspicion.

Again the reader is advised to have these, as well as all other tumors which are removed from the mouth, examined microscopically.

Treatment. Figure 13-118*A* to *E* illustrates the technique of removal of a fibropapilloma from the palate. It is important to include the mucosa from which the pedicle arose in the excising of these tumors if recurrence is to be prevented. It is not necessary to include or to destroy the periosteum.

ANGIOMAS

An angioma is a tumor of which the cells tend to form blood vessels or lymph vessels. When these tumors are made up of lymph vessels they are known as lymphangiomas; when composed of blood vessels, they are known as hemangiomas. Lymphangiomas are illustrated in Case Report Nos. 27 and 28. Hemangiomas are found on the labial and buccal mucosa, palate, tongue, and in the jaws (see case reports). They are covered by smooth epithelium, often nodular in form, and are dark blue if close to the surface (as most of these tumors are). Biopsy is contraindicated because of the hazard of profuse bleeding. Occasionally the surface is ulcerated. There are two types of hemangiomas: (1) capillary hemangiomas, which are composed of a stroma containing many small capillary blood vessels; (2) large cavernous hemangiomas, which appear microscopically to contain large endothelium-lined vascular spaces engorged with blood and blood elements. They are located peripherally in the soft tissue and centrally in bone.

PERIPHERAL HEMANGIOMA

Treatment. Small hemangiomas can be excised (see Figure 13-121). Large ones are treated by the injection of sclerosing solutions. The author's experience with the use of a sclerosing solution was not satisfactory. The hemangiomas were reduced in size, but not obliterated. In some cases the tumor is sclerosed, reducing its size, and then excised. Baurmash and Mandel report five minor cases of *small* hemangiomas 1 to 2 cm. in diameter successfully treated by the injection of 0.5 cc. of a 1 per cent solution of sodium tetradecyl sulfate (Sotradecol Sodium) into and around the mass. When all signs of inflammation subsided they reinjected, but not before a minimum of 2 weeks and at times 3 or 4 weeks.[6]

(*Text continued on page 818*)

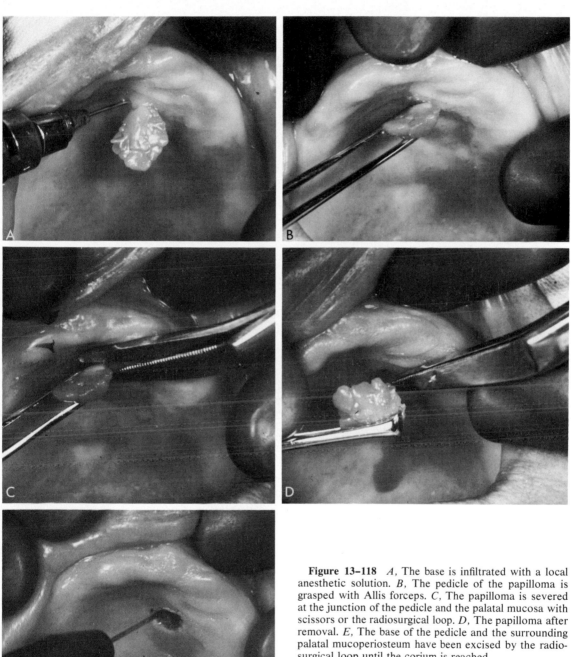

Figure 13–118 *A*, The base is infiltrated with a local anesthetic solution. *B*, The pedicle of the papilloma is grasped with Allis forceps. *C*, The papilloma is severed at the junction of the pedicle and the palatal mucosa with scissors or the radiosurgical loop. *D*, The papilloma after removal. *E*, The base of the pedicle and the surrounding palatal mucoperiosteum have been excised by the radiosurgical loop until the corium is reached.

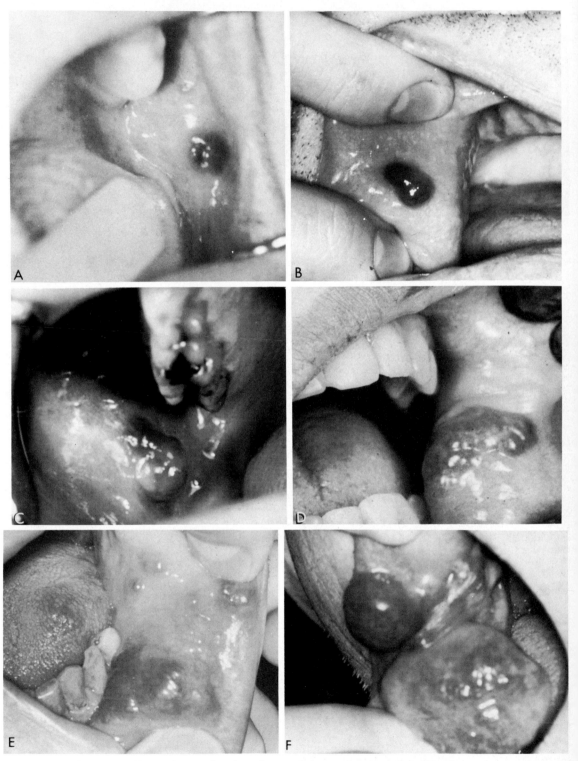

Figure 13–119 *A* to *D*, Hemangiomas of various sizes, and shapes of varices of the buccal mucosa.
E, Multiple separate varices of the buccal mucosa and a large hemangioma of the labial mucosa of the lower lip. *F*,
Massive hemangiomas of the buccal mucosa of the cheek and labial mucosa of the lower lip.

(*Figure 13–119 continued on opposite page*)

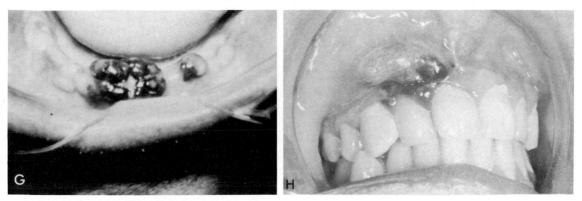

Figure 13–119 (*Continued.*) *G*, Vascular nevus on the crest of the mandibular ridge that is histologically similar to a hemangioma. *H*, A gingival hemangioma.

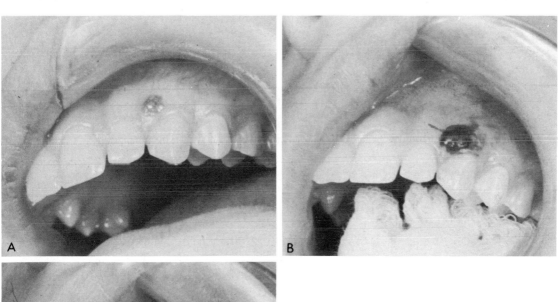

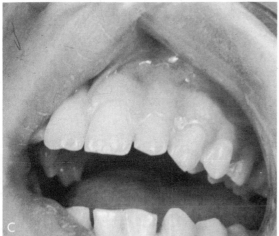

Figure 13–120 *A*, A small gingival varix in a 12-year-old girl. *B*, Superficially carefully cauterized with a silver nitrate stick several times 5 to 7 days apart so as not to destroy the thin, delicate gingival epithelial collar. *C*, End result. Varices usually start in this manner and gradually increase in size. Obviously, early treatment prevents what can develop into a monumental problem, as has been shown in previous figures.

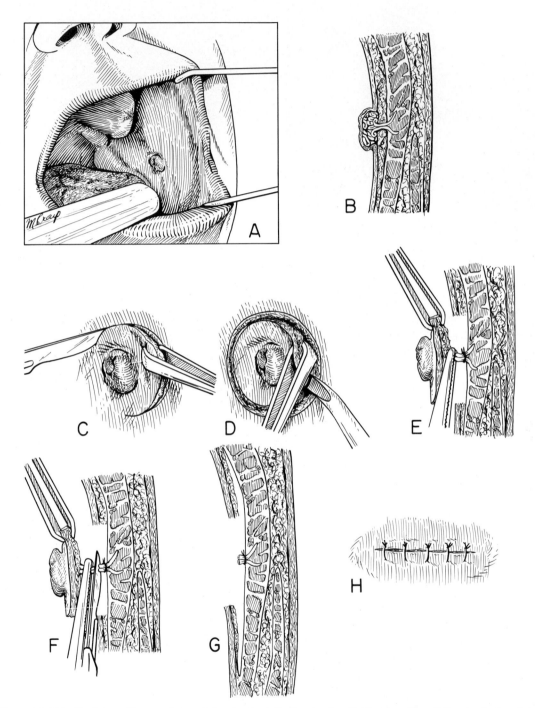

Figure 13–121   Excision of hemangioma of the cheek. *A*, Lesion *in situ*. *B*, Cross section of the cheek, showing the lesion with feeder vessels at the base extending into the muscular layer. *C*, The lesion is excised by a circumferential elliptical incision well beyond the base to prevent bleeding. An incision is made down to the buccinator muscle. *D*, The periphery is grasped and retracted with an Allis clamp, and the mucosa is bluntly dissected away up to the base of the lesion. *E*, The base of the lesion containing vessels is grasped with a hemostat, and a catgut ligature is placed around the vessels. *F*, Vessels are cut between the hemostat and the suture. *G*, The mucosa and submucosa are undermined in order to mobilize enough tissue for primary closure. *H*, Closure with interrupted sutures.

Case Report No. 24

VASCULAR HAMARTOMA OF THE CHEEK

MARVIN E. PIZER, D.D.S., M.S.

Patient. A healthy 9-year-old white female was admitted to National Orthopaedic and Rehabilitation Hospital for excision of tumors in the right cheek.

Chief Complaint. The patient had noticed

lumps in her right cheek; resultant cheek biting during eating had also become a problem.

History of Present Illness. These masses had first been noted 8 months previously, and, according to the patient's mother, they had doubled

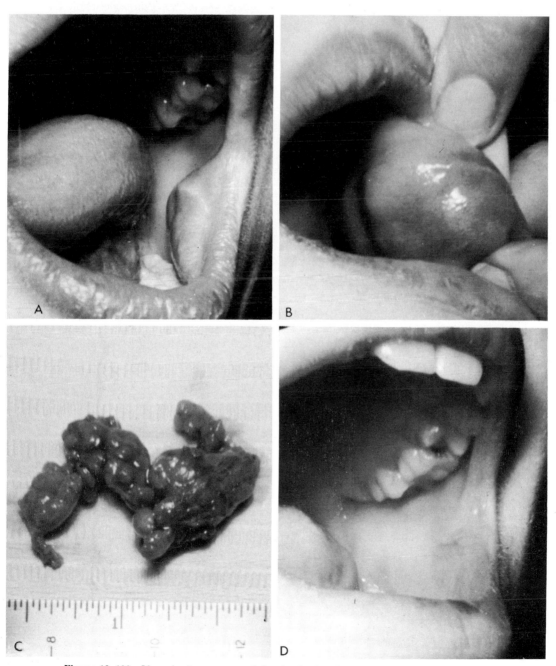

Figure 13–122   Vascular hamartoma of the cheek. (See Case Report No. 24 for details.)

in size in the last 2 months. There had been no pain.

Intraoral Examination. Firm nodules could be felt deep in the buccal mucosa. These were hard and painless on palpation. There was some thickening, probably scarring, of the mucosa overlying these masses from cheek biting. (See Figure 13–122*A* and *B*).

Extraoral Examination. Minimal asymmetry of the cheeks was seen that would probably not have been noted without knowledge of the palpable masses inside.

Physical Examination. Laboratory findings and those from the physical examination were all within normal limits.

Operative Technique. Under general endotracheal anesthesia, the patient was prepared and draped in the usual fashion, and the procedure that follows was performed. An elliptical incision was made in the buccal mucosa, beginning at the corner of the mouth and extending posteriorly 2½ to 3 inches. A segment of buccal mucosa was excised where the scarring had occurred. Then, by a combination of sharp and blunt dissection, the fibers of the buccinator muscle were divided and the nodules exposed. These nodules were found to be multiple, bluish-yellow, hard and varying in size from that of a BB to that of a pea. (See Figure 13–122*C*). These were all removed, and the wound was irrigated with normal saline; some of the nodules felt gritty. The wound was closed with 000 in-terrupted chromic catgut sutures. The patient tolerated surgery and anesthesia and left the operating room in good condition.

Pathology Report. *Macroscopic Description:* The specimen consists of a piece of fibroadipose tissue containing four shotty, hard lesions that cut with a gritty sensation and have on section a laminated structure, with calcific foci through the nodule. Each of the nodules measures about 0.4 cm. in diameter.

Microscopic Description: Sections show a number of rounded, hyalinized bodies that are surrounded in part by a muscular wall. These represent thrombotic and organized blood vessels. The adjacent tissue contains numerous endothelium-lined vascular spaces that are fairly closely apposed and render a pseudopapillary character to the lesion. There is a great deal of extravasated blood throughout the soft tissue, and here and there are deposits of hemosiderin. The origin of this lesion is not too clear, but it is consistent with some sort of atriovenous malformation.

Diagnosis: Vascular hamartoma of the cheek (Richard E. Palmer, M.D.).

Postoperative Course. The patient was discharged from the hospital on the second postoperative day and followed at the office periodically. She had an uneventful recovery. (See Figure 13–122*D*.)

Final Diagnosis. Vascular hamartoma of the cheek.

Shira injects boiling water into soft-tissue hemangiomas. He describes his technique as follows:

"Handling the boiling water for injection into cavernous hemangiomas does not present much of a problem. I keep the water boiling in a beaker on an electric stove just outside the operating room. When everything is ready to 'go' I put on three or four pairs of rubber gloves and then take sterile felt and

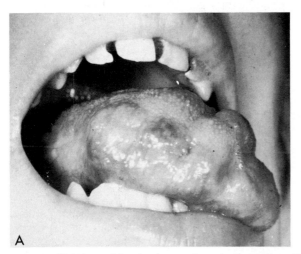

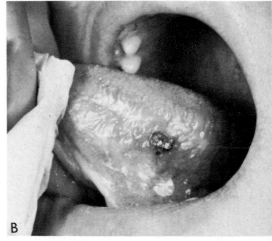

Figure 13–123 *A*, Massive hemangioma in the tongue. (Compare Figure 13–200). *B*, Small, discrete hemangioma that simulated a melanoma because of its jet black color.

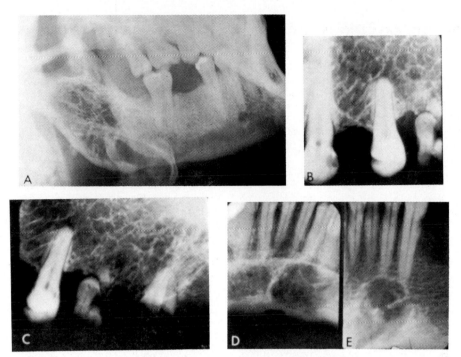

Figure 13–124 *A,* Cavernous hemangioma of the ramus of the mandible, showing coarse bone cancellations radiating from the center toward the periphery of the lesion. *B* and *C,* Cavernous hemangioma of the maxilla. Bone spicules extending at right angles to the bone and into the lesion can be seen at the anterior border of the lesion. *D* and *E,* Capillary hemangioma of the mandible. Well-circumscribed cavity in the bone with sclerotic borders. Within the lesion there is evidence of bone trabeculations that do not have a regular bone arrangement.

(*A,* Reproduced with permission from Stafne, E. C.: Value of roentgenograms in diagnosis of tumors of the jaws. Oral Surg., *6:*82–92 [Jan.], 1953. *B* and *C,* Reproduced with permission from Stafne, E. C.: Oral Roentgenographic Diagnosis. 4th ed. Philadelphia, W. B. Saunders Co., 1963. *D* and *E,* Reproduced with permission from Erich, J. B.: Central hemangioma of the mandible: Report of a case. Am. J. Orthod. [Oral Surg. Sect.] *33:*611–613 [Aug.], 1947.)

wrap it around the syringe. In this manner, the syringe is insulated and does not burn the hand. I inject the boiling water into several different areas of the tumor, depositing about 5 cc. in each site. The total amount utilized depends upon the size of the tumor. I then wait 3 months, and if there has not been sufficient sclerosing, I repeat the procedure. I have had good success in the management of this problem following this technique. It is a well-recognized method of treatment and has been used successfully by surgeons since the time of Wyeth."[79]

He also treats soft-tissue hemangiomas by radiation therapy as follows:

"I have used low-content radium needles with excellent results. The technique for utilizing radium needles for hemangiomas is the same as the use of radium for any other tumor. The size of the tumor is calculated, and radium is inserted to give a uniform exposure to all parts of the tumor, being careful to keep the needles sufficiently spaced to prevent 'hot spots' from developing. We have had no difficulty with postradiation slough."[79]

Electrodesiccation with a sharp needle electrode inserted directly through the mucosa into the hemangioma in many different areas is used by Figi and O'Brien[33] and Oringer.[58]

CENTRAL HEMANGIOMA

These rare tumors are fraught with great surgical danger because it is impossible to make a preoperative diagnosis from the roentgenogram unless the surgeon has a clue revealed by the roentgenogram (see Case Report No. 24). Of course the inability to make a diagnosis from the radiograph is common, and so some make their preoperative diagnosis by taking a biopsy. However, in the case of the central hemangioma, even this presumably innocuous procedure can result in a frightening hemorrhage difficult to control.

CENTRAL CAVERNOUS HEMANGIOMA OF THE MANDIBLE CAUSED BY A FOREIGN BODY

Patient. During routine oral radiographic examination of this 75-year-old male, a radiolucent area was found in the symphysis, and in it appeared to be a piece of metal (Figure 13–125). However, past experience prompted additional radiographs, which proved the foreign body to be in the soft tissues over the symphysis.

Operation. The mandible and soft tissues of the chin were anesthetized with right and left inferior alveolar nerve block injections and circumferential injections in the skin. Then a 21 gauge needle was passed through the skin into the mouth several times until the occlusal radiograph showed the guide needle to practically contact the foreign body (see Figure 13–126*A, B, C, D* and *E*). Cutting down alongside the needle orally, the foreign body, a piece of steel, was encountered and re-

moved. Then the mandible was exposed, an opening cut through the labial cortical plate and a very hemorrhagic fibrous tumor was, with difficulty, removed from the bony crypt.

Histopathologic Report. Cavernous hemangioma of the mandible.

The patient was a machinist and remembered that approximately 40 years earlier a piece of metal had struck him in the chin. He had had no symptoms then or since except a drop or two of blood on his chin at the time he was struck. Actually, he thought that what had hit him had glanced off. It is apparent, however, that this piece of steel penetrated the skin and struck the cortical plate hard enough to produce a hemorrhage in the cancellations and then the cavernous hemangioma was formed.

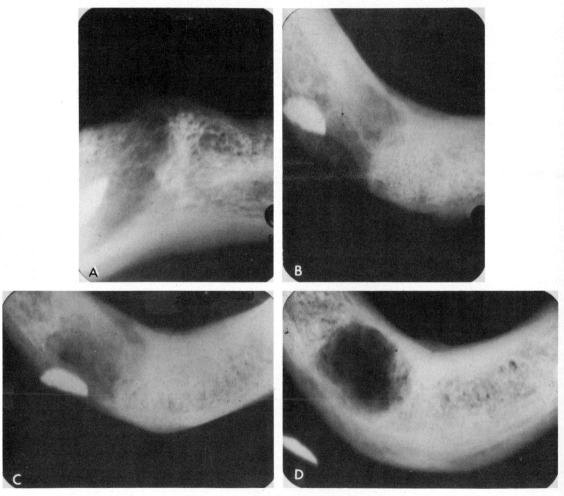

Figure 13–125 Various x-ray views taken to help locate this foreign body. (See Case Report No. 25.)

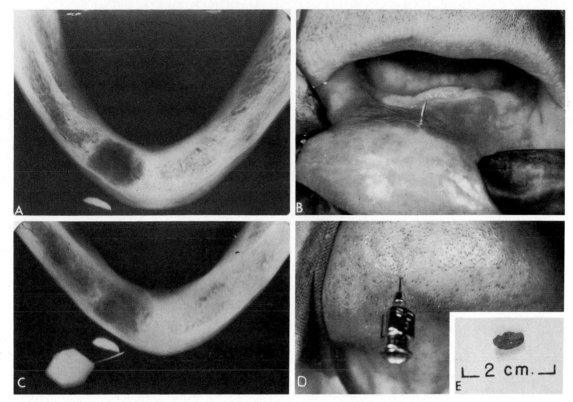

Figure 13–126 *A*, True occlusal view of cavernous hemangioma of the mandible and a foreign body. *B*, A 1½-inch 21 gauge needle used as a guide. *C*, Radiograph with guide needle in place. *D*, The needle was left in place while the oral tissues were cut and opened along the shaft of the needle until the metallic object was found. *E*, Piece of metal removed. (See Case Report No. 24 for details.)

Such major procedures as tying off the external carotid artery are not as effective as one might expect, because of the collateral blood supply from the opposite side. Incidentally, this fact must be borne in mind regardless of the reason for the ligation of the external carotid.

Shira establishes the diagnosis of central hemangiomas by the clinical and roentgenographic evidence as follows:

"A, spontaneous bleeding into the oral cavity, particularly noticeable at night; B, loose, depressible teeth; and C, honeycombed osteolytic lesions in the bone as visualized on the roentgenogram. If in doubt, I enter the lesion with a needle and aspirating syringe and see if I aspirate blood."[79]

Treatment. Concerning the treatment of central hemangiomas, Shira states: "In treating these lesions by external radiation, a dosage of 1800 to 2200 R. measured in air has been sufficient to bring about resolution of the lesions. With dosages in this range, osteoradionecrosis is no problem. Following radiation, the honeycombed osteolytic lesions

of the bone disappear and regeneration of normal bone is evident on the roentgenogram."[79]

Some surgeons excise these tumors. They state that the most important factor is adequate blood supply to replace that lost during surgery and the time consumed in controlling the hemorrhage. Packing, electrocoagulation and splinting can be tried, usually with poor results. It is obvious that coagulation in a pool of blood is ineffectual.

Our tumor was invasive and was extremely difficult to remove. In large central hemangiomas partial resection of the mandible has been advocated. This, in the author's opinion, is too radical, especially in view of the success of radiation therapy that Shira has reported.

Patients who present with a loose tooth or teeth and a history of spontaneous bleeding from the gingival tissue and whose radiographs reveal a radiolucent area with an irregular border most likely have a central hemangioma. (See Case Report No. 26 and Figure 13–127.)

Case Report No. 26

CENTRAL HEMANGIOMA OF THE MANDIBLE; DEATH FROM POSTOPERATIVE CORONARY EMBOLISM

P. L. KHURANA, D.D.S.

I was called at about 11 P.M. to examine a case of bleeding from the mouth. The patient, a girl of 11 years, had had three extractions performed by her local dentist earlier in the evening.

On clinical examination I noticed that the teeth extracted were three lower deciduous anteriors, and the area showed no bleeding. The lower left second deciduous molar was mobile, and there was definite oozing of blood every time I touched that tooth. There was a distinct swelling on the lower left side of the mandible. On questioning, she told me that the swelling had been there for about 6 months, and it had gradually increased in size. There was slight pain on palpation.

I presumed that the area was infected and did not take an x-ray at the time. I called the anesthetist for general anesthesia, and what I thought would be a very simple extraction turned out to be a nightmare.

The extraction itself was a minute's work, but immediately after I had removed the tooth, there was spurting of arterial blood that was almost uncontrollable. I tried to control it with digital pressure and packing the socket with gauze and cotton wool. As I was inserting the pack, I found a big cavity in the mandible in the area from which I had extracted the tooth. I packed the whole cavity, continued the digital pressure and sent for blood. The transfusion was started within 20 minutes. Bleeding was so profuse that in spite of packs, continued pressure and transfusion, it was 3 A.M. before it was checked. I moved the patient to the resuscitation ward with nasal oxygen and intravenous glucose-saline drip, and then, I decided to call it a day.

The next morning I examined the case. There was no bleeding, the pack was in position, and the intravenous glucose-saline drip was being continued, but oxygen had been stopped. An extraoral x-ray of the mandible was taken, and it showed a fairly large cavity in the lower left region of the mandible, with a partially developed molar in it. In view of the severe hemorrhage and the cavity in the mandible, I had made a provisional diagnosis of aneurysmal bone cyst of the mandible. See Figure 13–127A and B.

The next day, that is, the third, I decided to take the patient to the operation theater, arranged for more blood and called the surgeon to stand by in case of another hemorrhage. We started the blood transfusion, the patient was anesthetized, and I removed the pack. Unfortunately, blood shot out again. The surgeon came to my rescue; I assisted him in the ligation of the left external carotid artery. In spite of that, bleeding did not stop. Packs were put in. We ligated the right external carotid artery as well, continuing the transfusion throughout. I packed the cavity with beeswax and tried to persuade the surgeon to do a resection of the mandible, but he thought that there would be severe deformity in the girl when she grew up. As the bleeding had been controlled, we decided to leave the case and wait.

A curetted specimen from the cavity was sent for biopsy. The patient was again sent to the resuscitation ward, the blood transfusion being continued.

For the next 2 days there was no bleeding and no elevation of temperature, and the intravenous glucose-saline drip was continued intermittently.

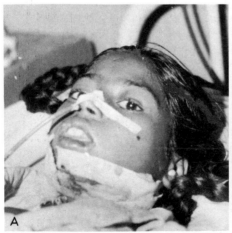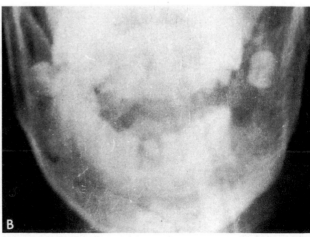

Figure 13–127 *A*, Patient with a central hemangioma of the mandible following initial surgery. She died from a coronary embolism after a second operation. *B*, View of the mandible (after the first operation), which revealed a partially formed third molar. (See Case Report No. 26 for details.)

On the sixth day the patient was shifted to the general ward, with strict instructions that she was not to be moved. Seven bottles of blood and four bottles of glucose-saline had been given to the patient by that time. On the seventh day, tragically, probably because of negligence on the part of the nursing staff, the patient, while getting up, fell off the bed and expired immediately.

Postmortem examination showed that death was due to a coronary embolism.

Resection of the mandible was done at autopsy. An x-ray was taken of the resected portion, but it did not help in diagnosis. The biopsy report came in a day later with the diagnosis of hemangioma of the mandible. It read as follows:

"Bony spicules in the hematoma, malformation and enlargement of blood vessels, in fibromuscular tissue. Arrangement of blood vessels is not normal."

The only possible source of the continued and excessive bleeding after the ligation of both the external carotid arteries, besides the bleeding of the hemangioma, could have been the presence of a collateral branch of the common carotid artery before its bifurcation into external and internal carotid arteries. This would not have been ligated.

To date, this is the seventh case recorded in dental literature.

LYMPHANGIOMA

Etiology. Two causes of lymphangioma are (*a*) trauma, seen most frequently in the lips, and (*b*) congenital, usually in the tongue or cheek.

Cahn[15] reports that this type of growth, while rare, is seen most commonly on the lip. He feels that it may start as a cracked lip which does not heal. New lymphatic channels accompany the new blood vessels that develop in injured tissue. If for some reason they are blocked, lymphangiectasis and edema take place. Interstitial fibrosis then follows, and the lips become thickened because of the semisolid mass akin to elephantiasis. In the patient described in Case Report No. 27 there was no evidence of previous history of cracked lips, although there are obvious scars in both lips.

Case Report No. 27

LYMPHANGIOMA OF THE LIPS

Patient. A male Negro aged 35 presented complaining that his lips were gradually increasing in size as he became older (Fig. 13–128).

Oral Examination. The lips were five times the usual size, normal in color, freely movable, non-painful and semisolid, although readily compres-

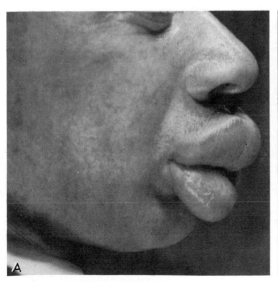
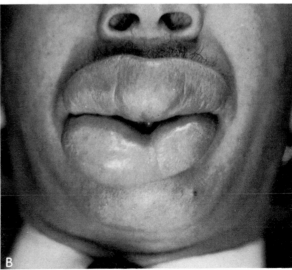

Figure 13–128 Lymphangioma of the lips. (See Case Report No. 27.)

sible. Scars are presented in the mucosa of both lips. There was no oral infection.

Physical Examination. Findings were essentially negative.

Diagnosis. Lymphangioma of the lips.

Case Report No. 28

LYMPHANGIOMA OF THE LIP

Patient. A boy aged 16 was admitted to the Magee-Women's Hospital complaining of a sore swollen lower lip of approximately 6 years' duration, which was increasing in size.

Oral Examination. Examination revealed a cracked, swollen, semisolid lower lip. The patient stated that the lip had been cracked almost as long as there had been swelling in the lip; it partially healed and then broke open again (Fig. 13–129).

Chronic gingivitis was present, owing to poor oral hygiene. Five chronically infected maxillary and mandibular teeth were present; these were extracted.

Physical Examination. Findings were essentially negative.

Blood Studies. The hemoglobin and differential count were normal. The white blood cells ran from 8800 to 12,000 per cubic millimeter over a 14-day period; otherwise the findings were normal. The blood chemistry was normal, as was the urine examination. Wassermann and Kahn tests were negative. The sedimentation time was over 90 minutes.

History. One month after a tonsillectomy, the patient first noticed that his lower lip was swollen. The initial swelling never disappeared, although there had been periods when the swelling was much less. However, the lip had gradually and consistently increased in size over the years. Since the onset he had noticed that damp weather or coryza caused an increase in size. There was no association between any particular food and degree of swelling.

Diagnosis. Lymphangioma of the lower lip.

Treatment. The recommended treatment for large lymphangioma is injection with sclerosing solutions or x-ray treatment. In both this and the preceding case x-ray treatment was started, but the patients failed to carry through with the treatment.

Following the above treatment, which has as its objective fibrosis of the vessels, normal contour of the part can be obtained by partial surgical excision or repeated insertions of an electrodesiccation needle into the tumor over a period of days.

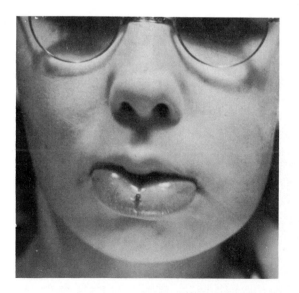

Figure 13–129 Lymphangioma of the lower lip. (See Case Report No. 28.)

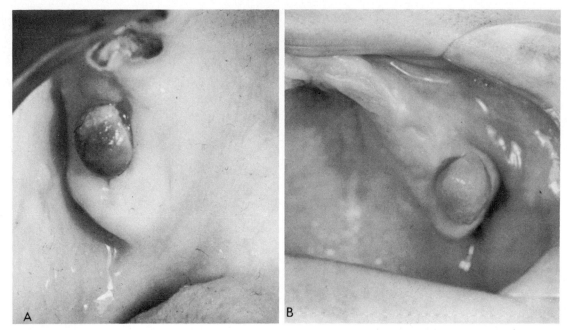

Figure 13–130 *A*, Herniation of the mucosa of the maxillary sinus originally diagnosed as a peripheral giant cell tumor. *B*, Similar appearing polyp from the maxillary sinus, which herniated through the alveolus following a molar extraction. (See Chapter 25 for treatment.)

INFLAMMATORY FIBROUS HYPERPLASIAS (EPULIS FISSURATA, REDUNDANT TISSUE, "DENTURE INJURY TISSUE")

One of the most common tumors in the oral cavity is that seen along the margins of ill-fitting dentures (see Figures 13–131 to 13–134). These really are not true neoplasms but are localized inflammatory hyperplasias. Frequently they are bifid, containing one or more fissures. These hyperplasias may be localized to one area of the denture, or might be extensive, involving one-half to three-fourths of the denture periphery. In the bottom of the valley of the folds there frequently is ulceration. These areas can become malig-

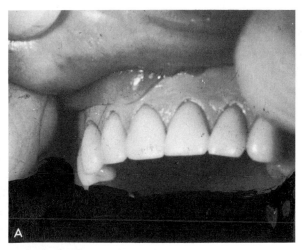
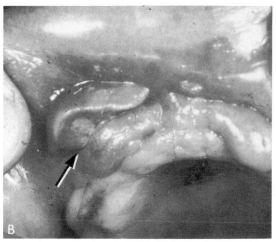

Figure 13–131 *A*, This patient wore the same denture for 25 years. Note how the hyperplastic fibrous fold of tissue hangs down over the labial flange of the denture. *B*, In the valley between the folds was an ulcerated area. Upon removal and biopsy a diagnosis of epidermoid carcinoma was made.

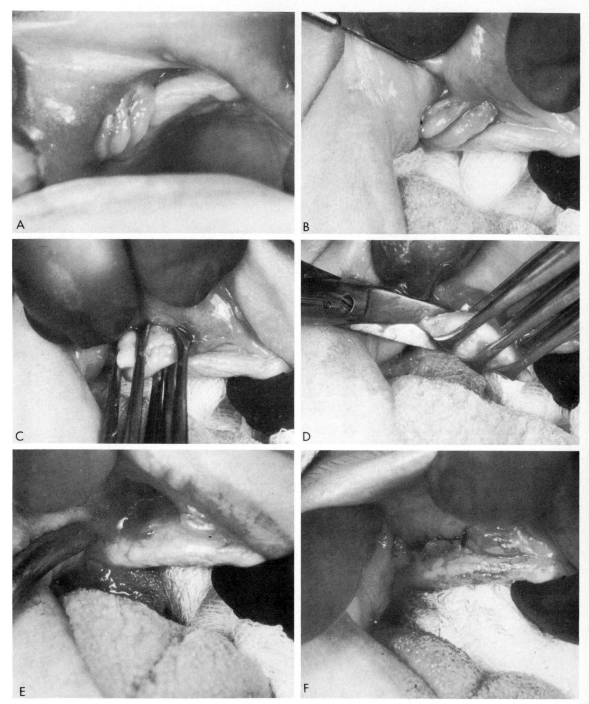

Figure 13–132 *A*, In this localized lobulated hyperplasia there are three folds of alveolar hyperplasia confined to the maxillary cuspid and bicuspid area. *B*, Anesthesia may be either local or general. In this case the patient is anesthetized with thiopental sodium, but it is the author's technique also to infiltrate the base of the tumor with a local anesthetic solution with a vasoconstrictor. *C*, The base of the tumor is carefully grasped with as many Allis forceps as are necessary to outline the base so that a line for cutting can be obtained which will permit complete excision of the tumor and still not involve the musculature of the lip or cheek. When the Allis forceps are in place, have the assistant hold the lip firmly while you place your finger over the skin on the opposite side from the tumor. Holding this finger in place, slowly move the tumor with the Allis forceps. If muscle tissue has inadvertently been caught between the beaks of the Allis forceps, the finger pressed against the skin will detect movement of the muscle tissue. If no muscle tissue is caught, then the finger will feel the tumor mass sliding over the muscles which do not move. *D*, Cut along the edge of the Allis forceps with a No. 9 Dean's scissors. Caution your assistant who is holding the Allis forceps *not* to move the forceps during this procedure. *E*, Wound after excision of the tumor. *F*, Edges of the mucosa are approximated with interrupted silk sutures.

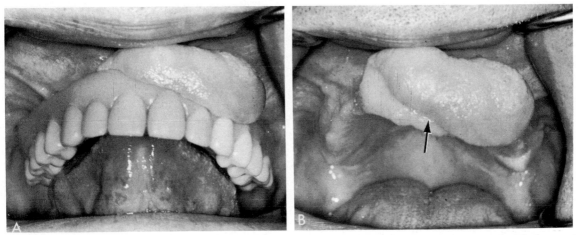

Figure 13–133 *A*, Massive fibrous epulis fissurata. *B*, With the denture removed the fissure created by the flange of the denture can be seen.

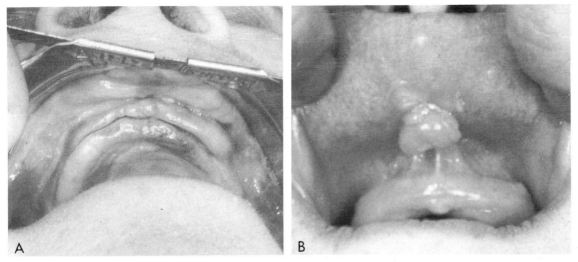

Figure 13–134 *A*, Inflammatory fibrous hyperplasia extending from the right maxillary bicuspid area to the left bicuspid area. The growth of this tumor was stimulated by the trauma exerted by the labial denture flange upon the mucosa of the sulcus as the alveolar ridge resorbed, permitting the dentures to settle. *B*, A nodule of fibrous hyperplasia whose formation was produced by the labial portion of the denture flange traumatizing the mucosa of the sulcus in the region of the labial frenum only.

nant. For this reason all such hyperplasias should be surgically excised, the tissue biopsied, and new dentures fitted.

Figure 13–132 illustrates the technique for excision of lobulated hyperplasia. For more information on this subject, see pages 169 to 171 in Chapter 3.

PYOGENIC GRANULOMA

The pyogenic granuloma is a tumor-like growth that occurs at all ages in both sexes. By far the most common site is the interdental gingiva, but the lesion may occur on the lips, on the tongue, and rarely on other areas of the oral mucous membrane. It presents as a soft pedunculated or broad-based growth that has a smooth red surface, is often ulcerated, bleeds easily, and may have a raspberry-like appearance.

The major mass of the "tumor" is composed of numerous small capillaries which are interspersed by edematous connective tissue with a mild to dense infiltration by polymorphonuclear leukocytes, plasma cells and lymphocytes.

Treatment consists of local excision. These growths will recur if the entire base is not included in the original excision or if the irritant is not removed.

Pregnancy Tumor. During pregnancy a pedunculated or sessile tumor, histologically identical with the pyogenic granuloma, may develop at the gingival line labially or buccally, and grow to the size of a walnut. Fre-

quently these tumors extend through the interseptal space and develop on both sides of the alveolar process. The tumor is covered with hyperplastic epithelium, is red, or purplish red, bleeds easily, and grows rapidly as compared with other oral tumors. As a rule the tumor starts in some area of the mouth where there is some form of irritation, such as an ill-fitting crown, an irregular filling or deposits of serumal calculus. This local irritation, which means inflammation, and the stimulating effect that the estrogenic hormones have on the growth of epithelium, are the two factors which result in the growth of the "pregnancy tumor." Because of the extreme vascularity of these tumors, they blanch on pressure.

TREATMENT. Surgical excision, with removal of the irritating cause and cauterization of the base should be carried out. If the tumor is removed and the cause left behind, there is a good possibility that the tumor will recur. The patient should be advised that there is a possibility of recurrence which may necessitate a second removal. It has been stated that these tumors disappear with the termination of the pregnancy. It is my observation that this does does not happen. (See Figures 13–135 to 13–137.)

Postextraction Pyogenic Granuloma. These growths are also seen in postextraction alveoli, and are the result of the presence in the socket of some foreign irritating material—for example, bits of tooth structure, enamel, dentine, filling material, calculus or a piece of dead bone. They may also possibly

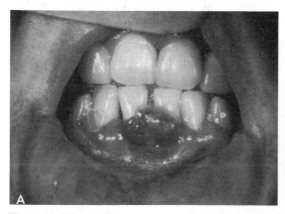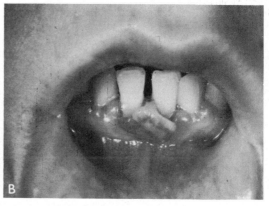

Figure 13–135 *A,* "Pregnancy tumor" (pyogenic granuloma) at 6 months. This tumor started about the end of the third month of pregnancy, and had been steadily growing larger. As can be seen, this patient had a clean mouth, but the separation of the central incisors permitted food to pack between these teeth with resultant irritation to the gingival tissue. With the onset of pregnancy, this tumor developed at the only point of inflammation in the mouth. *B,* "Pregnancy tumor" moved away from the teeth, showing the pedicle arising from the interseptal tissue. Surgical excision at the base with superficial cauterization to control bleeding is indicated. (See text.)

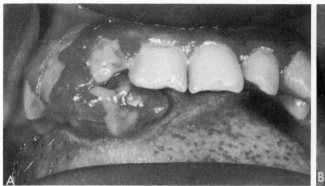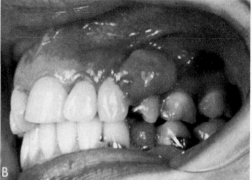

Figure   13–136   Two examples of pyogenic granulomas ("pregnancy tumors").

be an outgrowth of a periapical granuloma which was not removed at the time of extraction of the tooth.

In appearance they are masses of irregular mulberry-like reddish blue granulation tissue or a well-circumscribed, smooth, rounded tumor-like proliferation from the socket. An example of a pyogenic granuloma growing out of the alveolus after an extraction is shown in Figure 13–138. This latter entity must be differentiated from the herniation of the maxillary sinus mucosa or the herniation of a polyp from the maxillary sinus as described in Figure 13–130.

Pus is freely expressed when the surface is cut. Treatment consists of curettage and debridement of the socket to remove the foreign

material and the soft tissue of the pyogenic granuloma.

GIANT CELL TUMORS AND GIANT CELL REPARATIVE GRANULOMAS

These lesions are found either peripherally or centrally in the jaws. They are thought to be either (1) neoplastic in origin or (2) the result of trauma. Based on the following discussion they can be classified:

1. Peripheral lesions or peripheral giant cell tumors (see Figures 13–142 to 13–158 for examples and study the captions).

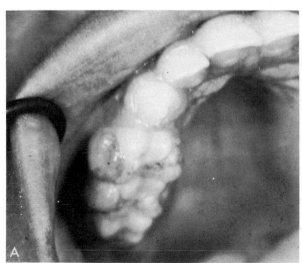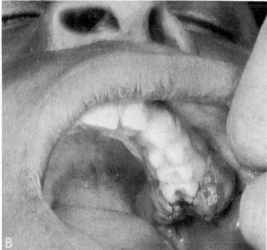

Figure 13–137   Two examples of "pregnancy tumors" (pyogenic granulomas) that extend through the interproximal spaces, forming large buccal and lingual masses which bleed freely when traumatized by eating and sometimes when talking. Treatment should be as indicated in previous figures and in the text. Good oral hygiene, including scaling, is a "must" during pregnancy.

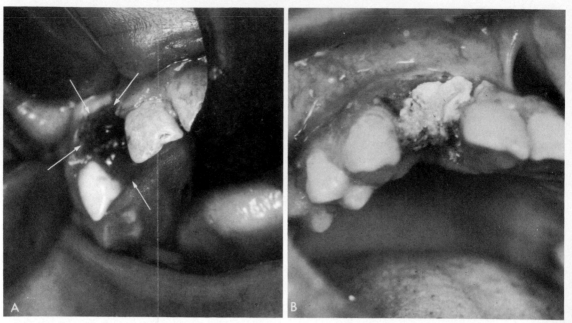

Figure 13–138 *A,* One week after the extraction of the right maxillary lateral incisor this hemorrhagic pyogenic granuloma extruded from the alveolus. Under general anesthesia the alveolus was thoroughly curetted to remove the pyogenic granuloma in its entirety. *B,* Bleeding was controlled by packing the alveolus with 1/4-inch iodoform gauze.

2. Central lesions or central giant cell tumors (see Figures 13–159 to 13–164).

Jaffe states that those lesions which have been listed as giant cell tumors in jaw bones are for the most part reparative granulomas, and so he suggests the term "giant cell reparative granuloma" for these central lesions. He believes them to be different from the true giant cell tumor, which is a neoplasm in the true sense, while the "granuloma" represents a local reparative reaction to trauma.[44]

Giant cell lesions are frequently seen in children between the ages of 8 and 15. The resorptive process associated with the roots of primary teeth may also be responsible for the formation of these reparative granulomas.

Bernier and Cahn agree with this theory following their review of 41 so-called peripheral "giant cell tumors" and have adopted Jaffe's term with the qualification of "peripheral."[8] Shafer, Hine and Levy have pointed out that since the lesion is not truly a "reparative" one, this term is frequently dropped.[75]

True giant cell tumors of the mandible and maxilla according to Jaffe are extremely rare. Histologically, he states, "in a lesion representing true giant cell tumor of bone, the lesional tissue shows large numbers of giant cells distributed more or less evenly through-out the tissue fields, and these giant cells are set in a rather cellular stroma of spindle-shaped or polyhedral cells. Furthermore, this lesion is one which recurs even after thorough curettage and requires removal of a section of bone and teeth to prevent further recurrence."[44]

The histologic pattern of the central giant cell reparative granuloma according to Jaffe is a rather characteristic one. "In a rather loose vascular stroma composed of small spindle-shaped cells, one notes a good deal of hemorrhagic extravasation. The multinuclear cells present are sparse, small and unevenly distributed, and often clumped in areas of hemorrhage. One will note also some microscopic lobules of this lesional tissue; one may see, here and there, some delicate trabeculae of newly formed bone."[44]

Others[12, 20] believe that the benign giant cell tumor of bone cannot be distinguished from the central giant cell reparative granuloma on the basis of microscopic examination.

True giant cell tumors rarely appear before the age of 20. When a giant cell lesion is found in the jaws, one should make certain that the patient is not suffering from hyperparathyroidism in which the so-called "brown tumor" is frequently found. Histologically it

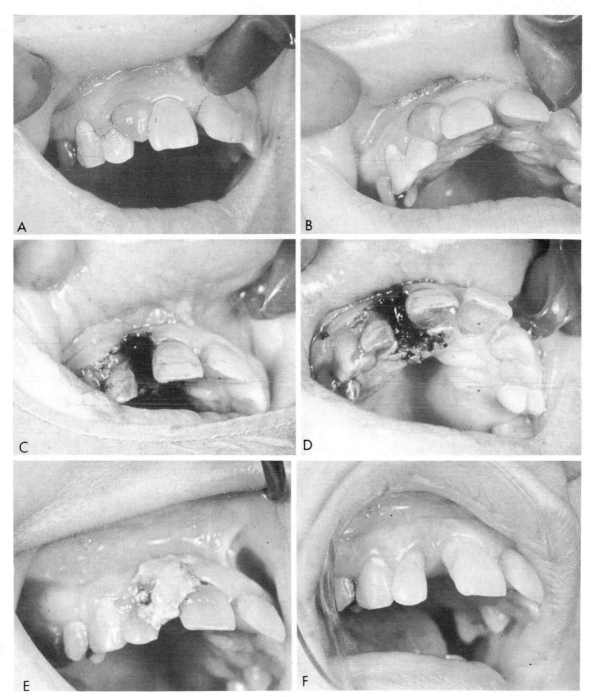

Figure 13–139 *A*, A peripheral ossifying fibroma that had been excised three times previously and that, from its history and appearance plus radiographic evidence of interseptal osseous destruction. I incorrectly diagnosed as a peripheral giant cell tumor. An excisional biopsy proved this to be a peripheral ossifying fibroma. *B*, Occlusal view. *C*, Tumor excised. *D*, Base cauterized. *E*, Zinc oxide and eugenol dressing applied for 1 week. *F*, Tissue healed. No recurrence has followed.

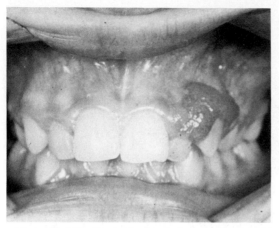

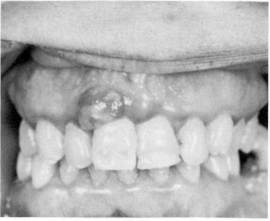

Figure 13–140 Hyperplastic gingival tissue in a 15-year-old girl that recurred four times after removal. This was undoubtedly associated with puberty. But why this bright red, soft, friable growth only involved the gingiva around the maxillary lateral incisor and cuspid is unknown. The excisions (excisional biopsies) were done to allay the fears of the parents that their daughter was developing a malignant tumor. The recurrence ceased when she passed puberty.

Figure 13–141 This lesion simulates somewhat the appearance of a peripheral giant cell tumor; however, on histologic examination it proved to be a pyogenic granuloma. While these lesions can be found on the mucosa, lips and tongue, they most frequently arise on the gingiva. They can be smooth or lobulated, with a pedicle or a sessile base. They are fragile and hemorrhage with the slightest injury. The cause is usually a minor trauma that permits the entrance of microorganisms, and these stimulate proliferation of the vascular endothelium. Treatment is surgical excision and mild cauterization of the base. Calculus is frequently found on the neck of the adjacent tooth or teeth and should be removed.

Photographic Case Report

INTERDENTAL PERIPHERAL GIANT CELL TUMOR

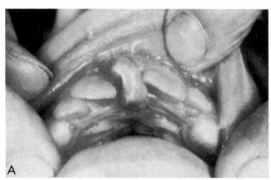

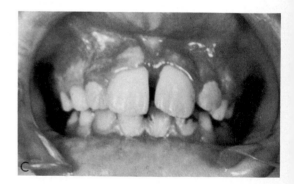

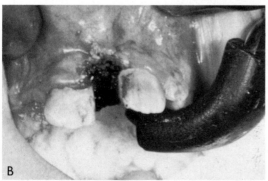

Figure 13–142 Peripheral giant cell tumor in a 12-year-old boy. *A,* Tumor arose from the interdental tissue, slowly separating the central incisors. *B,* Tumor excised and base cauterized. *C,* Five weeks postoperative appearance. Note the rapid closure of the diastema. Gingival tissues are contouring very well. Note improvement over *A.*

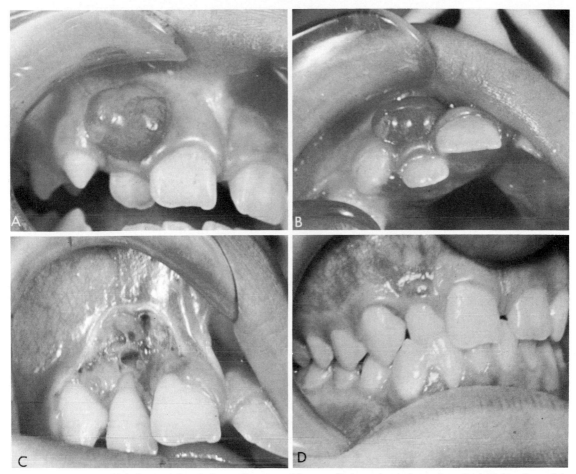

Figure 13–143 *A,* Globular peripheral giant cell tumor with a sessile base that is located on the labial surface of the maxillary mucoperiosteal membrane. *B,* Note that in this case it does not arise from the gingival tissues, which are the most common sites for these tumors. *C,* Nevertheless, because these tumors do recur, a few millimeters of tissue around the base are included when the tumor is excised with its underlying periosteum. As can be seen, the necks of the maxillary cuspid and central incisor are partly exposed labially, while the entire labial surface of the lateral incisor is exposed. Very slight coagulation was used to control the bleeding. *D,* Ten months later the labial mucoperiosteal membrane has covered the exposed labial bone and the gingiva has also been restored, covering the necks of the three teeth originally approximating the tumor base. When the giant cell tumor arises from the gingiva, frequently after removal and coagulation of the exposed bone, the gingiva does not return to its original insertion or contour and the necks of adjacent teeth are, unfortunately, exposed.

is practically impossible to differentiate these lesions. Biochemical determinations on the blood serum will rule out hyperparathyroidism. A serum calcium value of over 11.5 mg. per 100 cc. is of definite diagnostic significance in favor of hyperparathyroidism.

PERIPHERAL GIANT CELL TUMORS AND PERIPHERAL GIANT CELL REPARATIVE GRANULOMAS

Peripheral giant cell pedunculated or sessile tumors or peripheral giant cell granulomas are located on the alveolar process of the maxilla or mandible, and are generally found springing from the necks of the teeth or on the edentulous ridge. These painless swellings of bluish red color are slow-growing and are usually well circumscribed. The larger lesions become lobulated and separate the adjacent teeth.

Radiographs of the area in which peripheral giant cell tumors are located reveal a demineralization of the osseous structure at the base of the tumor.

Roentgenographs. Examination of good oral roentgenograms will help in determining preoperatively whether the tumor is a giant cell tumor or a giant cell reparative granuloma. If it is a giant cell tumor there will

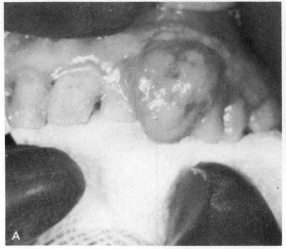

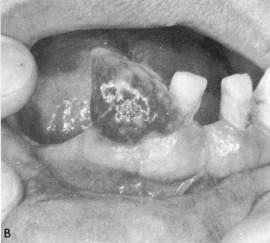

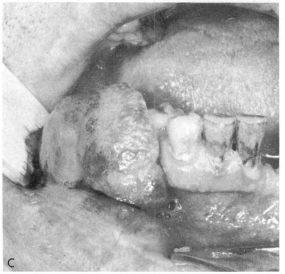

Figure 13–144 *A*, An example of a pedunculated peripheral giant cell reparative granuloma in a 25-year-old female. The pedicle arose from the interseptal tissue between the left lateral incisor and cuspid. It was treated by excision and cauterization of the base. *B*, Cone-shaped peripheral giant cell tumor whose pedicle arises from the gingiva of the mandibular right lateral incisor and cuspid. *C*, Very large and unusual pedunculated giant cell tumor (shaped like a doughnut without the hole) arising from the mandibular buccal mucoperiosteal membrane opposite the bicuspids.

usually be radiographic evidence of localized bone resorption (demineralization) below the tumor. Only occasionally is there radiographic evidence of localized bone resorption below giant cell reparative granulomas.

Treatment. Large tumors should be biopsied before they are excised and the extent of surgery is based on whether the tumor is a peripheral giant cell tumor or a peripheral giant cell reparative granuloma. Small tumors are conservatively excised down to bone with superficial cauterization of the base.

If the preoperative pathology report is *peripheral giant cell tumor*, we make a wider excision of the tumor and coagulate the base.

At this first operation we are still comparatively conservative. We are not dealing with a malignancy and one can always become more radical at subsequent operations. It is necessary to be more radical in your surgical approach to subsequent recurrences of peripheral giant cell tumors. (See Case Report No. 29.) Adjacent teeth have to be sacrificed and excision of alveolar process is necessary with more extensive coagulation of the remaining osseous tissue. This results subsequently in a sequestrum which eventually loosens and is lifted off.

In *peripheral giant cell reparative granulomas*, the first comparatively conservative

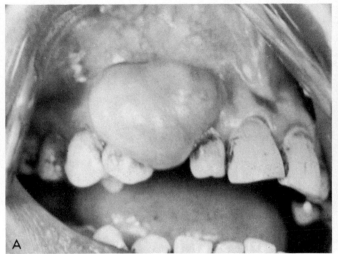

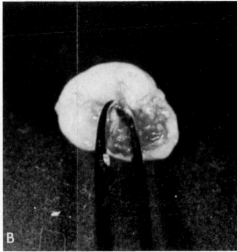

Figure 13–145 *A*, At first glance this tumor could be mistaken for a peripheral giant cell tumor. However, this was an unusual fibroma; it was triangle-shaped, as contrasted with the common globular shape, and had a pedicle base rather than a sessile base. It does have a smooth surface in contrast to the irregular nodular surface of the giant cell tumor as shown in *A* of Figure 13–144.

surgical excision with cauterization of the base is usually adequate to prevent a recurrence. If there is a recurrence more vigorous cauterization generally suffices. Never has the author found it necessary to extract adjacent teeth or remove large sections of alveolar bone to prevent recurrences of peripheral giant cell reparative granulomas.

Clinically it has been my observation that the more resorption of bone beneath either of these peripheral giant cell lesions or resorption of the roots of teeth in central giant cell lesions, the greater the possibility of recurrence. Repeated recurrences are a good indication that the lesion is a true giant cell tumor.

(*Text continued on page 845*)

Case Report No. 29

PERIPHERAL GIANT CELL TUMOR

History. This 15-year-old male stated that this tumor had been present for 4 years. During this time it was removed three times by the family physician and a surgeon. His mother brought with her three pathology reports in which the diagnosis was recorded as a giant cell tumor. This slow-growing tumor has separated the cuspid and bicuspid over 1 cm (Fig. 13–146*A* to *C*). The tumor is soft and friable, and so the surface is devoid of epithelium as the result of masticatory trauma.

Treatment. In view of the history of three recurrences and the pathology report, I advised radical surgery to include the extraction of teeth on either side of the tumor and the excision of alveolar bone and coagulation of the base. To this the mother objected. On her insistence, another conservative operation was performed, namely, wide excision of the tumor and coagulation of the base (Fig. 13–146*D*).

Subsequent Course. Over the next 18 months I excised this recurrent tumor four times, being more radical in the extraction of teeth and the removal and coagulation of bone at each subsequent operation. Figure 13–146*E* shows the final result: a marked loss of the alveolar ridge of the maxilla with a marked depression greater than what appears on the photograph, as well as the loss of the maxillary central and lateral incisors, the cuspid and the first and second bicuspids — all this before the tumor growth was stopped. Repeated recurrence is the typical history of a true giant cell tumor, peripheral or central.

(*Text continued on page 844*)

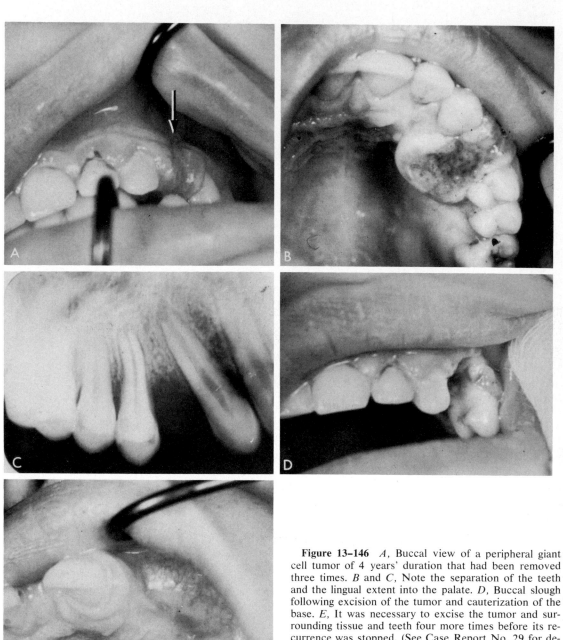

Figure 13–146 *A,* Buccal view of a peripheral giant cell tumor of 4 years' duration that had been removed three times. *B* and *C,* Note the separation of the teeth and the lingual extent into the palate. *D,* Buccal slough following excision of the tumor and cauterization of the base. *E,* It was necessary to excise the tumor and surrounding tissue and teeth four more times before its recurrence was stopped. (See Case Report No. 29 for details.)

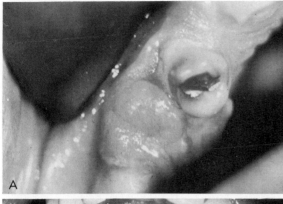

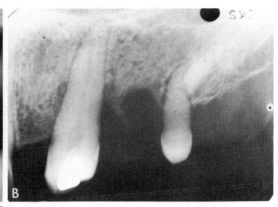

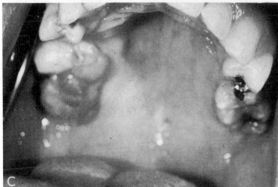

Figure 13–147 *A,* A sessile, lobulated peripheral giant cell tumor arising from the crest of the maxillary ridge distal to the second bicuspid in a male patient, aged 32. *B,* Periapical radiograph reveals invasion of the alveolar bone between the second bicuspid and the rudimentary tooth buried in the tumor. *Treatment:* Wide excision of the tumor and the two teeth was necessary because of the destruction of bone. Base was cauterized. *C,* A large multinodular, sessile peripheral giant cell tumor covering the maxillary tuberosity and partially covering the lingual surface of the maxillary second bicuspid. Treatment is excision, including the mucoperiosteal tissue for several millimeters around its base, and cauterization of the osseous tissue beneath the tumor.

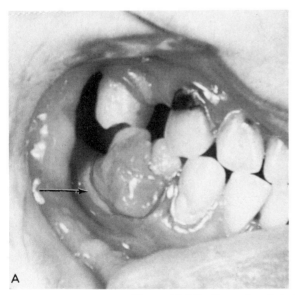

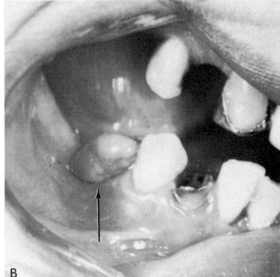

Figure 13–148 Examples of gingival peripheral giant cell tumors.

Photographic Case Report

EXCISION OF A SESSILE PERIPHERAL GIANT CELL TUMOR

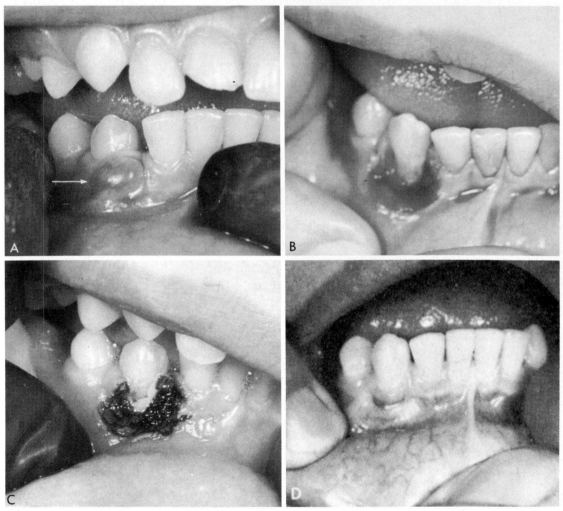

Figure 13–149 *A,* A 12-year-old boy presented with a bluish red sessile tumor at the neck of the right mandibular cuspid. This tumor had been slowly growing for approximately 6 months. It blanched on pressure. *Tentative diagnosis:* (1) Hemangioma, (2) peripheral giant cell tumor. *B,* Under local anesthesia the tumor was widely excised as shown. *C,* The base was widely and carefully cauterized but *not* the osseous tissue. *Pathology report:* Peripheral giant cell tumor. In view of our failure to excise the tumor down to bone and to cauterize the base (due to our impression that this was a hemangioma) we felt that a recurrence of the tumor was a certainty. We were pleasantly surprised. *D,* One year later there was no sign of recurrence.

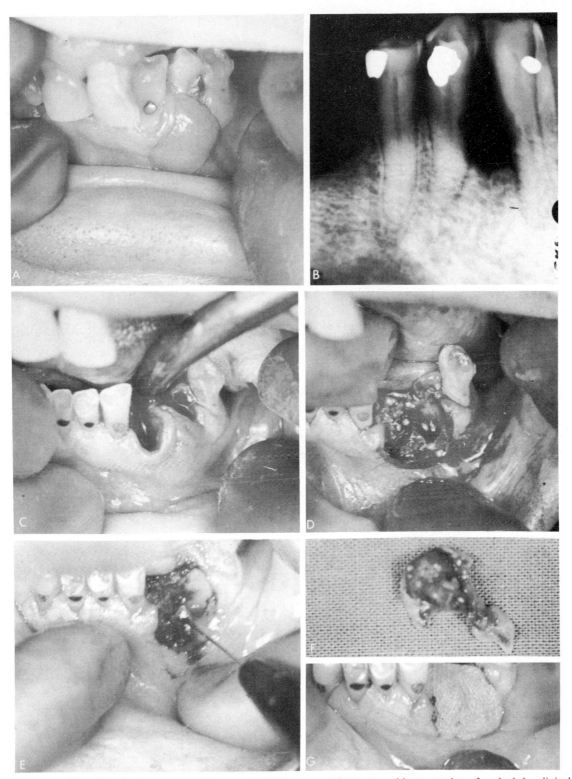

Figure 13–150 *A*, This slow-growing, firm, round, labially expanding tumor with a smooth surface had the clinical appearance of a fibroma. *B*, It is rare, however, to see resorption of bone beneath a fibroma. *C*, The adjacent teeth were extracted. *D*, A block section from buccal to lingual side was excised. *E*, The osseous tissue was coagulated. *F*, Resected specimen. *G*, Iodoform gauze sutured into the defect. *Diagnosis:* Invasive peripheral giant cell tumor.

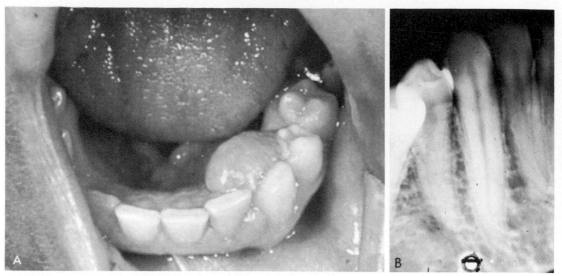

Figure 13–151 *A*, The clinical appearance of this mandibular lingual tumor with a sessile base was somewhat like that of the tumor in Figure 13–152. However, this was a hard tumor, compared to the softness of giant cell tumors, and there was not any radiographic evidence of bone resorption (*B*). Note also that this tumor had been subjected to considerable masticatory trauma, since it had been present for over 2 years, and did not show any sign of irritation or inflammation. Contrast this with the tumor shown in Figure 13–152.

Treatment: Excision of tumor, mild cauterization of the base.

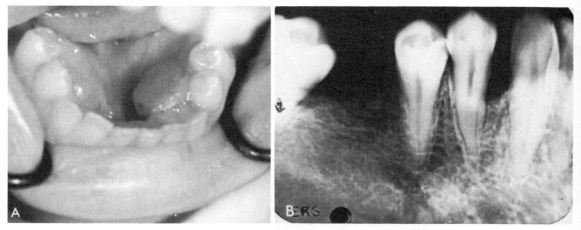

Figure 13–152 *A*, Gingival peripheral giant cell granuloma on the lingual side of the mandible. Note how masticatory trauma has worn down this friable tumor, as compared with a lingual fibroma, such as the dense, hard tumor shown in Figure 13–151*A*. Both are treated by excision and cauterization of the base. *B*, Note the interproximal loss of bone caused by the presence of this tumor between the mandibular cuspid and first bicuspid.

Photographic Case Report

EXCISION OF A PEDUNCULATED PERIPHERAL GIANT CELL TUMOR

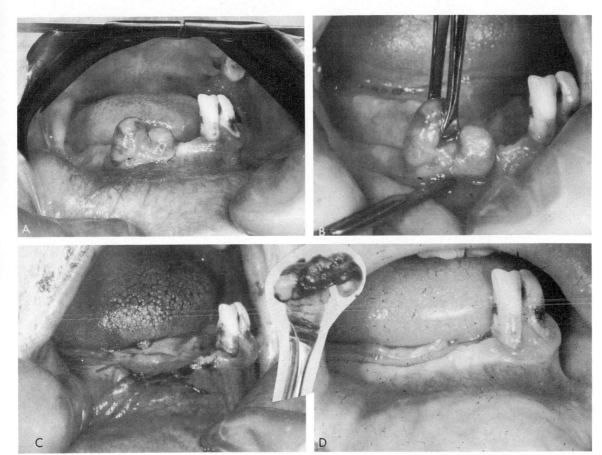

Figure 13–153 *A,* A 68-year-old woman who was completely edentulous except for the teeth shown in the photograph stated that the tumor on the crest of the mandibular ridge had been growing slowly for the past 5 years. The tumor was semisolid, pedunculated and lobulated, and in color varied from a bluish red to a light pink. *Operation:* wide excision and cauterization of the base.

B, The base was infiltrated with local anesthetic, and starting several millimeters beyond the pedicle, an incision was made completely through the mucoperiosteal membrane until bone was contacted; the incision was carried around the pedicle. Then with a periosteal elevator the tumor was stripped free from the crest of the ridge. The base was fulgurated thoroughly and several sutures placed across the wound to control hemorrhage, which persisted in spite of fulguration. *Histology report:* Giant cell tumor. *C,* Immediate postsurgical view showing cauterized base. *Inset,* Resected specimen. *D,* Ridge 3 months after operation. *Follow-up:* No recurrence 1 year later, and the patient did not return again. In this case a comparatively conservative original operative procedure was adequate.

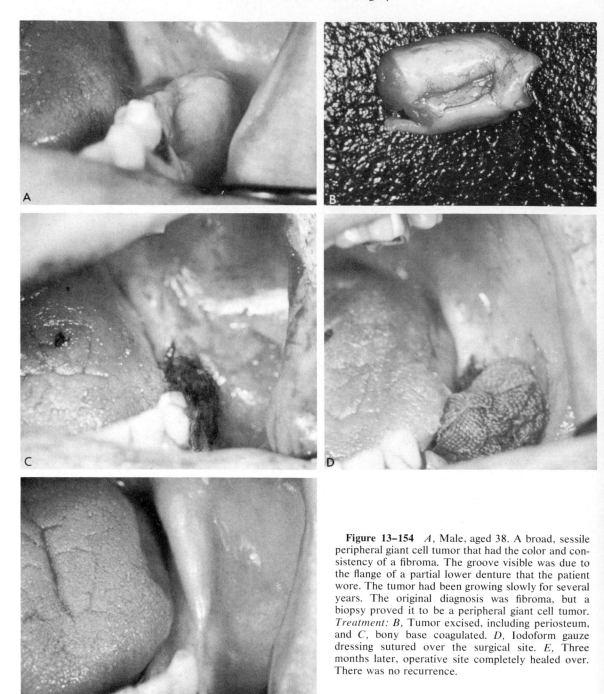

Figure 13–154 *A*, Male, aged 38. A broad, sessile peripheral giant cell tumor that had the color and consistency of a fibroma. The groove visible was due to the flange of a partial lower denture that the patient wore. The tumor had been growing slowly for several years. The original diagnosis was fibroma, but a biopsy proved it to be a peripheral giant cell tumor. *Treatment: B*, Tumor excised, including periosteum, and *C*, bony base coagulated. *D*, Iodoform gauze dressing sutured over the surgical site. *E*, Three months later, operative site completely healed over. There was no recurrence.

Figure 13–155 *A* and *B*, Seven-year-old boy with a large, multinodular sessile-based giant cell tumor covering the cuspid and bicuspid area. *C* and *D*, Tumor had separated the teeth and destroyed alveolar bone. The first bicuspid is missing. *E*, Tumor excised down to bone and the second bicuspid, which had lost most of its alveolar bone, was removed. The bony crypt was cauterized. *F*, Two postoperative recurrences developed, and at the second recurrence the first molar and the involved alveolar bone were excised and the bone cauterized. *G*, Nine months later. Bone had healed, although there was a concavity in the ridge, as can be seen in this radiograph. There were no further recurrences.

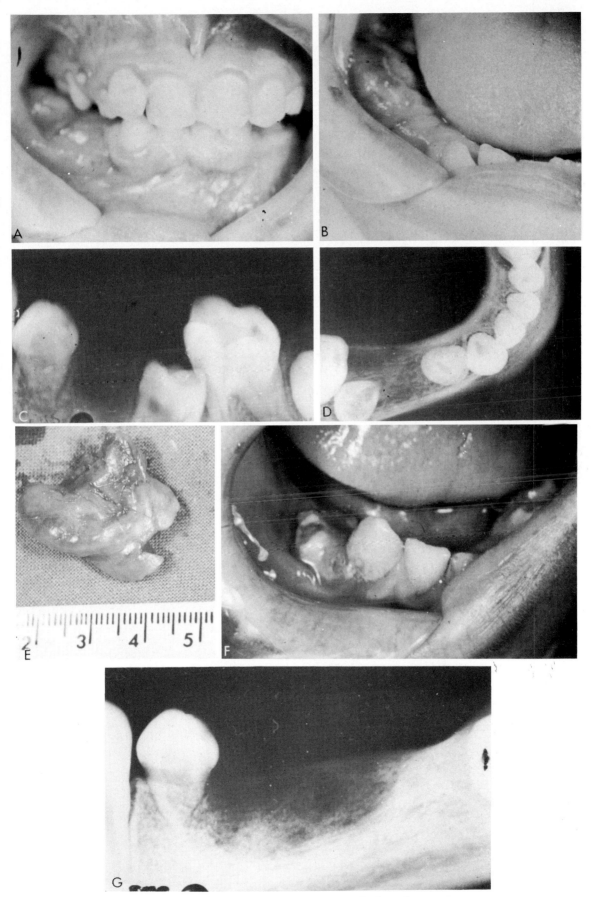

Figure 13–155 *See opposite page for legend.*

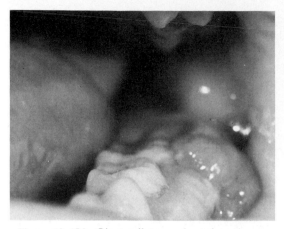

Figure 13–156   Giant cell tumor buccal to the mandibular third molar in an 18-year-old male.

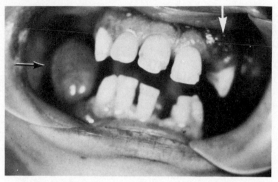

Figure 13–157   Oral tumor in a patient with myelogenous leukemia. Leukemic infiltration produced this large lobular tumor. Note hemorrhagic lesion on the left maxillary labial tissue.

Case Report No. 30

PERIPHERAL GIANT CELL TUMOR IN THE MIDLINE OF THE MAXILLA

H. Serrano Roa, D.D.S.

A 6-year-old girl was seen in the Department of Estomatology of the Roosevelt Hospital in Guatemala City, Central America, because of a swelling on the gingiva in the superior incisor region that had grown in 5 months. Examination showed a firm mass, 2 by 3 cm., over the occlusal surface of the teeth (Fig. 13–158A). It extended to the mucobuccal fold labially and as far as the palate. It was firmly attached with a wide base and appeared to involve the bone. The mass was purple in appearance and was ulcerated. It bled easily, especially at meal-time.

X-ray examination showed a large area of bone resorption around the unerupted teeth (Fig. 13–158B). Findings in the complete physical examination of the patient were negative. Under general anesthesia a circular incision was made around the tumor mass, with a margin of about 5 mm. The mass was shelled from the bone with periosteal elevators. The bone was smoothed, after which gel-

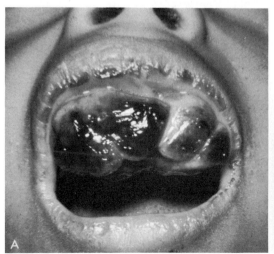

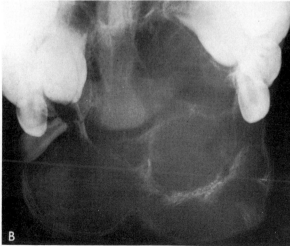

Figure 13–158   Peripheral giant cell tumor in the anterior midline of the maxilla. (See Case Report No. 30 for details.)

foam was placed to arrest hemorrhage. Petrolatum gauze was placed over this, and sutured. The patient was sent to the ward, with instructions for antibiotic therapy and a change of gauze every 24 hours. The new granulation tissue began to appear on the fourth postoperative day.

Pathologic diagnosis: Benign giant cell tumor.

CENTRAL GIANT CELL TUMORS

The central giant cell tumor is solitary or multilocular, forming in the spongiosa; as it gradually increases in size, it expands the bone. It may, and does in some cases, destroy the cortex, but it does not break through the periosteum. The teeth may become loose because of destruction of the supporting bone.

Should the teeth which appear to be involved in the tumor be extracted? If the teeth are loose, because of extensive loss of bony support, and are grossly displaced, they should be extracted. If the teeth are firm and in normal position in the arch, *do not extract them.* Root canal fillings can be inserted where

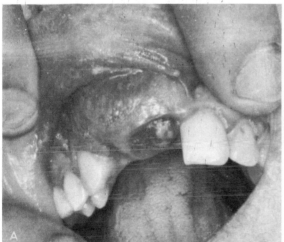
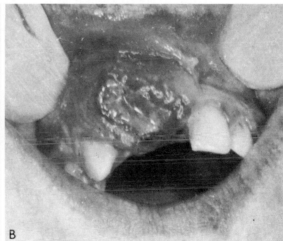

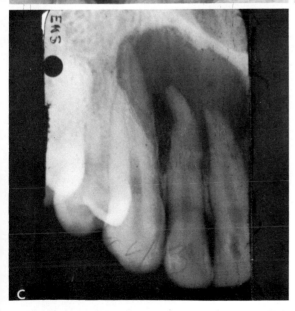

Figure 13–159 *A,* Central giant cell tumor in the anterior right maxilla of a 25-year-old woman. A diagnosis of a cyst *(C)* had originally been made, and the central and lateral incisors were extracted with the mistaken idea that this would permit drainage of the "cyst." When "drainage" failed to take place, the swelling increased and "pyogenic granulation tissue" appeared in the "alveolus," according to the referral note. The patient was sent to the clinic for diagnosis and treatment.

A wedge-shaped biopsy approximately 5 mm. wide was taken through the labial mucoperiosteal membrane into the tumor. When the patient was informed that the diagnosis was a benign giant cell tumor, she deferred surgical treatment until after her vacation. Three weeks later the patient returned with the large necrotic area shown in *B.* It was rationalized that the reduction of blood supply to this portion of the tumor, due to the mucoperiosteum-covered biopsy, had produced the necrosis of the labial portion of the tumor. The tumor was now completely excised from its crypt in the anterior maxilla.

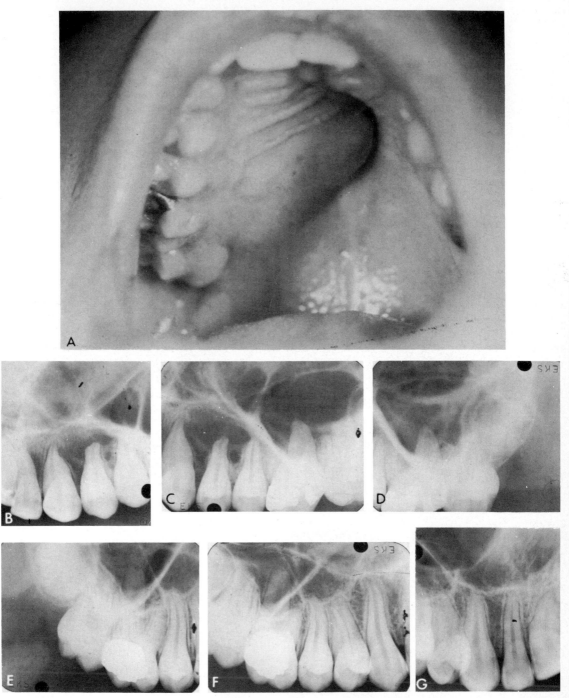

Figure 13-160   *A,* An example of expansion of the palatine process of the maxilla due to a central giant cell tumor. The cortical bone is intact. The patient was a 14-year-old male.

B to *D,* Radiographic appearance of a central giant cell tumor of the right maxilla. Note the resorption of the roots of the right bicuspids and first molar. There was no buccal expansion. Note the irregular, lobulated sclerotic outline about the apices of the right cuspid, bicuspid and molar teeth. Compare the right radiographs, *B* to *D,* with the left, *E* to *G.* *Treatment:* Because of the almost certain recurrence if the teeth were not removed, extraction of the teeth, excision of bone and tumor, and coagulation of the base were performed. In spite of this radical treatment, there were four additional operations to remove recurrent growths before this tumor stopped recurring. Compare these radiographs with those seen in Figure 13-161, and compare this history with the case report of that unusual central giant cell tumor and its conservative treatment.

necessary. The case described in Case Report No. 31 convinced the author years ago that it is not necessary to extract those teeth which appear to be involved in the tumor.

The central giant cell reparative granuloma radiographically appears as an oval or round area of increased radiolucency that is faintly trabeculated. The roots of the teeth are frequently resorbed. There is nothing definitive about the radiograph which would permit a preoperative diagnosis.

At operation the lesion is usually a reddish brown spongy mass of friable tissue that is shelled out readily (see Figure 13–164*I*). However, in the case shown in Figure 13–161, the lesion in parts had the color and consistency of large blood clots and was extremely friable (see Figure 13–161*K*).

If the lesion is a reparative central giant cell granuloma, simple curettage with a packing, to be described later, will suffice. (See Case Report No. 31 below.) It will recur if incompletely removed, but it does not become malignant.

Treatment. These tumors should be removed by thorough curettage, and the surrounding bone cauterized by thermal or chemical means in an attempt to destroy any tumor cells in the cancellous bony tissue. The application of a sclerosing solution such as Carnoy's,* with ferric chloride (this has moderate penetration with rapid local fixation and excellent hemostatic action which is a great help in controlling the bleeding from the bony crypt of these very vascular tumors) to the walls of the bony cavity is recommended. Phenol followed by 95 per cent alcohol may be used.

After the tumor is removed, 1/2-inch iodoform gauze is saturated with Carnoy's solution and the bony cavity filled completely with this gauze. Care is taken to protect the surrounding soft tissues from this solution-soaked gauze because of its escharotic action. Excess solution is removed by pressure of dry sponges; a dry sponge is placed over the dressing and sutured to place. This dressing is left in for 72 to 96 hours before removal. On removal the cavity is irrigated and dressed with an analgesic paste or iodoform gauze saturated with eugenol if necessary to control postoperative pain. As healing takes place possible recurrence is watched for. Radiation therapy is used by some in the treatment of central tumors.

---

*Absolute alcohol	6 ml.
Chloroform	3 ml.
Glacial acetic acid	1 ml.
Ferric chloride	1 gm.

Case Report No. 31

SURGICAL TREATMENT OF A LARGE CELL TUMOR OF THE ANTERIOR MAXILLARY REGION

Patient. An 18-year-old girl was admitted to the hospital because of bleeding into the nasal cavity, and protrusion of the upper lip as the result of expansion of the labial cortical plate. (See Figure 13–161*A* and *B*.)

Oral Examination. There was a marked bulging of the labial plate. Visual and digital examination of this area revealed a thin eggshell thickness of bone, which was readily compressed, giving rise to a sensation of "crackling." The anterior teeth all were vital, of good color, and had no fillings.

Radiographic Examination. This revealed a large radiolucent area about 3 cm. in width which appeared to involve the roots of the 4 upper anteriors and extended posteriorly and superiorly for a distance of approximately 5 cm., encroaching on the nasal cavity. Laterally, the cystic cavity approximated the maxillary sinus, there being only a thin layer of bone separating the two. (See Figure 13–161*C* to *F*.)

On visual examination, the nasal cavity revealed a slight rounded protuberance in the floor. It appeared that this was the probable area from which the patient had had periodic hemorrhages, as evidenced by blood clots which dropped back into the nasopharynx. Nose and throat consultation report was otherwise negative. No operation in the nasal cavity was indicated. Transillumination of the maxillary sinus was negative. Transillumination of the radiolucent area was definitely positive. This means a dark shadow was shown on the labial cortical plate, proving that solid material was in the radiolucent area and this blocked the passage of light rays which were placed in contact with the palatal tissue by means of a transillumination light.

A preliminary diagnosis of a "hemorrhagic cyst"

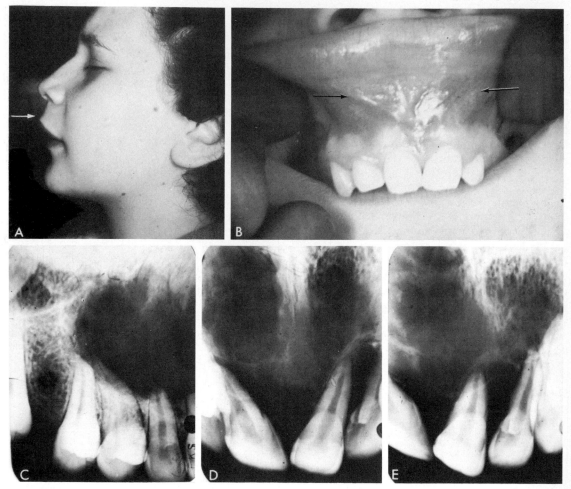

Figure 13–161 *A,* Central giant cell tumor of the maxilla. The patient noticed that her upper lip was gradually being pushed forward by the expansion of the anterior upper jaw. *B,* The upper anterior labial cortical plate was markedly expanded. *C* to *E,* Intraoral films revealed an extensive radiolucent area. All the teeth were vital according to the electric pulp tester.

(*Figure 13–161 continued on opposite page*)

was made, although the "cystic area" was not uniform in its shadows, there being a variation in the density of blacks and grays, which were irregular in outline.

The soft tissue overlying the center of the labial protuberance was anesthetized by infiltration anesthesia; then a trocar and cannula of approximately No. 12 gauge were passed through the soft tissue and labial plate into the center of the cystic cavity. The trocar was removed and a 5 cc. syringe was attached to the cannula. Unsuccessful attempts were made to aspirate fluid from the cystic cavity. Only 0.5 cc. of frothy, bloody fluid was obtained. This cast considerable doubt on the tentative diagnosis of a "hemorrhagic cyst"; however, it was reasoned that possibly, because of the communication of the cyst to the nasal cavity, there were partially organized blood clots filling the cavity.

Next an attempt was made to fill the cavity with iodized oil so that the outline might be clearly visualized radiographically. Four cubic centimeters were injected, but at the end of the first cubic centimeter the patient reported tasting the oil. Radiographic examination revealed only a small quantity of iodized oil remaining in the cavity. A second attempt to inject oil was equally unsuccessful (see Figure 13–161*G* and *H*). This proved that the cavity was filled with tissue, and a tentative diagnosis of central giant cell tumor was made.

The patient was informed as to our findings and recommendation for surgical excision of the maxillary tumor. She was also told that it would be necessary to extract at the time of operation at least her four maxillary incisors and perhaps more. She pleaded to retain her teeth, as she was to be married within 6 weeks and promised to return later for the extraction of her teeth, even though it

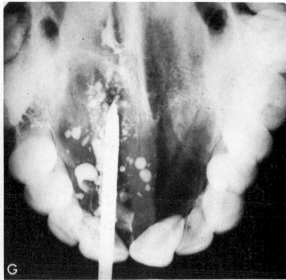

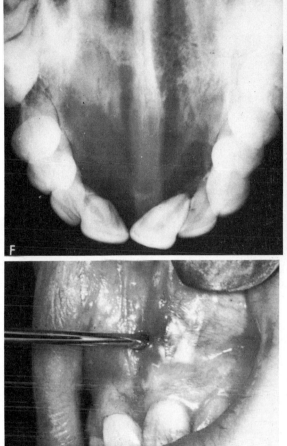

Figure 13–161 *(Continued.)* *F,* The occlusal view indicates the extent of the radiolucent area palatally. Note the absence of a clear-cut border to this radiolucent area such as is seen in palatal cysts. *G,* A cannula was inserted and an attempt to aspirate fluid was nonproductive. Then an attempt was made to inject a radiopaque oil. As seen on this occlusal view, only a few drops of the iodized oil were forced into this area. *H,* Cannula inserted into radiolucent area of the maxilla.

(Figure 13–161 continued on following page)

meant two operations. In view of these circumstances we agreed to postpone the extraction of her teeth at the operation for the removal of her tumor.

Operation. A semicircular incision was made starting over the apex of the upper right cuspid and curving down to 3 mm. from the gingival line at the centrals, then back up to the apex of the left cuspid. The tissue was reflected with a periosteal elevator, revealing a bulging area of labial plate about 5 cm. in diameter. This area was of eggshell thickness and was perforated in the center. With bone shears, periosteal elevators and hemostats this bone was removed to make an opening approximately 3 by 2 cm. (see Figure 13–161*I* and *J*). There was no cystic sac present. In the cavity was a large mass of purplish red granulation tissue (see Figure 13–161*K*). When this was cleaned out with curettes and hemostats, it was observed that the cavity extended back from the labial plate 3 cm. into the spongiosa of the palatine process of

the maxilla. It extended from the right second bicuspid area to the left second bicuspid area.

On the posterior-superior aspect of the cavity was a bulging into the nasal cavity through the bony plate of the floor of the nasal cavity with a perforation into the nasal cavity. This explained the nasal bleeding. Carnoy's sclerosing solution was swabbed over the bony crypt. About 12 inches of ½-inch iodoform gauze were worked into the cavity. The flap was ironed into position and sutured, allowing one end of the gauze to protrude slightly. The patient left the operating room in good condition.

Pathology Report. *Macroscopic:* The specimen consisted of numerous irregular pieces of soft, reddish, granular tissue forming a mass of 5 cm. in diameter. No cyst wall could be discerned.

Microscopic: The tumor was made up of dense fibrous tissue stroma arranged in whorls through which numerous large multinucleated foreign body giant cells were seen.

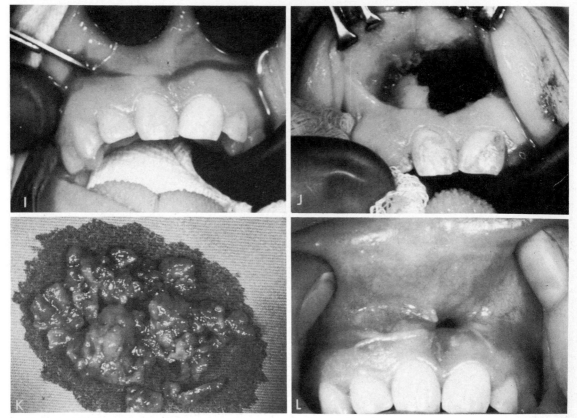

Figure 13–161 (*Continued.*) *I*, Under intravenous anesthesia a large semicircular incision was made and the muco-periosteal flap was reflected. *J*, The thin cortical plate was removed. Care was exercised not to expose any of the roots of the teeth that radiographically appeared to be involved, but were proved to be vital. *K*, A large quantity of yellowish red tissue was easily removed with a large-bowled curette. There was not a limiting capsule. The pathologist's report confirmed the diagnosis of central giant cell tumor. The area was treated with Carnoy's sclerosing solution and filled with iodoform gauze. *L*. The cavity in the maxilla and palate gradually filled in. Two years later there was no sign of recurrence.

(*Figure 13–161 continued on opposite page*)

Diagnosis: Central giant cell tumor.

Postoperative Course. The patient was checked by the otolaryngologist for evidence of any tumor growth in the nasal cavity. None was seen and since the excision of the tumor, no nasal clots had formed.

The patient reported regularly for postoperative irrigation of the maxillary cavity during the next 8 months. She refused extraction of her anterior teeth, and in view of the uneventful healing that was taking place, we adopted a watchful waiting attitude also. The extent of healing is shown at the end of 8 months in Figure 13–161*L*. At this time she and her husband moved to another city.

Here she periodically checked with her dentist, who annually sent me complete radiographs of her teeth and palatal process. Those taken 5 years after removal of the tumor are shown in Figure 13–161*M* to *R*. Furthermore, all her maxillary teeth are vital except the left maxillary central incisor. The radiographs of this tooth show the absence of a root canal!

In view of the postoperative history, this case apparently was a central giant cell granuloma.

Moral: Be conservative when operating on benign tumors. Remember, you can always be more radical at subsequent operations when or if they become necessary.

(*Text continued on page 857*)

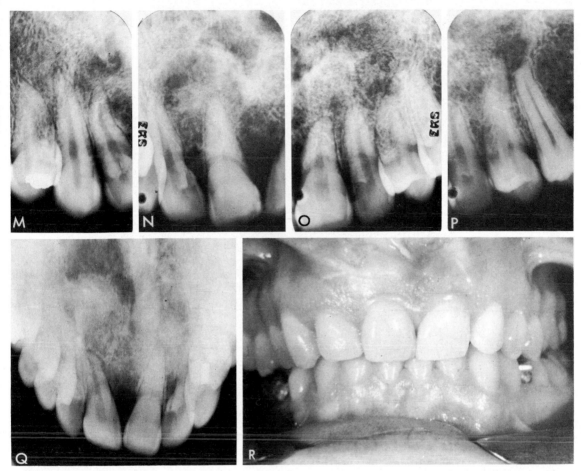

Figure 13–161 *(Continued.)* *M* to *P,* Periapical dental roentgenograms 5 years after surgery show condensed bone in the midline and normal cancellations in other areas. *Q,* Occlusal roentgenogram 5 years after surgery shows complete filling in of bone. Note that the left maxillary central incisor no longer has a root canal. Compare this tooth with its appearance 5 years previously as shown in *D. R,* Appearance of the teeth and labial tissues 5 years after surgery. (See Case Report No. 31 for details.)

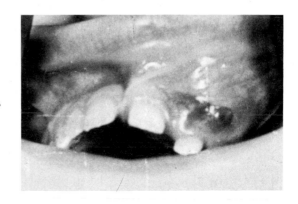

Figure 13–162 Central giant cell tumor in the maxilla of a 10-year-old boy. The tumor first expanded the labial cortical plate and then perforated it. The tissue at the point of penetration was purplish red.

RECURRENT CENTRAL GIANT CELL TUMOR

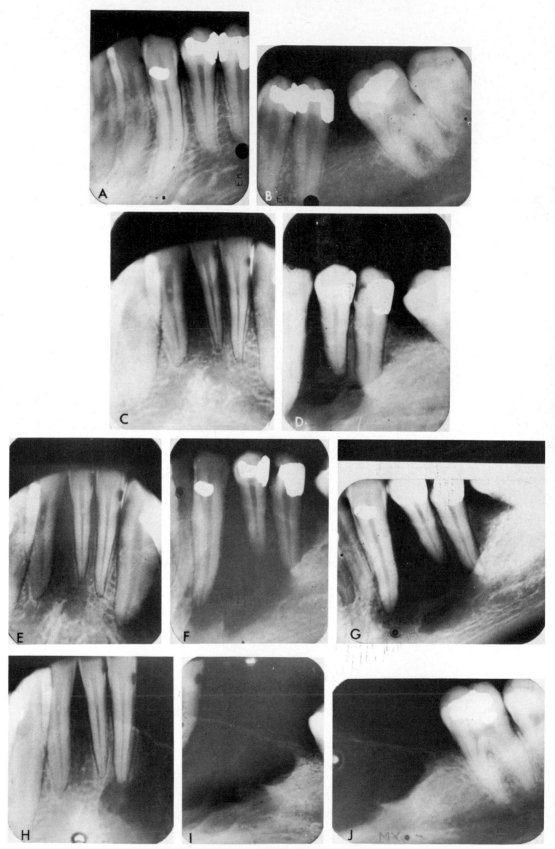

Figure 13–163 *See opposite page for legend.*

(Figure 13–163 continued on opposite page)

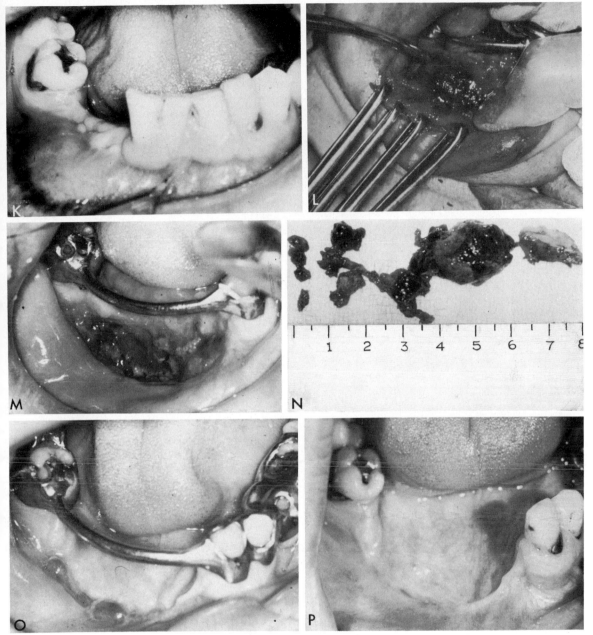

Figure 13–163 *(Continued.)*

Figure 13–163 *A* and *B*, Central giant cell tumor of the mandible. These oral radiographs from a complete routine oral radiographic examination of a young man, aged 24, do not reveal any noteworthy radiographic osseous changes. In the light of what subsequently developed, one might say that the large cancellations beneath the bicuspids might be early evidence of a central giant cell tumor. However, large cancellations are normal in this area.

C and *D*, Sixteen months later the patient returned with a complaint that he had noticed a painless round swelling about 1 cm. in diameter on the lingual surface of the left mandible. Radiographs were taken and an operation advised, but the patient failed to return.

E to *G*, A year after radiographs *C* and *D* were taken, the patient returned complaining of a gradually increasing swelling in the right mandibular cuspid and bicuspid region. These teeth were vital. Oral radiographs revealed the radiolucent areas shown above. There was no resorption of the roots. At this time at the regional V.A. clinic, the cuspid and bicuspids were extracted and the tissue in this area was curetted. The histopathologic report revealed central giant cell tumor.

H to *J*, Six months later the patient returned to the regional V.A. office complaining of a salty taste in his mouth and a large swelling at the operative site. He was sent to the V.A. hospital for treatment. Oral examination revealed marked swelling labially, buccally and lingually in the right mandible. (See *K*.) The radiographs revealed extensive destruction of the right mandible in the region of the incisors, cuspid, bicuspids and first molar. At this time the incisors and molar were extracted, and a block section containing the tumor was cut out of the mandible. Just the inferior border of the mandible was left. (See *L* to *O*.)

(Figure 13–163 continued on following page)

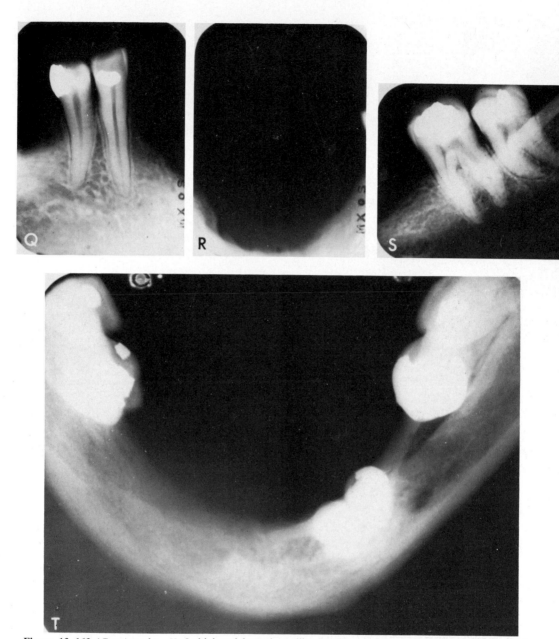

Figure 13–163 (*Continued.*)   *K,* Labial and buccal swelling. *L,* Tumor exposed. *M,* Postoperative defect 1 week later. A block section was excised from the mandible through the canal to the lower third of the mandible. For this reason a cast splint was cemented to the teeth to prevent a fracture. *N,* Reddish brown tumor and bone. *O,* Three-month postoperative view. *P,* Eighteen-month postoperative view. The tumor has not recurred. This is a typical series of events when treating a true central giant cell tumor if inadequate surgery is performed originally.

Q to *S,* Periapical radiographs 18 months postoperatively. *T,* Occlusal radiograph. No sign of recurrence in any of these films.

SURGICAL TREATMENT OF A CENTRAL GIANT CELL TUMOR OF THE MANDIBLE

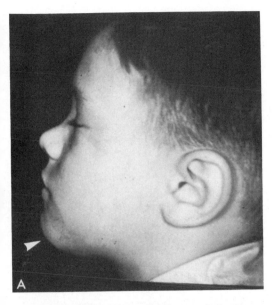

Figure 13–164 *A,* A boy, aged 6½, with an expanded symphysis of the mandible due to a central giant cell tumor. *B* to *D,* Periapical radiographs of the mandibular anterior teeth showing the osteolysis and displacement of the teeth by this central giant cell tumor. *E* and *F,* Two occlusal radiographs taken at different angles to ascertain the extent of destruction of bone.

(*Figure 13–164 continued on following page*)

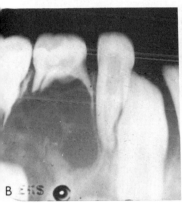

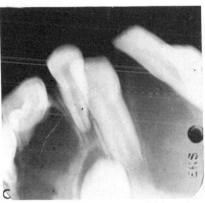

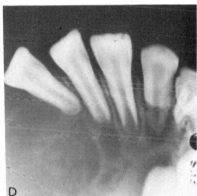

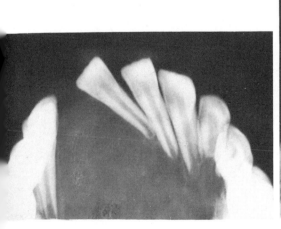

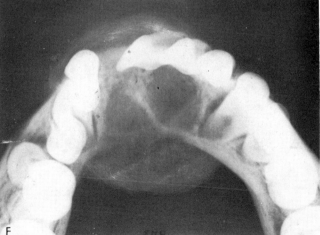

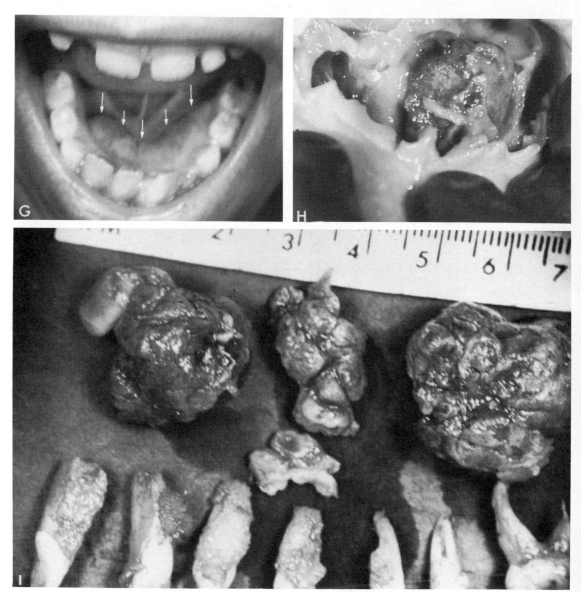

Figure 13–164 (*Continued.*)   Operative steps in the excision of a central lobulated giant cell tumor of the mandible: *G*, The teeth are separated and loose. The lingual cortical plate is thinned and expanded to the point where the lingual frenum originates in the tongue.

H, The teeth have been extracted and the thin cortical plate cut away, exposing the reddish brown tumor.

I, Central lobulated giant cell tumor of the mandible that "shelled out" easily in large and small masses. Note the adherence of tumor tissue to the roots of the deciduous and permanent teeth.

(*Figure 13–164 continued on opposite page*)

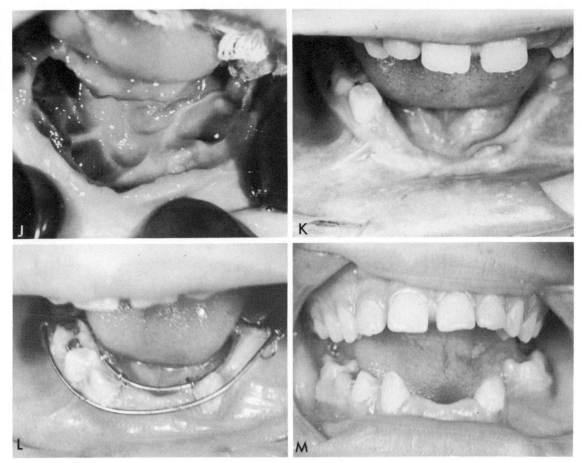

Figure 13–164 (*Continued.*) *J,* The tumor has been enucleated. As can be seen, it was lobulated with a "pseudo-capsule." All that remained of the symphysis of the mandible was the dense cortical bone of the inferior border. Neither of the uncrupted permanent cuspids was disturbed. The cavity was filled with iodoform gauze saturated at the bottom with Carnoy's solution.

K, Two years later, no recurrence and one cuspid is erupting.

L, To help guide the permanent cuspids into normal position, this orthodontic device was attached to the first permanent molars.

M, Two years later, size and contour of the symphysis of the mandible have been completely restored.

OSTEITIS DEFORMANS (PAGET'S DISEASE)

A discussion of the symptoms, diagnosis and treatment of osteitis deformans is included in the legend for Figure 13–165.

ENOSTOSIS, OSTEOSCLEROSIS, CONDENSING OSTEITIS

An enostosis of the mandible or maxilla is a deposit of new bone within the spongiosa. This growth is confined within the cortex, and the bone is not expanded.

The bone is denser than the surrounding normal bone, irregular in outline, and markedly radiopaque. These concentrations of bone have also been called bone whorls, sclerotic bone, osteosclerosis, and condensing osteitis.

In the interpretation of enostosis, it is necessary to exclude many other radiopaque changes that are similar in radiographic density, shape, size and location, such as exostosis, calcified cementoma, salivary stone and residual root. This differential diagnosis is discussed elsewhere in this book. Here we are concerned with the differential diagnosis between enostosis and condensing osteitis.

Pollia classifies condensing osteitis as (1) infective, (2) traumatic, (3) thermal, and (4) defensive.[63] It is the result of bone reaction to chronic inflammation or infection, whereas

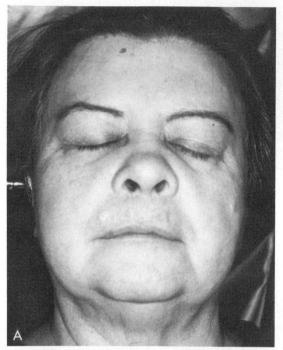

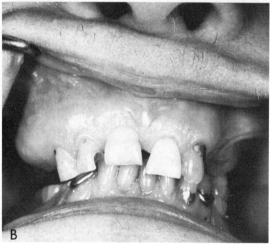

Figure 13–165 Osteitis deformans (Paget's disease). This chronic bone disease is usually found in patients past middle age and develops very slowly. There is progressive enlargement of the skull and jaws and deformities of other skeletal bones, such as the tibia, femur and spine. Fractures are not unusual because of increased fragility. Symptoms are: bone pain, severe headache, weakness, dizziness, mental disturbance and, due to osseous compression of nerves in their foramina, blindness, deafness or facial paralysis.

A, Note the enlarged skull with prominent frontal bones, zygomas and jaws. *B,* Both the maxilla and mandible are increasing in size, resulting in gradual but steady widening of spacing of the teeth. According to Stafne,[88] involvement of both jaws is a rare condition.

(Figure 13–165 continued on opposite page)

enostosis, according to Eselman,[32] is an abnormal anatomic variant of the internal structure of the cortex similar to the exostosis on the external cortex. If it is possible to obtain good occlusal radiographs, enostosis is diagnosed if it is shown that the radiopaque area arises from either the buccal or lingual internal cortex or the lamina dura. See Figure 13–166.

In addition, enostosis does not produce expansion of the cortex, nor does early condensing osteitis, but the author has seen at least one case of long-continued chronic in-

fection with condensing osteitis and buccal and lingual expansion (see Figure 13–169).

The teeth are vital in enostosis, unless the vitality has been lost from other causes. When the condensing osteitis is due to periapical infection, the teeth are nonvital; when due to trauma or thermal changes, the teeth are vital. Trauma can readily be determined by checking the bite; thermal changes are elicited by questioning the patient.

Treatment. Surgery is not indicated in enostosis or condensing osteitis of traumatic or thermal origin. In nonvital teeth with con-

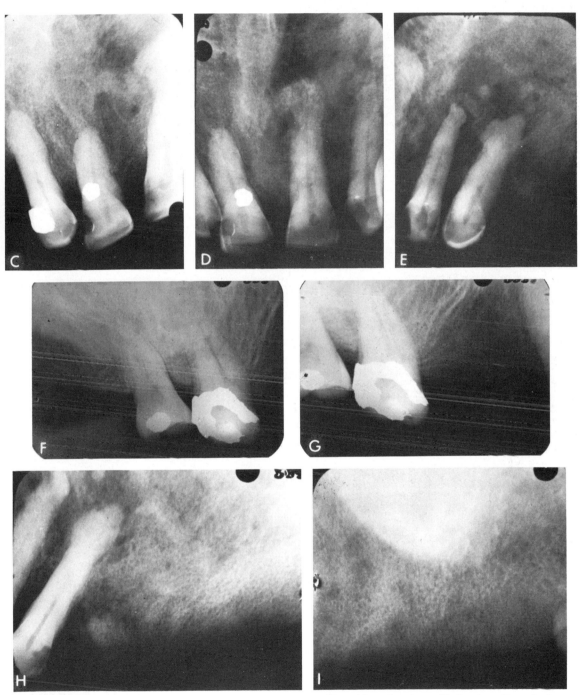

Figure 13–165   *(Continued.)*   *C* to *P*, Radiographs of the maxillary (*C* to *I*) and mandibular (*J* to *P*) teeth show a ground glass appearance of the trabecular pattern and an absence of the lamina dura. There are some root resorption and hypercementosis.

(Figure 13–165 continued on following page)

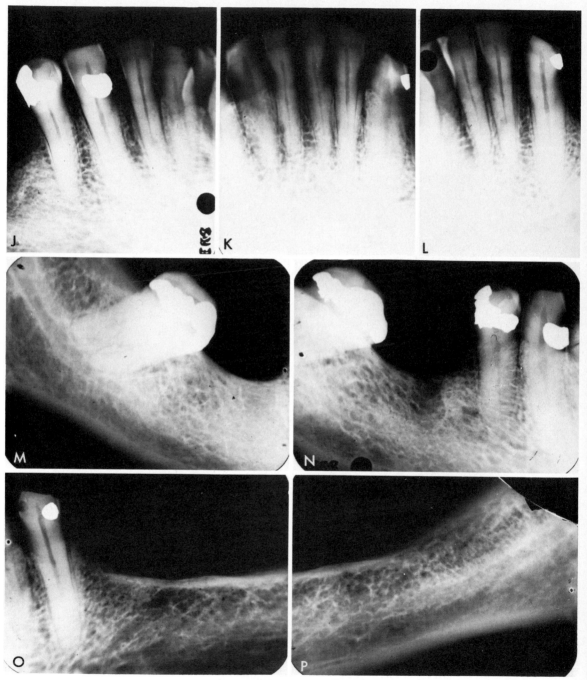

Figure 13–165   *(Continued.)*

(Figure 13–165 continued on opposite page)

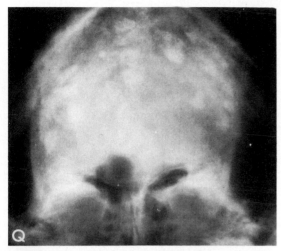

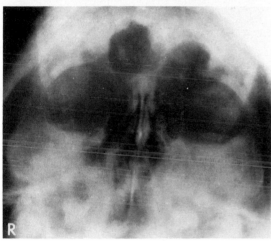

Figure 13–165 *(Continued.) Q,* Postero-anterior radiograph of the skull has the typical "snowball" or "cotton wool" effect due to alternating areas of osteoporosis and osteosclerosis.

R, Posteroanterior radiograph of the mid-face showing marked osseous enlargement of both zygomas and the maxilla, which on the right side has practically obliterated the maxillary sinus.

(Figure 13–165 continued on following page)

densing osteitis, extraction or endodontic therapy is indicated.

FIBRO-OSTEOMA, OSTEOFIBROMA, OSSIFYING FIBROMA, OSTEOID OSTEOMA, FIBROUS DYSPLASIA, LOCALIZED OSTEITIS FIBROSA, LOCALIZED OSTEODYSTROPHY

These benign tumors are found peripherally and centrally in bone, with the latter the most frequent. They are slow-growing and are symptomless. They may be found in the early forms by a routine oral radiographic examination (see Figure 13–172), but usually the patient notes an asymmetry of the face and presents for treatment with a history of a gradual unilateral expansion of the mandible or maxilla. These early forms radiographically simulate cementomas. (Compare Figures 13–78*A* and 13–172.)

These tumors result from the destruction of the normal spongiosa, which is then replaced with areas of fibrous connective tissue containing areas of osteogenesis.

Radiographically, there may be multilocular radiolucent areas with clear-cut margins as shown in Figure 13–173*G*. This is usually referred to as an ossifying fibroma and the encapsulated tumor shells out readily, thus removing the entire tumor with little chance of recurrence.

In the diffuse tumor, referred to as osteoid osteoma or fibrous dysplasia, there is a radiolucent area with areas of a ground glass appearance without a distinct margin. If there is advanced osteogenesis the area may be radiopaque (see Figures 13–177*C* and 13–179).

Treatment. The treatment is enucleation

(Text continued on page 867)

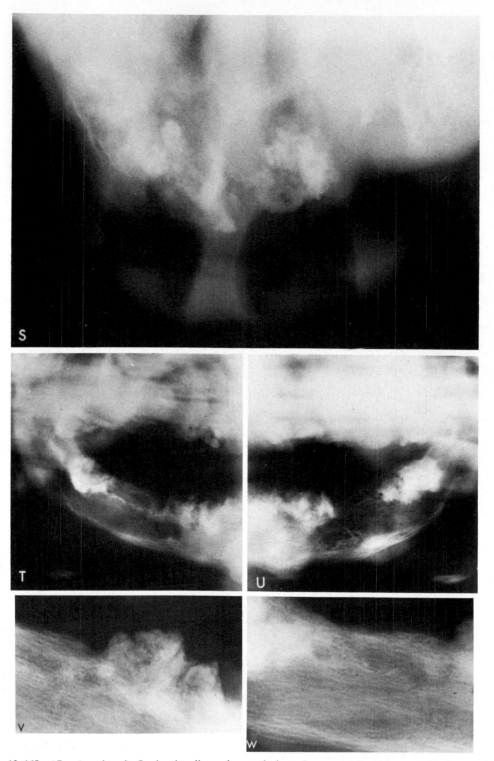

Figure 13–165 *(Continued.)* *S*, Occlusal radiograph reveals irregular osteosclerotic areas with intervening areas of osteoporosis in the anterior of the maxilla. The enlarged maxilla has practically obliterated the right maxillary sinus and to a lesser degree the left. No air chamber can be seen in either sinus.

T and *U*, Panoramic radiograph strikingly reveals the solid dense bone structure in the right half of the maxilla and to a lesser degree in the left midface. Osteoporosis is seen in the anterior maxilla. Both this view and the occlusal one show a smaller nasal cavity as the bone enlarges.

V and *W*, Intraoral radiographs of the dense, uniform "ground glass" osteosclerosis seen in another 70-year-old patient with osteitis deformans.

Treatment: There is no specific treatment. Death is rarely due to this disease. Dentoalveolar or other necessary oral surgery is not contraindicated. The patient who is, of necessity, made edentulous should be told that as the jaws slowly enlarge, new and larger dentures must be constructed.

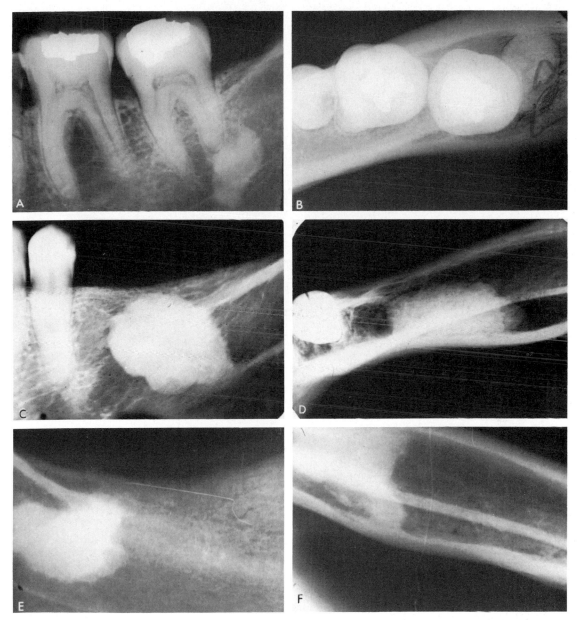

Figure 13–166 Three cases of enostosis. The occlusal radiographs, *B, D* and *F*, prove that the radiopaque areas shown in *A, C* and *E* arise from the cortex. (Read the text for a more detailed description.)

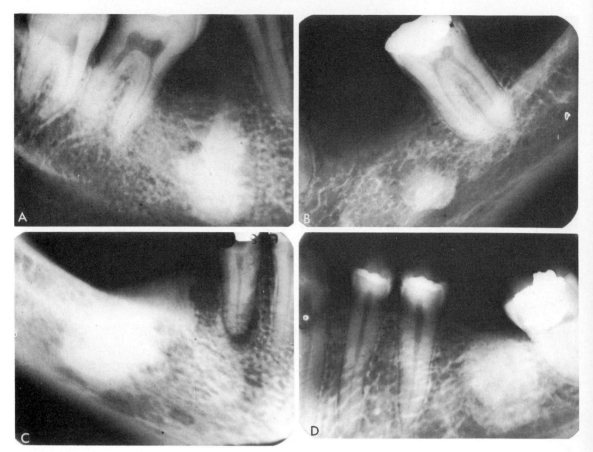

Figure 13-167　*A, B, C* and *D* illustrate various stages of developing areas of osteosclerosis. It is difficult in these cases to state definitely whether they are cementomas, because radiographically their appearance is quite similar to cementomas in various stages of calcification. The reader is referred to the illustrations on cementomas (Figs. 13-75 to 13-80). A point of differentiation is the rather definite radiolucent area that surrounds cementomas, contrasted with the diffuse radiolucent area that surrounds these osteosclerotic areas of infective osteitis.

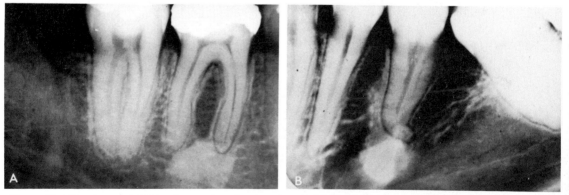

Figure 13-168　*A* to *F*, Additional examples of osteosclerosis. This condition was not caused by infection but may have resulted from a reparative process following a localized infection. However, in the example shown here all these teeth were vital. The cause of these osteosclerotic areas is not known.

(*Figure 13-168 continued on opposite page*)

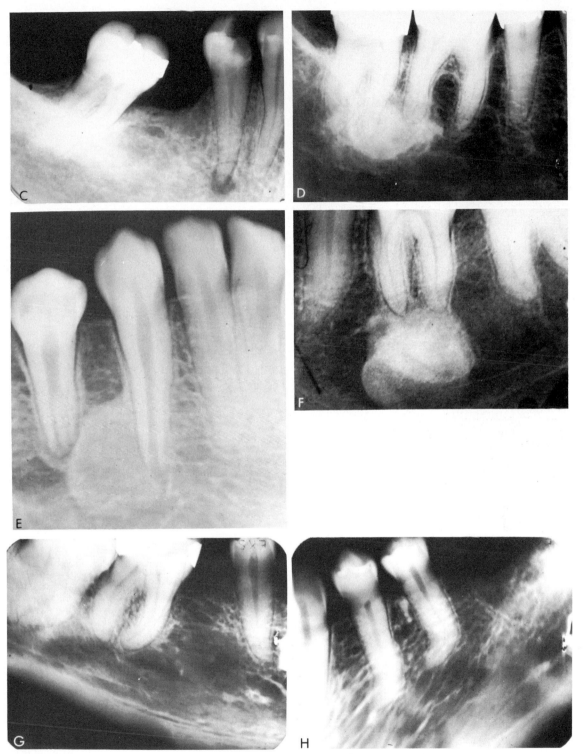

Figure 13–168   *(Continued.)*

G and *H*, Two examples of the opposite condition, osteoporosis, in which there has been a failure of the osteoblasts to lay down bone matrix. This condition may have been caused by disuse atrophy due to the absence of functional stress following the extraction of the first molar. However, the area of osteoporosis shown here extends too far for this to be a logical explanation in this case. Note in these two periapical radiographs the large cancellous area beneath the bicuspids, where functional stress is still present.

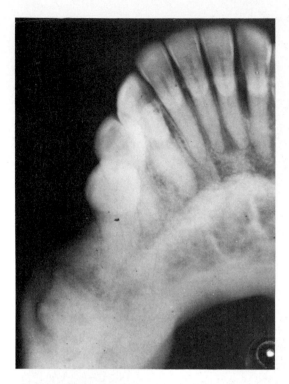

Figure 13–169 Condensing osteitis about retained mandibular molar roots, with evidence of infection, which has produced expansion of the buccal and lingual cortical bone.

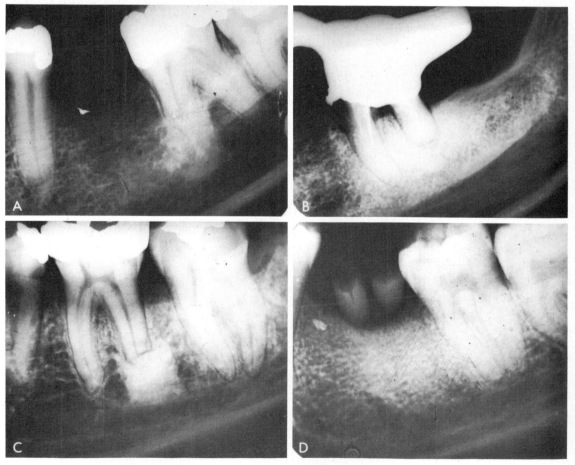

Figure 13–170 *See opposite page for legend.*

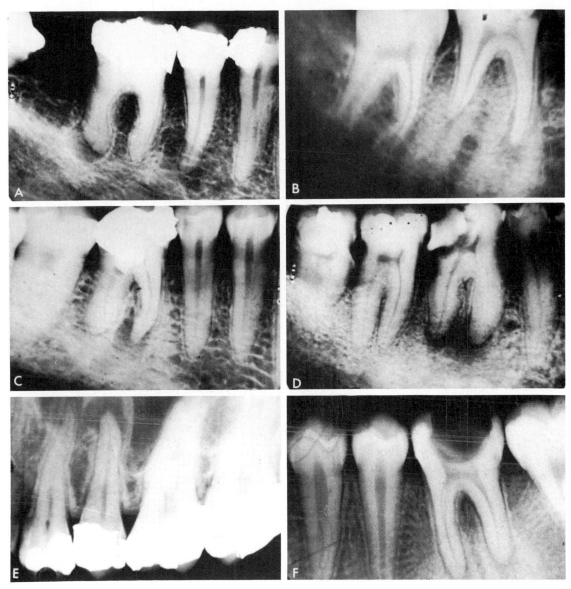

Figure 13–171 Additional examples of periapical defensive osteosclerosis.

Figure 13–170 Examples of condensing osteitis. *A,* Typical condensing osteitis that probably had its stimulus from an area of periapical infection. Note the irregular margin that helps differentiate these osteosclerotic areas from retained roots or calcified cementomas. *B,* Diffuse condensing osteitis about both roots of the first molar. Note resorption of the distal root. This is a form of defensive osteitis. It is also apparent here that trauma played a role in this osteosclerosis. *C,* Infective condensing osteitis about the mesial root of the second molar. Note sharp, well-defined resorption of the distal root. *D,* Note diffuse, extensive osteosclerotic bone beneath the remnants (apical thirds) of the mandibular first molar that are not even in bone but are suspended in the soft tissue.

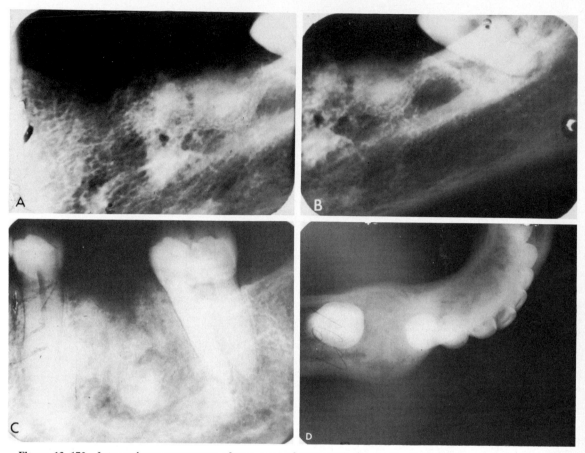

Figure 13–172　Intraoral roentgenograms of two cases of monostotic fibrous dysplasia of the mandible.

A and *B*, First case. Mottled appearance is evident in these dental radiographs because of the scattered calcified formations in an area of large bony trabeculae that probably represents the fibrous tissue matrix of the tumor.

C and *D*, Second case. *C*, Fine bony trabeculae in which there are calcified areas present in this tumor. *D*, The occlusal radiograph of this area reveals the same fine bony trabeculae that give this tumor the so-called ground glass appearance. Note the buccal expansion and the unusual slight bony expansion.

Treatment: In these single and fairly well delineated lesions surgical excision should be carried out. This is not indicated in large, diffuse lesions (see Figures 13–174 and 13–175) but is in cases of *well-circumscribed* fibro-osteomas (fibrous dysplasia), as demonstrated in Figure 13–173.

of the well-circumscribed ossifying fibromas, complete eradication by curettage of the small areas of fibrous dysplasia (localized osteitis fibrosa) and conservative reduction of the large non-encapsulated tumors purely for cosmetic reasons. Further operations may be necessary for these cases because of recurrence.

Figure 13–173　*A*, An enlarged deformed right horizontal ramus (body) of the mandible due to fibrous dysplasia (ossifying fibroma), which produced facial asymmetry in this 18-year-old male. (See Case Report No. 32 for details.)

B, The occlusal radiograph of the lesion area compared to the normal left mandible shows a thin expanded labial and lingual cortex, evidence of new bone formation with areas of increased density and the opposite, darker areas of reduced density where there are an increase in fibrous matrix and a reduction in osseous tissue.

C to *E*, The periapical dental radiographs show that there is a preponderance of fibrous tissue in this lesion with clearly defined borders.

Case Report No. 32

ENUCLEATION OF AN OSSIFYING FIBROMA OF THE MANDIBLE

History. Five years previously this patient, aged 18, had an infected deciduous molar extracted elsewhere. Since then there has been gradual swelling, despite the fact that over the past years his dentist extracted the cuspid, bicuspids and first molar in an attempt to control the gradually increasing swelling. Since the teeth have been extracted, incisions for "drainage" were made in his jaw and his family physician gave him a "series of penicillin shots," all to no avail as his jaw has continued to expand.

Oral and Radiographic Examination. There was a hard expansion of the right body of the mandible extending from the cuspid area to the second molar. Radiographs reveal well-circumscribed multilocular areas of radiolucency with striations and radiopaque areas throughout (see Figure 13–173A).

Impression. Ossifying fibroma, confirmed by biopsy.

Treatment. The tumor was enucleated. An incision was made along the crest of the tumor from the cuspid area to the distobuccal corner of the second molar, starting and ending in the mucobuccal fold. The mucoperiosteal flap was reflected and the thin expanded buccal cortical plate was re-moved with bone shears and rongeurs, exposing the multilobular fibrous tumor. This was cut into sections and removed with large-bowled curettes and periosteal elevators (see Figure 13–173H). The inferior alveolar canal was not exposed. The thin lingual cortical plate was not disturbed. The cavity was filled with 1-inch iodoform gauze which was saturated with Carnoy's solution (see formula on page 847).

To date, 5 years later, there has not been a recurrence.

Pathology Report: *Macroscopic:* The tissue submitted, 24½ grains, had been removed in a number of pieces. They ranged from 1 to 3 cm. in diameter. They were quite firm and cut with a very gritty and hard consistency as if they were producing osseous tissue, although the tissue itself was fibromatous; it had a grayish yellow color interspersed with some areas of red which suggested hemorrhage. Representative sections were submitted for decalcification and study.

Microscopic: This tissue showed whorls and trabeculae of spindle-shaped fibrous tissue cells. There was a uniform diffuse scattering of small bits of new bone.

Diagnosis. Ossifying fibroma.

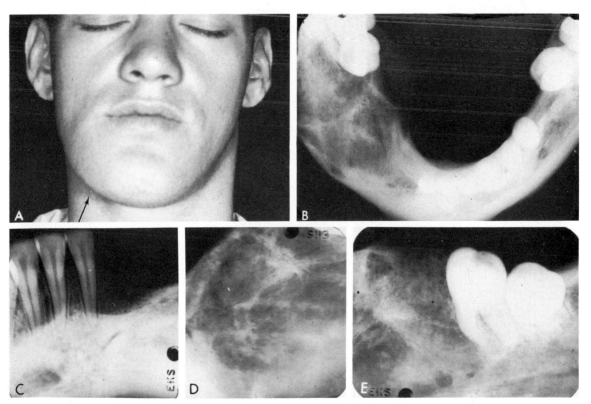

Figure 13–173 *See opposite page for legend.*

(Figure 13–173 continued on following page)

869

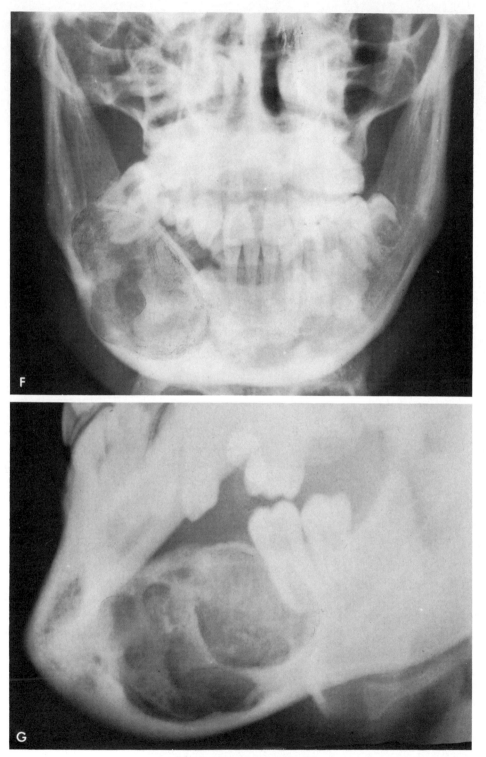

Figure 13–173   (*Continued.*)

(*Figure 13–173 continued on opposite page*)

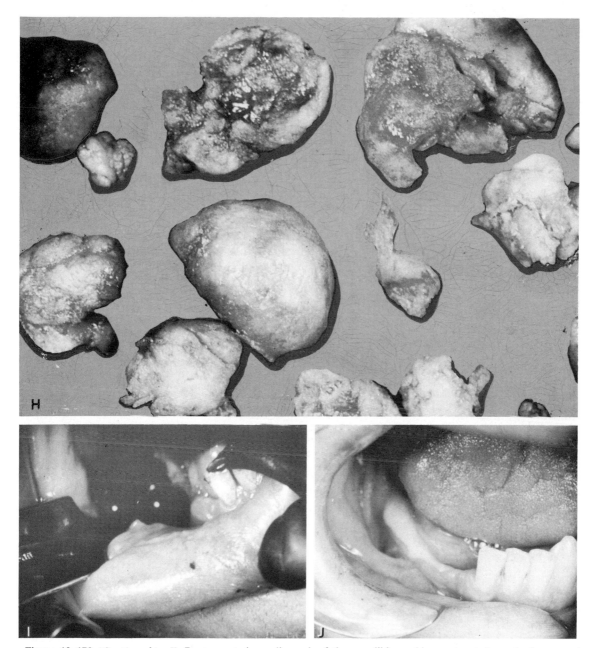

Figure 13–173 *(Continued.)* *F,* Posteroanterior radiograph of the mandible enables us to study again the normal left body of the mandible and the fibrous dysplasia (ossifying fibroma) of the right body. It is very obvious in this view and in *G,* the right lateral jaw radiograph, that in this particular clinical entity there are large, well-circumscribed, clearly defined masses of the "tumor," with clear-cut borders surrounded by normal osseous tissue. It is this type of lesion that can and should be enucleated in sections (see tumor sections in *H*), since this has produced a cure in the majority of the cases seen by the author.

I, View 1 week after surgery. *J,* Mandibular cavity gradually filling in with bone 4 months later. There has not been any recurrence.

These lesions should not merely be "carved back to the normal size for cosmetic reasons," since they obviously will continue to grow. Cases of *diffuse* fibrous dysplasia, in which there is *not* a clear line of demarcation between normal and osseous tissue and the lesion (such as is shown in Figures 13–174 and 13–175), do not permit definitive surgery aimed at a cure and so are treated by cosmetic surgical reduction of the abnormal growth, as periodically indicated.

REDUCTION OF AN OSTEOID OSTEOMA OF THE MANDIBLE FOR COSMETIC REASONS

History. This patient, aged 30, had observed a gradual enlargement of the right jaw for several years but thought that the growth had been accelerated the past year (see Figure 13–174A and B). She had lost the teeth in the bicuspid and molar areas because of caries.

Radiographic Examination. There was expansion of the right body of the mandible (horizontal ramus) from the cuspid to the third molar area (see Figure 13–174C). The normal cancellations had been replaced by an alternating pattern of osteolytic and osteosclerotic finely granular osseous structure, which in some areas had a ground glass appearance. The tumor did not have a limiting clear-cut border. This tumor appeared to be an osteoid osteoma. There was more osseous tissue than fibrous tissue (see Figure 13–174C to F).

Treatment. The tumor was widely exposed and reduced in size by chisels and bone shears, until a cosmetically acceptable contour was achieved. The tumor cut much more easily than did normal bone, and it did not bleed excessively. Soft tissues were replaced, trimmed and sutured.

Pathologic Report: *Macroscopic.* The tissue from the right mandible consisted of 2 pieces, the larger of which measured 1.8 by 1 by 0.4 cm., and the smaller of which measured 0.3 cm. in diameter. Both pieces were hard and bony and presented granular, grayish white to pink-red surfaces.

Microscopic. The tissue was composed of coarse spicules of bone, with a fibrous connective tissue stroma that was cellular but myxomatous, and it contained a few chronic inflammatory cells. Both osteoclasts and osteocytes were present.

Diagnosis: Osteoid osteoma of mandible.

(*Text continued on page 877*)

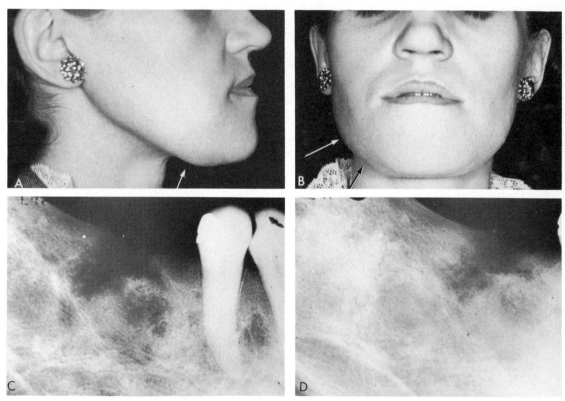

Figure 13–174 *A* and *B*, Bilateral osteoid osteoma of the mandible with greater expansion of the right body (horizontal ramus) than the left. It was this gradually increasing unilateral deformity in the right lower third of the face that prompted this patient to seek help. (See Case Report No. 33 for details.) *C* and *D*, In these two periapical radiographs, the mandibular right molar area of the roughly rectangular radiolucent area at the crest of the ridge is where an incisional biopsy was taken. The lesion was mottled with alternating areas of radiolucency and sclerosis. The latter areas have a "ground glass" appearance. This simultaneous process of resorption and repair accounts for the mottled appearance seen in these radiographs.

D, Posteroanterior radiograph of the mandible reveals a more active process of osteoporosis and osteosclerosis in the right body of the mandible. The "ground glass" texture of the osseous tissue in the left mandible, while there is enlargement, seems more stable.

(*Figure 13–174 continued on opposite page*)

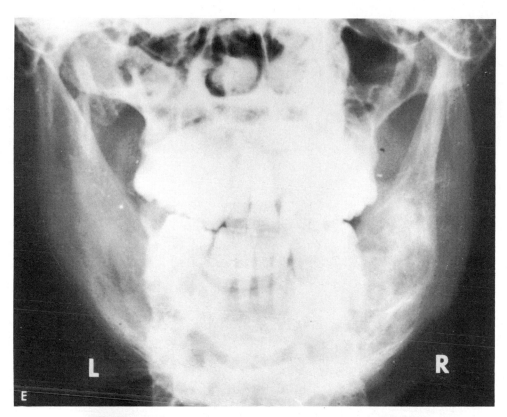

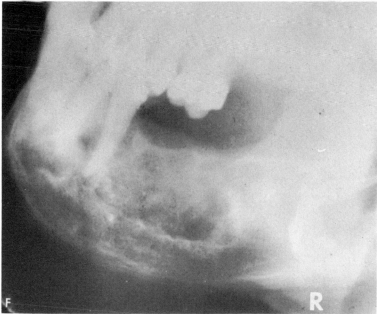

Figure 13–174 (*Continued.*)   *E,* Extensive enlargement of the right body of the mandible is apparent. This is a diffused lesion as compared with the circumscribed lesions shown in Figure 13–166, which had clearly defined borders or loculations, both large and small, in the bone of the body of the mandible. It is this "blending" of the "tumor" into the normal surrounding osseous tissue that makes excision practically impossible, and certainly sectioning of the mandible *is not indicated.* Rather, these lesions are reduced in size by reflecting the mucoperiosteal membrane and "carving" the bone to return it as nearly as possible to its original size and shape. As the lesion once more produces disfigurement, cosmetic surgery is again performed.

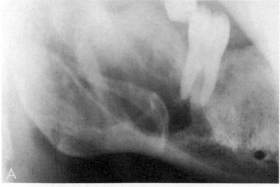

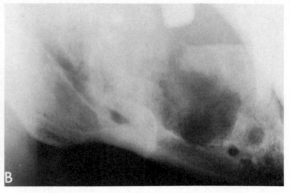

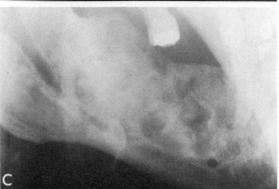

Figure 13–175 In lesions of fibrous dysplasia in which fibrous tissue is predominant, usually in younger patients, the area is radiolucent and resembles a cyst. For this reason it is often diagnosed as a cyst, as happened in this case. They may be monocystic or polycystic. (Also see Figure 13–176.) We did not see this patient, but the radiographs were loaned to us.

A, Left oblique radiograph of the left mandibular third molar area and vertical ramus. Tentative diagnosis was a radicular cyst or a follicular cyst from a supernumerary fourth molar follicle. The third molar was extracted and "nothing was found when the periapical space was explored with a curette." *B*, Follow-up radiograph 2 years later. The radiolucent area is "smaller." *C*, Four years later. "Radiolucent area completely filled in with bone."

Discussion: No histologic examination was made of this lesion, but it certainly appears to us to have been fibrous dysplasia in which the fibrous matrix in the lesion shown in radiograph *A* was, in 4 years, displaced by a lesion with more osseous than fibrous tissue. While there are still small radiolucent areas, the lesion has the typical "ground glass" appearance seen in the older lesions. We were unable to obtain a biopsy to confirm our diagnosis. We were told that the patient did not have a facial deformity, but there is a triangular projection of the lesion above the crest of the ridge, which appears to be larger in the last radiograph (*C*) than in the first (*A*).

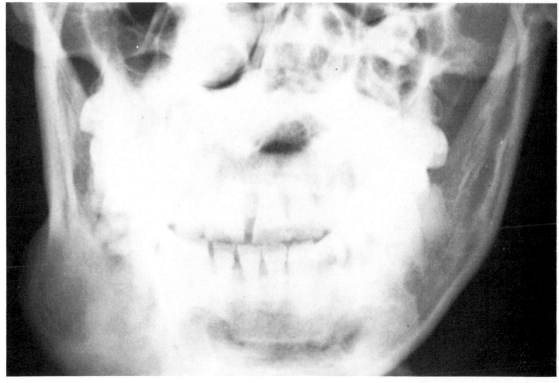

Figure 13–176 *See opposite page for legend.*

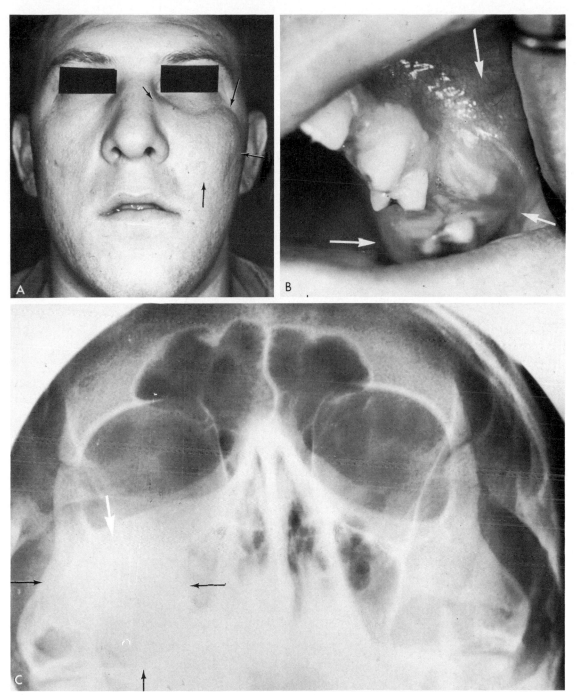

Figure 13–177 *A,* The left maxillary swelling is caused by monostotic fibrous dysplasia (ossifying fibroma) of the maxilla. *B,* Oral view showing buccal swelling. These tumors are reduced in size for cosmetic reasons. This is accomplished by the intraoral reflection of the soft tissues overlying the tumor, including the periosteum, and sculpturing the mass with chisels, burs and files to an acceptable shape. The mass should be reduced to a slightly smaller size than the opposite side to delay the time when a subsequent surgical procedure is necessary, because growth is slow but continuous in these tumors. *C,* Posteroanterior radiograph of the maxillary sinuses and maxilla. Note that practically the entire left maxillary sinus is obliterated by the tumor.

Figure 13–176 Gross asymmetry of the mandible due to expansion of the cortex by monostotic fibrous dysplasia, which in this case is unusually dense, as shown by the radiopacity of the tumor. These lesions are most often unilateral and usually arise in the posterior regions of the jaws.

Treatment: Reduction in size, as previously described, for cosmetic reasons.

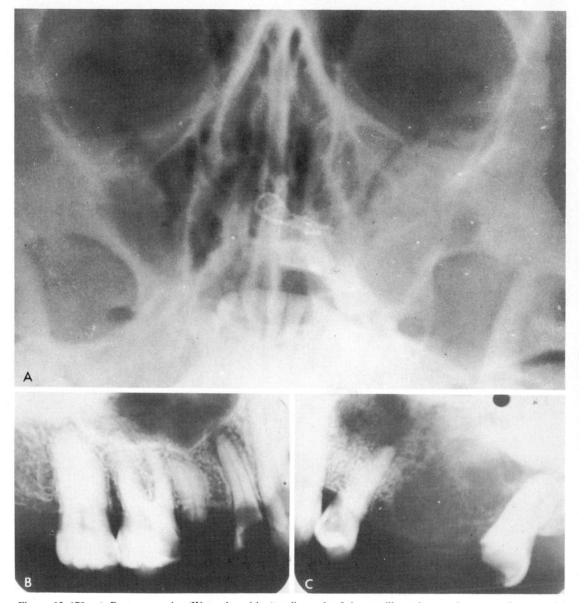

Figure 13–178 *A*, Posteroanterior (Waters' position) radiograph of the maxillary sinuses shows a radiopaque right maxillary sinus because it was filled with fibroma that also involved the right maxillary alveolar ridge, as shown in the periapical radiograph *(C)*. By contrast, the normal left alveolar ridge is shown in *B*, and the normal air-filled left maxillary sinus is shown in *A*.

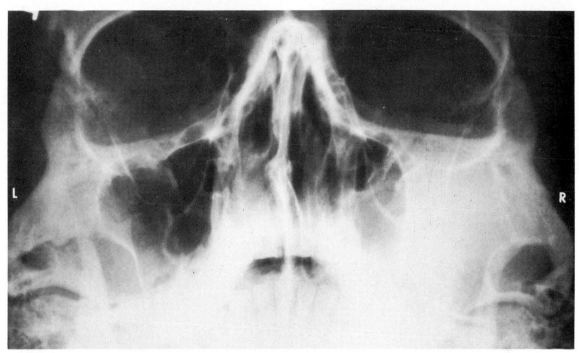

Figure 13–179 Posteroanterior radiograph showing extensive fibrous dysplasia (osteofibroma) of the maxilla that has materially reduced the size of the right maxillary sinus.

Case Report No. 34

FIBROUS DYSPLASIA OF THE MANDIBLE RESOLVES, PRODUCING AN IDIOPATHIC BONE CAVITY

H. Serrano Roa, D.D.S.

Patient. A 9-year-old girl was seen in the Department of Estomatology of the Roosevelt Hospital in Guatemala City, Central America, in October, because of a painful noninflammatory swelling in the left side of the mandible. The patient's mother said that the deformity had started about a year before, but it had not been painful until now.

Physical Examination. Examination revealed that the first lower permanent molar on the left side had extensive caries and pulpitis, which undoubtedly had produced the pain. The mandible was expanded in the molar area. The x-ray examination showed deep, extended caries in the first molar; the bone was rarefied, with irregular trabeculations; in the occlusal view the cortical bone was thinned and expanded.

The molar was extracted, and at the same time a biopsy of the osseous lesion was taken. The histopathologic diagnosis was fibrous dysplasia of the mandible. Because of the patient's age the lesion

was not treated but she was told to come back for periodic check-ups.

Six years later in November, this patient returned, complaining of pain in the still-expanded left mandible. With the impression that the diagnosis was the same as that of 6 years previously, the patient was prepared for surgical treatment for the fibrous dysplasia. The original radiographs taken in 1965 had been lost. When the mucoperiosteal flap was reflected, a very thin cortical bone was found, and inside, a large cavity that extended from the premolar area to the ascending ramus. (See Figure 13–180.) The cavity was empty, and the neurovascular bundle was seen exposed in its course along the lower portion of the cavity. No capsule was found. The cavity was filled with furasin gauze, to be extracted on various sessions later. The patient was kept under observation as the osseous tissue filled in the cavity.

DISCUSSION

In this reported case a bone cavity was apparently produced by resolution of fibrous dysplasia. In the author's opinion it is a very good possibility that this is the type of process causing these idiopathic bone cavities in the mandible that we have been calling "traumatic cysts," and "hemorrhagic cysts" (see Chapter 12).

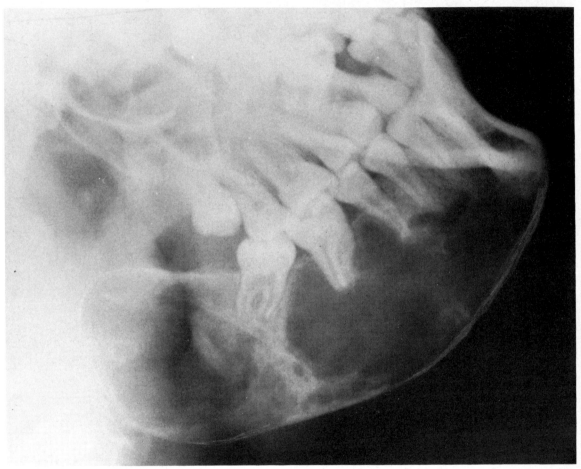

Figure 13–180   Idiopathic bone cavity apparently resulting from resolution of fibrous dysplasia of the mandible. (See Case Report No. 34 for details.)

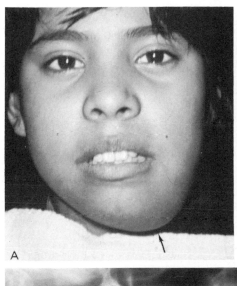
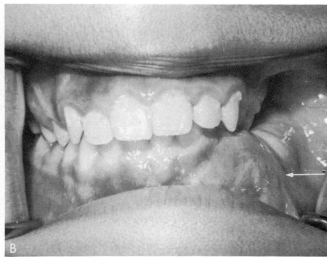
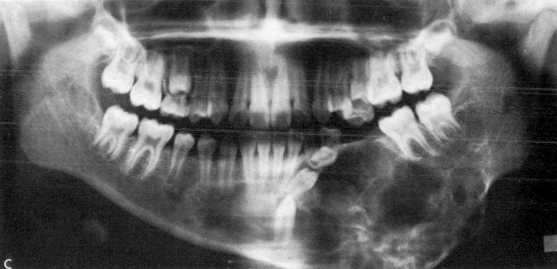

Figure 13–181 *A,* Twelve-year-old girl with deformed mandible resulting from fibrous dysplasia (ossifying fibroma). Very large buccal *(B)* and inferior *(C)* expansion of the body of the mandible.

The referral notes said, "This young Mexican-American girl, aged 12, was seen by me and is periodically being followed. She was operated on when she was 9 years old. An intraoral trim and biopsy were performed. The pathology report indicated ossifying fibroma. She will have definitive cosmetic surgery when she is in her mid or late teens."

When this patient was first seen by me, attention was called to the fact that the excellent radiograph *C* showed very clearly that this ossifying fibroma was the lobular type, wherein there are definite margins. In such cases the treatment of choice, because in most instances it is definitive and does not permit recurrence, should be an operation to remove this tumor, which could easily be accomplished by carrying out the technique described in Figure 13–173. The procedure of trimming and contouring when the lesion is circumscribed with clear-cut margins, in my experience, is not the best method of treatment. Enucleation of this tumor offers the near certainty of a cure as soon as the condition is diagnosed and the tumor removed. (Courtesy of Lawrence A. Saunders, D.D.S.)

BENIGN OSTEOBLASTOMA (GIANT OSTEOID OSTEOMA) OF THE MANDIBLE*

N. H. SMITH, M.D.S.

Patient. In May a boy, aged 7 years, presented with a hard, bony mass in the left body of the mandible. (See Figure 13–182*A* and *B*.) He complained that the mass was at times painful, especially at night, sometimes being severe enough to awaken him.

History. There was a history of a kick in the jaw in May of the previous year. The initial bruising had disappeared, but shortly afterward expansion of the jaw was noticed. The patient had consulted a surgeon, and that August the mass was explored. The specimen was reported on as follows: "The section shows a mass of exuberant periosteal bone formation akin to fracture callus." Healing was uneventful, but later the swelling recurred, this time the patient complaining of increasing pain in the region.

Physical Examination. Examination revealed a fit, well-developed boy with a noticeable facial asymmetry due to enlargement of the mandible extending from the midline to the left molar region. Intraorally, a normal transitional dentition was present, the teeth being well aligned and not mobile. The mandible was expanded, both buccally and lingually from the midline to the left first permanent molar, the swelling extending lingually almost to the midline. On palpation the mass was found to be hard and tender, with the overlying mucosa being distinctly hyperemic. There was no loss of sensation in the lower lip.

Radiographic Examination. Radiographs showed a somewhat spherical mass occupying the left body of the mandible, situated between the incisors and the first permanent molar. The lesion showed a marked irregularity in bone structure and was demarcated from normal bone by a narrow translucent zone. The permanent unerupted teeth adjacent to the mass were displaced away

from it, the cuspid being depressed toward the lower border of the mandible. (See Figure 13–182*C* and *D*).

Laboratory Findings. Findings in laboratory tests (complete blood count, serum alkaline phosphatase, calcium and phosphorus; and urine analysis) were within normal limits. Erythrocyte sedimentation rate was 17 mm. in 1 hour.

Operative Notes. On May 24, under general anesthesia, a biopsy was performed. A mucoperiosteal flap was raised from the central incisors to the left second deciduous molar, the incision being carried around the lingual aspect of the teeth. The shelf of abnormal bone thus exposed was removed. One piece of gelatin sponge was placed to control bleeding. Postoperatively, the wound healed well.

Pathology Report. The section shows two distinct zones. The outermost is composed of fine but densely packed bony trabeculae closely resembling much of the tissue in the previous biopsy. This zone is covered by periosteum, and the nearby trabeculae are being extended by osteoblastic activity. At the inner aspect of this zone the trabeculae are being eroded by osteoclasts.

This outer zone is clearly demarcated from the deeper zone, which is mainly fibrous, with irregularly arranged trabeculae of young bone and osteoid. The trabeculae are mostly covered by plump osteoblasts, but there are a few osteoclasts present. The trabeculae are not continuous across the tissue between the two zones.

---

*Adapted from Smith, N. H.: Benign osteoblastoma of the mandible: A case history. J. Oral Surg. *30*(4): 288–292 [Apr.], 1972. Copyright by the American Dental Association. Reprinted by permission.

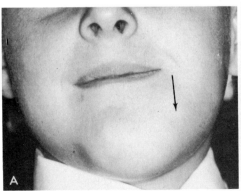
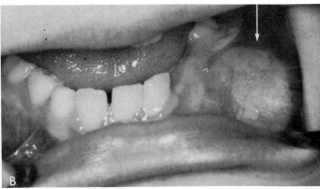

Figure 13–182 Benign osteoblastoma (giant osteoid osteoma) of the mandible. (See Case Report No. 35 for details of this successful conservative treatment.)

(*Figure 13–182 continued on opposite page*)

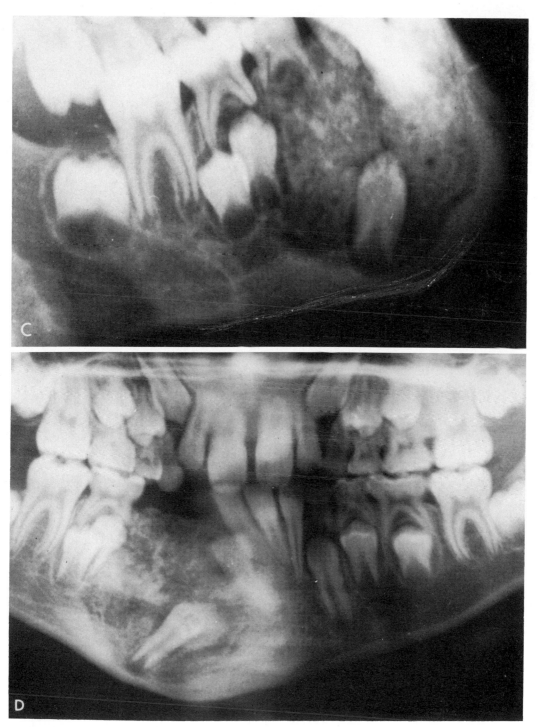

Figure 13–182 (*Continued.*)

(*Figure 13–182 continued on following page*)

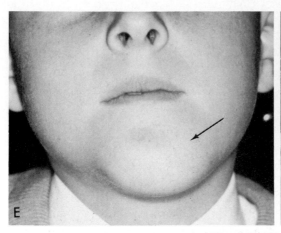

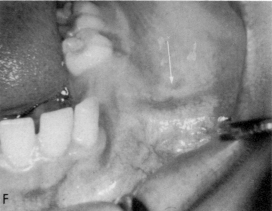

Figure 13–182 *(Continued.)*

The appearance of the deeper material and history of pain suggest osteoid osteoma. However, the activity in the outer zone is most unusual in osteoid osteoma, and this tumor is very rare in the jaws. There is no obvious inflammatory process, although there may be a deeper focus, and the lesion could be chronic osteitis resulting from the previous trauma. The lesion appears to be a reactive overgrowth of bone and not neoplastic. There is no evidence of malignancy.

Treatment. In the light of this report, and because an attempt to remove the entire lesional tissue would have probably resulted in a disfiguring facial deformity, it was decided to adopt a policy of watchful waiting. The patient was reviewed at regular intervals; but by March within 2 years of when I had first seen him, it became clear that the

lesion was continuing to expand, the patient also complaining of increasing pain. (See Figure 13–182D.)

As a prelude to surgery the biopsy slides, together with radiographs, were reviewed by a number of pathologists (including Dr. D. Dahlin, Mayo Clinic, Rochester, Minnesota, U.S.A.; Professor I. R. H. Kramer, Eastman Dental Hospital, London, England; Professor B. E. D. Cooke, Dental School, Cardiff, Wales), who agreed that the lesion was benign osteoblastoma.

Since the extent of the lesion was such that it probably could not be removed entirely without interrupting the continuity of the mandible, and in the light of published reports indicating healing of similar lesions following incomplete removal, it was decided to excise as much of the tumor as

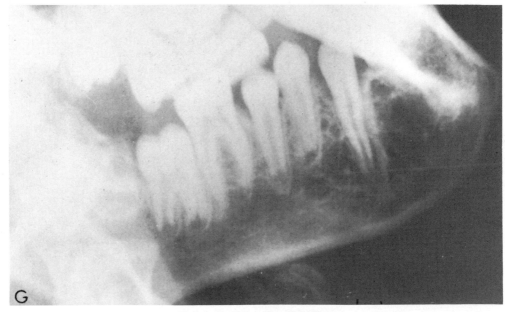

Figure 13–182 *(Continued.)*

(Figure 13–182 continued on opposite page)

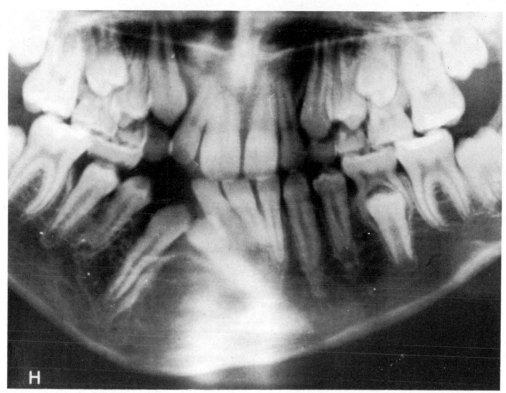

Figure 13–182   *(Continued.)*

possible without compromising the integrity of the jaw.

On the first day of May, under general anesthesia, a buccal mucoperiosteal flap was elevated, extending from the distal side of the permanent mandibular left first molar to the distal side of the right cuspid. A wafer thin shell of subperiosteal bone was thus exposed covering a mass of bony tissue projecting from the buccal aspect in the left canine premolar region. This proved to be soft and when cut by a chisel had a somewhat gritty consistency.

As the mass was pared down the deeper portion became harder and took on more the appearance of normal bone. Bleeding was free but not excessive, blood loss amounting to 200 ml. No evidence of encapsulation was seen. Excision continued to the point where a normal jaw outline was achieved, the final contouring being done with a file.

The postoperative course was uncomplicated and the wound healed well. When seen two months later the patient was free of pain and the

mucosa no longer appeared hyperemic. Radiographs taken in August of the year following the second admission showed a nearly normal contour of the mandible except at the lower border in the canine region where little surgical contouring had been done. Of even greater interest was the marked change in the trabecular pattern in the region formerly occupied by the lesion, the bone now appearing nearly normal in structure. With regard to the teeth that had previously been displaced, the first bicuspid had returned to its normal position and the cuspid was nearly upright and close to the crest of the ridge. The patient had no complaint of pain and the mucosa was of normal color and texture.

When the patient was seen the next April (2 years after the second admission), only slight evidence of mandibular fullness of the left side was discernible (see Figure 13–182E and F), and there was marked radiographic improvement, with a normal bone pattern developing in the region (see Figure 13–182G and H).

(Text continued on page 888)

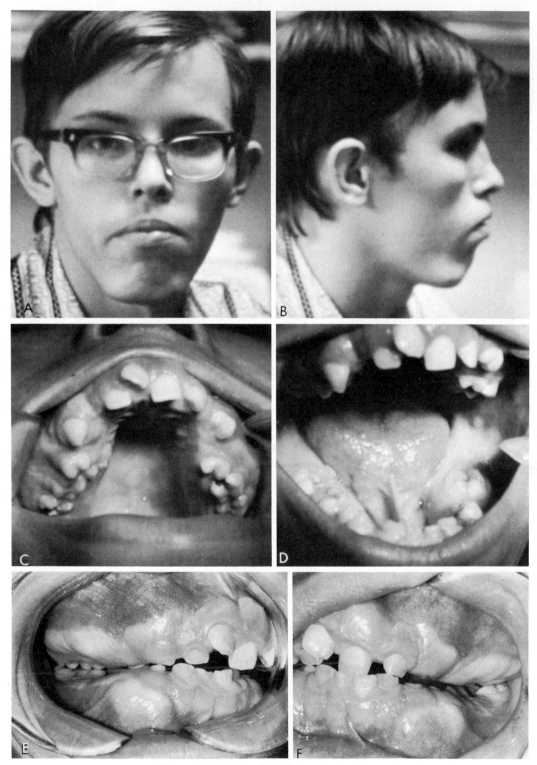

Figure 13–183 *See legend on opposite page.*

(*Figure 13–183 continued on opposite page*)

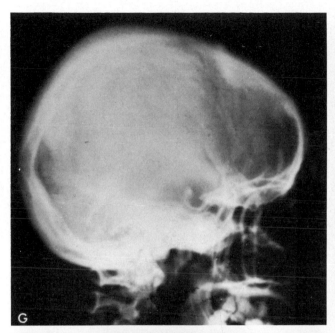

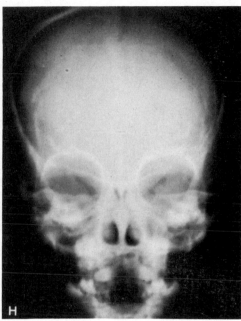

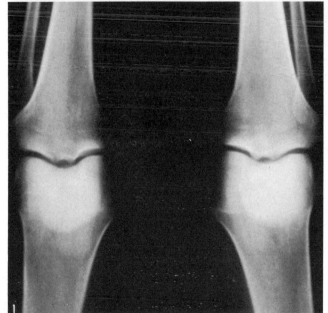

Figure 13–183 In the differential diagnosis of tumors of the jaws, congenital and other skeletal diseases must be eliminated. These are illustrations of a 16-year-old male with the abnormal oral bone growth seen in craniometaphyseal dysplasia.

Note especially such facial features as a scaphocephalic skull with prominent frontal and parietal bosses, dental malocclusion and unerupted, impacted teeth. (Note that this patient does not have hypertelorism or a broad, flat nasal bridge, which are frequent characteristics in these cases.) Diagnosis is aided by roentgenograms of the skull showing a fairly uniform hyperostosis or sclerosis, or both, and roentgenograms of long bones showing a flaring or splaying in the metaphyseal area. Goodman and Gorlin list these and other features.[34] (Courtesy of Dr. E. A. McDonald.)

OSTEOGENIC SARCOMA OF THE LEFT MANDIBLE

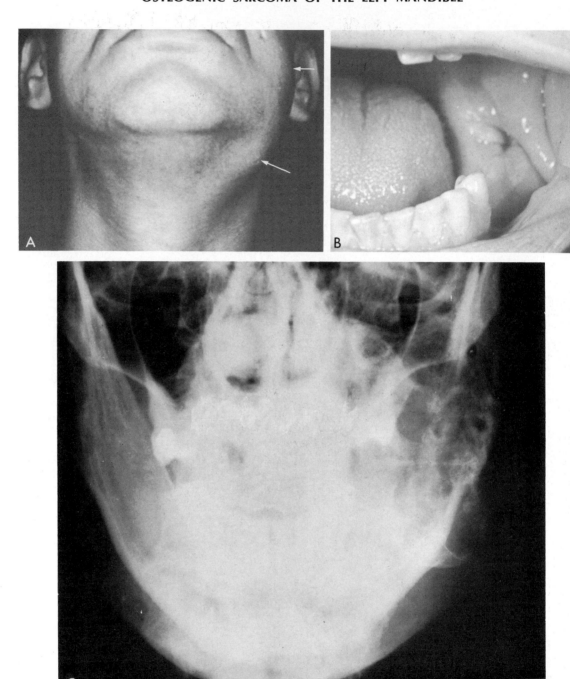

Figure 13–184 *A,* This patient, who has lateral swelling over the ramus and hard, swollen submandibular lymph nodes, was referred to us from another city for the treatment of "chronic osteomyelitis." He had been receiving treatment from his physician and a surgeon for over a year that included massive doses of penicillin and two surgical procedures to "remove sequestra and establish drainage."

B, Note the wide lingual and buccal expansion of the lingual cortex seen intraorally and the incision for "drainage." The diagnosis of "osteomyelitis" was made with the posteroanterior and lateral oblique roentgenograms *(C* and *D),* which accompanied the patient. Neither these nor our intraoral views *(E, F* and *G)* presented the typical radiographic picture seen in osteomyelitis. Actually, the latter radiographs had the appearance of fibrous dysplasia. Osteomyelitis was ruled out not only because of the radiographic findings but also because there was not a continuous free discharge of pus. Also, the former radiographs revealed the simultaneous resorption and building of bone, which is characteristic of some forms of fibrous dysplasia; however, one does not see hard lymph nodes in fibrous dysplasia.

(*Figure 13–184 continued on opposite page*)

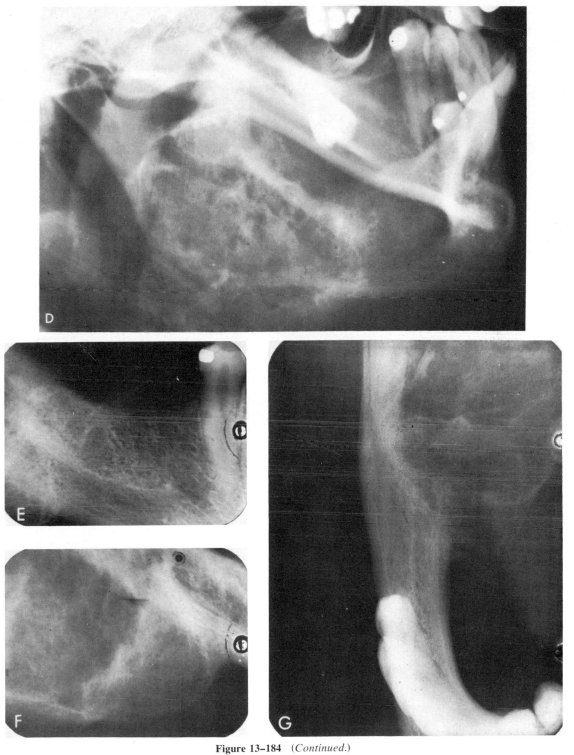

Figure 13–184   *(Continued.)*

(Figure 13–184 continued on following page)

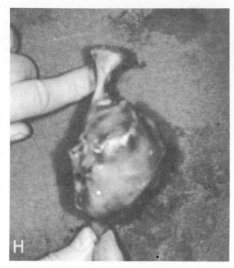 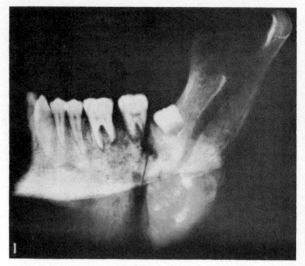

Figure 13–184 (*Continued.*)   A biopsy was taken, and the resultant diagnosis was osteogenic sarcoma. *H, Treatment:* Section and disarticulation of the left body and ramus of the mandible and neck dissection to remove the lymph nodes.

Note: Radiographically, two types of osteogenic carcinoma are seen: one in which bone destruction predominates (osteolytic), and the other in which the deposition of bone is greater (osteoblastic). A review of all these radiographs demonstrates that both processes were clearly shown. Stafne points out that in osteogenic sarcoma there is seen "extending downward from the lower border (of the mandible) evidence of periosteal bone formation which appears as spicules or lamellae situated at right angles to the surface of bone, producing a radiating sun-ray, or fan, appearance. This picture is characteristic of osteogenic sarcoma in many instances but is not peculiar to this condition alone."[87] There was no "sun-ray" effect in the radiographs of this case. According to statistics, osteogenic sarcomas of the mandible are rare.

I, Osteogenic sarcoma of the osteoblastic or sclerosing type. Roentgenogram of a resected mandible, showing at its inferior border periosteal bone formation that produces a characteristic sun-ray or fan appearance. (*I,* Reproduced with permission from Stafne, E. C.: Oral Roentgenographic Diagnosis. 4th ed. Philadelphia, W. B. Saunders Co., 1975.)

Case Report No. 36

ORAL LESIONS IN HYPERPARATHYROIDISM
H. Serrano Roa, D.D.S.

Patient. A female, 33 years old, came to the Department of Estomatology of the Roosevelt Hospital in Guatemala City, Central America, complaining of two growths, one in the maxilla and the other in the mandible, slowly growing for 3 years. Eight months previously, the rate of growth had increased. The mandibular tumor had been excised twice but rapidly grew back again.

Physical Examination. There was a facial deformity that had been created by the tumors. The patient's movements were slow, and she was nervous and difficult to communicate with. The oral examination revealed an expansive growth of about 4.5 by 3 cm. in the upper left maxilla. The cuspid and bicuspids were displaced labially and

buccally. The mucosa covering the tumor was red, with some pale areas. The mass was hard and not painful. The tumor arising on the midline of the edentulous mandibular alveolar ridge was 2.5 by 1.5 cm., mobile and soft. (See Figure 13–185A.)

Radiographic Examination. The radiograph showed an enlargement in the maxilla, with sharply defined round and oval radiolucent areas. (See Figure 13–185B). The mandibular occlusal radiograph (Fig. 13–185C) showed expansion of the labial cortical bone. The three displaced teeth did not have a lamina dura. With the clinical impression that both were giant cell tumors, calcium and phosphate in serum were checked. In two samples taken on different days the calcium was

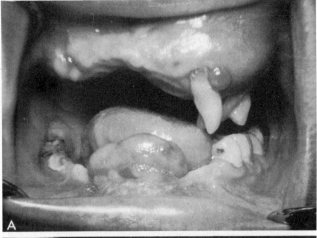

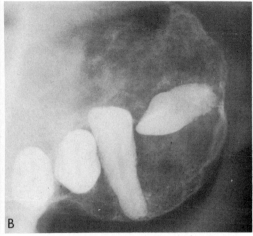

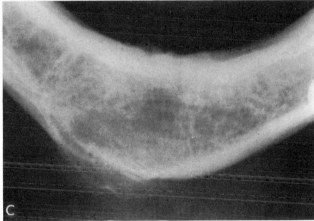

Figure 13–185 Oral lesions in hyperparathyroidism. (See Case Report No. 36 for details.) Compare also Figure 12–108.

down to 13.5 and 13.7 mg., and the phosphate was down to 3.3 and 3.5 mg. Radiographs of the cranium and hands showed osseous lesions, apparently giant cell tumors. Radiographs revealed nephrocalcinosis in the left kidney. There was bilateral renal insufficiency.

Treatment. The neck was explored, and a hyperparathyroid adenoma was found and removed. When the patient was stabilized, the tumors of the maxilla and mandible were excised.

Final Diagnosis. Hyperparathyroidism.

Case Report No. 37

MAXILLARY EXTRAMEDULLARY SOLITARY PLASMA CELL MYELOMA (PLASMACYTOMA)

H. Serrano Roa, D.D.S.

Patient. A 46-year-old male was seen in the Department of Estomatology in the Roosevelt Hospital of Guatemala City, Central America, because of a swelling in the left superior part of the maxilla. (See Figure 13–186A and B.) Eight months previously, the first and second molars had been extracted because they were painful. Follow-

ing the extractions, the present swelling began to grow to its present size.

Physical Examination. Examination showed a man in apparent good health, with asymmetry of the left face because of an enlargement. Intraorally, the tumor was hard, firm and painless. (See Figure 13–186E.) The x-ray examination

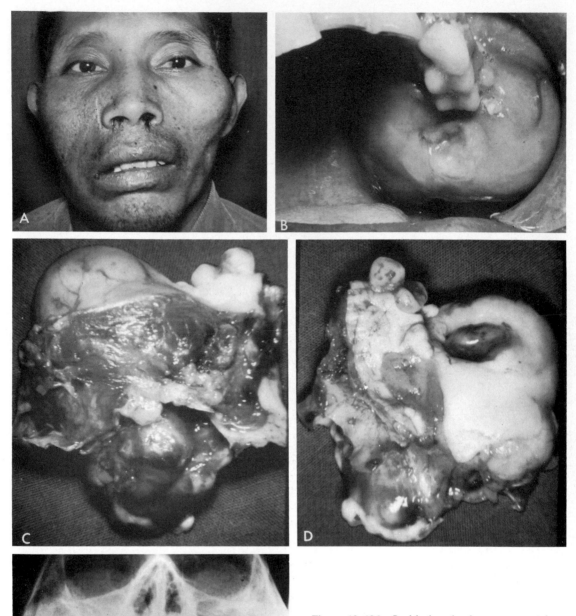

Figure 13–186 Oral lesions in plasmacytoma (plasma cell myeloma). (See Case Report No. 37 for details.) Compare also Figures 12–105 to 12–107.

showed an opacity in the left maxilla. The orbital floor and the interior of the maxillary sinus were not involved.

Pathology Report. A biopsy was taken, and the pathology report was extramedullary plasmacytoma in the maxilla. Because of the rareness of this tumor in this area, new biopsies were taken, and all confirmed the first diagnosis.

Treatment. Preoperative radiation was given (3000 R.), and 3 weeks later a maxillotomy was performed under general anesthesia. A Fergusson incision was made, and a section of the maxilla, along with the tumor, was resected. A skin graft was put inside of the cavity, and an immediate prosthetic support for the graft was inserted and retained for 5 days. The patient had an uneventful recovery and healed with a minor deformity in his mouth and face.

(*Text continued on page 899*)

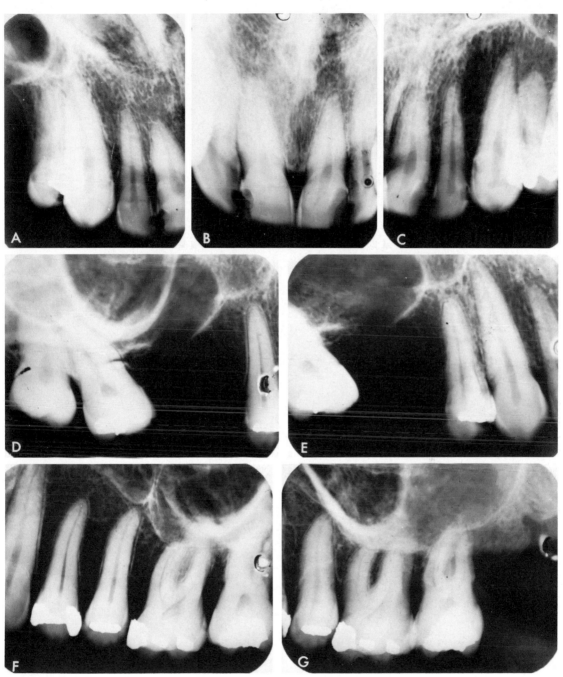

Figure 13–187 (1)

Figure 13–187 *1*, Complete dental radiographs of a 30-year-old male reveal the presence of a mesioangularly impacted right mandibular third molar and a horizontally impacted left third molar, with extensive loss of alveolar bone below the crowns of both third molars extending to the apical region of the distal roots of the second molars (*J* and *M*, on following page). The lower right mandibular bicuspids and first molars were extracted, according to the patient, because these teeth became loose from "pyorrhea." The left maxillary second bicuspid and first molar had been treated similarly. This seemed strange in view of the lack of evidence of periodontal disease in other areas of the jaws. The impacted mandibular third molars were excised and the unusually brownish "granuloma-like" tissue was sent for a histologic examination.

Diagnosis: Eosinophilic granuloma.

A skeletal survey revealed a moderate-sized osteolytic lesion in the patient's femur. The patient was referred to the roentgenologist for treatment.

(*Figure 13–187 continued on following page*)

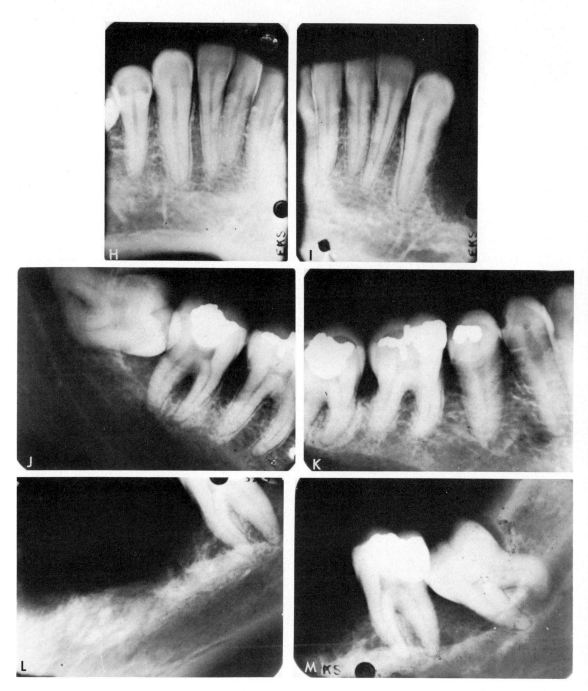

Figure 13–187 *(Continued.)* **(1)** *See legend on preceding page.*

(Figure 13–187 continued on opposite page)

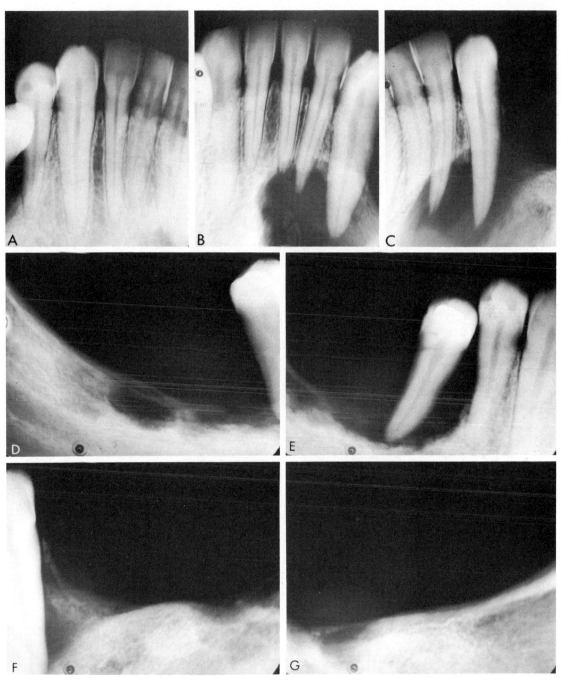

Figure 13–187   *(Continued.)*   **(2)**

Figure 13–187   *(Continued.) 2,* Dental radiographs during the next 27 months. In spite of what was considered to be adequate and "safe" radiation therapy, the lesion spread through the mandibular alveolar process, destroying it and the cortical bone and exfoliating all the remaining mandibular bicuspids and molars. Note the left second mandibular bicuspid "floating" in the soft-tissue lesion; also note the scalloped osteolytic lesions on the surface of the ridge in both mandibular molar areas. These were excised down to the bone, which was cauterized. In addition, an osteolytic lesion involves the apices of the mandibular right central and lateral incisors and the cuspid.

(Figure 13–187 continued on following page)

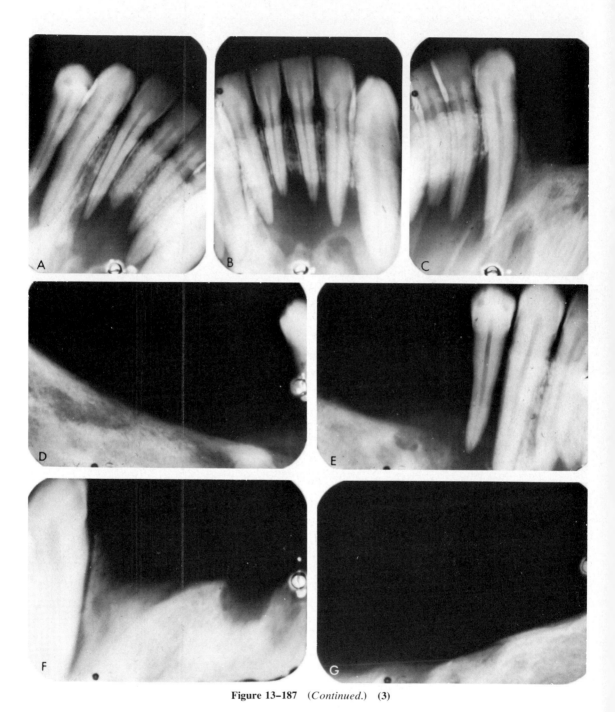

Figure 13–187   (*Continued.*)   **(3)**

Figure 13–187   (*Continued.*) *3,* Fourteen months later, mandibular periapical and occlusal radiographs were taken. The last remaining first bicuspid is "floating" in tissue, and the apex of the adjacent cuspid is involved. In addition, now all mandibular incisors as well as the left cuspid have an extensive loss of periapical bone, and the occlusal radiograph (see *6B*) shows that the very dense lingual cortical bone has been perforated.

(*Figure 13–187 continued on opposite page*)

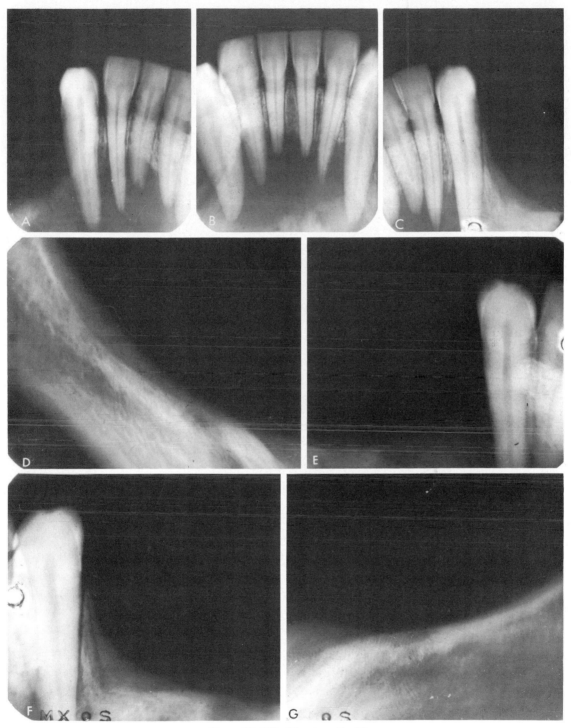

Figure 13–187 (*Continued.*) (**4**)

Figure 13–187 (*Continued.*) *4*, Fourteen months later, all the posterior mandibular teeth have been lost because of the complete destruction of the supporting alveolar bone by the eosinophilic lesions. The destruction of osseous tissue in the symphysis and around the apical thirds of all the anterior teeth is clearly demonstrated.

(*Figure 13–187 continued on following page*)

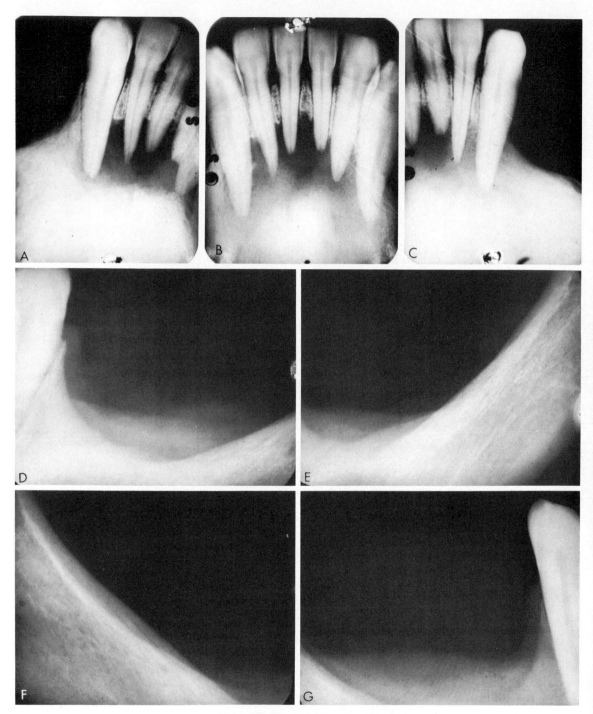

Figure 13–187   (*Continued.*)   **(5)**

Figure 13–187 (*Continued.*)   *5,* Ten months later we have the first radiographic evidence that the dissemination of the eosinophilic lesion has been stopped, and dense osseous tissue is slowly filling the osteolytic lesion about the apices of the remaining six mandibular anterior teeth. Note in the occlusal view (see *6C*) that the perforation through the dense lingual cortical bone has been closed with osseous tissue.

For reasons unknown, in spite of the rampant destruction of mandibular bone over a period of 65 months, not any maxillary teeth became involved in this destructive process, as can be seen in the maxillary periapical films shown in series *7,* taken the same day as series *5.* All the textbooks I have consulted state, with minor variations, that the prognosis of patients with eosinophilic granulomas is good, since "curettage or x-ray therapy or both are curative, symptoms usually subsiding within 2 weeks after treatment." Of course there is always included the escape clause, "in the majority of cases." In my *one case,* it took 260 weeks to stop the progress of the disease, let alone cure it.

(*Figure 13–187 continued on opposite page*)

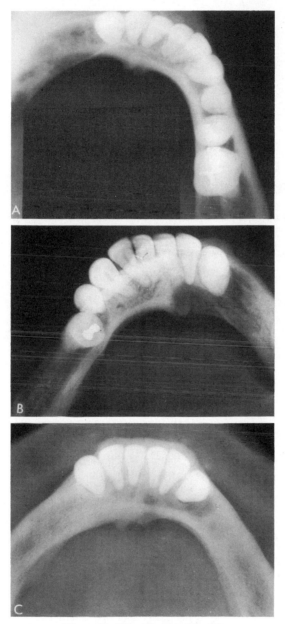

Figure 13–187 (*Continued.*) **(6)**

Figure 13–187 (*Continued.*) *6A*, No evidence of eosinophilic lesions in the symphysis. *B*, Destruction in the symphysis with perforation of the dense lingual cortical bone in the region of the right central and lateral incisors and cuspid. (See the periapical series in *3*.) *C*, Spontaneous healing. No treatment. (Compare the series in *5*.)

(*Figure 13–187 continued on following page*)

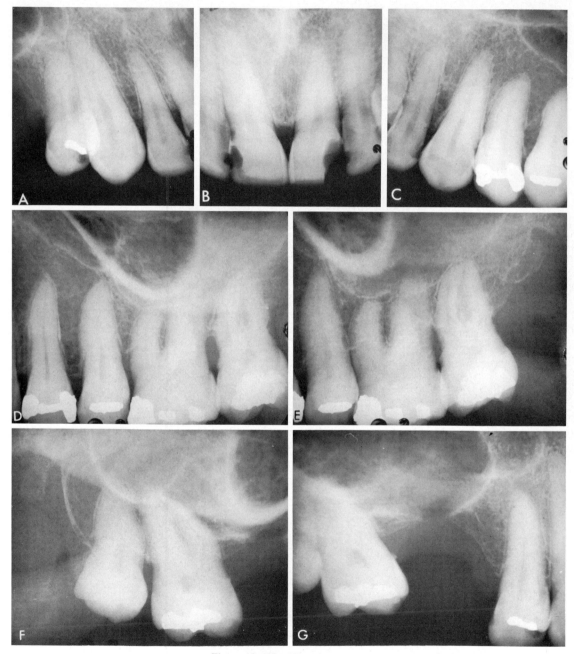

Figure 13–187   (*Continued.*)   **(7)**

Figure 13–187   (*Continued.*)   *7,* No evidence of eosinophilic destruction in the maxilla 65 months after the disease was first found in the mandible. No explanation is known.

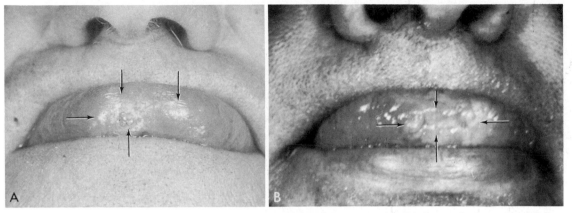

Figure 13–188   *A,* Smooth, thin leukoplakia with a few small nodules on the tip of a pipe smoker's tongue. Findings in an incisional biopsy were negative. The patient stopped smoking, and the lesion disappeared. *B,* Irregular, thick, fissured and nodular leukoplakia on the tip of another pipe smoker's tongue. Incisional biopsy was performed. *Diagnosis:* Epidermoid carcinoma.

LEUKOPLAKIA

A discussion of terms is definitely indicated before one can appreciate the seriousness of the lesions referred to as leukoplakia.

Leukoplakia in its simplest terms means "white plaque." Clinically this is the best definition and description of the entity. Microscopically, however, leukoplakia may appear as one of two distinct forms. The first is a benign hyperkeratotic lesion which shows a histologic picture of hyperkeratosis and orderly maturation of the cells of the epithelial layer. The second form shows the typical pattern of hyperkeratosis along with dyskeratosis and loss of the epithelial basement membrane.

A survey of oral pathologists by Sprague revealed that the great majority required, as a microscopic criterion for leukoplakia, the presence of dyskeratosis alone or with other microscopic features.[86]

Because of dyskeratosis and loss of the epithelial basement membrane, leukoplakia should be regarded as a potentially premalignant lesion and should be treated as such. Of 100 cases of leukoplakia studied by Mac-Keown, 30 showed epidermoid carcinoma.[49]

Leukoplakia is a disease marked by the development of white irregular patches, which may become thickened, fissured or verrucous in appearance, upon the mucous membranes, particularly those of the lips, cheeks, gingivae, palate, tongue or floor of the oral cavity.

Irritants such as smoke, snuff, or strong

(*Text continued on page 903*)

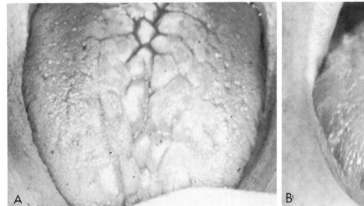
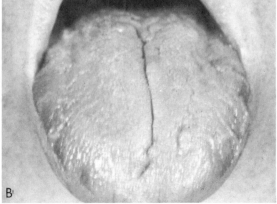

Figure 13–189   *A,* Leukoplakia on nodular congenital fissuring of the tongue. *B,* Deep midline fissure of the middle two-thirds of the tongue. This is uncommon and is the result of the failure of the two lateral halves of tongue to close completely on the dorsal surface. (*A,* Courtesy of H. G. G. Robinson, D.M.D.)

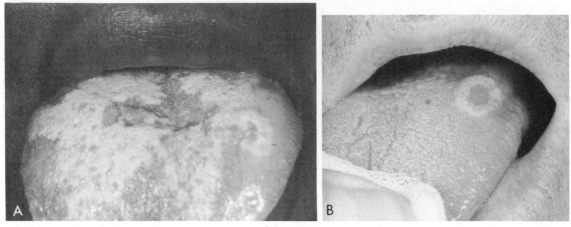

Figure 13–190 *A,* "Geographic tongue" consists usually of multiple zones of desquamation of the filiform papillae in irregularly shaped but well-demarcated areas that migrate across or around the surface of the tongue. They are symptomless and of unknown cause. *B,* Single area of desquamation of the filiform papillae with a slightly raised white border. In 4 days it disappeared.

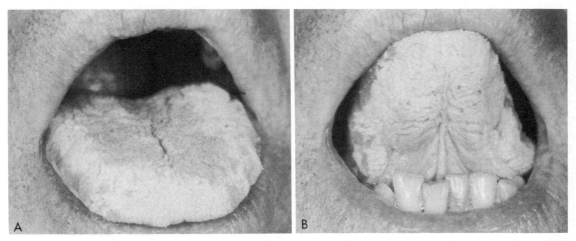

Figure 13–191 White sponge nevus of the mucosa of the dorsal (*A*) and ventral (*B*) surfaces of the tongue. These lesions are not commonly seen. They are usually widespread and may involve the cheeks, palate, gingiva, floor of the mouth, or portions of the tongue. The surface is covered with small papillary projections that give the mucosa a white spongy surface. It is a congenital disturbance of the oral mucosa.[62] (Also see Figure 13–223.) *Treatment:* None. The patient should be followed, although no case is recorded in which malignancy developed in these lesions.

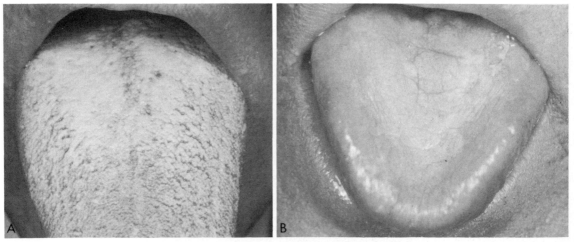

Figure 13–192 *See opposite page for legend.*

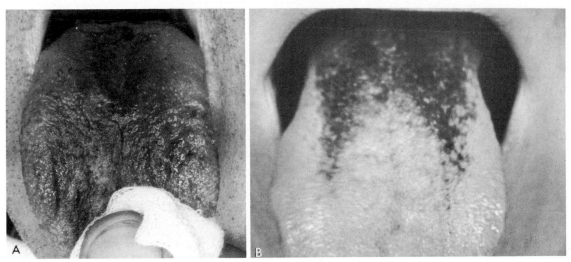

Figure 13–193 Brownish, black or yellow tongues have greatly elongated filiform papillae, which give the tongue the appearance of being hairy. Apparently, in these cases the tongue is invaded by pigment-producing bacteria, yeasts or fungi. These tongues can be associated with antibiotic therapy that is related to the predominance of fungi in the oral cavity. When this therapy is terminated, the oral flora becomes balanced and the tongue returns to normal.

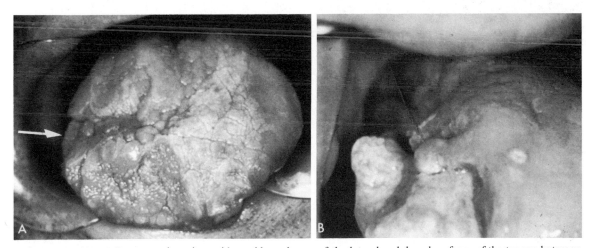

Figure 13–194 *A*, Recurrent invasive epidermoid carcinoma of the lateral and dorsal surfaces of the tongue between the anterior and middle thirds. Note the warty furrow with marked induration due to the downgrowth of the cancer into the musculature of the tongue. There were metastatic lesions. *B*, Four weeks later. Extensive necrosis is apparent.

Figure 13–192 *A*, Pseudoleukoplakia. This patient chewed "antacid stomach pills" daily that maintained this heavily coated white tongue.

B, The marked atrophy of both filiform and fungiform papillae produces this very smooth, bald, dorsal surface of the tongue. This is the result of long-standing malnutrition. It is commonly seen with iron deficiency anemia and pernicious anemia.

"Bald tongue" (atrophic glossitis) is also seen in patients with tertiary syphilis. Other tongue lesions associated with this disease are ulcerative glossitis, sclerotic glossitis and gummatous glossitis.

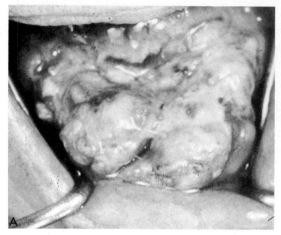
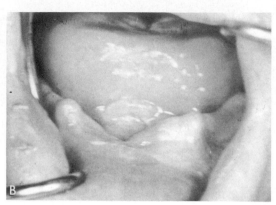

Figure 13–195 *A,* Fungating exophytic epidermoid carcinoma of the tongue with metastasis to the lungs. *B,* Solely for palliation, radiation therapy was administered to the tongue. These lesions "melt" rapidly. This is the healed post-radiation appearance.

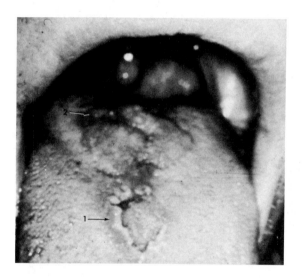

Figure 13–196 *1,* Tuberculous ulcer of the dorsum of the tongue with a typical ragged, undermined border. These are painful lesions and are usually associated with pulmonary tuberculosis.

2, Median rhomboid glossitis of the tongue. These are considered to be a developmental anomaly. This one has both depressed and elevated areas. These are usually symptomless, but occasionally patients will complain of a slight itching or burning sensation. (Courtesy of Dr. Carl Bender.)

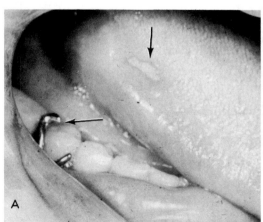
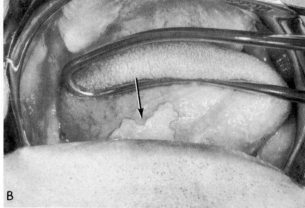

Figure 13–197 *A,* This small elongated white strip, leukoplakia, is the result of scratching of the lateral surface of the tongue by the poorly fitting clasp on the second bicuspid. *B,* Large elevated area of leukoplakia of unknown cause, with an irregular border on the ventral mucosa of the tongue. Findings in an incisional biopsy were negative.

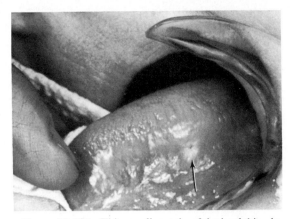

Figure 13-198 This small patch of leukoplakia, located on the mucosa of the ventral surface of the middle third of the tongue, clinically appears to be an innocent hyperkeratotic lesion. However, the small dark spot near the center is suspicious because it suggests a small ulcerous break-through of the basement membrane and invasion of the lamina propria. An excisional biopsy of the lesion was performed. *Diagnosis:* Epidermoid carcinoma (squamous cell carcinoma).

condiments may produce leukoplakia, as well as do alcohol, oral trauma from various dental sources, hot, spicy foods, allergy, avitaminosis A, galvanism and hypercholesterolemia. It has been called a precancerous lesion because of the frequency with which it becomes malignant.

Progressive changes occur in the leukoplakic area if the cause is not removed. The pearly white lesion becomes a light gray or brownish white, with fissuring of the surface, or a rough verrucous (warty) or papillomatous formation, and ultimately ulcerates. While ulceration is not necessary for malig-

nancy, when it occurs in an area of leukoplakia it is almost a certain objective proof of malignancy.

The size of the lesion varies from 0.5 cm. to a size covering the entire buccal mucosa or the dorsum of the tongue. The plaques may be confined to one area or they may be found in several locations. The margins are usually clear-cut and distinct, but occasionally, particularly in the early stages, they are vague and indefinite.[90]

Classification. Thoma[64] summarized the stages described by Prinz[64] and McCarthy[51] as follows:

Leukoplakia, Grade I. This type is characterized by the initial reaction of the mucous membrane to irritation. The mucosa presents a red, granular, sharply defined, slightly sensitive area, which remains in this stage of development but a short time before it becomes slightly whitish gray.

Leukoplakia, Grade II. This stage is described as the smooth tessellated type by Prinz. It is made up of a network of intense pearly white discolorations of diffuse opacity having a bluish tint. These patches are sharply outlined but without palpable induration, and look as if they were pasted on the mucous membrane. The smooth surface is frequently criss-crossed by irregular markings which radiate on the cheek in the form of a modified trident of a fan or form parquet-like subdivisions on the tongue. On palpation the finger will feel peculiar roughness of the affected part. If the disease is of extensive involvement, the patient may complain of dryness of the mouth, and the tongue, if affected, may be hindered in its movements.

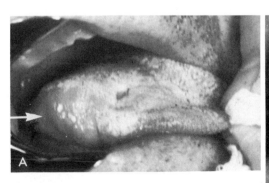

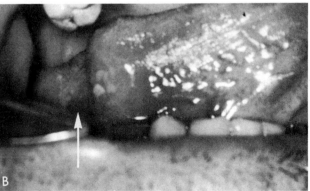

Figure 13-199 *A,* Base of the tongue, still mobile, with local swelling from an endophytic cancer. These are often overlooked. If the patient has an inability to protrude the tongue, or it deviates to one side when protruding, or the base is swollen or indurated or both, tumor must be ruled out. *B,* Later ulceration and sloughing will occur, as is shown in this second case. *Note:* Both these tongues were manually brought forward so that the bases could be seen.

Case Report No. 38

FIBROSARCOMA OF THE TONGUE

H. Serrano Roa. D.D.S.

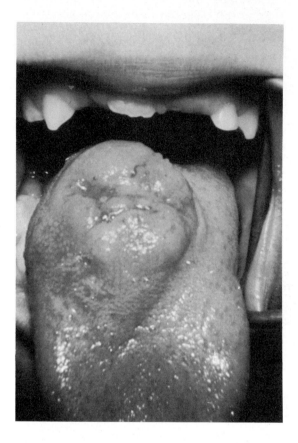

Patient. A 7-year-old girl was seen in the Department of Estomatology of the Roosevelt Hospital, Guatemala City, Central America, because of a tumor in her tongue of 1 year's known duration (Figure 13–200).

Physical Examination. Examination showed a tumor 3 by 3 cm. in the middle third, right side of the tongue. The growth was firm and painless and had a nodular surface. It did not interfere with swallowing or speech. A biopsy was taken.

Pathology Report. Fibrosarcoma.

Treatment. Under general anesthesia, the malignant tumor was excised. Histopathologic study confirmed the diagnosis. The follow-up of the patient for 1½ years showed that there was no evidence of recurrence, and the girl was in good health. Fibrosarcoma is a very rare lesion in the oral cavity.

Figure 13–200 Fibrosarcoma of the tongue. (See Case Report No. 38.)

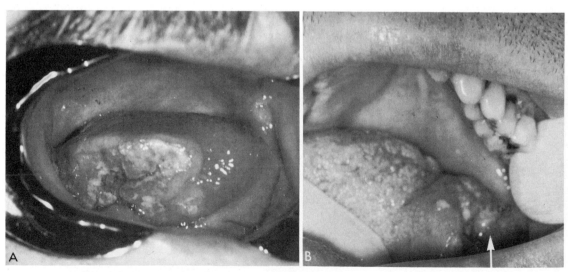

Figure 13–201 *A,* Invasive epidermoid carcinoma of the lateral anterior two-thirds of the tongue, which is markedly swollen with tumor. Note the fissured leukoplakia. *B,* Invasive epidermoid carcinoma of the base of the tongue, which is partially "frozen" by invasion of the musculature by the tumor.

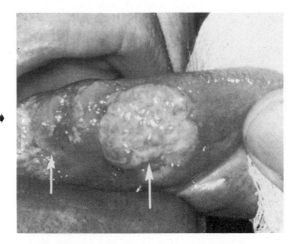

Figure 13–202 The anterior lateral tumor *(right arrow)* is an exophytic fungating globular epidermoid carcinoma. The posterior tumor *(left arrow)* is an invasive epidermoid carcinoma.

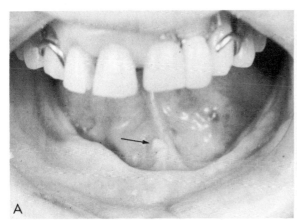

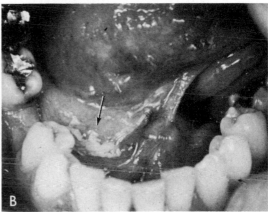

Figure 13–203 *A,* Solitary nodule of leukoplakia on the lateral surface of the lingual frenum. Findings in an excisional biopsy were negative. *B,* Irregular raised leukoplakia with rolled margins in the anterior floor of the mouth. Incisional biopsy was performed. *Diagnosis:* Epidermoid carcinoma.

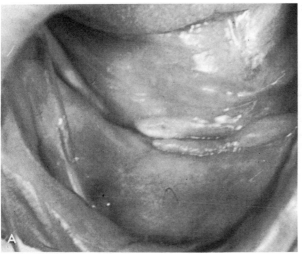

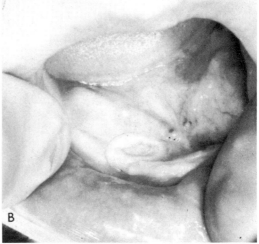

Figure 13–204 *A,* Small area of leukoplakia in the floor of the mouth containing an indurated ulcer with slightly raised borders. Excisional biopsy was performed. *Diagnosis:* Epidermoid cancer. *B,* A larger area of leukoplakia in the floor of the oral cavity. This lesion extends up over the crest of the edentulous alveolar ridge, where there is a much larger indurated ulcer with raised, rolled borders. Incisional biopsy was performed. *Diagnosis:* Epidermoid carcinoma.

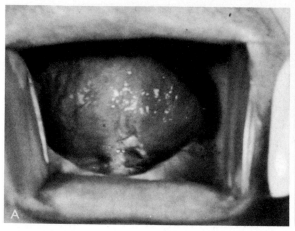
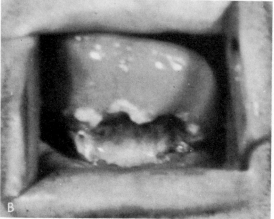

Figure 13–205 *A*, Irregular nodular leukoplakia of the anterior ventral surface of the tongue, with involvement of the lingual frenum and a small area of leukoplakia of the mucosa of the floor of the mouth. There is a fairly large invasive ulcer along the lateral border. Incisional biopsy was performed. *Diagnosis:* Epidermoid cancer. *B*, Two-week postradiation view showing the extent of slough and the postradiation edema of the tongue. (See Figures 13–206 and 13–208 for photographs of similar cases showing final healing. Read Chapter 29, "Radiation Therapy of Lesions of the Oral Cavity.")

LEUKOPLAKIA, GRADE III. When this stage is reached, leukoplakia is definite and easily recognized at a glance even by the layman. It presents indurated plaques of a milky white or pearly, silvery appearance, which are often raised and may cover a large area of the mouth. The lesion forms a harsh horny surface and tends to wrinkle and may form fissures.

LEUKOPLAKIA, GRADE IV. In this stage the lesion not only is markedly indurated and leathery, but also shows verrucous or papillomatous formations. It is, therefore, called the verrucous stage of leukoplakia by Prinz. The mucosa is covered by thick layers of keratinized epithelium which are often coated with a heavy fur. There are definite warty outgrowths which may form fairly large nodules. Fissures form with a downgrowth of epithelium causing localized induration. This stage has marked neoplastic potentialities and, therefore, is often called neoplastic leukoplakia. In such cases the tongue is materially handicapped in its movements and speech may become somewhat thick. Spontaneous desquamation and ulceration of the affected area may occur.

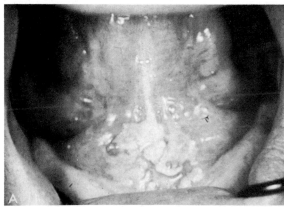
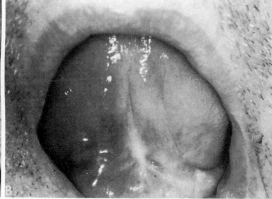

Figure 13–206 *A*, Large area of grayish white leukoplakia in the midline of the anterior floor of the mouth that is roughened, scaly, fissured and nodular in two areas. Incisional biopsy was performed. *Diagnosis:* Epidermoid carcinoma. *B*, Healed appearance following radiation treatment.

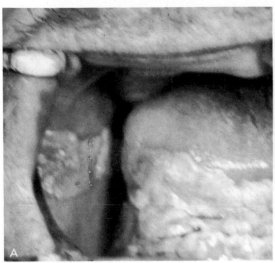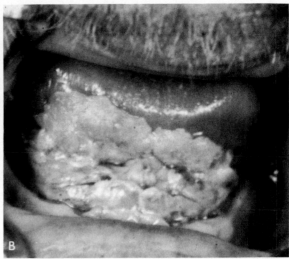

Figure 13–207 Chemical leukoplakia. This uremic patient, with the typical urinous, ammonia-like breath, had these grayish white thick, fissured, leathery areas on both cheeks *(A)*, beginning below the bilateral orifices of the parotid ducts, and on the anterior and lateral surfaces of the floor of the mouth and the ventral surface of the tongue *(B)*. These areas were bathed with saliva from the bilateral ducts from the submandibular glands and, of course, both cheeks from the parotid ducts. They are the result of continuous chemical burning by the caustic action of ammonia carbonate, which is formed from the salivary urea. Thus a coagulation necrosis results that appears like the thick, grayish white patches shown here.

Case Report No. 39

LIP SHAVE FOR LEUKOPLAKIA

Marvin E. Pizer, D.D.S., M.S.

Patient. An 89-year-old white male was admitted to Alexandria Hospital for a lip shave.

Chief Complaint. The patient had been experiencing pain in the midline of the lower lip at the mucocutaneous junction. A white lesion covered the exposed mucous membrane of the entire lower lip. (See Figure 13–209.)

History of Present Illness. One year prior to this admission the patient had had a lesion removed from the mucocutaneous region of the left lower lip. It was diagnosed by the pathologist as benign leukoplakia of the mucous membrane of the lip and senile keratosis of the skin of the left lower lip. The mucous membrane lesion had recurred, and the entire lower lip was now involved. There appeared to be a retention cyst in the midline of the lower lip at the mucocutaneous junction. The patient was put on vitamin A to see if any improvement would result. There being no improvement in 1 month, surgical excision was considered necessary.

Medical Evaluation. The patient had arteriosclerotic heart disease, which was demonstrated by physical examination, chest x-ray and electrocardiogram. He was on anticoagulants and a diuretic. Although there was no evidence that he had suffered myocardial infarction, he had had phlebitis 3 years previously and was on anticoagulant therapy prophylactically. Osteoarthritis and a questionable gastric ulcer were noted in the history. Findings in

blood and urine studies were within normal limits; however, the prothrombin time revealed the patient's blood to be well anticoagulated. We do not insist on discontinuation of anticoagulant therapy before oral surgery.

Operative Technique. Under local anesthesia, with 2 per cent carbocaine, bilateral mental nerve blocks were administered. A first incision was made from the commissure of the left lower lip along the mucocutaneous junction to the commissure of the right lower lip. A second incision was made posterior to this in the mucous membrane of the lip to encompass the white lesion, allowing a margin of about 1/2 cm. of normal tissue. With pickups the mucocutaneous lesion was elevated, and with traction and by sharp dissection the white lesion of the lower lip was completely removed. Four silk sutures were placed in the mucous membrane close to the site of excision, for traction. Then the mucous membrane of the inner aspect of the lower lip was undermined with small curved scissors down to the labial vestibule from one corner of the lip to the other. Following this, the undermined mucous membrane was transposed and sutured to the skin with 5–0 interrupted silk sutures. A pressure dressing was applied to the skin of the lower lip. The patient tolerated surgery and anesthesia and left the operating room in good condition.

Pathology Report. *Macroscopic:* The specimen

consists of the mucosal surface of the lower lip, measuring 6.0 by 1.2 cm., with submucosal tissue to a depth of 0.3 cm. attached to it. The mucosal surface is pinkish tan, with patchy areas of grayish tan. The specimen is multisectioned and designated. Also in the container are yellowish and pinkish tan rubbery tissue fragments aggregating 1.9 by 1.4 by 0.5 cm.

Microscopic: Multiple sections of the lower lip show small areas of epithelial atrophy with intervening areas of slight acanthosis. The surface shows hyperkeratosis, and there is subepithelial hyalinization. An inflammatory infiltrate, consisting primarily of lymphocytes, is present adjacent to the basal layer. An occasional epithelial cell in the basal layer shows slight dyskeratosis. Also submitted are fragments of voluntary muscle and fibroadipose tissue. Small foci of salivary gland tissue are present in the fat, and there are lymphocytes in the glandular stroma.

Diagnosis: Leukoplakia, lower lip. Salivary gland tissue showing slight inflammation, lower lip. Fragments of voluntary muscle, lower lip (Dee R. Parkinson, M.D.).

Postoperative Course. The patient had an uneventful recovery. Alternate sutures were removed on the fifth postoperative day and the remainder on the seventh postoperative day, at which time the patient was discharged from the hospital and followed in the office. He was given an antiactinic cream to wear on his lips when outside. The patient is comfortable and 1 year postoperatively is without recurrence.

Final Diagnosis. Leukoplakia, lower lip. Salivary gland tissue showing slight inflammation, lower lip. Fragments of voluntary muscle, lower lip.

COMMENT

Our decision to do this procedure was carefully weighed against the patient's medical history, as well as the recurrence of this condition on his lips. It was felt that incisional biopsy might not reveal the entire histologic picture, since the lesion was so widespread and no particular site could be designated as characteristic of this lesion for an incisional biopsy; therefore, complete surgical excision was considered the procedure of choice.

Differential Diagnosis. White lesions in the oral cavity which may simulate leukoplakia are: lichen planus (Fig. 13–214), senile keratosis, white sponge nevus (Figs. 13–191 and 13–223), carcinoma, traumatic lesions, pemphigus, erythema multiforme, herpes simplex, syphilis, chemical burns (Fig. 13–207), such as that seen from an aspirin tablet which has been allowed to dissolve against the mucosa, or strongly astringent mouthwash. Monilial stomatitis (thrush), which usually is seen in the young, can be seen in all age groups. Milky white patches are usually seen in the cheeks and tongue but they may involve the entire oral mucosa. Diagnosis is confirmed by microscopic examination of the scraping or by analysis of a culture.

(*Text continued on page 914*)

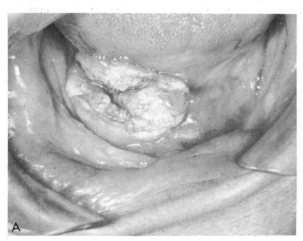
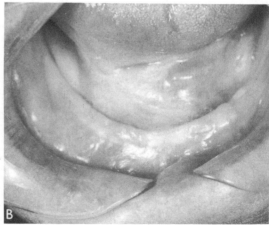

Figure 13–208 *A*, Large exophytic fissured epidermoid carcinoma in the floor of the mouth of an edentulous patient. *B*, Healed mucosa 3 years after radiation therapy.

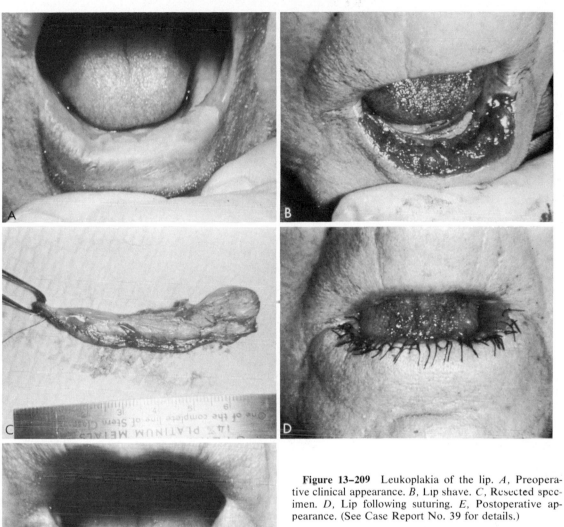

Figure 13–209 Leukoplakia of the lip. *A*, Preoperative clinical appearance. *B*, Lip shave. *C*, Resected specimen. *D*, Lip following suturing. *E*, Postoperative appearance. (See Case Report No. 39 for details.)

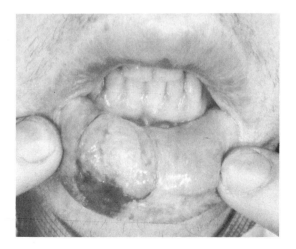

Figure 13–210 A rare neurotrophic "ulcer" of the lip in a 12-year-old boy, following local anesthesia of the inferior alveolar nerve. While they are called "ulcers," they are not painful, nor are they usually crater-like; rather they are elevated, circumscribed, pearly white lesions. However, giant ulcers of the side of the face following surgical ablation of the homolateral trigeminal nerve have been reported.[26, 41]

These are not to be confused with the postinjection ulcers produced by the patient's chewing of the numb lip; when seen, these are mostly in children. Neurotrophic ulcers should also be distinguished from lesions produced by the lips having been pinched between the handles of the forceps and the anterior teeth during extraction of teeth.

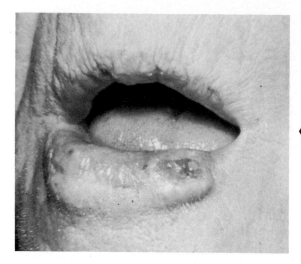

Figure 13–211 Superficial suppurative cheilitis glandularis of the lip. This painless, indurated swelling with crusting and ulceration had been present many months. *Treatment:* Nothing definitive, although some authorities consider this lesion premalignant.

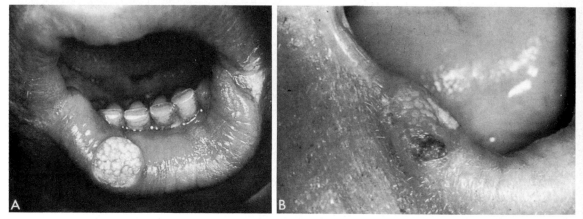

Figure 13–212 *A,* Verrucous carcinoma of the lip. *B,* Epidermoid carcinoma of the lip.

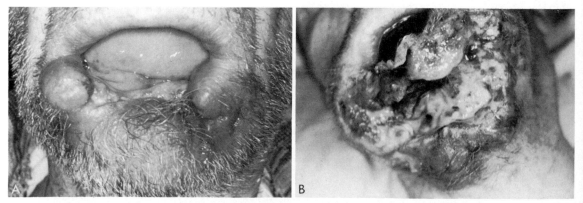

Figure 13–213 *A,* Recurrent extensive destruction of the lip from epidermoid carcinoma. *B,* At death.

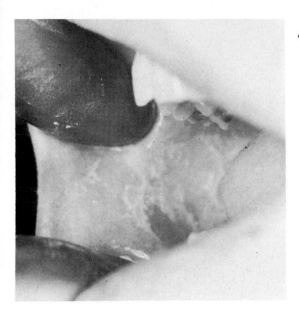

Figure 13–214 Reticular lichen planus of the buccal mucosa. Note the typical lace-like pattern. No specific treatment is used (see text).

Figure 13–215 Fordyce's granules or spots (Fordyce's disease). The latter is a misnomer, as this is not a disease but a developmental anomaly of sebaceous glands located in the buccal oral mucosa. This condition does not require treatment.

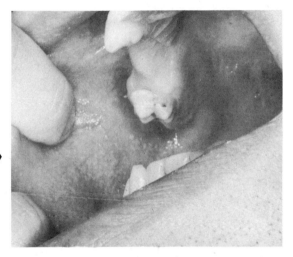

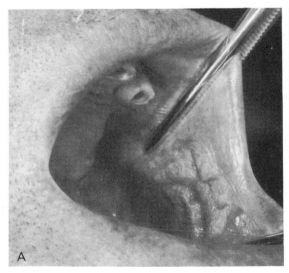

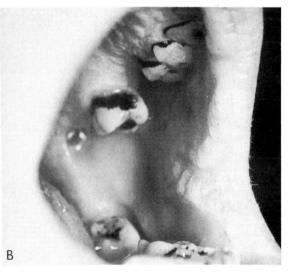

A   B

Figure 13–216 Hereditary benign intraepithelial dyskeratosis. These lesions are usually found on the buccal mucosa near the corners of the mouth (A and B). This white or grayish white, spongy, shaggy mucosa simulates white sponge nevus. According to Schafer and associates, "These patients also develop lesions of the eye characterized by superficial, foamy, gelatinous white plaques, sometimes producing temporary blindness. There is no increase in the death rate or in death from neoplastic disease in these patients."[75]

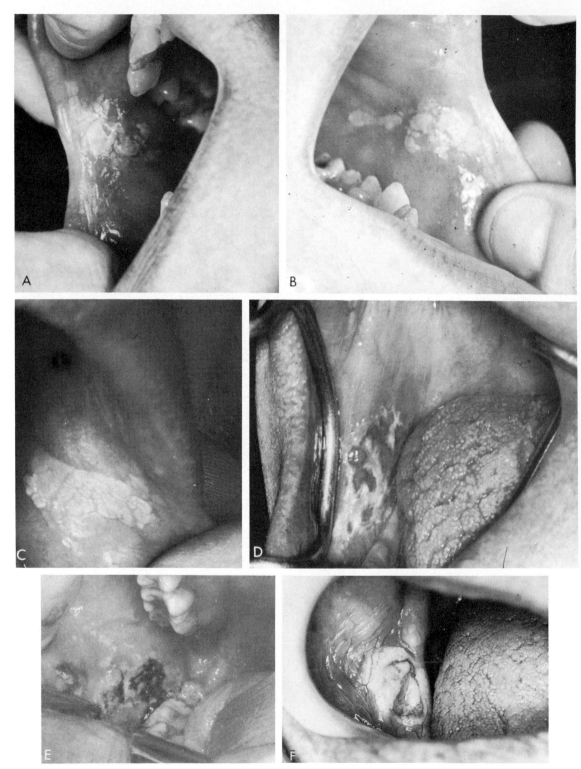

Figure 13–217 *A* to *C*, Examples of leukoplakia with indurated, raised pearly white plaques with definite margins and fissures. *D* to *F*, Leukoplakia with invasive epidermoid carcinoma.

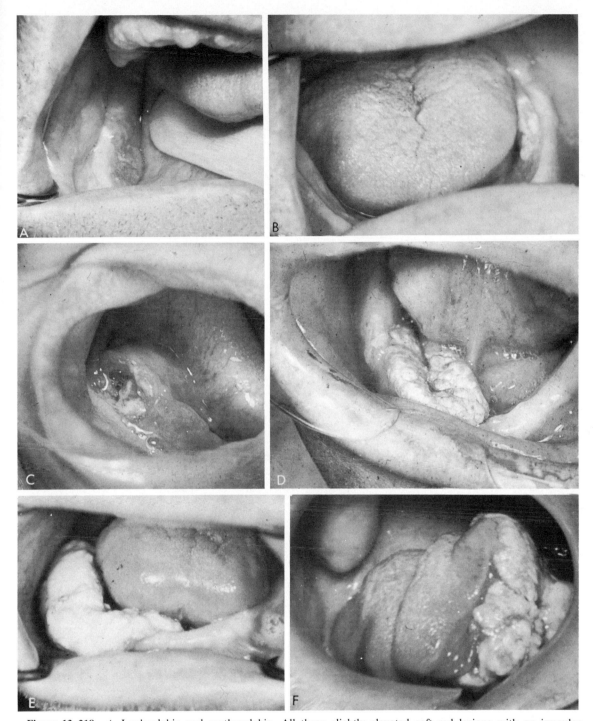

Figure 13–218 *A*, Leukoplakia and erythroplakia. All these slightly elevated soft red lesions with an irregular margin should be biopsied. According to Schafer and his colleagues, "The vast majority of cases of erythroplakia are histologically either invasive carcinoma or carcinoma *in situ* at the time of biopsy. The treatment is the same as that for any invasive carcinoma or carcinoma *in situ*."[75]

B, Epidermoid carcinoma *in situ*. *Treatment:* Regional upper block section of the area of the mandible.[1]

C, Invasive epidermoid carcinoma which developed in a lingual epulis fissurata produced by an overextended lingual flange of a full mandibular denture.

D, Verrucous carcinoma which also developed in an epulis fissuratum produced in the same manner as described in *C*.

E, Large exophytic verrucous carcinoma of the mandible. This lesion is slow-growing and only superficially invasive in its early stages. According to Schafer and associates, it "has a low metastatic potential and is amenable to local excision because of its relatively nonaggressive and protracted course."[75]

F, Another case of verrucous carcinoma with the same history as given in *C* and *D*.

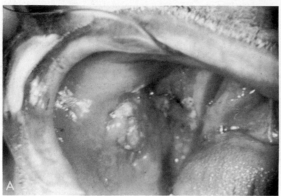
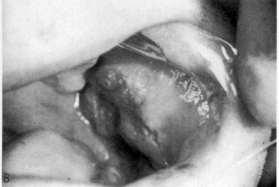

Figure 13–219 *A*, Exophytic epidermoid carcinoma of the buccal mucosa. *B*, Painful ulcerative invasive epidermoid carcinoma of the buccal mucosa.

Case Report No. 40

EPIDERMOID CARCINOMA OF THE MANDIBULAR GINGIVAE, TREATED BY SUBTOTAL RESECTION OF THE MANDIBULAR SEGMENT

H. Serrano Roa, D.D.S.

Patient.   A 55-year-old female was seen in the Department of Estomatology of the Roosevelt Hospital in Guatemala City, Central America, for a painful lesion of the palate, 8 days old.

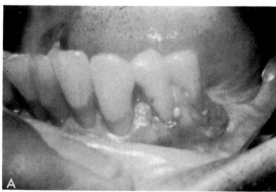
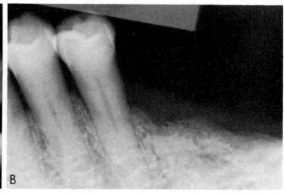

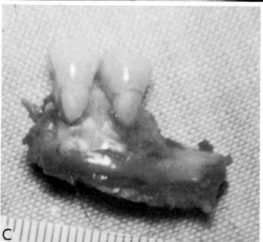

Figure 13–220 Epidermoid carcinoma of the mandibular gingivae. *A*, Preoperative clinical appearance. *B*, Intraoral radiograph. *C*, Resected specimen. (See Case Report No. 40 for details.)

Physical Examination. Examination of the oral cavity showed a small herpetic lesion in the middle of the palate and on the gingivae, from near the back of the mouth to the lower left cuspid. The lesion was 3 by 4 mm. and slightly elevated. The patient had been feeling pain when she used her partial denture.

Treatment. Medical treatment was given for both lesions. Three days later, the lesion on the palate had completely disappeared, but not the lesion on the gum. The patient did not have lymph-adenopathy. A biopsy was taken, and the pathology report indicated squamous cell carcinoma of the gum. Under local anesthesia a partial resection of the mandible was performed (Fig. 13–220).

Histopathology Report. The margins were free from disease, as were those of the bone resected. The gingival lesion was squamous cell carcinoma, well differentiated.

Subsequent Course. The patient has been followed, and she is in good health.

As an aid to differential diagnosis, some illustrations of leukoplakia demonstrating malignant changes and illustrations of more advanced cases of carcinoma are also included in this section. Study also Chapter 27, "The Diagnosis and Management of Oral Malignant Diseases."

Treatment of Leukoplakia. 1. Remove the factors of irritation. This includes the elimination of smoking, hot, spicy foods, ill-fitting full or partial dentures, sharp, carious teeth, cheek biting, galvanic sources and oral infections.

2. Make a thorough physical examination to discover and treat, if present, syphilis or avitaminosis A, systemic factors, such as hypercholesterolemia, allergies, or excessive estrogenic hormones.

3. If the lesion does not disappear within 2 weeks after the above treatment, then the lesion should be biopsied, and if nonmalignant it should be excised with a radiosurgical

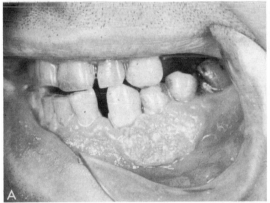
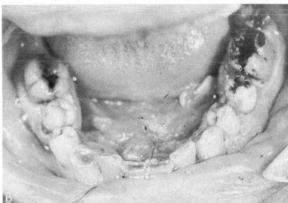
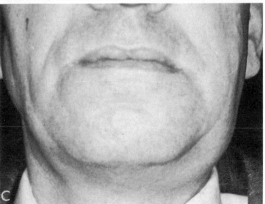

Figure 13–221 *A*, Epidermoid carcinoma of the gingiva. *B*, Extension through the interproximal space to the floor of the oral cavity. *C*, Metastasis to the neck nodes.

Treatment: resection of the mandible, floor of the mouth and neck nodes.

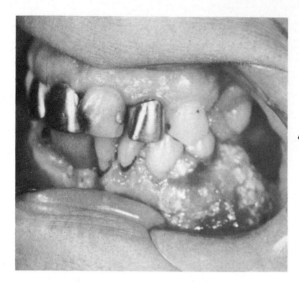

Figure 13–222   Fulminating exophytic epidermoid carcinoma of the gingiva.

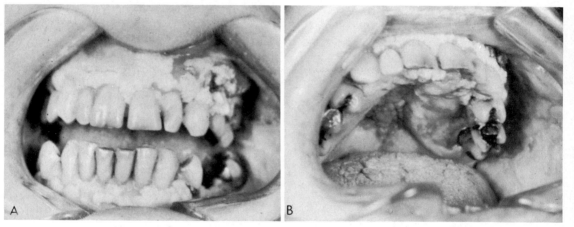

Figure 13–223   White sponge nevus of the gingiva and palatal tissue. (See Figure 13–191 and its legend.)

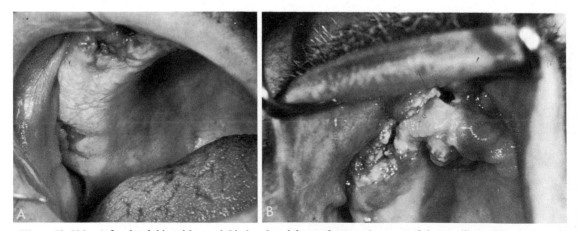

Figure 13–224   *A*, Leukoplakia with a wrinkled and nodular surface on the crest of the maxillary ridge. *B*, Invasive ulcerative epidermoid carcinoma of the anterior edentulous maxillary alveolar process.

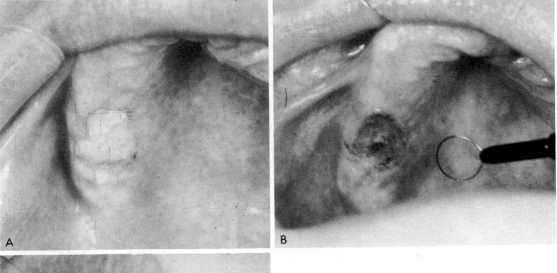

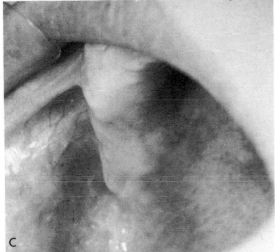

Figure 13–225 *A*, Leukoplakia with definite raised margins. *B*, Lesion excised with a radiosurgical loop. *C*, Healed ridge.

loop. *"Watchful wating" is not advisable!* If malignant it should be treated as such.

If malignant dyskeratosis is present, the lesion is widely excised. If dyskeratosis alone or with other microscopic features is present, excise the lesion with the knife or radiosurgical loop.

LICHEN PLANUS

Lichen planus is an uncommon inflammatory skin disease with flat, angular persistent papules occurring in circumscribed patches and usually with white, plaque-like lesions on the buccal mucosa.

The types of lichen planus that are seen clinically are annular, nodular and erosive. The oral lesions are made up by a coalescence of white pinhead papules. Beyond these plaques individual white papules are usually formed. This is an important diagnostic feature of this disease, which Darling and Crabb are convinced is found in the oral cavity more frequently without accompanying skin lesions than with them.[31]

The buccal mucosa and tongue are the usual sites for this disease, which is characteristically seen as lacework (see Figure 13–214), rings, irregular lines or starlike designs.

The oral lesions may be ulcerated. These lesions are not precancerous. If there is doubt as to whether the lesion is lichen planus, or leukoplakia, or any of the other entities which produce white lesions, a biopsy should be taken.

The etiology is unknown and treatment is empirical, aimed at improving the patient's general health.

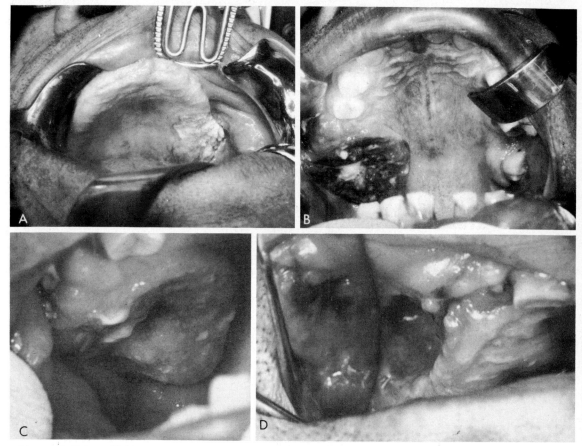

Figure 13–226 *A*, Verrucous carcinoma of the edentulous maxillary alveolar ridge. *B*, Expanding epidermoid carcinoma of the right maxilla. *C*, Necrosis in a large epidermoid carcinoma of the palate and maxilla. *D*, Opening into the necrotic center of an epidermoid carcinoma of the maxillary sinus.

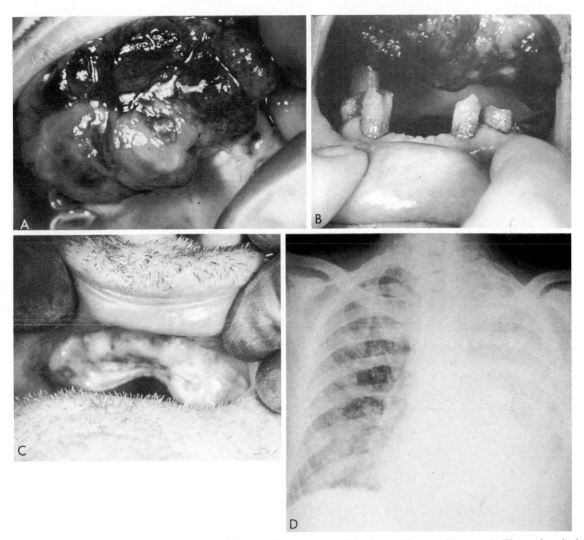

Figure 13–227 *A*, Rhabdomyosarcoma of the maxillary anterior ridge in an 80-year-old man. *B*, The patient had traumatized the edentulous anterior alveolar ridge during mastication for over 20 years. *C*, Tumor excised for palliation. *D*, Metastases to the right lung.

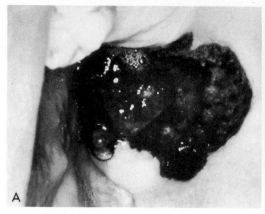

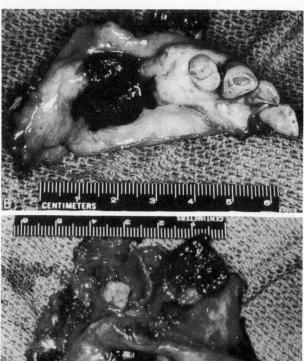

Figure 13–228   Malignant melanoma (melanocarcinoma) of the palate and crest of the alveolar ridge. *A,* Extent of the tumor on the palate and alveolar ridge. *B* and *C,* Resected section of the maxilla.

Malignant melanoma is a rare but very dangerous tumor. It is usually found, as shown here, on the maxillary alveolar ridge and palate. It is almost always fatal. *Treatment:* Radical surgical resection of the areas involved and regional node resection. (Courtesy of Ross P. Cafaro, Jr., D.D.S.)

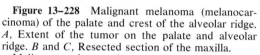

Case Report No. 41

MALIGNANT MELANOMA IN THE PALATE

H. Serrano Roa, D.D.S.

Patient.   A 27-year-old man consulted the Department of Estomatology at the General Hospital of Guatemala City, Central America, for a spot in the palate. He had first seen it 3 months pre-

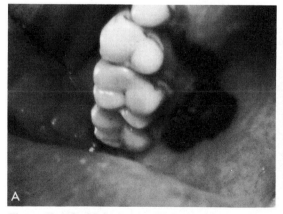

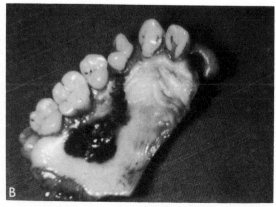

Figure 13–229   Malignant melanoma of the maxilla. *A,* Preoperative clinical appearance. *B,* Resected specimen. (See Case Report No. 41 for details.)

viously, and recently he had noticed a soreness when he took his meals.

Physical Examination. Examination showed a man in apparently good health. Intraorally, a blue-black spot was visible on the palate. It was slightly elevated and well defined. The patient had no palpable nodes, and roentgenograms of the skull, face and thorax appeared normal.

Treatment. Under general anesthesia a partial resection of the maxilla was performed (Fig. 13–229). A partial prosthesis was immediately inserted. The pathology report of the specimen indicated malignant melanoma in the palate. Three weeks later a radical neck dissection was performed.

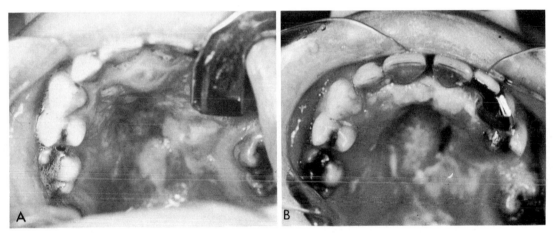

Figure 13–230 *A,* Reticulum cell sarcoma of the palate. This is an unusual sarcoma in the oral cavity. It was originally diagnosed as Vincent's infection. *B,* Three weeks later. There was wide dissemination of the disease, and the patient died 5 months later in spite of radiation therapy.

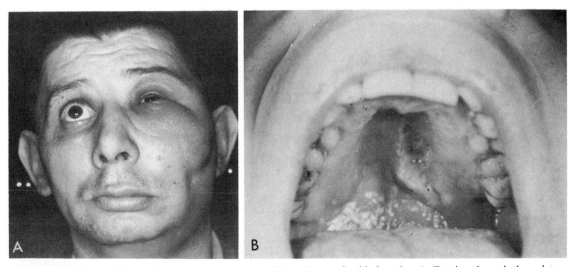

Figure 13–231 *A,* Epidermoid carcinoma of the maxillary sinus and orbital cavity. *B,* Erosion through the palate.

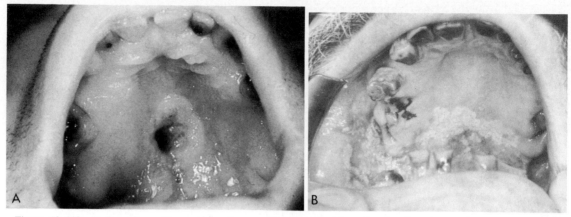

Figure 13–232 *A,* Invasive epidermoid carcinoma of the palate with perforation into the nasal cavity. *B,* Extension of epidermoid carcinoma from the esophagus to the buccal mucosa and soft palate.

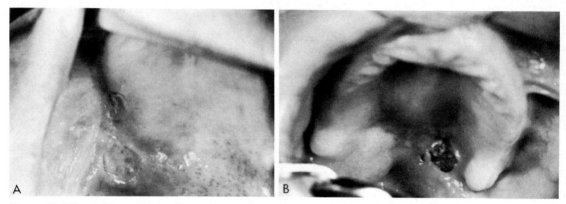

Figure 13–233 *A,* Mucoepidermoid carcinoma of the palate. *B,* Invasion of mucoepidermoid carcinoma of the palate.

REFERENCES

1. Alling, C. C., and Secord, R. T.: A technique for oral exfoliative cytology. Oral Surg., *17*:668–676 (May), 1964.
2. Archer, W. H.: Myxoma of left maxilla. Oral Surg., *13*:139–141 (Feb.), 1960.
3. Archer, W. H.: Ameloblastoma of symphysis of the mandible. Oral Surg., *12*:1055–1060 (Sept.), 1959.
4. Austin, L. T., Jr., Dahlin, D. C., and Royer, R. Q.: Giant-cell reparative granuloma and related conditions affecting the jaw bone. Oral Surg., *12*:1285–1295 (Nov.), 1959.
5. Bauer, W. H., and Bauer, J. D.: The so-called "congenital epulis." Oral Surg., *6*:1065, 1953.
6. Baurmash, H., and Mandel, L.: The non-surgical treatment of hemangioma with Sotradecol. Oral Surg., *16*:777 (July), 1963.
7. Bernier, J. L.: The Management of Oral Disease. St. Louis, C. V. Mosby Co., 1955.
8. Bernier, J. L., and Cahn, L. R.: The peripheral giant cell reparative granuloma. J.A.D.A., *49*:141 (Aug.), 1954.
9. Bernier, J. L., and Thompson, H. C.: Myoblastoma. Am. J. Dent. Res., *4*:158, 1949.
10. Bhaskar, S. N.: Synopsis of Oral Pathology. St. Louis, The C. V. Mosby Co., 1965.
11. Bhaskar, S. N., and Akamine, R.: Congenital epulis (congenital granular cell fibroblastoma). Oral Surg., Oral Med. & Oral Path., *8*:517, 1955.
12. Bhaskar, S. N., Bernier, J. L., and Godby, F.: Aneurysmal bone cyst and other giant cell lesions of the jaws: report of 104 cases. J. Oral Surg., *17*:30 (July), 1959.
13. Boyd, W.: Textbook of Pathology. 7th ed. Philadelphia, Lea & Febiger, 1961.
14. Cahn, L. R.: Dentigerous cyst as a potential adamantinoma. Dent. Cosmos, *75*:889, 1933.
15. Cahn, L. R.: Pathology of the Oral Cavity. Baltimore, Williams & Wilkins Co., 1941.
16. Cahn, L. R.: Personal communication.
17. Cahn, L. R., and Tiecke, R. W.: Oral Pathology. New York, McGraw-Hill Book Co., Inc., 1965.
18. Carr, B. M., and Mohnac, A. M.: Simple ameloblastoma within a follicular cyst of the maxilla; report of a case. Oral Surg., *15*:1136 (Sept.), 1962.

19. Caruso, W. A., and Itkin, A.: Ameloblastic odontoma: report of a case. Oral Surg., *16*:582 (May), 1963.

20. Chaudhry, A. P.: Personal communication.

21. Chaudhry, A. P., Robinovitch, M. R., Mitchell, D. F., and Vickers, R. A.: Chondrogenic tumors of the jaws. Am. J. Surg., *102*:403 (Sept.), 1961.

22. Chaudhry, A. P., Sabes, W. R., and Gorlin, R. J.: Unusual oral manifestation of chronic lymphatic leukemia. Oral Surg., *15*:446 (Apr.), 1962.

23. Chaudhry, A. P., Vickers, R. A., and Gorlin, R. J.: Intraoral minor salivary gland tumors, an analysis of 1414 cases. Oral Surg., *14*:1194 (Oct.), 1961.

24. Cheyne, V. D., Tiecke, R. W., and Horne, E. V.: A review of so-called mixed tumors of the salivary glands including an analysis of fifty additional cases. Oral Surg., *1*:359, 1948.

25. Christensen, R. W.: The treatment of oral hemangiomas: report of four cases. Oral Surg., *12*:912–921 (Aug.), 1959.

26. Cliff, I. S., and Demis, D. J.: Giant ulcer of the face following surgery for trigeminal neuralgia. Arch. Intern. Med., *119*:218–222 (Feb.), 1967.

27. Colby, R. A., Kerr, D. A., and Robinson, H. B. G.: Color Atlas of Oral Pathology. Philadelphia, J. B. Lippincott Co., 1961.

28. Crane, A. R., and Tremblay, R. G.: Myoblastoma. Am. J. Path., *27*:357, 1945.

29. Custer, R. P., and Fust, J. A.: Congenital epulis. Am. J. Clin. Path., *22*:1044, 1952.

30. Cutler, E. C., and Zollinger, R.: Sclerosing solution in the treatment of cysts and fistulae. Am. J. Surg., *19*:411, 1933.

31. Darling, A. I., and Crabb, H. S. M.: Lichen planus. Oral Surg., *7*:1276 (Dec.), 1954.

32. Eselman, J. C.: Personal communication.

33. Figi, F. A., and O'Brien, R. W.: Treatment of Angiomas. Plast. Reconstr. Surg., *18*:448–459 (Dec.), 1956.

34. Goodman, R. M., and Gorlin, R. J.: The Face in Genetic Disorders. St. Louis, The C. V. Mosby Co., 1970.

35. Gorlin, R. J., Chaudhry, A. P., and Pindborg, J. J.: Odontogenic tumors: classification, histopathology and clinical behavior in man and domesticated animals. Cancer, *14*:73–101 (Jan.-Feb.), 1961.

36. Gould, S. E., Hinerman, D. L., Batsakis, H. G., and Beamer, P. R.: Microscopic Pathology. Baltimore, The Williams & Wilkins Co., 1964.

37. Greuel, D.: Hemangiomas of the oral cavity: results of radiotherapy. Dtsch. Med. Wochenschr., *84*:2229–2234 (Dec.), 1959.

38. Hansen, E.: Lymphangioma of the tongue. Tandlaegebladet, *64*:359–365 (June), 1960.

39. Hellinger, M. J., Kardas, C. M., and Sellers, W.: A clinicopathologic correlation of oral white lesions: study of 45 cases. Oral Surg., *16*:1365 (Nov.), 1963.

40. Hooton, E.: On certain eskimoid characters in Icelandic skulls. Am. J. Phys. Anthropol., *1*:53, 1918.

41. Howell, J. B.: Neurotrophic changes in the trigeminal territory. Arch. Derm., *86*:442–449, 1962.

42. Hurst, D. W., and Meyer, O. O.: Giant follicular lymphoblastoma. Cancer, *14*:753–778, 1961.

43. Jackson, C., and Jackson, C. L.: Diseases of the Nose, Throat and Ear. 2nd ed. Philadelphia, W. B. Saunders Co., 1959.

44. Jaffe, N. L.: Giant cell reparative granuloma, traumatic bone cyst, and fibrous (fibro-osseous) dysplasia of the jaw bone. Oral Surg., *6*:159 (Jan.), 1953.

45. Kemperer, P.: Myoblastoma of the striated muscle. Am. J. Cancer, *20*:324, 1934.

46. Kerr, D. A.: Myoblastoma myoma. Oral Surg., *4*:158, 1949.

47. Kerr, D. A., and Weiss, A. W.: Pigmented ameloblastoma of the mandible: report of a case. Oral Surg., *16*:1339 (Nov.), 1963.

48. Kolas, S., et al.: Occurrence of torus palatinus and torus mandibularis in 2478 dental patients. Oral Surg., *6*:1134–1141 (Sept.), 1953.

49. MacKeown, J. L.: Leukoplakia, a precancerous condition: a statistical analysis of 100 cases. Thesis, Graduate School, University of Pittsburgh, 1948.

50. McCall, J. O., and Wald, S. S.: Clinical Dental Roentgenology. 4th ed. Philadelphia, W. B. Saunders Co., 1957.

51. McCarthy, F. P.: Etiology, pathology and treatment of leukoplakia buccalis. Arch. Dermat. & Syphilol., *34*:612, 1936.

52. Mason, M. H.: Lymphangioma of the tongue: treatment and appraisal of long-term results. Arch. Surg., *87*:761–767 (Nov.), 1960.

53. Millard, H. D.: Oral exfoliative cytology as an aid to diagnosis. J.A.D.A., *69*:547 (Nov.), 1964.

54. Miller, S. C., and Roth, H.: Torus palatinus: a statistical study. J.A.D.A., *27*:1950–1957 (Dec.), 1940.

55. Moore, C. H.: The incidence of torus palatinus in the newborn. Thesis, University of Pittsburgh School of Dentistry, 1959.

56. Northrop, P. M.: Complex composite odontoma: report of three cases. J. Oral Surg., *21*:492 (Nov.), 1963.

57. Olech, E.: Hemangioma of the cheek involving the opening of Stensen's duct treated by injection of a sclerosing solution. Oral Surg., *16*:641 (June), 1963.

58. Oringer, M. J.: Electrosurgery in Dentistry. 2nd ed. Philadelphia, W. B. Saunders Co., 1975.

59. Owen, N., and Stevenson, K. L.: Treatment of hemangioma. Plastic & Reconstr. Surg., *3*:109, 1948.

60. Pape, T. J., and Hawkins, D. B.: Congenital granular-cell myoblastoma of the oral cavity. Oral Surg., *15*:377 (Mar.), 1962.

61. Perez-Tamayo, R.: Mechanisms of Disease. An Introduction to Pathology. Philadelphia, W. B. Saunders Co., 1961.

62. Pindborg, J. J.: Atlas of Diseases of the Oral Mucosa. 2nd ed. Philadelphia, W. B. Saunders Co., 1973.

63. Pollia, J. A.: Fundamental Principles of Alveolo-Dental Radiology. New York, Dental Items of Interest Publishing Co., 1939.

64. Prinz, H.: Some common diseases of the oral mucous membrane and the tongue. Dent. Cosmos, *69*:53, 1927.

65. Rappaport, H., Winter, W. J., and Hickes, E. B.: Follicular lymphoma; a re-evaluation of its position in the scheme of malignant lymphoma, based on a survey of 253 cases. Cancer, *9*:792–821, 1956.

66. Robinson, M., and Slavkin, H. C.: Dental amputation neuromas. J.A.D.A., *70*:662 (Mar.), 1965.

67. Rosenberg, C. J., and Cruz, J.: The so-called adenoblastoma: report of two cases. Oral Surg., *16*:1459 (Dec.), 1963.

68. Rovin, S.: Cytology—Its value in the diagnosis of

oral cancer. Dent. Clin. North Am., *15*:807–815 (Oct.), 1971.

69. Rovin, S.: An assessment of the negative oral cytologic diagnosis. J.A.D.A., *74*:759–762 (Mar.), 1967.

70. Rovin, S.: The role of biopsy and cytology in oral diagnosis. Dent. Clin. North Am., 429 (July), 1965.

71. Ryba, G. E., and Kramer, I. R. H.: Continued growth of human dentine papillae following removal of the crowns of partly formed deciduous teeth. Oral Surg., *15*:867 (July), 1962.

72. Sandler, H. C., ed.: Oral exfoliative cytology: Veterans Administration cooperative study, 1962. Washington, Government Printing Office, 1963.

73. Sandler, H. C.: Reliability of oral exfoliative cytology for detection of oral cancer. J.A.D.A., *68*:489–499 (Apr.), 1964.

74. Schreiber, L. K.: Bilateral odontomas preventing eruption of maxillary central incisors. Oral Surg., *16*:503 (Apr.), 1963.

75. Shafer, W. G., Hine, M. K., and Levy, B. M.: A Textbook of Oral Pathology. 3rd ed. Philadelphia, W. B. Saunders Co., 1974.

76. Shapiro, B. L., and Gorlin, R. J.: An analysis of oral cytodiagnosis. Cancer, *17*:1477 (Nov.), 1964.

77. Shira, R. B.: Biopsy in oral diagnosis and treatment planning. Dent. Clin. North Am., 41–54 (Mar.), 1963.

78. Shira, R. B.: Treatment of benign soft tissue lesions. Dent. Clin. North Am., (July), 1964.

79. Shira, R. B.: Personal communication.

80. Shira, R. B., and Bhaskar, S. N.: Oral surgery-oral pathology conference No. 5 (Ameloblastoma). Oral Surg., *16*:1131 (Sept.), 1963.

81. Shira, R. B., and Bhaskar, S. N.: Oral surgery-oral pathology conference no. 7. (case report—amelo-blastic fibroma). Oral Surg., *16*:1377 (Nov.), 1963.

82. Shklar, G., and Meyer, I.: Neurogenic tumors of the mouth and jaws. Oral Surg., *16*:1075 (Sept.), 1963.

83. Sinkovits, V.: Facial hemihyperplasia. Stoma. *12*: 188–199 (Nov.), 1959.

84. Small, I. A., and Waldron, C. A.: Ameloblastomas of the jaws. Oral Surg., *8*:281, 1955.

85. Smith, J. F.: Rhabdomyosarcoma of lower lip. Oral Surg., *15*:454 (Apr.), 1962.

86. Sprague, W. G.: A survey of the use of the term leukoplakia by oral pathologists. Oral Surg., *16*:1067 (Sept.), 1963.

87. Stafne, E. C.: Oral Roentgenographic Diagnosis. 4th ed. Philadelphia, W. B. Saunders Co., 1975.

88. Stafne, E. C.: Paget's disease involving maxilla and mandible. Report of a case. J. Oral Surg., *4*:114–115 (Apr.), 1946.

89. Thoma, K. H.: Oral Surgery. 4th ed. St. Louis, C. V. Mosby Co., 1963.

90. Thoma, K. H.: Oral Pathology. St. Louis, C. V. Mosby Co., 1960.

91. Thoma, K. H., and Goldman, H. M.: Central myxoma of the jaw. Am. J. Orthod. (Oral Surg. Sect.), *33*:532, 1947.

92. Thoma, K. H., and Robinson, H. B. G.: Oral and Dental Diagnosis. 4th ed. Philadelphia, W. B. Saunders Co., 1955.

93. Waldron, C. A., Thompson, C. W., and Connor, W. A.: Granular-cell ameloblastic fibroma. Oral Surg., *16*:1202 (Oct.), 1963.

94. Woo, J.: Torus palatinus. Am. J. Phys. Anthropol., *8*(NS):81–111 (March), 1950.

95. Young, D. R., and Robinson, M.: Ameloblastomas in children. Oral Surg., *15*:1155 (Oct.), 1962.

96. Yrastorza, J. A.: Inflammatory papillary hyperplasia of the palate. J. Oral Surg., *21*:330 (July), 1963.

CHAPTER 14

AFFECTIONS OF THE SALIVARY GLANDS

Salivary glands may be affected by tumors, cysts, sialoliths (stones), sialadenitis from infection, sialoductitis with subsequent strictures of the ducts, avitaminosis A atrophy, or trauma. Mikulicz's disease, whose exact nature is unknown, has no one manifestation but is a chronic or recurrent enlargement of all the salivary and lacrimal glands due to an accumulation of lymphatic tissue there (see Figure 14–1). Sage regards total surgical excision of the glands as "unwarranted except in the most advanced stage of the disease with extensive destruction, chronic inflammation and serious symptoms." He uses "a combination of duct ligation and radiation therapy."[22]

Mixed tumors, carcinomas, or lymphoblastomas may affect the internal structure of the glands. Cysts are usually of the retention type

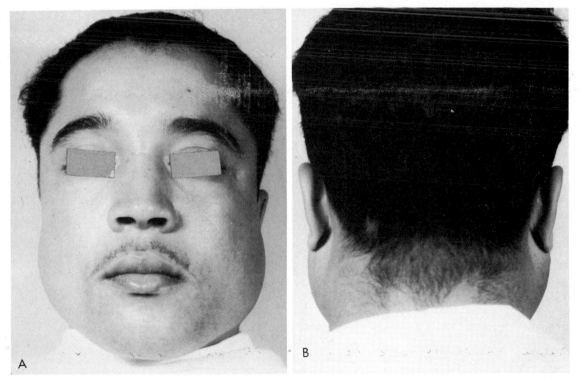

Figure 14–1 Bilateral swelling of the parotid, submaxillary and lacrimal glands in a rare case of Mikulicz's disease. There is an infiltration of, and replacement of, the normal gland structure by lymphoid tissue. It is associated with sarcoidosis, malignant lymphoma or collagen disease.

caused by stricture of the duct from trauma or infection, and these may be secondarily infected. Sialoliths may be found in any of the salivary glands, but they are more commonly found in the submandibular (submaxillary) gland and duct (Wharton's). Less frequently stones are found in the parotid gland or duct (Stensen's), and I have never seen one in the sublingual gland. The theoretical explanation of the latter is that the many short ducts prevent stasis of saliva in the sublingual gland or its ducts.

SIALOGRAPHY

Sialography is the roentgen demonstration of a salivary duct and gland by means of the injection of radiopaque solutions (Lipidol, Ethiodol, Hypaque, Sinografin, Pantopaque). The sialogram is a useful diagnostic aid which, however, has its limitations as indicated later. Feldman and others recommend "image intensification fluorosialography" because: "(1) Interstitial, extraductal injections can be detected immediately. (2) Filling of the duct and gland can be controlled without relying on a variable end-point determination or blind technique. (3) Radiographs can be obtained at optimal positions."[9]

Schulz and Weisberger[24] recommend the following views for the parotid: (1) True lateral jaw, (2) anteroposterior, and (3) fronto-submental. The lateral jaw radiograph should be taken last to prevent loss of the opaque contrast medium that has been injected into the salivary duct or gland. The views that best visualize the submandibular gland are the lateral oblique and true lateral views of the mandible. They summarize their article as follows:

"Encapsulated expanding tumors within the salivary glands, if large or favorably placed, may be demonstrated by sialography. The characteristic finding of a mixed tumor of the parotid is displacement or deformity of the duct system so that the radicles appear to be spread, kinked or pressed upon by the tumor. Small or peripheral tumors may not be recognized.

"The recognition of malignant and infiltrating tumors as such has been disappointing at this hospital, although other investigators report characteristic findings in the presence of an infiltrating lesion, such as carcinoma destruction of the duct system and evidence of infiltration of the small structures of the gland rather than displacement by an expanding encapsulated tumor.

"Extrinsic tumor masses may be shown by

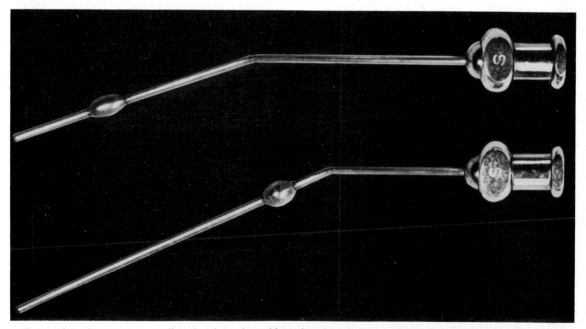

Figure 14–2 Intravenous needles that have been blunted and angled for sialography. Note the positions of the solder stoppers and the angulation. *Upper,* For the parotid duct. *Lower,* For the submandibular duct. (Reproduced by permission of R. Ollerenshaw, and the Department of Medical Illustrations, Manchester Royal Infirmary, Manchester, England.)

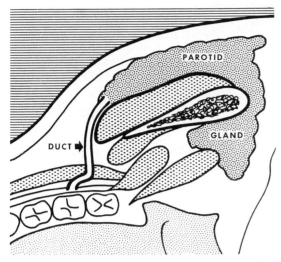

Figure 14–3 Cross section through the ascending mandibular ramus, showing the relation of the parotid gland to the bone, muscle and soft tissue. (Reproduced by permission of R. Ollerenshaw, and the Department of Medical Illustrations, Manchester Royal Infirmary, Manchester, England.)

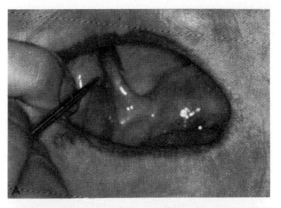

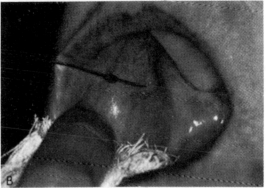

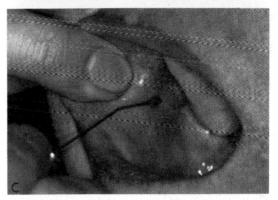

a displaced but otherwise normal gland or duct.

"Swellings of the salivary glands due to Mikulicz's disease or sarcoid have shown normal sialographic findings.

"Swellings due to inflammatory processes within the gland or duct, or due to obstruction by stricture or stone in the duct, almost constantly show characteristic findings.

"In chronic parotitis in one variety the acini seem to have coalesced, and many small, sharply defined cavities are seen distributed throughout the substance of the gland. Swinburne calls this *sialoangiectasis*

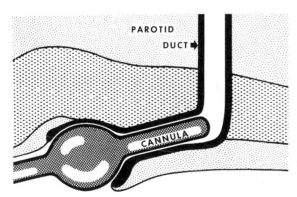

Figure 14–4 The parotid duct turns sharply through the buccinator muscle. The stopper on the needle seals the opening and holds the tip away from the duct wall. (Reproduced by permission of R. Ollerenshaw, and the Department of Medical Illustrations, Manchester Royal Infirmary, Manchester, England.)

Figure 14–5 *A*, Eversion of the cheek for injection of the parotid duct. The site of the papilla is indicated by the tip of the dilator. *B*, Insertion of the cannula. *C*, The stopper sealing the papillary orifice. (Reproduced by permission of R. Ollerenshaw, and the Department of Medical Illustrations, Manchester Royal Infirmary, Manchester, England.)

(see Figure 14–12). Patients with this condition have recurrent bouts of swelling with some chronic enlargement, and may or may not have a mucopurulent discharge from the duct. In the presence of chronic infection, the small cavities may coalesce, and the duct system appears widened and irregular. The characteristic roentgen findings are many globular collections of opaque medium, ranging from 1

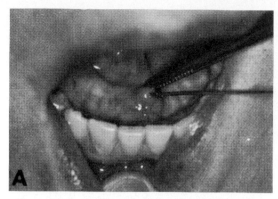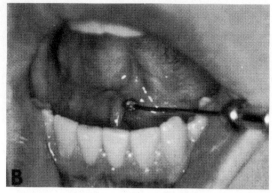

Figure 14–6 *A,* Fixation of the submandibular duct with a small hemostat and dilatation with a lacrimal duct dilator. *B,* Cannulation of the submandibular duct for injection of contrast media. (Reproduced by permission of R. Ollerenshaw, and the Department of Medical Illustrations, Manchester Royal Infirmary, Manchester, England.)

mm. to 3 or 4 mm. in diameter distributed over the substance of the parotid gland (see Figure 14–10). In some presumably early cases or in those in which the infection is minimal, the ducts are smooth, not displaced, and of normal width. More chronic cases show ragged and widened ducts. Multiple abscesses within the duct can be filled through the duct in most instances and appear on the roentgenogram as large, irregular cavities. Multiple strictures of the parotid (Stensen's) duct give the characteristic "sausage" appearance (see Figure 14–13). In swellings due to the presence of obstructing stones, the calculus can be shown in the duct."[25]

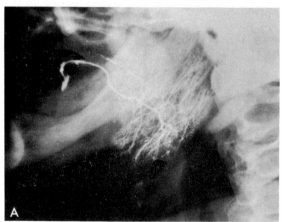

Figure 14–7 *A,* A sialograph of a normal parotid gland. Note the fine arborization, as visualized out to the very periphery of the gland. Note the uniform diameter of the lumen of the duct into the substance of the gland. *B,* A smaller normal parotid gland with an accessory gland (*arrow*) anterior to the main gland. *C,* Note the arrow that points to a stricture in the parotid duct. Posterior to this obstruction the lumen is enlarged. Excess iodized oil is on the inner surface of the cheek above and below the cannula.

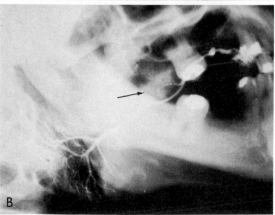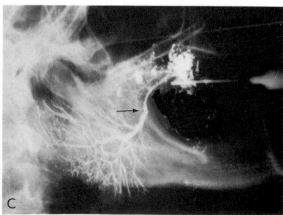

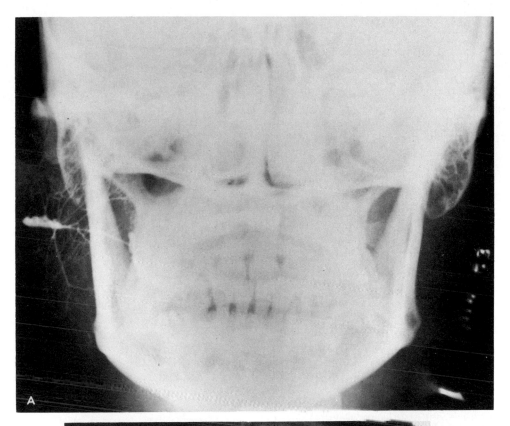

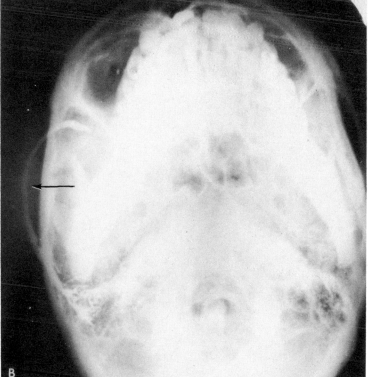

Figure 14–8   *A*, Normal posteroanterior sialograph of the parotid gland. *B*, Normal parotid duct.

TECHNIQUE OF INJECTION FOR SIALOGRAPHY

In all cases, routine radiographs are made before sialography to determine the presence of calculi and calcified glands.

Parotid Gland. Ollerenshaw and Rose recommend that a 5-cc. syringe be "fitted with a special cannula, made from a blunted intravenous needle that has been angled to about 140 degrees and on which a stopper has been formed by a blob of solder. The blunted point must be given a high polish to prevent trauma of the duct. The location of the stopper and the angulation are different in the needles used for the injection of the submandibular duct and for the parotid duct. The needle for the parotid duct has the shorter straight portion distal to the stopper (Fig. 14–2). This position of the stopper limits the distance that the cannula can advance and thus prevents impingement on the wall where the duct passes at an angle through the buccinator muscle (Fig. 14–4).

"The patient sits opposite the surgeon, with an assistant steadying the head. Gentle eversion of the cheek between finger and thumb (Fig. 14–5A) reveals the orifice of the parotid duct opposite the second upper molar. Massage, or a mouthwash of 0.5 per cent hydrochloric acid, if preferred, stimulates the flow of saliva and makes identification easy. The cannula is gently inserted in the line of the duct (Fig. 14–5B) and slid inward until the stopper impinges on the papilla (Fig. 14–5C). The stopper prevents reflux of contrast medium during the injection. There is no need for complex maneu-vers with the cannula in the duct. On completion of the injection the cannula is removed and a small swab is placed over the orifice to mop up any overflow that would otherwise spoil the radiograph. It is removed, of course, before an exposure is made. Excellent radiographs can be obtained up to 20 minutes after injection.

"Dilatation will probably be essential in cases of primary stenosis in the parotid duct. Overdilatation is to be avoided, as it tends to permit too rapid emptying of the gland before radiography is complete. In cases where simple probing is required, it is better to use the much finer lacrimal probes.

"Various statements have been made concerning the volume of the injection, the consensus being that 1.5 to 2 cc. is sufficient for the parotid gland."

Submandibular Gland. "The orifice of the submandibular duct is not so easy to locate, because it is situated on the tip of a very mobile papilla, which must be fixed by blunt forceps before cannulation is attempted (Fig. 14–6A). By keeping the papilla gently taut in the line of the duct, the long cannula will enter easily as far as the stopper, which again acts as a seal (Fig. 14–6B).

"Should it be necessary to dilate the orifice of the duct before cannulation, the best instrument for the purpose is a lacrimal duct dilator of suitable size. A set of these probes should be at hand."*

---

*Reprinted with permission from Ollerenshaw, R., and Rose, S.: Sialography: A valuable diagnostic method. Dent. Radiogr. Photogr., *29*(3), 1957.

Case Report No. 1

SUPPURATIVE PAROTITIS ASSOCIATED WITH CHRONIC DENTAL INFECTION

A year ago a 16-year-old patient noticed a swelling of his right face in front of his ear. He consulted his dentist, who found an abscessed maxillary molar. After the extraction of this molar the swelling gradually disappeared. Two weeks ago the patient again noticed that when he got up in the morning he had marked swelling in the right face and jaw in the region of the ramus and ear and has had a degree of fever. Although he did not have any pain and did not know of any infected teeth, he again saw his dentist, who referred him to me (Fig. 14–9A). Oral radiographs revealed a chronically abscessed right maxillary third molar.

Patient had marked swelling and tenderness all over the right parotid gland region. The orifice of Stensen's duct was red and swollen and on pressure pus exuded from the duct (Fig. 14–9B).

The right maxillary third molar was extracted. Aureomycin, 250 mg. every 6 hours straight for 7 days, was prescribed. The parotid (Stensen's) duct was gently dilated and more pus flowed freely from the gland. Following the extraction of the abscessed tooth the parotitis subsided quickly and within three weeks had completely disappeared. (Fig. 14–9C and D).

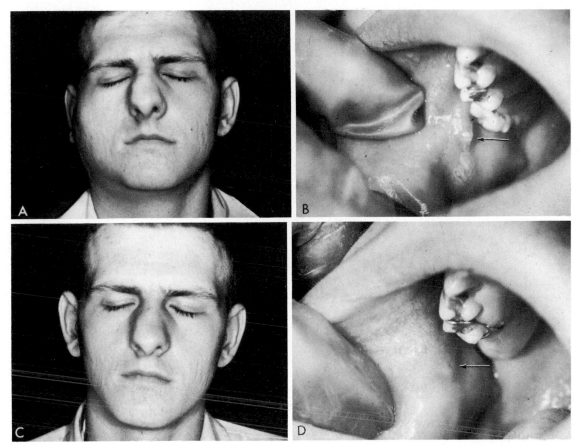

Figure 14–9 *A*, Parotitis from dental infection. (See Case Report No. 1 for details.) *B*, Thick pus flowing from the orifice of the parotid duct. *C*, Two weeks following the extraction of an infected right maxillary third molar and antibiotics, the parotid gland has returned to normal. *D*, There is no drainage from the duct, and inflammation has disappeared.

SUPPURATIVE SIALADENITIS

Sialadenitis (inflammation of a salivary gland) may chronically or acutely affect any of the salivary glands. While the parotid gland is the one (parotitis) usually affected, occasionally the submandibular gland may also be involved. The causes are:

1. Infections in or about the oral cavity (see Case Report No. 1 and Figure 14–9).
2. As a complication in conjunction with a general infection such as scarlet fever, smallpox, typhoid fever or pyemia (Fig. 14–10).
3. Following abdominal surgery, usually developing 5 to 7 days after the operation. Infection is generally due to staphylococci but, occasionally, streptococci may be found (Fig. 14–11).
4. Contagious or epidemic parotitis (mumps), an acute infectious and contagious disease caused by a virus, as a common disease of childhood.

Treatment. Acute cases of suppurative sialadenitis, with swelling, fever, lymphadenopathy and purulent drainage, usually occur in the parotid gland and respond quickly to the administration of penicillin or the broad-spectrum antibiotics. Irradiation is condemned by Welch and Trump[30] and Leake, Krakowiak and Leake.[14]

Culture the exudate from the duct and administer systemically the indicated antimicrobial for 5 to 7 days. *Staphylococcus aureus* is usually found in adults and *Streptococcus viridans* in children. The swelling gradually disappears in about 2 weeks, and salivary output returns. However, many of these patients have recurrent attacks of suppurative parotitis.

Prevention of Recurrence. Quinn and Graham advocate the use of systemic antibiotics

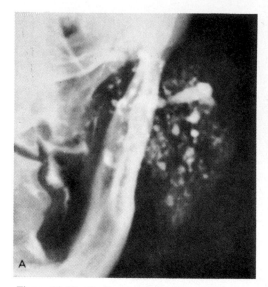
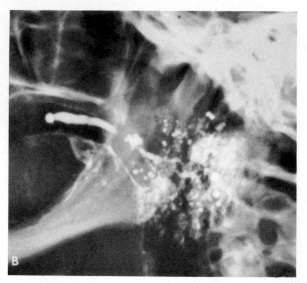

Figure 14–10   Radiographs showing abscess formation in a case of recurrent pneumococcal infection. *A*, Anteroposterior projection. *B*, Lateral projection. (Reproduced by permission of R. Ollerenshaw, and the Department of Medical Illustrations, Manchester Royal Infirmary, Manchester, England.)

and intraductal instillation of antibiotics to prevent recurrence of suppurative parotitis.[21] Specifically, during the acute stage of recurrent parotitis, patients are given antibiotics systemically for 5 to 7 days.

According to these researchers, "A sialogram is made to investigate changes within the gland after the acute phase has subsided. Some investigators have noted that sialography alone is therapeutic in some cases because it dilates the ducts and ductules and

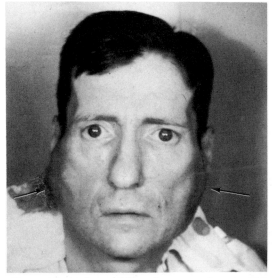

Figure 14–11   Acute bilateral suppurative parotitis with incision and drainage following abdominal surgery. This is a postsurgical complication whose etiologic cause is unknown.

flushes out the gland. If this is the patient's first episode of suppurative parotitis, the intraductal instillation of antibiotics may be deferred after the sialogram, until the next episode of gland infection."

METHOD OF INTRADUCTAL INSTILLATION OF ANTIBIOTICS.   "Polyethylene No. 50 tubing, or a syringe and blunted needle, with the same technique of cannulation as that used for sialography, is used for instillation of antibiotic solution. Before injecting the antibiotic solution, 2 per cent lidocaine hydrochloride (Xylocaine) is instilled and retained for at least 5 minutes to anesthetize the duct system and prevent a burning sensation. The antibiotic solution is mixed with 2 per cent lidocaine hydrochloride for the same reason. Tetracycline (Achromycin), 15 mg. per ml. 2 per cent plain lidocaine hydrochloride for adults and 10 mg. per ml. 2 per cent plain lidocaine hydrochloride for children, is used. Approximately 1.5 to 2.5 ml. is used to fill the gland in children and 3 to 4 ml. in adults. Obvious enlargement of the gland and the patient's discomfort indicate that the gland is full. The tetracycline solution should be retained 5 to 10 minutes, depending on the patient's tolerance. The dosages were empirically derived because higher doses caused an increased burning sensation; these levels proved adequate to prevent recurrence of the infection.

"This treatment is repeated daily for 5 consecutive days. The salivary exudate after the first treatment is usually yellow or milky and includes small flakes that indicate some retention of the antibiotic solution. The saliva gradually returns to normal in an additional 5 to 7 days.

"Systemic tetracycline or erythromycin (250 mg. four times a day for 10 days) is given concomitantly to assist in elimination of the infection. Erythromycin is given to young children instead of tetracycline to avoid staining of developing teeth."*

Quinn and Graham advise that other methods for the treatment of recurrent suppurative parotitis, such as radiation and ligation, have not been successful at their institution (Ochsner Clinic), nor has surgical excision of the superficial part of the gland, which they feel "is a rather radical approach to a disease that can be treated by medication."[21] If medication fails, then other methods mentioned obviously must be tried.

ABSCESS OF THE PAROTID TAIL

Small reported the value of sialography in disclosing a hidden abscess in the parotid tail that was responsible for a case of membranous glomerulonephritis. This young man was chronically and critically ill for 6 months when a dental consultation was requested on September 28. This consultation, "with reference to a persistent small, slightly tender, indurated area in the tail of the left parotid, resulted in the decision to obtain a sialogram to determine whether the swelling was extra- or intraglandular. This was done on October 2, with 1.5 cc. of a water-soluble contrast medium injected following duct dilatation with small bougies. The roentgenograms showed a normal duct and normal arborization of the frontal gland portion. There was pooling of contrast medium in the tail of the gland, which could be caused by overfilling or possibly by the filling of a cavity or abscess in the area. The filling defect was about 1 by 3 cm. in the area of presialogram tenderness. Following the sialographic procedure, the patient developed a tender swelling over the entire gland. In 24 hours the gland was markedly swollen and systemic toxicity was apparent. A diagnosis of sialadenitis was obvious, and a

regimen of local moist heat, tetracycline, penicillin, and parenteral fluids was instituted. The patient . . . responded dramatically to treatment, and the parotid became symptom-free on the day of the fourth treatment. On this same day the urine became protein-free and remained so. The patient has remained free of symptoms since his return to full duty.

"This case illustrates the value of sialography in disclosing a hidden abscess in the parotid tail which must be assumed to be responsible for this patient's severe kidney disease. It illustrates also the cooperation between hospital services in caring for the patient in an unusual case and shows that one must be prepared for an exacerbation of symptoms following sialography of a potentially infected salivary gland."*

OBSTRUCTIVE SIALADENITIS

Chronic intermittent swelling of one of the salivary glands, which is associated with eating is usually due to blockage of the duct by a sialolith (discussed later in this chapter).

Chronic intermittent swelling of the parotid gland not associated with eating is a frequent complaint. Many of these cases are caused by a stricture in the duct (see Figure 14–13) and are treated by repeated dilatation with graduated urethral whalebone filiform bougies or graduated silver probes. In a reasonably good percentage of cases this effects a cure.

In a series of 87 cases of chronic obstructive sialadenitis Eisenbud and Cranin in their excellent article report: "Initial response to dilatation and sialography was favorable in 80 per cent of the parotid cases and 72 per cent of the submandibular cases. Among 47 patients followed from 1 to 5 years after treatment, 83 per cent reported no recurrence of disease. No significant difference in the results of treatment was noted between parotid and submandibular cases. It is concluded that dilatation and sialography represents a clearcut therapeutic procedure that is beneficial in the majority of cases of chronic obstructive sialadenitis." In other cases there is apparently a low grade infection. These are

---

*From Quinn, J. H., and Graham, R.: Recurrent suppurative parotitis treated by intraductal antibiotics. J. Oral Surg., *31*:36–39 (Jan.), 1973. Copyright by the American Dental Association. Reprinted by permission.

*Reproduced with permission from Small, E. W.: Sialographic diagnosis of a parotid abscess in a case of membranous glomerulonephritis. Oral Surg., *20*:71 (July), 1965; copyrighted by The C. V. Mosby Co., St. Louis.

most difficult to cure. Many times the iodized oil used in sialography effects a cure. (See further discussion of submandibular stenosis on page 941.)

DENTAL CAUSES OF PAROTID SWELLING

Ollerenshaw and Rose state that "during the eruption of the second and third molar teeth, pain and discomfort may cause young patients to chew their food on the opposite side of the mouth, and the papilla of the parotid duct on the painful side tends to be sucked inward and bitten. Occasionally the initial lesion, an ulcer of the papilla in close relation to the teeth, is seen, but more usually there is an established terminal stenosis. Dental extraction or alteration of bite in the fitting of crowns may produce the same result. There is no sialangiectasis and the saliva is sterile.

"Older patients, invariably those wearing dentures, may complain of swelling after meals, often over a period of 6 months. In these cases, alveolar absorption has led to an ill-fitting denture that rides up into the alveobuccal sulcus, where it may have caused ulceration. The shifting of the denture during mastication causes nipping of the papilla; the consequent stenosis extends farther along the duct than it does in young patients in whom only the buccal portion is involved. Cultures of saliva from such patients are also sterile."[17] Treatment is the correction of the dental problems and dilatation of the ducts, as described later.

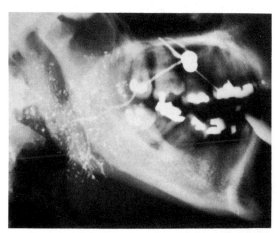

Figure 14–12 Radiographic appearance of an advanced case of terminal sialoangiectasis. (Reproduced by permission of R. Ollerenshaw, and the Department of Medical Illustrations, Manchester Royal Infirmary, Manchester, England.)

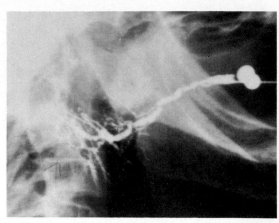

Figure 14–13 Typical recurrent obstructive parotitis. The main duct pattern has been called "sausage string." (Reproduced by permission of R. Ollerenshaw, and the Department of Medical Illustrations, Manchester Royal Infirmary, Manchester, England.)

TREATMENT OF SIALECTASIS (SIALOANGIECTASIS)

Prowler and associates state that sialectasis is not a primary disease but is secondary to duct obstruction.

"In the submandibular gland, it seems that the primary agent is intraductal calculus." They feel that in the parotid gland the parotid obstruction is primarily due to "infection, mucous plug, allergies or late sequelae of mumps and collagen diseases." While sialoliths are not commonly found in the parotid ducts, there are such cases, and three are illustrated later in this chapter.

If the removal of the cause is not curative, then more radical treatment is necessary, in their opinion. Therefore, they treat those cases in which the "salivary obstruction has produced irreversible parotid gland and duct changes that predispose to subsequent ... repeated painful swellings, infections and symptom complexes" with a "unique combined approach." When the patient is asymptomatic they give radiation therapy (1800 R. in nine treatments). When all radiation reaction is over, they occlude the parotid duct "with a No. 8 lachrymal duct probe for 5 minutes. After removal of the probe, if massage of the gland does not produce any ductal discharge, under local anesthesia [they] intraorally isolate the parotid duct, doubly ligate and cut it. The incision is closed with horizontal mattress sutures of silk. The sutures are removed on the seventh postoperative day."[18]

STRICTURE OF THE PAROTID DUCT

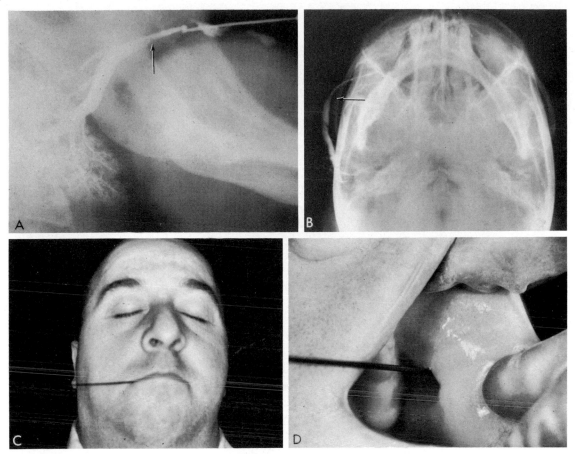

Figure 14-14 *A* and *B*, This patient had had recurrent parotid swelling because of a stricture in the parotid duct, clearly shown in the sialographs, about 1 inch from the orifice. Note the large dilatation of the main and accessory excretory ducts. *C* and *D*, This case was treated by repeated dilatation with filiform bougies of gradually increasing size; lacrimal duct probes can be used.

SIALODUCTITIS

Inflammation of a salivary gland (sialadenitis) is accompanied by inflammation of the duct (sialoductitis) in the majority of cases. During the acute phase, there is marked hyperemic pouting of the orifice of the duct, and drops of pus are readily expressed. The sequelae can be strictures at one or more points along the duct (Fig. 14–13). A single stricture of the parotid duct is shown in Figure 14–14*A* with dilatation of the duct posterior to the stricture. In Figure 14–15 a single stricture at the orifice of the parotid duct prevents the escape of saliva, which, damming up in the duct, has produced a dilated duct and the localized swelling in the cheek shown in this figure. Treatment here was the

excision of the strictured duct orifice. Multiple strictures produce a bead-like or sausage-like appearance of the duct, as shown in Figure 14–13.

In the chronic or subacute stages of sialadenitis, the gland is less swollen and not as tender, the pouting and redness of the orifice of the duct disappears and, when the duct is gradually enlarged by the insertion of a series of gradually increasing sizes of filiform bougies or lacrimal duct probes that have been lubricated with mineral oil, fairly large quantities of turbid saliva can be milked from the gland and out of the duct. This treatment is carried out every other day for a week, then once a week for about a month. Quinn suggests injecting 2 per cent lidocaine into the ductal systems and holding it there for 3

STRICTURE OF THE PAROTID DUCT WITH SEGMENTAL DILATATION

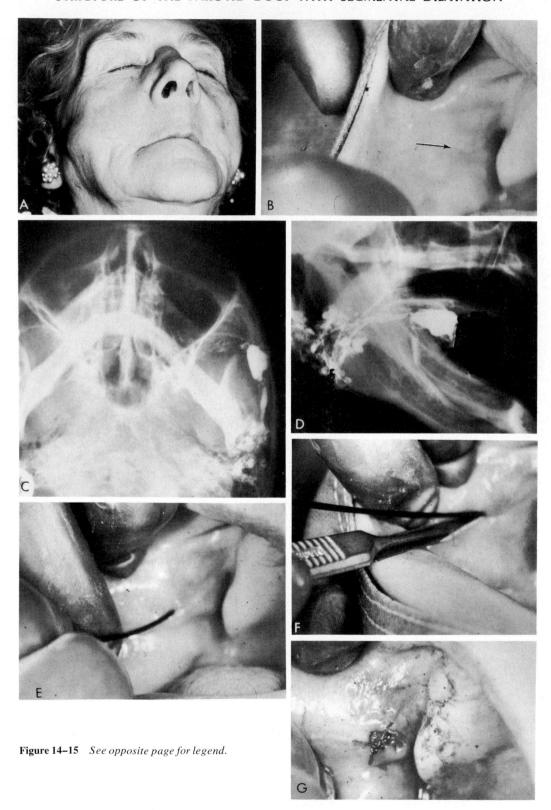

Figure 14–15   *See opposite page for legend.*

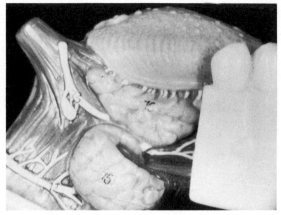

Figure 14–16 Anatomic model of the sublingual gland (at *76*) and submandibular gland (at *75*).

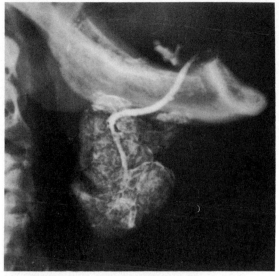

Figure 14–17 True lateral projection of a normal submandibular gland. The entire gland and its arborization of ducts is clearly seen. The right angle in the duct is the point at which the duct passes over the posterior border of the mylohyoid muscle. This is a frequent location of sialoliths. The comparative stasis of saliva at this point undoubtedly facilitates the formation of sialoliths. (Reproduced by permission of R. Ollerenshaw, and the Department of Medical Illustrations, Manchester Royal Infirmary, Manchester, England.)

minutes to minimize the pain of dilatation of the duct by the increasingly larger bougies.[20] As already described, he also suggests the intraductal instillation of antibiotics. Many of these cases then remain asymptomatic for a period of several months, when there is a recurrence of swelling and pain. If the patient reports promptly for dilatation (Fig. 14–18), the acute phase is avoided and the swelling and tenderness regress rapidly. In cases that do not respond to treatment as described, radiation of the gland with ligation of the duct, as previously described, or sialoadenectomy, is indicated. See Case Report No. 2 and Figures 14–19 and 14–20.

Case Report No. 2

SIALOADENECTOMY FOR CHRONIC SUPPURATIVE SIALADENITIS AND SIALODUCTITIS OF THE SUBMANDIBULAR GLAND AND DUCT

JOHN C. GAISFORD, M.D., AND W. HARRY ARCHER, D.D.S.

History. For a year prior to the present admission the patient, a 40-year-old woman, had had intermittent hard swelling and pain in the right area that, at first, was thought to be due to the chronically infected mandibular first and second molars. She did not recall a definite relationship between eating and the swelling. Two weeks following the extraction of the infected teeth, the hard, tender mass was still present beneath the body of the mandible and so she was admitted to another hos-

Figure 14–15 *A*, Gross localized segmental dilatation of the parotid duct due to stricture of the orifice. *B*, Atrophy of the papilla of the duct. Only with the greatest difficulty and by using magnification and fine lacrimal duct probes was the orifice located and gradually stretched with larger probes so that a cannula could be introduced and sialographs *C* and *D* made.

C, A basal sialograph reveals large segmental dilatation of the anterior third of the duct, beginning at the orifice. *D*, This lateral jaw sialograph shows the typical abscess formation seen in cases of recurrent pneumococcal infection.

E, A large dilator was introduced into the dilated area of the duct. *F*, A No. 11 knife blade was inserted alongside the probe, slitting the duct and oral mucosa into the dilated area. *G*, The oral mucosa was sutured to the duct wall, thus creating a large orifice.

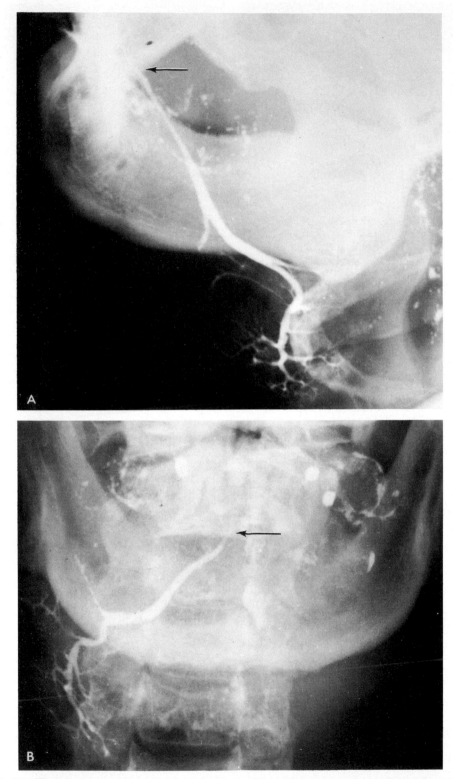

Figure 14–18 This patient complained about moderate swelling and discomfort in the right submandibular gland region when eating that gradually disappeared during mastication. The occlusal radiograph was negative for a sialolith and the oblique right sialogram (*A*), and the posteroanterior sialogram (*B*) did not reveal any sialolith in the deeper portions of the duct or in the gland. They did, however, show constriction of the terminus of this submandibular duct, which restricted the salivary flow rate. Treatment was dilatation of this area of the duct.

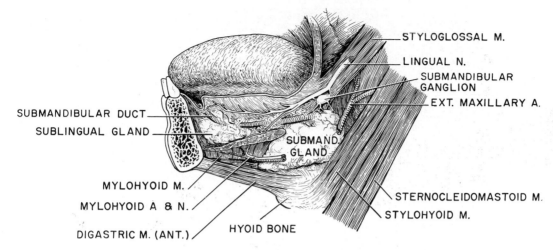

Figure 14–19 Section of the face showing anatomic positions of salivary glands and ducts. Note especially the relationship between the lingual nerve and the submandibular duct.

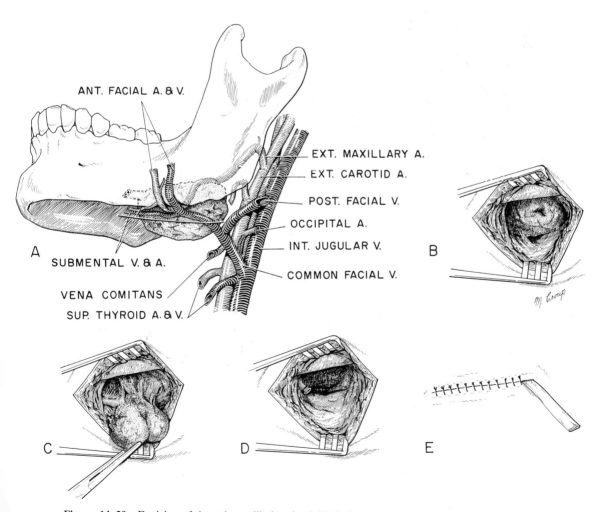

Figure 14–20 Excision of the submandibular gland. Technique is described in Case Report No. 2.

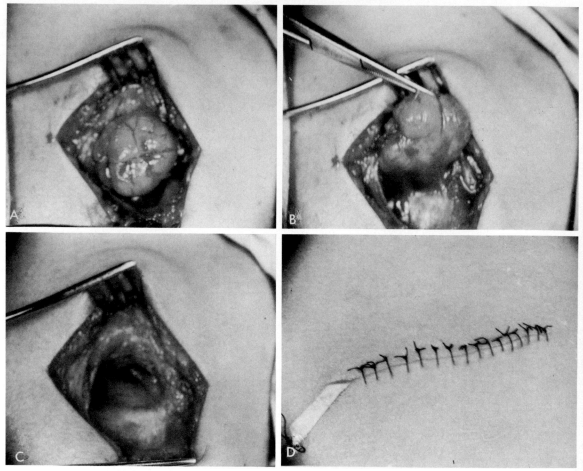

Figure 14–21   Sialoadenectomy for chronic recurrent sialadenitis. (See Case Report No. 2 for details.)

pital, where x-rays were taken. According to the patient, the x-rays showed nothing unusual and so she was discharged from the hospital.

Subsequently, the patient had several minor episodes of moderate swelling and pain in this area that lasted for only a few days. However, 5 weeks before the present admission she had had an acute episode, with extensive swelling, severe pain and a temperature of 102° F. At that time she was treated with antibiotics and the application of heat to her jaw for a period of 10 days, at which time the swelling and tenderness gradually subsided. Five days before this admission the swelling began to recur in the same area and she was referred to Dr. Archer, who diagnosed the case as chronic recurrent sialadenitis with sialoductitis, resulting in strictures of the submandibular duct. Attempts to dilate the submandibular duct were futile. The patient had never noticed pus, excess saliva or a "bad taste" in her mouth.

Examination. The right submandibular gland was very swollen, hard and exquisitely tender. The patient reported that this was the largest amount of

swelling she had ever had and, by far, the most painful.

Progress Notes. Four doses of codeine, $1/2$ grain, and aspirin compound, 10 grains, every 4 hours did not relieve her pain. The pain gradually decreased as the swelling in the gland diminished. She had complete relief of pain when, for the first time in the many episodes of swelling since the onset of this condition, she noticed a large amount of what she described as "slimy, salty fluid" in her mouth. Following this spontaneous discharge, the swelling and tenderness disappeared in the next 2 days. However, the gland remained hard and larger than normal.

Treatment. In view of the patient's history, sialoadenectomy was decided upon. This was done a week after the acute symptoms had subsided.

Technique. Following routine preparation, sterile drapes were applied. An incision was made just underneath the middle of the body of the right mandible approximately 4 to 5 cm. in length (see Figures 14–20 and 14–21). Bleeding points were clamped and ligated. The platysma muscle was incised; bleeding points were clamped and ligated. The deep cervical fascia was then dissected away from the gland, which was felt to be firm, hard, enlarged, but not attached to any surrounding structures. By blunt and sharp dissection, this gland was delivered into the wound (see Figure 14–20C and 14–21B). All bleeding points were clamped and ligated. The duct leading to the gland was clamped and doubly ligated, and the gland removed in its entirety (see Figure 14–20D). Following the removal of this gland, a rubber Penrose drain was inserted and the subcutaneous tissues were closed with 0000 chromic catgut. The skin was closed with 5–0 silk (see Figures 14–20E and 14–21D). A pressure dressing was applied and the patient was removed from the operating room in good condition.

Recovery was uneventful; there was no noticeable dryness (xerostomia) of the mouth. Extirpation of the submandibular gland does not materially reduce the quantity of available saliva, inasmuch as the parotid glands produce sufficient saliva to offset the small amount lost from the extirpated submandibular gland.

SURGICAL CORRECTION OF STENOSED SUBMANDIBULAR DUCTS BY INSTALLATION OF POLYETHYLENE TUBE*

SANFORD M. MOOSE, D.D.S.,
AND CHARLES W. SUMMERS, D.D.S.

Diagnostic procedures in the management of potential or questionable premalignant lesions of the floor of the mouth have stimulated work on the surgical correction of stenosed submandibular ducts to restore normal salivary flow. The generally accepted practice of "stripping" the mucous membrane of the floor of the mouth to eradicate premalignant lesions, such as leukoplakia, may result in duct occlusion. It is not uncommon for the duct of the submandibular gland to be surgically traumatized during the stripping operation. This often results in a stenosed salivary duct incapable of secreting the fluid of the submandibular salivary gland. The nonpatency of a duct must be evaluated carefully, and treatment must be instituted accordingly. Other causes of nonpatency must be considered and eliminated before the procedure to be described here is undertaken. Detailed methodical digital, visual, and x-ray examination, as well as a thorough history, will be necessary if one is to determine the exact cause of the stenosis and to rule out acute trauma, sialoliths, mucous plugs, sialadenitis, or other pathologic conditions that may occlude the lumen of the duct.

It is not the purpose of this article to go into detail concerning the various causes of occlusion and methods for correcting each. Rather, we will offer a method by which a duct occluded by the processes of healing following a traumatic episode can be surgically corrected to reestablish patency of the duct. It must be pointed out, however, that the injudicious incision to "drain the congested and distended duct," regardless of the original cause, may result in the formation of scar tissue and further aggravate the nonpatency.

Materials and instruments required for the operation are simple and readily available. The items required are (1) silk sutures, sizes 000 and 5–0, with appropriate needle holder and suture scissors; (2) malleable, blunt silver probes of various sizes; (3) local anesthetic; (4) Addison or other suitable tissue forceps; (5) an assortment of polyethylene tubing (No. 19 gauge is a good average); (6) a sharp scalpel with two or three replacement blades; (7) aspirator apparatus; and (8) sterile 2-inch by 2-inch gauze sponges. It may also be noted that the services of an assistant are necessary for this procedure to be executed properly. The mobility of the tissues, the salivation, and the patient's wandering tongue make it difficult for the surgeon to be successful without the aid of another pair of hands.

Technique. The patient should be adequately premedicated with a suitable agent to assure quiet cooperation and a stationary surgical operative site. Drugs should not be given to decrease the salivary flow prior to the operation, as the secretion of saliva from the duct is very helpful in identifying the duct. Anesthesia is obtained by blocking the lingual nerve and by local infiltration. The floor of the mouth is prepared and a 000 silk suture is placed well beneath the duct, and at right angles to it, in order to support, elevate, and stabilize the structure (Fig. 14–22). The suture is used for traction instead of a tenacu-

*Reproduced in part with permission from Moose, S. M., and Summers, C. W.: Surgical correction of stenosed submandibular ducts by installation of polyethylene tube. Oral Surg., *18*:563–568 (Nov.), 1964; copyrighted by the C. V. Mosby Co., St. Louis.

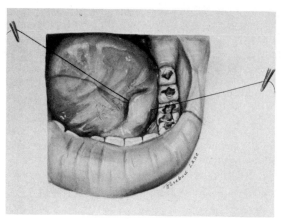

Figure 14–22 A suture placed well beneath the duct is used for traction. The suture ends are held wide apart and taut to elevate the structure for maximum access.

lum, tissue hook, or tissue forceps. The sutures are pulled taut to elevate the structure. This affords the surgeon maximum access and visibility. An incision is made over the duct and down through the old scar tissue until the duct is identified. The duct is isolated by means of sharp and blunt dissection. After the duct has been identified, a round-end silver probe should be inserted and passed down into the duct (Fig. 14–23). A tube of the largest diameter that can be inserted into the duct is selected, and a piece 1.5 to 2 cm. long is cut off. The end to be inserted is tapered slightly. A suture is then passed through the untapered end of the tube that is to protrude into the mouth. This will ultimately be used to anchor the tube to the floor of the mouth and prevent it from being propelled out of the duct. An incision is made

in the isolated duct to permit insertion of the polyethylene tubing. If scar tissue prevents total freeing of the duct, it should be excised to expose the lumen. The tube is now inserted into the opening of the duct while the latter is elevated for access by the previously inserted suture passed under the duct. When it is determined that the tapered end of the tube has entered the duct, its remaining length is gently inserted up to the anchoring suture on the distal end.

If difficulty is encountered in inserting the tube, force should not be applied. The tube should be withdrawn and the duct entered with a round-end malleable silver probe. Under such circumstances the polyethylene tube should be threaded over the silver probe and pushed well beyond that portion of the probe that will enter the duct and act as a pilot (Fig. 14–24). After the probe has been inserted the desired distance, the polyethylene tube is slipped down the probe and gently guided into the duct. The probe is then withdrawn while the tube is held in place.

The loose ends of the anchoring suture are now picked up, and one end is threaded into a suture needle. An encircling suture is passed deep into the tissues beneath the duct, brought around and under the tube two or three times, and tied securely (Fig. 14–25). It must be emphasized that these sutures may disengage very quickly if they are engaged only in the epithelium of the floor of the mouth. The objective is to keep the tube in the duct by means of sutures until the new orifice of this duct has healed around the tube, and invagination of the oral epithelium into the duct is complete. If the tube is removed

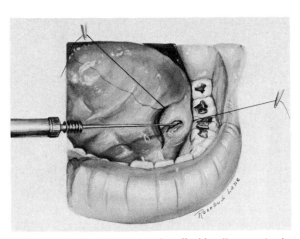

Figure 14–23 A round-end malleable silver probe is used to identify the duct lumen.

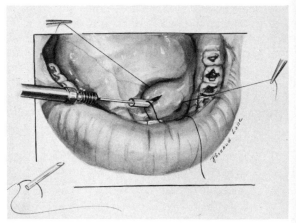

Figure 14–24 Note tubing on silver probe and anchor suture through tubing. This method of inserting the tube can be used if difficulty is encountered in inserting the tube alone.

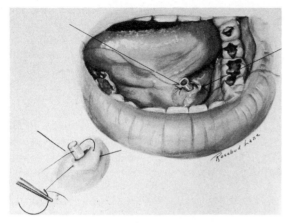

Figure 14–25 The silver probe has been withdrawn from the polyethylene tubing while it was held in place in the duct. The suture shown in Figure 14–24 has been used for a deep, encircling suture to anchor the tube.

3. The patient is requested to refrain from unnecessary talking and other activity that may require movement of the tongue and floor of the mouth. This cannot be overemphasized.
4. The patient is cautioned that swelling of the submandibular glands during the healing phase is to be expected.
5. Foods that are normally considered stimulating to the salivary gland are initially to be avoided.
6. Cannulating tubes are to remain in place as long as possible. Normal exfoliation of the sutures holding the tubes can be expected between 2 and 3 weeks after the operation.
7. Tubes are to be replaced immediately if they are lost before complete healing takes place.

too quickly, the surgically created orifice will collapse, and the unhealed edges will quickly unite again and occlude the duct. During the healing period drainage of the glands is not dependent upon maintenance of an open lumen of the tube. Very often the lumen becomes plugged with desquamated epithelium and by-products of surgery, even though the duct was patent at time of surgery. For this reason, the patient should be advised that during the period of healing the glands may fill quickly following stimulation and secrete their contents rather slowly. Normally, a functional gland will force a flow around the tube during the period of its retention.

Two to three weeks' retention of the primarily installed tubes may not provide sufficient time for epithelialization of the newly formed duct. On occasion a duct that appeared satisfactory at the time of removal of the polyethylene tube later becomes occluded, probably as the result of circumferential cicatricial tissue. It is therefore suggested that after removal of the primary cannula a second tube, one half the length of the first, be installed and retained until there is definite evidence of a well-epithelialized duct opening.

Postoperative Instructions.
1. The patient is requested to refrain from taking anything into the oral cavity while the area is still anesthetized to reduce the possibility of postoperative damage.
2. The patient is requested to maintain a soft, high-protein, high-calorie diet during the period that the tube is in place.

SALIVARY FISTULA

The most common causes of salivary fistulas are trauma and infection. (Fig. 14–26). Rarer causes are ulceration from gangrenous stomatitis, tuberculosis or syphilis. Ob-

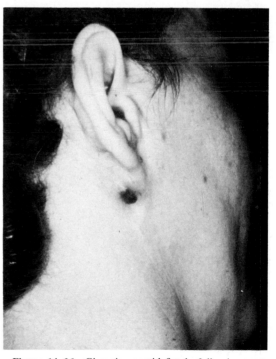

Figure 14–26 Chronic parotid fistula following acute parotitis in which the abscess ruptured and drained spontaneously. Several attempts were made by a general surgeon to close this fistula. The patient refused further surgery or a sialogram.

viously, those fistulas that drain orally do not need surgical correction. While all authorities mention trauma as one of the causes, the author is impressed with the fact that for 20 years, he has inserted hundreds of pins through the skin and parotid gland in the treatment of fractures of the mandible by the extraoral skeletal pin fixation method (see Chapter 18), and not once has a fistula developed following the insertion or removal of these pins.

Parotid ducts severed by penetrating wounds may be treated as described in Case Report No. 3 and shown in Figures 14–30 and 14–31. Extraoral fistulas of this duct may be closed by freeing the proximal end and transferring it to the buccal mucosa. Extraoral fistulas from the submandibular and sublingual glands may require excision of these glands.

Posterior extraoral persistent fistulas from the parotid gland, as shown in Figure 14–26, require excision of at least a portion of the gland.

Case Report No. 3

TRAUMA TO THE PAROTID GLAND, ITS DUCT AND RAMUS FROM A BULLET

A 32-year-old man was accidentally shot during a hunting accident, the bullet passing through the back of his neck, comminuting the ramus (see Figure 14–27), lacerating the parotid duct and passing through his cheek (Figures 14–29 and 14–31). When brought to the hospital 3 days after the ac-

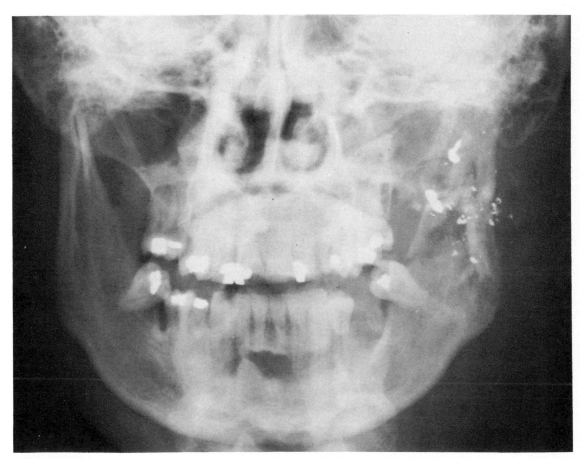

Figure 14–27 Fractured mandible, with the ramus comminuted by a bullet that also severed the parotid duct. (See Case Report No. 3 for details.)

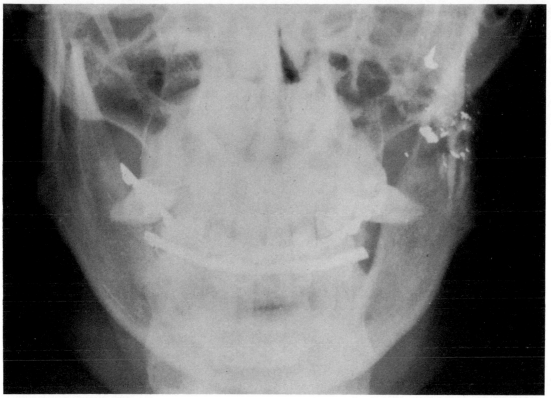

Figure 14–28 The fracture was reduced by intermaxillary elastics between maxillary and mandibular splints wired to the necks of the teeth, and manual manipulation of the fragments of the vertical ramus.

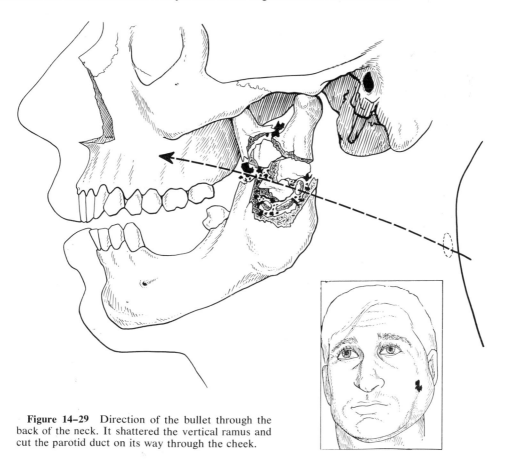

Figure 14–29 Direction of the bullet through the back of the neck. It shattered the vertical ramus and cut the parotid duct on its way through the cheek.

945

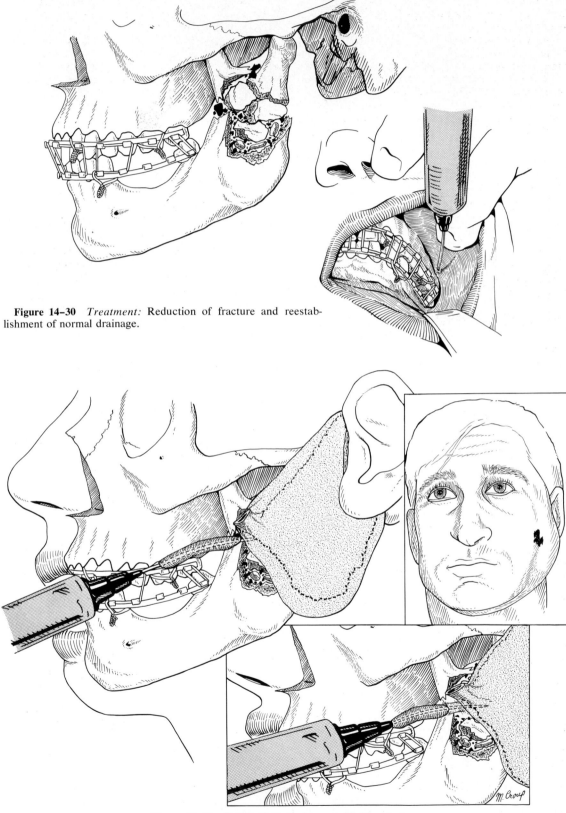

Figure 14–30 *Treatment:* Reduction of fracture and reestablishment of normal drainage.

Figure 14–31 Route of needle in reestablishing drainage.

cident, he had extensive swelling and discomfort in the left parotid gland region and malocclusion from the comminuted fracture. The fracture was reduced (see Figures 14–28 and 14–30). Several opinions were expressed concerning the treatment of the parotid gland. They were: (1) remove the gland, (2) irradiate the gland, and (3) our opinion to attempt to reestablish normal drainage through the parotid duct. While this was met with skepticism, it was agreed that nothing would be lost by such an attempt. The point of a 20 gauge needle was rounded off and attached to a 10 cc. syringe.

The needle was inserted into the parotid duct until resistance was encountered and overcome, at which point it was possible to aspirate 25 cc. of clear saliva slightly tinged with blood (see Figures 14–30 and 14–31). The swelling was considerably reduced. Each day thereafter the same procedure was followed, smaller quantities of saliva being obtained. After 7 days it was observed that saliva flowed freely from the parotid duct. The duct remained patent and the patient was discharged from the hospital.

SALIVARY GLAND TUMORS

Larson and Schmidt state that about 88 per cent of all tumors of the salivary glands occur in the parotid gland, 5 per cent or more in the submandibular gland and 5 per cent in the minor salivary and mucous glands, with the hard palate area the most frequent location. They advocate early resection because of an increase in the incidence of recurrence as the tumors increase in size, and because of their malignant potentialities.[13]

SURGICAL APPROACH FOR SALIVARY GLAND TUMORS

Garcelon, in his survey of 329 patients with salivary gland tumors over a 10 year period, found that 172 had mixed tumors and 98 had carcinoma. Carcinoma was diagnosed in 22 per cent of those patients with parotid gland tumors and in 52 per cent of those with submandibular gland tumors. He states that the most successful treatment of a mixed tumor of the parotid gland appears to be complete removal of the tumor with as generous a portion of the parotid gland as the situation permits. Mixed tumors of the submandibular gland are treated by total excision of the involved gland. This results in no disability. However, the lingual nerve is in this region and care should be taken to avoid severing or traumatizing it (see Figure 14–19). He also advocates radical neck dissection as the most successful initial treatment for carcinoma of the submandibular gland.[11]

Parotid Gland Tumors. According to Buxton and his associates, the presence of a new growth in the parotid gland is an indication for its removal. All parotid tumors, whether benign or malignant, should be treated by means of total parotidectomy.[5] James and

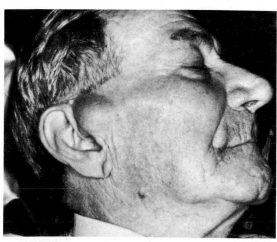

Figure 14–32 Pleomorphic adenoma (mixed tumor) of the parotid gland. The patient, aged 74, guessed it had been present over 10 years.

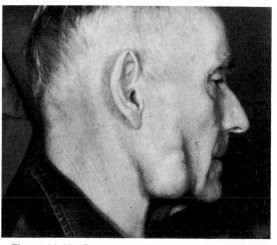

Figure 14–33 Recurrent (?) pleomorphic adenoma (mixed tumor) of the parotid gland. A benign mixed tumor had been excised from this area of the gland over 20 years earlier.

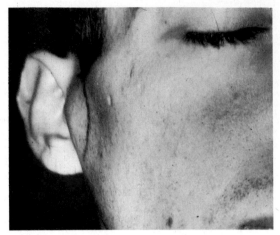

Figure 14-34 Malignant lymphoma simulates in appearance and location a pleomorphic adenoma. However, the typical hardness of the mixed tumor is absent.

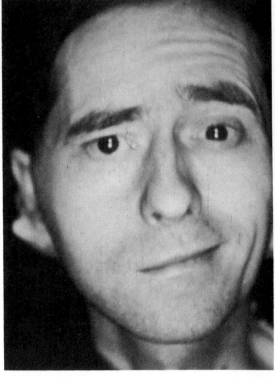

Figure 14-36 Malignant diffuse pleomorphic adenoma of the parotid gland with seventh nerve involvement.

Saleeby maintain that regardless of how benign, how encapsulatcd, or how superficially located the new growth may appear, the lesion is potentially dangerous.[12] Many malignant tumors are well encapsulated and show no evidence of local infiltration or regional spread. Although the accurate interpretation of benign or malignant histopathologic changes in parotid gland tumors is difficult and oftentimes impossible, the pathologic diagnosis should cause minimal concern if the parotid gland tumor is treated by total removal. In many cases of parotid gland cancer, total parotidectomy, despite loss of facial nerve function, has proved curative.

In general, if it is not feasible to eradicate tumor tissue completely by surgical means, radiation in the form of x-ray, radium or cobalt may be utilized; however, radiation therapy should play but a small role in the treatment of parotid gland tumors. Benign tumors are radioresistant and should therefore be treated by surgical excision; malig-

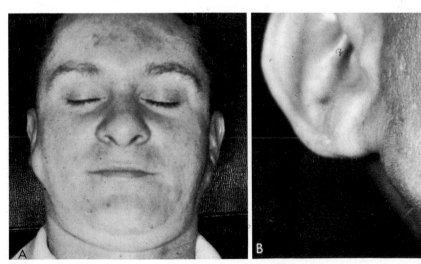

Figure 14-35 A sebaceous cyst that looks somewhat like a pleomorphic adenoma; however, it is soft, not hard.

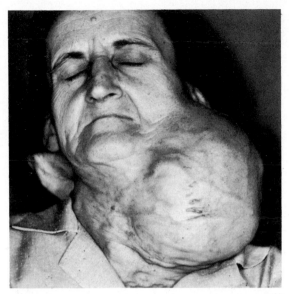

Figure 14–37 Pleomorphic adenoma (mixed tumor) of the parotid gland, which has slowly been growing for over 40 years. The patient permitted a biopsy many years ago. When she learned that the tumor was not malignant, she refused surgery, even though she was told that malignant transformation frequently took place in later years.

nant tumors are more responsive to roentgen-ray therapy, which is occasionally helpful. Roentgen therapy alone in the primary treatment of malignant tumors of the parotid gland rarely cures; it is an acceptable procedure when surgical intervention is contraindicated.

The prognosis for survival of patients with tumors of the parotid gland depends on the presence and degree of malignancy and on the completeness with which resection of the tumor can be accomplished. Since it is not always possible to differentiate benign from malignant lesions unless facial paralysis is present or unless distant metastases have occurred, early, complete removal of the tumor is imperative.

COMBINED SURGICAL AND RADIOTHERAPEUTIC APPROACH FOR PAROTID AND SUBMANDIBULAR TUMORS

Benign Tumors.* Smith and associates state, "From 1951 to 1961, 70 tumors of parotid and submandibular glands were seen at our Center,† 30 were benign mixed tumors and 40 were malignant.

"Many authors have advocated surgery alone for benign tumors. For many years, our treatment policy in benign salivary gland tumors has been a combined surgical and radiotherapeutic approach. In some instances, this included preoperative radiation to a tumor dose of 3000 rads in 3 weeks, followed in 4 to 6 weeks by enucleation of the tumor, and a radium-needle implantation into the tumor bed (3000 to 4000 rads). In others, enucleation is performed initially, and radium needles are implanted in the tumor bed to give a dose of 6000 to 7000 rads in 5 to 7 days.

"Our impression is that preoperative radiation reduces slightly the size of benign tumors and thickens the pseudocapsule of the tumor, thus facilitating enucleation.

"In patients referred postoperatively whose

---

*See Chapter 13 for a description of mixed tumors of the minor salivary glands and their treatment.

†The Ontario Cancer Foundation London Clinic, London, Canada.

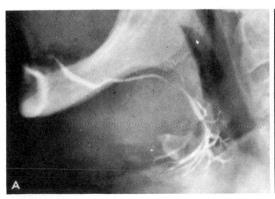
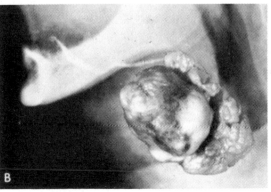

Figure 14–38 *A*, Radiograph showing displacement by a tumor but no interruption of the duct pattern. *B*, Composite illustration showing a photograph of the lipoma and resected submandibular gland superimposed on the sialograph of the same patient. (Reproduced by permission of R. Ollerenshaw, and the Department of Medical Illustrations, Manchester Royal Infirmary, Manchester, England.)

tumor had been small and superficial, radium-needle implantation is performed. If the tumor had been more extensive or situated deeply (with removal baring the facial nerve), or if the histologic study had shown a high degree of cellularity, postoperative radiation is given with cobalt-60 beam, using a pair of wedges to a tumor dose of 4000 rads in 3 weeks."[27]

Malignant Growths. Smith and associates find that "most carcinomas are seen postoperatively, after partial or complete excision. In some inoperable patients, the diagnosis is established by needle aspiration. A few present with recurrence after previous surgery.

"Generally, radium-needle implantation is unsuitable in this group, because an inadequate volume would be treated. We favor external radiation with cobalt-60 with a wedge pair in either the parotid or the submandibular region. The volume and depth of the area treated can be adjusted by varying the obliquity and the separation of the fields and the thickness of the wedges.

"Many of these tumors are radioresistant, and a tumor dose in the range of 5000 to 7000 rads in 4 to 6 weeks is necessary. Occasionally, in the elderly frail patient, a tumor dose of 3000 rads in 2 weeks will suffice to provide worthwhile growth restraint."[27]

SIALOLITHIASIS (SALIVARY STONES)

Salivary stones (salivary calculi) may be found in the salivary glands or in their ducts. They are yellowish white to brown in color and are either smooth or covered with fine to coarse nodules; the color darkens with the age of the stone. They are 75 per cent calcium carbonate and 10 per cent calcium phosphate. In some cases the salts are laid down in concentric layers. It is thought that they are formed around desquamated epithelial cells or bacteria in the glands that act as a nidus, and then they pass forward in the duct. The frequency with which multiple stones are found in the ducts lends credence to this theory.

Salley and associates[22] found that vitamin A deficiency produced, in the major and

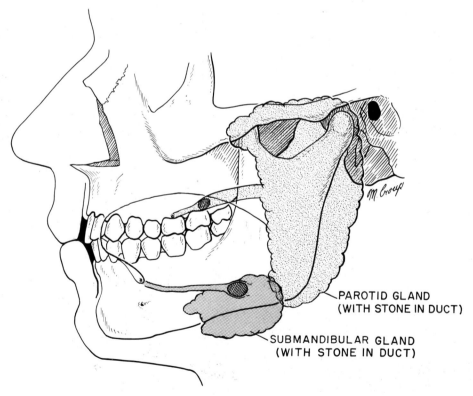

PAROTID GLAND
(WITH STONE IN DUCT)

SUBMANDIBULAR GLAND
(WITH STONE IN DUCT)

Parotid Gland – Lateral to mandible
Submandibular Gland – Medial to mandible

Figure 14–39 Positions of the parotid and submandibular glands and ducts; each duct contains one sialolith here.

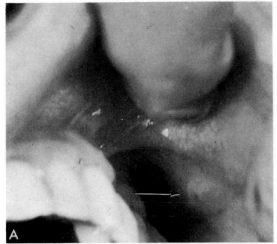

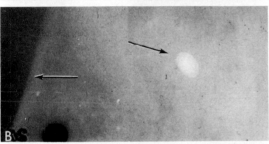

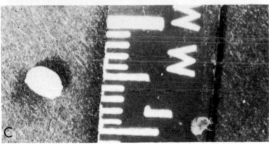

ton's) duct, or the submandibular gland itself. The parotid (Stensen's) duct or the parotid gland is the second most frequent location. The sublingual (Bartholin's) ducts or the sublingual gland itself is the rarest location for sialoliths. Rarely are sialoliths found in the sublingual gland because of the many short ducts (up to twenty) draining this gland (see

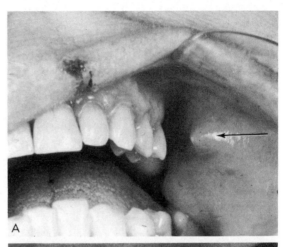

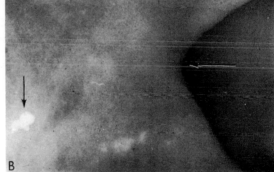

Figure 14–40 Sialolith in the parotid duct. *A,* Congested papilla with the dark, inflamed orifice of the parotid duct in the middle. *B,* Radiograph of a small sialolith at the orifice. A sialolith is best shown on underexposed periapical radiographic films held by the patient on the inside of the cheek along the course of the duct, beginning anterior to the duct's orifice. The arrow on the left indicates the edge of the cheek and lip. *C,* Small round, smooth sialolith removed by slitting the lumen through the orifice.

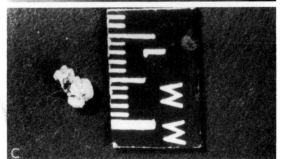

minor salivary glands of hamsters, "almost complete disappearance of secretory acini in replacement of gland parenchyma with infiltrates of acute and chronic inflammatory cells. Smaller ductal structures, likewise, are absent and the larger collecting ducts exhibit squamous metaplasia of ductal epithelium with large keratotic plugs."[23]

Location. The most common location of salivary stones is the submandibular (Whar-

Figure 14–41 A pebbled, irregular sialolith in the parotid duct. *A,* Swollen papilla with a drop of pus at the orifice. *B,* Sialolith at the left. Arrow on the right points to the juncture of the upper and lower lips. The stone was removed by slitting the lumen through the orifice. *C,* This sialolith was formed by the fusion of many tiny calcific units that formed in the gland or posterior duct and moved forward to join those particles already stalled at the orifice.

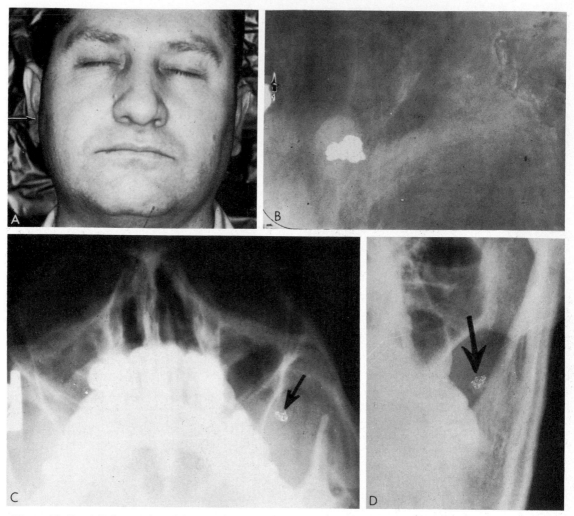

Figure 14-42 *A*, Inflammation of the parotid gland. *B*, Sialolith in the papilla of the duct, as revealed on this dental radiograph.

C and *D*, It is very difficult to visualize small sialoliths by extraoral films. The absence of a sialolith on such a film should not rule out the possibility of its presence. The most certain diagnostic radiograph is, as has been stated, the intraoral dental film held to the cheek.

Figure 14-16). Sialoliths are also rare in the multitude of minor salivary glands in the oral cavity.

The secretions from the parotid gland are serous or watery, while those from the submandibular and sublingual glands are viscid, owing to the presence of mucin. These factors help account for the greater percentage of sialoliths found in the submandibular duct and gland.

Symptoms. The principal symptoms of salivary stone are as follows: (1) Swelling that is exaggerated when eating. (2) Tenderness, and in some cases, pain in the region of the gland, when eating; the pain may radiate to the ear and the neck. (3) Swelling and pain disappear between meals as the dammed-up secretions gradually flow around the obstruction, and the pressure in the duct and gland is relieved. (4) Repeated inflammatory reactions in the mucosa of the orifice of the duct, simulating ulcers, are observed when the stone is located in or near the orifice of the duct (see Figure 14-32). (5) Small quantities of pus may be observed near the orifice as a result of infection in the injured mucosal lining of the canal. (6) Secondary infection may develop in the gland and a diffuse cellulitis may extend to and involve the tissues surrounding the gland and duct. Ludwig's angina (bilateral submandibular cellulitis) may originate in a virulent infection in the sublingual

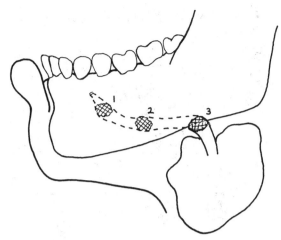

Figure 14–43 Most common locations of salivary stones in the submandibular duct.

or submandibular gland. These glands, having been traumatized by stones or the backed-up pressure of their own secretions, are susceptible to infection. (7) The patient notices a chronic swelling in the floor of the mouth. A large stone is easily felt by palpation.

Many salivary stones are symptomless. It is only when partial or complete obstruction of the duct occurs that symptoms develop. The obstruction is due to mechanical block-

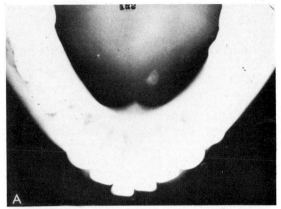

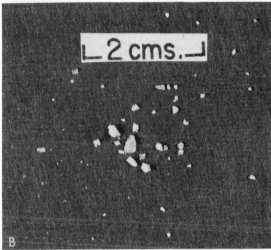

Figure 14–45 *A,* An occlusal radiograph, showing what appears to be one triangular sialolith, was made of a patient who had marked induration and edema of the left submandibular gland, and inflammation and swelling around the orifice of the submandibular duct. Instead of a single stone, multiple small salivary stones were evacuated from the duct, as shown in *B.* A moderate amount of flocculent material was also drained from the incised duct. It is apparent that this was not a solid stone, but rather a collection of small calcified particles, some held together by mucin, others loose in the fluid.

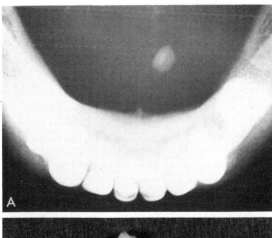

Figure 14–44 Salivary stone (sialolith) at the orifice of the submandibular (Wharton's) duct. There was a history of severe pain (burning) at mealtime. The patient did not recall any marked swelling of the submandibular gland. He had had inflammation periodically near the orifice of the duct.

age because of the stones, or to periductal infection, causing inflammatory edema that results in the occlusion of the lumen of the duct.

If the stones are *small,* about the size of a grain of wheat, and located in the anterior portion of the duct, dilatation of the duct orifice with graded whalebone rat-tail filiform bougies and manipulation of the stone along the duct may be sufficient to expel the stone. Lubricate the bougies with mineral oil; insert them gently until the stone is contacted. Allow each succeeding larger size to remain in position for 5 minutes; then attempt to milk the stone out of the duct. In all other cases, sialolithotomy is the method of choice for the removal of salivary stones.

RADIOGRAPHIC VISUALIZATION OF SIALOLITHS

While sialoliths may be revealed by the extraoral radiographs mentioned earlier, failure to visualize them does not prove their absence, particularly in the submandibular or parotid ducts. In all cases in which the possibility of sialoliths exists, an intraoral radiographic examination of the salivary ducts is made with occlusal and periapical dental films. The occlusal film is placed as far pos-

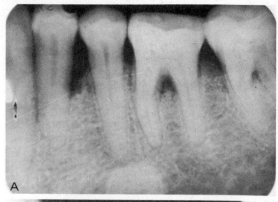

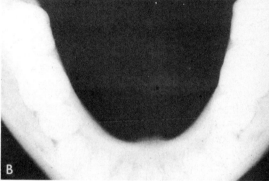

Figure 14–47 *A,* A radiopaque area on this dental radiograph might be osteosclerosis in the cancellous bone of the mandible or a superimposed sialolith. *B,* The underexposed occlusal radiograph ruled out the second possibility. (See also Figures 14–46 and 14–48 and their legends.)

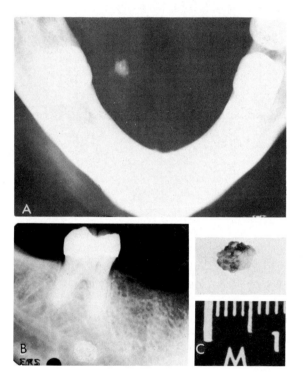

Figure 14–46 *A,* Occlusal radiograph of a sialolith in the submandibular duct midway between the gland and its orifice.

B, This radiopaque area, which had the appearance of a localized area of osteosclerosis, suggested also the possibility of the superimposition of a "salivary stone" on the periapical film. This can happen if the film is not held in contact with the lingual surface of the mandible but instead is only held against the lingual surfaces of the teeth, permitting the film to lie on the floor of the oral cavity, as happened in this case. This is proved by the occlusal film. When taking an occlusal radiograph to rule out or confirm the possibility of a sialolith, it is essential to underexpose the film so as not to "burn out" images of small or partially formed "stones." Note the marked underexposure of this occlusal film.

C, The sialolith after removal. The patient's history was only mildly suggestive of this possibility. This was a small stone, but "little stones become big stones." (See Figure 14–48.)

teriorly over the floor of the mouth as possible, keeping the tongue forward and beneath the film. The head is tilted back so that the central x-ray beam will strike the film at a right angle. The exposure time is reduced so that the images of small stones are not "burned out" by overexposure. Several films with varying exposure times should be made.

Radiographs of the sublingual gland and also the submandibular duct are made with intraoral periapical films by placing the film in the mouth so that the upper edge of the film is in contact with the teeth, while the lower edge extends over the mucosa of the floor of the mouth, forming a 45-degree angle with the lingual mandibular cortical plate. The central x-ray is then directed through the inferior border of the mandible at minus 15 degrees. Underexpose the films, taking several exposures with varying exposure times for the reason stated previously.

The panoramic films are not satisfactory for the diagnosis of sialoliths in the submandibular or sublingual ducts because the sialoliths in most cases would be superimposed on the mandible. (See Figure 14–62.) If these were large enough, they would give the appearance on the radiograph of osteosclerotic areas in bone. It would be advisable, when such areas appear on panoramic radiographs, for occlusal films to be taken to rule out the possibility of a sialolith in a submandibular duct and intraoral films on the inner surface of the upper cheek to rule out the possibility of a sialolith in the parotid duct.

To locate sialoliths in the parotid duct, fasten two periapical dental films together with tape and place them on the inner surface of the cheek over the parotid duct. The central x-ray is directed at a right angle through the cheek, and the exposure time is reduced accordingly.

Phleboliths, calcified lymph nodes and idiopathic calcified bodies have been found in the submandibular area in the cheek. This fact must be kept in mind when diagnosing salivary stones in the salivary ducts and glands. The subjective and objective symptoms of ductal obstruction plus the radiographic findings will aid in making a differential diagnosis.

TECHNIQUE FOR SURGICAL REMOVAL OF SALIVARY STONES IN THE SUBMANDIBULAR DUCT

Digitally palpate the oral tissues in that region in which the stone is presumed to be located, according to the radiographic findings, until the stone is distinctly felt by the tip of the index finger. *Do not operate until the stone is located digitally or with a probe.* Artifacts on x-ray films may simulate sialoliths.

Local or general anesthesia can be used. If the stone is in the submandibular (Wharton's) duct, and local anesthesia has been selected, the lingual nerve should be blocked, using the technique for blocking this nerve at the same time the inferior alveolar nerve is blocked; use 2 cc. of anesthetic solution. Nerve blocking is preferable to infiltration, because the latter distends the tissues in the operative field and interferes with digital palpation and instrument manipulation.

For local anesthesia of the tissues overlying the parotid (Stensen's) duct, infiltrate the anesthetic solution into the mucobuccal fold above the section of the duct in which the stone is located.

If general anesthesia is elected, then except for the simplest type of stones (*e.g.,* those located at the duct orifice or immediately beneath the mucosa at the terminal third of the duct), the patient should be hospitalized, and nasoendotracheal anesthesia should be administered.

The reader will find many case reports concerning the removal of sialoliths (salivary stones) in these pages. He is advised to study the illustrations and read the accompanying legends. (For the most part, material in the legends is not repeated in the text.)

Case Report No. 4

EXCISION OF A SUBMANDIBULAR SIALOLITH

The patient, a 42-year-old white man, was admitted to the Eye and Ear Hospital on January 29 at 6:25 P.M. because of a "growth under the tongue."

History. The patient had a sore mouth about 10 years ago, and a diagnosis of an oral ulcer was made at that time. He had first noticed a sublingual "growth" about 5 years ago. The swelling caused no pain, but the patient was told that it should be removed before dentures could be placed.

Oral Examination. See Figure 14–48A to C.

Physical Examination. There was evidence of cardiac enlargement and an apical systolic murmur. The blood pressure was 130/70. The mouth was completely edentulous.

Laboratory Report. All findings were within normal limits.

Course. The patient was scheduled for operation on January 30, but after a preoperative hypodermic injection of 100 mg. of Demerol and 1/150 grain of atropine sulfate he became very ill. He had nausea, vomiting, profuse perspiration and vertigo. The operation was cancelled for this day.

When the patient had recovered, an injection of atropine sulfate, 1/150 grain, was ordered. He showed no signs of an adverse reaction, so the previous reaction was attributed to Demerol. The operation was scheduled for the next day.

Operation. Under thiopental sodium anesthesia, two hemostats were placed, one anterior and

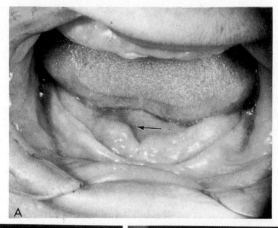

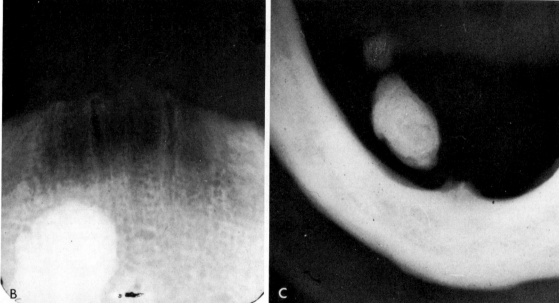

Figure 14–48 *A,* In this case the history of pain and swelling of the submandibular duct at mealtime, plus the objective symptom of a hard swelling at the terminus of the duct, practically "clinched" the tentative diagnosis of a sialolith. (See Case Report No. 4 for further details.) *B,* This large radiopaque area in this periapical radiograph could, of course, have been osteosclerosis. *C,* However, the occlusal film revealed not only one sialolith, but two.

D, The mouth prop has been placed, and a suture passed through the midline of the tongue, which is then lifted against the oropharyngeal partition. The mucosa overlying the duct and its stones is then grasped with hemostats on either side of the stones, and lifted. One or two sutures, as shown in Figure 14–50, is a better method of lifting and holding the duct and oral tissues. (Study the text.)

E, The mucosa is incised from hemostat to hemostat down to the duct, which is then opened longitudinally over the stones. With a large-bowled curette the stones are then lifted from their beds and removed.

F, The two salivary stones shown in *C.*

G, Stones shown in the radiograph. Note that in this one case we have a smooth small stone and a large fissured and rough stone covered with a fine, sandy surface.

H, An iodoform gauze drain is placed in the expanded duct. *I,* The iodoform gauze drain is sutured into the duct. *J,* About ½ inch of the gauze drain is allowed to protrude from the duct.

(Figure 14–48 continued on opposite page)

one posterior to the swollen area of the region containing the stones, and by extraoral finger pressure under the mandible by the anesthetist, whose arm passed underneath the sterile drapes, the area was raised from the floor of the mouth (Fig. 14–48D). An incision was made with a No. 15 blade across

this area, exposing the larger of two stones. A small quantity of pus escaped from the incision. This stone was easily removed with a periosteal elevator, using the wide end as a spoon. The smaller stone followed readily (Fig. 14–48E to G).

Approximately 2 inches of ½-inch iodoform

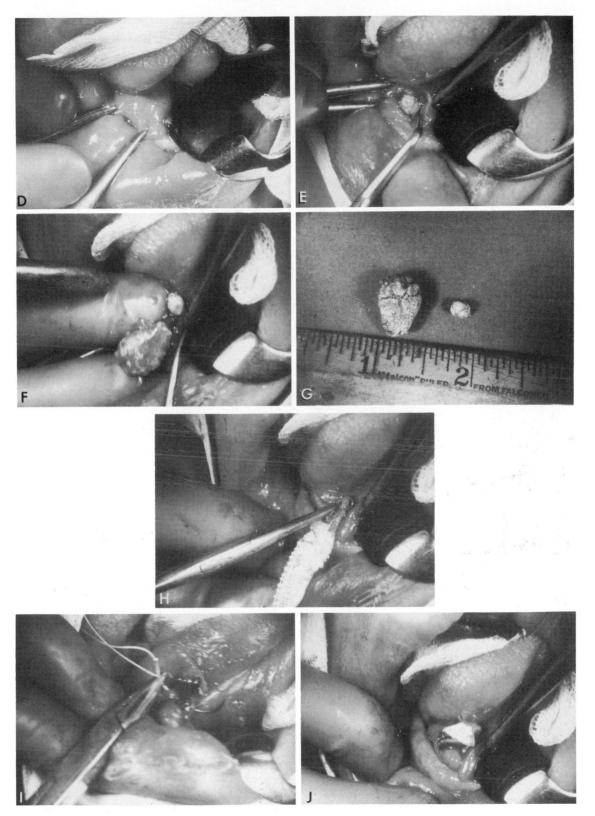

Figure 14-48 (*Continued.*)

gauze drain were placed in the space occupied by the stones, and a suture was placed to hold the drain in position (Fig. 14–48*H* to *J*).

Postoperative Course. Ice was applied to the face for the first 24 hours *only;* then infrared heat was used for 20 minutes three times a day. Penicillin, 400,000 units daily by intramuscular injection, was prescribed. Fluids were forced, 3000 cc. daily,

along with 100 mg. of ascorbic acid three times a day. A mouthwash of 10 drops of sodium hypochlorite in a glass of water was used four times a day.

The gauze drain was removed on the second postoperative day, and the patient was discharged on the third day after operation.

Salivary Stone Near the Orifice or in the Anterior Half of the Submandibular Duct

If the stone is just beneath the mucosa in the anterior half of the submandibular duct, force the structures in the floor of the oral cavity upward by finger pressure beneath the mandible, and maintain this pressure throughout the operation.

Pass a curved needle deep through the oral tissues distal to the stone so that the needle passes *beneath* the duct. The suture is then

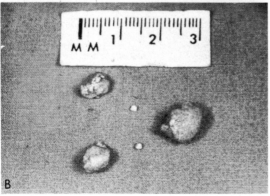

Figure 14–49 *A,* Marked terminal expansion of the submandibular duct. *B,* Expansion was caused by the presence of one large and two small sialoliths and scores of tiny wafers of semisolid material (two of which are shown here) in a flocculent fluid. It is interesting to note that there was no inflammation of the covering mucosa or duct orifice. In fact, the patient was symptomless.

used to lift and hold the duct and superficial tissues during surgery (see Figure 14–50). This will also prevent the stones from moving backward through the duct into the gland.

Locate the stone with the tip of the index finger, incise the mucosa overlying the duct and stone, expose and split the duct against the stone.

Lift the stone from its bed by a large-bowled curette. Pus is frequently observed around and distal to the stone.

Insert a wick of iodoform gauze or a rubber drain into the wound.

Pass a catgut or silk suture through the sides of the wound and through the drain to hold it in place.

Remove the hemostats.

Instruct the patient to use hypochlorite mouthwash (10 drops to a glass of lukewarm water) four times daily.

Allow the drain to remain in place for 48 hours.

Prefabricated Radiopaque Sutures in Ductal Sialolithotomy

Baurmash and Mandel use a radiopaque suture material (silk braided over a thin wire) to circumscribe, posteriorly and anteriorly, the submandibular duct with the sialolith between the two sutures.[3] These sutures are used for the purpose of localization of the sialolith, also as a means whereby the tissues in the floor of the oral cavity, including the duct, are raised and held during sharp and blunt dissection through the tissues until the stone is reached in the duct. The radiopaque sutures are inserted and radiographs are taken immediately to make certain that the sialolith is between the two sutures. If the sialolith is not between the two sutures, change the position of the radiopaque sutures and take another radiograph until the foreign material is found between the two sutures.

They state, "When the suture needle is introduced, initially, at the medial aspect of the

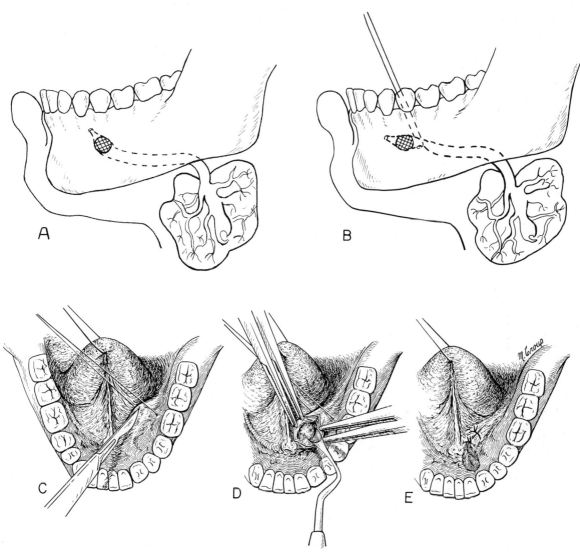

Figure 14–50 Surgical technique for removal of sialoliths from the terminus of the submandibular (Wharton's duct. *A,* Stone *in situ.* Notice proximal dilatation of the duct. A suture in the tongue is used for better control during an operation performed under general anesthesia. *B,* A transfixation suture is passed around the duct proximal to the stone to prevent it from slipping back into the gland. *C,* Gentle traction is applied to the transfixation suture, and an incision is made directly over the stone and directly down to it. The superior surface of duct is slit longitudinally over the stone. *D,* The stone is removed with a curette and the area cleansed of any small sialoliths. The transfixation suture is then removed, and the duct and gland are milked toward the incision to remove any debris. *E,* The incision is closed, with a drain in place.

plica, the possibility of injury to the blood vessels is minimized. It is true that the major vessels and nerves are, for the most part, located medial to the posterior portion of the sublingual gland and submandibular duct, but at the same time, the best and most accurate control of the needle is obtained during the first half of its introduction into the tissues.

"The silk-braided wire suture appears to have a definite superiority over plain wire ligature.* The ease in handling the suture, both during insertion and during the procedure, the ability to tie knots tightly, without slippage, and the opportunity to apply external tension without tearing the enclosed soft tissues are all obvious advantages."[3]

---

*AUTHOR'S NOTE: 28 gauge cable wire suture can be used very satisfactorily in the same manner.

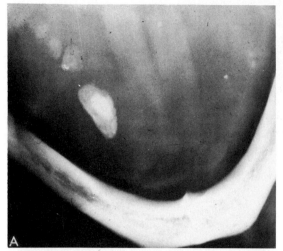

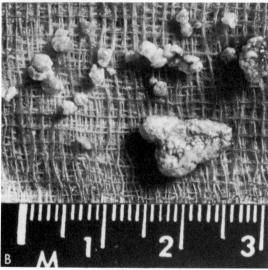

Figure 14–51 This patient for the previous 4 years had had repeated attacks of swelling and pain beneath the mandible and in the floor of the oral cavity. Originally the swelling and pain were associated with mealtimes, but not for the past 3 years. She had been treated symptomatically with antibiotics.

A, Occlusal film reveals multiple sialoliths, but many more "stones" were recovered at operation and are shown in *B.* Many are still "soft stones." A large quantity of pus and flocculent material drained from the distended duct when it was incised to remove the sialoliths. Many small sialoliths were removed during the aspiration of the pus.

Salivary Stone Located Deep in the Submandibular Duct or Gland

If the stone is in the posterior third of the submandibular (Wharton's) duct and deep in the floor of the oral cavity, the operation for the intraoral removal of the stone is much more difficult (study Figures 14–60 and 14–61).

Place the patient on rigorous oral hygiene,

including prophylactic treatment and the use of aqueous Merthiolate mouthwashes, 1:1000, instituted 2 days before the operation and just before the operation is undertaken. While we cannot sterilize the oral cavity, we can materially reduce the bacterial count in it.

Gently and carefully pass a small metal blunt probe into the duct until the gritty surface of the stone is contacted. This sensation is distinctly felt by the fingers holding the probe.

Keep the probe in position by wires attached to the incisor teeth.

Take a radiograph to determine whether or not the probe is in contact with the stone.

Now follow the technique shown in Figure 14–60.

With the probe still in place, elevate the
(*Text continued on page 967*)

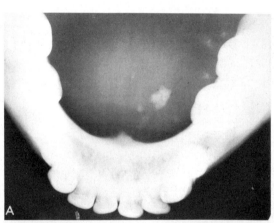

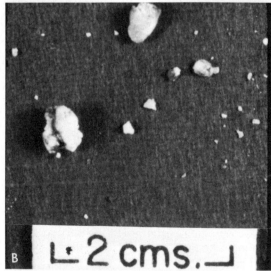

Figure 14–52 Multiple sialoliths in a widely dilated duct, as can be seen by the distribution of those "stones" that were large enough to be radiopaque. There was a considerable quantity of pus and thick flocculent fluid present.

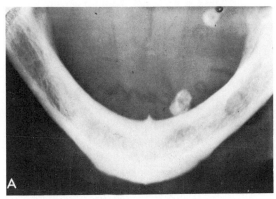

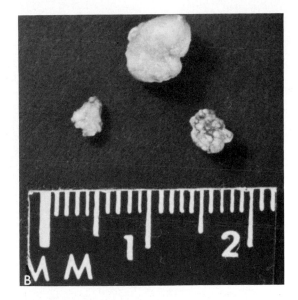

Figure 14–53 Another example of the various sizes and distribution of sialoliths in a submandibular duct. However, in this case very little flocculent fluid was present.

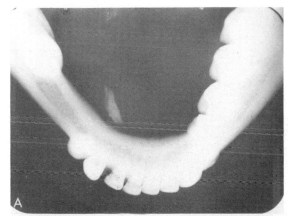

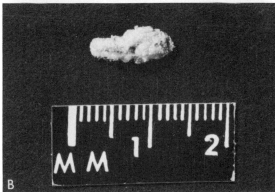

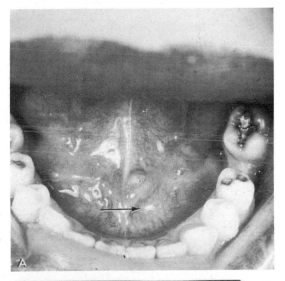

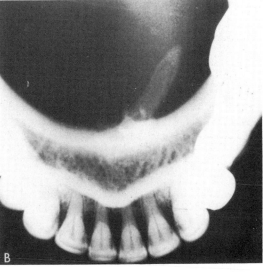

Figure 14–54 An isolated elongated, irregularly shaped sialolith (with a pitted and sandy surface) at the terminus of the submandibular duct. Such sialoliths usually produce considerable irritation and inflammation of the duct and its orifice, and pus is seen slowly draining.

Figure 14–55 *A,* Pus slowly but continuously discharged from the submandibular duct. Upon palpation of the floor of the oral cavity a spindle-type sialolith about 2 cm. long was easily felt lodged against the papillary orifice and extending posteriorly, as shown in *B.*

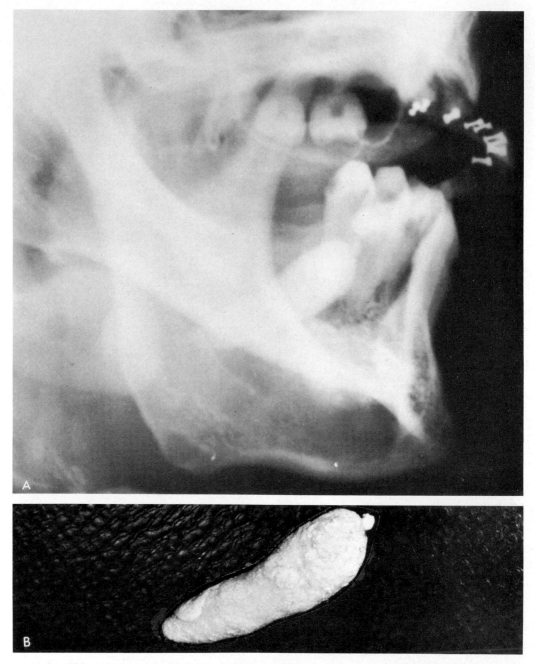

Figure 14–56 This patient sought relief from his physician for "mouth and jaw trouble." The medical roentgenologist took this extraoral oblique lateral jaw radiograph and made a diagnosis of an "unerupted impacted mandibular canine tooth of the mandible." On the basis of this "diagnosis," the patient was referred for the "removal of the impacted tooth"! The object does look somewhat like a cuspid, but obviously it was a large sialolith. This graphically points out what can happen when one of the most valuable and readily available diagnostic "tools," the index finger, is not used routinely to explore the soft tissues of the oral cavity. In this case the true identity of this object would easily have been established by palpation of the soft tissues in the floor of the mouth, supplemented with an occlusal radiograph. Much embarrassment, for all concerned, could have been avoided.

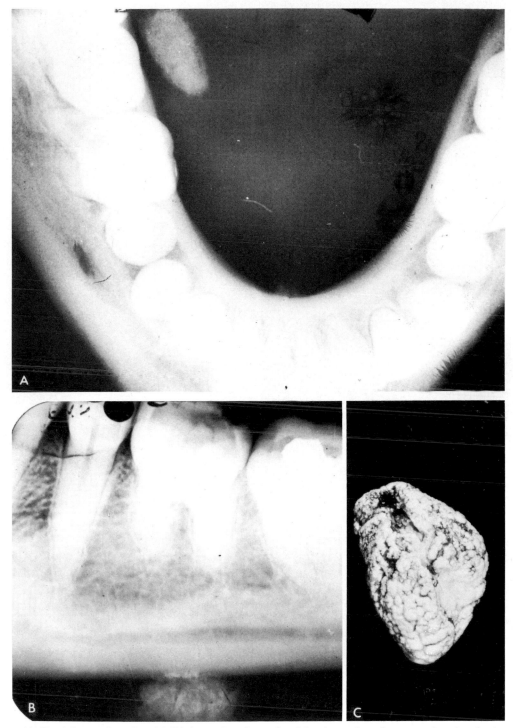

Figure 14–57   A large triangular sialolith located at the angle of the duct, where it turns rather sharply downward over the posterior border of the mylohyoid muscle.

EXCISION OF A SIALOLITH FROM THE SUBMANDIBULAR DUCT

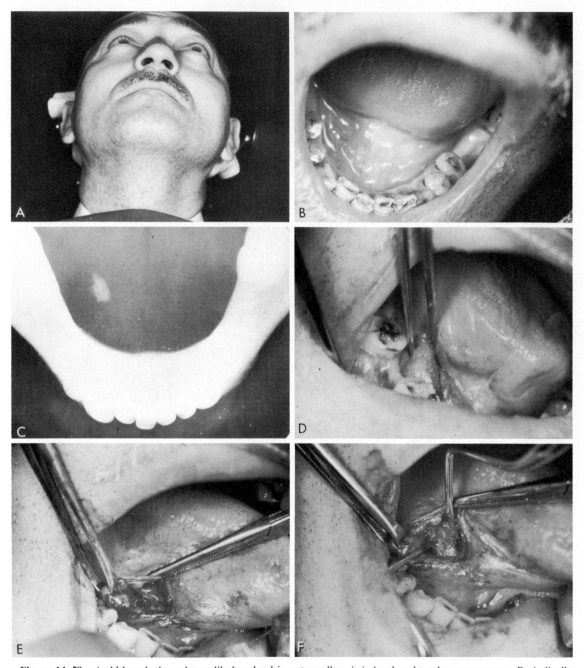

Figure 14–58 *A,* Although the submandibular gland is not swollen, it is hard and tender on pressure. Periodically the patient has pain and a feeling of fullness on the right side that is not related to eating.

B, The floor of the oral cavity, except for the slight dusky red color of the mucosa overlying the duct on the right side, is normal. On palpation a hard body about ½ inch long can be felt, and pain is produced by pressure.

C, The occlusal radiograph reveals a sialolith.

D, With blunt forceps the mucosa and duct distal to the sialolith are grasped and elevated.

E, The mucosa is incised and separated.

F, By blunt dissection the duct is exposed and elevated by two large-bowled curettes placed beneath the sialolith.

(*Figure 14–58 continued on opposite page*)

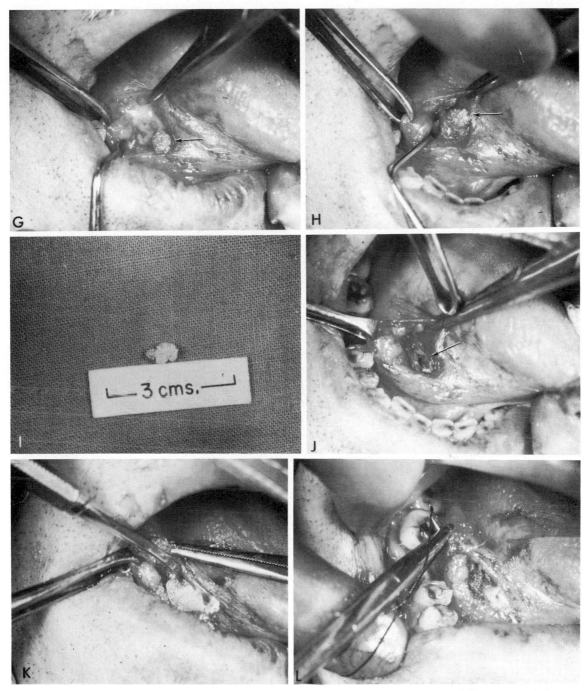

Figure 14–58 (*Continued.*)   *G*, The lumen of the duct over the stone is slit, exposing the sialolith and permitting the escape of flocculent fluid distal from the "stone."

H, After suctioning of the flocculent fluid, the sialolith is clearly visible.

I, The removed sialolith.

J, The exposed duct with the incision on the dorsal surface.

K, Iodoform gauze (¼-inch) is tucked into the lumen of the duct through the incision.

L, One black silk suture through the mucosa, anterior and posterior to the drain, closes the mucosa. The drain is removed in 24 hours and the sutures in 72 hours.

EXCISION OF A SIALOLITH FROM THE SUBMANDIBULAR DUCT

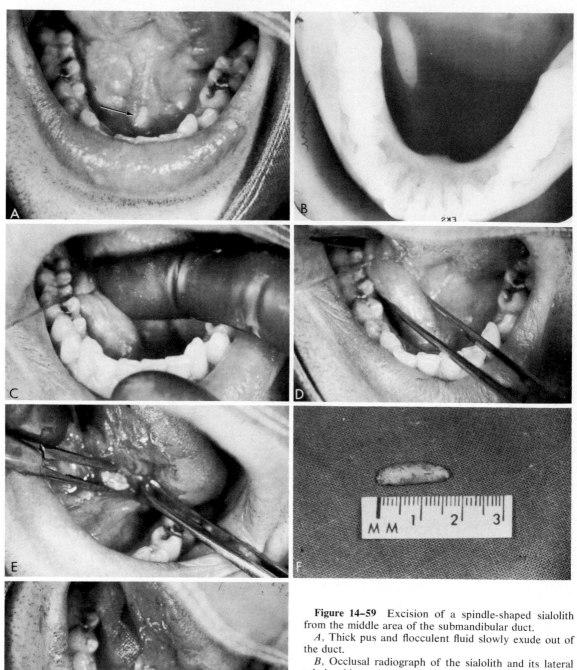

Figure 14–59 Excision of a spindle-shaped sialolith from the middle area of the submandibular duct.

A, Thick pus and flocculent fluid slowly exude out of the duct.

B, Occlusal radiograph of the sialolith and its lateral relationship to the mandible.

C, Palpation of the sialolith and stabilization with a suture through the mucosa, under the duct and back out into the oral cavity. This suture prevents the "stone" from moving posteriorly in the expanded duct during surgery, and it permits lifting and fixing the duct during surgery.

D, The covering mucosa, duct and contained sialolith are grasped with blunt forceps.

E, By sharp and blunt dissection the duct is exposed and opened, and the anterior end of the sialolith is exposed, grasped and removed.

F, Sialolith.

G, Iodoform gauze (¼-inch) is inserted, and mucosa only is closed on either side of the drain.

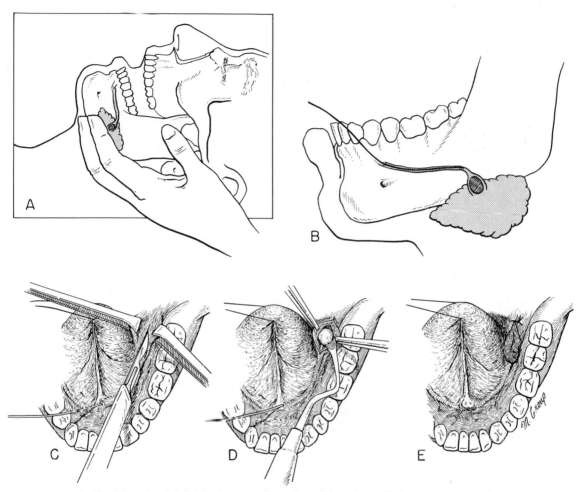

Figure 14–60 Excision of a sialolith in the posterior region of the submandibular (Wharton's) duct.

A, Position of the assistant's hand during operation. He must forcibly elevate the submandibular gland so that it projects into the mouth as far as possible.

B, A filiform bougie, or preferably a suitably sized silver lachrymal duct probe (Bowman's), is passed into the duct and the floor of the mouth retracted in order to tense the tissues over the duct. At the same time the assistant forcibly elevates the gland with his fingers.

C, The operator incises directly over the stone after it has been felt with the bougie. A No. 15 Bard-Parker scalpel is used to incise the oral mucosa, to expose the duct by blunt dissection (the probe in the duct makes this easier) and to split the duct wall over the stone. Constant pressure under the jaw so that the gland is pushed up during operation is very necessary for accessibility.

D, The stone is removed.

E, The incision is closed with a drain. (See Figure 14–62 for an illustration of a stone in this location.)

floor of the mouth by external finger pressure and make an incision *just through the mucosa,* 1 inch long, over the probe, and, as nearly as possible, above the stone. In making the incision, take care to avoid severing the lingual nerve.

Hold the tissues apart with Gardner retractors; use a weak suction constantly. A good headlight is essential.

Next carry out blunt dissection by hemostats and periosteal elevators through the structures in the floor of the oral cavity until the duct with the contained probe is exposed. Cut through the duct where the probe touches the stone so that the opening will permit delivery of the stone.

Remove the stone or stones with a curette or hemostat.

Insert a ½-inch strip of rubber dam or ½-inch iodoform gauze drain in the bottom of the wound.

Pass a 000 silk suture through the edges of the wound and through the drain material to insure its retention in the wound.

(*Text continued on page 974*)

EXCISION OF A SALIVARY STONE FROM THE SUBMANDIBULAR DUCT

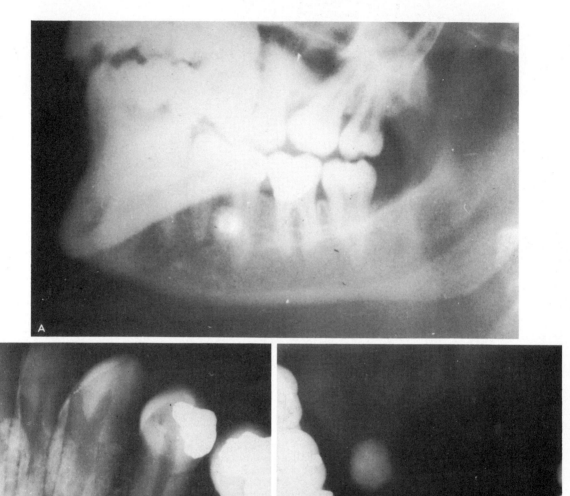

Figure 14–61 *A,* Oblique lateral jaw radiograph of a stone in the submandibular (Wharton's) duct. Note that in this film as well as in Figure 14–47*A,* the stone might be mistaken for an area of osteosclerosis. The patient's history, plus occlusal films, confirms the diagnosis. *B,* Small intraoral periapical radiograph of the sialolith shown in *A. C,* The occlusal film confirms the diagnosis of a salivary stone in the submandibular duct.

(Figure 14–61 continued on opposite page)

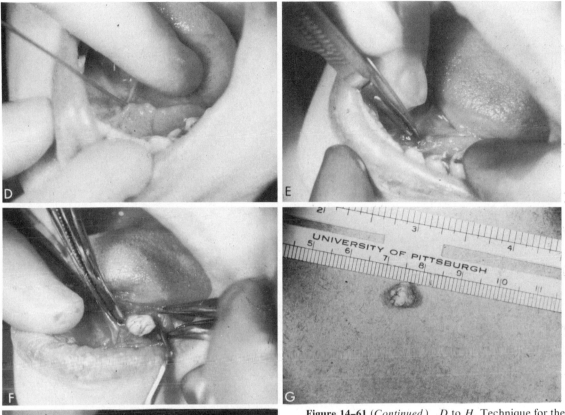

Figure 14–61 (*Continued.*)   *D* to *H*, Technique for the removal of a similar sialolith.

D, For sialoliths located in the posterior region of the submandibular duct, an appropriately sized silver lachrymal duct probe (Bowman's) is passed gently into the duct until the stone is contacted. Pressure should be exerted beneath the gland by the fingers of the assistant to force the gland up and forward. This will help prevent forcing the stone back into the gland. The duct, it must be remembered, is larger posteriorly than anteriorly, because posterior pressure of saliva behind the stone enlarges the duct from the stone back to the gland.

E, With the probe held in place in the duct, a spear-pointed scalpel is inserted into the duct alongside the probe, and the duct and overlying mucosa are split along the probe and grasped with hemostats until the stone is reached.

F, The cut edges are held apart with hemostats, and with continuing pressure beneath the gland, a large-bowled curette is inserted beneath the stone, which is lifted from its bed. The iodoform drain is inserted and the mucosa sutured.

G, The smooth stone after removal.

H, Four-week postoperative photograph. The duct is patent.

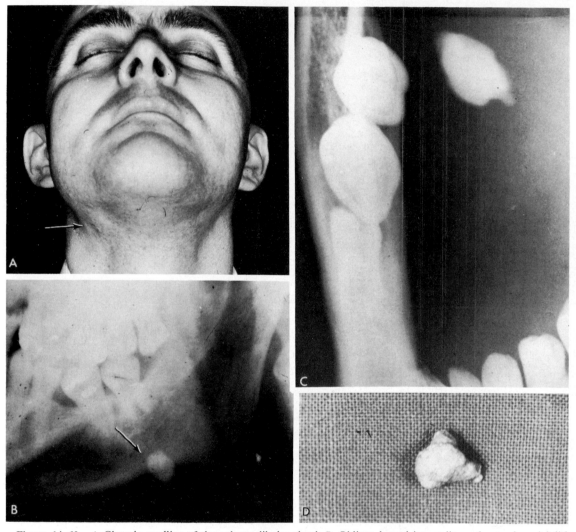

Figure 14–62   *A*, Chronic swelling of the submandibular gland. *B*, Oblique lateral jaw radiograph reveals a sialolith located at the junction of the duct and the gland, or just above the gland where the duct turns sharply forward over the distal border of the mylohyoid muscle. *C*, Occlusal radiograph reveals this stone only because the x-ray tube was moved laterally beneath the right third molar area and the central ray directed superiorly and anteriorly to project the image of the stone forward and upward onto the film. *D*, Sialolith which was removed by the technique shown in Figure 14–61.

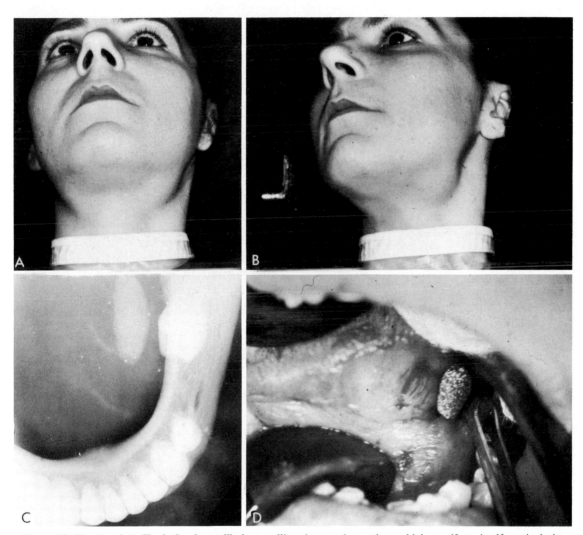

Figure 14–63 *A* and *B*, Typical submandibular swelling due to obstruction, which manifests itself particularly at mealtime. Note that the margins are very distinct. In chronic submandibular adenitis the swelling blends into the surrounding soft tissue, as is shown in Figure 14–58*A*. *C*, Modified occlusal film technique, as described in Figure 14–62. was used to visualize this sialolith. *D*, Large granular "stone" that was removed by the technique described in Figure 14–60.

EXCISION OF A SUBMANDIBULAR DUCT SIALOLITH

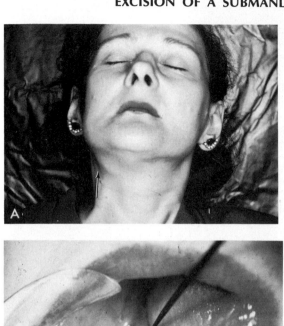

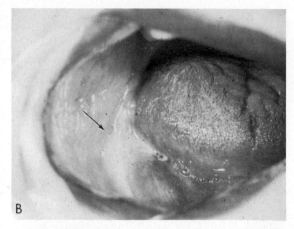

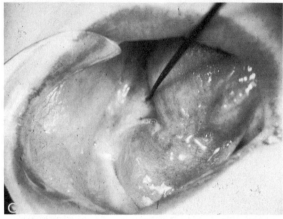

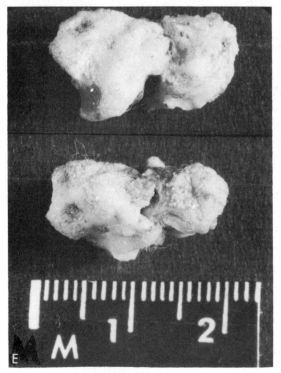

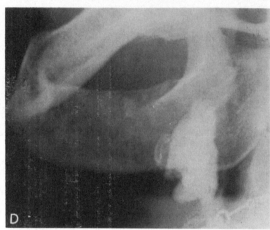

Figure 14–64 *A,* Chronic submandibular adenitis caused by massive sialoliths shown in *D* and *E*. During an acute episode of adenitis the patient suddenly had a "mouth full of pus" and immediate relief from her acute pain. Subsequently she noticed that daily thereafter she had drainage of the flocculent material shown in *B. C,* A probe in the fistula, surrounded by draining flocculent fluid, is in contact with one of the large sialoliths in the duct and submandibular gland shown in *D* and radiograph *E*. The technique for removal illustrated in Figure 14–61 was used to remove these sialoliths.

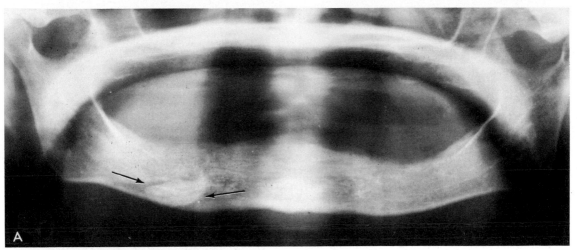

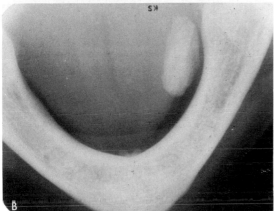

Figure 14–65 *A*, Panoramic radiograph showing an oblong radiopaque area that may be due to condensing osteitis or osteosclerosis, or a superimposed sialolith in the submandibular duct. *B*, The occlusal radiograph clearly demonstrates that there is a sialolith in the submandibular duct.

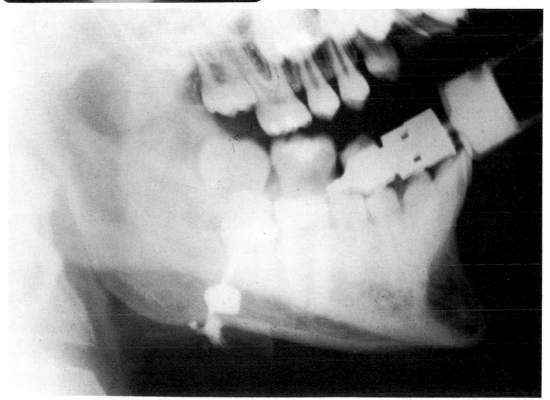

Figure 14–66 Sialolith at the origin of the duct of the submandibular gland. Note that it has practically completely blocked the duct, as very little of the radiopaque fluid has been forced around the salivary stone into the gland.

Use warm sodium hypochlorite mouth-washes (10 drops to $1/2$ glass of lukewarm water) every 3 hours.

Apply hot, wet dressings under the mandible continuously.

Sialoliths located in the submandibular gland should be removed by sialoadenectomy in most cases.

REFERENCES

1. Alexander, W. N., and Andrews, J. L.: Minor salivary gland sialolithiasis: Report of a case. J. Oral Surg., 23:461–462 (July), 1965.
2. Bach, H. G., and Buttenberg, D.: Postoperative parotitis. München Med. Wochenschr., 100:532 (Apr.), 1959.
3. Baurmash, H., and Mandel, L.: Pre-fabricated radiopaque sutures in ductal sialolithotomy. Oral Surg., 12:1296–1301 (Dec.), 1959.
4. Blatt, I. M., Denning, R. M., Zumberge, J. H., and Maxwell, J. H.: Studies in sialolithiasis: 1. The structure and mineralogical composition of salivary gland calculi. Ann. Otol. Rhinol. Laryngol., 47:595–617 (Sept.), 1958.
5. Buxton, R. N., Maxwell, H. H., and Cooper, D. R.: Tumors of the parotid gland. Laryngoscope, 59:565 (June), 1949.
6. Cheyne, V. D., Tiecke, R. W., and Horner, E. V.: A review of so-called mixed tumors of the salivary glands including an analysis of fifty additional cases. Oral Surg., 1:359 (Apr.), 1948.
7. Editorial: Tumors of parotid gland. J.A.M.A., 151(5):388 (Jan. 31), 1953.
8. Eisenbud, L., and Cranin, N.: The role of sialography in the diagnosis and therapy of chronic obstructive sialadenitis. Oral Surg., 16:1181 (Oct.), 1963.
9. Feldman, M. L.: Image-intensification fluorosialography. Oral Surg., 19:328–330 (Mar.), 1965.
10. Forsberg, A., Lagergren, C., and Lonnerblad, T.: Dental calculus: a biophysical study. Oral Surg., 13:1051–1060 (Sept.), 1960.
11. Garcelon, G. G.: Salivary gland tumors; management and results. Arch. Surg., 78:12–16 (Jan.), 1959.
12. James, A. G., and Saleeby, R.: The management of parotid gland tumors. Ohio State Med. J., 48:920 (Oct.), 1952.
13. Larson, D. L., and Schmidt, I. R.: Primary salivary gland tumors. Surg. Clin. North Am., 38:981–993 (Aug.), 1958.
14. Leake, D. L., Krakowiak, F. J., and Leake, R. C.: Suppurative parotitis in children. Oral Surg., 31:174–179 (Feb.), 1971.
15. Mandel, L., and Baurmash, H.: The role of sialography in extraparotid disease. Oral Surg., 31: 164–173 (Feb.), 1971.
16. Moose, S. M., and Summers, C. W.: Surgical correction of stenosed submandibular ducts by installation of polyethylene tube. Oral Surg., 18:563–568 (Nov.), 1964.
17. Ollerenshaw, R., and Rose, S.: Sialography: A valuable diagnostic method. Dent. Radiogr. Photogr., 29(3), 1957.
18. Prowler, J. R., Bjork, H., and Armstrong, G. F.: Major gland sialectasis. J. Oral Surg., 23:421–430 (July), 1965.
19. Quinn, J. H.: Calcified bodies (idiopathic) in the buccal soft tissues. Oral Surg., 19:292–294, 1965.
20. Quinn, J. H.: Intraductal anesthesia of salivary glands. J. Oral Surg., 29:230–231 (Mar.), 1971.
21. Quinn, J. H., and Graham, R.: Recurrent suppurative parotitis treated by intraductal antibiotics. J. Oral Surg., 31:36–39 (Jan.), 1973.
22. Sage, H. H.: Duct ligation and small-dose radiation: A new treatment for Mikulicz's disease. Oral Surg., 20:287–293 (Sept.), 1965.
23. Salley, J. J., Bryson, W. F., and Eshleman, J. R.: Effect of chronic vitamin A deficiency on dental caries in the Syrian hamster. J. Dent. Res., 38:1038–1043 (Sept.-Oct.), 1959.
24. Schulz, M. D., and Weisberger, D.: The sialogram in the diagnosis of swelling about the salivary glands. Surg. Clin. North Am., 27:1156, 1947.
25. Schulz, M. D., and Weisberger, D.: Personal communication.
26. Small, E. W.: Sialographic diagnosis of a parotid abscess in a case of membranous glomerulonephritis. Oral Surg., 20:71 (July), 1965.
27. Smith, I. H., et al.: Cobalt-60 Teletherapy. New York, Harper & Row, 1964.
28. Stafne, E. C.: Oral Roentgenographic Diagnosis. 4th ed. Philadelphia, W. B. Saunders Co., 1963.
29. Swinburne, G.: Sialoangiectasis. Br. J. Surg., 27:713, 1940.
30. Tyler, J. E., et al.: Tumors of the salivary glands, a review of 53 cases. Oral Surg., 16:623 (May), 1963.
31. Welch, K. J., and Trump, D. S.: The salivary gland. In Mustard, W. T., et al. (Eds.): Pediatric Surgery. 2nd ed. Vol. 1, pp. 215–231. Chicago, Year Book Medical Publishers, Inc., 1969.
32. Wuehrman, A. H., and Manson-Hing, L. R.: Dental Radiology. St. Louis, The C. V. Mosby Co., 1973.

CHAPTER 15

ORAL SURGERY AND THE GERIATRIC PATIENT

IRVIN V. UHLER, D.D.S.

Gerontology is the science and study of aging. Although the noun "geriatrics" defines that branch of the healing arts that deals with the structural changes, physiology, diseases and hygiene of old age, the adjective "geriatric" is applicable to the patient treated by any member of the health professions, for the problems to be treated in elderly persons cross all the specialty lines of medicine and dentistry. Today, there are two major subdivisions of gerontology. The first is the aging of the whole individual. This subdivision pertains to the overall clinical care and evaluation of the person. The second is the biologic processes of aging (senesence), affecting the various organs or structures of the individual.

When the geriatric patient develops a problem in the oral structures, it is often first referred to the oral surgeon because of his close daily hospital association with medical confreres. It has first been brought to the attention of the attending physician. As with any unusual problem, he, in turn, has referred it to an appropriate member of the hospital staff, in this instance, a member of the oral surgery service. This places a firm responsibility on the oral surgeon. Admittedly, many of these oral problems are nonsurgical in nature. Therefore, oral surgeons are morally bound to guide these exceptions into the appropriate hands for proper dental care; this may involve the periodontist, the prosthodontist, the endodontist or the general practitioner. The responsibility of oral surgeons entails a reasonable degree of follow-up, for

many in the profession are inexperienced in this sphere and are understandably reluctant to accept problems that cannot be solved in the environment of their own offices. Oral surgeons must patiently point the way, since members of their specialty at present are the only segment of the dental profession accustomed to working efficiently outside the confines of their offices. Already there are a minimum of 20 million people over 65 in the United States, and it is natural to conclude that a large percentage are unable to visit dental offices. Therefore, it is incumbent upon the aware members of the dental profession to educate all segments of the profes-

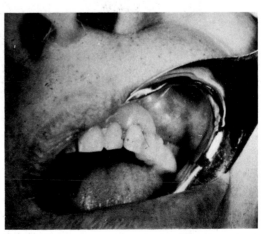

Figure 15–1 Unrecognized malignant growth in the left maxilla. The denture has been trimmed to accommodate the expanding neoplasm.

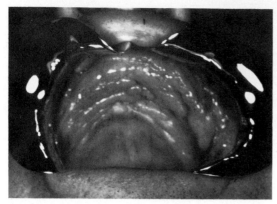

Figure 15–2 Massive hypertrophy of premaxillary area caused by wearing of the full upper denture against the six lower anterior teeth. (See Chapter 3 for other examples and surgical techniques.)

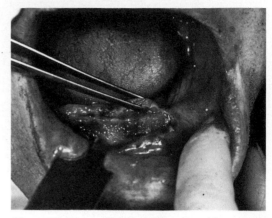

Figure 15–4 A knife-edged ridge caused by a denture uncorrected for the aging process. Excision of the sharp osseous projections and the hyperplastic tissue is indicated. (See Chapter 3.)

sion in rendering proper care to the senior citizens who are confined to their homes or an institution.

In the elderly patient, the most common problems involve irritation from dentures uncorrected to compensate for changes occurring in the alveolar structures because of deteriorations accompanying the aging process. These include massive hypertrophied tissue, sharp edentulous alveolar crests, sharp mylohyoid ridges, heavy muscle attachments from the denture-bearing regions, mandibles resorbed to the extent that the mental foramina and superior genial tubercles achieve the crest of the ridge. (In the older person the diminution in shape and size of the mandible

will often alter the facial appearance.) There are, of course, the all-too-frequent malignant diseases developing from denture irritation, again the result of the lack of compensation in the dentures for the normal aging changes of the denture-bearing tissues. Other conditions encountered are tori, expansile fibrous hypertrophy of the tuberosities, cysts, impacted teeth, retained roots, the results of external and internal trauma, salivary gland problems, leukoplakia, the effects of irradiation, acute and chronic periodontal problems, temporomandibular joint problems, neuritis, burning tongue and malnutrition. Most of these problems could be obviated in elderly persons if correct judgment were used and proper treatment urged when patients were younger. Measures to maintain proper vertical dimensions and occlusal harmony are most important in every stage of life. Correction of dentures to compensate for the aging process will prevent the formation of hypertrophied tissue, sharp edentulous alveolar crests, sharp mylohyoid ridges, and the formation of heavy muscle attachments. Tori should be removed when it becomes obvious that the patient will need replacement of missing teeth with prosthesis. Impacted teeth should be removed no later than the second decade of life. It is far more desirable to perform an elective procedure when the patient has youth on his side than to face a surgical emergency in the seventh or eighth decade of life. Notable among the conditions often neglected until surgery becomes imperative in later life are impacted teeth, retained roots, leukoplakia and cysts.

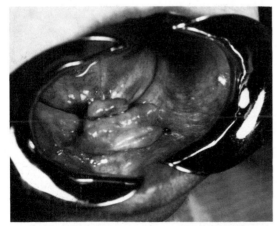

Figure 15–3 Hypertrophied tissue of symphysis area caused by ill-fitting denture that was not corrected for the aging process. (See Chapter 3.)

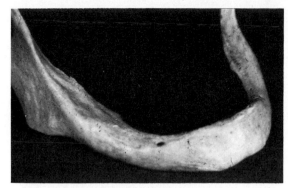

Figure 15–5 Mandible showing resorption to the extent that mental foramina have reached the crest of the ridge. Surgical repositioning is indicated to prevent trauma to the neurovascular bundle.

DIAGNOSIS IN THE OLDER PATIENT

Many of the disorders of the oral cavity begin insidiously and remain asymptomatic for years. Those that are symptomatic may be ignored by the patient, or overlooked through incomplete examination by the physician and dentist alike. A decade may pass before pain, asymmetry or dysfunction heralds something gone amiss. In undertaking treatment of conditions of the oral structures, the dentist must be alert for such systemic conditions as diabetes, arteriosclerosis, hypertension, arthritis, metastatic lesions, and malnutrition. Hence, anything but the team approach to the older patient is illogical.

In the area of diagnosis, the dentist must be aware of the physiologic changes occurring with the passage of time, or, to put it more bluntly, the manifestations of a prolonged period of degeneration. There is an appearance of generalized wasting, increased pigmentation of the exposed regions, decreased

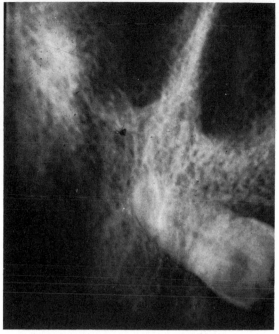

Figure 15–7 Impacted cuspid in an edentulous maxilla. The tissue surrounding the crown contained epithelial carcinoma.

water content, with drying and degenerative changes of sweat glands and a general loss of elasticity. There is greatly impaired regenerative capacity and loss of hair and teeth, with brittleness of the nails. All these are the more obvious signs. A major change, and one of importance to oral surgeons, is the osteoporosis, or atrophy that takes place in the bones. An old theory was that circulatory deficiency and depletion of calcium and phosphorus resulted in lack of organic material, with brittleness being the end result. Later views have been concerned with the reduction in the amount of organic matrix in the bones after increased protein breakdown that is an end result of androgen and estrogen deficiency. Osteoarthritic changes, as well, are common in the older patient. Oral surgeons see these changes reflected in the temporomandibular joint by hardening of the capsular ligament and stiffening of the interarticular disc. Fusion of the sternum is also common and impairs pulmonary ventilation through rigidity of the thorax, an important consideration in general anesthesia.

From the cardiovascular aspect, many factors must be kept in mind: A patient with a history of repeated angina attacks will have low coronary reserve and may produce an

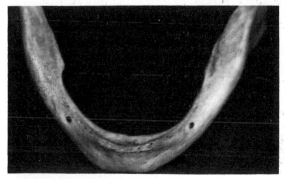

Figure 15–6 Extreme resorption of the mandible. A knife-edged ridge has developed, and mental foramina are on the crest of the denture-bearing area.

acute occlusion if the slightest degree of hypoxia occurs during anesthesia. The elderly person may manifest a hyperactive carotid sinus syndrome. If the patient has a history of tinnitus, blurring of vision, light-headedness, numbing and tingling in the extremities, he should undergo electrocardiographic and blood pressure studies before general anesthesia to check for this syndrome. However, the presence of heart disease does not mean that surgery must be withheld, for these patients typically improve with the elimination of infection. In the respiratory system, atrophy and fibrosis may reduce the lung fields as much as 25 per cent, and 35 per cent of the older persons show emphysematous changes. Blood values remain essentially unchanged in the geriatric patient. The foregoing diagnostic points again underscore the importance of the team approach in the management of the geriatric patient.

PREOPERATIVE CARE

Careful preoperative evaluation will reveal nutritional deficiencies that must be corrected before surgery is undertaken. Of prime urgency is correction of deficiencies in blood and protein. A rule of thumb holds that 500 cc. of whole blood is needed for every 3 points of deficit in the hematocrit under 50. Deficiencies in vitamins, calories and electrolytes must be restored preoperatively, except in the most extreme emergencies. In emergencies, the replacement of these factors

should be begun during surgery and be continued during and after the episode until corrected. Intravenous therapy must be carefully administered on the basis of cardiac deficiency, with constant vigilance for any sign of decompensation. Oral surgeons must always be alert for patients who have recently been on steroid therapy. They require 100 or 200 mg. of cortisone for several preoperative days, during surgery, and for several postoperative days, until the danger of shock is past.

If the surgery is to be undertaken for a malignant disease or if mutilating trauma will result in disfigurement, preoperative facial casts should be obtained. The anticipated loss should be reconstructed into a prosthesis in advance of surgery. Any deviation made necessary at surgery can be compensated for by use of self-curing acrylic resin. This immediate use of prosthesis will lessen the mental trauma to the patient, family and nursing staff alike. If the speech-producing organs will be rendered useless by surgery, a speech appliance such as the audio emitter may be incorporated into the patient's prosthesis, thus giving him immediate communication with those around him so he may easily make his needs known.

Careful preoperative consideration must involve everything possible to prevent the patient's postsurgical withdrawal from friends, family and society. No profession or specialty can cope single-handedly with such situations. The team approach involving multiple professions and disciplines coordinated in an orderly, long-range treatment plan is manda-

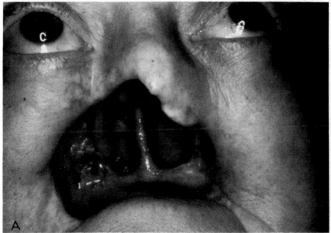
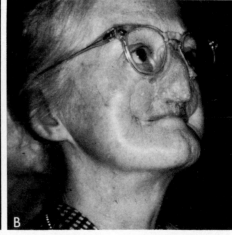

Figure 15–8 Mutilating surgery. Preoperative preparation of prosthesis prevents the patient's withdrawal from society. (Courtesy of Lancaster Cleft Palate Clinic.)

tory for a patient subjected to disfiguring orofacial surgery.

Included on the interdisciplinary team will be the oncologist, the oral pathologist, the oral surgeon, the radiologist and the internist (for the systemic care of the patient). There will be need for the prosthodontist, and there may be need for the periodontist or the endodontist. The speech therapist, the psychologist and the social worker as well may be needed to round out the team for total care.

ANESTHESIA

PREANESTHETIC MEDICATION

This is determined by the metabolic rate of the older patient. An older but vigorous patient may require and tolerate an adult dose, but the average older person will require only one third to one half the normal adult dose. The goal of premedication is relaxation, drying of secretions and lowering of the quantity of anesthetic agents required. The precautions necessary are avoidance of circulatory and respiratory depressions.

Narcotics. The narcotic drugs available are morphine, meperidine and pentazocine. Though morphine sulfate may be used with satisfactory results if the patient is in acute pain, the recommended dosage should not exceed 5 mg. Even this dosage may occasionally cause nausea, vomiting and depression of respiration and circulation. The cough reflex may also be depressed. In the event that morphine is used, the intravenous route is preferred, with the patient being watched carefully after each milligram is administered, because even small doses may give rise to circulatory or respiratory collapse. Another possibility is the postoperative occurrence of prolonged respiratory depression. Meperidine has the same indications as morphine. This drug, too, may depress responses of the central nervous system, as well as circulation and respiration. With the geriatric patient, no more than 10 mg. should be administered at one time, or profound circulatory collapse may occur. If the patient is on tranquilizers, meperidine should be used with caution. Pentazocine gives basically the same results as morphine. This drug, too, may cause nausea and dizziness, along with respiratory depression. It is used in the dosage of 20 to 30 mg. for the control of postoperative pain.

It must be emphasized that the use of a narcotic is not indicated in the aged patient unless he is in acute pain. The use of narcotics in preoperative and postoperative care of the aged definitely increases the hazards of a postoperative respiratory complication because of the depressant action upon respirations.

Barbiturates. These drugs are used principally for their hypnotic or sedative effect. Secobarbital or pentobarbital would be the drug of choice, given in a 30- to 60-mg. dose either intramuscularly or orally. If patients are agitated, this condition will be worsened by the use of these drugs. Primary contraindications to the preoperative use of the barbiturates are hepatic disease, cachexia, cardiovascular disease and pulmonary emphysema.

Anticholinergics. These prevent parasympathetic effects such as salivation and bradycardia. In most patients, these drugs will not be used, but when halothane or methoxyflurane is used, or endotracheal intubation is required, these drugs will help prevent bradycardia and cardiac arrest if given intravenously in concentrations over 0.4 mg.

Scopolamine. Because scopolamine causes depression of cortical impulses, this drug should not be used on elderly patients, since they become disoriented, have hallucinations and show increased motor activity.

Atropine Sulfate. This agent poses a parasympathetic blocking effect similar to scopolamine without producing cortical depression and is far more effective in blocking vagal effects. Respiration and tidal exchange are increased. Oral secretions are inhibited, and therefore atropine is an ideal drug for use prior to, and with, thiopental sodium–nitrous oxide–oxygen anesthesia. Cautious premedication based on the older patient's vigor and physical build will preclude the need for antagonists. However, when depression occurs as a result of poor tolerance on the patient's part, there is no substitute for oxygen administration with manual breathing assistance until the medication has run its course.

LOCAL ANESTHESIA IN GERIATRIC PATIENTS

Many procedures of a minor nature may be performed in the aged under local anesthesia, providing the patient is not hypertensive, does not have advanced arteriosclerosis and is not subject to agitation. Premedication is managed as outlined under Preanesthetic Medication. As in all procedures of a local anesthetic nature, total cooperation of the patient is of greatest importance. Fear and apprehension must be controlled. Although the oral route may be used to obtain sedation, better control and effectiveness are obtained by the intravenous route. Lidocaine, 1 in 100,000 dilution, is the anesthetic of choice, administered with a fine 26 gauge needle. Injections must be made slowly, as the fragile tissues of the elderly patient are prone to ballooning, with resultant hematomas, unless great gentleness is used. As the needle is advanced through the tissues, small amounts of the anesthetic should be injected as the needle progresses to its final destination. With effective nerve block or regional subperiosteal infiltration, or both, and a cooperative patient, most minor procedures in the field of oral surgery are possible.

CHOICE OF GENERAL ANESTHESIA

There is no universal anesthetic for any age group of patients, and no anesthetic is safer than the person administering it. Therefore, when a general anesthetic is indicated, there is the absolute necessity for an anesthesiologist to manage the patient, through the preoperative period, the episode of surgery and the postoperative period, until full recovery from the anesthetic is attained.

Unless contraindicated by liver damage, cardiac decompensation or allergic manifestations, an acceptable procedure involves fractional, symptomatic doses of 2 per cent thiopental sodium, supplemented with nitrous oxide and oxygen. Halothane may be added, if consistent with the patient's history, since it provides good muscular relaxation. Anesthesia is slowly induced with the intravenous agent in the senior patient, and when consciousness is lost, a full face mask is applied and 100 per cent oxygen is administered. This is important, as older patients are usually disturbed by application of a face mask while fully conscious.

Relaxation to accomplish intubation is achieved with succinylcholine chloride. This drug is preferable to curare, since its effect is of very short duration. The older patient is very slow to recover from the effects of curare. When intubation has been accomplished, anesthesia is maintained with a minimum of 50 per cent oxygen. In any event, even on the most vigorous patient, oxygen should not fall below the level existing in the environmental air. With the high oxygen concentration under controlled respiration technique, anesthesia is maintained by small intermittent supplementation of thiopental sodium given as needed.

MANAGEMENT DURING OPERATION

The geriatric patient does not tolerate even minimal blood loss without irreversible and irreparable damage. In delicate tissues, fine needles and fine suture material must be used. There is no point in using suture material of greater tensile strength than the tissues themselves. Mass ligation will produce necrosis, at best is insecure, and will reward the operator only with postoperative infection. Interrupted sutures will have less tendency to interfere with circulation and will result in better wound margins than continuous sutures. In the event of postoperative infection, drainage can be accomplished without disturbing the entire incision. Dead spaces must be prevented. Ignoring the foregoing will bring a postoperative legacy of thrombosis, circulatory impairment, infection and higher mortality.

Unless the surgery is lifesaving in nature, it will be assumed that all preoperative deficiencies have been met. Surgically, geriatric patients are likely to develop shock early, especially if not properly managed. Shock may be remedied primarily by the replacement of lost fluids and adequate oxygenation. Blood loss must be replaced drop for drop. Vasopressor drugs can be administered as a last resort. It cannot be compensated for by glucose or saline infusions, nor can shock be corrected in this way. Plasma expanders will do little, as they are incapable of oxygen and carbon dioxide transport. Strict attention must be given to all fluid loss. Too little replacement may lead to hyperpyrexia; excessive replacement may cause pulmonary edema, polyuria or circulatory collapse. Shock may be precipitated during surgery by exhaustion of the adrenocortical steroids. The patient often may be reclaimed by quick administration of corticosteroids. Falling blood pressure similarly may be stabilized by adrenal cortex extract in glucose in water. Hypoxia is inexcusable. Procedures in the older patient should be carried out as quickly as skill and good surgical principles will allow. After 1½ hours of surgery, mortality in geriatric patients increases 25 per cent.

POSTOPERATIVE MANAGEMENT

In the recovery room, the older patient's airway must be watched carefully. An oxygen supply, an airway device and suction apparatus must be at his side until he has recovered. Because of the debilities of old age, difficulties in clearing the airway of mucous secretions are ever present. If there is indication of respiratory distress, a tracheotomy is in order.

The patient should be continually urged to expectorate and to turn from side to side. When he reaches his room, this routine is continued. The geriatric oral surgery patient should be urged into ambulation within 24 hours to preclude circulatory, respiratory and urinary complications. Pain must be controlled without causing depression. Use of a sedative and an analgesic will give more efficacious pain relief with less respiratory depression than will a larger dose of a single analgesic. Routine antibiotic therapy is important; this procedure is defended on the basis that all oral surgical work on geriatric patients is done in a potentially infected field, in a patient who has a lowered resistance to infection. Fluids are replaced as deficiencies occur. Intake and output are measured. Postoperative feeding consists of fluids or soft diets. Deficiencies are overcome by use of protein hydrolysates, water-soluble vitamins, blood and serum albumin. If re-dressing or other phases of postoperative care will disturb the patient, pretreatment sedation and analgesia are in order. Use of the tranquilizing drugs will facilitate overall management of the tense or emotionally disturbed geriatric patient.

When an older patient has been discharged as cured, the obligation of the oral surgeon has not terminated. The postsurgical geriatric patient must be kept on an effective follow-up schedule. Tissues bordering the operative site must be inspected regularly, for in the late seventh, eighth and ninth decades, blood supply diminishes and nutritional and reparative processes are greatly diminished. If a postirradiation edentulous jaw shows evidence of sequestration but termination of exfoliation and infection is achieved, the oral surgeon cannot in good faith order the patient to leave his dentures out and dismiss him. Problems of malnutrition will take over that may become irreversible. Then, too, the postirradiation alveolar process is subjected to trauma unless covered with properly fitting dentures. Postoperative patients recovering from malignant disease must be on a regular review schedule, as must patients recovering from cysts with a recurrence potentiality.

Necessary precautions when outpatient premedication or general anesthesia is used. The ambulatory outpatient is not premedicated to the extent indicated for the hospitalized patient. In addition, he must be accompanied by a responsible adult, who will see him into his home. He must not drive an automobile for 24 hours, nor be around machinery that could cause injury. Alcohol must be restricted for 24 hours, and at home a responsible adult must be in attendance for a minimum of 24 hours.

CHAPTER 16

ORAL AND PANORAMIC RADIOGRAPHS AND LOCALIZATION

J. C. ESELMAN, D.D.S., W. J. UPDEGRAVE, D.D.S., and W. HARRY ARCHER, D.D.S.

The value of any diagnostic technique or instrument is judged by the amount and validity of the information that can be obtained from it. In dental radiography, the definitive and detailed information contained on periapical and bitewing films of good quality makes them indispensable in diagnosis. However, they are somewhat limited in their coverage. Occlusal and extraoral procedures can be utilized to cover a greater area, but at the sacrifice of some image detail and definition. Furthermore, there frequently is unavoidable distortion, enlargement, or superimposition of intervening anatomic structures, which often obscures information pertinent to the diagnosis. Panoramic radiography largely overcomes these limitations, and even though they lack the definition and detail of periapical radiographs, panoramic films contribute information that cannot be obtained by other conventional methods. When the panoramic radiograph is combined with a well-taken right-angle intraoral series, the scope of one complements the definition and detail of the other, resulting in a comprehensive and accurate radiographic survey of the maxillomandibular region. A complete radiographic examination, including both intra- and extraoral films, is an essential aid in diagnosis and treatment planning in oral surgery (Figs. 16–1, 16–2 and 16–3).*

---

*Adapted from Updegrave, W. J.: Visualizing the mandibular ramus in panoramic radiography. Oral Surg., *31*:422–429, 1971; and Updegrave, W. J.: The role of panoramic radiography in diagnosis. Oral Surg., *22*:49–57, 1966.

LOCALIZATION

When an oral procedure is indicated involving teeth or foreign bodies that are beneath the surface of the gingivae, it is imperative that the exact location of the body be determined, as an aid to the operator. Localization is indicated in the following instances: foreign bodies; broken needles; broken instruments; filling materials in the alveolar process; retained roots; impacted, supernumerary and unerupted teeth; calculi in a gland or duct of salivary glands; fractures of the maxilla and mandible; fracture of condyles; expansion of the alveolar process in cystic formation and intraosseous tumors. The following types of dental radiographic examinations are used in localization: periapical, bitewing and occlusal (topographical and cross-section). Extraorally the lateral jaw, oblique jaw, lateral head, posteroanterior (Waters' view) and panoramic radiographs are necessary to supplement intraoral radiographs. These radiographs are utilized in various ways in a number of localization techniques.

STEREOSCOPIC METHOD

This method is seldom used at the present time because of the development of more simplified and accurate methods.

Stereoscopic radiography consists of exposing and processing two films, one for each eye, by shifting the tube in a horizontal plane the distance between the pupils of the eye, then viewing these radiographs with a device known as a stereoscope. By this means two flat pictures are merged into one with depth and perspective (Fig. 16–7).

Dentists have failed to master this procedure because of the following technical difficulties: placing two films accurately in the same position in the mouth for two separate exposures; securing absolute immobilization of the patient's head between exposures; determining the proper vertical and horizontal angles of projection with two shifts of the tube; proper mounting of the films.

The problems of viewing stereoscopic films, the occasionally exaggerated stereoscopic effect, and the necessity of using a stereoscope also added to the difficulties in the development of this method.

SHIFT-SKETCH METHOD

This method is easily applied and gives sufficient information to be of practical value, but the occlusal method of localization (cross-section) remains the most accurate at the present time.

The technique of procedure is to expose and process two or more periapical radiographs of the same area, shifting the tube horizontally between exposures. As a result of the changes in horizontal angulation, the unerupted tooth or foreign body moves mesially or distally in relation to the other teeth or landmarks.

The rule governing the shift-sketch method is as follows: If the unerupted tooth or foreign body moves in the same direction in

(*Text continued on page 992*)

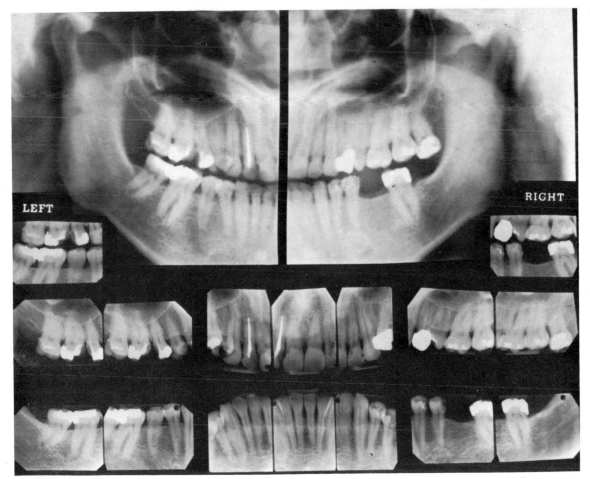

Figure 16–1 Panoramic and periapical films. One contributes to greater coverage, while the other shows definition and detail of the structures. (From Updegrave, W. J.: Visualizing the mandibular ramus in panoramic radiography. Oral Surg., *31*:422–429, 1971.)

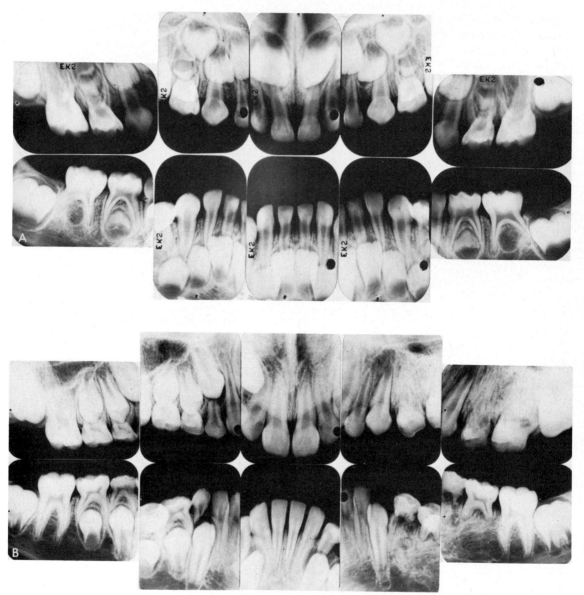

Figure 16–2   *A*, Patient 2½ years old. Perfect primary dentition, free of caries and with normal occlusion. Note the various stages of the formation of the permanent teeth at this age. *B*, Patient 8½ years of age with a mixed dentition. Also note the congenital absence of the right maxillary and mandibular permanent first and second bicuspids.

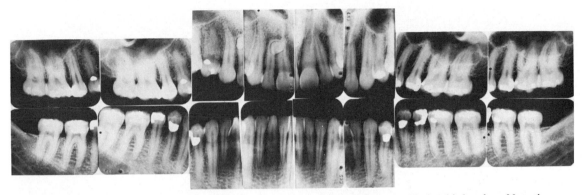

Figure 16–3 Patient 27 years of age with congenitally absent maxillary and mandibular third molars. Note the presence of a rudimentary maxillary central incisor.

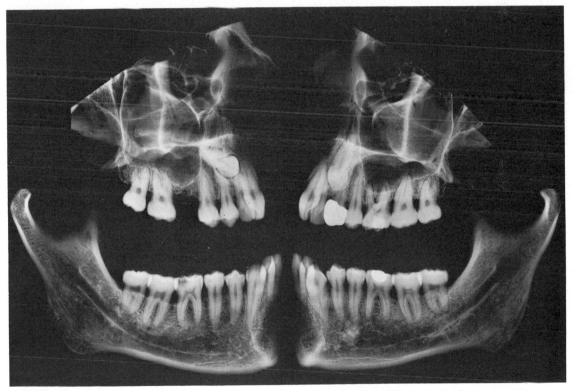

Figure 16–4 Lateral radiographs of each side of skull after sectioning. Note bilateral palatally impacted permanent cuspids.

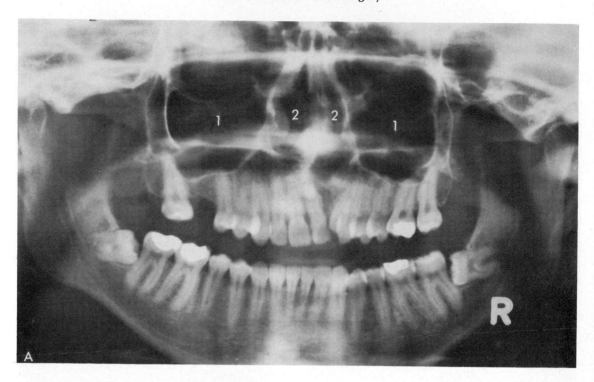

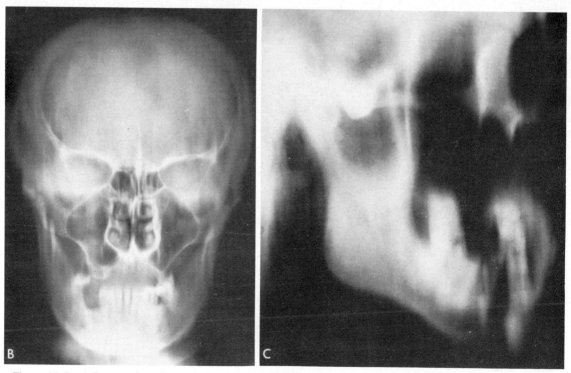

Figure 16–5   *A,* Panoramic radiograph showing the maxillary sinuses *(1)* and nasal cavity *(2). B,* Tomogram of maxillary and small frontal sinuses in an edentulous maxilla. Note how in this case the maxillary sinuses extend *beneath* the floor of the nasal cavity. This radiograph also shows the nasal cavity and turbinates in excellent cross-sectional detail. *C,* Tomogram of the temporomandibular joint. Better visualization can usually be obtained with the modified ramus panoramic view, as described later in the text.

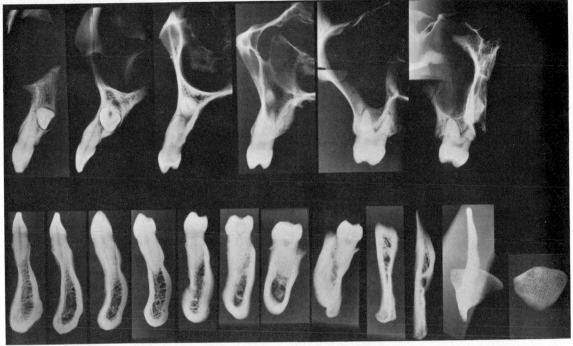

Figure 16–6 Radiographs made after additional vertical sectioning of one half of the skull.

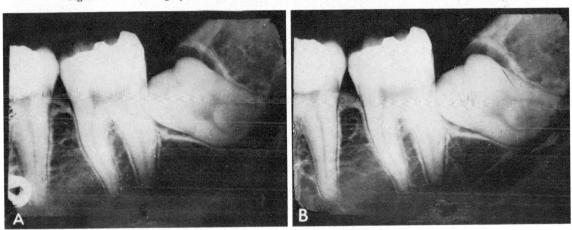

Figure 16–7 Two views for use in stereoscopic method.

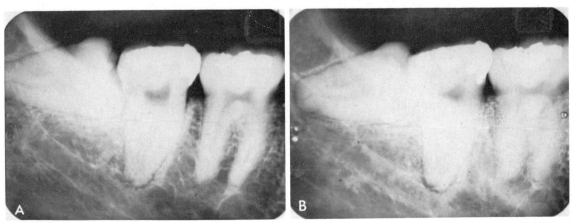

Figure 16–8 *A,* Lingual aspect of a horizontally impacted mandibular third molar. *B,* The tube is shifted to the left, and the impacted tooth moves to the right on the second molar; therefore, the impaction is on the buccal side.

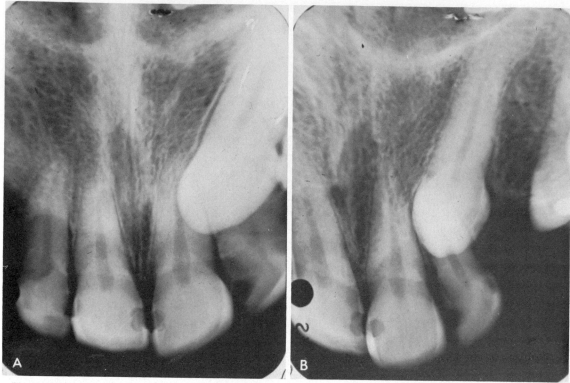

Figure 16–9 Lingual aspect. The tube is shifted to the right, and the impacted tooth moves to the right; therefore, the impaction is lingual.

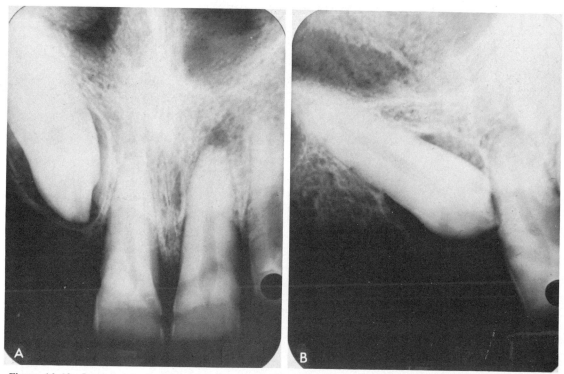

Figure 16–10 Impacted tooth, lingual aspect. *A,* The rays are projected straight through the central incisors, at the normal vertical angulation. *B,* The film and tube are shifted slightly to the observer's left, causing the impacted cuspid to move to the right and closer to the central incisor; therefore, it moves opposite to the direction in which the tube was shifted and is located to the labial side.

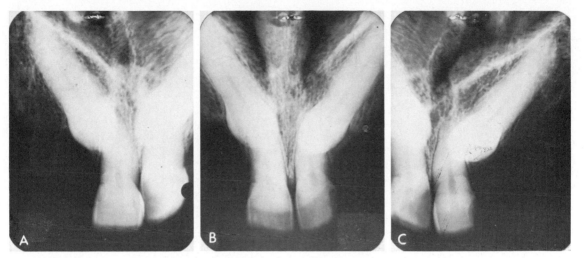

Figure 16-11 Impacted teeth, lingual aspect. *B,* The rays are directed straight through the central incisors, using normal vertical angulation. *C,* The tube is shifted to the right, and the impacted right cuspid moves in the same direction. *A,* The tube is shifted to the left, and the impacted left cuspid moves in the same direction; therefore, both cuspids are located to lingual.

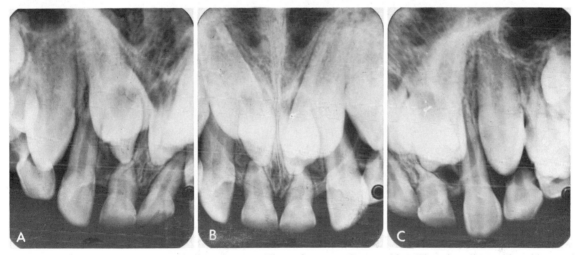

Figure 16-12 Supernumerary teeth, lingual aspect. The patient was 10 years old. *B,* There is radiographic evidence of two supernumerary teeth and impacted right and left central incisors. *C,* The tube was shifted to the right, the supernumerary tooth moved closer to the lateral incisor, and the central incisor moved away from the lateral incisor. *A,* The tube was shifted to the left, and the same movement of the corresponding teeth on the left side occurred; therefore, the impacted supernumerary teeth are located lingual to the impacted central incisors.

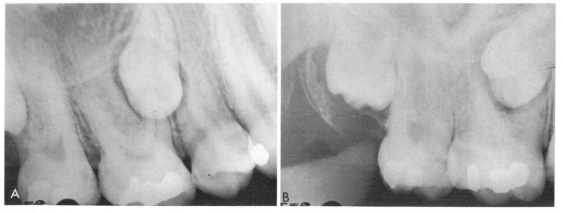

Figure 16-13 Radiograph *A* is made with the standard technique. *B,* The tube is shifted distally, and this area is radiographed with the standard technique. The unerupted second bicuspid has moved distally, the *same direction* that the tube was moved. This proves that the second bicuspid is on the lingual side of the arch.

which the tube is shifted, it (the unerupted tooth or foreign body) is located on the lingual side. If it moves in the opposite direction in which the tube is shifted, the location is on the labial or buccal side. This method can also be applied by changing the vertical angulation of the tube.

Diagrammatic and practical illustration of the shift-sketch method is shown in Figures 16–8 to 16–13.

OCCLUSAL METHOD (TOPOGRAPHICAL AND CROSS-SECTION)

Topographical occlusal views are indicated when the dentist desires to observe a gross view of a cystic area or an impacted tooth that has not been fully oriented on the periapical film.

For accurate localization the cross-section occlusal view should be used in combination with the periapical film, which extends the angle of projection to an arc ranging from zero to 90 degrees, depending on the region radiographed.

The vertical portion of the frontal bone is the greatest obstruction encountered in occlusal views (cross-section) of the anterior portion of the maxilla where it is parallel with the long axis of the anteriors. In certain cases some modification of the vertical angle is necessary to disclose this region.

The occlusal film is size 2¼ by 3 inches and is manufactured in regular and super-speed. The super-speed is the best film for occlusal views (cross-section) of the maxilla because of its extreme sensitivity. The intraoral cassette should be used with the super-speed films for occlusal views of the maxilla, since it decreases the time of exposure and chance of movement of the patient.

The technique of procedure is standardized and well illustrated in the textbooks of dental radiography. Figures 16–14 to 16–17 give examples of the topographical application of the occlusal method.

Figures 16–18 to 16–30 give examples of the cross-sectional application of the occlusal method.

EXTRAORAL METHOD

Extraoral radiographs will supplement the periapical and occlusal examinations for locations or areas that cannot be reached intraorally.

Extraoral radiographs are necessary to complete the radiographic survey in cases of impacted teeth, fractures, cysts, foreign bodies, and malformations.

The reader is referred to Chapter 17, "Roentgen Anatomy of the Facial Bones and Jaws," for detailed information on this subject.

The equipment should be available and the technical procedures well understood for extraoral examinations. Figures 16–31 to 16–36 illustrate the application of the extraoral method in various abnormalities of the maxilla and mandible.

CONTRAST MEDIA

Iodized oil and gutta percha are the materials used for contrast media and are indicated for use in the following conditions: in tracing fistulas that open into the oral cavity; to examine the depth of periodontal pockets; to show the outline of cysts; to follow the outline of ducts and glands in salivary disturbances.

Figures 16–37 to 16–39 illustrate the application of the situations in which contrast media are useful in oral radiographic localization.

WIRE CABLE SUTURES

See Chapter 4, page 246, for this technique.

PANOGRAPHY*

DEFINITION AND DETAIL

Since panography utilizes intensifying screens and an increased object-film distance, the definition and detail of the individual teeth and adjacent structures are inferior to those produced by periapical and bitewing radiographs of good quality (see Figure 16–1). Caries is not as sharply demarcated in panography, and incipient interproximal lesions are sometimes obscured in the posterior regions because of overlapping images.

(*Text continued on page 1006*)

*Adapted from Updegrave, W. J.: Visualizing the mandibular ramus in panoramic radiography. Oral Surg., *31*:422–429, 1971; and Updegrave, W. J.: The role of panoramic radiography in diagnosis. Oral Surg., *22*:49–57, 1966.

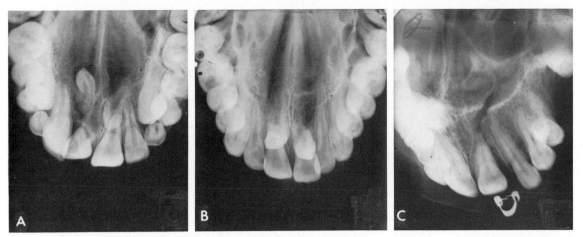

Figure 16–14 Supernumerary teeth and fracture of maxilla, lingual aspect. *A* and *B,* Views of supernumerary teeth in the anterior portion of the maxilla. *C,* Fracture of the maxilla extending along the distal edge of the upper right central incisor, through the floor of the nose and distal to the second molar.

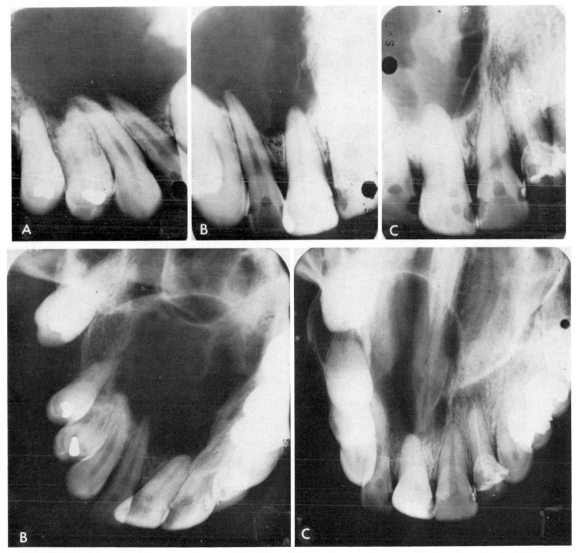

Figure 16–15 Cyst, lingual aspect. The periapical films show a large cystic area extending from the left side of the median line to the upper right second molar, involving the maxillary sinus. The topographical occlusal views show the complete cystic outline. Note that the occlusal views give additional information about the areas shown in the correspondingly labeled periapical films.

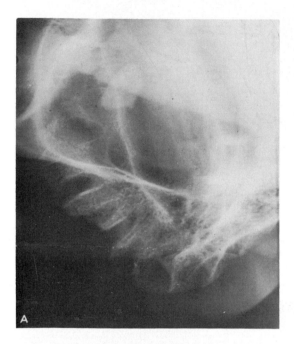

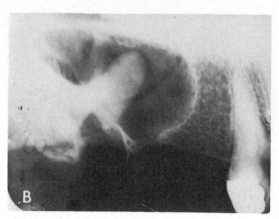

Figure 16–16   Fractured root, lingual aspect. An illustration of the lingual root forced into the maxillary sinus *(A)*, with an occlusal topographical view as a supplement *(B)*. Many times root tips in the sinus will not show on the periapical film and can be located only with the use of the topographical view. Note the fractured lingual root.

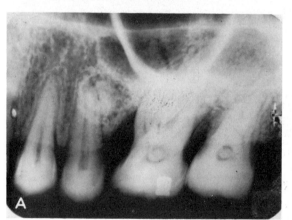

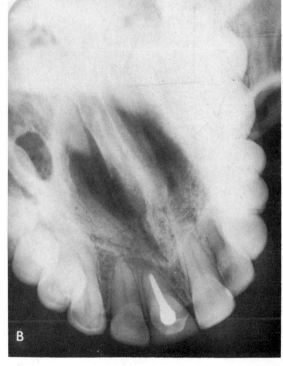

Figure 16–17   Fractured root, lingual aspect. *A,* The periapical radiograph of this case shows a small radiopaque area near the apex of the upper right second bicuspid. *B,* A topographical view shows it to be a root tip under the zygomatic process. The patient's history revealed difficulty during extraction of the upper right first molar 10 years previously.

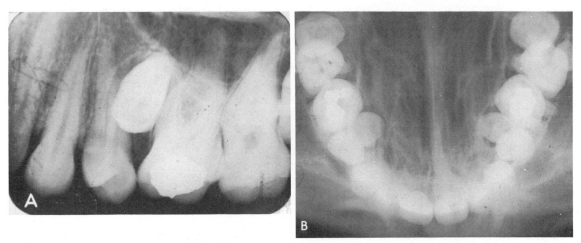

Figure 16-18 Impacted and supernumerary teeth, lingual aspect. *A,* The upper right second bicuspid is impacted. *B,* Occlusal view showing the upper right second bicuspid located in a horizontal position with the apex extending out the buccal side, between the roots of the right first bicuspid and molar. The upper left second bicuspid is impacted, but is not in a true horizontal position. Note the supernumerary teeth on either side in the molar region, in buccal location.

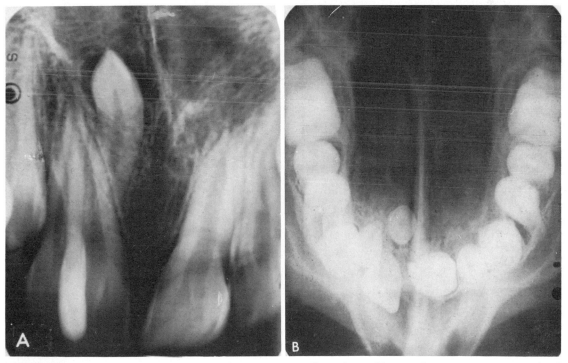

Figure 16-19 Supernumerary tooth, lingual aspect. *A,* Radiographic evidence of a supernumerary tooth. *B,* Occlusal view showing lingual location. This is an excellent illustration of definite localization. Application of the shift-sketch method in this case would reveal the supernumerary tooth in lingual location, but not as accurately as the occlusal view.

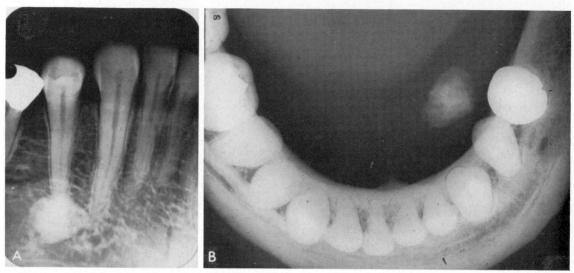

Figure 16–20 Salivary stone, lingual aspect. *A,* Radiopaque area at the apex of the lower left first bicuspid, which could be mistaken for an area of condensing osteitis. *B,* Occlusal view showing this area to be a salivary calculus in Wharton's duct.

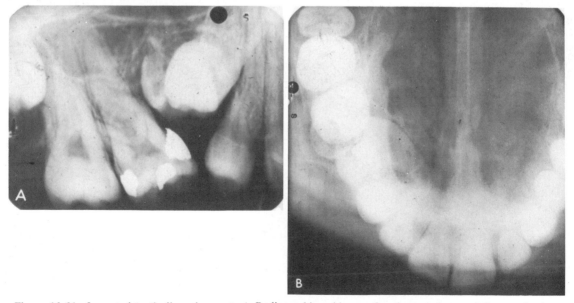

Figure 16–21 Impacted teeth, lingual aspect. *A,* Radiographic evidence of an impacted upper left second primary molar and second bicuspid. *B,* Occlusal view showing accurate localization; the primary molar shows buccal location, and the upper second bicuspid is in lingual location, with the apex toward the anterior teeth.

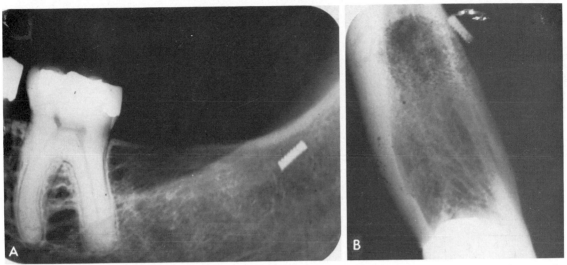

Figure 16–22   Foreign body, lingual aspect. *A,* Radiographic evidence of a crosscut fissure bur in the lower molar region. *B,* Occlusal view of the same region, showing the bur on the lingual side in soft tissue. This illustration should convince the reader that depth is not present on the radiograph. From *A* alone the interpreter is unable to tell whether the bur is on the buccal side, in the alveolar bone or on the lingual side. The supplemental occlusal view is necessary for accurate interpretation. (See Chapter 25 for more examples of foreign bodies and the techniques for their removal when indicated.)

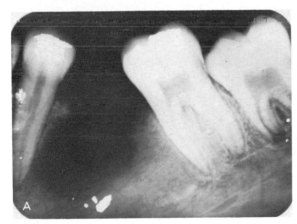

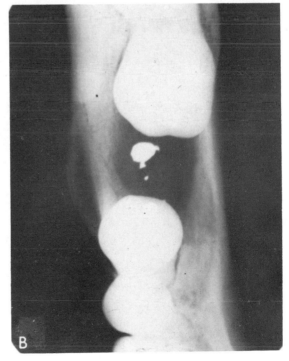

Figure 16–23   Foreign body with a cystic area, lingual aspect. *A,* Radiographic evidence of a foreign body with cystic formation in the lower first molar region. *B,* Definite localization of the foreign body, with cystic expansion of the alveolar bone on the buccal side; the thin radiopaque (white) line is the interpretive feature of how much expansion has occurred.

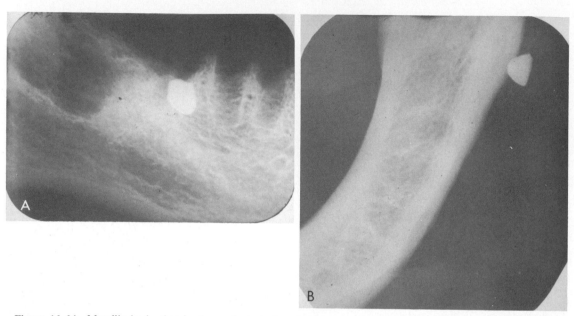

Figure 16-24   Metallic body that in the periapical view *(A)* appears to be in the cancellous bone. The occlusal radiograph *(B)* proves otherwise.

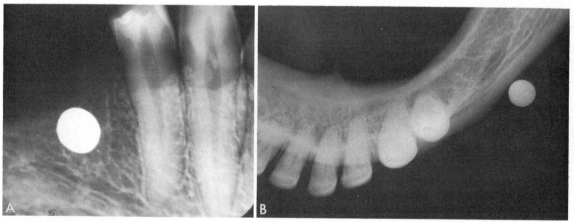

Figure 16-25   *A*, BB shot appears on the periapical film to be contained in the bone. *B*, Occlusal film shows it actually to be in the buccal soft tissue.

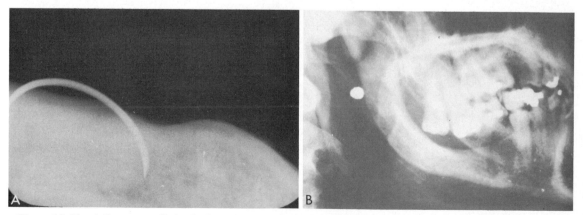

Figure 16-26   *A*, Suture needle in the buccal soft tissue. *B*, Left oblique radiograph of the mandible with a foreign body distal to the ramus.

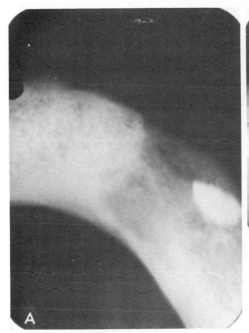

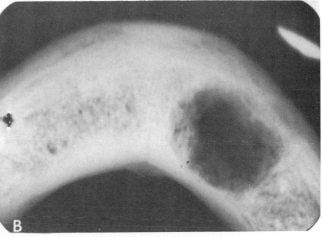

Figure 16–27 *A*, Periapical film shows a metallic body that appears to be in the osseous tissue of the mandibular right bicuspid area. *B*, The occlusal film reveals its presence in soft tissue of the lip. (See Chapter 25 for technique of its removal.)

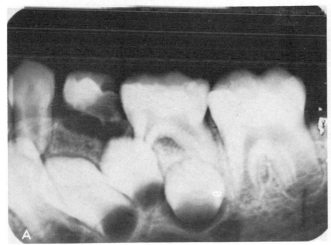

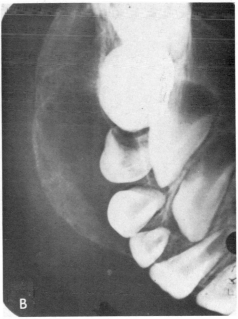

Figure 16–28 Cystic expansion of the alveolar bone, lingual aspect. The patient was 5 years old. *A*, Evidence of the succedaneous teeth in a slightly abnormal erupting position. *B*, Occlusal view showing marked expansion of the alveolar bone on the buccal and lingual sides. The thin radiopaque (white) line is the interpretive feature.

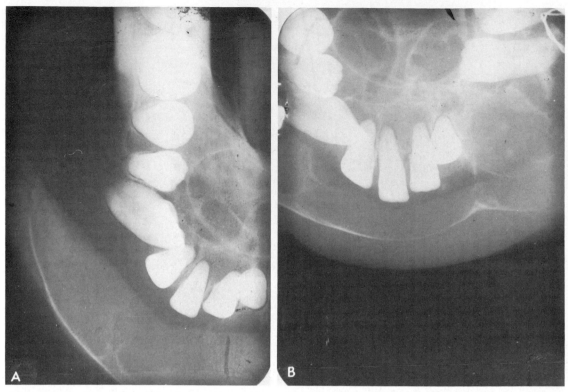

Figure 16–29 Expansion of the alveolar bone with cystic formation. Occlusal films of the anterior portion of the mandible of the same patient as shown in Figure 16–28, showing a severe expansion of the alveolar bone, with cystic formation and displacement of certain teeth.

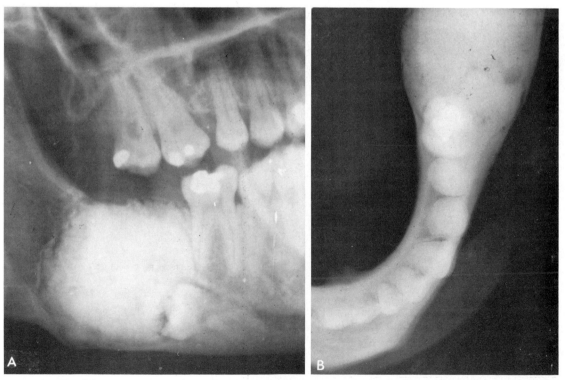

Figure 16–30 Odontoma. *A,* Lateral jaw film showing radiographic evidence of an odontoma. Note the position of the second molar. *B,* Occlusal film showing a marked expansion of the alveolar bone, with the inverted second molar in a buccal location.

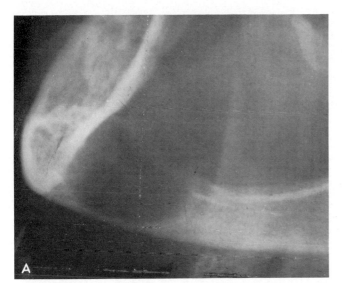

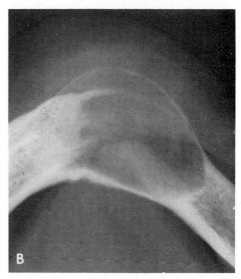

Figure 16–31 A cyst in the anterior portion of the mandible. *A*, Oblique jaw radiograph showing a cystic area in the anterior portion of the mandible. *B*, Occlusal film showing a marked expansion of the labial cortical bone.

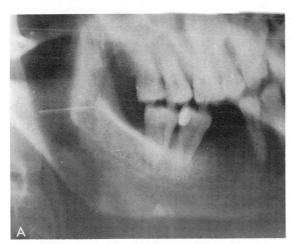

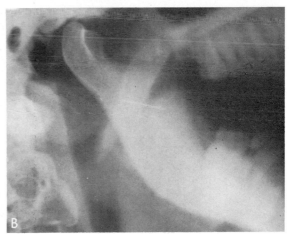

Figure 16–32 Broken needle. *A*, Oblique jaw radiograph with broken needle from a mandibular injection, the teeth being in normal occlusion. *B*, Lateral head radiograph with the mouth opened, giving a more accurate position of the needle. The modified ramus technique No. 1 or No. 2, as described in this chapter, will have less distortion and should be used if possible.

A different method that will aid the operator is to insert another needle in correct position for the mandibular injection, and take a lateral head radiograph, with the mouth open. This will reveal whether the broken needle is above or below the correctly inserted needle. (See also Chapter 25.)

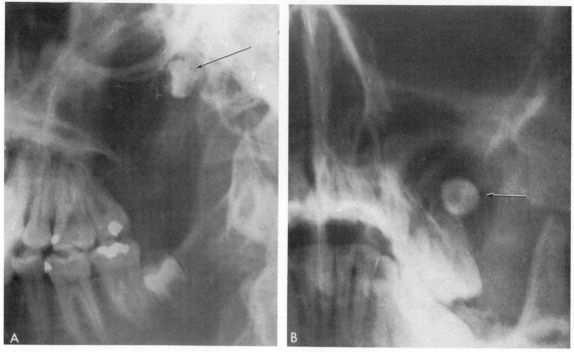

Figure 16–33 Impacted and misplaced tooth with cystic formation. *A*, Oblique jaw radiograph showing an upper right third molar in abnormal position. *B*, Posteroanterior radiograph showing the third molar in buccal location, with a cystic area and expansion of the alveolar process.

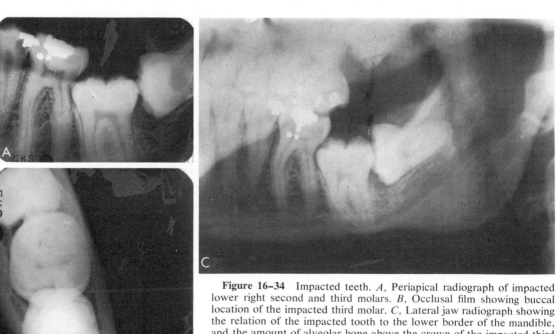

Figure 16–34 Impacted teeth. *A*, Periapical radiograph of impacted lower right second and third molars. *B*, Occlusal film showing buccal location of the impacted third molar. *C*, Lateral jaw radiograph showing the relation of the impacted tooth to the lower border of the mandible, and the amount of alveolar bone above the crown of the impacted third molar. The reader should note that each type of radiographic examination has added information to aid the operator.

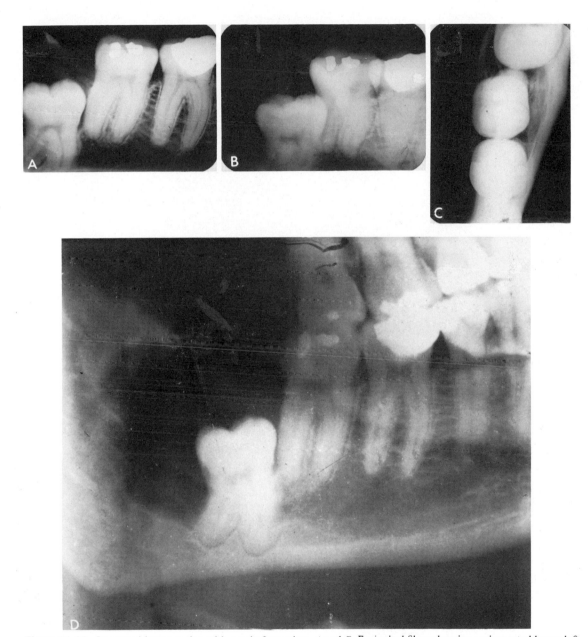

Figure 16–35 Impacted lower molar with cystic formation. *A* and *B*, Periapical films showing an impacted lower left third molar with cystic formation. *C*, Occlusal view showing buccal location of the impacted tooth. *D*, Lateral jaw radiograph adding information which aids the operator: the relation of the impacted tooth to the lower border of the mandible and the complete outline of the cystic area in the ramus.

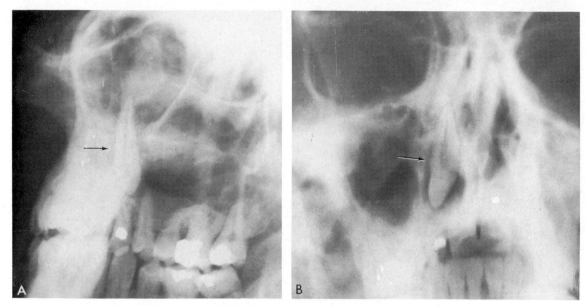

Figure 16–36 Impacted cuspid. *A*, Lateral head radiograph showing an impacted cuspid. Note the high position of the crown in relation to the apices of the other teeth. *B*, Posteroanterior film (Waters' position) showing location of the impacted cuspid in relation to the nasal cavity and maxillary sinus.

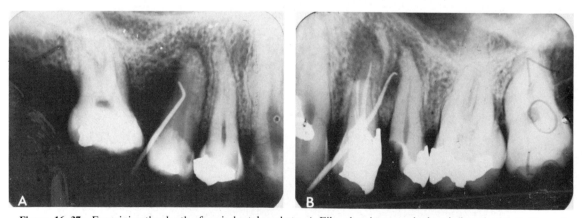

Figure 16–37 Examining the depth of periodontal pockets. *A*, Film showing a marked periodontal pocket. The gutta percha points are of greatest value in determining the depth of periodontal pockets on the buccal and lingual sides of the roots. *B*, Gutta percha point placed in a fistula and following a tract distally to the second bicuspid.

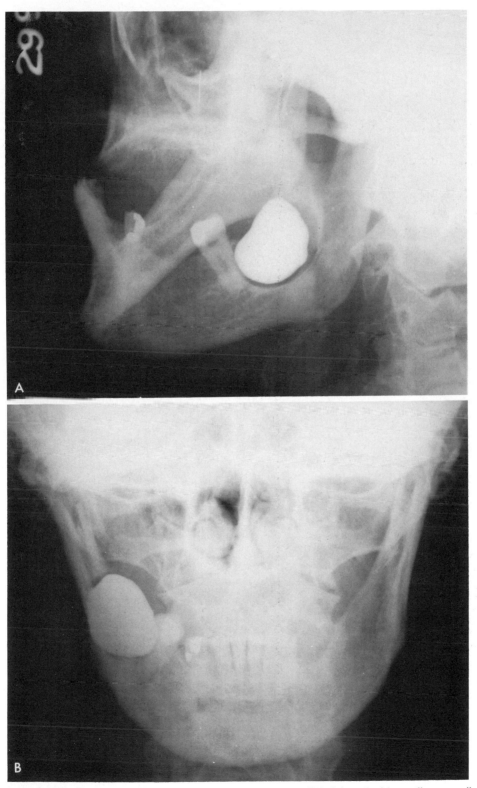

Figure 16-38   Residual cyst of the body and ramus of the mandible injected with a radiopaque oil.

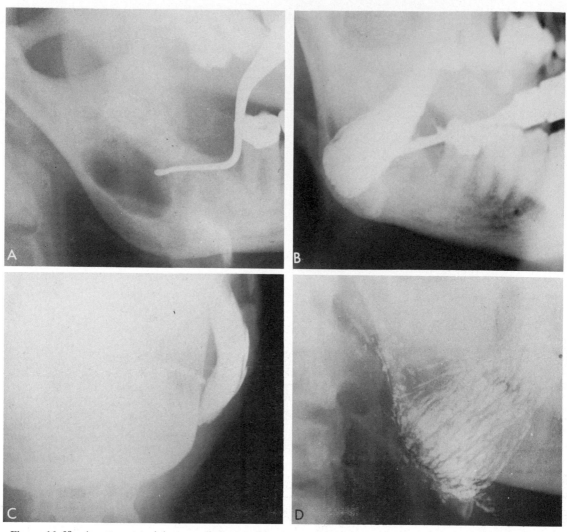

Figure 16–39 An attempt to inject a radiopaque oil into a cyst failed *(A)* because the syringe with the dye inadvertently penetrated the thin overlying lateral bone *(B)* and injected the dye into the masseter muscle *(C)*. Seven months later the dye is still present and distributed throughout the entire muscle *(D)*. The patient was symptom-free from the time of the original injection.

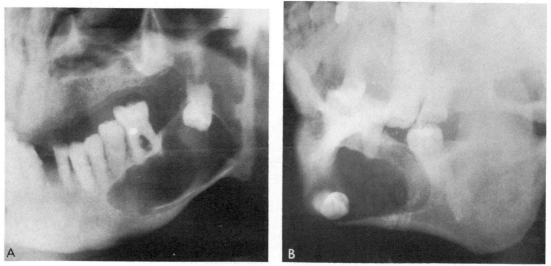

Figure 16–40 The panoramic radiograph of the dentigerous cyst shown in *A* is relatively free of the obvious distortions that are shown in *B*, which was an oblique radiograph of the mandible.

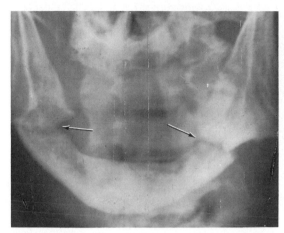

Figure 16–41 Bilateral fracture of an edentulous mandible. This posteroanterior view shows both posterior fragments rotated toward the median line and the anterior fragment pulled back and down. This view should alway supplement a lateral jaw radiograph of either side.

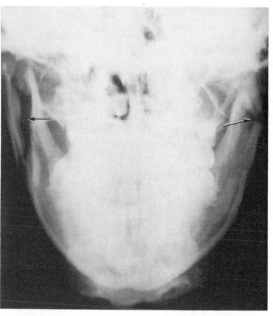

Figure 16–42 Nose-chin position for this posteroanterior radiograph of the mandible, which reveals a right subcondylar fracture and a vertical fracture of the left mandibular ramus.

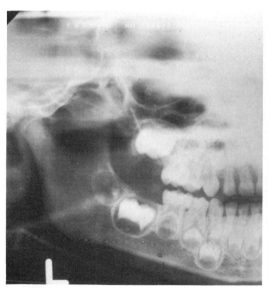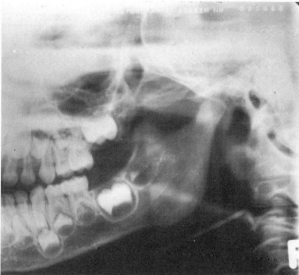

Figure 16–43 Panoramic radiograph of 4½-year-old patient. (From Updegrave, W. J.: Visualizing the mandibular ramus in panoramic radiography. Oral Surg., *31*:422–429, 1971.)

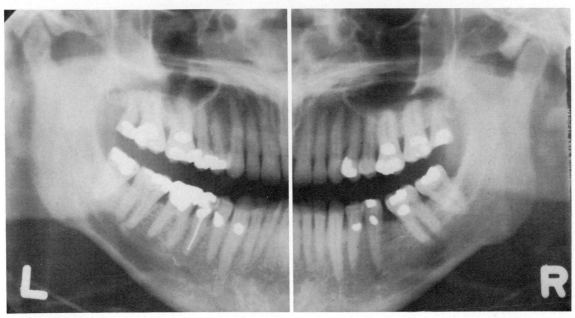

Figure 16–44 Panoramic radiograph of an adult, taken in the conventional position. (From Updegrave, W. J.: Visualizing the mandibular ramus in panoramic radiography. Oral Surg., *31*:422–429, 1971.)

The periapical bone pattern is also less definitive on the panograph, and in periodontal lesions fine details of importance to the diagnosis are sometimes lost. However, the continuity of projection of the alveolar bone may have some advantage over the segmented projection seen on periapical and bitewing radiographs. Definition and detail of the trabecular bone pattern are also superior on intraoral radiographs. The importance of this is evident in conditions of periapical pathosis, in which the differential diagnosis often hinges on the radiographic characteristics of the lesion. However, panography is not intended to be a substitute for periapical radiography; rather, it should be considered as a supplementary examination technique that supplies additional information for diagnosis. It is gross visualization of the entire maxillomandibular region that directs attention to areas requiring further detailed study.[10]

ADVANTAGES

One of the great advantages of panoramic radiography is its coverage. In addition to the teeth and supporting tissues, the maxillary region, extending to the superior third of the orbits, is visualized, and the entire mandible, extending distally to the temporomandibular joint region, is also included in the examination. Such broad coverage is essential when a lesion extends beyond the range of conventional radiographic procedures (Fig. 16–44).

Panography is sometimes referred to as a radiographic hemisection that produces the same result as a conventional radiograph of separated sides of a sectioned skull (see Figure 16–4). This makes the anatomic structures more identifiable and orients the teeth in their correct relationship to adjacent structures and to each other (Fig. 16–45).

In patients with limited opening of the jaws, or none, due to trauma, ankylosis, trismus from acute infection or pain in temporomandibular joints, panography is clearly indicated.

DISTORTION

Some degree of *inherent* distortion is present in all panoramic radiographs. This is unavoidable, since a fixed beam-film relationship is utilized to project structures that vary greatly in the same individual and between individuals. Differences in conformity and size of the jaws and teeth, variations in arrangement of the teeth in the jaws, and asymmetry between the right and left sides all contribute to some degree of distortion. In periapical radiography adjustments in film positioning and angulation are made to compensate for those differences, but in panography adjustment is limited to positioning of the patient's head.

Lineal distortion of the teeth, recorded as foreshortening, elongation, magnification, or reduction in size, may occur in panoramic radiography. This will be exaggerated if the patient's head is incorrectly positioned. To minimize this, the following rules should be observed when using the panoramic radiographic unit:

1. Align the midsagittal plane with the vertical center line of the chin support (Fig. 16–46A).
2. Center the lower border of the mandible on the chin support, equidistant from each side.
3. Parallel the occlusal plane of the teeth (tragus-ala line) with the floor (Fig. 16–46A).

If the midsagittal plane is off center, or if the mandible is incorrectly positioned on the support, the image of the side that is farthest from the film will be enlarged, while that of the opposite side will be reduced in size. Patients with marked asymmetry may require a different head position for each side, making it necessary to take separate exposures to avoid a similar distortion.

The occlusal plane of the teeth should be parallel to the floor (Fig. 16–46A). If the occlusal plane is positioned upward from this parallel position, the shadow of the hard palate is projected over the apices of the maxillary teeth. In addition, the maxillary molars are elongated and enlarged, while the mandibular molars are slightly reduced in size, with less distinct profiles (Fig. 16–46C and E).

If the occlusal plane is positioned downward from a position parallel to the floor, the mesiodistal aspects of all teeth become narrowed, and their relationships are crowded. In addition, there is an overall loss of definition in the teeth (Fig. 16–46D and F).

In addition to lineal distortion, there is a 7 to 12 per cent overall enlargement of the radiographic image because of the varying object-film distances and the fixed anode-film distance. However, enlargement sometimes serves the purpose of drawing attention to conditions that conceivably could be overlooked in a routine intraoral examination.

Distortion of Mandibular Rami. The oral surgeon is vitally and continuously concerned with the mandibular rami because of the frequency of impactions, cysts, fractures, tumors and temporomandibular dysarthroses in this anatomic area. The structures that exhibit the greatest distortion and indistinctness on the conventionally taken panoramic radiograph are the mandibular rami with their condyloid and coronoid processes. If this problem is eliminated, the value of panoramic radiography as a diagnostic adjunct would be further enhanced. The modified technique described in following paragraphs will accomplish this.

(*Text continued on page 1011*)

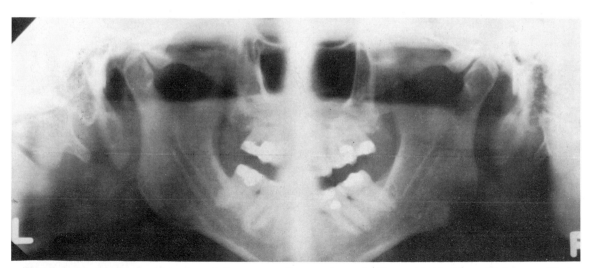

Figure 16–45 Modified ramus view of the same patient as shown in Figure 16–44. (From Updegrave, W. J.: Visualizing the mandibular ramus in panoramic radiography. Oral Surg., *31*:422–429, 1971.)

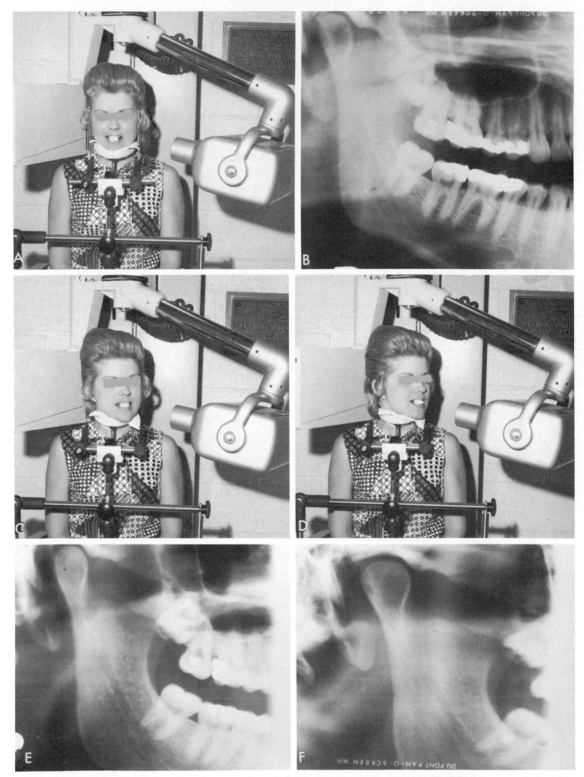

Figure 16–46 *A* and *B*, Conventional panoramic technique, right mandible. *C* and *E*, Modified ramus technique No. 1 of right mandible. *D* and *F*, Modified ramus technique No. 2 of right mandible. (From Updegrave, W. J.: Visualizing the mandibular ramus in panoramic radiography. Oral Surg., *31*:422–429, 1971.)

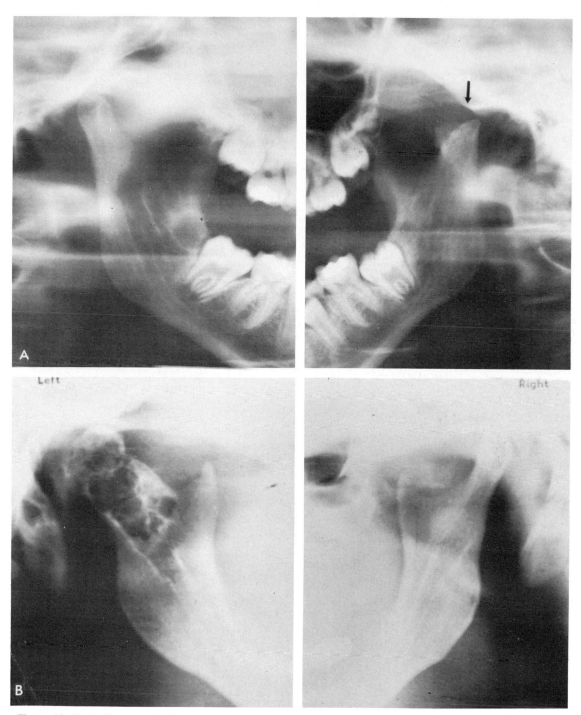

Figure 16–47 *A*, Ramus technique disclosing fracture of right condyle. *B*, Myxoma of left condyle. (From Updegrave, W. J.: Visualizing the mandibular ramus in panoramic radiography. Oral Surg., *31*:422–429, 1971.)

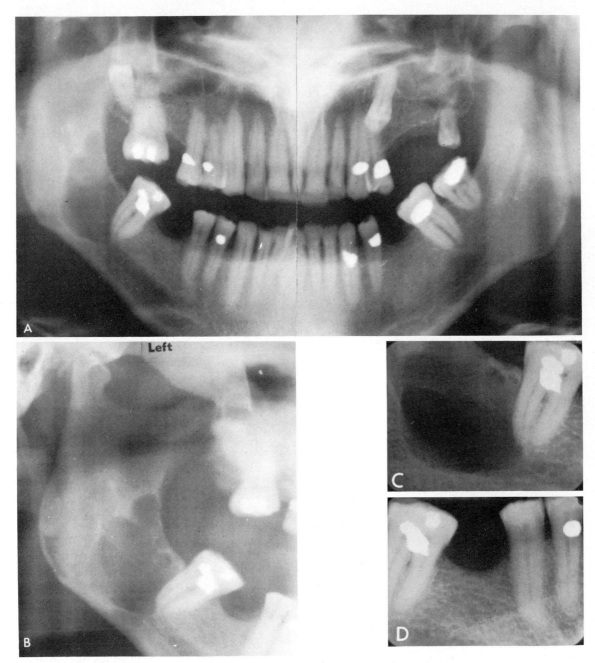

Figure 16–48   Dentigerous cyst. *A*, Conventional panoramic radiograph. (Also of interest is the inverted molar in the left maxilla.) *B*, Ramus technique panoramic radiograph. *C* and *D*, Intraoral periapical radiographs.

There are two basic reasons for distorted images of the mandibular ramus on the conventional panoramic radiograph:

1. The ramus is positioned outside the focal trough or plane.

2. The ramus is positioned diagonally rather than perpendicularly to the x-ray beam.

To correct these factors, the two techniques that follow may be used.

RAMUS TECHNIQUE NO. 1.   For the average head size ramus technique No. 1 is most useful (Fig. 16-46C and E).

1. The right and left sides are recorded as individual exposures on the same film.

2. The operator positions the condyles anterior and inferior to their fossae by having the patient protrude the mandible into an edge-to-edge incisal relationship. To open beyond this, a block of any desired thickness can be inserted between the anterior teeth.

3. The head is brought forward to a position in which the mandible is anterior to and rests upon the chin stop. Then the head is rotated *away* from the side to be radiographed, so that the midline is aligned with a point midway between the center line on the chin stop and the edge nearest the tube head. The back of the patient's head should be in contact with the cassette carrier (Fig. 16-46C and E).

4. The cassette carrier is adjusted until its base is at the level of the mandibular angle.

5. Referring to the thickness of the patient's head to determine the kilovoltage, the operator begins exposure and allows it to continue until chair shift begins. At this point, the *radiation switch* should be shut off, but completion of the rotational cycle should be permitted. This exposes one side.

6. To radiograph the opposite side on the same film, the procedure is repeated with the patient's head repositioned for the unexposed side. *(Caution:* One should remember to *turn on* the radiation switch at the beginning of the exposure and to *turn it off* when the chair begins to shift.)

RAMUS TECHNIQUE NO. 2.   When the patient's head is rather large, ramus technique No. 2 is used (Fig. 16-46D and F).

1. Everything is similar to the technique just described except for positioning of the patient's head.

2. The head is rotated away from the side being radiographed, so that the *midline is aligned with the edge of the chin stop* nearest the tube head. This rotates the mandible to a more anterior position, bringing the ramus closer to the focal plane and into better alignment with the x-ray beam.

The value of these techniques in visualizing the mandibular ramus for various conditions is demonstrated in Figure 16-47. Comparisons of the conventional technique with the modified ramus techniques are seen in Figures 16-48 to 16-51.

THE RADIATION FACTOR

Patient Dosage.   According to Kite and associates, "The total calculated skin dose ranges from 15 to 22 roentgens per film with an unfiltered tube head."[5]

Gonadal dose to the patient is also minimal in panography. Measurements by Jung of radiation delivered to the gonadal area (lap doses) by three types of panoramic units ranged from 0.5 to 0.48 mR. Since these were "lap dose" measurements, Jung states that the actual gonadal dose would amount to less than one tenth of these figures, a relatively insignificant amount.

Jung found that a 15-film intraoral examination using films with an "A.S.A. rating of 12" delivered a gonadal area dose ranging from 0.7 to 1.21 mR., more than three times the amount received from the panographic examination.[4] These are also "lap dose" measurements; therefore, the actual gonadal dose for the intraoral examination would also be insignificant.

Operator Dosage. Kite and associates found that the maximum radiation received by the operator in an unshielded position was 5 to 10 mR. per hour. This indicates that he could make 10 hours of exposure in one week, which, on the basis of 22 seconds per exposure, would amount to more than 1500 exposures and still not exceed the 100 mR. per week maximum permissible dose. Kite relates that his two technicians took 800 panoramic films in a single month, resulting in an exposure of only 10 mR. as recorded on film badges worn by each.[5]

It appears that the leakage and scatter radiation from panographic units are well within acceptable limits.

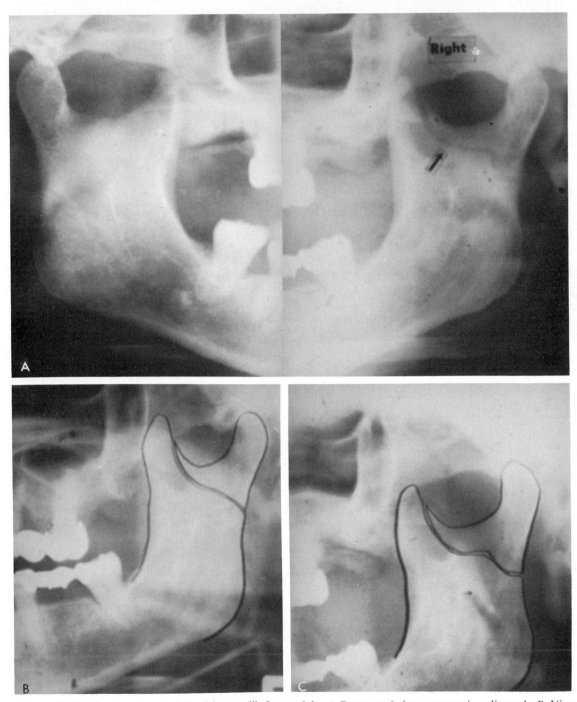

Figure 16–49   Fractured neck of the right mandibular condyle. *A*, Ramus technique panoramic radiograph. *B*, View with conventional panoramic technique (traced). *C*, View with ramus technique (traced). *D* and *E*, Transorbital technique.

(*Figure 16–49 continued on opposite page*)

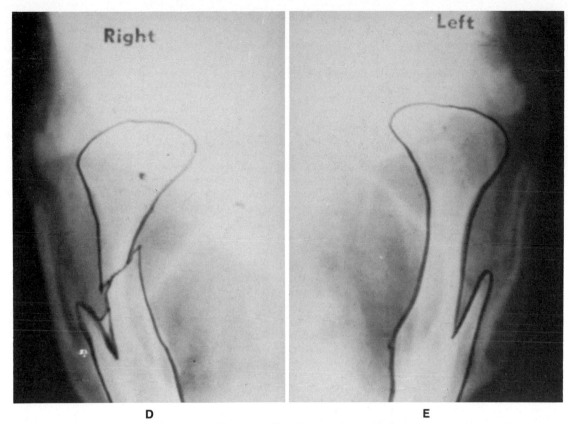

D

E

Figure 16–49 *(Continued.)*

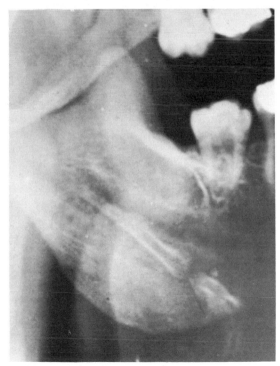

Figure 16–50 An example of distortion of the mandibular ramus (foreshortened and widened) and superimposition of the hyoid bone on it when an oblique radiographic view was taken. Mistakenly the superimposed hyoid bone was diagnosed as an elongated styloid process.

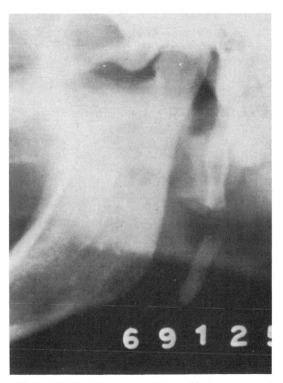

Figure 16–51 The panoramic modified ramus technique, as described previously, produces a much more accurate radiograph of the ramus and reveals a true enlarged styloid process.

REFERENCES

1. Blackman, S.: Panography. Oral Surg., *14*:1178–1189, 1961.
2. Blackman, S.: Rotational tomography of the face. Br. J. Radiol., *33*:408–418, 1960.
3. Christen, A. G., and Segreto, V. A.: Distortion and artifacts encountered in Panorex radiography. J.A.D.A., *77*:1096–1101, 1968.
4. Jung, T.: Gonadal doses resulting from panoramic x-ray examinations of the teeth. Oral Surg., *19*:745–753, 1965.
5. Kite, O. W., Swanson, L. T., Levin, S., and Bradbury, E.: Radiation and image distortion in the Panorex x-ray unit. Oral Surg., *15*:1201–1210, 1962.
6. Kumpula, J. W.: Present status of panoramic roentgenography. J.A.D.A., *63*:194–200, 1961.
7. Paatero, Y. V.: Pantomography and orthopantomography. Oral Surg., *14*:947–953, 1961.
8. Updegrave, W. J.: Visualizing the mandibular ramus in panoramic radiography. Oral Surg., *31*:422–429, 1971.
9. Updegrave, W. J.: The role of panoramic radiography in diagnosis. Oral Surg., *22*:49–57, 1966.
10. Updegrave, W. J.: A comprehensive dental radiographic examination. Bull. Phila. County Dent. Soc., *29*:11–12, 1964.
11. Updegrave, W. J.: Panoramic dental radiography. Dent. Radiogr. Photogr., *36*:75–83, 1963.

CHAPTER 17

ROENTGEN ANATOMY OF THE FACIAL BONES AND JAWS

LEWIS E. ETTER, M.D.

No fundamental understanding of distorted anatomic features is possible without a detailed knowledge of the normal anatomy of the part under consideration. There are many confusing structures in the skull, roentgenologically considered, but these may often be clarified by analysis of individual bone components and what each of these contributes to the whole image in a given x-ray projection.[3, 4, 5]

The orbits are two pyramidal cavities lying below the forehead, and are formed by the frontal, zygomatic, maxillary, lacrimal, ethmoid, palatal and sphenoid bones. Each is pierced by an optic foramen, a superior and inferior orbital fissure, infraorbital foramen and canal, and supraorbital notch or foramen. Study of an oblique posteroanterior view (Waters' view) of the skull (Fig. 17–1) shows features contributed by the several bones composing the orbit. These are clearly labeled for study.* Attention should also be given to the several radiologic lines forming the upper margin or roof of the orbit and to the oblique orbital line, which is seen to have a frontal

and sphenoid bone component. Also to be noted are the parts contributed by the malar bone, which can best be distinguished when that bone is separated from the remainder, as in Figure 17–2, and again when restored in the skull, as in Figure 17–3.

Similarly, examination of the disarticulated maxillae and zygomatic bones in the posteroanterior and Waters' projections reveals exactly what these bones contribute to a roentgen image of these parts. Note especially how the infraorbital canal and foramen are projected into the floor of the orbit in each case (Figs. 17–4 and 17–5). In the film of the living subject (Fig. 17–6) the relation of the infraorbital canals and foramina of the maxillae is shown with the foramina rotunda and ovale of the sphenoid. Also to be noted is an oblique line forming the lateral wall of the antra and representing a cross-sectional projection of the infratemporal surface of the maxilla, in some skulls appearing to be a downward extension of the oblique orbital line.

Another view, complementary to this, and of great value to the oral surgeon, is the so-called basal view (Fig. 17–7) or verticosubmental view of Hirtz. This projection shows structures in the anterior and middle cranial fossae and particularly well those surrounding the antra and orbits. The infraorbital

*Exposure technique required for the regular dental x-ray unit to produce the various radiographs illustrated in this chapter was prepared by Raymond W. Clark, R.T., A.R.R.T., Chief Radiology Technician of the Department of Radiology, School of Dental Medicine, University of Pittsburgh.

(Text continued on page 1020)

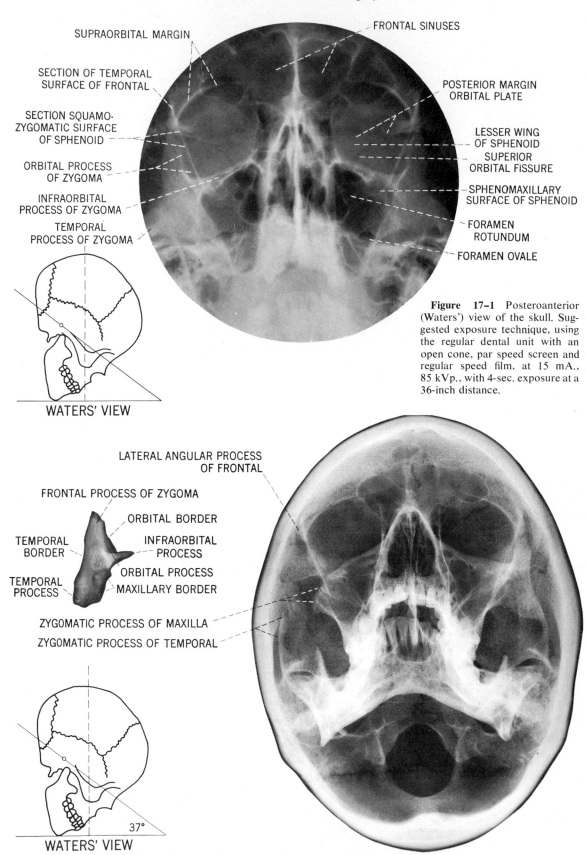

SUPRAORBITAL MARGIN

FRONTAL SINUSES

SECTION OF TEMPORAL
SURFACE OF FRONTAL

POSTERIOR MARGIN
ORBITAL PLATE

SECTION SQUAMO-
ZYGOMATIC SURFACE
OF SPHENOID

LESSER WING
OF SPHENOID

SUPERIOR
ORBITAL FISSURE

ORBITAL PROCESS
OF ZYGOMA

SPHENOMAXILLARY
SURFACE OF SPHENOID

INFRAORBITAL
PROCESS OF ZYGOMA

FORAMEN
ROTUNDUM

TEMPORAL
PROCESS OF ZYGOMA

FORAMEN OVALE

WATERS' VIEW

Figure 17–1 Posteroanterior (Waters') view of the skull. Suggested exposure technique, using the regular dental unit with an open cone, par speed screen and regular speed film, at 15 mA., 85 kVp., with 4-sec. exposure at a 36-inch distance.

LATERAL ANGULAR PROCESS
OF FRONTAL

FRONTAL PROCESS OF ZYGOMA

ORBITAL BORDER

TEMPORAL
BORDER

INFRAORBITAL
PROCESS

ORBITAL PROCESS

TEMPORAL
PROCESS

MAXILLARY BORDER

ZYGOMATIC PROCESS OF MAXILLA

ZYGOMATIC PROCESS OF TEMPORAL

37°

WATERS' VIEW

Figure 17–2 Same exposure technique as that shown for Figure 17–1.

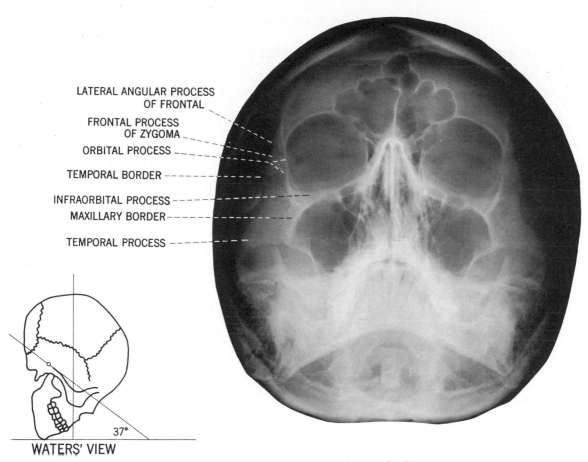

LATERAL ANGULAR PROCESS
OF FRONTAL

FRONTAL PROCESS
OF ZYGOMA

ORBITAL PROCESS

TEMPORAL BORDER

INFRAORBITAL PROCESS

MAXILLARY BORDER

TEMPORAL PROCESS

37°

WATERS' VIEW

Figure 17–3 Same exposure technique as that shown for Figure 17–1.

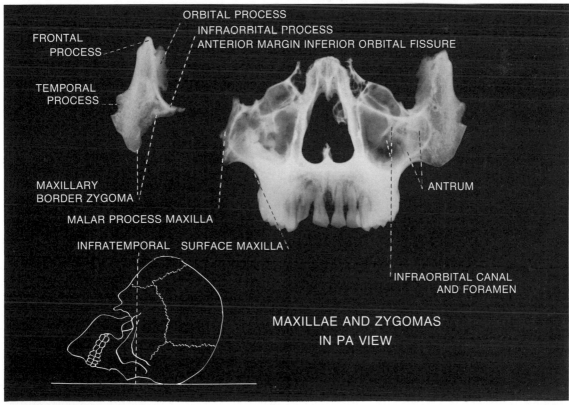

ORBITAL PROCESS
INFRAORBITAL PROCESS
ANTERIOR MARGIN INFERIOR ORBITAL FISSURE

FRONTAL
PROCESS

TEMPORAL
PROCESS

ANTRUM

MAXILLARY
BORDER ZYGOMA

MALAR PROCESS MAXILLA

INFRATEMPORAL   SURFACE MAXILLA

INFRAORBITAL CANAL
AND FORAMEN

MAXILLAE AND ZYGOMAS
IN PA VIEW

Figure 17–4

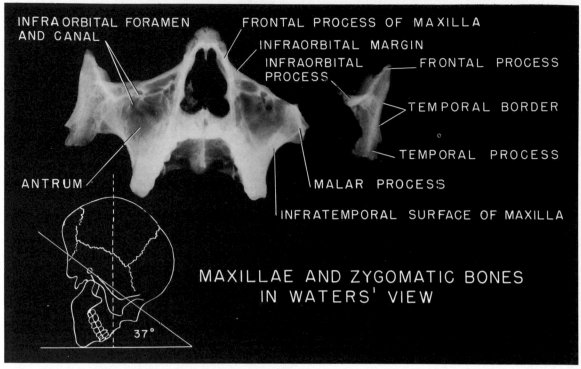

Figure 17–5

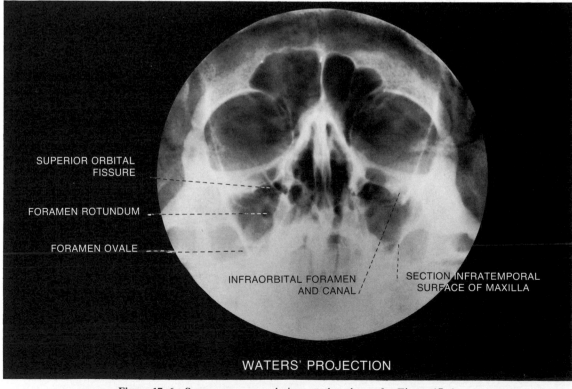

Figure 17–6   Same exposure technique as that shown for Figure 17–1.

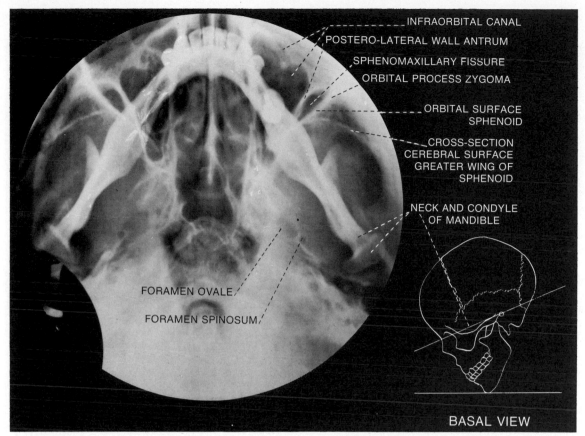

INFRAORBITAL CANAL
POSTERO-LATERAL WALL ANTRUM
SPHENOMAXILLARY FISSURE
ORBITAL PROCESS ZYGOMA

ORBITAL SURFACE
SPHENOID

CROSS-SECTION
CEREBRAL SURFACE
GREATER WING OF
SPHENOID

NECK AND CONDYLE
OF MANDIBLE

FORAMEN OVALE

FORAMEN SPINOSUM

BASAL VIEW

Figure 17–7 Suggested exposure technique, using the regular dental unit with an open cone, par speed screen and regular speed film, at 15 mA., 85 kVp., with 4- to 5-sec. exposure at a 36-inch distance.

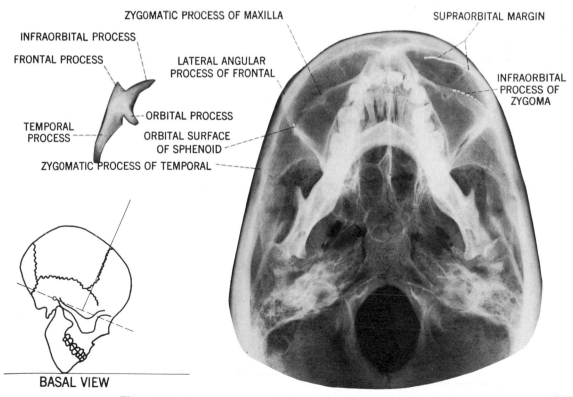

ZYGOMATIC PROCESS OF MAXILLA
SUPRAORBITAL MARGIN

INFRAORBITAL PROCESS
FRONTAL PROCESS
LATERAL ANGULAR
PROCESS OF FRONTAL

INFRAORBITAL
PROCESS OF
ZYGOMA

TEMPORAL
PROCESS
ORBITAL PROCESS
ORBITAL SURFACE
OF SPHENOID
ZYGOMATIC PROCESS OF TEMPORAL

BASAL VIEW

Figure 17–8 Same exposure technique as that shown for Figure 17–7.

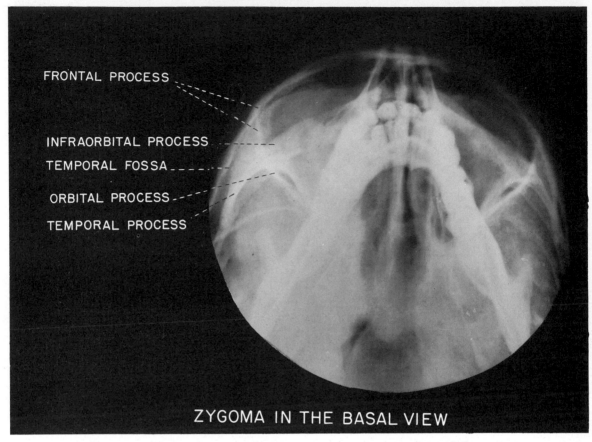

FRONTAL PROCESS

INFRAORBITAL PROCESS

TEMPORAL FOSSA

ORBITAL PROCESS

TEMPORAL PROCESS

ZYGOMA IN THE BASAL VIEW

Figure 17–9 Same exposure technique as that shown for Figure 17–7.

canal again can be identified, as well as the floor of the orbit and the posterolateral wall of the antrum, where it forms the anterior wall of the sphenomaxillary fossa. Likewise, parts of the zygoma, especially its orbital process, which articulates with the orbital surface of the greater wing of the sphenoid, are shown, as well as the zygomatic arch.

In Figure 17–8 the zygoma is shown separated from the skull in order to delineate its component parts better and so that it can be completely visualized in the living subject (Fig. 17–9). The basal view is of especial interest to oral surgeons because an excellent view of the mandible is obtained in this position. The condyles and temporomandibular joints are also clearly demonstrated (Fig. 17–10).

If it is desired to demonstrate the zygomatic arch in its entirety and thrown clear of the temporal bone, the position indicated in Figure 17–11 should be used. Varying degrees of obliquity will be required, depending upon

whether the skull under study is of the narrow or broad type.

An example of the use of the basal view in fracture of the maxilla is given in Figure 17–12. Here the posterolateral wall of the antrum is seen to be the site of a comminuted fracture that also involves the infratemporal surface of the maxilla and the zygomatic arch. In the complementary view for study of this area of the face, the fracture is also shown in the Waters' projection, but most complete understanding of the fracture is obtained by studying the two views, which serve to supplement each other (Fig. 17–13).

In about 7 per cent of basal views an important anomaly of interest in connection with injection of the mandibular branch of the trigeminal nerve from the lateral approach is the pterygoalar bar[1] (Fig. 17–14). This anatomic variant likely represents an ossified pterygoalar ligament and extends from the root of the lateral pterygoid lamina to the undersurface of the greater wing of the sphen-

(*Text continued on page 1030*)

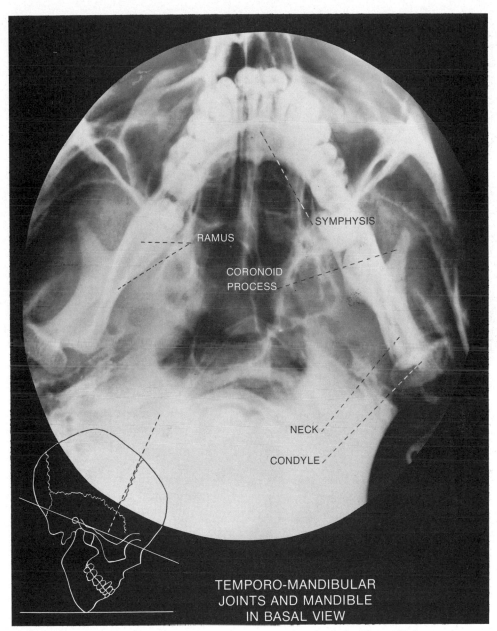

Figure 17–10 Same exposure technique as that shown for Figure 17–7.

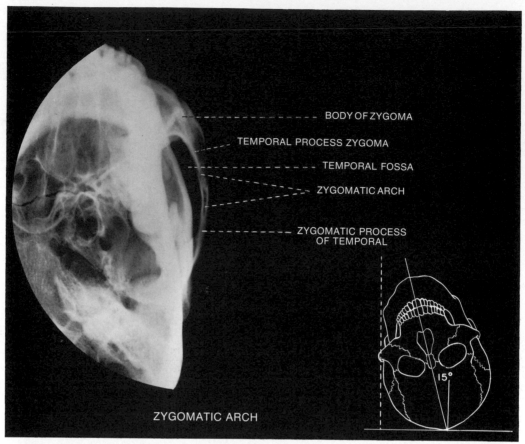

Figure 17–11 Suggested exposure technique, using the regular dental unit with an open cone, par speed screen and regular speed film, at 15 mA., 85 kVp., with ⁵⁄₁₀-sec. exposure at a 36-inch distance.

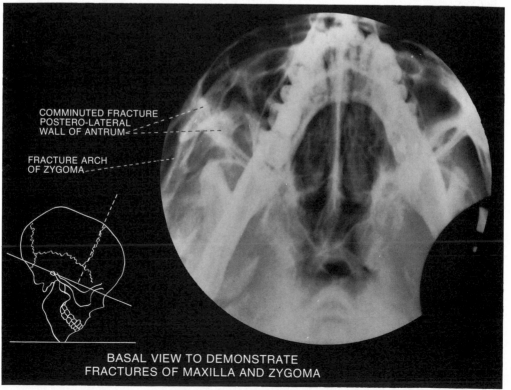

Figure 17–12 Same exposure technique as that shown for Figure 17–7.

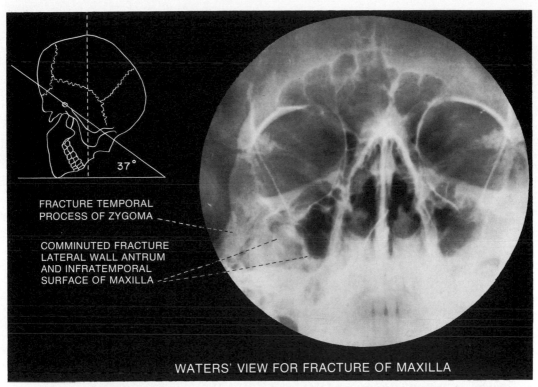

FRACTURE TEMPORAL
PROCESS OF ZYGOMA

COMMINUTED FRACTURE
LATERAL WALL ANTRUM
AND INFRATEMPORAL
SURFACE OF MAXILLA

WATERS' VIEW FOR FRACTURE OF MAXILLA

Figure 17–13 Same exposure technique as that shown for Figure 17–1.

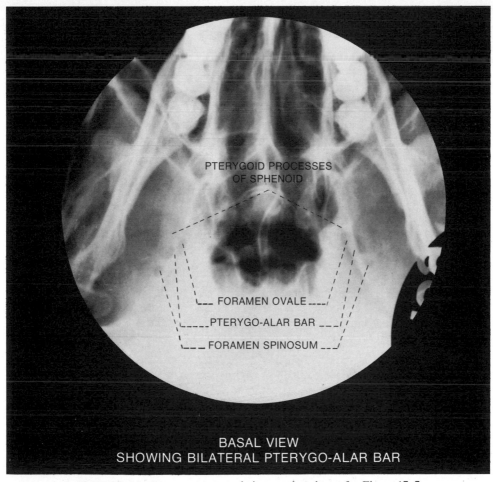

PTERYGOID PROCESSES
OF SPHENOID

FORAMEN OVALE

PTERYGO-ALAR BAR

FORAMEN SPINOSUM

BASAL VIEW
SHOWING BILATERAL PTERYGO-ALAR BAR

Figure 17–14 Same exposure technique as that shown for Figure 17–7.

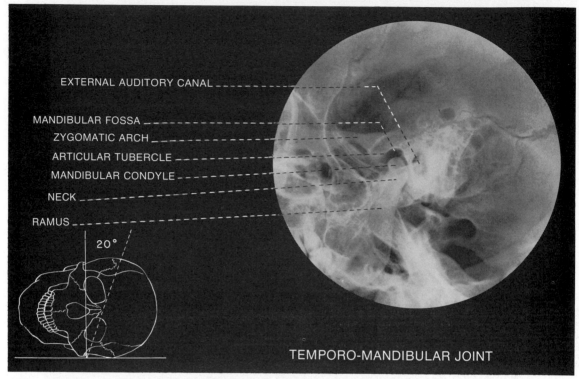

Figure 17–15   Suggested exposure technique, using the regular dental unit with an open cone, par speed screen and regular speed film, at 15 mA., 85 kVp., with ⁵/₁₀-sec. exposure at a 24-inch distance.

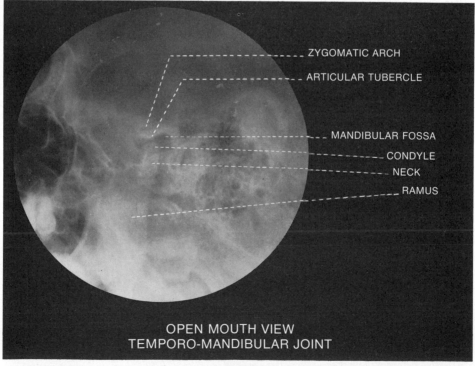

Figure 17–16   Same exposure technique as that shown for Figure 17–15.

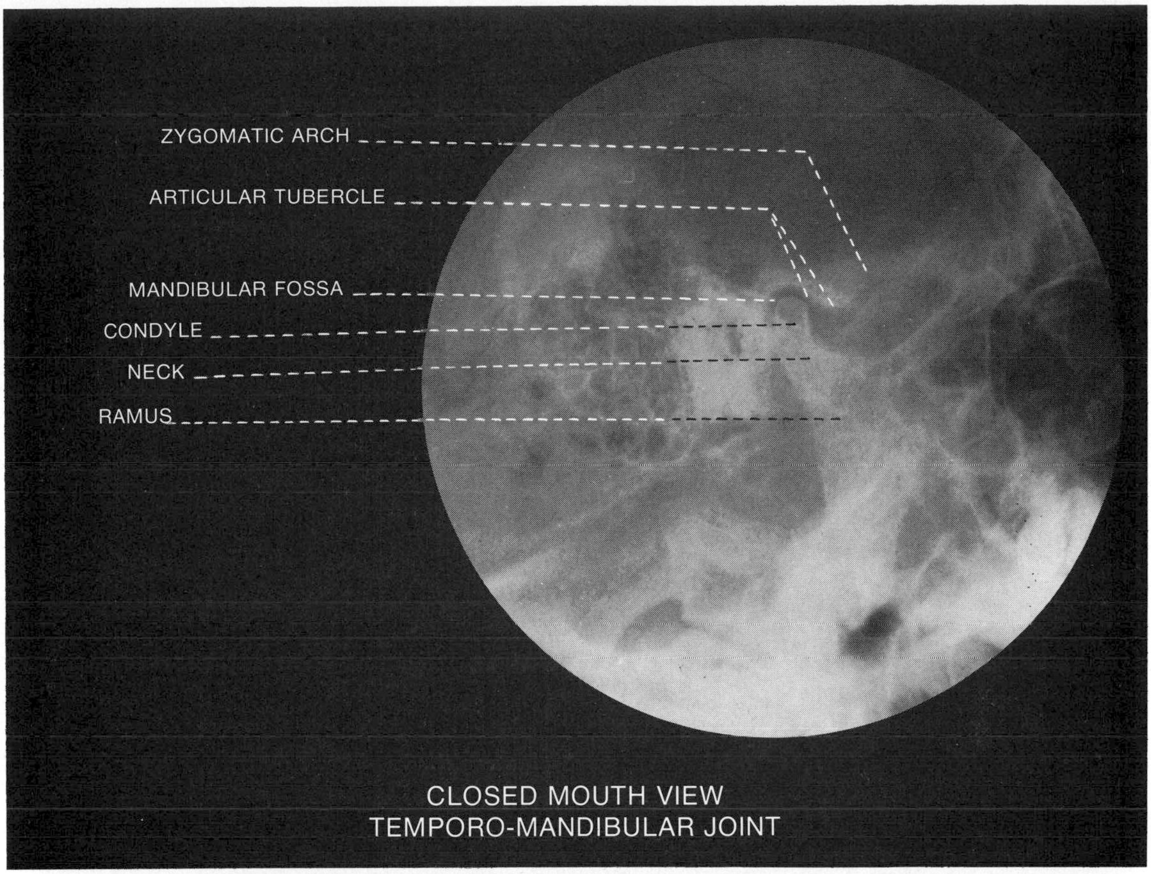

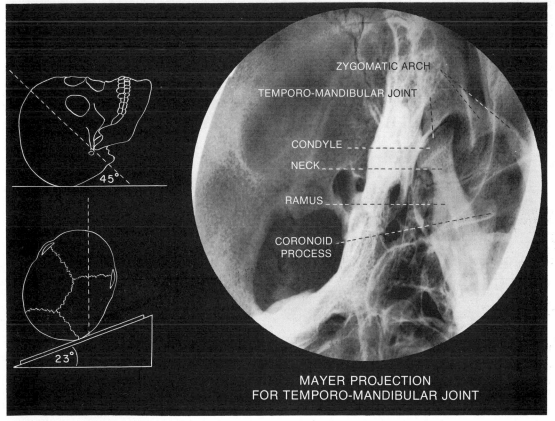

ZYGOMATIC ARCH
ARTICULAR TUBERCLE
MANDIBULAR FOSSA
CONDYLE
NECK
RAMUS

CLOSED MOUTH VIEW
TEMPORO-MANDIBULAR JOINT

Figure 17–17 Same exposure technique as that shown for Figure 17–15.

ZYGOMATIC ARCH
TEMPORO-MANDIBULAR JOINT
CONDYLE
NECK
RAMUS
CORONOID
PROCESS

45°

23°

MAYER PROJECTION
FOR TEMPORO-MANDIBULAR JOINT

Figure 17–18 Suggested exposure technique, using the regular dental unit with an open cone, par speed screen and regular speed film, at 15 mA., 85 kVp., with 1- to 2-sec. exposure at a 24-inch distance.

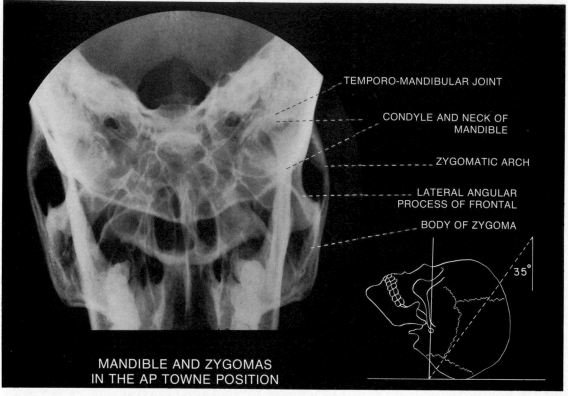

TEMPORO-MANDIBULAR JOINT

CONDYLE AND NECK OF MANDIBLE

ZYGOMATIC ARCH

LATERAL ANGULAR PROCESS OF FRONTAL

BODY OF ZYGOMA

35°

MANDIBLE AND ZYGOMAS IN THE AP TOWNE POSITION

Figure 17–19   Same exposure technique as that shown for Figure 17–1.

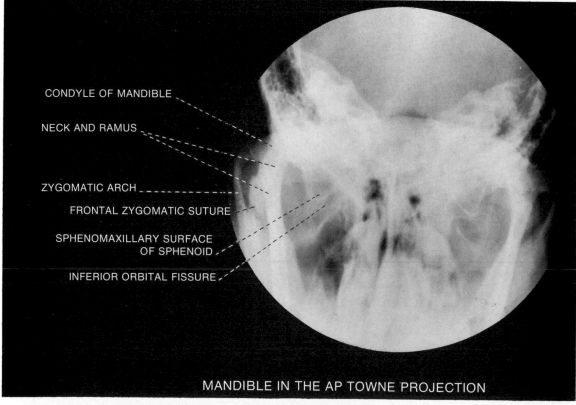

CONDYLE OF MANDIBLE

NECK AND RAMUS

ZYGOMATIC ARCH

FRONTAL ZYGOMATIC SUTURE

SPHENOMAXILLARY SURFACE OF SPHENOID

INFERIOR ORBITAL FISSURE

MANDIBLE IN THE AP TOWNE PROJECTION

Figure 17–20   Same exposure technique as that shown for Figure 17–1.

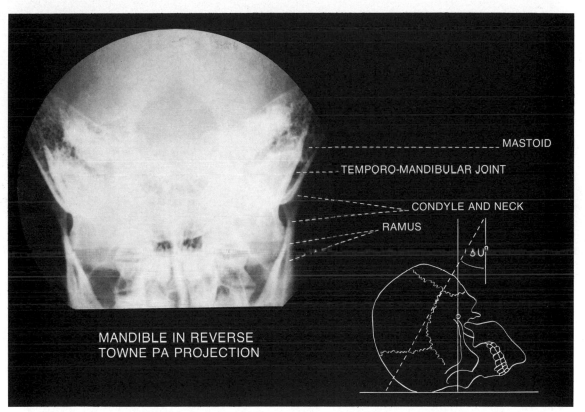

Figure 17–21   Same exposure technique as that shown for Figure 17–1.

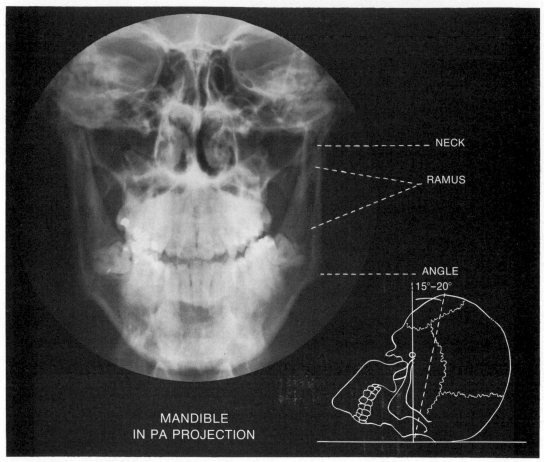

Figure 17–22 Suggested exposure technique, using the regular dental unit with an open cone, par speed screen and regular speed film, at 15 mA., 85 kVp., with 1⁵/₁₀ to 2-sec. exposure at a 36-inch distance.

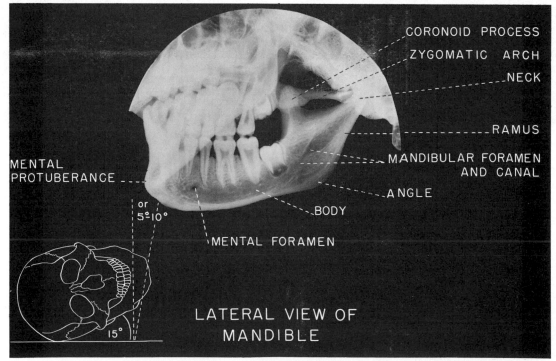

Figure 17–23 Suggested exposure technique, using the regular dental unit with an open cone, par speed screen and regular speed film, at 15 mA., 85 kVp., with ⁴/₁₀-sec. exposure at a 36-inch distance.

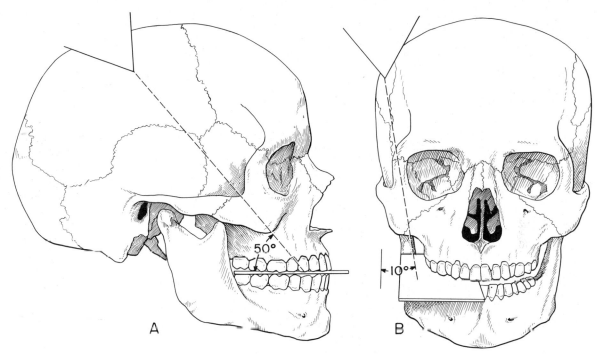

Figure 17–24 The zygomatic occlusal radiograph is designed to show the zygomatic arch. This arch includes the zygomatic process of the temporal bone and the temporal process of the zygomatic bone. This view is not considered adequate to depict the body of the zygomatic bone. (See Figures 17–13 and 17–19 for radiographic technique to show the zygomatic bone.)

Technique: The patient's head is positioned so that the occlusal plane of the maxillary teeth is parallel to the floor. A standard occlusal film is placed lengthwise in the patient's mouth and then moved laterally to the side to be radiographed. The posterior border of the film should contact the anterior border of the mandibular ramus. The patient is instructed to close the mouth, and the film is again adjusted so that its posterior border rests on the anterior border of the ramus (*A*), and the medial border of the film bisects the interseptal space of the maxillary central incisors (*B*). This position is for adult patients.

In positioning the film in a child's mouth the same technique is used except for the position of the medial border of the film. In these cases the medial border of the film is placed to bisect the cuspid of the opposite side being radiographed.

The machine head is positioned to form a plus 50-degree vertical angle and a 10-degree horizontal angle toward the midline. The position of the head of the machine is 3 inches above the ear on the side to be radiographed. The distance between the cone and the film is 8 inches.

In the postatomic era a new concept has emerged in radiographic techniques. This has come about through the development of more refined machines and highly sensitive film coatings. The combination of high-speed and ultra-speed films in conjunction with machines producing high kilovoltages (kV.) and milliampere (mA.) levels has markedly reduced exposure time and the resultant radiation. The modern dental radiographic unit is designed to operate at 100 kV./15 mA. and 90 kV./10 mA., with electronic timers functioning precisely enough to measure $\frac{1}{60}$-second intervals and the radiation beam being filtered through 0.25 mm. of aluminum. These factors permit the above film to be taken at an exposure time of between $\frac{1}{20}$ and $\frac{1}{10}$ of a second. This makes the marked reduction of radiation exposure to the patient quite apparent. (Technique devised by George E. Fuller, D.D.S.)

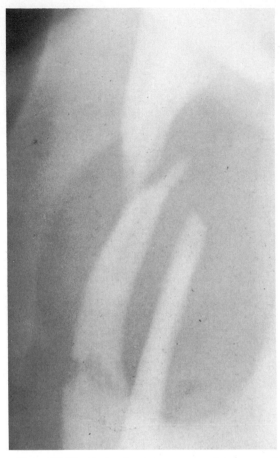

Figure 17–25 Occlusal roentgenogram of a segmental fracture of the left zygomatic arch made with the Fuller technique. The coronoid process is seen medial to the fracture. It can readily be seen how a more medially displaced fragment or fragments would impede the movements of the coronoid process during speech or mastication.

mouth views (Figs. 17–15 to 17–17). An additional projection of great value to gain a slightly different oblique view is the projection of Mayer, which is used frequently in mastoid study (Fig 17–18). This gives an excellent view of the condyle and mandibular fossa, as well as the zygomatic process of the temporal bone and the neck and ramus of the mandible. Additional useful views for both rami and temporomandibular joints are the anteroposterior Towne projection (Figs. 17–19 and 17–20) and the basal views already described. It will be seen how well the condyles, necks and rami are shown in this projection and how easily any lateral displacement in a fracture can be detected. In some cases it may be desirable to try a reverse Towne projection to delineate the temporomandibular joints, condyles and necks of the mandible. Figure 17–21 indicates the position of the skull for this view, which may be varied from 20 to 35 degrees, as found best to show the structures desired. It is also best to complete the examination with a posteroanterior projection of the skull to give a view of the rami and angles in the sagittal plane (see Figure 17–2).

Simple lateral views of the mandible are also frequently needed in fractures and for pathologic diagnoses. The principal features of the bone in this projection are shown in Figure 17–23.

oid, barring the lateral approach to the foramen ovale. This anomaly is clearly shown in Figure 17–15 and should be looked for when injection of the mandibular nerve at the foramen ovale is contemplated. As pointed out by Sweet, the number of complete injections into both the second and third divisions of the trigeminal is increased to over 95 per cent with use of radiographic control.[8]

In a study of the temporomandibular joints and mandible, several views are required to give the most complete information. First, a lateral oblique projection using a 20-degree angle is needed with both open- and closed-

REFERENCES

1. Chouké, K. S., and Hodes, P. J.: The pterygo-alar bar and its recognition by roentgen methods in trigeminal neuralgia. Am. J. Roentgenol., 65(2): (Feb.), 1951.
2. Etter, L. E.: Atlas of Roentgen Anatomy of the Skull. Springfield, Ill., Charles C Thomas, 1955.
3. Etter, L. E.: Radiographic anatomic studies of the skull. Med. Radiogr. Photogr., 27:1951.
4. Etter, L. E.: X-ray studies of the disarticulated skull. N.Y. State J. Med., 49:2808–2810 (Dec. 1), 1949.
5. Etter, L. E.: New method for roentgen anatomical study of the skull. Radiology, 53:394–402 (Sept.), 1949.
6. Etter, L. E., and Priman, J.: Importance of skull variations in blocking the trigeminal nerve and its branches for anesthesia of the head and face. Anesthesiology, 22:1 (Jan.-Feb.), 1961.
7. Etter, L. E., and Priman, J.: The pterygospinous and pterygo-alar bars. Med. Radiogr. Photogr. 35:1, 1959.
8. Sweet, W. H.: Trigeminal injection with radiographic control. J.A.M.A., 42:392–396, 1950.

INDEX

In this index *italic* page numbers indicate illustrations,
and (t) indicates a table; "vs." is used to
mean "differential diagnosis from."

Lip(s) (*Continued*)
 lower, cancer of, 1735, 1783–1785, *1784–1785,* 1808
  epidermoid carcinoma of, *1808*
  U resection of, 1736, *1738*
  vermilionectomy of, *1738*
 lymphangioma of, *823, 824*
 melanoma of, 1736
 normal, anatomic landmarks of, *1832*
 papilloma of, *811*
 pinching by forceps, 1579, *1579*
  vs. neurotrophic ulcer, *909*
 pleomorphic adenoma of, 718, *719,* 720, 721
 pyogenic granuloma of, 1743
 squamous cell carcinoma of, 1807
 stitch abscess of, 1746
 surgery of, anesthesia for, 1741, 1743, 1746, 1748
 upper, cancer of, 1736, 1785–1787, *1786,* 1808
Lip flap, mobilization and rotation of, 1745
Lip shave, for carcinoma, 1736
Lipoma(s), *805,* 806, *806*
 treatment of, 806
Liver, cirrhosis of, and oral surgery, 19
 disorders of, bleeding in, 1563, 1569–1571
  history taking and, 423
Localization, of infection, heat therapy and, 446
 radiographic, 982–1014
  contrast media in, *849,* 990, *1002–1004*
  extraoral method of, 990, *999–1002*
  occlusal method of, 990, *991–998*
   cross-section, 990, *993–998*
   topographical, 990, *991–992*
  shift-sketch method of, 983, *987–989*
  stereoscopic method of, 982, 983, *987*
  wire sutures in, 958, 959
Lock stitches, 102, 103
Loose teeth, causes of, 29
Ludwig's angina. See *Angina, Ludwig's.*
Lues, and osteomyelitis, 502, *1641*
Luxation, and dislocation, of mandible, 1644
 and penetration of maxillary sinus, 32, 1605
 of teeth, dentist's hand position during, 43
Lymph nodes, calcified, vs. sialoliths, *955*
 cervical, in physical examination, 424
 metastases in tongue cancer, 1812
Lymphadenitis, tuberculous, *477*
Lymphangioma(s), 823, *823,* 824, *824*
 etiology of, 823
Lymphoma, 807
 giant follicular, 807, *807*
 malignant, *948*
  and Bell's palsy, 1667, *1667*
  and Mikulicz's disease, *925*
  vs. pleomorphic adenoma, *948*
Lyons, C. J., 3

Macfee parallel transverse neck incision, *1796*
Malaria, history taking and, 423
Malassez, rests of, in cyst formation, 524
Malignant disease(s), oral, 1732–1805. See also *Cancer* and specific diseases.
Malignant lesions, of oral cavity, 1806–1807
Mallet, surgical, *30, 36*
 in extraction, 32, 35–37
Mallett, S. P., 8
Malnutrition, and bald tongue, *900*
 and impaction, 255

Malnutrition (*Continued*)
 in geriatric patient, 976, 977
Malocclusion. See also *Orthopedics, dentofacial.*
 and prostheses, *136*
 Angle's classification of, 1430
 Class I, 1430, *1431, 1437*
  treatment of, 1442–1444
 Class II, Division 1, *1379, 1380, 1382,* 1430, *1432, 1437*
   alveolectomy and dentures for, 183, *184, 186,* 187
   segmental surgery for, *1384,* 1395–1405, *1396–1407*
  Division 2, 1430, *1432, 1437*
   segmental surgery for, 1408, 1409, *1408–1410*
 Class III, *1379, 1383,* 1430, *1433, 1437*
  orthodontic treatment of, 1441, 1442
  ostectomy for. See *Ostectomy.*
  osteotomies for. See *Osteotomy.*
  segmental surgery for, *1384,* 1411–1421, *1412–1421*
   bilateral crossbite in, *1416–1418,* 1418
   chin protrusion in, 1418, *1419*
   open bite in, *1420,* 1421
   unilateral crossbite in, 1419–1421, *1420, 1421*
 classification of, 1429, 1430
 description of, 1429
Malposed teeth, and extraction, 16
 and odontectomy, 32
 definition of, 250(t)
 postoperative treatment for, 388, 389
 removal of, complications from, 386–388
Mandible, atrophic. See *Mandible, pipe-stem.*
 body of, cancer of, *1789*
 bone of, replacement of, *1801*
 cancer of, surgical treatment of, *1789*
 carcinoma of, *913, 914, 915*
 dislocation of, 1644–1655. See also *Dislocation, of mandible.*
 fractures of, 1073–1156. See also *Fracture(s), of mandible.*
 infection of, *1825*
 malignant lymphoma of, 1773–1774, *1774*
 malignant tumors of, 1772–1773, *1772*
 marginal resection of, 1755
 micrognathic, 1448. See also *Orthopedics, dentofacial.*
 muscles of, *1065–1069*
 osteoradionecrosis of, 1823, *1824, 1825*
  with spontaneous fracture, 1823
 pathologic fracture of, *1810, 1825*
 pipe-stem, *151*
  and odontectomy, 32
  fracture of, 1097
  treatment of, 1104
   complications in, 1100–1104, *1101–1103*
 prognathic, 1448. See also *Orthopedics, dentofacial.*
 radionecrosis of, treatment of, 1823
 reconstruction of, following resection, 1788
 resection of. See *Resection, of mandible.*
 resorption of. See *Resorption, of alveolar ridges.*
 spontaneous fracture of, 1823
 vascular nevus of, *815*
 visualization of, anteroposterior position in, Towne, *1026,* 1030, 1061
  basal view in, 1020, *1021*

Osteitis (*Continued*)
  condensing, diagnosis of, *27*
    treatment of, 858, 861
      vs. enostosis, 857, *858*, 861, *863–867*
      vs. osteosclerosis, vs. submandibular sialolith, *973*
      with osteomyelitis, *504*
    defensive, and root breakage, 28
Osteitis deformans, 857, *858–862*
Osteitis fibrosa, localized. See *Fibroma, ossifying.*
Osteitis fibrosa cystica. See *Hyperparathyroidism.*
Osteoarthritis, in geriatric patient, 977
Osteoarthrotomy, 1655–1662. See also *Condylectomy.*
Osteoblastic carcinoma, *887*
Osteoblastoma, benign, cysts vs., 635
Osteochondroma, maxillary, *714, 715,* 716
  treatment of, 716
Osteodystrophy, localized. See *Fibroma, ossifying.*
Osteoectomy. See *Ostectomy.*
Osteofibroma. See *Fibroma, ossifying.*
Osteofibrosis, vs. cementomas, *784*
Osteogenesis imperfecta, and pathologic fractures, 1047
Osteogenic carcinoma, *887*
Osteogenic sarcoma, of mandible, *886–888*
Osteoid osteoma. See *Fibroma, ossifying.*
Osteolytic carcinoma, *887*
Osteolytic osteosarcoma, cysts vs., 635
Osteoma(s), chisel technique in, *200*
  in maxillary sinus, *713*
  mandibular. See *Torus mandibularis.*
  of vertical ramus, *714*
  osteoid. See *Fibroma, ossifying.*
  palatal. See *Torus palatinus.*
  recurrent, *711*
Osteomalacia, and pathologic fractures, 1047
Osteomyelitis, 502, 1630–1644, *1631–1643*
  acute, 1633
  and ankylosis, of temporomandibular joint, 1528
  and chronic fistula, *497*
  and pathologic fractures, 1047, 1642–1644, *1643*
  antibiotic therapy for, 417, 1635
  bacteriology in, 1632
  chronic, 499–502, *499–504,* 1636–1640, *1637–1640*
    definition of, 1633
  cysts vs., 636
  definition of, 1630–1632
  diffuse, 499–501, *499–504*
    definition of, 1633
  diffuse fulminating, 1633
  etiology of, 1632
  extractions and, 1636–1642
  fractures and, 1146–1155, *1148–1151,* 1333, 1334
  heat therapy in, 446
  hemorrhagic. See *Aneurysmal bone cyst.*
  kinds of, 1633, 1634
  localized, 1633, 1634, *1641.* See also *Alveolalgia.*
  lues and, 502, *1641*
  postextraction. See *Alveolalgia.*
  radionecrosis and, 1813
  symptoms of, 1634
  treatment of, 1635–1644, *1637–1643*
  with condensing osteitis, *504*
Osteonecrosis, radiation and, 1812. See also *Osteoradionecrosis.*
Osteopetrosis, and root breakage, 28
  diagnosis of, 25, *26*
Osteoporosis, *865*
  and pathologic fractures, 1047

Osteoporosis (*Continued*)
  in geriatric patient, 977
  in osteitis deformans, *862*
Osteoporotic bone marrow defect, vs. cysts, 635
Osteoradionecrosis, *1823*
  antibiotics in prevention of, 1823
  intraoral mandibulectomy for, *1826–1827*
  of mandible, 1823, *1824, 1825*
  pain as sequela of, 1823
  pathogenesis of, 1823
  prevention of, 1758
Osteosarcoma, osteolytic, cysts, vs., 635
Osteosclerosis, *864, 867*
  diagnosis of, 25, *26,* 28
  vs. condensing osteitis, vs. submandibular sialolith, *973*
  vs. enostosis, vs. condensing osteitis, 857, 858, 861, *863–867*
  vs. retained roots, *247*
  vs. submandibular sialolith, *954, 968, 973*
Osteotomy, Le Fort I, 1498–1506. See also *Osteotomy, maxillary, total.*
  in segmental surgery, 1426
  maxillary, 1498–1508
    for diastema, *1507, 1508*
    total, 1498–1506
      anesthesia in, 1499–1501
      applications of, 1503
      complications in, 1503, 1506
      surgical technique in, 1501–1503
  of ramus, curved-line, *1450*
    in ankylosis, of temporomandibular joint, 1531
    oblique (vertical), 1445, *1445,* 1446, *1446, 1451,* 1490–1498, *1490–1496*
      case assessment in, 1489
      complications in, 1449
      for micrognathism, 1494–1498, *1494–1496*
      for prognathism, 1490–1494, *1490–1493*
      with horizontal osteotomy, of coronoid process, *1450*
    reverse L, *1497*
    sagittal-split, *1450, 1451*
      complications of, 1449, 1452
    subapical. See *Segmental surgery.*
    subcondylar, *1450,* 1478–1487, *1480–1489*
      case assessment in, 1478
      complications in, 1449, 1479
      relapses in, 1479
      technique in, 1479, *1480, 1481*
    vertical, of mandibular body. See *Ostectomy, of mandibular body.*
      of mandibular rami. See *Osteotomy, of ramus, oblique (vertical).*
Otalgia dentalis, styloid process pain and, 1728
Otitis, in cleft palate surgery, 1858
  in impaction, 258
Otitis media, and ankylosis, of temporomandibular joint, 1528
Outgrowths, osseous, removal for dentures, 179–206
Overbite, 183, *184.* See also *Malocclusion, Class II, Division 1.*
  definition of, 182
Overjet, 183, *184.* See also *Malocclusion, Class II, Division 1.*
  definition of, 182
  removal of, 196

Index